PAEDIATRIC SURGERY:
A COMPREHENSIVE TEXT
FOR AFRICA

EDITORS:

EMMANUEL A. AMEH
STEPHEN W. BICKLER
KOKILA LAKHOO
BENEDICT C. NWOMEH
DAN POENARU

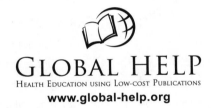

GLOBAL HELP
HEALTH EDUCATION USING LOW-COST PUBLICATIONS
www.global-help.org

Table of Contents: Volume I

TABLE OF CONTENTS: VOLUME II

CONTRIBUTING AUTHORS

Francis A. Abantanga, MD, Cert Paed Surg, PhD, FWACS,
   Cert Cardio Surg, FGCS
Associate Professor, Head, Department/Directorate of Surgery
School of Medical Sciences/Komfo Anokye Teaching Hospital
College of Health Sciences
Kwame Nkrumah University of Science and Technology
Kumasi, Ghana

Hesham M. Abdelkader, MD, MRCS, FEBPS
Lecturer of Pediatric Surgery
Division of Pediatric Surgery
Ain Shams University
Cairo, Egypt

Lukman O. Abdur-Rahman, MBBS, MPH, FWACS
Senior Lecturer and Consultant Paediatric Surgeon
Paediatric Surgery Unit, Department of Surgery
College of Health Sciences, University of Ilorin and University of Ilorin
Teaching Hospital
Ilorin, Nigeria

Auwal M Abubakar, MBBS, FWACS, FICS
Associate Professor and Consultant Paediatric Surgeon
Paediatric Surgery Unit, Department of Surgery
College of Medical Sciences, University of Maiduguri and
   University of Maiduguri Teaching Hospital
Maiduguri, Borno State, Nigeria

Adesoji O. Ademuyiwa, MBBS, FWACS, FMCS (Nig)
Lecturer and Consultant Paediatric Surgeon
Paediatric Surgery Unit, Department of Surgery
College of Medicine, University of Lagos
Lagos, Nigeria

James O. Adeniran, MBBS (Ib), FRCS (Glasg), FWACS,
   Dip Paed Surg (Lond)
Professor of Paediatric Surgery
Paediatric Surgical Unit
University of Ilorin and University of Ilorin Teaching Hospital
Ilorin, Nigeria

Frank Agada, FRCS Ed
Department of ENT, Head and Neck Surgery
York Hospital
York, U.K.

Sunday Olusegun Ajike, BDS, FWACS, PGDPA
Associate Professor and Consultant Maxillofacial Surgeon
Department of Dental Surgery
Ahmadu Bello University and Ahmadu Bello University Teaching Hospital
Zaria, Nigeria

Jennifer H. Aldrink, MD
Assistant Professor of Clinical Surgery
The Ohio State University College of Medicine
Division of Pediatric Surgery
Nationwide Children's Hospital
Columbus, Ohio, U.S.

Christopher C. Amah, MB ChB, FWACS
Senior Lecturer & Consultant Pediatric Surgeon
Department of Pediatric Surgery
University of Nigeria and University of Nigeria Teaching Hospital
Enugu, Nigeria

Emmanuel A. Ameh, MBBS, FWACS, FACS
Professor and Consultant Paediatric Surgeon
Chief, Division of Paediatric Surgery, Department of Surgery
Ahmadu Bello University and Ahmadu Bello University Teaching Hospital
Zaria, Nigeria

Nkeiruka Ameh, MBBS, FWACS
Senior Lecturer and Consultant Obstetrician and Gynecologist
Reproductive Endocrinology & Infertility Unit
Department of Obstetrics & Gynecology
Ahmadu Bello University and Ahmadu Bello University
   Teaching Hospital
Zaria, Nigeria

Manali S. Amin, MD, FACS
Instructor, Department of Otology and Laryngology
Harvard Medical School
Associate in Otolaryngology, Department of Otolaryngology
   and Communication Disorders
Children's Hospital Boston
Boston, Massachusetts, U.S.

Safwat S. Andrawes, MBChB, MMed Surgery, MSc Urology,
   FICS, FCS (ESCA)
Consultant Paediatric Surgeon and Paediatric Urologist
Gertrude's Children Hospital
Nairobi, Kenya

William Appeadu-Mensah, MB, CHB, FWACS, FGCS
Paediatric Surgery Unit, Department of Surgery
University of Ghana Medical School
Korle-Bu Teaching Hospital
Accra, Ghana

Marion Arnold, MBChB, DCH (SA)
Division of Pediatric Surgery
University of Stellenbosch
Tygerberg, South Africa

Johanna R. Askegard-Giesmann, MD
Clinical Research Fellow
Department of Pediatric Surgery
Nationwide Children's Hospital
The Ohio State University
Columbus, Ohio, U.S.

Jane P. Balint, MD
Associate Professor of Clinical Pediatrics
The Ohio State University College of Medicine
Director, Intestinal Support Service
Division of Pediatric Gastroenterology, Hepatology, and Nutrition
Nationwide Children's Hospital
Columbus, Ohio, U.S.

Behrouz Banieghbal, MB, BCh, BAO, FRCSI,
   FRC (SA) Paed Surg
Paediatric Surgeon and Senior Lecturer
Division of Paediatric Surgery
Johannesburg General Hospital
University of the Witwatersrand
Johannesburg, South Africa

Nick Bauman, MD, FRCSC
BethanyKids at Kijabe Hospital
Kijabe, Kenya

Peter Beale, FCS (SA); M Med Chir (Pret), FRCS (Edin)
Head of Paediatric Surgery Division
University of the Witwatersrand
Johannesburg, South Africa

Stephen W. Bickler, MD, DTM&H, FACS, FAAP
Professor of Surgery & Pediatrics
University of California, San Diego
Attending Pediatric Surgeon
Children's Hospital of San Diego
San Diego, California, U.S.

Christopher Bode, MBCHB, FWACS, FMCS (Nig)
Associate Professor and Consultant Paediatric Surgeon
Paediatric Surgery Unit, Department of Surgery
Lagos University and Lagos University Teaching Hospital
Lagos, Nigeria

Laura Boomer, MD
Resident in General Surgery
University of Nevada School of Medicine
Las Vegas, Nevada, U.S.

Eric Borgstein, MD, FRCS (Edin), FCS (ECSA)
Professor of Surgery
Consultant Paediatric Surgeon
College of Medicine, University of Malawi
Queen Elizabeth Central Hospital
Blantyre, Malawi

Richard Bransford, MD, FACS
Program Director
BethanyKids at Kijabe Hospital
Kijabe, Kenya

Mairo Adamu Bugaje, MBBS (ABU), FWAC-Paed
Senior Lecturer and Consultant Paediatrician
Head, Department of Paediatrics
Ahmadu Bello University and Ahmadu Bello University Teaching Hospital
Zaria, Nigeria

Brian H. Cameron, MD, FRCSC, FACS
Associate Professor of Pediatric Surgery
McMaster Children's Hospital
Hamilton, Ontario, Canada

Louise Caouette-Laberge, Paediatric Plastic Surgeon
    and Professor of Surgery
Hospital Sainte-Justine
Université de Montréal
Montréal, Qubec, Canada

Richard F. Carter, MD
Senior Resident, General Surgery
Department of Surgery
Virginia Commonwealth University School of Medicine
Richmond, Virginia, U.S.

John Chinda, MBBS, FWACS
Lecturer and Consultant Paediatric Surgeon
Paediatric Surgery Unit, Department of Surgery
University of Maiduguri and University of Maiduguri Teaching Hospital
Maiduguri, Nigeria

Lohfa B. Chirdan, MBBS, Dip Paed Surg (Lond), FWACS
Associate Professor and Consultant Paediatric Surgeon
Paediatric Surgery Unit, Department of Surgery
University of Jos and Jos University Teaching Hospital
Jos, Nigeria

Andrew Coatesworth, FRCS (ORL-HNS)
Department of ENT, Head & Neck Surgery
York Hospital
York, U.K.

Oriana D. Cohen, BA
Department of Surgery, Division of Pediatric Surgery
New York University Langone Medical Center
New York, New York, U.S.

Sharon Cox, MBChB, FCS (SA), Cert Paed Surg (SA)
Senior Consultant in Paediatric Surgery
Department of Pediatric Surgery
School of Child and Adolescent Health and Red Cross War Memorial Children's Hospital
University of Cape Town, Rondebosch
Cape Town, South Africa

Olamide O. Dairo, MD
Assistant Professor of Anesthesiology
The Ohio State University
Attending Anesthesiologist
Nationwide Children's Hospital
Columbus, Ohio, U.S.

Osarumwense David Osifo, MBBS, FWACS, FICS
Lecturer/Consultant Paediatric Surgeon
University of Benin Teaching Hospital
Benin City, Nigeria

Miliard Debrew, MD, FRCS (Eng), FCS (ECSA)
Assistant Professor of Paediatric Surgery
Black Lion Hospital, Addis Ababa University
Addis Ababa, Ethiopia

Ashish Desai, FRCS, FEBPS, MCh Paed, DNB Paed Surg
Consultant Paediatric Surgeon
King's College Hospital
London, U.K.

David P. Drake, MA, MB, BChir, FRCS, DCH
Consultant Paediatric Surgeon
Department of Paediatric Surgery
Great Ormond Street Hospital for Children
London, U.K.

Felicitas Eckoldt-Wolke, Professor of Pediatric Surgery
Chair and Chief of Clinic of Paediatric Surgery
Jena University Hospital
Friedrich Schiller University of Jena
Jena, Germany

Stella A. Eguma, MBBS, DA, FWACS
Professor of Anaesthesia
Ahmadu Bello University
Consultant Anaesthetist
Ahmadu Bello University Teaching Hospital
Zaria, Nigeria
Consultant Anaesthetist
John F Kennedy Memorial Hospital
Monrovia, Liberia

Sebastian O. Ekenze, MBBS, FWACS
Senior Lecturer & Consultant Pediatric Surgeon
Department of Pediatric Surgery
University of Nigeria and University of Nigeria Teaching Hospital
Enugu, Nigeria

Khalid A. ElAsmar, MBBCH, MS, MRCS
Division of Pediatric Surgery
Ain Shams University
Cairo, Egypt

Hesham Soliman El Safoury, MD
Professor of Pediatric Surgery
Ain-Shams University
Cairo, Egypt

Charles F.M. Evans, BSc, MBBS, MRCS (Eng), MD
Department of Paediatric Surgery
Oxford Children's Hospital
John Radcliffe Hospital
Oxford, U.K.

Iyekeoretin Evbuomwan
Professor and Consultant Paediatric Surgeon
Department of Surgery
University of Benin and University of Benin Teaching Hospital
Benin, Nigeria

Renata Fabia, MD, PhD, FACS
Assistant Professor of Clinical Surgery
The Ohio State University
Director of Burn Unit
Nationwide Children Hospital
Columbus, Ohio, U.S.

Julia B Finkelstein
New York University Langone School of Medicine
New York, New York, U.S.

Andrew P Freeland, FRCS
Consultant ENT Surgeon
John Radcliffe Hospital
Oxford, U.K.

Howard B Ginsburg, MD
Director
Division of Pediatric Surgery, Department of Surgery
New York University Langone School of Medicine
New York, New York, U.S.

John R. Gosche, MD, PhD
Chief, Division of Pediatric Surgery
Professor of Surgery, Department of Surgery
University of Nevada School of Medicine
Las Vegas, Nevada, U.S.

Hugh W. Grant, BSc, MB ChB, MD, FRCS (Edin), FRCS (Eng)
Consultant Paediatric Surgeon
John Radcliffe Hospital
Oxford, U.K.

Jonathan I. Groner, MD, FACS, FAAP
Professor of Clinical Surgery
The Ohio State University College of Medicine
Interim Chief, Department of Pediatric Surgery
Trauma Medical Director
Nationwide Children's Hospital
Columbus, Ohio, U.S.

Devendra K Gupta, MBBS, MS MCh, FAMS, FRCS,
  DSc (Honoris Causa)
Professor and Head, Department of Pediatric Surgery
All India Institute of Medical Sciences
New Delhi, India

Ahmed T. Hadidi, MB, BCh, MSc, MD, FRCS (Eng, Glasgow),
  FA (Germany), PhD
Professor of Pediatric Surgery
Chairman of Pediatric Surgery Dept. Offenbach Hospital, Offenbach
Chairman of Pediatric Surgery Dept., Emma Hospital, Seligenstadt
Frankfurt, Hessen, Germany

Larry Hadley, MB.CHB.,FRCS (Edin),FCS (SA)
Professor and Head of Department of Paediatric Surgery
Nelson Mandela School of Medicine
University of KwaZulu-Natal
Durban, South Africa

Alaa F. Hamza, MD, FRCS, FAAP (Hon)
Professor of Pediatric Surgery
Head of Liver Transplantation Unit
Division of Pediatric Surgery
Ain Shams University
Cairo, Egypt

Edward Hannon, BSc (Hons), MBChB (Hons), MRCS
Specialist Registrar in Paediatric Surgery
Oxford Children's Hospital
Oxford, U.K.

Sameh Abdel Hay, MD
Professor and Chief, Pediatric Surgery Unit
Ain Shams University
Cairo, Egypt

Hugo A. Heij, MD, PhD
Professor of Paediatric Surgery and Head
Paediatric Surgical Centre of Amsterdam
Emma Children's Hospital AMC and VU University Medical Centre
Amsterdam, The Netherlands

Chris Heinick, Paediatric Surgeon
Klinik für Kinderchirurgie der Friedrich-Schiller Universität
Jena, Germany

Afua A. J. Hesse, MB.ChB FRCS (Ed), FWACS, FGCS,
  Cert,HMPP (Leeds)
Associate Professor and Consultant Paediatric Surgeon
Head, Department of Surgery
Korle-Bu Teaching Hospital and the University of Ghana Medical School
Accra, Ghana

Rowena Hitchcock, MB BCh, MA, MD, FRCS
Consultant Paediatric Urologist
Oxford Children's Hospital
Oxford, U.K.

Piet Hoebeke, MD, PhD
Head of Department of Urology
Paediatric Urology and Urogenital Reconstruction
Ghent University Hospital
Ghent, Belgium

Sarah Howles, MRCS (Eng), MA
Department of Paediatric Surgery
Oxford Children's Hospital
Oxford, U.K.

Amy Hughes-Thomas, BSc (Hons), MBBS, MRCS (Eng)
Specialist Registrar Paediatric Surgery
The Children's Hospital, John Radcliffe NHS Trust
Oxford, England

Akanidomo J. Ibanga, BSc, MSc (Clin Psych)
School of Psychology
University of Birmingham
Birmingham, West Midlands, U.K.

Hannah B. Ibanga, MBBS, FWACP (Paeds), Child Psychology (Dip)
Emergency Department
Birmingham Children's Hospital
Birmingham, West Midlands, U.K.

Rebecca Inglis, BM BCh, MA (Cantab)
Junior Research Fellow
Department of Paediatric Surgery
John Radcliffe Hospital
Oxford, U.K.

Sha-Ron Jackson, IeMD
Pediatric Surgery Research Fellow
Children's Hospital Los Angeles
Keck School of Medicine
University of Southern California
Los Angeles, California, U.S.

Iftikhar Ahmad Jan, MBBS, FCPS, FRCS (Eng + Edin), FACS, FEBPS
Professor of Pediatric Surgery
The Children's Hospital
PIMS Islamabad and National Institute of Rehabilitation Medicine
Islamabad, Pakistan

Jayaratnam Jayamohan, MBBS, FRCS, BSc
Consultant Paediatric Neurosurgeon
Oxford Children's Hospital
Oxford, U.K.

V. T. Joseph, FRCS, MD
Consultant Paediatric Surgeon
John Radcliffe Hospital
Oxford, U.K.

Jonathan Karpelowsky, MBBCh, FCS (SA), Cert Paed Surg (SA)
Senior Specialist
Department of Paediatric Surgery
Red Cross War Memorial Children's Hospital
Cape Town, South Africa

Brian D. Kenney, MD
Assistant Professor of Clinical Surgery
Department of Pediatric Surgery
Nationwide Children's Hospital
The Ohio State University
Columbus, Ohio, U.S.

John Kimario, MMed
Consultant ENT Surgeon
Muhimbili National Hospital
Dar es Salaam, Tanzania

Sharon Kling, FCPaed (SA), MMed (Paed), M Phil
Tygerberg Children's Hospital and Stellenbosch University
Cape Town, South Africa

Sanjay Krishnaswami, MD, FACS, FAAP
Educational Director, Pediatric Surgical Residency
Assistant Professor, Division of Pediatric Surgery
Oregon Health & Science University
Portland, Oregon, U.S.

Neetu Kumar, MBBS, MRCS
Jenny Lind Children's Department
Norfolk & Norwich University Hospital
Norwich, U.K.

Jean-Martin Laberge, MD, FRCSC, FACS
Paediatric Surgeon and Professor of Surgery
Division of Pediatric General Surgery
The Montreal Children's Hospital of the McGill University Health Center
Montreal, Québec, Canada

Kokila Lakhoo, PhD, FRCS (Eng + Edin), FCS (SA), MRCPCH (U.K.), MBCHB
Consultant Paediatric Surgeon and Senior Lecturer
Children's Hospital Oxford and University of Oxford
Oxford, U.K.
African Affiliation: KCMC Tanzania

Richa Lal, MS, MCh
Additional Professor and Head
Department. of Pediatric Surgery
Sanjay Gandhi Post Graduate Institute of Medical Sciences
Lucknow, Uttar Pradesh, India

David A. Lanning, MD, PhD
Surgeon-in-Chief, Children's Hospital of Richmond
Associate Professor of Surgery and Attending Pediatric Surgeon
Department of Surgery
Virginia Commonwealth University School of Medicine
Richmond, Virginia, U.S.

Michael Laschat, MD
Consultant, Paediatric Anaesthesia
Children`s Hospital
Cologne, Germany

Mohammed A. Latif Ayad, MD
Consultant of Pediatric Surgery
Division of Pediatric Surgery
Ain Shams University
Cairo, Egypt

John Lazarus, MBChB, FC UROL (SA), MMed (Urology)
Paediatric Urologist
Red Cross War Memorial Children's Hospital
University of Cape Town
Cape Town, South Africa

Jacob N. Legbo, MBBS, FWACS, FMCS (Nig), FRCSEd, FICS
Senior Lecturer and Consultant Plastic and Reconstructive Surgeon
Plastic Surgery Unit, Department of Surgery
Usmanu Danfodiyo University and Usmanu Danfodiyo University Teaching Hospital
Sokoto, Nigeria

Katrine Lofberg, MD
Surgical Resident
Oregon Health & Science University
Portland, Oregon, U.S.

Muhammad Raji Mahmud, MBBS, FWACS
Lecturer and Consultant Neurosurgeon
Division of Neurosurgery, Department of Surgery
Ahmadu Bello University and Ahmadu Bello University Teaching Hospital
Zaria, Nigeria

Amaani K. Malima, MD (Bulgaria), MMed (Orthop-Tumaini), FCS (ECSA)
Head, Department of Surgery
Temeke Municipal Hospital
Dar es Salaam, Tanzania

N. Marathovouniotis, MD
Department of Paediatric Surgery and Paediatric Urology
Childrens Hospital
Town of Cologne, Germany

Franklin C. Margaron, MD
Senior Resident, General Surgery
Department of Surgery
Virginia Commonwealth University School of Medicine
Richmond, Virginia, U.S.

Maurice Mars, MBChB, MD
Department of TeleHealth
Nelson R Mandela School of Medicine
University of Kwa-Zulu Natal
Durban, South Africa

Ruth D. Mayforth, MD, PhD
Consultant Paediatric Surgeon
BethanyKids at Kijabe Hospital
Kijabe, Kenya

Hyacinth N. Mbibu, BSc, MBBS, FWACS
Professor and Consultant Urologist
Division of Urology, Department of Surgery
Ahmadu Bello University and Ahmadu Bello University
    Teaching Hospital
Zaria, Nigeria

Merrill McHoney, MB, BS, FRCS (Paeds), PhD
Academic Clinical Lecturer
Department of Paediatric Surgery
Oxford Radcliffe Hospital
Oxford, U.K.

Vivien M McNamara, BM, BS, FRCS (C/Th), FRCS (Paed Surg)
Department of Paediatric Surgery
Great Ormond Street Hospital for Children
London, U.K.

Alice Mears, MBCHB, FRCS
Paediatric Surgery Specialist Registrar
Oxford Children's Hospital and University of Oxford
Oxford, U.K.

Donald E. Meier, MD, FACS, FWACS
Professor and Endowed Chairman
Division of Pediatric Surgery
Texas Tech University Health Sciences Center, El Paso
El Paso, Texas, U.S.
Consultant Surgeon
Baptist Medical Centre
Ogbomoso, Nigeria
Honorary Professor of Pediatric Surgery
Addis Ababa University
Addis Ababa, Ethiopia

Ronald Merrell, MD
Department of Surgery
Virginia Commonwealth University School of Medicine
Richmond, Virginia, U.S.

Alastair J.W. Millar, FRCS, FRACS (Paed Surg), FCS (SA), DCH
Charles F.M. Saint Professor of Paediatric Surgery
University of Cape Town and Red Cross War Memorial
    Children's Hospital, Rondebosch
Cape Town, South Africa

Ashish Minocha, MBBS, MS, MCh, DNB, MNAMS, FICS
Consultant Paediatric and Neonatal Surgeon
Jenny Lind Children's Department
Norfolk & Norwich University Hospital
Norwich, U.K.

Catherine Mngongo, MMED Surg (KCMC), MBBCH (Tanzania)
Consultant Surgeon
Tumaini University
Kilimanjaro Christian Medical Centre
Kilimanjaro Moshi, Tanzania

Charles N. Mock, ScB, MPH, MD, PhD, FACS
Professor, Department of Surgery, and Professor of Epidemiology
University of Washington, Seattle, Washington, U.S.
Visiting Senior Lecturer
Department of Surgery
School of Medical Sciences/Komfo Anokye Teaching Hospital
College of Health Sciences, Kwame Nkrumah University
    of Science and Technology
Kumasi, Ghana

Sam W. Moore, MBChB, FRCS, Doctor of Medicine (MD)
Division of Pediatric Surgery
Tygerberg Hospital
University of Stellenbosch
Tygerberg, South Africa

Paul J. Moroz, MD, MSc, FRCSC, FAAOS
Assistant Professor
Department of Pediatric Orthopaedic Surgery
University of Ottawa and Children's Hospital of Eastern Ontario
Ontario, Ottawa, Canada
African affiliation: Department of Surgery, Kilimanjaro Christian
    Medical Centre,
Moshi, Tanzania

Philip M Mshelbwala, MBBS, FWACS
Consultant Paediatric Surgeon and Senior Lecturer
Division of Paediatric Surgery, Department of Surgery
Ahmadu Bello University and Ahmadu Bello University
    Teaching Hospital
Zaria, Nigeria

David Msuya, MD, MMED surgery, FCS (ECSA)
Consultant Surgeon
Kilimanjaro Christian Medical Centre and Tumaini University
Moshi, Tanzania

Evan P. Nadler, MD
Co-Director, Children's National Obesity Institute
Children's National Medical Center
Associate Professor of Surgery, Pediatrics, & Integrative
    Systems Biology
The George Washington University School of Medicine
    & Health Sciences
Washington, DC, U.S.

Abdulrasheed A. Nasir, MBBS, FWACS
Consultant Paediatric Surgeon
Division of Paediatric Surgery
University of Ilorin Teaching Hospital
Ilorin, Nigeria

Mark Newton, MD, FAAP
Associate Professor of Pediatric Anesthesiology
Vanderbilt University Medical Center
Nashville, Tennessee, U.S.
Consultant Anesthesiologist and Director of Kenya Registered Nurse
Anaesthetist Program
Kijabe Hospital
Kijabe, Kenya

Phuong D. Nguyen, MD
Department of Surgery, Division of Pediatric Surgery
New York University Langone Medical Center
New York, New York, U.S.

Paul T. Nmadu, FMCS (Nig), FWACS, FICS
Professor and Consultant Paediatric Surgeon
Division of Paediatric Surgery, Department of Surgery
Ahmadu Bello University and Ahmadu Bello University Teaching Hospital
Zaria, Nigeria

Peter M. Nthumba, MBChB, MMed (Surgery), FCS (ECSA)
Plastic, Reconstructive and Hand Surgeon
AIC Kijabe Hospital
Nairobi, Kenya

Alp Numanoglu
Red Cross War Memorial Children's Hospital
Cape Town, South Africa

Benedict C. Nwomeh, MD, MPH, FRCS (Eng, Ed, Glas),
    FACS, FAAP, FWACS
Associate Professor of Clinical Surgery
The Ohio State University
Director of Surgical Education
Department of Pediatric Surgery
Nationwide Children's Hospital
Columbus, Ohio, U.S.

Andrew Gustaf Nyman, MBBCh, MRCPCH
Paediatric Intensive Care Registrar
Oxford Children's Hospital
Oxford, U.K.

Modupe Odelola
Imperial College NHS Trust
St. Mary's Hospital
Praed Street
London

Michael O. Ogirima, FMCS, FWACS, FICS, FAOI
Associate Professor and Chief Consultant
Department of Orthopaedics and Trauma Surgery
Ahmadu Bello University and Ahmadu Bello University
    Teaching Hospital
Zaria, Nigeria

G. Olufemi Ogunrinde, MBBS, FWACP
Senior Lecturer and Consultant Paediatrician
Department of Paediatrics
Ahmadu Bello University and Ahmadu Bello University
    Teaching Hospital
Zaria, Nigeria

Adekunle O. Oguntayo, MBBS, FWACS, FICS
Senior Lecturer and Consultant Obstetrician and Gynecologist
Gynaecologic Oncology Unit
Department of Obstetrics and Gynecology
Ahmadu Bello University Teaching Hospital
Zaria Nigeria

Philemon E. Okoro, MBBS, FWACS
Lecturer and Consultant Paediatric Surgeon
University of Port Harcourt and Port Harcourt University
    Teaching Hospital
Port Harcourt, Nigeria

Peter F. Omonzejele, PhD
Department of Philosophy
University of Benin
Benin-City, Nigeria

Richard Onalo, MBBS, FMCP
Consultant Paediatrician
Department of Paediatrics
Ahmadu Bello University Teaching Hospital
Zaria, Nigeria

G. Ifeyinwa Onimoe, MBBS, FAAP
Clinical Fellow
Department of Hematology/Oncology/Bone Marrow Transplant
Nationwide Children's Hospital
Ohio State University
Columbus, Ohio, U.S.

Iyore A. Otabor, MD, MALD
Clinical Instructor and Research Fellow
Department of Pediatric Surgery
Nationwide Children's Hospital
The Ohio State University
Columbus, Ohio, U.S.

Dakshesh Parikh, MBBS, MS, FRCS (Paed), MD
Consultant Paediatric General and Thoracic Surgeon
Birmingham Children's Hospital NHS Foundation Trust
Birmingham, U.K.

Graeme Pitcher, MBBCh, FCS (SA)
Adjunct Professor
Department of Surgery
University of the Witwatersrand
Head, Paediatric Surgery
Chris Hani Baragwanath Hospital
Johannesburg, South Africa

Dan Poenaru, MD, MHPE, FRCSC, FACS, FCS (ECSA)
Consultant Paediatric Surgeon
BethanyKids at Kijabe Hospital
Kijabe, Kenya
Honorary Professor of Surgery
Aga Khan University
Nairobi, Kenya
Adjunct Professor of Surgery and Paediatrics
Queen's University
Kingston, Ontario, Canada

Jean Heuric Rakotomalala, MD
Paediatric Surgery Fellow (COSECSA)
BethanyKids at Kijabe Hospital
Kijabe, Kenya

Ashley Ridout, BM BCh, MA (Oxon), MRCS (Eng)
Oxford Deanery School of Surgery
Oxford, U.K.

Dorothy V. Rocourt, MD
Chief Fellow in Pediatric Surgery
Nationwide Children's Hospital
The Ohio State University
Columbus, Ohio, U.S.

Bankole S. Rouma, MD
Professor, Pediatric Surgery
University Hospital of Treichville
Abidjan, Côte d'Ivoire

Avraham Schlager, MD
Division of Pediatric Surgery, Department of Surgery
New York University School of Medicine
New York, New York, U.S.

Kant Shah, MBBS MRCS
Research Fellow
Department of Paediatric Surgery
Oxford Children's Hospital
Oxford, U.K.

Shilpa Sharma, MBBS, MS, M.Ch, DNB, Ph.D
Assistant Professor
Department of Pediatric Surgery
Post Graduate Institute of Medical Education and Research
Dr RML Hospital
New Delhi, India

Alison Shefler, MD, FRCP (C)
Consultant in Paediatric Intensive Care
Oxford Children's Hospital
Oxford, U.K.

Bello Bala Shehu, MBBS, FRCS, FACS, FWACS
Professor and Consultant Neurosurgeon
Chief, Regional Centre for Neurosurgery
Usmanu Danfodiyo University Teaching Hospital
Sokoto, Nigeria

Daniel Sidler, MD, M.Phil, FCS (SA)
Associate Professor of Paediatric Surgery and Senior Lecturer
Department of Paediatric Surgery
Tygerberg Children's Hospital, Stellenbosch University
Cape Town, South Africa

Michael Singh, MBBS; FRCS (Paed)
Consultant Paediatric General and Thoracic Surgeon
Birmingham Children's Hospital NHS Foundation Trust
Birmingham, U.K.

Saurabh Sinha, MBBS,FRCS
Fellow in Neurosurgery
Oxford Children's Hospital
Oxford, U.K.

Oludayo Adedapo Sowande, MBChB, FRCSEd, FWACS
Senior Lecturer and Consultant Paediatric Surgeon
Paediatric Surgery Unit, Department of Surgery
Obafemi Awolowo University Teaching Hospital
Ile Ife, Nigeria

Helen Sowerbutts, BA, BABCh Oxon
Speciality Trainee (ST1) in Paediatrics
Northwick Park Hospital
London, U.K.

Emily Stamell
Division of Pediatric Surgery, Department of Surgery
New York University School of Medicine
New York, New York, U.S.

Ronald S. Sutherland, MD, FACS, FAAP
Pediatric Urology
Professor of Surgery & Pediatrics (Clinical)
University of Hawaii, John Burns School of Medicine
Honolulu, Hawaii, U.S.

Atonasio Taela
Department of Surgery
Eduardo Mondlane University
Maputo Central Hospital
Maputo, Mozambique

Erin A. Teeple, MD
Bariatric/Minimally Invasive Surgery Fellow
Department of Pediatric Surgery
Nationwide Children's Hospital
The Ohio State University
Columbus, Ohio, U.S.

Ralf-Bodo Troebs, MD
Professor of Pediatric Surgery
Department of Pediatric Surgery
Catholic Foundation Marienhospital Herne
Ruhr University of Bochum
Herne, Germany

Nyaweleni Tshifularo, MBChB, FCS (SA)
Tygerberg Hospital
University of Stellenbosch
Stellenbosch, South Africa

Francis Aba Uba, MB ChB, FMCS, FWACS
Associate Professor of Surgery and Consultant Paediatric Surgeon
Paediatric Surgery Unit, Department of Surgery
University of Jos and Jos University Teaching Hospital
Jos, Nigeria

Jeffrey S. Upperman, MD, FACS, FAAP
Associate Professor of Surgery
Keck School of Medicine
University of Southern California
Director of Pediatric Trauma
Children's Hospital of Los Angeles
Los Angeles, California, U.S.

Usang E. Usang, FWACS, FMCS (Nig), FICS
Lecturer and Consultant Paediatric Surgeon
University of Calabar and Calabar University Teaching Hospital
Calabar, Nigeria

A.B. (Sebastian) van As, MBChB, MMed, MBA, FCS (SA), PhD
Professor and Head, Trauma Unit
Red Cross War Memorial Children's Hospital
Department of Paediatric Surgery
School of Child and Adolescence Health, University of Cape Town
Cape Town, South Africa

Stefan Wolke
Clinic of Paediatric Surgery
Jena University Hospital
Friedrich Schiller University of Jena
Jena, Germany

George G. Youngson, CBE, PhD, FRCS Ed
Professor and Consultant Paediatric Surgeon
Department of Paediatric Surgery
Royal Aberdeen Children's Hospital
Aberdeen, Scotland
African affiliation: External Examiner, University of Malawi

Nathan R. Zilbert
Division of Pediatric Surgery, Department of Surgery
New York University School of Medicine
New York, New York, U.S.

FOREWORD

Paediatric surgery has come of age with the publication of this landmark textbook directed to the African continent. A comprehensive textbook of this nature is long overdue and undoubtedly will serve as a basic reference tome, practical manual, and stimulus for innovative research for generations to come. Most current textbooks are written with an emphasis on surgical conditions and remedies commonly encountered in the developed world. However, in many developing countries, the aetiology, incidence, pathogenesis, clinical manifestations, investigations, treatment, and outcomes for common diseases, as well as diseases endemic to these regions, are different. Hence the need for a textbook to look beyond current texts and address diseases in a more comprehensive way.

The development of paediatric surgery as a speciality in Africa is relatively recent. In many areas, it is still compromised by a lack of demographic information, infrastructure, and trained surgeons familiar with the special needs of children, as well as limited anaesthetic services and fiscal deficiencies. Life for children on the African continent is therefore not easy. It is a constant battle against poverty, parasitic and other infections and diseases, trauma, debilitating congenital and central nervous system abnormalities, and many other factors impairing their growth and development.

Many of the same surgical diseases seen in the developed world must be diagnosed and treated in Africa under substantially less favourable and often adverse circumstances. The morbidity and mortality rates remain unacceptably high, with wide disparities between countries as well as between urban and rural communities. It is in this setting that this textbook will make a valuable contribution toward expanding knowledge and achieving improved surgical outcomes for all children.

Authorship was wisely chosen: each chapter is written by an acknowledged international expert and an African counterpart who has extensive experience. This daunting task is an affirmation of the specific need to address the often neglected surgical diseases of the region and their special circumstances. This collaboration also recognises the important contributions made by surgeons from Africa. They have a breadth of knowledge and experience to help unlock the doors of ignorance and to contribute to setting a standard of quality care. Many of the authors have earned national and international professional distinction as surgeons, teachers, innovative researchers, and leaders.

People often question the relevance of surgery on a continent where so many other issues are a priority. The estimated accumulative risk for a child to have a condition requiring surgical input is 85% by the age of 15 years, making it a significant public health problem. Obstacles to improve paediatric surgical care include a general lack of interest in surgical conditions affecting children, its poorly defined role, and a lack of political commitment. Surgical training in Africa is also very variable and beset with multiple challenges, which further compound the already suboptimal standard of surgical care. Sick children therefore are found on the doorsteps of health care workers, but the only way they can get their rightful due is to have knowledgeable and skilled surgeons caring for them.

This textbook, as a rich source of information, will consequently contribute significantly to paediatric surgical education in Africa, combining home-grown knowledge on the care of children with surgical conditions. Although this book is directed to the needs of surgeons working in Africa, it may also be of great help to those treating children from Africa somewhere in the developed world. Diseases know no boundaries.

Emeritus Professor Heinz Rode
Red Cross War Memorial Children's Hospital
University of Cape Town, South Africa

A NOTE FROM THE PUBLISHER

We are very pleased to partner with the authors to publish this entirely new and important book: *Paediatric Surgery: A Comprehensive Text For Africa*. This is a major achievement resulting from the contributions of many individuals.

All of the authors contributed their time, experience, and expertise, and for busy clinicians, writing is done at great personal sacrifice. Only by knowing the importance of a project do physicians elect to allocate such time for new material. We acknowledge the special contribution of Dr. Emmanuel Ameh for initiating and coordinating the entire undertaking. Please review the list of the text's contributors and note their diversity and impressive credentials.

Our staff also made this publication a priority. Deborah Cughan organized the project and used her graphic skills to integrate the text and illustrations for publication as well as to design the cover. Sandra Rush edited and indexed the book at a reduced non-profit rate. Additionally, Dean Carlson, our manager and web-master, helped to facilitate all aspects of the project.

Friends of the Global HELP Organization covered the cost of producing this book. Expenses include editing, indexing, formatting, web-site management, CD-Rom Library duplication, and hardcopy printing. Scores of generous people made donations and the major contributors were Henry & Cindy Burgess, George Hamilton, Paul & Suzanne Merriman, and Lana & Lynn Staheli.

We plan to distribute this publication as widely as possible. Along with the printed version, the full text is available on low-cost CD-Roms and may be downloaded in PDF format from our web-site without charge or restrictions.

For any new editions of the publication, please visit our web-site at www.global-help.org.

Lynn Staheli, MD, 2011
Founder and Volunteer Director,
Global HELP Organization
Paediatric Orthopaedist
Professor Emeritus, University of Washington
Seattle, Washington, USA

PREFACE

Paediatric surgery has become an established specialty in many parts of Africa and other developing countries. However, the surgical care of children continues to pose significant challenges in these settings, due partly to the enormous disparity between the large volume of patients and the few available paediatric surgical specialists. In addition, many patients present late, frequently with advanced diseases, and, unfortunately, available medical facilities are often suboptimal.

Although a number of good paediatric surgical textbooks are currently in use worldwide, few address the peculiar needs of surgeons in the developing world. Even though most aspects of paediatric surgical care are standard worldwide, in many cases, the approach, methods, and techniques described in Western textbooks may not be applicable to the African setting. Most existing textbooks are written by surgeons who assume a Western audience in their discussion of incidence rates, demographics, and socioeconomic aspects. Discussion of available treatment options and reference to "standard of care" assume a Western level of technology. Understandably, conditions common in Western countries are treated with greater emphasis while those commonly seen in Africa may not be discussed at all. This book presents a comprehensive overview of paediatric surgery that is most relevant to African children and their surgeons. When used along with the already available textbooks, it will provide a more balanced perspective to anyone interested in paediatric surgery in Africa

The authors of this book are primarily reputable paediatric surgeons with vast experience working in Africa, but also include those from developed countries, whose contributions will add the expertise gained from experience in state-of-the-art facilities. It is hoped that this collaboration will provide the reader with a safe approach to surgical care of children under difficult situations as well as up-to-date information on various aspects of paediatric surgery.

Africa is currently experiencing a severe shortage of paediatric surgical specialists, and a significant proportion of surgery on African children is still performed by general surgeons. Therefore, this book is targeted at trainees in both paediatric surgery and general surgery in Africa and similar settings as well as practising surgeons. Undergraduate medical students, paediatricians, and other paediatric health care practitioners will also find this book a useful reference. The recent increase in the numbers of charitable medical missions from Western countries will continue to bring surgeons from developed countries to Africa. These much-needed doctors will find the book an essential accessory to their work in Africa. Ultimately, we hope the children of Africa will be the final beneficiaries.

The Editors,

E. A. Ameh, Zaria, Nigeria
S. W. Bickler, San Diego, California, USA
K. Lakhoo, Oxford, UK
B. C. Nwomeh, Columbus, Ohio, USA
D. Poenaru, Kijabe, Kenya

Paediatric Surgery: A Comprehensive Text for Africa is published by the Global HELP Organization.

Seattle, WA, USA

ISBN 978-1-60189-129-7

Stomach, Duodenum, and Small Intestine

CHAPTER 59
INFANTILE HYPERTROPHIC PYLORIC STENOSIS

Lohfa B. Chirdan
Emmanuel A. Ameh
Amy Hughes-Thomas

Introduction

Infantile hypertrophic pyloric stenosis (IHPS) is a common surgical cause of vomiting in infancy in the Western world.[1,2] Historically, it was described as a disease entity in 1888 by Harald Hirschsprung.[3] Gastrojejunostomy was used to treat this disease until 1912, when extramucosal muscle-splitting pyloromyotomy was described by Ramstedt.[4] This procedure has dramatically changed the outcome of infants with IHPS.

Demographics

The reported incidence of IHPS in the Western world is 1–4 per 1,000 live births.[5] There is a male-to-female ratio of 4:1, with reported ratios ranging from 2.5:1 to 5.5:1.[6]

Pyloric stenosis appears to be more common in infants of caucasian descent and is less common in India and among black and Asian populations, with a frequency that is one-third to one-fifth that in the white population.[7]

In about 6–33% of infants with IHPS, associated anomalies have been described in the central nervous system (CNS), gastrointestinal tract (GIT), and urinary tract.[8]

Aetiology

Despite the frequency of pyloric stenosis, the aetiology remains unclear. Genetic predisposition acting in conjunction with environmental factors is the most widely accepted explanation; however, debate still continues as to whether it is a congenital or acquired disease.[9–11] Breast-feeding has been suggested as offering some immunity to the disease.[12]

First-born children have been noted to be more likely affected, and a familial link is seen with a greater than fivefold increase in the risk in first-degree relatives. The genetics explaining this are likely to be polygenic, as no single locus has been identified.[6] Male and female children of affected mothers carry a 20% and 7% risk, respectively, of developing the condition, whereas male and female children of affected fathers carry a 5% and 2.5% risk, respectively. Furthermore, an association is seen in twins, with concordance among monozygotic twins of 0.25–0.44, and in dizygotic twins of 0.05–0.10.[13]

Pathophysiology

Pyloric stenosis is characterized by hypertrophy of the pyloric musculature, leading to a mechanical obstruction of the gastric outlet in the affected infant. Thus, hypertrophied pyloric antral muscle fibres protrude distally into the duodenal lumen, producing a reflection of duodenal mucosa.

Infants with a diagnosis of pyloric stenosis will show characteristically low chloride and hydrogen ions as measured in the serum. The loss of gastric secretions secondary to protracted vomiting will result in dehydration. As a result, through aldosterone-stimulated absorption, potassium is excreted in the urine in an attempt to conserve sodium. As potassium depletion worsens, sodium resorption across the renal tubule is then achieved in exchange for a hydrogen ion, thereby creating paradoxical aciduria. Classically, this results in the occurrence of a hypochloraemic hypokalaemic metabolic alkalosis. In severe cases with diagnostic delay, hypoglycaemia and hypoalbuminaemia can be observed.

It is known that the pyloric hypertrophy will eventually resolve, but this takes a long period of time; the infant would usually succumb to the electrolyte derangement and dehydration before this happened.

Clinical Presentation

Infants with pyloric stenosis usually present with a gradual onset of worsening nonbilious vomiting, beginning between 3 to 6 weeks of age. The pattern of vomiting can vary, but often it progresses to the characteristic "projectile" vomiting. Infants may present in the early stages of the disease and be treated for reflux disease or undergone numerous formula changes before the diagnosis is made. Delay in diagnosis can result in significant electrolyte imbalance, weight loss, and failure to thrive.

The typical clinical features include the following:

- Nonbilious vomiting is usually forceful and postprandial.
- The infant is hungry after vomiting and eager to feed, only to vomit again.
- Weight loss occurs in severe cases.
- Signs of dehydration present in cases of repeated vomiting.
- Scaphoid abdomen especially noted after recent vomiting.
- Visible peristalsis may be observed in the upper abdomen, usually moving from the left hypochondrium towards the right side.
- A palpable mass is present in the right upper quadrant (90% in experienced hands); this is best appreciated while the infant is being fed with clear fluid.

Differential Diagnosis

The differential diagnosis of pyloric stenosis includes:

- gastro-oesophageal reflux;
- viral enteritis;
- pylorospasm;
- duodenal stenosis/duodenal web; and
- raised intracranial pressure.

Evaluation

Clinical Diagnosis

Depending of the time to presentation, the clinical picture can vary enormously from a well-hydrated baby to an emaciated infant. Weight loss and dehydration coupled with an insatiable appetite lead to a characteristic facies, with a furrowed brow, wrinkled appearance, and prominent sucking pads. In some infants, the distended stomach may be identifiable in the hypochondrium, with active peristaltic activity visible through the thin abdominal wall. On examination, a mobile, ovoid mass, commonly referred to as an "olive", is palpable in the epigastrium or the right upper quadrant.

If the pylorus is palpated by an experienced clinician, no further imaging is necessary. In some cases, however, other structures may be confused with hypertrophied pylorus, including the caudate lobe of the liver, the right kidney, the vertebrae, or an orogastric tube in the distal stomach. If there is any doubt, or in the absence of a palpable "olive", diagnostic imaging can be helpful.

Ultrasonography

In situations where doubt exists, examination by ultrasound (US) should be performed. This would normally confirm the presence of a pyloric "tumour". The characteristic appearance of pyloric stenosis on ultrasound is that of a "doughnut" or "bull's eye" on cross section of the pyloric channel. Pyloric dimensions with positive predictive value greater than 90% are muscle thickness greater than 4 mm and a pyloric channel length greater than 17 mm.[14] These limits may be lower in infants younger than 30 days of age (Figure 59.1).

An experienced sonographer will recognize periods of relaxation in infants with pylorospasm, commonly confused with pyloric stenosis at examination. Pylorospasm has been hypothesized to be an early stage of IHPS, but this has not been proven.

Upper Gastrointestinal Contrast Study

In an occasional case where doubt still persists after US examination, an upper gastrointestinal (UGI) series may be done. The UGI series would show a narrow pyloric channel, the so-called "string sign" and the "shoulder sign", caused by the impression of the pylorus into the stomach (Figure 59.2).

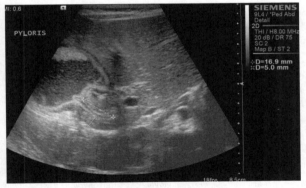

Figure 59.1: Ultrasound features of pyrolic stenosis.

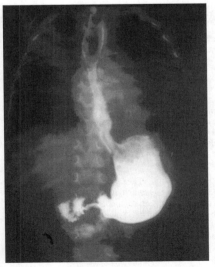

Figure 59.2: UGI contrast showing pyloric stenosis.

Serum Electrolytes

Serum electrolytes should be measured immediately when the patient arrives in hospital. If vomiting has been ongoing for several days, serum electrolytes are frequently deranged. The nature of derangement is a spectrum,[15,16] ranging from mild to severe hyponatraemia, hypochloraemia, hypokalaemia, and metabolic alkalosis. The degree of elevation of serum urea is directly related to the severity of dehydration.

Haemogram/Full Blood Count

Infants presenting late are often malnourished and may have some degree of anaemia, which may require correction. Therefore, a haemogram and full blood count are warranted.

Treatment

Correction of Electrolyte and Fluid Depletion

Patients with pyloric stenosis may have severe electrolyte disturbances, so the serum electrolytes should always be estimated. Mild electrolyte disturbances can be corrected preoperatively with 0.45% normal saline with 5% dextrose solution. Severe disturbances require correction with 0.9% normal saline bolus of 10 to 20 ml/kg, followed by administration of 0.9% saline in 5% dextrose solution. Potassium can be added if necessary when adequate urine output (1.5–2 ml/kg per hour) is established and under electrocardiogram (ECG) monitor. Fluid should be administered at a rate of 25–50% above maintenance.

Following resuscitation and correction of electrolyte imbalance, maintenance IV with 0.45% saline in 5% dextrose with 20 mmol potassium chloride should be given at 25-50% above the standard rate.

Meticulous care and time should always be taken to correct fluid and electrolyte depletion before any surgical correction. It is important to emphasize that mortalities from pyloric stenosis are attributable to fluid and electrolyte problems.

Nasogastric Decompression

Once diagnosis is made, all feeds are stopped. It is helpful to aspirate all gastric content by nasogastric tube (NGT). Frequently, this content comprises milk curds, which may require lavage with saline to adequately evacuate the stomach. Keeping the stomach empty would help prevent aspiration from vomiting. Once the stomach is emptied, the NGT is either closed off or removed to avoid worsening electrolyte depletion by aspirating gastric content.

In the West, gastric lavage is not routinely performed. An NGT is passed, size 8 Fr or above. Gastric losses are monitored and replaced milliliter for milliliter with 0.9% saline. To avoid iatrogenic hyperkalaemia, no potassium is added to the replacement fluid.

Surgical Correction

Surgical correction of pyloric stenosis is not an emergency, and therefore the electrolyte disturbances can and should be meticulously corrected before operation. Occasionally, children with pyloric stenosis will have jaundice due to a transient impairment of glucuronyl transferase activity. This is self-limited once postoperative feeding is initiated.

Infants undergoing pyloromyotomy are assumed to have a full stomach and the anaesthesiologist should keep this in mind. Both the anaesthesiologist and surgeon should be vigilant during the operation to prevent aspiration of gastric juice. The stomach must be evacuated in the operating room, particularly if NGT had not been inserted earlier.

Preoperative antibiotics are controversial; data supporting their use with the standard right upper quadrant incision are scant. They may be of benefit when performing the operation through the umbilical skinfold.

Operative Details

The standard operation is the Ramstedt pyloromyotomy. Classically, the operation has been approached through a right upper quadrant muscle-splitting approach[17]. Alternatively, the approach may be via a supra-umbilical transverse skinfold incision.

1. Once the peritoneum is entered, the omentum is retrieved into

the wound and elevated to lift the transverse colon. This manoeuvre enables the surgeon to identify the antrum of the stomach. The lower third of the stomach is then gently elevated using moist gauze to deliver the pyloric mass into the wound (Figure 59.3).

2. A vertical incision is then made into the mid anterior surface through the serosa and superficial muscularis, beginning about 1–2 mm from the pyloroduodenal junction to a point 0.5 cm into the lower antrum.

3. The underlying firm fibres are then divided using blunt dissection with a clamp, rounded end of a scalpel blade, or special Benson's pyloromyotomy spreader. Special care is taken to prevent mucosal perforation, especially at the lower end of the incision. Upward protrusion of the gastric mucosa indicates relief of the obstruction (Figures 59.4 and 59.5).

Mucosal perforation usually occurs at the duodenal end and is indicated by the appearance of bilious fluid. When this occurs, repair is done by using interrupted fine monofilament long-term absorbable sutures placed transversely and covered with omentum. If the closure of the mucosal perforation compromises the pyloromyotomy, which rarely happens, a fresh pyloromyotomy is done at about 45°–90° of the first incision. Air is then instilled through the NGT to check the integrity of the duodenal mucosa.

Use of a laparoscopic approach is increasing, with evidence supporting its benefits emerging.[18,19] A recent study has shown a safe alternative with a decreased time to full feeds postoperatively.[20]

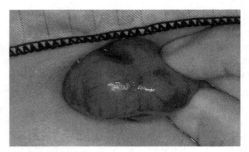

Figure 59.3: Operative view of pyloric mass.

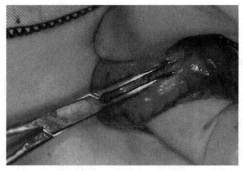

Figure 59.4: Spreading of the divided pyloric muscle.

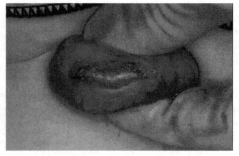

Figure 59.5: Myotomy with mucosal bulge.

Postoperative Management

Postoperative nasogastric decompression is not necessary unless the mucosa has been entered and repaired. Several feeding schedules have been advocated after surgery. Traditional structured feeding regimens as opposed to more rapid initiation and advancing feeding schedules are probably unnecessary. Feedings are begun 4 to 6 hours after operation, normally with low-volume balanced electrolyte or dextrose solution initially, rapidly advanced to full feeds of formula over the next 12- to 24-hour period. If the patient vomits, which is common after this procedure, the same volume feed that caused the emesis can be repeated. The patient is usually discharged the day after operation.

Surgical Complications

Intraoperative risks include bleeding, infection, and mucosal perforation. Postoperative complications include wound infection and dehiscence in about 1%. Persistent vomiting beyond 48 hours, thought to be due to gastric atony, occurs in about 3%. Unrecognized perforation during pyloromyotomy is a serious but rare problem demanding immediate reoperation.

Outcome

The majority of infants go on to make a full recovery postoperatively and need no further medical input. After a surgical pyloromyotomy, the pyloric muscle subsides to a normal size and, when viewed during subsequent operations, is usually visible only as a fine line over the pylorus at the site of the myotomy.

Incomplete pyloromyotomy may occur, but it is difficult to diagnose in the early postoperative phase. Imaging studies done postoperatively are difficult to interpret and usually not helpful. If complete gastric-outlet obstruction is present on a contrast study, repeated pyloromyotomy is necessary.

Mortality is rare, but when it occurs, it is usually from fluid and electrolyte depletion in infants presenting late, and inadequately corrected electrolyte problems before surgery.

Evidence-Based Research

Evidence on the management of pyloric stenosis in African children is rare, so clinicians have to depend on literature from the West, where the disease is more frequent. Table 59.1 presents the results of a survey on the management of IHPS conducted in the United Kingdom and Ireland.

Table 59.1: Evidence-based research.

Title	Surgical practice for infantile hypertrophic pyloric stenosis in the United Kingdom and Ireland—a survey of members of the British Association of Paediatric Surgeons
Authors	Mullassery D, Perry D, Goyal A, Jesudason EC, Losty PD
Institution	Academic Department of Pediatric Surgery, The Royal Liverpool Children's Hospital (Alder Hey), University of Liverpool, United Kingdom
Reference	J Pediatr Surg 2008; 43:1227–1229
Problem	Current practice amongst paediatric surgeons on the management of infantile hypertrophic pyloric stenosis.
Outcome/ effect	More than half of the surgeons surveyed used umbilical incision for pyloromyotomy, whereas only 15% do the pyloromyotomy laparoscopically. Fewer than 10% of surgeons surveyed use the classical right upper quadrant incision for pyloromyotomy. The study also showed that about half of the surgeons do not use antibiotics; however, 70% of those using the umbilical incision use antibiotics. The study concluded that umbilical incision and laparoscopic incisions are benchmarks for surgeons caring for children with infantile hypertrophic pyloric stenosis.
Historical significance/ comments	Acknowledging that IHPS may not be a major workload for the paediatric surgeon practicing in Africa, patients with this condition do come in occasionally, especially in major centres, so paediatric surgeons need to be aware of the current practices amongst paediatric surgeons who care frequently for these patients; hence, the importance of this article. Although there are a lot of variations in the practice, pyloromyotomy through whatever route remains the gold standard for caring for these group of patients.

Key Summary Points

1. Infantile hypertrophic pyloric stenosis affects infants 2–8 weeks of age, often presenting with repeated vomiting.

2. Although the disease may not be common in African children, practitioners may encounter the condition.

3. The aetiology is not clear, but pyloric muscle hypertrophy leading to mechanical obstruction of the pylorus is the endpoint.

4. The disease can be self-limiting, but the infant would succumb to dehydration and electrolyte imbalance if not treated.

5. Care should be taken to correct any fluid and electrolyte depletion before embarking on any surgical correction.

6. Extramucosal pyloromyotomy, introduced about a century ago, still remains the gold standard for surgical management of IHPS.

References

1. Hirschsprung H. Falle von angeborener pyloric stenose. Jb Kinderheik 1888; 27:61.

2. Ramstedt C. Zur operation der angeborenen pylorus-stenose. Med Klin 1912; 8:1702–1705.

3. Spicer RD. Infantile hypertrophic stenosis: a review. Br J Surg 1982; 69:128–135.

4. Stringer MD, Brereton RJ. Current management of infantile hypertrophic pyloric stenosis. Br J Hosp Med 1990; 43:266–272.

5. To T, Wajja A, Wales PW, et al. Population demographic indicators associated with incidence of pyloric stenosis. Arch Pediatr Adolesc Med 2005; 159:520–525.

6. Michel LE, Risch N. The genetics of infantile hypertrophic pyloric stenosis: a reanalysis. Am J Dis Child 1993; 147:1203–1211.

7. Klein A, Cremin BJ. Racial significance in pyloric stenosis. S Afr Med J 1970; 44:1130–1134.

8. Bidair M, Kalota SJ, Kaplan GW. Infantile hypertrophic pyloric stenosis and hydronephrosis: is there an association? J Urol 1993; 150:153–155.

9. Ohshiro K, Puri P. Pathogenesis of infantile pyloric stenosis: recent progress. Pediatr Surg Int 1998; 13:243–252.

10. Abel RM, Bishop AE, Doe CJ, et al. A quantitative study of the morphological and histochemical changes within the nerves and muscle in infantile hypertrophic pyloric stenosis. J Pediatr Surg 1998; 33:682–687.

11. Sherwood W, Choudhry M, Lakhoo K. Infantile hypertrophic pyloric stenosis: an infectious cause? Pediatr Surg Int 2007; 23:61–63.

12. Osifo DO, Evbuomwan I. Does exclusive breastfeeding confer protection against infantile pyloric stenosis? A 30 year experience in Benin City, Nigeria. J Trop Pediatr 2009; 55:132–134.

13. Carter CO, Evans KA. Inheritance of congenital pyloric stenosis. J Med Genet 1969; 6:233–254.

14. Hernanz-Schulman M. Infantile hypertrophic pyloric stenosis. Radiology 2003; 227(2):319–331.

15. Nmadu PT. Alterations in serum electrolytes in congenital hypertrophic pyloric stenosis: a study in Nigerian children. Ann Trop Paediatr 1992; 12:169–172.

16. Touloukian RJ, Higgins E. The spectrum of serum electrolytes in hypertrophic pyloric stenosis. J Pediatr Surg 1983; 18(4):394–397.

17. Fonkalsrud EW. Hypertrophic pyloric stenosis. In O'Neil Jr JA, Grosfeld JL, Fonkalsrud EW, Coran AG, Caldamone AA (eds). Principles of Pediatric Surgery, 2nd ed. Mosby, 2003, Pp 467–470.

18. van der Bilt JD, Kramer WL, van der Zee DC, Bax NM. Laparoscopic pyloromyotomy for hypertrophic pyloric stenosis: impact of experience on the results in 182 cases. Surg Endosc 2004; 18(6):907–909. Epub 27 Apr 2004.

19. Mullassery D, Perry D, Goyal A, Jesudason EC, Losty PD. Surgical practice for infantile hypertrophic pyloric stenosis in the United Kingdom and Ireland—a survey of members of the British Association of Paediatric Surgeons. J Pediatr Surg 2008; 43:1227–1229.

20. Hall NJ, Pacilli M, Eaton S, Reblock K, Gaines BA, et al. Recovery after open versus laparoscopic pyloromyotomy for pyloric stenosis: a double blind multi centre randomized controlled trial. Lancet 2009; 373:390–398.

CHAPTER 60
PEPTIC ULCER DISEASE IN CHILDREN

Oludayo Adedapo Sowande
Jennifer H. Aldrink

Introduction

Peptic ulcer disease (PUD) results from a disruption in the mucosal lining of the stomach or duodenum, allowing penetration through the muscularis mucosa. Over the years, the causative role of *Helicobacter pylori* in the etiology of primary PUD has been proven. Despite increasing attention to PUD as a cause of abdominal pain in children, many cases of PUD in children are not recognized until they are complicated by haemorrhage, perforation, or gastric outlet obstruction. This is invariably associated with an increase in morbidity and mortality.

Demographics

PUD is an uncommon disease of childhood, with an estimated frequency of 1 case in 2,500 hospital admissions in the United States. Data for developing countries, especially from Africa, are scarce, but peptic ulceration is being increasingly recognized in children in the developing world. A prevalence rate of 2% has been found among children presenting with abdominal pain. The majority of cases are duodenal ulcers.

The male-to-female ratio for all childhood PUD is 1.5:1. However, no sex difference in the incidence of primary PUD has been noted in infants or young children.

Aetiology

Peptic ulcer diseases in children and adolescents can be classified into two aetiologies, primary and secondary.

Primary PUD is commonly associated with *H. pylori* infection. Primary ulcers are more likely to be chronic, more common in blood group O and may be familial in 30–40% of PUD cases. It may be associated with elevated serum gastrin level, but this finding is inconsistent in children.

Secondary PUD occurs as a result of accompanying stressful medical or surgical conditions. It may follow severe burns (Curling's ulcer), severe head injury (Cushing's ulcer), and ingestion of nonsteroidal anti-inflammatory drugs (NSAIDs). Mucosal ischaemia, in association with increased gastric acid and pepsin production, and with decreased prostaglandins and mucus production, has been implicated in the development of secondary PUD.

In general, PUD results from an interaction between protective forces that prevent a breach in the integrity of the gastric and duodenal mucosa and those that contribute to mucosal inflammation and ulceration (Table 60.1).

Table 60.1: Protective and disruptive mechanisms for PUD.

Protective Mechanisms	Disruptive Mechanisms
1. Secretion of water-insoluble gastric mucus and bicarbonate	1. Gastric hyperacidity
2. Protective phospholipids	2. Acid-dependent pepsin
3. Rapid turnover of gastric mucosal cells	3. Mucosal ischemia
4. Normal mucosal blood flow	4. *Helicobacter pylori* infection
5. Inhibited acid secretion	5. Sepsis
	6. Traumatic injuries and burns
	7. Drugs (steroids)
	8. Alcohol
	9. Cigarette smoking
	10. Stress

Helicobacter pylori and Peptic Ulcer Disease

H. pylori, a gram-negative microaerophilic spirochete, has been implicated in the development of gastritis and peptic ulcer disease in both adults and children in the presence of acid and pepsin. *H. pylori* infection is mainly acquired during childhood. In India, almost 80% of the population has been infected by the age of 10 years, compared to less than 10% of the population in developed countries. *H. pylori* infection is thought to be transmitted mainly through the faecal-oral route in developing countries. Most infected individuals are asymptomatic; approximately 15% develop peptic ulcer disease and 1% develop gastric cancer. The organism has a unique ability to survive in the harsh acidic environment of the stomach by producing the enzyme urease, which allows it to alkalinize its microenvironment and survive for long periods of time. The organism also produces myriad other virulence factors such as catalase, vacuolating cytotoxin, and lipopolysaccharide. The organism has been classified as a class A carcinogen by the World Health Organization (WHO) because it has been causally associated with gastric carcinoma and lymphoproliferative disorders.

Clinical Presentation

History

A detailed history and physical examination are the mainstays of diagnosis, supplemented by diagnostic investigations where available. The most common symptom in PUD is abdominal pain. A high index of suspicion is necessary in children because abdominal pain is a common complaint; distinguishing the pain of PUD from other causes of abdominal pain is a major challenge. The child's inability to describe the symptoms very well may hinder the diagnosis. Not uncommonly, the diagnosis is not considered at all in children because PUD is thought largely to be a disease of adults.

The pain of PUD in toddlers and preschool age children is usually dull and vague, quite unlike what is described in adults, and may or may not be aggravated by food intake. The older child and adolescent may, however, present in the typical adult fashion with sharp and burning pain localized to the periumbilical or epigastric regions. The pain may exhibit periodicity with frequent exacerbations and remissions over weeks to months. There may be recurrent vomiting, leading to poor weight gain. Vomiting of food ingested over a few days should raise the suspicion of gastric outlet obstruction. A possibility of a family history of peptic ulceration should be sought as well as a history of ingestion of NSAIDs.

As in adults, PUD may be complicated by perforation, gastrointestinal tract (GIT) bleeding (hematemesis with melena), and gastric outlet obstruction. These complications may occur even in the absence of pain. Presentation in infants, particularly in neonates, is usually acute and may manifest as acute perforation or haemorrhage, even in the absence of recognizable stress.

The natural history of peptic ulcers in children has been well correlated with age. In early life (2–6 years), there is a tendency towards bleeding and perforation. In the age group of 7–11 years, the ulcers are usually acute, often perforate, and only rarely bleed or become chronic. In children older than 11 years of age, the behavior of the ulcers approximates that seen in adults.

Physical Examination

A general physical examination in uncomplicated cases is usually not informative. Pallor may suggest blood loss. A combination of chronic epigastric or periumbilical pain and anaemia should raise a suspicion of PUD in a child. Careful inspection, auscultation, and palpation of the abdomen, including rectal examination, are important, although findings may be normal. Haemorrhage accompanies PUD in 15–20% of patients and may be severe enough to require blood replacement. Shock may result from haemorrhage.

Peritonitis resulting from perforation of the GIT occurs in about 5% of children with PUD.

Investigations

Due to the cost and lack of availability of resources, investigating a child with abdominal pain should be focused and targeted. The following investigations may be indicated:

- The haemoglobin level is used to diagnose anaemia and determine its severity. A blood film appearance may show hypochromic, microcytic cells suggestive of iron deficiency anaemia. Sophisticated laboratory tests to diagnose iron deficiency anaemia in chronic cases may not be available in the developing world settings.

- Oesophagogastroduodenoscopy (EGD) is the procedure of choice for detecting PUD in children and adolescents but is often unavailable in most African hospitals. An endoscopy can be performed safely in all paediatric age groups. It allows for direct visualisation of the ulcers; the location and the number can be determined and biopsy can be taken where necessary. In children with severely deformed duodenum or pylorus, there may be some difficulty in visualisation of the duodenum. Urease activity can also be assessed by EGD. Therapeutically, EGD allows for control of bleeding ulcers by using vasoconstricting agents such as epinephrine or by using a heater probe to coagulate the bleeding vessels. Monitoring of response and efficacy of medical treatment can also be done via endoscopy. For peptic ulcer disease in children, a definitive endoscopic and microbiological diagnosis is advisable.

- An upper GI series is an alternative to EGD where such facilities are not available, but it has a high false positive rate of up to 30%. Diagnosis is based on the demonstration of an ulcer crater and deformity of the duodenal cap.

- Serum gastrin estimation may be useful in cases of suspected Zollinger-Ellison syndrome.

Diagnosis of *Helicobacter pylori* Infection

Invasive and noninvasive tests are available for diagnosing *H. pylori* infection. Invasive tests require endoscopy and include rapid urease test (RUT), histopathology, and culture of gastric biopsy. The noninvasive tests, such as urea breath test and stool antigen detection, are used to determine eradication of infection following treatment, whereas serology is used for epidemiological studies but may be unreliable in children.

Medical Care

The initial treatment of PUD in children is medical. The treatment of PUD, as in adults, encompasses eradication of *H. pylori*. This is accomplished by a combination of medications to reduce acid production and/or improve the mucosal defense in combination with antibiotics. The success of histamine-2 receptor blockers and proton pump inhibitors (PPIs), and the eradication of *H. pylori*, has virtually eliminated the need for elective ulcer surgery. Although colonisation by *H. pylori* may be high, there is no evidence that eradication in an asymptomatic patient is warranted. PPIs have been found to be safe in children.

Sucralfate, which is an aluminum salt of sulfated sucrose, may also be used. In the presence of acidic pH, sucralfate forms a complex, paste-like substance that adheres to the damaged mucosal area. This forms a protective coating that acts as a barrier between the lining and gastric acid, pepsin, and bile salts.

Recommended Eradication Therapies for *H. pylori* Disease in Children

First-line therapy is the use of one PPI and two antibiotics for 10 to 14 days. This can be either:

- omeprazole + amoxicillin + clarithromycin; or

- omeprazole + amoxicillin + metronidazole; or

- omeprazole + clarithromycin + metronidazole.

Second-line therapy is employed when there is no response to first-line therapy. It consists of either

- omeprazole + bismuth subsalicylate + metronidazole + amoxicillin or tetracycline for 14 days; or

- ranitidine + bismuth citrate + clarithromycin + metronidazole for 14 days.

Other drug combinations and durations of treatment are currently being evaluated.

For children in the developing world, cost may be a significant consideration in the treatment options available.

Management of Complications of PUD in Children

Surgical intervention is required in a small percentage of infants and in children with complications of PUD that include perforation, obstruction, intractable pain, and bleeding unresponsive to medical or endoscopic therapy.

Bleeding Peptic Ulcer Disease

Bleeding is the most common complication of PUD in children. Most cases are self-limiting and subside with conservative treatment. However, in an acute bleed, the most important clinical step is resuscitation and the restoration of blood volume. The following steps are critical:

1. Two large-bore intravenous catheters are inserted.

2. A bolus fluid of 20 ml/kg of crystalloid is infused rapidly to combat shock, and is repeated as necessary pending availability of cross-matched blood.

3. An appropriately sized urethral catheter is inserted to monitor urinary output. The urinary output, which may be all that is available in most centres in Africa, gives an estimation of organ perfusion as a response to the fluid resuscitation. An output of 1–2 ml/kg is considered satisfactory but should be used in concert with other clinical parameters. A central venous pressure monitor can be inserted where available. Complete blood counts and chemistry values are also determined.

4. A nasogastric tube (NGT) is placed as a way of performing lavage, preventing aspiration, and monitoring ongoing haemorrhage.

With these initial measures (steps 1–4), most bleeding peptic ulcers will subside.

5. Perform an endoscopy, if available, as soon as the patient is stable, usually within 24 hours of admission. Endoscopy confirms the diagnosis and may be therapeutic. Vasoconstrictive agents, such as epinephrine, 1 in 10,000 dilution, can be injected, and use of a heater probe, electrocoagulation, or photocoagulation can also be employed.

6. Angiography may be necessary in patients with a massive GI bleed in whom endoscopy cannot be performed. Angiography can depict the source of the bleeding, and allow for the direct injection of

vasoconstrictive agents. This is rarely available in resource-poor settings.

Rebleeding is reported to occur in 10–30% of cases and usually occurs within the first week after primary therapeutic endoscopy. Endoscopic treatment can be repeated for rebleeding.

Indications for surgery in bleeding PUD include:

1. failed endoscopic treatment;

2. identified arterial bleeding;

3. identified vessels at the base of the ulcer;

4. rebleeding; and

5. loss of more than 50% of the patient's estimated blood volume in a short period (i.e., 8–24 hours).

Choice of Surgery

Simple plication or oversewing of the bleeding source is usually all that is needed for peptic ulcers. A more definitive procedure, such as vagotomy and pyloroplasty, may be added if the patient is stable and fit. In patients with stress ulcers related to brain injury or burns, the procedure of choice may be vagotomy and antrectomy. Total gastrectomy is rarely performed to treat multiple gastric ulcers in paediatric patients.

Perforated Peptic Ulcer Disease in the Child

When perforation occurs, it is usually on the anterior wall of the first part of the duodenum, resulting in both chemical and bacterial peritonitis. Perforation is accompanied by the sudden onset of abdominal pain, vomiting, and generalised abdominal distention. Shoulder pain may be present due to diaphragmatic irritation. Examination of the acutely ill child reveals evidence of peritonitis with board-like rigidity and diminished bowel activity. In the infant, perforation may occur in the absence of any recognizable stress.

A plain abdominal x-ray may be helpful, as it may reveal pneumoperitoneum.

Late presentations are not uncommon in developing countries because of a lack of suspicion and poor access to health care. Late-presenting patients may be severely toxic and dehydrated, requiring urgent fluid resuscitation and correction of electrolytes and acid-base disorder. An NGT and urinary catheter should be inserted. The child should be started on broad-spectrum antibiotics. Surgery is performed as soon as the child is stabilized.

Operative repair of perforated ulcers may be performed by using a simple closure or oversewing. Where available, this may be accomplished laparoscopically. An omental patch (Graham patch) may be used to cover the area of perforation. This treatment should be followed by medical therapy. In a stable patient with chronic ulcer, a selective vagotomy or a bilateral truncal vagotomy with pyloroplasty may be added.

Gastric Outlet Obstruction

Gastric outlet obstruction occurs following chronic inflammation with fibrosis at the pylorus. This is often accompanied by acute inflammation and mucosal oedema, leading to luminal obstruction. Gastric outlet obstruction is an uncommon complication of PUD in children. It is characterized by recurrent episodic vomiting. The vomitus usually contains food residues eaten over the previous few days. The vomiting is characteristically projectile in nature. Weight loss is not uncommon, and in late presentation the child is severely dehydrated and pale.

Serum electrolytes characteristically show hypochloremic alkalosis with hyponatraemia and hypokalaemia. Blood gas analysis shows a base excess of more than +3. There may be hypoproteinaemia as a result of the malnutrition.

Diagnosis is usually confirmed by upper gastrointestinal series or endoscopic gastroduodenoscopy. A dilated stomach with narrowing of the pylorus and deformity of the duodenal bulb is typically demonstrated.

Treatment consists of aggressive resuscitation with crystalloid, ensuring adequate urinary output. Nasogastric decompression and lavage is necessary while the hypoproteinaemia and anaemia are

corrected. In some instances, the nasogastric decompression and treatment with antiulcer drugs will allow oedema to subside enough for gradual introduction of oral feeds. Definitive therapy consists of bilateral truncal vagotomy with pyloroplasty or in the presence of severe fibrosis gastrojejunostomy.

Prognosis and Outcomes

Peptic ulcer is usually a benign disease without a high mortality if diagnosed and treated early. With modern therapy and eradication of *H. pylori*, the cure rate is more than 90%. Mortality rates remain highest in neonates as well as in infants and children with systemic illness or injury who present with acute bleeding or perforation.

Prevention

Prevention involves the avoidance of predisposing factors, such as ingestion of NSAIDs, coffee, smoking, and alcohol in older children and adolescents. Secondary peptic ulceration in severely stressed and traumatized patients can be prevented by prophylactic antacids and H_2-receptor blockers or PPIs. Early recognition and evaluation of abdominal pain will prevent the development of complications of PUD.

Evidence-Based Research

Table 60.2 presents a retrospective study of 45 years of data on surgical treatment of peptic ulcer disease in children.

Table 60.2: Evidence-based research.

Title	A 45-year experience with surgical treatment of peptic ulcer disease in children
Authors	Azarow K, Kim P, Shandling B, Ein S
Institution	Division of General Surgery, The Hospital for Sick Children and University of Toronto, Toronto, Ontario, Canada
Reference	J Pediatr Surg 1996; 31(6):750–753
Problem	The role of the proton pump inhibitor on the incidence of surgery for complications of PUD and the outcome of surgical treatment in complicated PUD in children was investigated.
Comparison/ control (quality of evidence)	This is a retrospective study of all patients who required operations for PUD between 1949 and 1994 (n = 43). The patients were classified into three groups: A (n = 38): pre–H_2 receptor blocker era (1949–1975); B (n = 3): pre–proton pump inhibitor era (1976–1988); and C (n = 2): proton pump inhibitor era (1989–1994). The incidence of surgery for complicated PUD in children and the outcome of surgical intervention were compared across the three eras.
Outcome/ effect	The authors concluded that although the incidence of surgery for PUD has declined, the incidence of surgery for obstruction secondary to PUD has not. The obstruction probably is related to scarring from long-standing disease. *H. pylori* may be a risk factor in the development of obstruction. Lesser procedures, such as vagotomy and pyloroplasty for bleeding PUD, simple oversewing of a perforation, and vagotomy plus a drainage procedure for gastric outlet obstruction, may be sufficient with appropriate ulcer medical treatment postoperatively, especially in those who did not have definitive ulcer surgery.
Historical significance/ comments	This study provides indirect evidence that medical treatment has significantly reduced the incidence of complications of PUD, especially bleeding in children. In Africa and developing countries with a low index of suspicion and poor access to health care facilities, this may not be the case. In an environment where late presentation may be the case, the clinical state should determine the surgical approach to those presenting with complicated PUD; extensive surgery may not be indicated and simple surgery as practiced in this study may suffice

Key Summary Points

1. Peptic ulcer disease in children is being recognized increasingly worldwide, including developing countries.

2. A high index of suspicion is necessary to distinguish PUD in children from other causes of abdominal pain.

3. *Helicobacter pylori* is an important aetiological factor in PUD in children.

4. Peptic ulcer may present with such complications as haemorrhage, perforation, and gastric outlet obstruction, even in the absence of pain.

5. Newborns and infants tend to present with acute complications such as haemorrhage or perforation.

6. Oesophagogastroduodenoscopy is the main diagnostic investigation and is safe in the paediatric age group.

7. The mainstay of management of paediatric PUD is medical, consisting of a combination of PPI, sucralfate, or bismuth with two antibiotics.

8. Surgery is indicated only for complications such as uncontrolled haemorrhage, perforation with peritonitis, and gastric outlet obstruction.

Suggested Reading

Bittencourt RF, Rocha GA, Penna FJ, Queiroz DM. Gastroduodenal peptic ulcer and *Helicobacter pylori* infection in children and adolescents. J Pediatr Rio J 2006; 82:325–334.

Bourke B, Ceponis P, Chiba N, Czinn S, Ferraro R, Fischbach L, et al. Canadian Helicobacter Study Group Consensus Conference: Update on the approach to *Helicobacter pylori* infection in children and adolescents—an evidence-based evaluation. Can J Gastroenterol 2005; 19:399–408.

Drumm B, Koletzko S, Oderda G. *Helicobacter pylori* infection in children: a consensus statement. Medical position paper: Report of the European Pediatric Task Force on *Helicobacter pylori* on a consensus conference, Budapest, Hungary, September 1998. J Pediatr Gastroenterol Nutr 2000; 30:207–213.

Gold BD, Colletti RB, Abbott M, Czinn SJ, Elitsur Y, Hassall E, et al. *Helicobacter pylori* infection in children: recommendations for diagnosis and treatment. Medical position statement: The North American Society of Pediatric Gastroenterology and Nutrition. J Pediatr Gastroenterol Nutr 2000; 31:490–497.

Hassall E. Clinical practice guidelines for suspected peptic ulcer disease in children. BC Med J 1994; 36(8):538–539.

Hua M-C, Kong M-S, Lai M-W, Luo CC. Perforated peptic ulcer in children: A 20-year experience. J Pediatr Gastroenter Nutr 2007; 45:71–74.

Karlstron F. Peptic ulcer in children in Sweden during the years 1953–1962. Ann Paediatr 1964; 202:218–221.

Kawakami E, Machado RS, Fonseca JA, Patrício FRS. Clinical and histological features of duodenal ulcer in children and adolescents. J Pediatr (Rio J). 2004; 80:321–325.

Poddar U, Yachna SK. *Helicobacter pylori* in children: an Indian experience. Indian Pedatr 2007; 44:761–770.

Tsang TM, Saing H, Yeung CK. Peptic ulcer in children. J Paediatr Surg 1990; 25:744–748.

CHAPTER 61
NEONATAL INTESTINAL OBSTRUCTION

Daniel Sidler
Miliard Debrew
Kokila Lakhoo

Introduction

Neonatal intestinal obstruction (NIO) is one of the most common emergency conditions a paediatric surgeon is called upon to assess during the neonatal period. Successful management of NIO depends on timely diagnosis and referral for therapy. The diagnosis is based on history (symptoms) and physical examination (signs) confirmed by some investigations such as radiographic and histopathological studies. Catastrophic events such as volvulus, ischaemic loop of bowel, pneumoperitoneum, and/or pneumonia from aspiration and malnutrition could be overcome through efficient and timely resuscitation and urgent transport to a specialised unit.

The desired goal of healthy survival of neonatal intestinal obstruction requires a coordinated interaction of medical, nursing, and rehabilitative specialties in an organised team. Early surgical intervention is paramount and may mean all the difference between intestinal salvage and crippling short gut syndrome. The typical case of neonatal bowel obstruction is generally straightforward, and the outcome is potentially excellent. Only very preterm babies and those of extremely low birth weight may succumb. However, in Africa, late presentations and poor resources lend to a mortality of up to 50%.[1] Few dedicated paediatric hospitals exist in developing countries.[2]

Intestinal obstruction can be complete (atresia, anorectal malformation (ARM)) or incomplete (stenosis, web). Obstruction may be intraluminal (meconium ileus or meconium plug syndrome) or functional (Hirschsprung's disease (HD)). Proximal obstruction presents with earlier vomiting and less abdominal distention, whereas distal bowel obstruction lends itself to late emesis and greater abdominal distention. This chapter provides an overview on neonatal bowel obstruction. Each specific condition is covered in chapters elsewhere in this book, specifically, Chapter 58 (inguinal and femoral hernias and hydroceles), Chapter 62 (duodenal atresia and stenosis), Chapter 63 (intestinal atresia and stenosis), Chapter 65 (intestinal malrotation and midgut volvulus), Chapter 67 (meconium disease), Chapter 76 (Hirschsprung's disease), and Chapter 77 (anorectal anomalies).

Demographics

The incidence of NIO is approximately 1 in 5,000 live births. The true incidence in Africa is unknown, but a recent report from Tanzania has shown that it is still the most common neonatal surgical emergency.[1] Many cases still die undiagnosed and untreated.

Aetiology/Pathophysiology

Neonatal intestinal obstruction has varied aetiology, so the pathophysiology is diverse.

The gastrointestinal tract (GIT) arises from the yolk sac. At 3 to 4 weeks' gestation, it becomes a distinct entity. A connection, the vitelline (omphalomesenteric) duct, may persist as a Meckel's diverticulum. The alimentary tube is divided according to its blood supply into the foregut, midgut, and hindgut.

The foregut comprises the oesophagus, stomach, and duodenum. These are vascularised by multiple sources—the thyrocervical, intercostal, celiac axis, and superior mesenteric vessels.

The midgut comprises the jejunum and ileum as well as the ascending and proximal transverse colon. These are supplied by the superior mesenteric vessels.

The hindgut comprises the distal colon, which is supplied by the inferior mesenteric vessels, and the rectum, which is supplied by the internal iliac vessels.

Aberrations of foregut formation include duodenal stenosis, duodenal atresia, and annular pancreas. Maldevelopment of the midgut includes malrotation as well as jejunal and ileal atresia. Meconium ileus involves the distal ileum. Hirschsprung's disease (aganglionic megacolon), meconium plug syndrome, and imperforate anus involve the hindgut. Enteric duplications occur in all three locations.

Jejunoileal atresia is a condition acquired during foetal development due to disruption of the mesenteric blood supply. In their classic work on foetal dogs in 1955, Louw and Barnard from Cape Town, South Africa, clarified the pathophysiology of jejunoileal atresia.[3] Other abdominal conditions occurring in utero, such as gastroschisis, volvulus, or intussusception, may be associated with intestinal atresia due to kinking, stretching, or otherwise disrupting the blood flow to the foetal bowel. Chromosomal anomalies are rare (<1%) in babies with jejunoileal atresia.

Meconium ileus is the earliest manifestation of cystic fibrosis (CF), an autosomal recessive condition characterised by abnormalities in cellular membrane physiology and chloride ion transport that contribute to progressive respiratory failure, derangements in cellular secretory patterns, and diminished mucosal motility. In developed countries, 10–20% of newborns with CF present with meconium ileus, an association first described by Landsteiner in 1905.[4] A cystic fibrosis gene that is different from that in the caucasian population has been identified in the black African population;[5] however, the incidence in Africa is much reduced, and in many sub-Saharan countries, the disease is not reported.[6]

Abnormalities in the cystic fibrosis transmembrane regulator (CFTR) disrupt transmembrane flux of the chloride ion, which subsequently affects sodium transport as well. The meconium of affected babies is thick and sticky; this, coupled with the poor motility of an immature intestine, leads to intraluminal obstruction of the terminal ileum. A contrast enema might reveal the characteristic finding of a microcolon. It is essential to push the contrast up to the level of obstruction, namely, the distal ileum to be therapeutic by flushing out the meconium plugs (Figures 61.1 to 61.4).

Meconium plug syndrome refers to inspissated meconium obstructing the colon; it may denote HD but not CF. Conditions that predispose to dysmotility of the neonatal bowel (e.g., maternal pre-eclampsia, diabetes mellitus, administration of magnesium sulfate, prematurity, sepsis, and hypothyroidism) may be responsible for the formation of the meconium plug. A water-soluble contrast enema can be both diagnostic and therapeutic for this condition.

Hirschsprung's disease is a disorder of the neuroenteric pathways in the distal colon that results in a bowel that is tonically contracted. Bowel peristalsis is controlled by neuroenteric ganglion cells, which

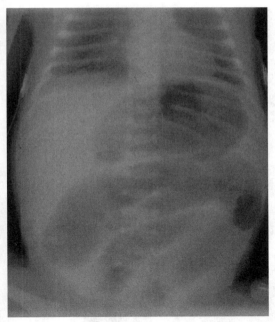

Figure 61.1: Radiograph showing ground-glass appearance of meconium ileus.

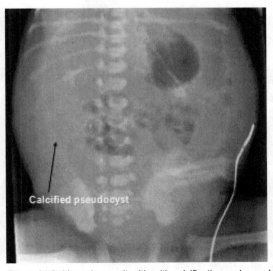

Calcified pseudocyst

Figure 61.2: Meconium peritonitis with calcification and pseudocyst due to in utero perforation.

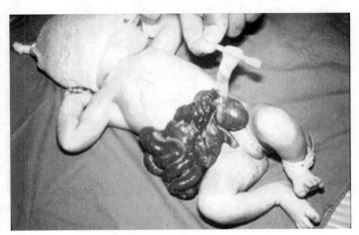

Figure 61.3: Meconium ileus with perforation.

are present in the submucosal layer of the intestine and migrate from the neural crest distally along the bowel to reach the rectum at about 7–10 weeks' gestation. HD is the congenital absence of neuroganglion cells; consequently, the peristaltic relaxation phase is absent distally, and the affected intestine does not appropriately relax, causing a functional obstruction. The extent of the aganglionic segment varies with each patient, but extends from the distal rectum proximally. The level at which the proximal but healthy bowel starts to dilate is called the transition zone (Figure 61.5).

The genetic defects responsible for HD consist of abnormalities on more than one chromosome and include the RET proto-oncogene, located at chromosome 10q11.21. RET interacts with a protein termed EDNRB, encoded by the gene EDNRB, which is located on chromosome 13.

Anorectal malformation

At 4 to 6 weeks' gestation, the hindgut separates into the urogenital sinus and the anorectum, which then undergoes canalisation. The distal third of the anus develops from ectoderm and becomes the anal pit, whereas the proximal portion of the anal canal is derived from mesoderm. An anal membrane covers the canal until 8 weeks' gestation, when it perforates and becomes a patent anus. Imperforate anus results if this sequence of events occurs improperly.

In summary, conditions of NIO include:

- hernia (inguinal, internal);

- atresia, stenosis, web (oesophageal, duodenal, jejunoileal, colonic);

- anorectal malformation;

- Hirschsprung's disease;

- meconium ileus or plug; and

- malrotation with midgut volvulus.

Clinical Presentation

History

The history of NIO is typical for the level (high/ low) and type (mechanical, functional) of obstruction. High intestinal obstruction presents with early vomiting, whereas low intestinal obstruction presents with abdominal distention and later onset vomiting. Feeding intolerance with bile-stained vomiting, absent meconium, and abdominal distention are therefore paradigmatic. With late presentation, the symptom presentation might change due to complications and malnutrition.

On antenatal ultrasound, polyhydramnios is a common feature. Intrauterine bowel dilatation may also be noted if scanned after 24 weeks' gestation.

Physical Examination

Depending on the level of intestinal obstruction, the physical finding is that of a distended abdomen. Within the African context, these babies often present late with aspiration pneumonia, malnutrition, and final events such as intestinal perforation and sepsis. A careful examination and search for typical signs (e.g., abdominal distention, peristaltic waves across the abdomen, absent anus or perianal fistulas, severe distention, and malnutrition in HD) usually reveal the appropriate suspected diagnosis.

Investigations

The most important and useful test in any NIO is the abdominal radiograph (AXR). A single supine and lateral shoot-through is usually sufficient. The distribution of the air contrast directs one to the appropriate diagnosis. Very distended loops of bowel are indicative of atresia. Long-standing drainage from a nasogastric tube (NGT), however, could make such a diagnosis difficult. A duodenal atresia could in this way be missed purely by the duodenal bulb being collapsed from the ongoing drainage. A repeat radiograph with injection of some air through the NGT facilitates the diagnosis.

Once a diagnosis is suspected, contrast studies may help in assessing the rest of the bowel and/or be therapeutic. Such investigation is paramount for the demonstration of the anatomy in ARM after a colostomy has been performed and to assess the length and level in HD (see Figure 61.5). A water-soluble contrast enema will help to clear the thick meconium in meconium ileus.

Further radiological studies have to be requested to assess associated abnormalities such as those included in the acronym VACTERL (vertebral, anorectal, cardiac, tracheo-oesophageal, renal, and limb).

Blood tests are needed to facilitate and modulate resuscitation. Depending on the severity of the condition and its delayed presentation, blood products might be needed for the surgery.

Management

Preoperative Treatment

All conditions need fluid resuscitation and nasogastric decompression. Broad-spectrum antibiotics should be started prophylactically.

Condition-Specific Management

Duodenal atresia

Evaluate for trisomy 21. Because duodenal atresia is considered a midline defect, an evaluation for associated anomalies should include echocardiography, head and renal ultrasonography, and vertebral skeletal radiography.

Jejunoileal atresia

Intraoperatively distal atresias can be identified by flushing the distal intestinal lumen with warm saline to confirm intestinal continuity down to the level of the rectum.

Meconium ileus

The traditional gastrografin enema has been replaced with a water-soluble contrast enema, which is equally effective in loosening the meconium impaction. The enema fluid must be refluxed into the terminal ileum.

N-acetylcysteine may be administered by NGT to further loosen the meconium.

Hyperosmolar enemas may increase the risk of hypovolaemic shock and injury to the intestine with perforation. The risk of perforation is reportedly 3–10%.

Meconium plug syndrome

A gentle rectal washout with temperate normal saline might alleviate the obstruction immediately. A rectal suction biopsy and or a contrast enema should rule out HD.

Full-thickness rectal muscle biopsy is recommended where there is no frozen section or histochemical assay available

Hirschsprung's disease

Initial rectal washout will alleviate the obstruction. Rectal suction biopsy or full thickness biopsy will confirm the diagnosis. A contrast enema will show the level of disease.

Imperforate anus

An 18-hour plus AXR, which is the time required for swallowed air to reach the level of obstruction, will help to show the level of abnormality.

Operative Therapy

Duodenal atresia

A diamond-shaped or side-to-side duodenoduodenostomy is an easy procedure to bypass the obstruction.

Malrotation with volvulus

Malrotation with midgut volvulus (Figure 61.6) is a true surgical emergency in the newborn. Delay in operation may result in catastrophic loss of the bowel and death.

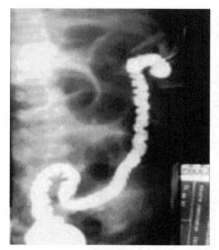

Figure 61.4: Contrast enema study showing microcolon.

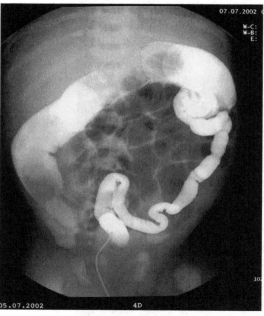

Figure 61.5: Contrast enema in Hirschsprung's disease showing diseased narrow bowel, transition zone, and dilated normal bowel.

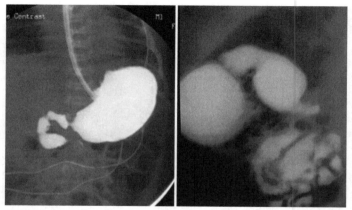

Figure 61.6: Contrast study showing malrotation with volvulus.

Assess the stage of ischaemia and derotate counterclockwise if the bowel seems viable. Inform the anaesthetist about the manoeuvre because there will be a flush of intravenous endotoxins.

Depending on the viability of the bowel, continue on to a Ladd's procedure, in which an extensive mobilisation of the mesentry is performed.

Removal of the appendix is controversial and a surgical choice.

Jejunoileal atresia
Surgery for jejunoileal atresia involves resection of the most distended proximal bowel and primary anastomosis. A diverting ostomy is avoided if possible. As with surgery for duodenal atresia, resection or tapering of the proximal dilated segment is occasionally necessary to limit the dysmotility that occurs in grossly dilated bowel. The ileocaecal valve is preserved if possible because this prevents egress of bacteria from the colon into the small intestine with resultant bacterial overgrowth and malabsorption.

Meconium ileus
Calcification on AXR (see Figure 61.2) indicates that an intestinal perforation occurred in utero and spontaneously sealed; if not, the extruded meconium is walled off by adjacent intestine to form pseudocysts.

These babies have meconium peritonitis, and their appearance is unmistakable; these are babies who are born with (as opposed to those who develop) a distended, erythematous abdomen.

A laparotomy is undertaken with drainage of the meconium pseudocyst and identification of the site of the perforation, which is converted to an enterostomy.

In uncomplicated meconium ileus, an enterostomy with irrigation of the bowel contents may successfully loosen the meconium and permit its evacuation and facilitate the closure of the enterostomy over a t-tube. Postoperatively, after a contrast study shows distal patency, the t-tube can be removed for the controlled fistula to close without further need of surgery. Rarely, some patients might need an ostomy for diversion and access for proximal and distal irrigation with N-acetyl cysteine.

Hirschsprung's disease
The treatment of Hirschsprung's disease is primarily surgical, except in instances of enterocolitis.

Patients with HD are treated with a colostomy near the transition zone (level of beginning of dilatation). If histological leveling is not possible in emergency cases, a right transverse diverting colostomy is safe. It is sometimes difficult to visualise the transition zone in a neonate.

A pull-through procedure is performed after the child is feeding and gaining weight or at least 6 weeks after enterocolitis.

Different procedures have been described as one- or two-stage procedures and are increasingly performed at a younger age.

The most recent innovations include minimally invasive techniques, such as the transanal pull-through using laparoscopy in cases in which the transition zone is not located in the distal sigmoid colon.

Imperforate anus
Low lesions with fistulous connections to the perianal skin can be repaired primarily by anoplasty.

If the fistula runs from the rectum to the vagina or urethra or urinary bladder, the imperforate anus is classified as high, and the infant should undergo a colostomy.

Definitive repair of the imperforate anus is classically performed by posterior sagittal anorectoplasty, in which the rectum is situated within the striated muscle complex and anal sphincter.[7]

The laparoscopic pull-through using three ports has become a favoured procedure for high anorectal malformations.

Increasingly, laparoscopic techniques have been used to repair the above-mentioned conditions. A good alternative for Africa is the minimal approach described by Banieghbal and Beale,[8] whereby access is gained through the umbilicus. Such an approach leaves a virtually unrecognisable scar.

General Postoperative Care
Modern supportive care in the intensive care unit (ICU) with continuing fluid resuscitation, parenteral nutrition, and respiratory support have been the bases for the increased survival rate. In countries where parenteral nutrition is not available, transanastomotic tubes have been tried with indefinite success for the purpose of early feeding. This postoperative management will make all the difference to the survival of children in Africa.

Two weeks after anorectoplasty, serial anal dilatations should start by using anal dilators of increasing size. Within Africa, the child should be kept hospitalised until the mother is comfortable with digital dilatations.

In all of these conditions, the neonatologist and paediatric surgeon must work together in a coordinated fashion, allowing the diagnosis to be quickly established and therapy to be rapidly implemented. In conditions of the intestine that are known to be associated with systemic disease, such as duodenal atresia (trisomy 21) and meconium ileus (cystic fibrosis), appropriate consultation should be obtained early, and the continued involvement of appropriate specialists may be warranted long after the baby has recovered from the initial hospitalisation.

Postoperative Complications
Postoperative complications pertain to factors of

- total parenteral nutrition (cholestasis and hyperalimentation hepatitis);

- central venous access (pneumo/hemothorax, catheter embolus); and

- catheter sepsis.

Postoperative Stricture and/or Adhesions
Anastomotic stricture is a complication after surgery. Postoperative adhesions can occur after any laparotomy. They may be caused by peritonitis from leaking anastomosis. A recent study of 1,541 children who had intestinal surgery showed an adhesion rate of almost 10% in the operative site and a rate of approximately 5% elsewhere.[9]

Decreased Gut Motility
Poor motility is often observed following repair of atresias. Chronic dilatation of the intestine proximal to the obstruction may alter normal peristalsis across that segment of bowel, even after the obstruction has been relieved.

Malabsorption
Short gut syndrome results when the length of intestine that remains postoperatively cannot sustain normal absorption of nutrients. The normal length of the small bowel in a term infant is approximately 250 cm. The estimated minimum jejunoileal length for sufficient bowel function in a term infant is around 75 cm. Resection of more than 60% of the small bowel or resection that removes crucial anatomic segments, such as the ileocaecal valve, predisposes to malabsorption.

Bacterial overgrowth may contribute to malabsorption and subsequent failure to thrive. Probiotics have been shown in some studies to normalise bowel flora and improve outcomes. Bowel-lengthening procedures and hormonal bowel manipulation may help wean the patient with short gut syndrome from dependence on parenteral nutrition.

Newer techniques, such as the serial transverse enteroplasty procedure (STEP), may offer improved bowel function and length in some patients. Small bowel transplant, with or without other viscera such as liver and pancreas, is being performed in select centres in the United States and United Kingdom with varying results.

Prognosis and Outcomes

The prognosis for babies with these conditions depends entirely on the delay at presentation, appropriateness of resuscitation, operative and anaesthetic expertise, and most of all on the postoperative care available. Unless there is a neonatal ICU (NICU), outcome is inevitably poor. All efforts in Africa should be spent on improving transport to hospital and postoperative care.

Prevention

The improvement of antenatal care and early transport to a tertiary centre may improve the management and outcome of babies with the above-mentioned congenital abnormalities. There seems to be some evidence that folic acid may decrease the incidence of ARM.

Evidence-Based Research

Table 61.1 presents a comparative analysis of neonatal patients with intestinal obstruction in two groups treated during five-year consecutive periods to track the trends in management.

Table 61.1: Evidence-based research.

Title	Trends in neonatal intestinal obstruction in a developing country, 1996–2005
Authors	Ekenze SO, Ibeziako SN, Ezomike UO
Institution	Department of Surgery, University of Nigeria Teaching Hospital, Enugu, Nigeria
Reference	World J Surg 2007; 31:2405–2409
Problem	Outcome of neonatal intestinal obstruction is poor in Africa compared to the rest of the world.
Intervention	Better resources and expertise and referral to a tertiary centre may improve results.
Comparison/ control (quality of evidence)	A comparative analysis was performed involving 128 consecutive NIO cases managed from January 1996 to December 2005 at the University of Nigeria Teaching Hospital, Enugu, in southeast Nigeria. Fifty-five (43.0%) neonates were managed in the first five years (group A), and 73 (57.0%) in the last five years (group B). The aetiology of obstruction did not vary significantly in the two groups. Average duration of symptoms before presentation fell from 5.9 days (group A) to 4.7 days (group B). With the exception of Hirschsprung's disease, all other cases required operative treatment. In HD, the colostomy rate declined from 44.4% (group A) to 26.7% (group B). More neonates in group B were managed with general anaesthesia and perioperative third-generation cephalosporin antibiotics (p = 0.01). Although the complication rate did not vary significantly in the two groups (group A, 42%; group B, 40.3%), survival improved (group A, 61.8%; group B, 72.6%). Earlier presentation, improved manpower, and use of potent antibiotics may have contributed to the improved outcome.
Outcome/ effect	Challenges in the form of lack of neonatal intensive care facilities and dearth of qualified personnel persist. There is a trend toward earlier presentation and increased survival of babies with NIO. Improving the existing facilities and trained manpower, and establishing collaboration with centres that have excellent results may further encourage the trend.
Historical significance/ comments	Survival of neonates in Africa with intestinal obstruction can improve from 50% to above 90%, as reported in the well-resourced part of the world, if the above challenges are met.

Key Summary Points

1. Neonatal intestinal obstruction is one of the most common neonatal surgical emergencies.

2. Successful management of NIO depends on timely diagnosis and referral for therapy.

3. The diagnosis is made based on clinical findings of bile-stained vomiting, degrees of abdominal distention, and failure to pass meconium.

4. Plain radiographs assist in most diagnoses.

5. Radiological contrast and histopathological studies further aid in the diagnoses.

6. Catastrophic events such as volvulus, ischaemic loop of bowel, pneumoperitoneum, and or pneumonia from aspiration and malnutrition, could be overcome through efficient and timely resuscitation and urgent transport to a specialised unit.

7. Outcomes are resource- and expertise-dependent.

References

1. Mhando S, Young B, Lakhoo K. The scope of emergency paediatric surgery in Tanzania. Pediatr Surg Int 2008; 24(2):219–222.

2. Pitcher G. Trends in neonatal intestinal obstruction in a developing country. World J Surg 2007; 31(12):2410–2411.

3. Louw JH, Barnard CN. Congenital intestinal atresia: observations on its origin. Lancet 1955; 269:1065–1067.

4. Busch R. On the history of cystic fibrosis. Acta Univ Carol 1990; 36(1-4):13–15.

5. Padoa C, Goldman A, Jenkins T, et al. Cystic fibrosis carrier frequencies in populations of African origin. J Med. Genet 1999; 36:41–44.

6. Westwood T, Brown R. Cystic fibrosis in black patients: Western Cape experiences. S Afr Med J 2006; 96:288–289.

7. Pena A. Anorectal malformations: experience with the posterior sagittal approach. In: Stringer MD, Oldham KT, Howard ER, eds. Pediatric Surgery and Urology: Long Term Outcomes. WB Saunders, 1998, 376–386.

8. Banieghbal B, Beale PG. Minimal access approach to jejunal atresia. J Pediatr Surg 2007; 42(8):1362–1364.

9. Grant HW, Parker MC, Wilson MS, et al. Adhesions after abdominal surgery in children. J Pediatr Surg 2008; 43(1):152–157.

CHAPTER 62
DUODENAL ATRESIA AND STENOSIS

Felicitas Eckoldt-Wolke

Afua A.J. Hesse

Sanjay Krishnaswami

Introduction

Congenital duodenal obstruction may be due to intrinsic or extrinsic lesions. Intrinsic duodenal obstruction may be caused by duodenal atresia, stenosis, diaphragm with or without perforation, or by a wind-sock web or membrane that balloons distally. Extrinsic duodenal obstruction may be caused by malrotation with Ladd's bands or a preduodenal portal vein or annular pancreas. The annular pancreas itself is not believed to be the cause of obstruction, as there is usually an associated atresia or stenosis in these patients.

Duodenal obstructions usually occur in the second part of the duodenum. They are believed to result from a developmental error during early foetal life within the area of intense embryological activity involved in the creation of the biliary and pancreatic structures. Thus, the obstruction usually occurs at or below the ampulla of Vater.

Duodenal obstruction is associated with prematurity (46%) and maternal polyhydramnios (33%).[1] In addition, there is a high incidence of specific associated anomalies, including Down syndrome (>30%), malrotation (>20%), congenital heart diseases (20%), and other gastrointestinal tract (GIT) and renal anomalies. Along with prematurity and low birth weight, these associated anomalies are known to be significant risk factors contributing to mortality in patients with duodenal atresia. Of note, the presence of Down syndrome itself does not influence the outcome of these babies.

Demographics

Although detailed statistics are not available in much of Africa, the incidence of duodenal obstruction is reported to be 1 in 5,000–10,000 births in most reports.[2] Duodenal obstruction and jejunoileal atresia rank among the two most common causes of intestinal obstruction in large series in the African population.[3]

Aetiology

It has been demonstrated that from gestational weeks 5 to 10, the duodenum is a solid chord. Intrinsic obstructions result from failure of vacuolization and recanalization. An annular pancreas results from fusion of the anterior and posterior anlage, forming a ring of pancreatic tissue that surrounds the second part of the duodenum. Extrinsic obstructions result from a variety of disorders of embryologic development specific to the pathology.

Clinical Presentation

Prenatal

Duodenal obstruction is readily diagnosed by prenatal ultrasound. Antenatal care with prenatal ultrasonography should therefore be offered to pregnant women in all circumstances. Duodenal obstruction presents up to gestational week 20 with a double-bubble phenomenon due to the simultaneous distention of the stomach and the first part of the duodenum. In more than 30% of cases, maternal polyhydramnios is present, and in some cases, serial amniotic aspiration has been reported as necessary. In facilities where ultrasound is not available, a high index of suspicion must be maintained in cases of maternal polyhydramnios. Pregnancy can last near to maturity, and spontaneous delivery is usually the case.

Postnatal Symptoms and Signs

Most women in Africa do not avail themselves of prenatal care, so the majority of duodenal obstructions present only after birth. Furthermore, because up to 60% of births occur outside health institutions, these cases often present very late. The most common presenting features are bilious vomiting and feeding intolerance. Dehydration and electrolyte depletion rapidly ensue if the condition is not recognized and intravenous therapy is not begun. Aspiration and respiratory failure may follow. Repeated nonbilious vomiting is seen in cases of supra-ampullary obstruction (20%). Patients with a web or partial stenosis can survive to present in a much delayed fashion.[2]

Physical signs are nonspecific but can include upper-abdominal distention with scaphoid lower abdomen. Additionally, in the appropriate clinical context, observation of typical Down syndrome features should raise suspicion towards duodenal obstruction as the cause for neonatal intestinal obstruction. Finally, a careful physical exam should concentrate on recognizing signs of significant congenital heart disease (e.g., cyanosis, murmurs), which could complicate perioperative management

Investigation

In tertiary perinatal centres where a prenatal diagnosis has already been established, no further diagnostic work-up is typically necessary.

In doubtful cases or in other settings, a plain abdominal x-ray is the key method for diagnosis. An x-ray showing double-bubble gas shadows is essentially pathognomonic for duodenal obstruction (Figure 62.1). If no double bubble is seen, instillation of 10–15 ml of air immediately prior to a plain abdominal radiograph may help to demonstrate these findings. In cases of stenosis or perforated membranes, air may be seen in the distal GIT. Water-soluble contrast radiography is confirmatory, but it is generally needed only in cases of incomplete obstruction. Radiographic findings of annular pancreas are usually indistinguishable from other forms of duodenal obstruction.

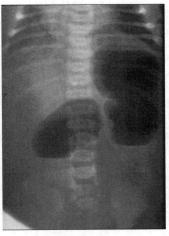

Figure 62.1: Double-bubble sign on plain x-ray. Note the lack of distal gas.

The most important differential diagnosis is duodenal obstruction due to malrotation, resulting in volvulus of the midgut loop or extrinsic compression related to Ladd´s bands across the duodenum. When no prenatal diagnosis is available, contrast radiography may be helpful to differentiate between these entities and can demonstrate the absence of the normal C-shaped curve of the duodenum or a classic "bird's-beak" shape secondary to a volvulus. When the diagnosis still remains in doubt, prompt laparotomy is warranted because undiagnosed volvulus can result in gangrene of the entire midgut within hours.

If available, in cases of incomplete obstruction, oesophagogastro-duodenoscopy (EGD) can be done to prove the existence of an intrinsic obstructing membrane. An endoscopic approach to membrane resection can be utilized.

Management

Preoperative Care

The intensity of preoperative care is typically proportionate to the time from birth until hospital presentation. Initial therapy consists of nasogastric decompression and appropriate replacement of fluid and electrolytes. Most of these newborn patients are premature and small for their gestational age, so special care must be taken to preserve body heat and to avoid hypoglycaemia, especially in cases of very low birth weight, congenital heart disease, and respiratory distress syndrome. When incubators are unavailable, the "kangaroo" method of nursing these children offers the best hope for survival.

General Intraoperative Considerations

General anaesthesia with endotracheal intubation is required. The most commonly utilized incision is a muscle-cutting, transverse, right upper quadrant incision. However, some centres are now employing minimal access laparoscopic methods for repair of duodenal obstruction.

A side-to-side duodenoduodenostomy is the standard repair for duodenal stenosis, atresia, or obstruction due to a preduodenal portal vein. In 1977, Kimura and colleagues described a modification of this procedure, known as the diamond-shaped duodenoduodenostomy.[4] In this technique, a horizontal incision is made across the distal aspect of the proximal, dilated bowel, and a lengthwise incision is made along the proximal aspect of the distal, small-calibre bowel. This can achieve a greater diameter of the anastomosis for better emptying of the upper duodenum. In some cases, duodenojejunostomy can be an alternative and may afford an easier repair with minimal dissection. The choice of surgical procedure is largely based on the preference of the surgeon.

When an annular pancreas associated with duodenal obstruction is encountered (Figure 62.2), the treatment of choice is performance of a duodenoduodenostomy between the segments of duodenum above and below the area of the ring of pancreas. One should never consider division of the pancreatic ring because that could result in a pancreatic fistula while the underlying stenosis or atresia of the duodenum would remain unchanged.

In the case of an endoluminal membrane, duodenotomy and resection of the membrane can be done after localisation of the ampulla of Vater. Alternatively, bypass of the membrane can be performed via a duodenoduodenostomy, if desired. As seen in Figure 62.3, fenestrated membranes may be amenable to an endoscopic approach to resection in centres where this facility is available.[5]

Operative Details

Once the abdomen is entered, the hepatic flexure of the colon is mobilised. The duodenum is adequately mobilized by a Kocher manoeuvre. The ligament of Treitz is divided as needed. A transpyloric tube passed via the nose or mouth is helpful at this stage. Air or saline can be passed into the second part of duodenum to assess the nature and level of obstruction.

The dilated proximal duodenum and collapsed distal duodenum are approximated by using stay sutures.

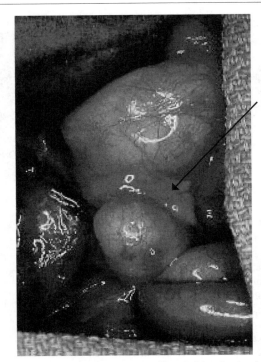

Annular pancreas across duodenum

Figure 62.2: Annular pancreas with underlying duodenal stenosis.

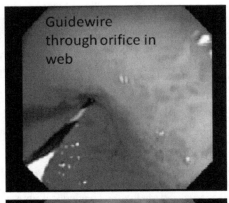

Guidewire through orifice in web

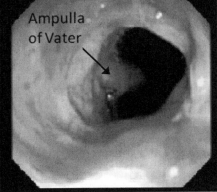

Ampulla of Vater

Figure 62.3: Endoscopic view of duodenal web before and after endoscopic dilatation and fenestration of the membrane.

For side-to-side anastomosis, interrupted Lembert sutures (4-0 or 5-0 vicryl or monocryl) start the dorsal part of anastomosis if a two-layer closure is desired. A transverse duodenotomy is made in the proximal segment, 1 cm above the stenosis, to avoid injury of the pancreatico-biliary system. Easy retrograde passage of a tube into the stomach rules out a duodenal web proximal to the duodenotomy. A parallel incision is made in the distal duodenum. The posterior layer of anastomosis is completed by inverting interrupted or continuous sutures of 4-0 or 5-0 vicryl or monocryl. A transanastomotic nasoduodenal silicone tube can be inserted to allow very early enteral feeding beginning at day one or two after surgery. The anterior layer of the anastomosis is completed in the same way. A few Lembert sutures may be used to complete the anastomosis.

For diamond-shaped duodenoduodenostomy, a little more mobilization is needed to bring the redundant proximal duodenal wall down to overlie the proximal portion of the distal segment. Then a transverse incision in the proximal and a longitudinal incision in the distal duodenum are made. The papilla of Vater is located by gentle pressure on the gallbladder. Stay sutures approximate the parts in corresponding points, as shown in Figure 62.4, and the remainder of the anastomosis and placement of a transanastomotic tube is carried out as previously described. Figure 62.5 shows intraoperative photos before and after duodenoduodenostomy.

For a duodenal web, the membrane is usually located in the second part of the duodenum. Localization of the membrane can be assisted by passage of a nasogastric tube (NGT) into the duodenum down to the level of the membrane. Care is to be taken to identify the so-called wind-sock phenomenon, which refers to a proximally attached, lax membrane that bulges into the distal duodenum, making the obstruction point appear more distal than it actually is. This can be identified by looking for a dimpling of the duodenal wall at the attachment point of the membrane more proximal than the distal tip of the NGT.

For membrane resection, a longitudinal incision is made, bridging between the wide and the narrow segments, or at the level of duodenal attachment of the membrane in the case of a wind-sock deformity. It is important to note that the ampulla of Vater may open directly into any membrane or close to it in its posterior-medial part. Therefore, identification of the ampulla is mandatory before excision of the membrane. Excision begins with a radial incision starting in the central ostium and leaving a rim of 1–2 mm of tissue at the duodenal wall. Once again, great care is to be taken to avoid damage to the ampulla of Vater. The resection line is oversewn with continuous suture vicryl 5-0. Before closing the duodenum transversely, patency of the distal duodenum is to be proven with a small silicon catheter and saline.

Postoperative Considerations and Complications

Intravenous infusions are continued for the postoperative period. Using a transanastomotic tube laying deep in the jejunum, feeding can be started as early as 48 hours postoperatively. Where available, parenteral nutrition via a central or peripherally inserted catheter can be very effective for longer-term nutritional support if transanastomotic enteral feeding is inadequate, not feasible, or not tolerated by the patient. All patients have a prolonged period of bile-stained gastric aspirate. This is mainly due to the ineffective peristalsis of the distended upper duodenum. The commencement of oral feeding is dependent upon a decrease in the volume of gastric aspirate and is often delayed for up to several weeks. Patients who have a severely prolonged return of duodenal function and have exceptionally marked dilatation of the proximal duodenum may benefit from reoperation and tapering of the proximal segment, although this is rare.

Anastomotic leak, intraabdominal sepsis, and wound complications also are rare.

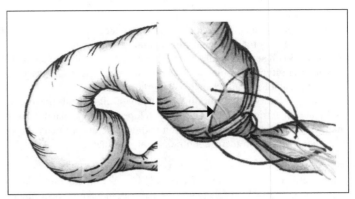

Figure 62.4: Diamond-shaped duodenoduodenostomy.

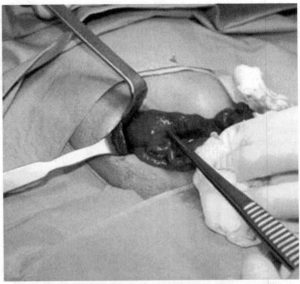

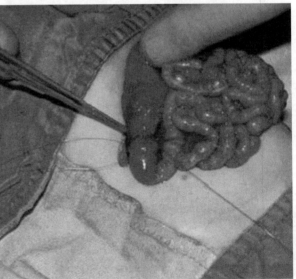

Figure 62.5: Intraoperative photo of duodenal atresia before (top) and after (bottom) duodenoduodenostomy.

Prognosis

Although prognosis of intestinal atresia in general is good, an overall mortality of 7% for duodenal obstruction is shown in large series.[6] Associated congenital anomalies are identified as an independent risk factor for an impaired clinical course. Low birth weight and the problems of prematurity further increase mortality risk.

The morbidity and mortality of neonatal intestinal obstruction is higher in Africa (40%) than in developed countries and is most likely due to late patient presentation and poor neonatal intensive care facilities available in many countries in the continent.[3]

Conclusion

The morbidity and mortality of intestinal obstruction can be improved with earlier referral to specialty centres and with meticulous resuscitation before surgery. Duodenoduodenostomy or duodenotomy with membrane resection in the appropriate circumstance are the typical operations of choice and produce good results with minimal short- or long-term operative-related morbidity. Problems of late presentation and poor neonatal intensive care facilities constitute the basis for the variance in outcomes in Africa when compared to those in developed countries.[7]

Nevertheless, even in Europe and North America, the outcome for children with duodenal obstruction is basically influenced by the degree of prematurity and the presence of associated anomalies.

Evidence-Based Research

Table 62.1 is an observational 15-year retrospective study of the use of diamond-shaped anastomosis for duodenal atresia.

Table 62.1: Evidence-based research.

Title	Diamond-shaped anastomosis for duodenal atresia: an experience with 44 patients over 15 years
Authors	Kimura K, Mukohara N, Nishijima E, Muraji T, Tsugawa C, Matsumoto Y
Institution	Department of Surgery, Kobe Children's Hospital, Kobe, Japan
Reference	J Pediatr Surg 1990; 25(9):977–979
Problem	Role of diamond-shaped anastomosis in the treatment of duodenal atresia and stenosis.
Intervention	Duodenoduodenostomy via diamond-shaped anastomosis.
Comparison/control (quality of evidence)	In this retrospective observational study, 44 patients over a 15-year period were examined for outcome after diamond shaped anastomosis. All patients underwent this method of repair, so there was no control group.
Outcome/effect	In all patients, oral feedings were commenced 3.66 ± 1.4 days postoperatively (range, 2 to 6). There was no operative-related mortality. Twenty-one patients had long-term follow-up from 6 months to 15 years. All patients had normal body weight for their age at last record, and current upper GI contrast study (done in 19 of 21 patients) revealed normal calibre of duodenum and anastomosis in all studied cases.
Historical significance/comments	This study, reported by the originator of the diamond-shaped anastomosis, states the efficacy of this technique in duodenal atresia. Given the relative rarity off the disorder, this report offers a substantial collection of patients with a prolonged follow-up period. Although a comparison group who underwent traditional side-to-side anastomosis was not included here, the results compare favorably to previously published reports of side-to-side anastomotic techniques. Because of its technical ease and its potential to allow early recovery of enteral function without excessive late complications, this technique may be of particular use in undeveloped regions where opportunity for follow-up care is limited.

Key Summary Points

1. Obstructions of duodenum can be intrinsic or extrinsic.

2. There is a high incidence of prematurity and associated anomalies, including cardiac and renal defects as well as Down syndrome.

3. Prenatal ultrasound can be very helpful and may reveal maternal polyhydramnios or a "double-bubble".

4. Physical signs are nonspecific but can include upper-abdominal distention with scaphoid lower abdomen.

5. The most important differential diagnosis to consider is duodenal obstruction due to malrotation, resulting in volvulus of the midgut loop

6. Postnatal plain radiograph revealing a double bubble (distended stomach and proximal duodenum) without evidence of distal gas in the appropriate clinical setting is essentially pathognomic for duodenal atresia.

7. Repair for all forms of duodenal obstruction can be accomplished through side-to-side or diamond-shaped anastomosis proximal and distal to the obstruction. Additionally, duodenal webs can be approached through partial resection of the membrane itself.

References

1. Dalla Vecchia LK, Grosfeld JL, West KW, Rescorla FJ, Scherer LR, Engum SA. Intestinal atresia and stenosis: a 25-year experience with 277 cases. Arch Surg 1998; 133:490–496; discussion, 496–497.

2. Millar, AJW, Rode H, Cywes S. Intestinal atresia and stenosis. In: Ashcraft KW, ed. Pediatric Surgery. 4th ed. Elsevier-Saunders, 2005.

3. Ameh EA, Chirdan LB. Neonatal intestinal obstruction in Zaria, Nigeria. East Afr Med J 2000; 77:510–513.

4. Kimura K, Tsugawa C, Ogawa K, Matsumoto Y, Yamamoto T, Asada S. Diamond-shaped anastomosis for congenital duodenal obstruction. Arch Surg 1977; 112:1262–1263.

5. Blanco-Rodríguez G, Penchyna-Grub J, Porras-Hernández JD, Trujillo-Ponce A. Transluminal endoscopic electrosurgical incision of fenestrated duodenal membranes. Pediatr Surg Int 2008; 24:711–714. Epub, 15 April 2008.

6. Piper HG, Alesbury J, Waterford SD, Zurakowski D, Jaksic T. Intestinal atresias: factors affecting clinical outcomes. J Pediatr Surg 2008; 43:1244–1248.

7. Ademuyiwa AO, Sowande OA, Ijaduola TK, Adejuyigbe O. Determinants of mortality in neonatal intestinal obstruction in Ile Ife, Nigeria. Afr J Paediatr Surg 2009; 6:11–13.

CHAPTER 63
INTESTINAL ATRESIA AND STENOSIS

Alastair J. W. Millar

John R. Gosche

Kokila Lakhoo

Introduction

Atresias of the jejunum and ileum are common causes of bowel obstruction in the neonate, with a third of infants born prematurely or small for their gestational age. Stenoses are much less common and seldom present in the newborn period due to delay in diagnosis. Whereas these conditions are associated with excellent prognoses in developed countries, delayed presentation and limitations in resources to support patients with delayed return of intestinal function contributes to overall lower survival rates in many African countries.[1–4] Early recognition and proper surgical management are vitally important to improving survival in countries with limited access to health care resources.

Demographics

The incidence of intestinal atresia in the United States is approximately 1 in 3,000 live births, but may be more frequent in Africa, with a reported incidence of less than 1 in 1,000 live births, with types III and IV (see next section) comprising 35% of the total number. Two reports from Nigeria[1,2] have shown that intestinal atresias are less common than imperforate anus, but occur with similar frequency to Hirschsprung's disease. Published reports suggest a higher prevalence of jejunoileal atresia among African American children in the United States,[5] but no racial predilection has been identified by authors from African countries. Nearly all infants with intestinal atresias develop symptoms within hours after birth. However, several publications have documented that neonates in African countries often do not reach definitive medical care for several days.[2,4] Unlike atresias, many patients with intestinal stenoses are not diagnosed until well beyond the neonatal period.

Aetiology/Pathophysiology

Our present understanding of the aetiology of intestinal atresias is based upon the classic experimental work of Louw and Barnard reported in 1955.[6] These investigators observed that ligating mesenteric vessels and causing strangulated obstruction in foetal dogs resulted in atretic lesions of the small intestine that were similar to those observed clinically in human neonates. Thus, atresias and stenoses of the small intestine are believed to be due to an ischaemic insult. This aetiologic mechanism explains the frequent association of atresias with mesenteric defects and with other conditions that may cause strangulated obstruction of the intestinal tract (e.g., volvulus, intussusception, internal hernias, and gastroschisis). An ischaemic aetiology may also explain why intestinal atresia is associated with maternal smoking and vasoconstrictor drug exposure during pregnancy.

The morphological classification into four types has both prognostic and therapeutic implications (Figure 63.1):

- Stenoses occurs in 11%.

- Type I atresia (23%) is a transluminal septum with proximal dilated bowel in continuity with collapsed distal bowel. The bowel is usually of normal length.

- Type II atresia (10%) involves two blind-ending atretic ends separated by a fibrous cord along the edge of the mesentery with mesentery intact.

- Type IIIa atresia (15%) is similar to type II, but there is a mesenteric defect and the bowel length may be foreshortened.

- Type IIIb atresia (19%) ("apple peel" or "Christmas tree" deformity) consists of a proximal jejunal atresia, often with malrotation with absence of most of the mesentery and a varying length of ileum surviving on perfusion from retrograde flow along a single artery of supply.

- Type IV atresia is a multiple atresia of types I, II, and III, like a string of sausages. Bowel length is always reduced. The terminal ileum, as in type III, is usually spared.

The immediate consequence of an atresia is dilatation of the bowel for a variable distance proximal to the first occlusion encountered. This dilated bowel, even when the obstruction is relieved by resection and anastomosis or stoma formation, remains dilated, having inefficient prograde peristalsis. Surgical strategies to overcome this include back resection of this bowel to a normal-calibre intestine or reduction in diameter by various tapering manoeuvres.

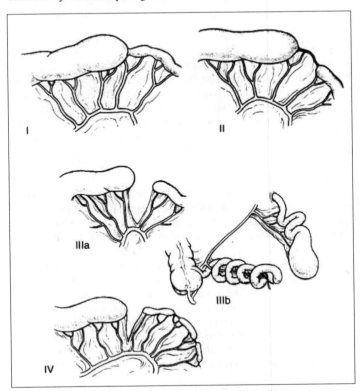

Source: Grosfeld JL, et al. Operative management of intestinal atresia and stenosis based on pathological findings. J Pediatr Surg 1979; 14:368.

Figure 63.1: Classification of intestinal atresia (see text for explanation of types I–IV).

History

Clinical Presentation

Intestinal atresias in Africa are usually not diagnosed prenatally. However, atresias of the proximal jejunum are frequently associated with polyhydramnios. Therefore, many of these patients are born prematurely and often are small for their gestational age, the latter due to inability to absorb nutrients from the amniotic fluid in patients with proximal intestinal obstructions.[7]

Intestinal atresia should be suspected in any newborn showing evidence of bowel obstruction (bilious vomiting, abdominal distention, and failure to pass meconium). Aspiration of >25 ml of fluid from the stomach via a nasogastric tube (NGT) is very suggestive of obstruction. Antenatal ultrasound scanning may show dilated loops of bowel with vigorous peristalsis, which is diagnostic of obstruction. Polyhydramnios may develop but it is more commonly seen in duodenal and oesophageal obstructions. The more distal the atresia, the more generalized the abdominal distention. After aspiration of gastric contents, the abdomen will be less distended and visible peristalsis may be observed. There is usually a failure to pass meconium, and typically small-volume gray mucoid stools are passed. Abdominal tenderness or peritonitis develops only with complications of ischaemia or perforation. This commonly occurs with a delay in diagnosis and is due to increased intraluminal pressure from swallowed air and secondary volvulus of the bulbous blind-ending bowel at the level of the first obstruction.

Physical Examination

Findings on physical examination are frequently not very revealing. Most patients will have some degree of abdominal distention. The amount of distention will vary, depending upon the level of obstruction. Patients generally do not have abdominal tenderness or an abdominal mass. Therefore, the presence of these findings suggests a complicated obstruction associated with ischaemia or prenatal perforation, or that the cause of obstruction may be malrotation with midgut volvulus.

Investigations

In most patients, a simple abdominal x-ray with anteroposterior (AP) and either cross-table or left lateral decubitus projection are adequate to make the diagnosis based upon the presence of dilated, air-filled intestinal loops and air-fluid levels (Figure 63.2). In addition, plain abdominal x-rays will suggest the level of obstruction based upon the number of dilated bowel loops. The presence of multiple dilated bowel loops without air-fluid levels suggests the possibility of meconium ileus, particularly if the intestinal content has a "ground glass" appearance. A single very dilated loop with a large fluid level is often indicative of atresia.

The differential diagnosis includes other causes of intestinal obstruction in the neonate. In patients with evidence of a proximal complete obstruction, the differential diagnosis is limited and no additional diagnostic studies are required. In patients with multiple dilated bowel loops, suggesting a distal obstruction, the differential diagnosis includes several conditions for which surgical intervention may not be required. Therefore, in these patients a contrast enema may be helpful to look for evidence of a meconium plug or meconium ileus, which may respond to nonoperative management. In addition, a contrast enema may demonstrate findings suggestive of Hirschsprung's disease, which would direct initial management towards obtaining confirmatory tests for this disease. A contrast enema showing a patent colon is helpful in that demonstration of colonic patency by injection of saline at operation—a sometimes tedious procedure—is not required (Figure 63.3).

In patients with intestinal stenoses, plain abdominal x-rays may demonstrate proximal bowel dilatation; however, in most patients a gastrointestinal contrast meal or enema is required to confirm and locate the site of partial obstruction.

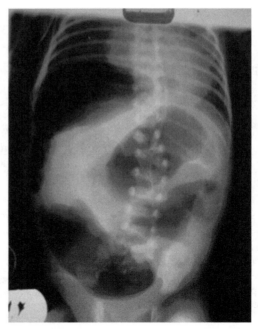

Figure 63.2: Abdominal radiograph showing several dilated gas-filled bowel loops in a jejunal atresia.

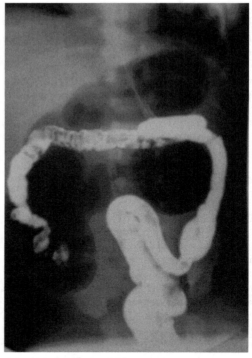

Figure 63.3: Contrast enema showing normal colon with dilated proximal small bowel in an infant with jejunal atresia.

Management

All patients should receive judicious fluid hydration prior to operative intervention. In addition, a nasogastric or orogastric tube should be passed to empty the stomach and decrease the risk of vomiting with aspiration. In general, patients with intestinal atresias have a low risk of associated cardiac anomalies, so that preoperative special investigation is not required unless the patient has clinical evidence of a serious cardiac defect.

At exploration, the site of the most proximal atresia is readily identified as the site of marked change in intestinal calibre. The outer wall of the intestine at the site of obstruction may appear intact or there may be an associated defect in continuity of the intestine and the mesentery (Figure 63.4). Generally, surgical treatment requires excision of the ends of the intestine involved in the atresia. It is also important to look for distal sites of obstruction, which can occur in up to 20% of patients and may not be immediately obvious due to lack of calibre change beyond the proximal atresia. These distal points of obstruction can be identified by flushing the distal intestinal lumen with saline to confirm intestinal continuity to the level of the rectum.

After resection of the atretic segment, the surgeon is faced with the difficult task of re-establishing continuity between intestinal segments with marked size discrepancies. Another consideration is the potential dysmotility of the proximal markedly dilated segment, which may result in delayed intestinal function and problems with bacterial overgrowth. Therefore, in patients with a relatively short segment of severely dilated proximal intestine, resection of the dilated segment with re-establishment of continuity by end-to-end anastomosis is a good option. However, in patients with long segments of proximal intestine that are significantly dilated, resection of the whole involved segment may result in inadequate remaining intestinal length to allow absorption of enteric nutrients (i.e., short bowel syndrome). Therefore, these patients frequently are treated by either imbrication or tapering enteroplasty of the proximal dilated segment. To date, no randomized studies have compared the outcomes for patients with intestinal atresias with or without the addition of an enteroplasty or plication. In patients for whom the atresia is just distal to the duodenojejunal flexure, it may be advantageous to resect the dilated bowel, derotate, and taper the duodenum with primary anastomosis. This facilitates passage of a transanastomotic feeding tube and early restoration of foregut function. The total residual length of bowel should be measured with a tape and recorded, as this gives some guidance as to prognosis.

Patients who have multiple atresias (type IV) or an apple-peel deformity (type IIIb) present particularly challenging management problems (Figures 63.5 and 63.6). These patients may require multiple anastomoses and frequently will experience long-term delays in return of intestinal function. In addition, many of these patients will have short bowel syndrome due to inadequate residual intestinal length. In general, the formation of stomas is unnecessary and should be avoided because dilated bowel does not reduce in caliber, and fluid and electrolyte losses may be severe.

Postoperative Complications

The most common postoperative complication is a functional obstruction at the site of anastomosis. Unfortunately, this complication may be due to the underlying intestinal dysmotility associated with this anomaly and may not be preventable by changes in surgical technique. Other less commonly observed complications include anastomotic leak and adhesive obstructions. Obstructions due to missed distal unrecognized atresias should not occur and can be prevented by proper evaluation at the time of the initial operation.

Prognosis and Outcomes

Most patients with intestinal atresia do not have associated life-threatening anomalies. Therefore, the primary factor that impacts mortality is the ability to support the nutritional needs of the patient during the postoperative period while awaiting adequate bowel function to allow enteral alimentation. In centres where parenteral nutritional support is feasible, these patients can be supported for prolonged periods of time while awaiting gastrointestinal function. However, in centres without these resources, patient mortality will be higher and primarily attributable to malnutrition. The judicious use of nasojejunal or gastrostomy transanastomotic feeding tubes for enteral feeding may be life saving.

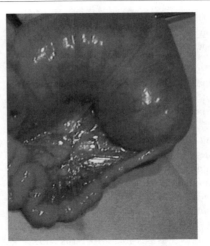

Figure 63.4: Type I jejunal atresia. Membrane occlusion without mesenteric defect or loss of intestinal length.

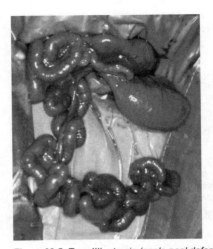

Figure 63.5: Type IIIb atresia (apple peel deformity). Note proximal jejunal atresia, malrotation, and mesenteric defect with a single artery of supply from the middle and right colic vessels with significant loss of intestinal length.

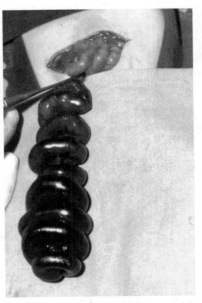

Figure 63.6: Type IIIb atresia with antenatal volvulus of the "apple peel" leading to short bowel.

Prevention

Unfortunately, there are no options at present for prevention because these anomalies are usually not recognized prior to birth.

Ethical Issues

In resource-poor regions without recourse to intensive care and parenteral nutrition, infants with ultra-short bowel resulting from congenital atresia may have to be managed conservatively. Discussion around parental expectations and centre outcomes should be part of the informed consent. Nursing staff and other caregivers should also be party to the decision-making process. Withdrawal of treatment that is thought to be futile is often difficult to institute. If there are choices to be made based on allocation of limited resources, then infants with the potential for good outcomes may be given preference for meagre resources. However, it is only the infrequent case of intestinal atresia that develops intestinal failure, and with prompt operation and preservation of as much functioning bowel as possible, prognosis should be excellent.

Evidence-Based Research

Table 63.1 presents a study of the change in mortality rates from jejunoileal atresia and stenosis over a nearly 50-year period.

Table 63.1: Evidence-based research.

Title	Jejuno-ileal atresia and stenosis
Authors	Rode H, Millar AJW
Institution	Red Cross Children's Hospital, Cape Town, South Africa
Reference	In: Prem Puri, ed. Newborn Surgery, 2nd ed. Arnold, 2003, Pp 445–456
Problem	Late presentation of jejunoileal atresia and stenosis in Africa.
Intervention	Surgery is curative if presentation is early enough.
Comparison/ control (quality of evidence)	Before 1952, the mortality for jejunoileal atresia alone was 90%. Between 1952 and 1955, the mortality was 80% when primary anastamosis was performed without bowel resection. Between 1955 and 1958, the mortality decreased to 22% due to liberal resection of the dilated loop and primary anastomosis. From 1959 to 2000, the mortality has decreased to 10%. Factors contributing to mortality were type III atresia, proximal bowel infarction, peritonitis, anastomotic leaks, missed distal atresias, short bowel syndrome, sepsis, and human immunodeficiency virus (HIV) infection.
Outcome/ effect	The survival rate is more than 90% in well-resourced countries, but 40–50% in Africa, where no nutritional support is available and presentation is late.
Historical significance/ comments	No advancement on vascular theory for aetiology. A variant of multiple intestinal atresias may have a familial/genetic cause.

Key Summary Points

1. Intestinal atresia may occur at any level of the gastrointestinal tract.

2. Small bowel atresia in most cases is due to an antenatal ischaemic insult to a segment of intestine. Resorption of the infarcted segment leads to occlusion of the lumen, with a varying degree of dilatation of the proximal blind end.

3. One-third of infants with intestinal atresia are born prematurely.

4. Differential diagnoses include midgut volvulus, meconium ileus, extensive aganglionosis, and intussusception.

5. The primary surgery for intestinal atresia consists of a generous back resection of the bulbous blind end and an end-to-end anastomosis.

6. Outcomes are generally good if sufficient bowel length remains.

7. Stomas should be avoided.

8. The mortality rate depends on birth weight, residual bowel length, the degree of dysmotility, associated anomalies, and septic complications.

References

1. Adeyemi D. Neonatal intestinal obstruction in a developing tropical country: patterns, problems and prognosis. J Trop Pediatr 1989; 35:66–70.

2. Ameh EA, Chirdan LB. Neonatal intestinal obstruction in Zaria, Nigeria. East Afr Med J 2000; 77:510–513.

3. Barrack SM, Kyambi JM, Ndungu J, Wachira N, Anangwe G, Safwat S. Intestinal atresia and stenosis as seen and treated at Kenyatta National Hospital, Nairobi. East Afr Med J 1993; 70:558–564.

4. Chirdan LB, Uba AF, Pam SD. Intestinal atresia: management problems in a developing country. Pediatr Surg Int 2004; 20:834–837.

5. Cragan JD, Martin ML, Moore CA, Khoury MJ. Descriptive epidemiology of small intestinal atresia, Atlanta, Georgia. Teratology 1993; 48:441–450.

6. Louw JH, Barnard CH. Congenital intestinal atresia: observation on its origin. Lancet 1955; 269:1065–1067.

7. Surana R, Puri P. Small intestinal atresia: effect on fetal nutrition. J Pediatr Surg 1994; 29:1250–1252.

8. Millar AJW, Rode H, Cywes S. Intestinal atresia and stenosis. In: Ashcraft KW, Holder TM, eds. Pediatric Surgery, Saunders, 2000, Pp 406–424.

CHAPTER 64
VITELLINE DUCT ANOMALIES

Bankole S. Rouma

Kokila Lakhoo

Introduction

Vitelline duct or omphalomesenteric duct anomalies are secondary to the persistence of the embryonic vitelline duct, which normally obliterates by weeks 5–9 of intrauterine life. These anomalies occur in approximately 2% of the population and may remain silent throughout life, or may present incidentally sometimes with an intraabdominal complication. Although Meckel's diverticulum is the most common vitelline duct anomaly (Figure 64.1(G)), a patent vitelline duct (Figure 64.1(A)) is the most common symptomatic presentation in developing countries.[1]

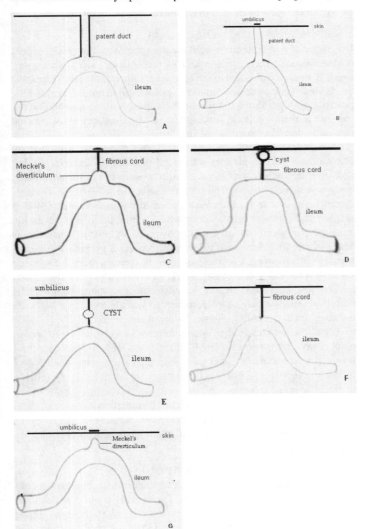

Figure 64.1: Remnants of the omphalomesenteric duct: (A) patent vitelline duct; (B) patent vitelline duct covered by skin; (C) Meckel's diverticulum with fibrous cord; (D) cyst with fibrous cord; (E) cyst; (F) fibrous cord; (G) Meckel's diverticulum.

Demographics

The most frequent malformation is Meckel's diverticulum, with an incidence of 2–3% of the population, but it is one of the most unlikely to cause symptoms. About 4% of children with a Meckel's diverticulum develop symptoms, and more than 60% of those who develop symptoms are younger than 2 years of age.[2–5] The male-to-female complication rate ratio is about 3:1.[3]

Embryology

During week 3 of gestation, the midgut is open into the yolk sac, which does not grow as rapidly as the rest of the embryo. Subsequently, by week 5, the connection with the yolk sac becomes narrowed and is then termed a yolk stalk, vitelline duct, or omphalomesenteric duct. Normally, the vitelline duct disappears by gestational week 9, just before the midgut returns to the abdomen. Persistence of some portion of the vitelline duct results in a number of congenital anomalies, of which Meckel's diverticulum is the most common. This anomaly is variable in length and location, but most often it is observed as a 1–5 cm intestinal diverticulum projecting from the antimesenteric wall of the ileum within 100 cm of the caecum. It possesses all three layers of the intestinal wall and has its own blood supply. The connection in a patent vitelline duct is usually to the ileum, but less commonly may be to the appendix or colon.[1] In other cases, part of the vitelline duct within the abdominal wall persists, forming an open omphalomesenteric fistula, an enterocyst, or a fibrous band connecting the small bowel to the umbilicus.[2–7]

Pathophysiology

Vitelline duct malformations comprise a wide spectrum of anatomic structures, depending on the degree of involution of the vitelline duct. The most common anomaly is Meckel's diverticulum, described as being 60 cm from the ileocaecal valve, 2 cm in diameter, 3 cm in length, and not attached to the abdominal wall. Most complications of these abnormalities are related to ectopic tissue (gastric, pancreatic, colonic, endometriosis, or hepatobiliary).[7]

Ectopic gastric tissue usually causes bleeding from ulceration of the adjacent ileal mucosa. The ileal mucosa is not equipped to buffer the acid produced by the ectopic gastric mucosa and thus is prone to ulceration. The site of the ulceration is most often at the junction of the normal ileal mucosa and the ectopic gastric mucosa. Some studies have shown a very low colonisation rate with *Helicobacter pylori* in children with ulcerative bleeding of Meckel's diverticulum.[3]

Intestinal obstruction may be caused by a Meckel's diverticulum attached to the umbilicus by a fibrous cord or by a fibrous cord between the ileum and the umbilicus. This may lead to a volvulus around the fibrous cord. A persistent vitelline artery, an end artery from the superior mesenteric artery, may cause obstruction and volvulus. Bowel obstruction can also occur by intussusception with the diverticulum as a lead point or by herniation or prolapse of the bowel through a patent omphalomesenteric fistula (with a characteristic "ram's horn" appearance).[5] Obstruction may be caused by phytobezoar.[6,7]

Like the appendix, a Meckel's diverticulum can become inflamed when the lumen is obstructed, resulting in decreased mucosal perfusion, tissue acidosis, and bacterial invasion of the wall. This can lead to progressive inflammation, with tissue gangrene and perforation. It is possible that the gastric or pancreatic mucosa contributes to the luminal obstruction, or the gastric mucosa can lead to ileal mucosal ulceration first, which facilitates bacterial invasion. Rarely, foreign bodies and parasites may be trapped within the diverticulum and cause obstruction of the diverticulum as does an enterolith.[7,8] Diverticular torsion leads to secondary ischaemia and inflammatory change.[7]

Anomalies of the omphalomesenteric duct can result in umbilical drainage from granulation tissue. Other anomalies include a duct extending to the umbilicus but covered with skin (Figure 64.1(B)); diverticulum attached to the umbilicus with a fibrous cord (Figure 64.1(C)), Littre's hernia, and intraabdominal cystic mass (Figure 64.1(D,E)).

Some tumours can be found in ectopic tissues, such as nesidioblastosis in ectopic pancreas tissue of a Meckel's diverticulum or tumours such as carcinoid, leiomyoma, neurofibroma, and angioma.[6–9]

Associated congenital anomalies include cardiac defects, congenital diaphragmatic hernia, duodenal atresia, esophageal atresia, imperforate anus, gastroschisis, malrotation, omphalocele, Hirschsprung's disease, and Down syndrome.

Clinical Presentation

The clinical presentation of vitelline duct abnormalities is variable and depends on the configuration of the remnant of the vitelline duct and whether it contains ectopic gastric or pancreatic tissues. In developed countries, the main forms of presentation are haemorrhage in 40–60%, obstruction in 25%, diverticulitis in 10–20%, and umbilical drainage.[3–5]

The classic presentation is an older infant or young child with painless rectal bleeding. This usually consists of a large volume of bright red bleeding but can occasionally also present as dark, tarry stools in small amounts. The bleeding is often massive and frequently requires transfusion. Melena may be episodic and usually ceases without treatment; sometimes the melena is insidious and not appreciated by the family. In a young child with haemoglobin positive stools and a chronic iron deficiency anaemia, the diagnosis of Meckel's diverticulum should be considered.

Intestinal obstruction, usually due to intussusception, is the most typical presentation in newborns and infants. The symptoms include crampy abdominal pain, bilious vomiting, currant-jelly stools, and abdominal distention. Intestinal obstruction may also be caused by a volvulus or arterial band. Because the volvulus usually involves the distal small bowel and the obstruction is most often a closed loop, there may be little emesis until late in the course. The sequelae of intestinal ischaemia, such as acidosis, peritonitis, and shock, may occur first, and can be fatal in infants.

Patients with Meckel's diverticulitis often have symptoms that resemble appendicitis. They are usually older children. Periumbilical pain is the first symptom. They usually do not have the same amount or intensity of vomiting and nausea as do children with appendicitis. On physical examination, their point of maximal tenderness may migrate across the abdomen as the child moves. About the same percentage of patients with diverticulitis will present with perforation. A perforated Meckel's diverticulum is potentially more serious than a perforated appendix because the former is more difficult to wall off due to its more mobile position. This may explain why perforated diverticulitis is more likely to result in diffuse peritonitis and pneumoperitoneum detectable on abdominal radiographs. For this reason, it is imperative to search carefully for a perforated Meckel's diverticulum as the cause of peritonitis when no inflamed appendix is discovered at appendectomy.

Other types of symptomatic omphalomesenteric duct malformations can result in umbilical drainage as well. The quantity and character of the drainage may indicate the origin of the lesion. Clear drainage or yellowish drainage signifies a probable urachal anomaly, whereas

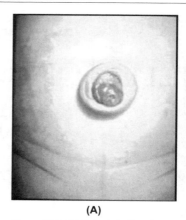 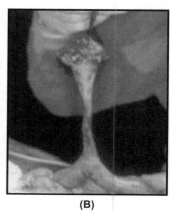

(A) (B)

Figure 64.2: (A) Patent vitelline duct; (B) vitello-intestinal communication.

an omphalomesenteric duct remnant manifests as faeculent drainage (Figure 64.2). The most common umbilical lesion is an umbilical granuloma, which secretes a mucoid material. If the drainage persists despite cauterization of the presumed granuloma with silver nitrate, or if the drainage is copious, imaging studies are indicated. Prolapse of the ileum into the duct at the anterior abdominal wall presents as a discoloured, mucosa-covered mass situated at the umbilicus.

Diagnosis

Diagnosis of a symptomatic vitelline duct malformation is dependent on the anatomic configuration and its presentation, signs, and symptoms. History and physical examination are important for the diagnosis. Some abnormalities are evident on physical examination (faecal fistula, prolapse of ileum through a patent duct, and umbilical granulation tissue with a small fistula). A fistulogram may be necessary to identify the part of the intestine involved preoperatively.

A complete description of the quality and frequency of the bloody stools is necessary in patients with rectal bleeding. Rectal examination and lower endoscopy is useful to identify other causes of lower bleeding (polyps and rectal tears). The test of choice for a bleeding Meckel's diverticulum is a technetium-99m pertechnetate isotope scan (Meckel scan), which preferentially concentrates the isotope in ectopic gastric mucosa. The specificity of scintigraphy is 95%, but the sensitivity is 85%.[7] A negative scan result does not, however, exclude a bleeding Meckel's diverticulum. Capsule endoscopy has proven to be of diagnostic value in some cases of bleeding Meckel's diverticulum, but the reports are very few. These tests are rarely available in developing countries. The best diagnostic test may be a laparotomy to visually look for a Meckel's diverticulum in children with unexplained rectal bleeding.

If obstruction from either intussusception or volvulus is suspected, plain x-rays may reveal dilated bowel loops and multiple air-fluid levels. An air enema or upper gastrointestinal study with small bowel follow-through is suggestive. Ultrasonography remains fairly reliable to diagnose intussusception.

A sinogram will exclude intestinal communication in umbilical sinuses, and abdominal ultrasonography should localise a cyst.[1] Inflammatory symptoms are similar to those of appendicitis and are diagnosed clinically.

Treatment

Symptomatic children with omphalomesenteric duct remnants should be resuscitated before intervention. Those with significant haemorrhage should be transfused. Patients with obstructive symptoms should be resuscitated as rapidly as possible to obviate the need for ischaemic bowel resection. The incision chosen varies with the symptoms and the age of the patient. Children with faeculent umbilical drainage (see Figure 64.2) or prolapse of the omphalomesenteric duct remnant can be explored by a small infraumbilical incision.

Children with Meckel's diverticulitis or a bleeding Meckel's diverticulum are operated on by using a transverse appendectomy incision with medial extension if necessary. Patients with suspected intestinal obstruction should be explored through a generous laparotomy incision.

An open diverticulectomy includes the following steps:

1. A transverse appendectomy incision or subumbilical incision is made.

2. The caecum and ileum are identified.

3. The ileum is followed proximally to find Meckel's diverticulum, approximately 60 cm from the ileocaecal valve.

4. The diverticulum with the ileum are delivered into the wound.

5. The diverticulum is excised with the adjacent ileum and primary ileal end-to-end anastomosis is fashioned.

In developed countries, some surgeons use linear staplers applied to the base of the anomaly, allowing complete amputation of the diverticulum without narrowing the lumen of the ileum. When ectopic gastric or pancreatic tissues are present near the base of the diverticulum, or if the base is wide, inflamed, or perforated, resection of the involved ileum is required with an end-to-end anastomosis.[2–5,10] If perforation has occurred, thorough peritoneal toileting is done after segmental ileal resection. The use of laparoscopy for resection of Meckel's diverticula has been reported by many authors.[11]

Controversy exists about what should be done when a Meckel's diverticulum is encountered during a laparotomy for unrelated symptoms. The debate focuses on the probability of the Meckel's diverticulum becoming symptomatic in the future weighed against the possibility of complications associated with resection.[2,4,5,7,10–13] Lesions with palpable ectopic mucosa (the consistency of gastric or pancreatic tissue differs sharply from that of ileal, jejunal, or colonic mucosal lining), a prominent vitelline artery, a fibrous vitelline artery remnant, evidence of inflammation, or a narrow base may all increase the chance of bleeding, obstruction, or diverticulitis and should be resected when encountered. In patients who have abdominal pain, it is prudent to resect a discovered diverticulum or any lesion with attachments to the umbilicus (to prevent ileal volvulus). Some authors suggest that resection of asymptomatic vitelline remnants in early childhood is reasonable at the time of laparotomy for other conditions.[10–13] In developing countries incidental Meckel's diverticulum should be removed in children to prevent later complications. If the diverticulum is left in place, it is imperative to alert the patient's family and the primary care physician about the presence of the lesion and its possible symptoms.

Postoperative Complications

Postoperative complications are generally the same as that of other operations: bleeding, infection, intraabdominal abscess formation, wound dehiscence, incisional hernia, and postoperative adhesive intestinal obstruction.

Evidence-Based Research

The study presented in Table 64.1 is a systematic review that addresses the management of incidentally detected Meckel's diverticulum.

Table 64.1: Evidence-based research.

Title	Incidentally detected Meckel diverticulum: to resect or not to resect?
Authors	Zani A, Eaton S, Rees CM, Pierro A
Institution	Department of Paediatric Surgery, Institute of Child Health, London, England
Reference	Ann Surg 2008; 247(2):276–281
Problem	The management of incidentally detected Meckel's diverticulum (MD) remains controversial.
Intervention	The aims of this paper were to establish the prevalence of MD, and the morbidity and mortality due to MD.
Comparison/ control (quality of evidence)	The prevalence of MD is 1.2%, and historical mortality of MD was 0.01%. The current mortality from MD is 0.001%. The number of MD resections per year per 100,000 population decreased significantly after the paediatric age range (P < 0.001). Resection of incidentally detected MD has a significantly higher postoperative complication rate than leaving it in situ (P < 0.0001). The long-term outcome of patients with incidentally detected MD left in situ showed no complications. To prevent one death from MD, 758 patients would require incidentally detected MD resection.
Outcome/ effect	The prevalence of MD is 1.2%, and historical mortality of MD was 0.01%. The current mortality from MD is 0.001%. The number of MD resections per year per 100,000 population decreased significantly after the paediatric age range (P < 0.001). Resection of incidentally detected MD has a significantly higher postoperative complication rate than leaving it in situ (P < 0.0001). The long-term outcome of patients with incidentally detected MD left in situ showed no complications. To prevent one death from MD, 758 patients would require incidentally detected MD resection.
Historical significance/ comments	MD is present in 1.2% of the population, it is a very rare cause of mortality, and it is primarily a disease of the young. Leaving an incidentally detected MD in situ reduces the risk of postoperative complications without increasing late complications. A large number of MD resections would need to be performed to prevent one death from MD. The above evidence does not support the resection of incidentally detected MD, in developed countries.

Key Summary Points

1. A patent vitelline duct with umbilical faecal drainage is the most symptomatic presentation of vitelline duct anomalies in developing countries.

2. In developed countries, the main forms of presentation are haemorrhage in 40–60%, obstruction in 25%, diverticulitis in 10–20%, and umbilical drainage.

3. The most common umbilical lesion is an umbilical granuloma, which secretes a mucoid material.

4. If the umbilical drainage persists despite cauterization of the presumed granuloma with silver nitrate, or if the drainage is copious, imaging studies are indicated.

5. In African children, an incidental Meckel's diverticulum must be resected because of the difficulties to rapidly access paediatric surgical heath facilities in case of complications.

6. Resection of asymptomatic vitelline remnants in early childhood at the time of laparotomy or laparoscopy for other conditions is indicated.

7. When ectopic gastric or pancreatic tissues are present near the base of the diverticulum, or if this base is wide, inflamed, or perforated, resection of the involved ileum is required with an end-to-end anastomosis.

8. If the indication of diverticulectomy is bleeding, then segmental ileal resection should be performed.

References

1. Ameh EA, Mshelbwala PM, Dauda MM, Sabiu L, Nmadu PT. Symptomatic vitelline duct anomalies in children. South Afr J Surg 2005; 43:84–85.

2. Vane DW, West KW, Grosfeld JL. Vitelline duct anomalies: experience with 217 childhood cases. Arch Surg 1987; 122:542–547.

3. Kurt P, Schropp, MD. Meckel's diverticumum. In: Ashcraft K, Holcomb GW III, Murphy JP, eds. Pediatric Surgery. Elsevier Saunders, 2005, Pp 553–557.

4. Moore TC. Omphalomesenteric duct malformations. Sem Pediatr Surg 1996; 5:116–123.

5. Vil D, Brandt ML, Panic S, Bensoussan AL, Blanchard H. Meckel's diverticulum in children: a 20 year review. J Pediatr Surg 1991; 26:1289–1292.

6. Sawin RS. Appendix and Meckel diverticulum. In: Oldham KT, Colombani PM, Foglia RP, eds. Surgery of Infants and Children. Lippincott-Raven, 1997, Pp 1215–1228.

7. Kumar SR, Kumar JV . Emergency surgery for Meckel's diverticulum. World J Emerg Surg 2008; 3:27.

8. Chirdan LB, Yusufu MD, Ameh EA, Shehu SM. Meckel's diverticulitis due to *Taenia sagginata*: case report. East Afr Med J 2001; 78:107–108.

9. Moore T, Johnston OB. Complications of Meckel's diverticulum. Br J Surg 1976; 63:453–454.

10. Varcee RL, Wong SW, Taylor CF, Newstead GL. Diverticulectomy is inadequate treatment for short Meckel's diverticulum with heterotopic mucosa. ANZ J Surg 2004; 74:869–872.

11. Mckay R. High incidence of symptomatic Meckel's diverticulum in patients less than fifty years of age: an indication for resection. Am Surg 2007; 73:271–275.

12. Marinaccio F, Romondia A, Nobili M, Niglio F, La Riccia A, Marinaccio M. Meckel's diverticulum in childhood, the authors' own experience. Minerva Chir 1997; 52:1461–1465.

13. Bani-Hani KE, Shatnawi NJ. Meckel's diverticulum: comparison of incidental and symptomatic cases. World J Surg 2004; 28:917–920.

CHAPTER 65
INTESTINAL MALROTATION AND MIDGUT VOLVULUS

Johanna R. Askegard-Giesmann

Christopher C. Amah

Brian D. Kenney

Introduction

Malrotation is a spectrum of anatomic abnormalities of incomplete rotation and fixation of the intestinal tract during foetal development. Disorders of intestinal rotation and fixation are of paramount importance to the paediatric surgeon because they are most commonly seen in infancy and childhood and can have catastrophic consequences when midgut volvulus occurs. Early diagnosis and surgical treatment of this disorder can be life saving.

Demographics

Malrotation is thought to occur in approximately 1 in 500 live births.[1,2] The exact incidence is not known because many patients may live their entire lives without experiencing problems or consequences from their malrotation. Approximately 80% of patients with malrotation will present within the first month of life, and of those, most will present within the first week of life.[1-4]

Embryology/Pathophysiology

Embryology

The adult midgut extends from the second portion of the duodenum to the proximal third of the transverse colon, and is derived from the embryologic midgut loop. The normal development of the human intestine involves two processes: rotation of the midgut and the subsequent fixation of the colon and mesentery. These processes occur in three stages.

Stage 1 consists of umbilical cord herniation, lasting from approximately weeks 5 to 10 of embryonic development. The midgut lengthens disproportionately during this period and undergoes rotation around the superior mesenteric artery (SMA) axis for a total of 270° in the counterclockwise direction. Stage 2 is the return of the midgut loop back into the abdomen; it occurs at approximately weeks 10 to 11. As the intestines re-enter the abdominal cavity, the cephalad midgut completes its 270° counterclockwise rotation as the caudad midgut also completes its rotation, resulting in the duodenum coursing inferior and posterior to the SMA and the caecum located in the right lower quadrant. When completed, this rotation ensures that the attachment of the base of the midgut loop is spread along a diagonal stretching from the ligament of Trietz on the left upper quadrant to the ileocecal junction in the right lower quadrant of the abdomen. Stage 3 is the period of fixation, and lasts from the end of stage 2 until just after birth. The descending and ascending colon mesenteries fuse with the retroperitoneum, and the small bowel is fixed by a broad mesentery from the duodenojejunal junction in the left upper quadrant to the ileocecal valve in the right lower abdomen. The broad base of the small bowel mesentery stabilises its position and prevents volvulus.[5,6]

Malrotation can be grouped into syndromes arising from anomalies of three categories: migration, rotation, and fixation.

Anomalies of Migration

Omphalocele

Return of the midgut from the yolk sac back into the abdominal cavity is usually completed by week 12 of intrauterine life. This enables the anterior abdominal wall mesodermal folds to meet at the central umbilical ring, thereby closing the anterior abdominal wall. When the return of the midgut is delayed or arrested, the anterior abdominal wall folds fail to meet, and an omphalocele in the central umbilical area of the abdomen is the result.

Congenital diaphragmatic hernia

If return of the midgut into the abdominal cavity, which divides the celomic cavity into peritoneal and pleural compartments, occurs before the closure of the pleuroperitoneal membrane at 8 weeks gestation, part of the returning midgut loop may herniate into the pleural cavity. This occurs usually in the posterolateral position on the left side.

Subhepatic appendix

With completion of the 270° rotation of the ileocecal limb of the midgut loop, the caecum is brought to the right upper quadrant of the abdomen. The caecum with the attached appendix then further descends down to the right lower quadrant position in the right iliac fossa and becomes fixed to the posterior abdominal wall. The caecum and appendix may fail to migrate and remain in that subhepatic position. This condition may cause a serious diagnostic dilemma in acute appendicitis.

Anomalies of Rotation

Nonrotation

Nonrotation may occur when the midgut returns to the abdominal cavity en masse without rotating. Then, the first and second parts of the duodenum are situated normally but the third and fourth parts descend vertically downward along the right side of the superior mesenteric artery. The small bowel lies on the right and the colon is doubled on itself to the left of midline.[7]

Reversed rotation

Reversed rotation has the caecum and colon positioned posterior to the superior mesenteric vessels, and the duodenum subsequently crosses anterior to it.

Malrotation

Malrotation is a spectrum of abnormalities that occurs when the normal process of rotation is arrested at various stages. Most frequently, the duodenojejunal flexure is located inferiorly and to the right of the midline. In addition, the caecum has failed to reach its normal position in the right iliac fossa and lies in a subhepatic or central position.

Anomalies of Fixation

Volvulus neonatorum

A normal fixation of the midgut loop results in a broad diagonal attachment of the loop to the posterior abdominal wall, extending from the ligament of Trietz to the ileocecal junction. With malfixation, the distance between these two points of attachment may become shortened, leaving the midgut loop hanging on a narrow and unstable pedicle that easily predisposes to twisting (volvulus) and strangulation.

Ladd's bands

When the caecum has failed to descend from the right upper quadrant to the right iliac fossa, anomalous fixation may occur, whereby dense fibrous bands (Ladd's bands) extend from the caecum and right colon across the duodenum to the retroperitoneum of the right upper quadrant. These bands may cause duodenal obstruction via extrinsic compression; however, the obstruction of the duodenum is most commonly caused by torsion at the base of the midgut mesentery. Bands may also form between the colon and the duodenum, drawing them closer together and predisposing the midgut towards volvulus.

Mobile caecum

Failure of fixation of the caecum to the posterior abdominal wall results in a floating caecum that may predispose to cecal volvulus.

Internal hernias

Failure of fixation of the mesentery of the duodenum, right colon, or left colon may result in the formation of potential spaces for internal or mesocolic hernias. Internal hernias are associated with partial bowel obstructions, as there may be recurrent entrapment of bowel, which may eventually lead to obstruction and strangulation.[5]

Other Associated Anomalies

Malrotation may be present in patients with heterotaxy syndrome (asplenia or right isomerism and polyspenia or left isomerism). Patients presenting with this syndrome should be investigated for the possibility of malrotation. Malrotation may also be seen in conjunction with intestinal atresias and may be the cause for developing atresias in some of these patients. Vecchia et al., in a large series, found that 28% of infants with duodenal atresias had malrotation and 19% of infants with jejunoileal atresia had malrotation.[8]

Clinical Presentation

The classic presentation of malrotation with acute midgut volvulus is a neonate with bilious emesis. The point of obstruction is typically beyond the ampulla of Vater, as demonstrated by the bilious emesis. However, this symptom is not synonymous with the diagnosis of malrotation. A majority (around 60%) of infants with bilious emesis will prove to have no anatomic obstruction, but imaging is necessary to exclude the potentially catastrophic event of midgut volvulus as a consequence of malrotation. Most patients with malrotation and many with volvulus have a normal history and have a normal physical exam. Other acute symptoms that may occur with malrotation are intermittent abdominal pain, diarrhoea, constipation, and haematochezia. The latter involves 10–15% of patients and is associated with a poorer prognosis because it is indicative of bowel ischemia).9 Patients presenting with peritonitis, abdominal distention, bloody stools, and haemodynamic instability (signs and symptoms of shock) have a much worse prognosis; the clinician may be misled from the diagnosis of malrotation with volvulus due to the other symptoms related to sepsis..

Malrotation may present in an insidious manner with chronic symptoms that develop over days, months, and even years. In one series by Spigland et al., when malrotation presented beyond the neonatal period, the delay in diagnosis was a mean of 1.7 years.[10] Chronic symptoms include intermittent pain, intermittent vomiting, malabsorption, and failure to thrive. Patients may be chronically misdiagnosed with other abdominal pain syndromes, "cyclic vomiting," or even psychologic disorders.[11] Howell et al. noted that 70% of children

presenting with malrotation had clinical evidence of malnutrition.[12]

Physical Examination

There are often very few, if any, diagnostic physical exam findings with malrotation and midgut volvulus. Late presentations may have abdominal distention and abdominal tenderness, and some patients may have haemodynamic instability if bowel necrosis and sepsis have occurred. The herald sign is bilious emesis and requires prompt diagnostic studies in order to prevent bowel ischaemia and necrosis.

Investigations

Imaging

It is reasonable to start with abdominal radiographs as the initial evaluation of a patient with biliary emesis or suspected malrotation. Patients should have two views of the abdomen: an anteroposterior supine view and either an anteroposterior upright view or a cross-table lateral view. Rarely do the radiographs suggest the diagnosis of malrotation. Instead, they help to exclude other aetiologies for the patient's symptoms and serve to guide further imaging. The most common bowel gas pattern in the setting of malrotation is normal. Findings suggestive of an abnormal location of bowel include

• the presence of proximal small bowel on the right; and

• a disproportionate dilatation of the duodenum with a "double bubble"—this may be seen with severe duodenal obstruction due to volvulus or bands.[1]

Upper Gastrointestinal Series

An upper gastrointestinal (UGI) series is the preferred test for radiographic diagnosis of malrotation and volvulus (Figures 65.1 and 65.2). It is usually performed with barium, except in cases of a very sick infant or child in whom the presence of infarcted bowel or perforation is possible, in which case water-soluble contrast is used. It is important to document the first bolus of contrast medium through the duodenum in the anteroposterior as well as the lateral projection. This can be done by quickly rotating the patient to the lateral position once the duodenojejunal junction is reached. The main radiographic signs of malrotation are[1]

• lateral radiograph suggesting that the distal duodenum is not attached in the retroperitoneum;

• low or medial position of the duodenojejunal junction;

• spiral "corkscrew" or Z-shaped course of the duodenum and proximal jejunum; and

• location of the proximal jejunum in the right abdomen.

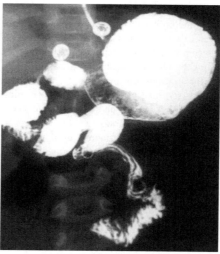

Figure 65.1: UGI depicting malrotation with abnormally low position of the ligament of Treitz.

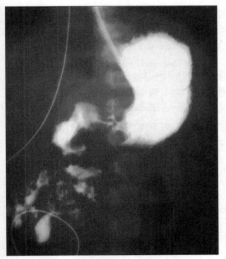

Figure 65.2: UGI depicting malrotation with all of the small bowel on the right side of the abdomen.

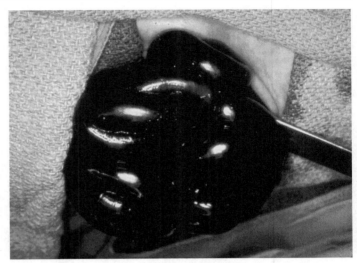

Figure 65.3: Severe small bowel ischaemia due to volvulus.

Ultrasound

Ultrasound is not the preferred imaging modality for malrotation, but it may be useful for some physicians with limited imaging modalities. Ultrasound can be used to evaluate other abdominal abnormalities and may be used to visualise the position of the mesenteric vessels. Normally, the superior mesenteric vein is to the right of the artery. In malrotation, the vein is frequently on the left, or it may rotate completely around the artery. These findings are neither sensitive nor specific for malrotation or volvulus, and should be further evaluated with additional diagnostic imaging studies, typically a UGI.

In resource-poor settings in most developing parts of Africa, where diagnostic facilities are limited or unavailable, it is safer to assume and handle all cases of bilious vomiting in a neonate as a potential malrotation syndrome with midgut volvulus. Such babies should be vigorously resuscitated and explored to avert the catastrophe of an entire midgut strangulation and gangrene, leading to short bowel syndrome.

Management

Preoperative Management

Preoperative management is focused on stabilising the patient and preparing for prompt surgery. The patient should be resuscitated with isotonic fluid (lactated Ringer's or normal saline) with an intravenous (IV) fluid bolus of 20 ml/kg, then kept on isotonic maintenance fluids, nothing by mouth (NPO), and nasogastric tube (NGT) decompression until surgery. The patient's urine output should be monitored; fluid resuscitation may depend on urine output or haemodynamics.

Operative Management and Technique

Ladd's procedure, first described in 1936, corrects the fundamental abnormality associated with malrotation and volvulus. The procedure consists of laparotomy with the following steps:[13,14]

1. The bowel is eviscerated and the entire bowel and mesenteric root are inspected.

2. The midgut volvulus, if one exists, is derotated in a counterclockwise direction.

3. Ladd's bands are lysed and the duodenum is straightened.

4. An appendectomy is performed.

5. The bowel is returned into the abdominal cavity with the caecum in the left lower quadrant.[13,14]

A laparoscopic approach may be feasible in older patients, but availability and technical comfort with this operation may be less than optimal.

Complicated cases with significant bowel ischaemia still demand an open approach.

The occurrence of an entire midgut strangulation and gangrene should be considered a disaster that must be prevented, especially in resource-poor settings where total parenteral nutrition (TPN) is neither available nor affordable (Figure 65.3). If widespread ischaemia of the midgut is observed at laparotomy, limited bowel resection and a second-look exploration 48 to 72 hours later to confirm viability of the remaining bowel are advised.

Postoperative Complications

Postoperative complications are similar to other surgical procedures and include infection and ileus. Patients with malrotation have been known to have postoperative intestinal dysmotility (pseudo-obstruction) that may delay return of the bowel function and contribute to their postoperative ileus. Normalisation of gut function occurs slowly in some children. Some reports in the literature suggest that there is an underlying functional abnormality of gut innervation associated with or as a consequence of malrotation.[15,16]

If the patient had bowel necrosis and required a resection, depending the length of residual viable bowel, the patient may have short bowel syndrome. This condition can be quite difficult to handle, and typically requires parenteral nutrition for at least the short term, and potentially long term.

Patients may also have strictures, either from their resection with anastomosis, or potentially from areas of ischaemia that did not require resection. These patients may not require additional surgeries, or they may require subsequent bowel resection of the stricture and/or revision of the strictured anastomosis.

Prognosis and Outcome

Survival of children with malrotation and volvulus is high (>80%); however, despite prompt diagnosis and surgery, a significant minority of patients still die or suffer substantial morbidity due to loss of intestines.

Factors associated with an increased mortality include:

• younger age (especially less than 30 days old);[17]

• other clinical abnormalities; and

• bowel necrosis.[4,17]

Prevention

There are no preventive measures to take regarding this disease process. Early detection and treatment are the only measures to help prevent a poor outcome from malrotation with volvulus.

Ethical Issues

The patient with short bowel syndrome as a result of malrotation with volvulus that occurred either in utero or in the neonatal period presents a real treatment challenge in the industrialised nations and may be even more difficult in countries where resources are more limited. These patients require TPN and significant medical care to prevent dehydration and failure to thrive. In addition, these patients require central lines for prolonged periods of time and are often plagued by complications from the central lines.

Evidence-Based Research

In the absence of comparative studies, a recent review of malrotation and volvulus is shown in Table 65.1.

Table 65.1: Evidence-based research.

Title	Malrotation and volvulus in infancy and childhood
Authors	Millar AJW, Rode H, Cywes S
Institution	University of Cape Town and Red Cross Children's Hospital, Rondesbosch, Cape Town, South Africa
Reference	Sem Pediatr Surg 2003; 12:229–236
Problem	Review of malrotation and volvulus.
Intervention	Diagnostic radiology and surgical treatment.
Comparison/control (quality of evidence)	Comparison of recent cases with previously published cohort.
Historical significance/comments	A large series of patients reviewed for presenting symptoms, evaluation, and surgical management.

Key Summary Points

1. Malrotation is a spectrum of anatomic abnormalities related to fixation of the intestinal tract.

2. Bilious emesis in a newborn should be considered midgut volvulus until proven otherwise.

3. A prompt diagnostic UGI study should be done on any newborn with bilious emesis to rule out malrotation with midgut volvulus.

4. If investigative studies cannot be done, then the patient should have fluid resuscitation and prompt surgical exploration to prevent the catastrophic complications of midgut volvulus.

5. Ladd's procedure for malrotation includes detorsion of volvulus if one is present, lysis of dense fibrous bands (Ladd's bands), placement of small bowel and large bowel in abdomen in nonrotated manner, and appendectomy.

6. There is an increased mortality for malrotation in younger patients, patients with clinical abnormalities, or those with bowel necrosis.

7. Patients may have a delay in the return of bowel function after surgery, especially if volvulus was present.

References

1. Strouse PJ. Disorders of intestinal rotation and fixation ("malrotation"). Pediatr Radiol 2004; 34:837–851.

2. Torres AM, Ziegler MM. Malrotation of the intestine. World J Surg 1993; 17:326–331.

3. Filston HC, Kirks DR. Malrotation—the ubiquitous anomaly. J Pediatr Surg 1981; 16:614–620.

4. Berdon WE, Baker DH, Bull S, et al. Midgut malrotation and volvulus: which films are most helpful? Radiology 1970; 96:375–383.

5. Smith SD. Disorders of intestinal rotation and fixation. In: Grosfeld JL, O'Neill Jr. JA, Fonkalsrud EW, Coran AG, eds. Pediatric Surgery. Mosby, 2006, Pp 1342–1357.

6. Iken JJ, Oldham KT. Malrotation. In: Ashcraft K, Holcomb III GW, Murphy JP, eds. Pediatric Surgery. Saunders, 2005, Pp 435–447.

7. Millar AJW, Rode H, Cywes S. Malrotation and volvulus in infancy and childhood. Sem Pediatr Surg 2003; 12:229–236.

8. Vecchia LKD, Grosfeld JL, West KW, et al. Intestinal atresia and stenosis. Arch Surg 1998; 133:490–497.

9. Bonadio WA, Clarkson T, Naus J. The clinical features of children with malrotation of the intestine. Pediatr Emerg Care 1991; 7:349.

10. Spigland N, Brandt ML, Yazbeck S. Malrotation presenting beyond the neonatal period. J Pediatr Surg 1990; 25:1139–1142.

11. Amah CC, Agugua-Obianyo NEN, Ekenze SO. Intestinal malrotation in the older child: common diagnostic pitfalls. W Afr J Radiol 2004; 11:33–37.

12. Howell CG, Vozza F, Shaw S, et al. Malrotation, malnutrition, and ischemic bowel disease. J Pediatr Surg 1982; 17:469–473.

13. Ladd WE. Surgical diseases of the alimentary tract in infants. N Engl J Med 1936; 215:705–708.

14. Mazziotti MV, Strasberg SM, Langer JC. Intestinal rotation abnormalities without volvulus: the role of laparoscopy. J Am Coll Surg 1997; 185:172–176.

15. Devane SP, Coombes R, Smith VV, et al. Persistent gastrointestinal symptoms after correction of malrotation. Arch Dis Child 1992; 67:218–221.

16. Feitz R, Vos A. Malrotation: the postoperative period. J Pediatr Surg 1997; 32:1322–1324.

17. Messineo A, MacMillan JH, Palder SB, et al. Clinical factors affecting mortality in children with malrotation of the intestine. J Pediatr Surg 1992; 27:1343–1345.

CHAPTER 66
GASTROINTESTINAL DUPLICATIONS

Auwal M Abubakar
Ralf-Bodo Troebs

Introduction

Gastrointestinal duplications (GIDs) are rare congenital malformations. They can arise anywhere from the mouth to the anus.[1] Due to the rarity of these lesions, they frequently present both diagnostic and therapeutic challenges. They may be unexpectedly encountered intraoperatively, and appropriate surgical management requires that the attending surgeon be familiar with the pathology and clinical characteristics of GID.

Demographics

Gastrointestinal duplications occur with a prevalence of 1:4,500 births.[2] In most series, there is no sex predilection. Even though GID is rare, many reports exist with large numbers of patients accumulated over long periods.[3–8] Few reports, however, come from Africa.[9–11]

About 60–70% of patients present before the age of 2 years.[6,8,12] In Africa, due to more difficulties with diagnosis, patients may present at an older age.[11]

Embryology

There are many theories on the embryology of GID. None of these theories, however, is able to explain all types of duplication. The presence of heterotopic tissue in duplications and the consistent mesenteric location of duplications has put many of these theories to question.

These embryological theories include the following:

- *Split notochord syndrome:*[13,14] GID is related to the development of neuroenteric canals, which is related to the thoracic duplications that have associated abnormalities of the cervical and thoracic vertebrae.

- *Abnormalities of recanalisation of the solid stage:*[15] It is only some part of the foregut that undergoes recanalisation, and this process occurs on both the mesenteric and antimesenteric sides of the bowel, whereas duplications are found only on the mesenteric side.

- *Remnants of embryologic diverticula:*[16] This may explain the higher frequency of GID found in the terminal ileum because there are usually numerous diverticula found during development. The presence of heterotopic mucosa, the mesenteric location of GID, and the presence of tubular duplications puts this theory to question.

- *Partial twinning:*[17] This can explain duplications of the hindgut. These are usually associated with malformations of the genitourinary tract.

- *Environmental factors such as trauma or hypoxia:*[18,19] In early foetal development, environmental factors may lead to duplications, and duplications may, in fact, be a part of the spectrum of intestinal atresias.

Pathology

Gastrointestinal duplications are rare congenital malformations. They generally have the following characteristics irrespective of location:

- They are in or adjacent to the wall or part of the gastrointestinal tract and are consistently on the mesenteric side.

- They share a common blood supply with the native bowel.

- They have a definite smooth muscle coat and are lined by alimentary tract mucosa that may be similar to the adjacent bowel or heterotopic tissue.

The most common site of GID is the ileum, followed by the oesophagus, colon, and jejunum (Table 66.1).

Grossly, GIDs are spherical (Figure 66.1) in 82% of the cases; these are the most prevalent type at all levels[20] and do not commonly communicate with the adjacent bowel. The remaining GIDs are tubular, more extensive, more likely to have heterotopic gastric mucosa, and usually communicate with the adjacent bowel, most commonly

Table 66.1: Summary of distribution of locations of 431 gastrointestinal duplications in 395 patients from six studies.

Location	Bower et al. (1978)[6]	Hocking et al. (1981)[7]	Holcomb et al. (1989)[8]	Stringer et al. (1995)[9]	Karnak et al. (2000)[10]	Pulgandla et al. (2003)[11]	Totals (%)
Oropharyngeal	0	–	0	2	1	–	3 (<1)
Oesophagus	15	8	21	15	7	–	66 (15)
Stomach	8	8	8	10	1	6	41 (10)
Duodenum	4	1	2	3	3	7	20 (5)
Jejunum/ileum	34	32	47	21	17	51	202 (47)
Colon	12	4	15	10	9	5	55 (13)
Rectum	2	5	5	6	2	4	24 (6)
Thoracoabdominal	1	2	3	6	2	0	14 (3)
Others	2	0	0	4	0	0	6 (1)
Totals (duplications/ patients)	(78/64)	(60/53)	(101/96)	(77/72)	(42/38)	(73/72)	431 (100)

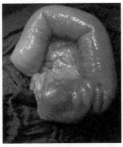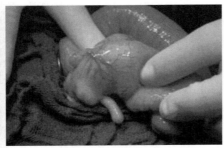

Figure 66.1: Spherical duplication of the ileocaecal area in an 8-month-old child.

in the small and large bowels. The lining mucosa is usually the same as the adjacent normal bowel, but can be heterotopic, such as gastric, squamous, transitional, ciliated columnar mucosa, pancreas, lymphoid aggregates resembling Peyer's patches, and ganglion cells. Others include heterotopic lung tissue or thyroid stroma.[12] However, heterotopic gastric and pancreatic tissues are the ones of significant clinical importance due to the risk of peptic ulceration and pancreatitis. Even though GID in children is benign, malignant transformation has been described in adults.[21]

Diagnosis

Clinical Features
There is no common clinical pattern of signs and symptoms of duplications. They present with a variety of symptoms or sometimes as masses found incidentally during routine examinations or investigations, or they are encountered during an operation for other problems.

Most patients present before the age of 2 years,[11,12] but presentation during adulthood has been described.[4,22] The clinical presentation also varies according to the age of the patient, location of duplication, type of mucosal lining, duration of disease, and presence of complications. The clinical presentation may be due to the pressure effect of the duplication. Feeding difficulties are associated with masses in the floor of the mouth. In thoracic duplications, this leads to respiratory distress or dysphagia. Other symptoms in the chest include recurrent pneumonia and failure to thrive. In the abdomen, GID causes intestinal obstruction but may also cause ureteric, biliary, or even vena caval obstruction. Pancreatitis can arise from pressure on the pancreas. Duplications in the abdomen commonly present with pain, vomiting, and abdominal mass.

The clinical presentation may also be secondary to complications of the duplications. These include intussusception,[12] volvulus,[8] perforation,[23] bleeding (related to ectopic gastric mucosa), peptic oesophageal stricture, and malignant transformation, as seen in adults.[21]

Prenatal Diagnosis
Prenatal diagnosis of GIDs is becoming widespread in the Western world. This ability to accurately identify GID has provided an opportunity to intervene. In cases of nonimmune hydrops in thoracic duplications, thoracoamniotic shunting is carried out in utero in some centres with experience in foetal treatment.[24] This is done in the immediate postnatal period before the onset of symptoms or the development of complications.[2]

Investigations

In the management of GID, accurate preoperative diagnosis is difficult. This is because GID is very rare, and the clinical presentation is nonspecific.

In Africa, where resources are limited, the more expensive investigations, such as computed tomography (CT) scan and magnetic resonance imaging (MRI), should be reserved for the very difficult cases. The most common investigations carried out are ultrasonography (US) and contrast medium examinations.

Ultrasonography
US is the most common modality used and should be the first choice. It typically shows a double-layered wall (inner echogenic mucosa and outer sonoluscent muscular layer). When this double-layered pattern is present on US, a GID is confirmed and there is no need for further radiologic evaluation.[25,26]

Plain X-Rays
A plain chest x-ray (plain abdominal/lateral) will be able to detect foregut duplications in the chest in up to 90% of cases. Plain abdominal x-ray may show evidence of intestinal obstruction.

Contrast Medium Studies
Contrast medium studies may reveal compression or displacement of the adjacent organ. Rarely, it will show communication with the adjacent native organ, but it does not specify the nature of the duplication.

CT Scan or MRI
A CT scan or MRI is employed in difficult cases. It is noninvasive and has the advantage of demonstrating the exact location and relationship to adjacent normal structures. It may also reveal other duplications. It is particularly useful in thoracic, pelvic, and the rare large retroperitoneal duplication cysts. A spinal MRI will outline the relationship of the cyst with the spinal column and spinal canal.

Technetium 99m Pertechnetate Scintigraphy Scan
This scan indicates the definite existence of GID when it contains ectopic gastric mucosa. This is especially useful in oesophageal, duodenal, and tubular small bowel duplications with a high incidence of heterotropic gastric mucosa.

Laparoscopy
Laparoscopy is useful in cases when all the above investigations are not conclusive.

Treatment
The goal is to make a prompt diagnosis and provide treatment before the onset of symptoms or the development of complications. The ideal treatment for GID is complete excision. However, GID in children is a benign disease, and any treatment should not be more radical than to eliminate the patient's complaints and prevent further recurrence.

Important points to be considered in the surgical treatment of GID include:

1. the nature of the blood supply shared between the duplication and native bowel;

2. the presence of heterotopic gastric mucosa, which will negate internal drainage due to the risk of peptic ulceration; and

3. the relationship with adjacent structures, such as the biliary tract in duodenal duplications.

The treatment of GID is best considered by location of the duplication. However, in selected cases, an intraoperative frozen section may give further information on the absence or presence of heterotopic components.

Oropharynx
Oropharyngeal duplications are rare and constitute less than 1% of duplications. They may contain ectopic gastric or colonic mucosa. These cysts are excised by an intraoral incision.

Oesophagus
Oesophageal duplications are related to the right side of the oesophagus and are best approached through a right posterolateral thoracotomy. A supraclavicular approach is used for those located in the cervical region. These lesions should be completely excised due to the high incidence of gastric heterotopia in this location. Where facilities are available, a thoracoscopic approach is preferable for isolated lesions.[27]

Thoracoabdominal

Thoracoabdominal cysts are not intimately adherent to the oesophagus but are usually to the posterior right side of the chest and may have communication through the right crus of the diaphragm to the pylorus, duodenum, jejunum, or ileum. They are often lined by ectopic gastric mucosa. It is also important to ensure that there is no neuroenteric communication. If present, this should be excised in consultation with a neurosurgeon. Incomplete excision will lead to meningitis. The best approach here is the use of separate posterolateral thoracotomy and abdominal approaches. Depending on the extent of the lesion and the patient's condition, it may be carried out at the same surgery or staged. For isolated lesions, thoracoscopic resection is becoming the preferred treatment.

Gastric

Gastric duplications represent 8% of duplications. Unlike other duplications, these are more common in girls.[28] Most of these duplications are on the greater curvature, but they can rarely be on the lesser curvature or the pylorus. They usually do not communicate with the stomach, and complete excision is possible. More extensive lesions are excised with a limited partial gastrectomy.

Duodenum

Duodenal duplications also are rare. The treatment of choice for duodenal duplications is complete excision with preservation of the duodenum. However, this total excision is not always possible if the cyst is in close proximity to the pancreas or the biliary or pancreatic ducts.

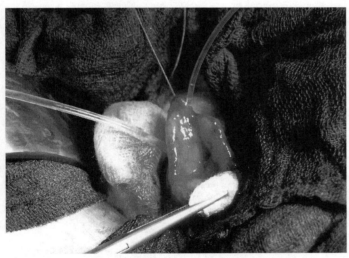

Figure 66.2: Communicating cystic duplication of the duodenum. Exposure after duodenotomy. The upper tube is within the major papilla; the lower one intubates the cyst.

The walls of the ducts may be included in the thickness of the wall of the duplication and may also share the same blood supply with the cyst (Figure 66.2). In these cases, the options include:[29]

- partial resection of part of the cyst wall but including the mucosal lining; or
- internal drainage through a wide cystoduodenal anastomosis or a cystojejunal Roux-en-Y anastomosis.

Small Bowel

The small bowel (jejunum/ileum) is the site of about half of all GIDs. The cystic types of duplications are sometimes easily shelled out, but most are resected with primary end-to-end anastomosis to restore bowel continuity. A laparoscopic approach may be effective to identify the lesion and minimize the abdominal wall incision by lifting up the affected bowel segment.

The tubular type of GID can involve the whole ileum. It has an 80% incidence of gastric heterotopia. Extensive resections will lead to short bowel syndrome, and drainage into the adjacent normal bowel is not encouraged due to the risk of peptic ulceration. In these cases, the multiple stepwise stripping of the mucosa is as described by Wrenn,[30] but anastomosis of the duplication to the stomach has also been tried.[31]

Colon

Colonic duplications rarely contain ectopic gastric mucosa. The rare complete colorectal duplication may be associated with doubling anomalies of the genitourinary organs, such as the bladder and vagina.[17] Cystic duplications can be shelled out or resected with primary colocolostomy. Tubular duplications of the colon have one or more communications with the native bowel. If it is extensive, a distal communication is created with the colon or rectum.

Rectum

Rectal duplications are usually presacral. In 90% of cases, there is no communication with the rectum. The posterior sagittal approach is preferred. It gives good exposure, facilitates safer removal and repair, and prevents entering or compromising the rectal lumen. Laparotomy is preferable, however, for the rare anterior duplications.[32]

Prognosis and Outcome

The outcome of surgical treatment of duplications is good. Poor outcomes are observed when there are associated severe malformations, which in themselves carry a high morbidity and mortality.

Evidence-Based Research

GIDs are very rare anomalies, so most large series are accumulated over three to four decades from big referral centres. It is difficult to have randomized studies.

Key Summary Points

1. Gastrointestinal duplications are rare.

2. GIDs can arise from the mouth to the anus.

3. The aetiology of gastrointestinal duplications is heterogenous.

4. About half of all duplications are located in the small bowel.

5. The clinical features of gastrointestinal duplications is nonspecific; a high index of suspicion is required for prompt diagnosis.

6. Most patients with gastrointestinal duplications will present before 2 years of age, but presentation during adulthood, as well as late malignant transformation, has been described.

7. The presence of ectopic gastric mucosa, especially in tubular duplications, should be documented, as it has an impact on the approach to management.

8. Ultrasonography should be the first line of investigation.

9. The ideal treatment is total excision; however, in children, GID is a benign disease, and therapy should not jeopardise the integrity of the adjacent normal bowel.

10. The results of surgical treatment are good.

References

1. Ladd WE, Gross RE. Surgical treatment of duplications of the alimentary tract enterogenous cysts, enteric cysts or ileum duplex. Surg Gynecol Obstet 1940; 70:295–307.

2. Schalamon J, Schleef J, Hollwarth ME. Experience with gastrointestinal duplications in childhood. Langenbeck's Arch Surg 2000; 385:402–405.

3. Bower RJ, Sieber WK, Kiesewetter WB. Alimentary tract duplications in children. Ann Surg 1978; 188:667–674.

4. Hocking M, Young DG. Duplications of the alimentary tract. Br J Surg 1981; 68:92–96.

5. Holcomb GW III, Gheissari A, O'Neill JA Jr, Shorter NA, Bishop HC. Surgical management of alimentary tract duplications. Ann Surg 1989; 209:167–174.

6. Stringer MD, Spitz L, Abel R, et al. Management of alimentary tract duplications in children. Br J Surg 1995; 82:74–78.

7. Karnak I, Ocal T, Senocak ME, Tanyel FC, Buyukpamukcu N. Alimentary tract duplications in children: report of 26 years' experience. Turk J Pediatr 2000; 42:118–125.

8. Pulingandla PS, Nguyen AS, Flageole H, et al. Gastrointestinal duplications. J Pediatr Surg 2003; 38:740–744.

9. Oluwole SF, Adekunle A. Rectal duplication in chronic large bowel obstruction. Can J Surg 1987; 30:419–420.

10. Adejuyigbe O, Hameed AO, Fadiran OA. Gastric duplication: case report and review of literature. Niger Med J 1988; 18:357–361.

11. Adejuyigbe O, Olayinka OS, Sowande OA, Abubakar AM. Gastrointestinal duplications in Ile-Ife, Nigeria. East Afr Med J 2002; 79:134–136.

12. Ildstad ST, Tollerud DJ, Weiss RG, et al. Duplications of the alimentary tract: clinical characteristics, preferred treatment and associated malformations. Ann Surg 1988; 208:184–189.

13. Stern LE, Warner BW. Gastrointestinal duplications. Semin Pediatr Surg 2000; 9:135–140.

14. Bentley JFR, Smith JR. Developmental posterior enteric remnants and spinal malformations. Arch Dis Child 1960; 35:76–86.

15. Bremer JL. Diverticula and duplications of the intestinal tract. Arch Patholog 1952; 38:132–140.

16. Lewis FT, Thyng FW. Regular occurrence of intestinal diverticula in embryology of pig, rabbit and man. Am J Anat 1908; 7:505–519.

17. Ravitch MM. Hind gut duplication, doubling of colon and genital urinary tracts. Ann Surg 1953; 137:588–601.

18. Mellish RWP, Koop CE. Clinical manifestations of duplication of the bowel. Pediatrics 1961; 27:397–407.

19. Favara BE, Franciosi RA, Akers DR. Enteric duplications: thirty-seven cases. A vascular theory of pathogenesis. Am J. Dis Child 1971; 122:501–506.

20. Macpherson RI. Gastrointestinal tract duplications: clinical, pathologic, etiologic and radiologic considerations. Radiographics 1993; 13:1063–1080.

21. Orr MM, Edwards AJ. Neoplastic change in duplication of the alimentary tract. Br J Surg 1975; 62:269.

22. Simsek A, Zeybek N, Yagli G, et al. Enteric and rectal duplication and duplication cysts in the adult. ANZ J Surg 2005; 75:174–176.

23. Piolat C, N'die J, Andrini, P, et al. Perforated colon: a rare cause of meconium peritonitis with prenatal diagnosis. Pediatr Surg Int 2005; 21:110–112.

24. Ferro MM, Milner R, Voto L, et al. Intrathoracic alimentary tract duplication cysts treated in utero by thoracoamniotic shunting. Fetal Diagn Ther 1998;13:343–347.

25. Barr LL, Hayden CK, Stanberry D, et al. Enteric duplication cysts in children: are their ultrasonographic wall characteristics diagnostic? Pediatr Radiol 1990; 20:326–328.

26. Deftereos S, Soultanidis H, Limas C, et al. Duodenal duplication: is ultrasonographic appearance enough to confirm diagnosis? Rom J Gastroenterol 2004; 23:345–347.

27. Bratu I, Laberge J, Flageole H, Bouchard S. Foregut duplications: is there an advantage to thoracoscopic resection? J Pediatr Surg 2005; 40:138–141.

28. Lewis PL, Holder I, Feldman M. Duplication of the stomach: report of a case and review of the English literature. Arch Surg 1961; 82:634–640.

29. Merrot T, Anastasescu R, Pankevych T, et al. Duodenal duplications: clinical characteristics, embryological hypothesis, histologic findings, treatment. Eur J Pediatr Surg 2006; 16:18–23.

30. Wrenn EL Jr. Tubular duplications of the small intestine. Surgery 1962; 52:494–498.

31. Jewett TC Jr, Walkner AB, Cooney DR. A long term follow up on duplication of the entire small intestine treated by gastroduplication. J Pediatr Surg 1983; 18:185–188.

32. La Quaglia MP, Feins N, Eraklis A, Hensen WH. Rectal duplications. J Pediatr Surg 1990; 25:980–984.

CHAPTER 67
MECONIUM ILEUS

Felicitas Eckoldt-Wolke

Auwal M. Abubakar

Introduction

Neonatal bowel obstruction by a thick and tenacious meconium is known as meconium ileus. Meconium abnormalities cause multiple neonatal intestinal obstructive disorders of varying severity, ranging from the benign meconium plug syndrome to the complicated meconium ileus associated with cystic fibrosis (CF). The largest group of patients presenting with meconium ileus are children who suffer from CF, accounting for 75% of all caucasian patients with meconium ileus.

In the last 20 years, a specific type of meconium ileus, not associated with CF, has been described in premature neonates with very low birth weights. Meconium ileus, however, does occur in up to 20% of neonates with CF and is the earliest manifestation of the disease.

Demographics

Cystic fibrosis is the most common serious inherited defect affecting the caucasian population. It is transmitted as an autosomal recessive condition with a 5% carrier rate and an incidence of approximately 1:2,500 live births. Hamish et al. reported the incidence of CF in live-born babies in America to be lower in blacks (1:15,000).[1] The cystic fibrosis transmembrane conductance regulator (CFTR) is located on the long arm of chromosome 7. The delta F508 mutation is the most common mutation among caucasians. There are, however, great differences between populations. For example, delta F508 mutation is present in 70% of CF alleles in caucasians in the United States, but accounts for only 43% in African Americans.[2] In the literature, a great racial variation is assumed.[3] Meconium ileus is reported to be a rare finding in African populations.[4–7]

Premature and very low birth weight (VLBW) babies can suffer from a condition resembling meconium ileus called meconium ileus equivalent (Figure 67.1). Babies at risk for meconium ileus equivalent usually can survive only in intensive care units with ventilation therapy.[8] Such units are rare in Africa, and this may be the reason why meconium ileus equivalent is not described in large studies of neonatal paediatric surgical care in Africa.

Aetiology

The intraluminal obstruction in meconium ileus is due to abnormally thick and tenacious meconium (Figure 67.2). It becomes inspissated in the distal ileum, blocking the lumen. Abnormally dilatated mucous glands in the distal ileum secrete mucus with a very high protein content containing an abnormal mucoprotein, which is responsible for the tenaciousness of the meconium. In VLBW babies, the problem seems to be the disproportion between the tenaciousness of normal meconium and the underdevelopment of the contractility of the bowel. In both cases, meconium is strongly attached to the wall of the distal ileum, creating pellets of white meconium in a narrow lumen.

Classification

The clinical presentation varies depending on the type of meconium ileus. Instances of meconium ileus can be classified into uncomplicated and complicated types.

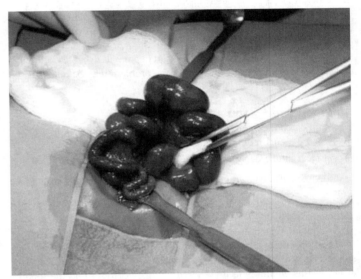

Figure 67.1: Meconium ileus in a low birth weight baby.

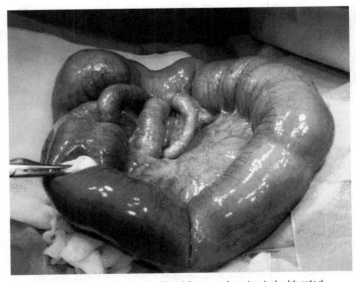

Figure 67.2: Meconium ileus with dilated ileum and contracted, obturated terminal ileum.

Uncomplicated Form

The neonate may appear relatively normal for the first 12–18 hours of life. However, as the proximal bowel fills with air, abdominal distention, emesis (later bilious), and failure to pass meconium are noted. On examination, distended loops of intestine may be visible. Bowel sounds are present but sluggish. Mucosal plugs may be evacuated on rectal examination after withdrawal of the finger.

Complicated Form

About half of meconium ileus patients have a complicated form, associated with volvulus, perforation, or atresia. Massive distention, tenderness, or erythema indicates the presence of complications. There are no bowel sounds; vomiting is usually bilious. The child is in a critical condition.

Investigations

Plain abdominal radiographs show a distended intestine. Air-fluid levels may or may not be present. A "soap bubble" appearance in the right lower quadrant may be the result of air mixed with the meconium.

The initial diagnostic test is a contrast enema. In the case of a meconium ileus, it shows a microcolon. Meconium pellets in the distal ileum can also be determined. This diagnostic investigation also enables one to exclude colonic atresia and rotation anomalies. The main differential diagnosis is Hirschsprung´s disease. This will need to be excluded by suction rectal biopsies.

The same diagnostic methods are used in premature babies, although due to the prematurity, recognition of the problem may be delayed.

Treatment

Nonoperative Treatment

Uncomplicated meconium ileus may be successfully treated nonoperatively. All patients require standard supportive care:

• oral gastric tube decompression;

• intravenous fluids to replace deficits and counteract ongoing losses; and

• meticulous attention to the acid-base balance.

In uncomplicated cases, a gastrografin enema (dilution 3:1) is the treatment of choice.[9] It can be accompanied by use of N-acetylcysteine/saline (1:5) in several enemas and in addition to the oral tube. The effect of this enema is to draw large volumes of fluid into the lumen. Therefore, the child must be well-rehydrated prior to this procedure. The child's pulse rate and urine output have to be carefully monitored. This procedure is successful in more than 50% of affected children. The patient should evacuate spontaneously over the next 6–8 hours. If the patient fails to evacuate or if a complicated meconium ileus is present, a surgical procedure must be carried out.[7]

Operative Treatment

Operative treatment is indicated when the nonoperative treatment fails or is associated with complications such as perforation or in the complicated type of meconium ileus. In all cases, a supraumbilical transverse incision is used.

Three procedures can be used:

1. enterostomy and decompression;

2. resection and stoma formation; or

3. resection and anastomosis.

Enterostomy

Enterostomy is performed by opening the bowel on the antimesenteric border proximally where the dilated bowel tapers down. A size 10 catheter is pulled upwards, and the sticky meconium is washed out by using gastrografin or a 1:5 solution of acetylcysteine/saline. Patience is required during this procedure; it takes a considerable amount of time because one has to work carefully. Further, the distal plugs have to be washed out. When the small bowel is empty, the enterostomy can be closed in the usual way.[10]

Resection

Resection and formation of a stoma is the most common form of management. Several forms of stoma are possible, with the most wide-spread being the Bishop-Koop type anastomosis (Figure 67.3).[11] The most distended part of the ileum is resected. An end–to-side anastomosis is constructed about 3 cm distal to the resection margin. The open end is brought out as a stoma and sutured to the skin. In critical cases, a double-barrel stoma may be the best option.

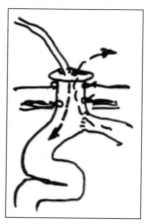

Figure 67.3: Bishop-Koop anastomosis for irrigation.

Postoperative Complications

General supportive care is provided as after any major laparotomy. The oral gastric tube is left in place until bowel function returns. Use of N-acetylcysteine via the oral tube, or a stoma, or by enema may further aid passage. Oral feeding is started with pancreatic enzyme supplementation.

CF is confirmed or ruled out by determining the sweat chloride level. Close attention has to be given to pulmonary care in CF children.

Weaning is often not a problem. Extended physiotherapy and specific attention to pulmonary infections and general growth of the child are decisive for the quality of the child's further life.

In some cases, the Bishop-Koop anastomosis closes by itself. In other cases, special attention has to be paid to clearance of the obstructed segment. After this, closure of the enterostomy can be carried out. In CF, distal ileum obstruction tends to recur, so special care has to be taken to ensure normal bowel movements.

Prognosis

The prognosis for children suffering from CF has improved in the developed countries due to neonatal care, general nutrition, treatment of pulmonary infections, and specific antibiotics.

Neonates with very low birth weight require a specific type of treatment. Their survival depends on intensive neonatal care with ventilation, broad spectrum antibiotics, and a specific enteral nutrition.

Ethical Issues

In developed countries, CF is a genetic-based diagnosis. Specific care has to be given to children with CF. This has enabled the life-span of CF sufferers to be extended to 30 to 40 years, whereas historically in Europe these children died at about age 20. One of the main procedures that has made this improvement possible is the gastrografin enema developed by Helen Noblett.[9] In combination with this, use of N-acetylcysteine often makes it possible to avoid having to perform a laparotomy. If the combination fails, surgery and enterostomy have to be carried out.[2]

Evidence-Based Research

The condition is uncommon, and relevant studies of surgical treatment with a significant number of patients are not available.

Key Summary Points

1. Meconium ileus is very rare in Africa.

2. Among Caucasians, 75% of meconium ileus is associated with cystic fibrosis.

3. A rare variant of meconium ileus not associated with cystic fibrosis has been described in premature very low birth weight babies.

4. The patients present as uncomplicated or complicated meconium ileus.

5. The treatment of uncomplicated cases is nonoperative by gastrografin enema.

6. In complicated and failed nonoperative treatment cases, operative intervention is required.

7. The prognosis of children with meconium ileus has improved with advances in supportive care in the developed countries.

References

1. Allan DL, Robbie M, Phelan PD. Familial occurrence of meconium ileus. Eur J Pediatr 1981; 135:291–292.

2. Nandi B, Mungongo C, Lakhoo L. A comparison of neonatal surgical admissions between two linked surgical departments in Africa and Europe. Pediatr Surg Int 2008; 24:939–942.

3. Naguib ML, Schrijver I, Gardner P, et al. Cystic fibrosis detection in high-risk Egyptian children and CFTR mutation analysis. J Cyst Fibros 2007; 6:111–116.

4. Adeyemi SD. Neonatal intestinal obstruction in a developing tropical country: patterns, problems, and prognosis. J Trop Pediatr 1989; 35:66–70.

5. Barrack SM, Kyambi JM, Ndungu J, et al. Intestinal atresia and stenosis as seen and treated at Kenyatta National Hospital, Nairobi. East Afr Med J 1993; 70:558–564.

6. Mutesa L, Azad AK, Verhaeghe C, et al. Genetic analysis of Rwandan patients with cystic fibrosis–like symptoms: identification of novel cystic fibrosis transmembrane conductance regulator and epithelial sodium channel gene variants. Chest 2009; 135(5):1233–1242. Epub 18 November 2008.

7. Rescorla FJ, Grosfeld JL. Contemporary management of meconium ileus. World J Surg 1993; 17:318–325.

8. Emil S. Meconium obstruction in the very low birth weight premature infant. Pediatrics. 2004; 114:1367; author reply, 1367–1368.

9. Noblett HR. Treatment of uncomplicated meconium ileus by gastrografin enema: a preliminary report. J Pediatr Surg 1969; 4:190–197.

10. Millar AJW, Rode H, Cywes S. Management of uncomplicated meconium ileus with T tube ileostomy. Arch Dis Child 1988; 63(3):309–310.

11. Jawaheer J, Khalil B, Plummer T, et al. Primary resection and anastomosis for complicated meconium ileus: a safe procedure? Pediatr Surg Int 2007; 23:1091–1093.

CHAPTER 68
INTUSSUSCEPTION

Afua A.J. Hesse
Francis A. Abantanga
Kokila Lakhoo

Introduction

Intussusception is the most common type of intestinal obstruction seen in the paediatric age group, especially in infants and toddlers. It is an occlusive-strangulation type of intestinal obstruction, and all necessary measures should be taken early to ensure prompt diagnosis and treatment in order to prevent ischaemia and necrosis of bowel. Intussusception occurs when a portion of the proximal bowel (usually referred to as the intussusceptum) telescopes into a segment of the adjoining distal bowel (known as the intussuscepiens). The intussusceptum is propelled further into the intussuscepiens by peristalsis and eventually becomes thickened, oedematous, and swollen, leading to blockage of its lumen (occlusion) and subsequent pinching off of its mesentery (strangulation).

Children with intussusception in the African subregion, as a rule, present late to hospital for management[1,2,3] as a result of lack of knowledge on the part of parents, who try assorted local remedies before bringing the child to hospital.

Diagnosis of the condition can be difficult and tricky,[4] sometimes causing diagnostic confusion with other conditions, such as enterocolitis, dysentery, and gastroenteritis, further delaying the diagnosis. When the diagnosis is made late (meaning more than 48 to 72 hours after symptoms develop), surgery is usually the only option left to most surgeons. About 90–95% of intussusceptions occur in children between the ages of 3 months and 3 years,[5,6] and usually do not have a pathological lead point (i.e., they are idiopathic in nature).[6]

Demographics

Intussusception is known to occur among children in Africa, but unfortunately its true incidence is not known. It is seen with striking variation in frequency in various parts of the world. Worldwide, the incidence is estimated to be approximately 2–4 cases per 1,000 children, with a male-to-female ratio ranging from 1.4:1 to 3:2.[1-4,7-9] The male preponderance is more remarkable in the latter months of infancy. Intussusception tends to occur in well-nourished infants, around the time of weaning of the infant; its incidence in malnourished children is less than 30%, as quoted in the literature from Africa.[10] No paediatric age group is exempt from having intussusception, but it is more common in infants and toddlers. After 3 years of age, anatomically identifiable pathological lead points (PLPs) may be the cause of an intussusception in about 1.5% to 12% of children.[9,11]

Aetiology

In most childhood intussusceptions, the cause is usually unknown; this type of intussusception is referred to as idiopathic. This is the case in 90–95% of intussusceptions found in infants and toddlers. In this group of children, there may be hypertrophy of the mural lymphoid tissues, known as Peyer's patches, in the terminal ileum as a result of a viral illness (caused by adenovirus or rotavirus) with a history of acute gastroenteritis and/or respiratory tract symptoms. Operative findings in these children often include enlarged mesenteric lymph nodes and Peyer's patches.[11,12] In others, a mobile caecum is found. In most hospital-based studies in the subregion, in children younger than 3 years of age with intussusception, 10–30% were found to have had gastroenteritis.[1,10]

The most common PLP in the causation of nonidiopathic intussusception, especially in older children, is Meckel's diverticulum,[4,13–15] followed by polyps of the small intestine and colon.[11,12,14,15] Other PLPs include intestinal duplications, lymphomas, haemangiomas, lymphosarcomas, enteric cysts, Henoch-Schönlein purpura with submucosal haematomas, cystic fibrosis with inspissated meconium, benign intestinal neoplasms, Peutz-Jeghers familial polyposis, ectopic gastric mucosa, ectopic pancreatic mucosa, and worm infestations (especially *Ascaris lumbricoides*). The proportion of intussusceptions with a PLP increases with age.[13] Intussusception may also occur in children as a result of trauma, such as a postoperative complication after abdominal surgery,[3,12,13] especially retroperitoneal surgery, and after immunization with rotavirus vaccine.[10]

Pathophysiology

An imbalance of the longitudinal forces along the intestinal wall is believed to be the cause of intussusception.[9,11] This lack of homogeneity of longitudinal forces along the intestinal wall can be caused by a mass acting as a lead point or may result from a disorganized pattern of peristalsis. Because of the imbalance between the contractions of the circular muscles perpendicular to the axis of the longitudinal forces, a kink develops in the abnormal portion of the intestine, thus creating a fulcrum for infolding of this area, resulting in its invagination into the adjacent distal bowel (Figure 68.1). The telescoped intestine then acts as the apex of the intussusception (known as the intussusceptum) and completely invaginates into the distal portion of the bowel that receives it (the intussuscipiens) (Figure 68.2). The process of invagination continues, the mesentery is pulled along with the intussusceptum and can travel all the way to the rectum, and as the intussusceptum progresses, the lymphatic return is first impeded and eventually venous drainage is impaired as a result of increased pressure in the wall of the intestine, leading to congestion and oedema of the intussusceptum.

Eventually, the arterial blood supply to this segment of bowel is obstructed. The mucous membrane, which is very sensitive to ischaemia, sloughs off first and is passed out as mucous stools initially; the ischaemic mucosa bleeds when it sloughs off in the end, and this

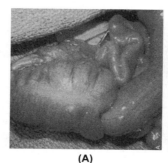 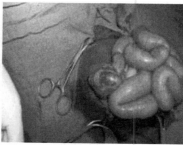

| (A) | (B) |

Figure 68.1: Two infants with manually reduced intussusception: (A) infolding or indentation of the terminal ileum where the intussusceptum started; (B) infolding of the caecum, resulting in a caeco-colic intussusception.

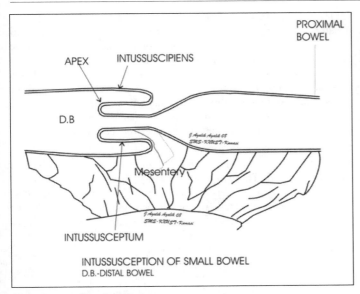

Source: Courtesy of Francis A. Abantanga.

Figure 68.2: Diagrammatic representation of an idiopathic intussusception. The apex is the lead point of the intussusception

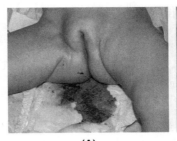 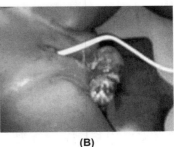

(A)　　　　　　　　　　　**(B)**

Figure 68.3: (A) Red current jelly stool 8 hours post presentation. (B) A prolapsed necrotic intussusception, which was found to be ileo-ileocolic intraoperatively. A right hemicolectomy was carried out, and the child survived.

blood mixes with the mucosa and mucus to give the classic "red currant jelly stools".

If the swelling, oedema, and ischaemia are not relieved, the lumen of the bowel will become completely occluded, and transmural necrosis of the intussusceptum will set in, leading to fluid sequestration, translocation of intestinal bacteria into the peritoneal cavity, perforation of the bowel, and possibly peritonitis.

Clinical Presentation

The usual presentation is of a healthy, well-fed infant aged between 6 and 9 months on average.

History

There may or may not be an antecedent infection (e.g., a viral infection). A good history eliciting the following findings will most often suggest the diagnosis.

1. There is a sudden onset of uncontrollable/inconsolable crying, which occurs intermittently every 10 to 30 minutes and lasts for a few seconds or so. This coincides with the sudden onset of colicky abdominal pains, when the intussusceptum together with the mesentery and nerves are drawn into the intussuscipiens. The screaming is high-pitched in nature and is unexpected.

2. The child stops screaming and plays normally in between attacks until the next occurrence of colicky abdominal pain sets in. This type of abdominal pain is pathognomonic of intussusception in infants because the pattern in which that the child cries for some time, stops and plays, and starts crying again, is rarely seen in other conditions.

3. During the periods when the child screams, he or she frequently draws up the lower limbs to the abdomen as if to reduce the pain. Between the colicky episodes, the child may appear listless and frequently pale.

4. Vomiting sets in. Vomiting tends to begin earlier in infants and is reflex in nature. Vomiting due to intestinal obstruction is a late sign, and the vomitus may be bilious.

5. Stools may at first be mucoid (the sloughed-off mucosa). Blood in stools may appear as early as within the first 6 hours, but it may also be absent until a day later. Blood mixed with mucus, giving the characteristic appearance of red currant jelly stools of intussusception, is present in only about 30% of cases (Figure 68.3(A)). There are occasions when the bloody mucoid stools are first noticed only after a digital rectal examination (DRE) of the child.

6. The triad of intermittent abdominal pain, vomiting, and bloody stools is encountered in about 30% of infants with intussusception.[10,11]

7. A history of diarrhoea or constipation may be given. However, the parents may give a history of diarrhoea only just before the onset of the bloody mucoid stools. This may lead to confusion in the diagnosis because medical conditions such as dysentery will usually be the first thing to come to mind. As a result, there is a delay in diagnosis, especially if the first-line medical caregiver has a low index of suspicion for intussusception.

8. There may be a history of a recent immunisation using rotavirus vaccine[5,10] or of a viral illness.[3]

9. In older children, the major symptom is abdominal pain, which is present in almost all cases. Bloody stools and vomiting are reported in about 25%. The triad of abdominal pain, bloody stools, and vomiting is a rare combination in this age group, and these are nonspecific symptoms.[14]

Physical Examination

Physical examination will reveal a healthy-looking child, especially if the patient is brought for consultation within the first few hours of the occurrence of the intussusception. In the presence of the typical triad of intermittent abdominal pains, vomiting, and bloody mucoid stools, there is the need to examine the child thoroughly in order to make the right diagnosis.

Infants and toddlers who present late (i.e., after 24 hours), which is the rule and not the exception in the African subregion) will be irritable, weak, and lethargic. To avoid delays in making a clinical diagnosis, the presence of pallor and lethargy in a child who has cried for several hours to days should alert the clinician to these subtle features of intussusception in addition to the presence of any one or two symptoms of the classical triad mentioned above.

The late-presenting child also will be dehydrated, or frankly in shock with cold clammy extremities (typical of late presentation and/or late diagnosis). The degree must be assessed rapidly and corrected appropriately. In addition, the child will be febrile or anaemic.

In those who present early, an abdominal mass may be palpable, if present. In late presenters, the abdomen is distended (sometimes grossly) and tender, and it is difficult to palpate any intraabdominal masses. If the abdomen is tender, with rebound tenderness and guarding, one should suspect the presence of peritonitis and therefore treat it appropriately (see the section "Treatment" later in this chapter).

If the abdomen is not distended (i.e., it is flat or scaphoid), the right iliac fossa feels empty—this is the Dance's sign.

On digital rectal examination, the rectum may be empty or one may palpate the intussusceptum or the lead point of the intussusception in the rectum, and on withdrawal of the examining finger, there may be passage of only mucus or bloody mucoid stools; the finger may or may not be stained with blood. In the late presentations, the chances of passage of blood per rectum are high due to possible necrosis of the bowel. There may be prolapse of the intussusceptum through the anal orifice in those who present very late (Figure 68.3(B)).

Investigations

In resource-poor settings, the physician may not have access to the investigations described here, in which case a high clinical acumen and index of suspicion is the next best alternative. Our management algorithm for the child with intussusception is illustrated in Figure 68.4.

Characteristically, diagnostic investigations include abdominal ultrasound (US) scans in axial and longitudinal views. This is accurate in detecting intussusception with a certainty of up to 100% and can also show additional pathologies such as the presence of a PLP.[6,15,16] It also allows the operator to be able to say whether the intussusception is in the small intestine or the large bowel.

In the axial/transverse view, the intussusception is seen as a target lesion or has a doughnut sign (Figure 68.5). In the longitudinal view, there is a pseudokidney or sandwich appearance. When the radiologist or ultrasonographer sees these two signs, the abdominal mass is likely an intussusception. In most cases, the radiologist is able to tell whether there is a PLP or not.

There are definite signs on US that will influence nonoperative management (i.e., hydrostatic or pneumatic reduction); the details of these are beyond the scope of this book but can be obtained from the literature.[17–23] Ultrasound may pick up a PLP (Figure 68.6).

Generally, trapped fluid[17,18] on US scan and the absence of blood flow at Doppler imaging,[6,17,24,25] where available, are indicators of ischaemia, and irreducibility of the intussusception and should be carefully considered in any further management of the lesion.

In the absence of ultrasound, other investigations can be used.

Contrast Enema Examination

The contrast most frequently used is barium solution, but an air enema can also be used. The two main classic signs of intussusception at enema examination are the meniscus sign produced by the rounded apex of the intussusceptum protruding into the column of contrast material and the coiled spring sign formed when the oedematous mucosal folds of the returning limb of the intussusceptum are outlined by contrast material in the lumen of the colon.[6]

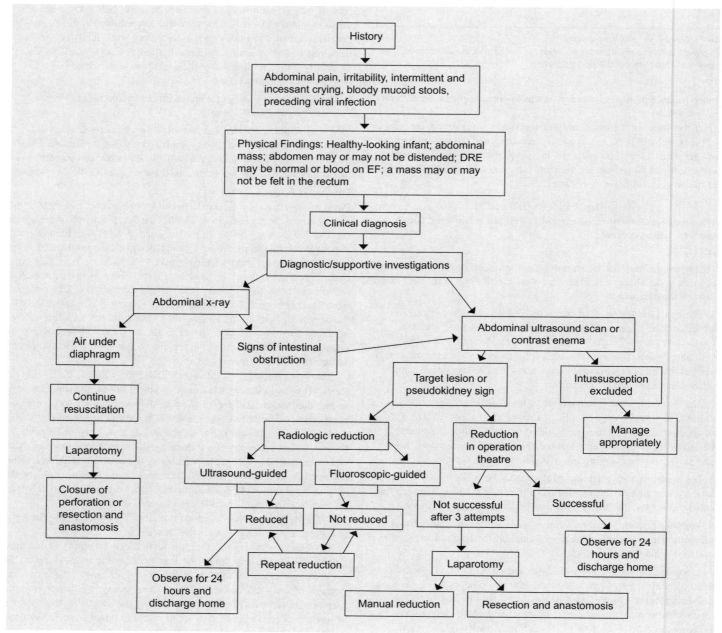

(DRE = digital rectal examination; EF = examining finger)

Figure 68.4: Algorithm for the management of a child with intussusception

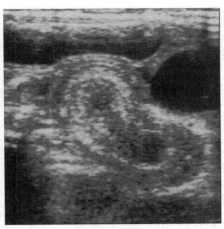

Figure 68.5: Ultrasound scan showing the doughnut appearance (target lesion) of an intussusception.

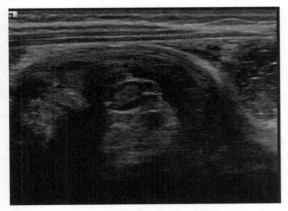

Figure 68.6: Intussusception with lead point.

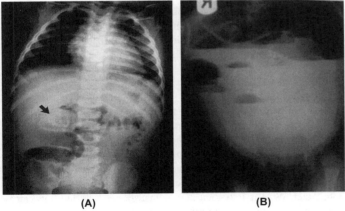

(A) (B)

Figure 68.7: (A) Intussusception on plain abdominal x-ray showing the target sign. (B) Plain erect abdominal radiograph of a 6-month-old child with intussusception, showing multiple air-fluid levels consistent with intestinal obstruction.

Plain Abdominal Radiographs

Plain abdominal radiographs can also be used to diagnose intussusception because there are a number of radiographic signs of intussusception, but they have a poor sensitivity of about 45%. These signs include a soft tissue mass seen at the right upper quadrant, reduced air in the small intestine or a gasless abdomen, and air in a displaced appendix.[6] The two more specific radiographic findings of intussusception are (1) the target sign, seen in Figure 68.7(a) at the right upper quadrant over the kidney, which consists of a soft tissue mass with concentric circular

areas of lucency due to mesenteric fat of the intussusceptum; and (2) the meniscus sign (a crescent of gas in the colonic lumen outlining the intussusceptum).

Plain radiographs most often display multiple air-fluid levels indicating intestinal obstruction (Figure 68.7(b)). These are usually late signs. Sometimes, a plain abdominal radiograph in the presence of intussusception may be unremarkable, however.[26]

If the caecum is found to be filled with gas or faeces in its normal position on a plain abdominal radiograph, then intussusception can often be excluded. Plain abdominal radiographs are done to exclude pneumoperitoneum, especially in children who present late with intussusception. Once one or two of the cardinal signs of intussusception are present, however, the radiograph can be used, if available, to help confirm the diagnosis.

Computed Tomography

Computed tomography (CT) scan and magnetic resonance imaging (MRI) very rarely are used for the diagnosis of intussusception, especially in poorly resourced countries. They are of use when the diagnosis of intussusception is in doubt, or the presentation is atypical of intussusception, or when the child has vague abdominal complaints of unknown cause. Also, in a few cases where the US scan is inconclusive or atypical, then either a CT scan or an MRI can be used to make the diagnosis. The presence of a bowel-within-bowel configuration with inclusion of mesenteric fat and/or mesenteric vessels is pathognomonic for intussusception on MRI or CT scan.

Other Investigations

Other supportive investigations include a full blood count (FBC), and blood urea, creatinine, and electrolytes to assess the extent of dehydration.

By using the various investigations (e.g., plain radiography, abdominal ultrasonography, barium enema, CT scan, and MRI), and finally after laparotomy, intussusception can be classified as:[1,25]

• *Enterocolic:* ileocolic (the most predominant type of intussusception seen in infants and toddlers); ileo-ileocolic; ileocaecal;

• *Enteroenteric:* jejunojejunal, jejunoileal, ileo-ileal; or

• *Colocolic:* caecocolic, colocolic.

• Special forms of intussusception include the following:

• *Retrograde intussusception:*[14,16] Invagination of the distal bowel (intussusceptum) into the proximal bowel (intussuscipiens).

• *Postoperative intussusception:* Complicates the postoperative period in about 0.5–16% of laparotomies.[11,12] A majority of cases occur after retroperitoneal dissection or extensive bowel manipulation.

• *Spontaneous reduction of intussusception:* More than half of intussusceptions are asymptomatic and are frequently diagnosed during ultrasonography, barium enema examinations, or CT scan for one reason or another.

• *Other:* Intussusceptions can occur around different catheters (e.g., various feeding tubes such as gastrojejunostomy tubes, nasojejunal tubes,[14] etc.).

Treatment

The treatment of intussusception in children is an emergency, by either nonoperative or operative methods. Delay in treatment will lead to ischaemia and necrosis of the intestine, bowel perforation, peritonitis, shock, and possibly death. Nonoperative reduction (NOR) is the first line of approach where facilities are available; if that fails, the next logical step is operative management.

Contraindications to the use of NOR in the treatment of a child with intussusception are obvious peritonitis,[16,26] pneumoperitoneum secondary to bowel perforation,[16] shock,[16] a grossly distended abdomen (relative contraindication), small-bowel intussusception such as ileo-ileal or ileo-ileocolic, and a long duration of symptoms before admission to hospital (>24 hours).

Before any mode of treatment is decided upon, the child must be vigorously resuscitated with fluids, including blood if the need arises. A nasogastric tube (NGT) is used to decompress the stomach, an intravenous (IV) line with a large-bore paediatric cannula appropriate for the age is set up, and a urethral catheter is passed into the bladder to monitor the effectiveness of the resuscitative measures by aiming at obtaining 0.5–2 ml of urine per kilogram body weight per hour. Broad-spectrum antibiotics must be started.

Give 20 ml/kg body weight of IV fluids (normal saline (NS) or Ringer's lactate (RL)) in a minimum of 30–45 minutes to a maximum of 1 hour. Repeat this until the child is well hydrated, then put on maintenance fluids using 4.3% or 10% dextrose in one-fifth NS (see Chapter 5, Fluid and Electrolyte Management). The maintenance fluid (NS or RL) is given as 4 ml/kg/hr for the first 10 kg, then 2 ml/kg/hr for the next 10 kg, up to 20 kg and 1 ml/kg/hr for anything more than 20 kg, all in 24 hours. Thus, a 25-kg child will receive: (4 × 10 × 24) + (2 × 10 × 24) + (1 × 5 × 24) = 960 + 480 + 120 = 1,560 ml of fluid in 24 hours as maintenance fluid.

As stated above, childhood intussusceptions can be managed nonoperatively or surgically. Nonoperative reduction of intussusception is now considered by most paediatric surgeons as the method of choice for its treatment and involves the use of various agents, gaseous or fluid. NOR can be carried out by using fluids such as barium,[6,17,27] normal saline,[6,24] and water-soluble contrast media.[6] This method is referred to as hydrostatic, as opposed to pneumatic or air enema reduction (AER), in which only air[4,18] is used. These agents may be used under either fluoroscopic or ultrasound guidance. Note, however, that barium can induce chemical peritonitis when it leaks through a bowel perforation into the peritoneal cavity. Water is not suitable because it will be absorbed should the procedure be prolonged and cause water intoxication.

The Procedure for NOR

Nonoperative reduction is usually performed in the radiology unit by (paediatric) radiologists with a paediatric surgeon in attendance. The procedure can also be performed by a paediatric surgeon trained in ultrasonography. The procedure involves allowing the fluid (barium solution, water-soluble contrast medium, or NS) to flow at a height of about 100 cm above the level of the buttocks into the rectum and further up the colon to meet the intussusceptum and, under sustained pressure, to reduce it. This is all done under fluoroscopy or US guidance, and the process of reduction is followed carefully. The reduction is considered successfully if there is reflux of fluid back into the terminal ileum through the ileocaecal valve (Figure 68.8(a)).

Air can also be used for reduction of the intussusception. Fluoroscopy-guided or US-guided pneumatic reduction of the intussusception is considered superior to hydrostatic reduction because it is safer, faster, and cleaner, and it requires less radiation. Also, pneumatic reduction has a higher success rate than hydrostatic reduction. It is advisable to use pressures not exceeding 120 mm Hg for the pneumatic reduction of intussusceptions in children. Pressures less than 80 mm Hg are noneffective.

After a successful enema reduction (hydrostatic or pneumatic), the child should be kept in hospital for a period of 24 hours for observation and then can be discharged home. Feeding can also be resumed immediately after the procedure.

The recurrence rate of NOR is less than 10%. Recurrence may be due to incomplete reduction (but under fluoroscopy- or US-guided reduction, that is less likely) or due to the presence of a PLP. A recurrent intussusception should be treated by first trying NOR again; if that fails or a PLP is observed, then surgery is advised.

It is recommended that if the first attempt at enema reduction of the intussusception fails, two or three more attempts can be made, and if these fail to reduce the intussusception, the child should undergo

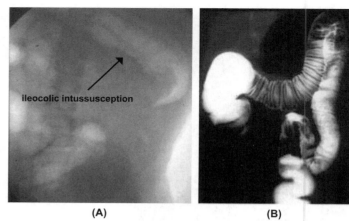

Figure 68.8: (A) Air reduction of an ileocolic intussusception. (B) Barium enema showing intussusceptum in the distal ascending colon.

surgical reduction. Surgery is also advised if there is leakage of fluid into the peritoneal cavity as a result of perforation of the bowel. Leakage of air can cause gross abdominal distention, splinting of the diaphragm resulting in acute respiratory distress, and a life-threatening abdominal compartment syndrome.[28] The pneumoperitoneum thus caused is readily recognizable, and immediate intervention in the form of abdominal paracentesis using a large-bore needle (gauge 14 or 16) in the radiology unit before transporting the patient to the operation theatre can be life saving.

We believe that the best results are obtained following NOR of intussusception.

Alternative Methodology

In the absence of a fluoroscope and/or US facilities in an institution, air enema reduction of intussusception can be done in the operating room with the child under anaesthesia.[29] This method has been developed locally, and we attest to its safety and suitability for poorly resourced regional or district hospitals in West Africa, where children with intussusception are brought very late to hospital.[30]

The AER method involves submerging the free end of the NGT in a kidney dish filled with water and inserting a 20 or 22 Fr Foley catheter into the rectum (fully blowing up the balloon). An aneroid sphygmomanometer is attached to the Foley catheter (Figure 68.9(A–D)), and air is then insufflated into the rectum between pressures of 80 to 140 mm Hg. Before insufflating air into the rectum, the surgeon first palpates the abdomen under anaesthesia, since the child is now completely relaxed, and determines the position of the mass in the peritoneal cavity. As the air is insufflated, the surgeon continuously palpates and follows the progress of the mass from wherever it was proximally. When the intussusception is completely reduced, air flows proximally into the small intestines and into the stomach. The air passes through the NGT and is noticed as a continuous flow of bubbles in the kidney bowl filled with water. What is important here is that the air flow into the kidney dish must be continuous, which confirms that the intussusceptum has reduced. The balloon of the Foley catheter is deflated and the catheter removed; some of the air will escape through the anal orifice, resulting in the abdomen becoming soft again and less tense.

Then, the abdomen is again examined to feel for the mass. Normally, one cannot palpate the intussusception after a successful reduction (except for the palpation of the reduced oedematous bowel, which requires some experience for one to accept that it is oedematous bowel and not the intussusception that one is feeling beneath the fingers).

The patient is sent to the recovery ward to recover from anaesthesia and can be fed 3 hours after the procedure. The patient is observed for 24 hours, within which period a repeat ultrasound scan is done to confirm the successful reduction of the intussusception or, in the absence of an ultrasound machine, about 10 to 20 ml of barium solution is given orally (through the NGT, if still in place). This is usually observed in the stools within 24 hours, when the patient can then be discharged home.

If reduction fails after two to three attempts (i.e., the mass is still palpable and its reduction is not progressing), or if there is a suspicion of a perforation of the bowel (air escapes freely and easily into the peritoneal cavity, the abdomen becomes grossly distended, and after removing the Foley catheter no air escapes from the anal orifice), the NOR procedure is immediately suspended and a laparotomy is performed. As a precaution, the instruments for a laparotomy are always set on a tray, and the theatre nurse is scrubbed and gowned, ready and waiting. By using this method in our institution, we have had 59.1% successful reduction rates.[30]

Surgical management is reserved for children with failed hydrostatic or pneumatic reduction of the intussusception; those who develop leakage of fluid into the peritoneal cavity during enema reduction; those in whom free air, peritonitis, or shock was present on admission; or those in whom PLP (e.g., a polyp, enterogenic cyst, etc.) was detected during investigations or after NOR.

Surgical Management

Access into the peritoneal cavity is usually through an above or below transverse umbilical incision. The intussusception (Figure 68.10) is delivered into the wound, and an attempt is made to reduce it manually by a combination of milking and squeezing of the intussusceptum by the surgeon and gentle tugging on the free limb of the intussusceptum by the assistant. If the manual reduction is successful, the operation ends there. Some surgeons will fix the caecum if it is found to be very mobile, and others will perform an appendectomy, depending on which incision was used, to prevent any future confusion should the patient present again later with suspected appendicitis.

If an attempt at manual reduction fails as a result of tears or a perforation in the bowel, or if the intussusception is deemed to be gangrenous from inspection at the beginning of the surgery, or if a PLP is found, then segmental resection is performed with re-establishment of bowel continuity by an end-to-end anastomosis.

Another operative method for reduction of intussusception is by laparoscopic surgery,[31] during which the intussusceptum is pulled out of the intussuscipiens. All the manoeuvres carried out by the open method can be done laparoscopically, including resection and anastomosis.

Postoperative Complications

Postoperative complications include recurrence of the intussusception, perforation of the bowel during NOR of the intussusception, surgical site infection, anastomotic leak, anastomotic breakdown, enterocutaneous fistula (especially if the patient is poorly nourished), postoperative adhesive intestinal obstruction, and incisional hernias.

Prognosis and Outcome

Prognosis is usually excellent if diagnosis is early, resuscitation is carried out thoroughly, and treatment is started early, especially with successful nonoperative reduction of the intussusception. Worldwide, the overall mortality of intussusception is about 1%, and near zero with NOR of the intussusception.

On the African continent, however, mortality is very high, ranging from 12.1% to 35.1%.[2,3,7,9] Recurrence rates following NOR range from 5% to 20%[15,16] with a mean of about 10%.[16] After surgical reduction, recurrence rates range from 1% to 4%.[32]

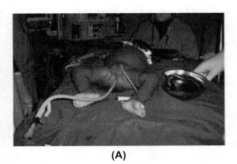

(A)

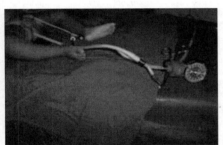

(B)

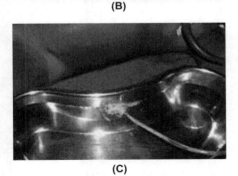

(C)

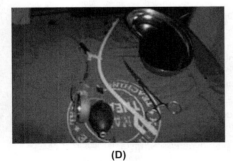

(D)

Source: Courtesy of Francis A. Abantanga.

Figure 68.9: Theatre setup for pneumatic or air enema reduction of an intussusception in a 7-month-old child. (A) The child is anaesthetized and ready for AER; (B) close-up view of the setup; (C) the continuous bubbling of air into the kidney dish with water, indicating that the intussusception has been reduced; (D) the complete set of requirements.

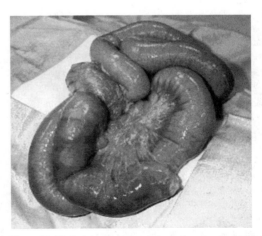

Figure 68.10: An intraoperative picture of an ileo-ileal intussusception in a child. Note the oedematous and inflamed intussuscepiens and the enlarged mesenteric lymph nodes.

Prevention

In the main, the majority of intussusceptions in children, especially infants and toddlers, are idiopathic and difficult to prevent. Hence, prevention is aimed at educating parents or caregivers about the disease and its potential hazard so that children will be brought early to hospital. Primary medical caregivers also need to be educated to increase their index of suspicion for earlier diagnosis and intervention.

Table 68.1: Evidence-based research.

Title	Sonographic features indicative of hydrostatic reducibility of intestinal intussusception in infancy and early childhood
Authors	Mirilas P, Koumanidou C, Vakaki M, Skandalakis P, Antypas S, Kakavakis K
Institution	Agia Sophia Children's Hospital, Goudi, Athens, Greece
Reference	Eur Radiol 2001; 11: 2576–2580
Problem	To find out which sonographic patterns of intussusception are indicative of reducibility by hydrostatic reduction in children.
Intervention	All children with intussusception underwent sonographic examination of the abdomen using transverse and longitudinal scans. The sonograms were evaluated for (a) a target lesion with multiple concentric rings surrounding an echogenic centre, (b) a doughnut-like mass in the transverse plane in which the thickness of the hypoechoic external ring was measured, (c) appearance of trapped fluid in the doughnut-like or target-like mass, and (d) coexistence of free fluid in the peritoneal cavity.
Comparison/ control (quality of evidence)	The hydrostatic reduction rate was 100% when the head of intussusception appeared as a target lesion; with a thickness of the hypoechoic external ring of the doughnut ≤ 7.2 mm, the reduction rate was 100%; if the thickness was between 7.5 and 11.2 mm, the reduction rate was only 68.9%; if the thickness of the hypoechoic external ring of the doughnut-like mass was more than 14.0 mm, surgical reduction was required.
Outcome/ effect	Wall thickness was found not to be a significant prognostic factor in the reducibility of intussusception, trapped fluid was found to be consistently a poor prognostic feature of reducibility of an intussusception, and free fluid in the peritoneal cavity did not have any adverse effect on air-reduction prognosis.
Historical significance/ comments	This paper is significant in the sense that if one can get a report of the ultrasonographic patterns of the intussusception, it is possible to decide beforehand which intussusceptions will easily reduce without much effort and which ones will need more effort to reduce them or even which ones should not undergo hydrostatic or pneumatic reduction for fear of causing a perforation or reducing a gangrenous bowel.

Evidence-Based Research

Table 68.1 presents a study to find out which sonographic patterns of intussusception are indicative of reducibility by hydrostatic reduction in children. Table 68.2 presents a 10-year-study to determine whether nonoperative management of intussusception is effective and safe in children age 3 years or older.

Table 68.2: Evidence-based research.

Title	Is non-operative intussusception reduction effective in older children? Ten-year experience in a university affiliated medical center
Authors	Simanovsky N, Hiller N, Koplewitz BZ, Eliahou R, Udassin R
Institution	Hadassah Medical Center, Jerusalem, Israel
Reference	Pediatr Surg Int 2007; 23:261–264
Problem	Nonoperative management of intussusception in children aged 3 years or more in order to determine its efficacy and safety in this age group.
Intervention	Clinical features of intussusception were collected from this group of children, recording the age, predisposing factors, symptoms, and signs, with a review of the sonographic and fluoroscopic images to assess the degree of intussusception and possible underlying PLP.
Comparison/ control (quality of evidence)	An abdominal ultrasound scan was done in all 24 children with 26 intussusceptions revealing a pseudokidney sign of intussusception in all and mesenteric lymphadenopathy in 10. Image-guided reduction was attempted in all except one with a small bowel obstruction; in two, barium enema reduction was attempted; and in 23, air enema reduction was performed.
Outcome/ effect	In four children, a PLP was the cause of the intussusception: one Meckel's diverticulum and three Burkitt's lymphoma. Air enema reduction in two of the last three and barium enema reduction in the last one failed to reduce the intussusceptions. Four children failed nonoperative management of their intussusceptions: three by pneumatic reduction and one by barium enema reduction, but when surgery was performed, no PLP was found in any of them. Finally, 18 patients with intussusception confirmed by ultrasound scan, who did not have PLP, were successfully reduced by using air enema.
Historical significance/ comments	This paper confirms the notion that all intussusceptions in children, regardless of age, should be managed by using nonoperative methods (pneumatic or hydrostatic) first. It is only when this fails that surgery should be considered.

Key Summary Points

1. Intussusception is an occlusive-strangulation type of intestinal obstruction that requires early diagnosis and treatment.

2. more than 90% of intussusception cases occur in the age range from 3 months to 3 years, and they are usually idiopathic in nature.

3. Intussusception with a pathological lead point occurs more in the older age group, but can be seen in infants and toddlers.

4. Intussusception is rare but possible in neonates, so clinicians should have a high index of suspicion if there is a prolapsed rectal mass in such children.

5. Diagnosis is clinical and confirmed by ultrasound scan of the abdomen looking for a target lesion/doughnut sign in the axial view and the pseudokidney/sandwich appearance in the longitudinal view.

6. An erect plain abdominal radiograph may be requested for exclusion of pneumoperitoneum, but it is not a routine investigation for diagnosing intussusception. The radiograph will, however, inform one about the presence of intestinal obstruction.

7. Once the diagnosis is confirmed, it is necessary to resuscitate the child for an attempt at hydrostatic or pneumatic reduction under either fluoroscopy or ultrasound guidance first. A maximum of three attempts should be made to reduce the intussusception.

8. All nonoperatively reduced intussusceptions should be observed for a minimum of 24 hours in hospital before being discharged.

9. All patients who are haemodynamically unstable, are in shock, have peritonitis, have bowel perforation either on admission or during nonoperative reduction of the intussusception, are suspected of having a gangrenous bowel (see Figure 68.3) and those who have failed pneumatic reduction should undergo open surgery and an attempt at manual reduction or segmental resection and end-to-end anastomosis.

References

1. Abantanga FA, nii-Amon-Kotei D, Ayesu-Offei H. Intussusception in Kumasi, Ghana: analysis of 84 cases. JUST 1996; 16:95–98.

2. Abdul-Rahman LO, Yusuf AS, Adeniran JO, Taiwo JO. Childhood intussusception in Ilorin: a revisit. Afr J Paediatr Surg 2005; 2:4–7.

3. Bode CO. Presentation and management outcome of childhood intussusception in Lagos: a prospective study. Afr J Paediatr Surg 2008; 5:24–28.

4. Blanch AJM, Perel SB, Acworth JP. Paediatric intussusception: epidemiology and outcome. Emergency Med Australasia 2007; 19:45–50.

5. Kombo LA, Gerbers MA, Pickering LK, et al. Intussusception, infection, and immunization: summary of a workshop on rotavirus. Pediatr 2001; 108:e37.

6. del-Pozo G, Albillos JC, Tejedor D, et al. Intussusception in children: current concepts in diagnosis and enema reduction. Radiographics 1999; 19:299–319.

7. Keita M, Barry OT, Doumbouya N, et al. Acute intussusception in childhood. Aspects of epidemiologic, clinical features and management at Children's Hospital, Donka, Guinea, Conakry. Afr J Paediatr Surg 2006; 3:1–3.

8. Ravitch MM. Intussusception. In: Ravitch MM, Welch KJ, Benson CD, Aberdeen E, Randolph JG, eds. Pediatric Surgery. Year Book Medical Publishers, Inc., 1984, vol. 2, Pp 989–1003.

9. Carneiro PMR, Kisusi DM. Intussusception in children seen at Muhimbili National Hospital, Dar-es-Salam. EAMJ 2004; 81:439–442.

10. Bines JE, Ivanoff B. Acute intussusception in infants and children. Incidence, clinical presentation and management: a global perspective. A report prepared for the steering committee on diarrhoeal diseases, vaccines and vaccine development. In: Vaccines and Biologicals. World Health Organization, 2002.

11. Doody DP, Foglia RP. Intussusception. In: Oldham KT, Colombani PM, Foglia RP, Skinner MA, eds. Principles and practice of pediatric surgery. Lippincott Williams & Wilkins, 2005; Vol. 2, Pp 1297–1305.

12. Ein SH, Daneman A. Intussusception. In: Ziegler MM, Azizkhan RG, Weber TR, eds. Operative Pediatric Surgery. McGraw Hill Professional, 2003, Pp 647–655.

13. Blakelock RT, Beasley SW. The clinical implications of non-idiopathic intussusception. Pediatr Surg Int 1998; 14:163–167.

14. Navarro O, Daneman A. Intussusception. Part 3: Diagnosis and management of those with an identifiable or predisposing cause and those that reduce spontaneously. Pediatr Radiol 2004; 34:305–312.

15. Chahine AA. Intussusception. Available at: http://emedicine.medscape.com/article/930708 (accessed 25 December 2008).

16. Ko HS, Schenk JP, Troger J, Rohrscheider WK. Current radiological management of intussusception in children. Eur Radiol 2007; 17:2411–2421.

17. Mirilas P, Koumanidou C, Vakaki M, et al. Sonographic features indicative of hydrostatic reducibility of intestinal intussusception in infancy and early childhood. Eur Radiol 2001; 11:2576–2580.

18. Britton I, Wilkinson AG. Ultrasound features of intussusception predicting outcome of air enema. Pediatr Radiol 1999; 29:705–710.

19. del Pozo G, Gonzalez-Spinola J, Gomez-Anson B, et al. Intussusception: trapped peritoneal fluid detected with US—relationship to reducibility and ischemia. Radiology 1996; 201:379–383.

20. Reijnen JAM, Festen C, van Roosmalen RP. Intussusception factors related to treatment. Arch Dis Child 1990; 65:871–873.

21. Lee HC, Yeh HJ, Leu YJ. Intussusception: the sonographic diagnosis and its clinical value. J Pediatr Gastroenterol Nutr 1989; 8:343–347.

22. McDermott VC, Taylor T, Mackenzie S, et al. Pneumatic reduction of intussusception: clinical experience and factors affecting outcome. Clin Radiol 1994; 49:30–34.

23. Stephenson CA, Seibert JJ, Strain JD, et al. Intussusception: clinical and radiographic factors influencing reducibility. Pediatr Radiol 1989; 20:57–60.

24. Krishnakumar, Hameed S, Umamaheshwari. Ultrasound guided hydrostatic reduction in the management of intussusception. Indian J Pediatr 2006; 73:217–220.

25. Saxena AK, Seebacher U, Bernhardt C, Höllwarth ME. Small bowel intussusception: issues and controversies related to pneumatic reduction and surgical approach. Acta Paediatrica 2007; 96:1651–1654.

26. Simanovsky N, Hiller N, Koplewitz BZ, Eliahou R, Udassin R. Is non-operative intussusception reduction effective in older children? Ten-year experience in a university affiliated medical center. Pediatr Surg Int 2007; 23:261–264.

27. Atalabi OM, Ogundoyin OO, Ogunlana DI, et al. Hydrostatic reduction of intussusception under ultrasound guidance: an initial experience in a developing country. Afr J Paediatr Surg 2007; 4:68–71.

28. Ng E, Kim HB, Lillehet CW, Seefelder C. Life threatening tension pneumoperitoneum from intestinal perforation during air reduction of intussusception. Pediatr Anaesthesia 2002; 12:798–800.

29. Cheung ST, Lee KH, Yeung TH, et al. Minimally invasive approach in the management of childhood intussusception. ANZ J Surg 2007; 77:778–781.

30. Abantanga FA, Amoah M, Adeyinka AO, Nimako B, Yankey KP. Pneumatic reduction of intussusception in children at the Komfo Anokye Teaching Hospital, Kumasi, Ghana; East Afr Med J 2008; 85:550–555.

31. Wiersma R, Hadley GP. Minimizing surgery in complicated intussusception in the Third World. Pediatr Surg Int 2004; 20:215–217.

32. Irish MS. Intussusception: surgical perspective. Available at: http://emedicine.medscape.com/article/937730 (accessed 25 December 2008).

CHAPTER 69
MISCELLANEOUS CAUSES OF INTESTINAL OBSTRUCTION

Lohfa B. Chirdan

Sanjay Krishnaswami

Introduction

Various causes of mechanical bowel obstruction, such as intestinal atresias, intussusception, meconium ileus, external herniations, and midgut volvulus, have been covered elsewhere in this book. This chapter is concerned with the various other causes of obstruction that could be encountered in children in Africa. These conditions include peritoneal adhesions, parasites, foreign bodies, sigmoid volvulus and ileosigmoid knotting, internal herniations, external compression from abdominal masses, faecal impaction, and paralytic ileus. A summary of the important features and investigations of these conditions is outlined in Table 69.1.

Peritoneal Adhesions

Adhesions are internal fibrous, band-like scars occurring after injury to the peritoneum and are the result of biochemical and cellular responses attempting to repair the peritoneum. Although this process is beneficial, it could also have detrimental effects, one of which is small bowel obstruction (SBO). The most common cause of adhesions is iatrogenic, secondary to previous abdominal operations. The data on postoperative adhesions in children are sparse, and most of what we know about adhesions is extrapolated from adult series. An estimated 93% of adults undergoing laparotomy eventually develop adhesions, although only a fraction of these will become symptomatic.[1] Grant et al. reported that 1.1% of children younger than 16 years of age undergoing lower abdominal surgery would be admitted as a direct consequence of adhesions and 8.3% would have a readmission that may be related to adhesions four or more years from the time of initial surgery.[2]

In developed countries, strategies to reduce postoperative adhesions, such as the use of talc-free gloves, improved suture and prosthetic materials, and especially minimal access surgery, are commonly utilized. Many of these resources are not available in developing countries, however.[3] Therefore, it appears that the burden of morbidity due to adhesions may gradually shift to developing countries where open laparotomies are still the norm in children.[4–6]

Apart from postoperative adhesions, inflammatory diseases and trauma can cause peritoneal adhesions, leading to bowel obstruction in children. SBO from inflammatory adhesions may sometimes be seen soon after operation for such suppurative conditions of the abdomen as ruptured appendix and typhoid intestinal perforations or in patients with solid organ injury due to trauma who were managed either operatively or nonoperatively.[4–7] Note that other causes of postoperative bowel obstruction, such as intussusception (classically seen after large retroperitoneal operations), can exist, and the treatment of these may differ from adhesion-related SBO.

Clinical Features

The clinical features of bowel obstruction from peritoneal adhesions could include vomiting, abdominal distention, abdominal pain, constipation, and fever. While the other signs may be seen even early in the disease course, fever usually occurs in children with bowel gangrene or perforated bowel and should therefore be taken seriously if pres-

Table 69.1: Summary of features of intestinal obstruction from various causes.

Aetiology	Important features	Important investigations	Treatment
Peritoneal adhesions	Abdominal scars or history of surgeries, trauma, or acute abdomen in the past	Multiple air-fluid levels on plain x-ray of abdomen; contrast study of GI tract in doubtful cases	Nasogastric decompression, intravenous fluids and antibiotics for 24–48 hours; exploratory laparotomy if child is not improving
Bezoars/foreign bodies	History of ingestion of foreign bodies or psychological condition; vomiting, failure to thrive; abdominal mass that may be palpable	Plain abdominal films and contrast studies; computed tomography (CT) scan if available	Endoscopic removal; use of pancreatic enzymes; laparotomy
Faecal impaction	History of constipation or motility disorder	Plain x-ray of abdomen	Repeated rectal washout; manual evacuation
Parasites	Endemic area, passage of worms per rectum or vomiting of worms	Stool examination, plain x-ray of abdomen	Antihelminthic; laparotomy
Sigmoid volvulus and ileosigmoid knotting	Rapid onset of abdominal distention	Plain x-ray of abdomen; contrast enema, lower endoscopy in doubtful cases	Laparotomy and sigmoidectomy
Pseudo-obstruction (Ogilvie's syndrome)	History of chronic constipation; sickle cell disease	Plain x-ray	Neostigmine
Internal herniation	Recurrent abdominal pains	Plain x-ray; contrast study or CT scan in some cases	Laparotomy
External compression	Abdominal mass	Plain x-ray; CT scan	Laparotomy and removal of mass
Paralytic ileus	Usually postoperative, sepsis or severe hypokalaemia/ hypomagnesaemia	Urea and electrolyte estimation; plain x-ray of abdomen, presence of rectal gas	Nasogastric decompression; intravenous fluids; electrolyte replenishment

ent. Other signs of advanced disease, such as rectal bleeding, may be encountered frequently. This was a presenting feature in 10% of children with adhesive bowel obstruction in one series from Nigeria.[4]

Investigations

The diagnosis of bowel obstruction is usually clinical. In a few patients who have bowel perforation, plain chest x-ray may show gas under the diaphragm. Plain abdominal films may show dilated loops of bowel and multiple air-fluid levels. Prominent valvulae conniventes suggest small bowel obstruction, and marked haustrations may occur in large bowel obstruction. However, although these bowel markings readily appear in adults and older children, they may be absent in infants and younger children. In fact, it may be impossible to distinguish between small and large intestines on plain films in infants.

In patients with previous adhesive SBO who have signs of incomplete obstruction or others in whom the diagnosis is in doubt, a contrast examination of the gastrointestinal tract is useful, although barium contrast may occasionally cause impaction above the obstruction. Failure of the contrast to pass into the distal small bowel suggests intestinal obstruction. The average transit time for oral contrast to reach the colon is 3–4 hours, but this time could be significantly longer when there is obstruction. If the patient's clinical status allows, contrast progression can be followed by plain x-rays up to 12–24 hours later. Contrast enema (typically with water-soluble contrast) may be useful in children with distal obstruction. A complete blood count, grouping and cross matching, and serum chemistry are done in all patients.

Management

Management involves resuscitation and correction of fluid and electrolyte deficits by administration of intravenous (IV) fluids. Nasogastric decompression is then instituted, and broad spectrum antibiotics may be started. If the condition does not improve on the above management after 48 hours, laparotomy should be considered.[8-11] Early operative intervention is preferred for children, especially infants, because the already nutritionally compromised child has less tolerance compared to adults for the 48-hour starvation period. In children who present with features of bowel strangulation and gangrene, laparotomy should be undertaken immediately after adequate resuscitation (Figure 69.1).

At operation, adhesions can be single, multiple, or dense. Single adhesions are divided (Figure 69.2). In patients with multiple adhesions, it is important to identify all offending bands. Some surgeons believe that it is important to free the entire peritoneal cavity of all adhesions, whereas others believe that only the adhesions that obstruct the intestine should be divided because the other adhesions have fixed the remaining bowel in an unobstructed position. In most instances, it is wiser to remove only the offending bands because trauma may trigger another episode of adhesions. Adhesions are divided sharply, aided by countertraction from the assistant. Bowel gangrene is a common finding, especially in Africa.[4] In this situation, bowel resection with end-to-end bowel anastomosis is done (Figure 69.3).

Repeated adhesions can be a major problem, and therefore many mechanical and chemical approaches have been developed. Internal stenting using long tubes such as the Baker or Leonard tubes can be of help, and intestinal plication may help to fix the bowel in the unobstructed position.[7] Chemical methods have evolved over the years to deal with or reduce the incidence of peritoneal adhesions. These chemical agents include heparin, fibrinolytic compounds, nonsteroidal anti-inflammatory drugs (NSAIDs), low molecular weight dextran solutions, antihistamines, prokinetic agents, calcium channel blockers, and steroids.[3-7] As evidenced by the multiplicity of these methods, none of these techniques has been shown to completely eliminate the problem of adhesions. Meticulous handling of tissues and careful surgery with the use of talc-free gloves as well as minimally invasive abdominal surgery, where possible, may cause less tissue injury and lead to fewer adhesions.

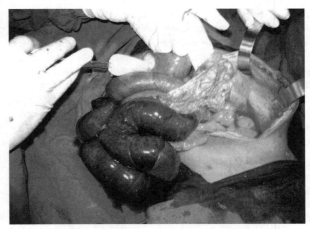

Figure 69.1: Bowel gangrene from postoperative adhesion SBO.

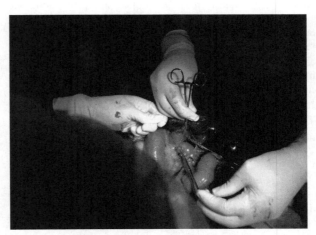

Figure 69.2: Dividing the adhesions.

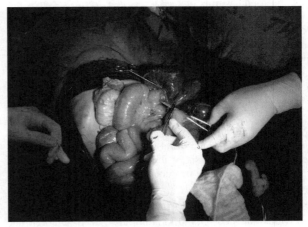

Figure 69.3: Resection of gangrenous bowel.

Foreign Bodies and Bezoars

Foreign bodies (FBs) of the aerodigestive tract can be involved in causing intestinal obstruction in children of all ages. There is a tendency for children to put everything in their mouths, so ingestion of an FB is a major problem, especially in Africa, where poverty and hunger may be contributory. Below the level of the oesophagus and stomach, ingested FBs may be impacted in the C-loop of the duodenum, at the ligament of Treitz, Meckel's diverticulum, or the ileocaecal valve, causing intestinal obstruction. Perforation with peritonitis may cause secondary obstruction.

Bezoars are masses of solidified ingested materials (organic or inorganic) found in the stomach or small intestines that can cause intestinal obstruction in children.[7,12] They are of many types. Trichobezoars are seen in the mentally retarded as well as in emotionally disturbed children, typically teenage girls, and usually consist of swallowed hair or random ingested objects. Phytobezoars are made of vegetable material and usually obstruct the distal ileum, or stomach, especially postvagotomy. Lactobezoars are usually observed in premature infants receiving early feeding of undiluted milk. They can be caused by powdered formulas mixed inappropriately.

Presentation and diagnosis

Children usually present with vomiting and failure to thrive. An epigastric mass, often in the shape of the stomach, may be palpable on physical examination. Plain films of the abdomen are often diagnostic, but upper gastrointestinal contrast study may be needed in some cases.

Management

Bezoars in the stomach may be broken apart by using an endoscope. This may be facilitated by introducing pancreatic enzymes. Laparotomy with gastrostomy or enterostomy may be needed to remove hairs that cause complete obstruction. Care must be taken to remove the entire bezoar because it can fragment on removal and be lodged more distally, causing further problems. In cases of colonic obstruction, colostomy may be needed. The underlying disorder resulting in bezoar formation, such as a psychological problem, must be managed appropriately.

Parasites

Parasites can cause intestinal obstruction, generally in the mid or distal small bowel, but can even occur in the large bowel. In the tropics, *Ascaris lumbricoides* is the most common parasite involved. These worms usually get entangled in the small intestine, producing a mass that could lead to intestinal obstruction. Although the majority of children present with a subacute course, about a quarter present with features of acute intestinal obstruction, including vomiting, abdominal distention, and constipation.[13–15] Some children may present with vomiting of the round worms or passage of the worms through the rectum. Investigations include plain abdominal x-ray in additional to stool examination for evidence of parasites. The plain roentgenogram of the abdomen may show a typical "whirlpool" pattern that indicates intraluminal worms in most cases. Children with subacute intestinal obstruction usually respond to the administration of an oral antihelmintic such as piperazine and management of pain using antispasmodics such as Buscopan®.[15] Patients with acute intestinal obstruction should be quickly resuscitated by using intravenous fluids and then undergo emergency laparotomy. At laparotomy, the worms should be disimpacted and milked into the distal colon. In cases of bowel gangrene, resection and anastomosis of the bowel is done. However, in the latter situation, note that worms could migrate into the peritoneal cavity through the anastomosis site.

Sigmoid Volvulus and Ileosigmoid Knotting

Sigmoid volvulus and ileosigmoid knotting are rare in children but can cause intestinal obstruction with lethal consequences.[16] The main predisposing factor to sigmoid volvulus is a large redundant sigmoid colon with a narrow base, which then acts as a fulcrum for the sigmoid colon to twist, usually in a counterclockwise direction. Ileosigmoid knotting involves the twisting of the small bowel and sigmoid mesenteries around each other. The mechanism for ileosigmoid knotting is unclear. An excessively mobile small bowel due to an elongated mesentery, combined with a long sigmoid colon on a narrow mesenteric pedicle, along with the ingestion of a bulky diet in the presence an empty small bowel have been suggested as a possible mechanism.[17,18]

The main presenting feature of either sigmoid volvulus or ileosigmoid knotting is acute onset of abdominal distention and pain followed by obstipation. In ileosigmoid knotting, however, the abdominal distention may not be remarkable. Vomiting may be also be present. Investigations include plain abdominal x-ray, which may show a bent inner-tube sign. The classic features of sigmoid volvulus on plain abdominal films are not as obvious in ileosigmoid knotting. Contrast enema studies occasionally can be helpful in doubtful cases. However, such investigations, as well as small bowel follow-through studies, should be used judiciously because they could precipitate intestinal perforation, especially in ileosigmoid knotting.[16] After the diagnosis is made, laparotomy should not be delayed once fluid and electrolytes status has been corrected and broad spectrum antibiotics administered.[16,17] Bowel gangrene is common, and resection with anastomosis of the bowel should be done in these cases.

Internal Herniation

Bowel herniation into abnormal or normal peritoneal recesses could lead to acute intestinal obstruction in children.[19] Herniation could occur into normal, anatomic duodenal, or caecal recesses, leading to intestinal obstruction. Postoperative defects in the mesentry can also lead to herniation of the bowel and subsequent obstruction and strangulation.[19] Other abnormal sites for herniation of the bowel leading to obstruction include the falciform ligament, if a defect is present, and the foramen of Winslow.[20,21] A high index of suspicion is needed for prompt diagnosis and subsequent treatment because delay usually leads to bowel gangrene, which increases the mortality rate.

Other Causes

External abdominal masses such as intraabdominal tumours, faecal impaction, paralytic ileus, and benign bowel tumours can result in intestinal obstruction in children.

Evidence-Based Research

Articles on adhesive bowel obstruction in children in Africa are scanty. Prospective studies are few, and available guides have to be based on retrospective studies, many of which are from the West. Table 69.2 presents a large series involving postoperative bowel obstruction in newborns and infants.

Table 69.2: Evidence-based research.

Title	High incidence of post-operative adhesions in newborns and infants
Authors	Young JY, Kim DS, Muratore CS, Kurkchubasche A, Tracy TF Jr, Luks FI
Institution	Division of Pediatric Surgery, Brown Medical School, Providence, Rhode Island, USA
Reference	J Pediatr Surg 2007; 42:962–965
Problem	The incidence of, risk factors for, and need for operative intervention in postoperative bowel obstruction in children.
Comparison/ control (quality of evidence)	The authors reviewed children who had laparotomy or laparoscopy to determine the incidence of small bowel obstruction due to adhesions. They also compared the incidence in older children to that in infants and neonates.
Outcome/ effect	Of 2,187 abdominal operations performed in children, 61 (2.8%) had postoperative bowel obstruction, 70.5% of these requiring reoperation. Postoperative bowel obstruction was more common in children younger than 1 year of age compared to older children (P = 0.01). Infants are significantly more likely to require operative intervention compared with older children (P = 0.01).
Historical significance/ Comments	This large series supports previous evidence that nonoperative management of adhesive small bowel obstruction often fails in infants and younger children. A laparotomy is often needed when postoperative obstruction occurs in this age group, and it should be performed with minimum delay.

Key Summary Points

1. Apart from the classical causes of mechanical bowel obstruction, other pathologic entities may lead to bowel obstruction in children.

2. As techniques to decrease postoperative adhesions, such as minimally invasive surgery, become more widespread in the developed world, the burden of adhesions may begin to shift to Africa.

3. Children with adhesive intestinal obstruction should be meticulously followed; delay in operative intervention should be avoided.

4. A high index of suspicion is needed for the diagnosis of foreign bodies and bezoars in children, and psychiatric evaluation should be part of the postoperative work-up.

5. The mainstay of management of patients with parasitic obstruction is medical (antihelminthic); however, patients with acute symptoms should be explored immediately after adequate resuscitation.

6. Sigmoid volvulus and ileosigmoid knotting, although rare in children, can be fulminant, making early resuscitation and laparotomy the keys to a successful outcome.

References

1. Menzies D, Ellis H. Intestinal obstruction from adhesions: how big is the problem? Ann R Coll Surg Engl 1990; 72:60–63.

2. Grant HW, Parker MC, Wilson MS, Menzies D, Sunderland G, Thompson JN, Clark DN, Knight AD, Crowe AM, Ellis H. Adhesions after abdominal surgery in children. J Pediatr Surg 2008; 43:152–157.

3. Attard JP, MacLean AR. Adhesive small bowel obstruction: epidemiology, biology and prevention. Can J Surg 2007; 50:291–300.

4. Ameh EA, Nmadu PT. Adhesion obstruction in children in Northern Nigeria. Trop Doct 2004; 34:104–106.

5. Olumide F, Adedeji A, Adesola AO. Intestinal obstruction in Nigerian children. J Pediatr Surg 1981; 16:225–229.

6. Adejuigbe O, Fashakin EO. Acute intestinal obstruction in Nigerian children. Trop Gastroenterol 1989; 10:33–39.

7. Schwartz MZ. Disorders of the peritoneum and peritoneal cavity. In: O'Neil JA, Rowe MI, Grosfeld JA, Fonkalsrud EW, Coran AJ, eds. Pediatric Surgery. Mosby St Louis, 1998, Pp 451–455.

8. Young JY, Kim DS, Muratore CS, Kurkchubasche AG, Tracy TF Jr, Luks FI. High incidence of post-operative bowel obstruction in newborns and infants. J Pediatr Surg 2007; 42:962–965.

9. Choudhry MS, Grant HW. Small bowel obstruction due to adhesions following neonatal laparotomy. Pediatr Surg Int 2006; 22:729–732.

10. Vijay K, Anindya C, Bhanu P, Mohan M, Rao PL. Adhesive small bowel obstruction (ASBO) in children—role of conservative management. Med J Malaysia 2005; 60:81–84.

11. Akgur FM, Tanyel FC, Buyukpamukcu HI. Adhesive small bowel obstruction in children: the place and predictors of success for conservative treatment. J Pediatr Surg 1991; 26:37–41.

12. Eitan A, Katz IM, Sweed Y, Bickel A. Fecal impaction in children: report of 53 cases of rectal seed bezoars. J Pediatr Surg 2007; 42:1114–1117.

13. Villamizar E, Mendez M, Bonilla E, Varon H, de Onatra S. Ascaris lumbricoides infestation as a cause of intestinal obstruction in children: experience with 87 cases. J Pediatr Surg 1996; 31:201–205.

14. Mukhopadhyay B, Saha S, Maiti S, Mitra D, Banerjee TJ, Jha M, Mukhopadhyay M, Samanta M, Das S. Clinical appraisal of Ascaris lumbricoides, with special reference to surgical complications. Pediatr Surg Int 2001; 17:403–405.

15. Salman AB. Management of intestinal obstruction caused by ascariasis. J Pediatr Surg 1997; 32:585–587.

16. Chirdan LB, Ameh EA. Sigmoid volvulus and ileosigmoid knotting in children. Pediatr Surg Int 2001; 17:636–637.

17. Shepherd JJ. Ninety-two cases of ileosigmoid knotting in Uganda. Br J Surg 1967; 54:561–566.

18. Akgun Y. Management of ileosigmoid knotting. Br J Surg 1997; 84:672–673.

19. Fan HP, Yang AD, Chang YJ, Juan CW, Wu HP. Clinical spectrum of internal hernia: a surgical emergency. Surg Today 2008; 38:899–904.

20. Gingalewski C, Lalikos J. An unusual cause of small bowel obstruction: herniation through a defect in the falciform ligament. J Pediatr Surg 2008; 43:398–400.

21. Mboyo A, Goura E. Massicot R, Flurin V, Legrand B, Repetto-Germaine M, Caron-Bataille S, Ndie J. An exceptional cause of intestinal obstruction in a 2 year old boy: strangulated hernia of the ileum through Winslow's foramen. J Pediatr Surg 2008; 43:e1–e3.

CHAPTER 70
NECROTISING ENTEROCOLITIS

Avraham Schlager
Marion Arnold
Samuel W. Moore
Evan P. Nadler

Introduction

Necrotising enterocolitis (NEC) is a disease of the infant gastrointestinal tract (GIT) most commonly found in premature newborns. Although the aetiology and pathogenesis of the disease is not fully understood, in its most severe cases, NEC rapidly progresses from bacterial invasion of the intestinal wall to full-thickness bowel necrosis, leading to perforation and subsequent peritonitis, sepsis, and possibly death.[1] The elusive nature, unpredictable onset and progression, as well as the fragile nature of the affected patient population, combine to make NEC one of the leading causes of morbidity and mortality in neonatal intensive care units (NICUs) globally.[2,3]

Although technological advances, such as the advent of the modern intensive care unit (ICU), initially yielded fairly dramatic improvements in the survival of patients with NEC,[4,5] the condition is still associated with a sustained high mortality (19–50%), even in developed countries,[6] with little improvement over the last two decades.[7] These advances have been accompanied by a dramatic rise in the cost of treating patients with NEC. As a result, the challenges facing clinicians in First World nations are magnified in developing countries, where medical care is often constricted by dilemmas of triage and allotment of limited resources.

Demographics

Necrotising enterocolitis is the most common cause of death in surgical neonates worldwide.[8] Although the prevalence of NEC varies geographically and temporally, sometimes occurring in clusters or epidemics, the overall incidence in the United States is estimated to be 1–3 cases for every 1,000 live births.[9] Due to improvements in technology and perinatal care and the concomitant increase in survivability of neonates, the incidence of the disease appears to be increasing in Western nations.[10] Interestingly, there appears to be an overall increase in NEC prevalence in developing countries in recent years as well. This may be partly attributed to factors such as the increased survival of very small premature infants, the increasing drug abuse culture, and the high incidence of preterm labour (especially in developing countries), as well as the impact of the HIV epidemic currently sweeping over sub-Saharan Africa, where an increase in severity can probably be anticipated. Accurate statistical analysis of the disease in continental Africa is not feasible because the poor access to antenatal diagnosis, primary health care, transport facilities, and low survival of infants with delayed presentation significantly contribute to the decreased number of recorded admissions with the diagnosis of NEC.[11]

Epidemiology and Incidence

NEC is the most frequent and most lethal disease affecting the GIT of premature infants.[12] The disease appears to display no particular ethnic predilection. Prematurity remains the most consistent risk factor for developing NEC, with incidence and mortality from NEC both inversely related to birth weight and gestational age.[13] Approximately 7–10% of very low birth weight (VLBW) infants (<1,000 g) suffer from NEC, and almost 20% of these newborns experience a period of suspected disease known as an "NEC scare" at some point during their postnatal care.[7,14] Additionally, several reports have suggested that there may be an inverse relationship between gestational age and the age at onset of the disease.[15,16] Snyder et al. have recently reported that VLBW infants developed NEC later than their higher-weight cohorts, which may suggest that birth weight and age at the onset of disease may also be inversely related.[16]

Although the disease does not exclusively affect premature infants, nearly 90% of patients who develop NEC are premature. When NEC does occur in term infants, it is almost always associated with comorbidities that promote intestinal ischaemia (e.g., congenital heart disease, neonatal asphyxia, maternal pre-eclampsia, and diabetes) or causes of intestinal obstruction such as Hirschsprung's disease.

Reported NEC mortality in the United States ranges from 15% to 30%, with smaller infants, infants with more extensive disease, and infants requiring surgery at the greatest risk.[7] Although the mortality rates in industrialised nations have been decreasing over the past 30 years due to early detection, implementation of preventive measures, and upgrading of intensive care support facilities, this success has not been shared by developing countries due to limited resources.[17]

Aetiology/Pathophysiology

Despite extensive research in the field, an adequate understanding of the aetiology and pathophysiology of NEC remains elusive. Current knowledge of the cause and course of NEC has been confined to associated risk factors and recognised patterns of pathophysiologic change. Although any portion of the intestinal tract may be involved, NEC most commonly affects the terminal ileum. Its frequent distribution to the distal ileum and right side of the colon suggests a local vascular component because this area is most removed from the blood supply.

The histologic hallmark of NEC is a "bland infarct," which is characterised by full thickness coagulation (ischaemic) necrosis, a paucity of acute inflammatory cells (neutrophils), and a predominantly lymphocytic infiltrate (Figure 70.1).[18] Santulli and colleagues described a classic triad of pathological events leading to the development of NEC, including (1) intestinal ischaemia, (2) colonisation by pathogenic bacteria, and (3) excess protein substrate in the intestinal lumen.[19] Using this triad, Kosloske et al. hypothesised that quantitative extremes of two out of three of these factors is sufficient to cause NEC.[20]

Mucosal ischaemia arises from a neonatal insult resulting from factors such as a decrease in end diastolic blood flow, foetal distress, cold exposure, asphyxia, hypotension, congenital heart disease, or sepsis. Intestinal ischaemia results in local production of free radicals and initiates a cytokine cascade within the gut wall.

Novel treatments are currently being developed to abrogate the toxic effects of some of the local factors at play in the inflammatory process.[21] As a result of the mucosal damage, bacterial translocation can occur through the intestinal wall, and systemic infection may follow, leading to further ischaemia and necrosis of the bowel wall, progression to perforation, peritonitis, overwhelming septicaemia, and possible multiorgan failure and death.

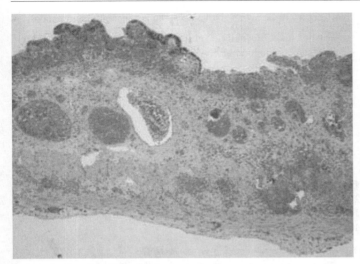

Figure 70.1: Small intestine showing necrosis, haemorrhage and congestion with a focal area of re-epithelisation of the mucosa (right). Original magnification, 20x.

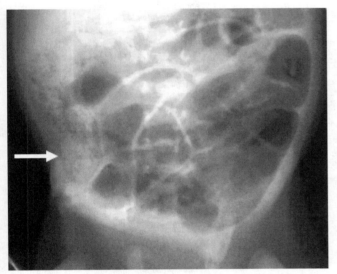

Figure 70.2: Frontal abdominal radiograph showing pneumatosis intestinalis in the right colon (arrow).

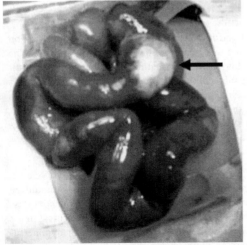

Figure 70.3: Segments of small bowel showing hyperaemia and an area of full-thickness necrosis (arrow).

Among the most accepted and consistently recognised risk factors for developing NEC are prematurity and timing and content of gastrointestinal feeding (i.e., formula concentration). Certain aspects of prematurity have been recognised that would appear to place these children at increased risk for NEC development. Among these are immaturity of gastrointestinal motility, digestive ability, circulatory regulation, intestinal barrier function along with abnormal colonisation by pathologic bacteria, and underdeveloped intestinal defense mechanisms.[22] Other risk factors implicated in the pathogenesis of NEC include bacterial infection,[23] the presence of pathogenic bacteria in the ICU (the so-called NEC epidemics), intestinal ischaemia,[24,25] certain pharmacologic agents,[26,27] and a host of inflammatory mediators,[28,29] although their relative contributions remain unclear. Other factors particularly pertinent to developing nations include antenatal factors, such as impaired umbilical artery flow, multiple pregnancy, and maternal infections, including HIV.[30] Nevertheless, despite these numerous recognised associations, no clear pathway of pathogenesis has been identified.

Pathology

NEC usually begins in the mucosal layer of the bowel. Intramural progression may be recognised by the frequent association of pneumatosis intestinalis, which represents bacterial hydrogen gas in the intestinal wall (Figure 70.2). This gas may extend into the vessels and into the portal vein and may be visualised radiographically as portal venous gas. Macroscopically, there is considerable variation in the degree of bowel involvement from a fairly minor inflammatory response of the bowel to full thickness necrosis, which may involve large segments of intestine (Figure 70.3). The terminal ileum and caecum are most commonly affected, but NEC represents a spectrum of disease; in its severest form, it may affect the entire bowel and parts of the stomach (NEC totalis). The affected bowel frequently extends beyond the macroscopic disease seen at surgery.

At surgery, the serosal surface is characterised by patches of full-thickness necrosis, oedema, and subserosal haemorrhages in affected portions of bowel. Pneumatosis intestinalis may be seen and felt in the bowel wall and may extend into the mesentery. Perforation of transmural necrotic patches is common, with subsequent gross contamination and peritonitis. Surgical intervention is required in at least 40% of patients with NEC due to intestinal necrosis with or without perforation. The objectives of surgical management are to remove the necrotic bowel, preserve bowel length, divert the faecal stream if required, and control sepsis.

Clinical Presentation

Infants with acute NEC usually present with both specific gastrointestinal signs as well as nonspecific physiologic signs often indicative of generalised infection. The classic history for a patient with NEC is a premature infant within 2 weeks of delivery who begins to develop feeding intolerance, distention, and/or blood per rectum after the initiation of formula feeds. The most common gastrointestinal signs reported are abdominal distention and blood per rectum. Others include feeding intolerance, bilious emesis, haematemesis, and guaic positive stools. Some of the nonspecific signs include lethargy, temperature and glucose instability, hypotension, and apnoeic spells associated with bradycardia (Table 70.1).

Initial physical exam findings are often subtle, significant only for mild distention and tenderness. As the disease progresses, the abdominal exam often reveals significant tenderness, palpable bowel loops, and an inflammatory mass, along with erythema or oedema of the abdominal wall.

Table 70.1: Specific and nonspecific signs of NEC.

Gastrointestinal signs	Nonspecific physiologic signs
Feeding intolerance	Hypotension
Abdominal distention	Temperature instability
Blood per rectum	Apnoeic spells (with bradycardia)
Bilious emesis	Lethargy
Haematemesis	Glucose instability

Laboratory Testing and Imaging

A complete blood count often demonstrates thrombocytopaenia and may show leukocytosis or, more commonly, leukopaenia.[31] Blood gas analysis (arterial, venous, or capillary) may demonstrate a significant base deficit due to metabolic acidosis associated with hypoperfusion, but is not necessarily indicative of intestinal necrosis. Because the initial history, physical exam, and laboratory findings in patients with NEC are often nonspecific, sepsis from a source other than the GIT is the most common diagnosis that needs to be excluded in cases of suspected NEC. Other diagnoses that may be included are malrotation of the intestines with midgut volvulus, gastroenteritis, Hirschsprung's disease, intestinal atresia, intussusception, and, less commonly, gastro-oesophageal reflux disease.

Plain radiography remains the imaging modality of choice in the diagnosis of NEC. In 70% of cases, the diagnosis is established by the presence of pneumatosis intestinalis on plain abdominal radiograph. Other radiographic findings in infants with NEC include air in the portal vein, a ground-glass appearance suggestive of ascites, pneumoperitoneum (Figure 70.4), and the "fixed-loop" sign, which is the defined as one or several loops of dilated small intestine that remain unchanged in position on x-ray over 24 to 36 hours. The fixed loop sign is suggestive of a nonperistalsing segment of intestine due to necrosis. Whereas contrast studies of the GIT, such as computed tomography (CT) and magnetic resonance imaging (MRI) scans, have not been proven to be clinically useful in the evaluation of patients with NEC,[32–35] a recent study has suggested a possible role for sonography due to its increased ability to detect intraabdominal fluid, bowel wall thickness, and bowel wall perfusion.[36] The resources available in developing countries may limit the applicability of ultrasound in such regions.

Radiologic features commonly associated with NEC include:

• thickened, distended bowel loops;

• pneumatosis intestinalis, or gas in the bowel wall;

• pneumoperitoneum, which indicates intestinal perforation;

• portal venous air (a severe infection that is not an absolute indication

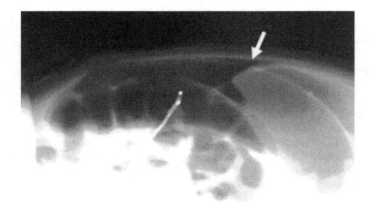

Figure 70.4: Decubitis abdominal radiograph demonstrating pneumoperitoneum (arrow); Rigler's sign is also seen.

for surgery in its own right as it may be a transient phenomenon);

• constant ("fixed") small bowel loop present on serial x-rays, which indicates necrotic loop of bowel;

• ascites;

• thickening of the abdominal wall due to cellulitis;

• outline of falciform ligament highlighted by intraperitoneal air ("football sign"); and

• outlining of the intestinal wall between two gas lucencies ("Rigler's sign").

Bell Staging System

Based on this initial work-up, patients with a presumed diagnosis of NEC can be classified into one of three clinical stages, as described by Bell et al.[37] (Table 70.2).

Table 70.2: Simplified Bell staging system for NEC..

Stage	NEC involvement	Manifestations	Radiographic signs
I	Infants with mild features suggestive, but not diagnostic, of NEC	Gastrointestinal, includes feeding intolerance, abdominal distention, blood per rectum, etc.; systemic includes temperature instability, lethargy, bradycardia, etc.	Abdominal radiograph with nonspecific ileus pattern
II	Infants with definitive NEC but without indication for surgical intervention	Persistent or marked gastrointestinal or systemic manifestations	Abdominal radiograph with pneumatosis intestinalis
III	Infants with more advanced NEC, defined by intestinal necrosis, signs of clinical deterioration or intestinal perforation	Above signs with deteriorating vital signs, evidence of septic shock or marked gastrointestinal haemorrhage	Above radiographic signs with pneumoperitoneum or other signs suggestive of intestinal necrosis

Source: Kliegman RM, Fanaroff AA. Necrotizing enterocolitis. N Engl J Med 1984; 310:1093–1103.

Differentiation of NEC from Spontaneous Intestinal Perforation

Spontaneous intestinal perforation (SIP) or focal intestinal perforation (FIP) have been reported as disease entities different from NEC. The aetiology, pathophysiology, and best treatment of spontaneous intestinal perforation remain subjects of ongoing research, but the principles for the management of NEC mostly apply. Similar to NEC, FIP presents with the sudden onset of a pneumoperitoneum. However, unlike NEC, FIP often represents a small isolated perforation, which may spontaneously seal without surgery in the very low weight infant (<1,000 g).

Management

Initial management of acute NEC consists primarily of supportive care. If patients are receiving enteral alimentation, the feedings should be discontinued and an orogastric tube should be placed to decompress the stomach. Aggressive intravenous fluid resuscitation is critical in the early phase of NEC to prevent exacerbation of intestinal hypoperfusion, and a catheter may be inserted into the bladder to help monitor urine output and adequacy of resuscitation. Blood and urine cultures should be obtained, and broad-spectrum antibiotics should be administered. Currently, the recommended antibiotic therapy regimen includes ampicillin, gentamicin, and clindamycin or metronidazole to cover gram-positive, gram-negative, and anaerobic bacteria, respectively. In a series reported by Chan et al., several gram-negative bacteria resistant to ampicillin or gentamicin were isolated.[38] Thus, depending on the antimicrobial profile of the institution, different antibiotic strategies may be required to treat the emerging strains of bacteria.

In addition to clinical exams and continued haemodynamic monitoring, disease progression should be monitored by using serial abdominal radiographs, ideally obtained every 6 to 8 hours. Daily and as-needed x-rays may be sufficient, however, if that is all the resources will allow. Imaging protocols should include both vertical and horizontal beam radiographs to ensure adequate sensitivity for signs of disease progression. Many institutions use supine abdominal images along with cross table lateral images, which allow the infants to remain supine, thereby minimising repositioning of the unstable patients.[24] Alternatively, decubitus films often more clearly demonstrate pneumoperitoneum. If repeat radiographs display an unchanged or improving pattern of pneumatosis intestinalis, then expectant management may be continued, provided that the infant remains haemodynamically stable.

Acute Medical Management Summary

In the absence of surgical indications, acute medical management of patients with suspected NEC includes the following:

1. Resuscitation: intravenous fluids, nasogastric decompression, careful control of acid-base balance, and correction of electrolyte abnormalities.

2. Cessation of oral feeds and medications.

3. Broad-spectrum antibiotics: guided by cultures and local microbiological profile.

4. Management of thrombocytopaenia and abnormal clotting profile; important due to the potential for cerebral bleeds.

5. High index of suspicion for complications: frequent monitoring and reassessment as well as x-ray monitoring in the acute patient to look for pneumoperitoneum (6 to 8 hourly or as clinically indicated).

6. Early surgical consultation.

Surgical Indications

Indications for surgical intervention focus on signs of perforation or impending perforation. Development of pneumoperitoneum on abdominal radiograph is considered an absolute indication for surgical intervention. Other signs, such as a fixed loop on abdominal radiographs, an abdominal mass or erythema of the abdominal wall on physical exam, positive paracentesis, or little to no clinical improvement despite optimal medical management, are considered relative indications. Some authors argue that portal venous air on radiography should also mandate surgical intervention due to its associated poor prognosis (70% mortality in some series), although this is not a universally accepted view.[39,40] With the exception of evidence of pneumoperitoneum, the timing and method of surgical intervention must be made based on individual cases.

Exploratory Laparotomy versus Primary Peritoneal Drainage

Although there is a general consensus regarding the factors and relative indications for surgical intervention, in the setting of acute NEC, controversy persists regarding the optimal surgical strategy. Some authors have advocated primary peritoneal drainage alone as definitive therapy for advanced NEC.[41,42] Primary peritoneal drainage is performed by using a 0.5–1–cm incision to evacuate the peritoneum of all faecal and purulent content followed by aggressive irrigation and placement of a drain. Advocates of primary laparotomy argue that many patients with NEC treated initially with peritoneal drainage require subsequent

laparotomy[43,44] and therefore primary laparotomy would minimise the number of surgical interventions in these patients. A recent multicentred, prospective randomised trial comparing laparotomy to primary peritoneal drainage in patients weighing less than 1,500 g with perforated NEC showed no significant difference in survival, dependence on parenteral nutrition, or length of hospital stay.[43] It has also been suggested that peritoneal drainage may be particularly suited to the treatment of infants less than 26 weeks gestational age or who weigh less than 1,000 g because isolated intestinal perforations are more frequently encountered in this patient population.[44] In regions with scarce resources and a shortage of skilled personnel, primary peritoneal drainage may be the best initial option for all NEC patients who meet the criteria for surgical intervention.

Extent of Surgical Intervention

Most authors agree that the extent of surgical intervention should be determined by the degree of bowel involvement encountered at laparotomy. Approximately 50% of infants with acute NEC present with focal disease, and the other 50% present with multiple areas of involvement.[43] Nearly 20% of infants treated surgically for NEC are found to have pan-involvement, which is defined as disease encompassing greater than 75% of the total intestine.[34]

Focal Perforation

Exploratory laparotomy with limited resection and creation of an enterostomy remains the standard of care for infants with NEC found to have a focal perforation. Recently, some authors have advocated intestinal resection with primary anastomosis as an alternative to enterostomy, citing the high morbidity associated with enterostomies in the newborn population.[43,45,46] Additionally, they argue, primary anastomosis affords the possibility of avoiding a second surgery. Advocates of resection and enterostomy creation maintain that the majority of stomal complications are minor and easily managed.[47] Additionally, early ostomy closure has been shown to be well-tolerated in this patient population[48] and therefore does not justify the added risk inherent in primary anastomosis. Cooper et al. reported their experience with primary anastomosis as compared to resection and diversion at the Children's Hospital of Philadelphia.[49] They reported that overall survival for infants who underwent intestinal diversion was 72%, compared to only 48% for patients with primary anastomosis. Postmortem examination of 7 out of the 14 patients who died after primary anastomosis revealed two anastomotic leaks and a gangrenous anastomosis that was easily disrupted during the postmortem exam. The authors of that study concluded that primary anastomosis is not comparable, much less superior, to intestinal diversion.

Principles of Surgery

NEC with pan-involvement carries the highest mortality rates;[50] infants who survive often develop short-bowel syndrome and long-term TPN dependence with associated complications.[1,33] As such, surgical strategies have focused on minimising the extent of bowel resection without compromising patient outcome. One such strategy is primary peritoneal drainage as a temporising measure to allow the infant time to regain haemodynamic stability and perfuse viable bowel, thus saving bowel that may have been resected with initial laparotomy.[51] Some surgeons even suggest that peritoneal drainage may, in fact, serve a definitive therapy for some cases of NEC, particularly for VLBW (<1,000 g) infants.[52,53] Nevertheless, the majority of infants treated with peritoneal drainage require subsequent laparotomy in some series.[54] Currently, peritoneal drainage is considered by many as an initial approach in haemodynamically unstable VLBW infants with NEC to allow resuscitation and stabilisation prior to definitive laparotomy.[46]

When initial laparotomy is employed, the overriding consideration is to spare as much bowel as possible to prevent short bowel syndrome. Aggressive resection of all diseased segments leads to sacrifice of intestine with borderline viability, and creation of multiple ostomies results in loss of intestinal length at the time of stoma closure. For this reason, a second-look laparotomy after proximal diversion has been proposed as an alternative to initial extensive resection. Weber and Lewis[55] reported their results of 32 infants with acute NEC who underwent operative intervention with resection of only frankly necrotic bowel and proximal diversion. Survival of the 14 infants who met criteria and underwent a second-look surgery was similar to that of the infants who underwent only one procedure. The authors concluded that a second-look strategy results in survival rates similar to a single-stage procedure while potentially sparing intestinal length.

Surgical Indications in Developing Nations

Much of the success over the years in the treatment of NEC has been afforded by supportive care and sophisticated ICUs and therefore has not been manifest in segments of the developing world. Banieghbal and colleagues have suggested the institution of more aggressive surgical protocols in developing nations that do not have modernised intensive care unit capabilities may lead to improved survival in those regions.[17] In their prospective study, conducted at a single institution in Johannesburg, South Africa, 450 neonates with NEC were treated with a more aggressive surgical protocol, and results were compared to prior data collected using the more classic criteria described by Kosloske.[56] The aggressive surgical protocol consisted of:

1. Laparotomy is undertaken in all patients with radiological perforation within 8 hours.

2. Any neonate with peritonitis on clinical exam is actively resuscitated and re-examined in 4–6 hours. Continuing peritonitis is an indication for laparotomy within 4 hours.

3. If the main area of disease is found to be in the ileocolic region, extended colonic resection for all macroscopic disease is performed with ileostomy creation.

4. In the cases of multiple areas of perforation/necrosis, only the most obvious necrotic/perforated bowel is excised with anastomosis or enterostomy, and a second-look laparotomy is performed in 3–4 days. The authors reported an overall decrease in mortality rate from 82% to 48%, with the institution of the more aggressive surgical protocol. Infants with active disease involving a limited length of the terminal ileum and/or colon derived the greatest benefit from the more aggressive protocol. Each individual hospital/region must decide whether this protocol or one using primary peritoneal drainage is suitable for the local resources available.

Postoperative Complications

The overall mortality rate for NEC is 15–30%. Smaller infants, infants with a larger proportion of diseased intestine, and infants undergoing surgery have the highest mortality rates. With improvements in supportive care and monitoring, the survival rate for patients with NEC has been increasing, calling attention to the issue of postoperative complications in those survivors. Overall, infants <28 weeks gestation had a significantly higher complication rate (47%) compared to those further along in gestation (29%).[57] Complications of NEC can be separated into early or predischarge complications and late, usually chronic, complications.

Early Complications

A multiinstitutional observational study reported that 39% of NEC patients who underwent surgery had some type of stomal or wound complication.[57] One multicentred prospective cohort study reported the overall incidence of postoperative intestinal stricture at 10.3% and an intraabdominal abscess occurred in 5.8%, with no difference between the initial laparotomy versus the initial drainage group.[58] Laparotomy was found to have a 7.9% incidence of wound dehiscence as compared to a 1.3% incidence in the initial drainage group. The overall rate of prolonged parental nutrition, defined as lasting >85 days, is 11% and was similar for the drainage and laparotomy groups.

Late Complications

Late, or postdischarge, complications of NEC are often chronic in nature. Infants with stage II or greater NEC are reported to have a significantly higher risk of long-term neurodevelopmental impairment compared to similar infants without NEC.[59] Additionally, surgery for NEC has been shown to be an independent risk factor for physical, psychomotor, and neurodevelopmental impairment compared to VLBW infants without NEC.[60] Although the reason for this increased risk of neurodevelopmental delay is not entirely clear, some studies suggest that increased duration of parenteral nutrition may render the neonate particularly susceptible to this issue.[61] Due to the high risk of preterm infants with NEC developing neurodevelopmental disability, most units now recommend close follow-up for all ≤1,250-gram infants who develop stage II or III (clinical) NEC.

Prevention Strategies

Treatment strategies to reduce the incidence of NEC have targeted some of the perinatal insults believed to contribute to its pathogenesis, such as bacterial colonisation, immaturity of the neonatal defense system, and formula feeding.[62] Some approaches include (1) administration of prophylactic oral antibiotics to decontaminate the gut[63–65]; (2) administration of glucocorticoids to accelerate epithelial cell maturation;[66–68] and (3) administration of human (breast) milk, which is replete with substances that are both immunologically active as well as trophic for the intestinal mucosa.[69,70]

Oral Antibiotics

The use of prophylactic oral antibiotics for the prevention of NEC has met with mixed results. The theory behind the proposed efficacy of antibiotic treatment is that gut decontamination may prevent potential pathogens from invading the bowel wall after mucosal breakdown. Indeed, results of one trial suggested early introduction of such antibiotics as gentamicin and amoxicillin in cases of suspected NEC have been shown to have a protective effect.[71] However, subsequent trials failed to demonstrate a reduced incidence of NEC in patients receiving prophylactic antibiotics.[72] As such, the issue of prophylactic antibiotics in the prevention of NEC remains controversial and is not commonly practiced due to the inherent risks of antibiotic resistance and pseudomembraneous colitis. A new area of study that is being actively researched is administering probiotic bacteria in an effort to prevent pathogenic bacteria from colonising the intestine.[73]

Corticosteroids

A large multicentred trial reported a decreased incidence of NEC in infants of mothers who received prenatal steroids.[57] Similarly, a 12-day course of postnatal steroids reduced the incidence of NEC in newborn infants with respiratory distress syndrome.[74] These results, however, are called into question as a meta-analysis performed by the Cochrane Database of 15 randomised trials of postnatal steroids demonstrated no benefit in the prevention of NEC. Thus, the question of whether steroids should be used in the prevention of NEC remains unresolved.[75]

Human Breast Milk

Studies have shown that neonates fed with human breast milk are 10 times less likely to develop NEC, although the exact mechanism of this protective affect is unknown.[76,77] Possible protective factors present in breast milk include macrophages, neutrophils, lymphocytes, lactoferrin, oligosaccharides, growth factors, and immunoglobulins.[60] In a landmark study by Eibl et al.,[78] supplementation of standard formula with IgA and IgG reduced the incidence of NEC in a cohort of premature infants. Subsequent trials using monomeric IgG supplementation alone showed conflicting results.[79,80] Ultimately, the question regarding the mechanism by which breast milk exerts its protective effect is yet to be elucidated.

Ethical Issues

Many of the ethical issues involved in the treatment of NEC in developing nations relate to the challenge of proper and efficient allocation of scarce resources. The survival rate of the disease often relies on prolonged, intensive, and costly ICU care, so the question arises as to the advisability of expending precious time and money on aggressive interventions only to yield poor survival rates. Additionally, a high percentage of the survivors of NEC in these regions end up with long-term complications that cannot be adequately managed, which leads to further morbidity and mortality. These issues must be evaluated based on the resources of each individual region.

Table 70.3: Evidence-based research.

Title	Laparotomy versus peritoneal drainage for necrotizing enterocolitis and drainage
Authors	Moss RL, Dimmitt RA, Barnhart DC, Sylvester KG, Brown RL, Powell DM, et al.
Institution	Yale University School of Medicine, New Haven, Connecticut, USA; among others
Reference	N Engl J Med 2006; 354(21):2225–2234
Problem	Evaluation of primary peritoneal drainage versus laparotomy in infants with perforated necrotising enterocolitis.
Intervention	Laparotomy, primary peritoneal drainage.
Comparison/ control (quality of evidence)	The population was 117 preterm infants (delivered before 34 weeks of gestation) with birth weights less than 1,500 g and perforated NEC at 15 paediatric centres randomised to undergo primary peritoneal drainage or laparotomy with bowel resection. Postoperative care was standardised. The primary outcome was survival at 90 days postoperatively. Secondary outcomes included dependence on parenteral nutrition 90 days postoperatively and length of hospital stay.
Outcome/ effect	At 90 days postoperatively, there was no significant difference in mortality between the drainage and laparotomy groups (34.5% versus 35.5%, P = 0.92). There was also no significant difference in dependence on parental nutrition (47.2 % versus 40.0%, P = 0.53) or mean length of stay (126±58 days and 116±56 days, respectively; P = 0.43).
Historical significance/ comments	This randomised, prospective trial suggests that treatment with primary peritoneal drainage and laparotomy with bowel resection are comparably efficacious in the treatment of perforated NEC. Mortality in this patient population was found to be ~35%. Although 5 out of the 30 patients (16.7%) in the primary peritoneal drainage group subsequently required laparotomy for clinical deterioration, drainage obviated the need for laparotomy in the remaining infants without any discernible increase in mortality.

Evidence-Based Research

Table 70.3 presents a study that compares primary peritoneal drainage and laparotomy in infants with perforated NEC. Table 70.4 revisits indications for surgery in NEC.

Table 70.4: Evidence-based research

Title	Indications for operation in necrotizing enterocolitis revisited
Authors	Kosloske AM
Institution	Department of Surgery, Ohio State University College of Medicine, Columbus, Ohio, USA: University of New Mexico Hospital, Albuquerque, New Mexico, USA
Reference	J Pediat Surg 1994; 29(5):663–666
Problem	Evaluation of 12 criteria as predictors of intestinal gangrene in patients with necrotising enterocolitis.
Comparison/ control (quality of evidence)	A series of 147 infants treated for NEC was analysed to evaluate the accuracy of 12 proposed findings as indicators of intestinal gangrene. These findings included pneumoperitoneum, portal venous gas, fixed loop, fixed abdominal mass, erythema of abdomen, positive paracentesis, severe pneumatosis, clinical deterioration, low platelet count, severe gastrointestinal haemorrhage, abdominal tenderness, and gasless abdomen/ascites. Operation was performed (usually resection and enterostomy) for evidence of intestinal perforation or gangrene. Intestinal gangrene was documented for all infants by either operation, autopsy, or radiographic findings of pneumoperitoneum or intestinal stricture.
Outcome/ effect	The findings of pneumoperitoneum, portal venous gas, and positive paracentesis each had specificities and positive predictive values approaching 100% with a prevalence greater than 10%. Pneumoperitoneum had a prevalence of 48%. The findings of a "fixed-loop," palpable abdominal mass and erythema of the abdominal wall also had specificities and positive predictive values approaching 100% but had a prevalence below 10%. Severe pneumatosis had a specificity of 91%, and positive predictive value of 94% and a prevalence of 20%. The remaining five findings all had specificities below 90%, positive predictive values below 80%, and prevalence ranging between 2% and 28%.
Historical significance/ comments	Although no single finding is particularly sensitive for intestinal necrosis, the findings of pneumoperitoneum, portal venous gas, positive paracentesis, fixed-loop sign, palpable abdominal mass, and erythema of the abdominal wall all had specificities approaching 100% and may be used as an indication for surgical intervention. Severe pneumatosis was also found to have a fair specificity for intestinal necrosis. The remaining findings had poor specificity and positive predictive value. Although seven of these findings were highly specific for intestinal necrosis, the prevalence of these signs were low. As such, the absence of these findings cannot rule out intestinal necrosis, and the decision for surgical intervention will often rely on clinical judgment of the managing surgeon.

Key Summary Points

1. Necrotising enterocolitis occurs in 1–3 infants per 1,000 live births.

2. Ninety percent of cases occur in premature infants.

3. Mortality rates range between 15% and 30%.

4. The aetiology and pathophysiology of the disease is not well understood.

5. Prematurity as well as timing and content of gastrointestinal feeding are the most consistent risk factors associated with NEC.

6. Human breast milk has been shown to be protective against the development of NEC.

7. NEC presents with both specific gastrointestinal signs of vomiting, distention, and blood per rectum as well as nonspecific signs of haemodynamic instability.

8. Abdominal radiography is the primary imaging tool in establishing the diagnosis of necrotising enterocolitis.

9. Pneumoperitoneum is an absolute indication for surgical intervention; relative indications include a fixed-loop on abdominal radiographs, an abdominal mass or erythema of the abdominal wall on physical exam, positive paracentesis, and whether there is little or no evidence of clinical improvement.

10. Primary peritoneal drainage and laparotomy are comparable treatments for perforated necrotising enterocolitis.

11. Surgical goals focus on resection of frankly necrotic bowel with an effort to preserve intestinal length.

12. Advances in intensive care unit facilities in developed nations have translated into improved survival in patients with NEC.

13. More aggressive surgical protocols may improve survival in developing nations that lack modern intensive care unit facilities.

References

1. Kliegman RM, Fanaroff AA. Necrotizing enterocolitis. N Engl J Med 1984; 310:1093–1103.

2. Hsueh W, Caplan MS, Qu XW, et al. Neonatal necrotizing enterocolitis: clinical considerations and pathogenetic concepts. Pediatr Dev Pathol 2003; 6:6–23.

3. Amoury RA. Necrotizing enterocolitis—a continuing problem in the neonate. World J Surg 1993; 17:363–373.

4. Grosfeld JL, Cheu H, Schlatter M, et al. Changing trends in necrotizing enterocolitis. Experience with 302 cases in two decades. Ann Surg 1991; 214:300–306.

5. Kosloske AM, Musemeche CA, Ball WS Jr, et al. Necrotizing enterocolitis: value of radiographic findings to predict outcome. Am J Roentgenol 1988; 151:771–774.

6. Rees CM, Eaton S, Kiely EM, et al. Peritoneal drainage or laparotomy for neonatal bowel perforation? A randomized controlled trial. Ann Surg 2008; 248:44–51.

7. Guner YS, Chokshi N, Petrosyan M, et al. Necrotizing enterocolitis—bench to bedside: novel and emerging strategies. Semin Pediatr Surg 2008; 17:255–265.

8. Amoury RA. Necrotizing enterocolitis—a continuing problem in the neonate. World J Surg 1993; 17:363–373.

9. Newell SJ. Gastro intestinal disorders: necrotizing enterocolitis. In: Rennie JM, Roberton NRC, eds. Textbook of Neonatology, 3rd ed, Churchill Livingstone, 1999, 747–755.

10. Luig M, Lui K. Epidemiology of necrotizing enterocolitis—Part I: Changing regional trends in extremely preterm infants over 14 years. J Paediatr Child Health 2005; 41:169–173.

11. Nandi B, Mungongo C, Lakhoo K. A comparison of neonatal surgical admissions between two linked surgical departments in Africa and Europe. Pediatr Surg Int 2008; 24(8):939–942.

12. Ford HR, Sorrells DL, Knisely AS. Inflammatory cytokines, nitric oxide, and necrotizing enterocolitis. Semin Pediatr Surg 1996; 5:155–159.

13. Lin PW, Nasr TR, Stoll BJ. Necrotizing enterocolitis: recent scientific advances in pathophysiology and prevention. Semin Perinatol 2008; 32:70–82.

14. Uauy RD, Fanaroff AA, Korones SB, et al. Necrotizing enterocolitis in very low birth weight infants: biodemographic and clinical correlates. National Institute of Child Health and Human Development Neonatal Research Network. J Pediatr 1991; 119:630–638.

15. Teasdale F, et al. Neonatal necrotizing enterocolitis: the relationship of age at the time of onset and prognosis. Canad Med Assoc J 1980; 123:387.

16. Snyder CL, Gittes GK, Murphy JP, et al. Survival after necrotizing enterocolitis in infants weighing less than 1,000 g: 25 years' experience at a single institution. J Pediatr Surg 1997; 32:434–437.

17. Banieghbal B, Schoeman L, Kalk F, et al. Surgical indications and strategies for necrotizing enterocolitis in low income countries. World J Surg 2002; 26:444–447.

18. Ballance WA, Dahms BB, Shenker N, et al. Pathology of neonatal necrotizing enterocolitis: a ten-year experience. J Pediatr 1990; 117:S6–S13.

19. Sántulli TV, Schullinger JN, Heird WC, Gongaware RD, Wigger J, Barlow B, Blanc WA, Berdon WE. Acute necrotizing enterocolitis in infancy: a review of 64 cases. Pediatrics 1975; 55(3): 376–387.

20. Kosloske AM. Epidemiology of necrotizing enterocolitis. Acta Paediatr Suppl 1994; 396:2–7.

21. Guner YS, Chokshi N, Petrosyan M, et al. Necrotizing enterocolitis—bench to bedside: novel and emerging strategies. Semin Pediatr Surg 2008; 17:255–265.

22. Srinivasan PS, Brandler MD, D'Souza A. Necrotizing enterocolitis. Clin Perinat 2008; 35:251–272.

23. Scheifele DW. Role of bacterial toxins in neonatal necrotizing enterocolitis. J Pediatr 1990; 117:S44–S46.

24. Kliegman RM. Models of the pathogenesis of necrotizing enterocolitis. J Pediatr 1990; 117:S2–S5.

25. Martinez-Tallo E, Claure N, Bancalari E. Necrotizing enterocolitis in full-term or near-term infants: risk factors. Biol Neonate 1997; 71:292–298.

26. Hufnal-Miller CA, Blackmon L, Baumgart S, et al. Enteral theophylline and necrotizing enterocolitis in the low-birthweight infant. Clin Pediatr (Phila) 1993; 32:647–653.

27. Grosfeld JL, Chaet M, Molinari F, et al. Increased risk of necrotizing enterocolitis in premature infants with patent ductus arteriosus treated with indomethacin. Ann Surg 1996; 224:350–355; discussion 355–357.

28. Ford H, Watkins S, Reblock K, et al. The rolwe of inflammatory cytokines and nitric oxide in the pathogenesis of necrotizing enterocolitis. J Pediatr Surg 1997; 32:275–282.

29. Caplan MS, Hsueh W. Necrotizing enterocolitis: role of platelet activating factor, endotoxin, and tumor necrosis factor. J Pediatr 1990; 117:S47–S51.

30. Desfrere L, de Oliveira I, Goffinet F, et al. Increased incidence of necrotizing enterocolitis in premature infants born to HIV-positive mothers. AIDS 2005; 19:1487–1493.

31. Hutter JJ, Hathaway WE, Wayne ER. Hematologic abnormalities in severe neonatal necrotizing enterocolitis. J Pediatr 1976; 88:1026.

32. Buonomo C. The radiology of necrotizing enterocolitis. Radiol Clin North Am 1999; 37:1187–1198.

33. Kao SC, Smith WL, Franken EA Jr, et al. Contrast enema diagnosis of necrotizing enterocolitis. Pediatr Radiol 1992; 22:115–117.

34. Rencken IO, Sola A, al-Ali F, et al. Necrotizing enterocolitis: diagnosis with CT examination of urine after enteral administration of iodinated water-soluble contrast material. Radiology 1997; 205:87–90.

35. Maalouf EF, Fagbemi A, Duggan PJ, et al. Magnetic resonance imaging of intestinal necrosis in preterm infants. Pediatrics 2000; 105(3, pt 1):510–514.

36. Epelman M, Daneman A, Navarro OM, et al. Necrotizing enterocolitis: review of state-of-the-art imaging findings with pathologic correlation. Radiographics 2007; 27:285–305.

37. Bell MJ, Ternberg JL, Feigin RD, et al. Neonatal necrotizing enterocolitis. Therapeutic decisions based upon clinical staging. Ann Surg 1978; 187:1–7.

38. Chan KL, Saing H, Yung RW, et al. A study of pre-antibiotic bacteriology in 125 patients with necrotizing enterocolitis. Acta Paediatr Suppl 1994; 396:45–48.

39. Kosloske AM. Epidemiology of necrotizing enterocolitis. Acta Paediatr Suppl 1994; 396:2–7.

40. Rowe MI, Reblock KK, Kurkchubasche AG, et al. Necrotizing enterocolitis in the extremely low birth weight infant. J Pediatr Surg 1994; 29:987–990; discussion 990–991.

41. Moss RL, Dimmitt RA, Barnhart DC, et al. Laparotomy versus peritoneal drainage for necrotizing enterocolitis and drainage. N Engl J Med 2006; 354:2225–2234.

42. Cass DL, Brandt ML, Patel DL, et al. Peritoneal drainage as definitive treatment for neonates with isolated intestinal perforation. J Pediatr Surg 2000; 35:1531–1536.

43. Parigi GB, Bragheri R, Minniti S, et al. Surgical treatment of necrotizing enterocolitis: when? how? Acta Paediatr Suppl 1994; 396:58–61.

44. Albanese CT, Rowe MI. Necrotizing enterocolitis. Semin Pediatr Surg 1995; 4:200–206.

45. Ade-Ajayi N, Kiely E, Drake D, et al. Resection and primary anastomosis in necrotizing enterocolitis. J R Soc Med 1996; 89:385–388.

46. Hofman FN, Bax NMA, van der Zee DC, et al. Surgery for necrotizing enterocolitis: primary anastomosis or enterostomy? Pediatr Surg Int 2004; 20: 481–483.

47. Weber TR, Tracy TF, Jr, Silen ML, et al. Enterostomy and its closure in newborns. Arch Surg 1995; 130:534–537.

48. Gertler JP, Seashore JH, Touloukian RJ. Early ileostomy closure in necrotizing enterocolitis. J Pediatr Surg 1987; 22:140–143.

49. Cooper A, Ross AJ, O'Neill Jr JA, et al. Resection with primary anastomosis for necrotizing enterocolitis: a contrasting view. J Pediatr Surg 1988; 23:64–68.

50. Holman RC, Stehr-Green JK, Zelasky MT. Necrotizing enterocolitis mortality in the United States, 1979–85. Am J Public Health 1989; 79:987–989.

51. Rovin JD, Rodgers BM, Burns RC, et al. The role of peritoneal drainage for intestinal perforation in infants with and without necrotizing enterocolitis. J Pediatr Surg 1999; 34:143–147.

52. Cheu HW, Sukarochana K, Lloyd DA. Peritoneal drainage for necrotizing enterocolitis. J Pediatr Surg 1988; 23:557–561.

53. Dimmitt RA, Meier AH, Skarsgard ED, et al. Salvage laparotomy for failure of peritoneal drainage in necrotizing enterocolitis in infants with extremely low birth weight. J Pediatr Surg 2000; 35:856–859.

54. Ahmed T, Ein S, Moore A. The role of peritoneal drains in treatment of perforated necrotizing enterocolitis: recommendations from recent experience. J Pediatr Surg 1998; 33:1468–1470.

55. Weber TR, Lewis JE. The role of second-look laparotomy in necrotizing enterocolitis. J Pediatr Surg 1986; 21:323–325.

56. Kosloske A. Indications for operation in necrotizing enteroclitis revisited. J Ped Surg 1994; 29:5 663–666.

57. Chwals WJ, Blakely ML, Cheng A, et al. Surgery-associated complications in necrotizing enterocolitis: a multiinstitutional study, J Pediatr Surg 2001; 36:1722–1724.

58. Blakely ML, Lally KP, McDonald S, et al. Postoperative outcomes of extremely low birth-weight infants with necrotizing enterocolitis or isolated intestinal perforation: a prospective cohort study by the NICHD Neonatal Research Network. Ann Surg 2005; 241:984–994.

59. Schulzke SM, Deshpande GC, Patole SK. Neurodevelopmental outcomes of very-low-birth-weight infants with necrotizing enterocolitis: a systematic review of observational studies, Arch Pediatr Adolesc Med 2007; 161:583–590.

60. Hintz SR, Kendrick DE, Stoll BJ, et al. Neurodevelopmental and growth outcomes of extremely low birth weight infants after necrotizing enterocolitis, Pediatrics 2005; 115:696–703.

61. Neubauer AP, Voss W, Kattner E. Outcome of extremely low birth weight survivors at school age: the influence of perinatal parameters on neurodevelopment. Eur J Ped 2008; 167:87–95.

62. Vasan U, Gotoff SP. Prevention of neonatal necrotizing enterocolitis. Clin Perinatol 1994; 21:425–435.

63. Fast C, Rosegger H. Necrotizing enterocolitis prophylaxis: oral antibiotics and lyophilized enterobacteria vs oral immunoglobulins. Acta Paediatr Suppl 1994; 396:86–90.

64. Egan EA, Mantilla G, Nelson RM, et al. A prospective controlled trial of oral kanamycin in the prevention of neonatal necrotizing enterocolitis. J Pediatr 1976; 89:467–470.

65. Siu YK, Ng PC, Fung SC, et al. Double blind, randomised, placebo controlled study of oral vancomycin in prevention of necrotising enterocolitis in preterm, very low birthweight infants. Arch Dis Child Fetal Neonatal Ed 1998; 79:F105–F109.

66. Bauer CR, Morrison JC, Poole WK, et al. A decreased incidence of necrotizing enterocolitis after prenatal glucocorticoid therapy. Pediatrics 1984; 73:682–688.

67. Halac E, Halac J, Begue EF, et al. Prenatal and postnatal corticosteroid therapy to prevent neonatal necrotizing enterocolitis: a controlled trial. J Pediatr 1990; 117:132–138.

68. Israel EJ, Schiffrin EJ, Carter EA, et al. Cortisone strengthens the intestinal mucosal barrier in a rodent necrotizing enterocolitis model. Adv Exp Med Biol 1991; 310:375–380.

69. Pitt J, Barlow B, Heird WC. Protection against experimental necrotizing enterocolitis by maternal milk. I. Role of milk leukocytes. Pediatr Res 1977; 11:906–909.

70. Goldman AS, Thorpe LW, Goldblum RM, et al. Anti-inflammatory properties of human milk. Acta Paediatr Scand 1986; 75:689–695.

71. Krediet TG, van Lelyveld N, Vijlbrief DC, et al. Microbiological factors associated with neonatal necrotizing enterocolitis: protective effect of early antibiotic treatment. Acta Paediatr 2003; 92: 1180–1182.

72. Hansen TN, Ritter DA, Speer ME, et al. A randomized, controlled study of oral gentamicin in the treatment of neonatal necrotizing enterocolitis. J Pediatr 1980; 97:836–839.

73. Hoyos AB. Reduced incidence of necrotizing enterocolitis associated with enteral administration of Lactobacillus acidophilus and Bifidobacterium infantis to neonates in an intensive care unit. Int J Infect Dis 1999; 3:197–202.

74. Tapia JL, Ramirez R, Cifuentes J, et al. The effect of early dexamethasone administration on bronchopulmonary dysplasia in preterm infants with respiratory distress syndrome. J Pediatr 1998; 132:48–52.

75. Halliday HL, Ehrenkranz RA. Early postnatal (<96 hours) corticosteroids for preventing chronic lung disease in preterm infants. Cochrane Database Syst Rev 2, 2000.

76. Buescher ES. Host defense mechanisms of human milk and their relations to enteric infections and necrotizing enterocolitis. Clin Perinatol 1994; 21:247–262.

77. Schnabl KL, Van Aerde JE, Thomson AB, et al. Necrotizing enterocolitis: a multifactorial disease with no cure. World J Gastroenterol 2008; 14: 2142–2161.

78. Eibl MM, Wolf HM, Furnkranz H, et al. Prevention of necrotizing enterocolitis in low-birth-weight infants by IgA-IgG feeding. N Engl J Med 1988; 319:1–7.

79. Rubaltelli FF, Benini F, Sala M. Prevention of necrotizing enterocolitis in neonates at risk by oral administration of monomeric IgG. Dev Pharmacol Ther 1991; 17:138–143.

80. Richter D, Bartmann P, Pohlandt F. Prevention of necrotizing enterocolitis in extremely low birth weight infants by IgG feeding? Eur J Pediatr 1998; 157:924–925.

CHAPTER 71
SHORT BOWEL SYNDROME

Alice Mears
Kokila Lakhoo
Alastair J. W. Millar

Introduction

Short bowel syndrome (SBS) is defined as intestinal failure due to a loss of intestine resulting in inadequate length of bowel for maintaining the nutrition and hydration of the individual without either intravenous or oral supplementation.

With some reported exceptions, the minimum length of small bowel required for infant survival on enteral feeds is generally 25 cm in the presence of an intact ileocaecal valve (ICV) and colon, and 40 cm without an ICV and large bowel. Note that norms of intestinal length vary considerably, with a range of 250 cm to 300 cm of small bowel at term. The estimated length in a preterm infant of 26 and 32 weeks gestation is 70 cm and 120 cm, respectively. Thus, gestational age is an important factor. However, an infant is considered to have SBS when he or she behaves as if SBS is present, and the infant should be treated as such.

The intestine has the ability to adapt over time such that up to half of patients with SBS who initially require total parenteral nutrition (TPN) may be weaned off and gradually gain independence from TPN. However, in the absence of the availability of TPN, SBS carries a dismal prognosis. The management of SBS is resource-intense, requiring the availability of intensive care, TPN, and expert medical and surgical intervention. Even in optimal settings, infants and children with SBS suffer extensive morbidity and mortality. In most countries in Africa where TPN is not available, the outcomes are poor.

Demographics

Short bowel syndrome is mercifully rare. In Europe, the incidence is estimated to be approximately 2 per million. According to Gupta et al.,[1] the incidence of SBS in neonates is around 3 per 100,000 births per year. In Africa, the incidence is unknown because survival is close to zero.

Aetiology

Some of the common causes of short bowel syndrome are shown in Table 71.1. SBS can be congenital, but is more generally acquired from surgical resection of bowel. Of the congenital bowel atresias type 3b ("apple peel" type) and type 4 (multiple atresias, "string of sausages" type) are most likely to result in SBS. Functional SBS can also occur where there is severe malabsorption despite adequate bowel length or intact bowel.

Table 71.1: Common causes of short bowel syndrome.

Congenital	Acquired
Atresia	Midgut volvulus
Gastroschisis	Mesenteric infarction (e.g., sickle cell crisis)
Hirschsprungs disease (long segment)	Necrotising enterocolitis; adhesive band obstruction/strangulation
	Trauma

Pathophysiology

The effects of loss of bowel length depend on the type and length of bowel remaining.[1]

Small bowel motility is three times slower in the ileum than in the jejunum. The ileo-caecal valve also slows transit. The colon has the slowest transit time, between 24 and 150 hours. The efficiency of salt and water absorption also varies in the different parts of the intestine. The jejunum is very inefficient, with an efficiency of water absorption of 44% compared to 70% in the ileum and greater than 90% in the colon. The corresponding estimates for efficiency of salt absorption are 13% in the jejunum, 72% in the ileum, and greater than 90% in the colon.

Jejunum

If the jejunum alone is lost, there is no permanent defect in absorption—the ileum will take over. However, the jejunum normally releases the hormones cholecystokinin, serotonin, gastric inhibitory peptide, and secretin. Lower secretion of these hormones due to absence of the jejunum will result in decreased pancreatic secretion, gallbladder contraction, and gastric hypersecretion.

Ileum

The ileum is unique in absorbing vitamin B_{12} and bile salts. Absorption of nutrients takes place throughout the small bowel. Ileal resection results in decreased transit times and salt and water absorption. A larger than normal volume of fluid and electrolytes enters the colon. The reabsorption of bile salts is decreased and so their synthesis is increased. The flow of unabsorbed bile salts into the colon irritates the colon and impairs its ability to absorb salt and water, leading to choleretic diarrhoea. The depletion of the bile salt pool leads to cholelithiasis and fat malabsorption, resulting in steatorrhoea.

The degree of fat and carbohydrate malabsorption is related to the length of ileum resected. There is also reduced absorption of essential minerals, including calcium, magnesium, zinc, and phosphorus. Furthermore, there is an excessive loss of zinc in diarrhoea, leading to immune deficiency.

Ileocaecal Valve

Loss of the ICV reduces gut transit time. The loss of this barrier between the small and large bowel also leads to bacterial overgrowth of the remaining gut.

Colon

It is thought that the colon in SBS is important for driving adaptation of the gut as well as assuming an increased importance in absorption of water, potassium, and sodium as well as carbohydrates. Without the colon and ICV a longer length of ileum is required for survival.

Intestinal Adaptation

Intestinal adaptation[2] is the process whereby the intestine adjusts to its loss of length through hyperplasia of the mucosal surface in an effort to increase its absorptive capacity. The bowel dilates, lengthens, and thickens to increase the efficiency of absorption per unit length. There is an increase in the number of cells in the proliferating zones of the crypts, and villus height increases, resulting in an increased surface area for absorption. Histological evidence of adaptation can be seen from 48 hours after bowel resection, and diarrhoea is seen to decrease over the first 3 months. Early adaptation may take years and is greater with proximal than distal bowel resection.

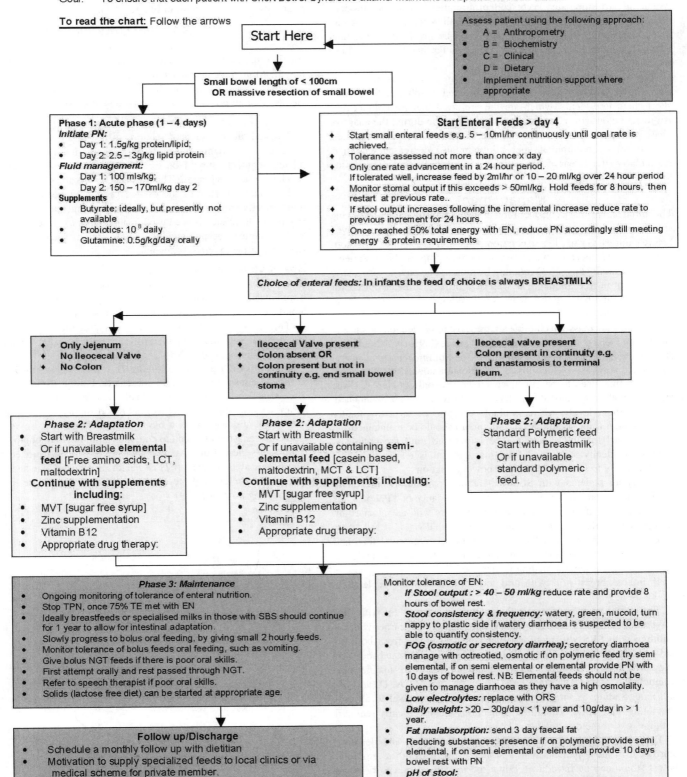

Management of Short Bowel Syndrome

Goal: To ensure that each patient with Short Bowel Syndrome attains/ maintains an optimal nutrition status.

To read the chart: Follow the arrows

Start Here

Assess patient using the following approach:
- A = Anthropometry
- B = Biochemistry
- C = Clinical
- D = Dietary
- Implement nutrition support where appropriate

Small bowel length of < 100cm
OR massive resection of small bowel

Phase 1: Acute phase (1 – 4 days)
Initiate PN:
- Day 1: 1.5g/kg protein/lipid;
- Day 2: 2.5 – 3g/kg lipid protein
Fluid management:
- Day 1: 100 mls/kg;
- Day 2: 150 – 170ml/kg day 2
Supplements
- Butyrate: ideally, but presently not available
- Probiotics: 10^8 daily
- Glutamine: 0.5g/kg/day orally

Start Enteral Feeds > day 4
- Start small enteral feeds e.g. 5 – 10ml/hr continuously until goal rate is achieved.
- Tolerance assessed not more than once x day
- Only one rate advancement in a 24 hour period.
- If tolerated well, increase feed by 2ml/hr or 10 – 20 ml/kg over 24 hour period
- Monitor stomal output if this exceeds > 50ml/kg. Hold feeds for 8 hours, then restart at previous rate..
- If stool output increases following the incremental increase reduce rate to previous increment for 24 hours.
- Once reached 50% total energy with EN, reduce PN accordingly still meeting energy & protein requirements

Choice of enteral feeds: In infants the feed of choice is always BREASTMILK

- **Only Jejenum**
- **No Ileocecal Valve**
- **No Colon**

- **Ileocecal Valve present**
- **Colon absent OR**
- **Colon present but not in continuity e.g. end small bowel stoma**

- **Ileocecal valve present**
- **Colon present in continuity e.g. end anastamosis to terminal ileum.**

Phase 2: Adaptation
- Start with Breastmilk
- Or if unavailable **elemental feed** [Free amino acids, LCT, maltodextrin]
Continue with supplements including:
- MVT [sugar free syrup]
- Zinc supplementation
- Vitamin B12
- Appropriate drug therapy:

Phase 2: Adaptation
- Start with Breastmilk
- Or if unavailable containing **semi-elemental feed** [casein based, maltodextrin, MCT & LCT]
Continue with supplements including:
- MVT [sugar free syrup]
- Zinc supplementation
- Vitamin B12
- Appropriate drug therapy:

Phase 2: Adaptation
Standard Polymeric feed
- Start with Breastmilk
- Or if unavailable standard polymeric feed.

Phase 3: Maintenance
- Ongoing monitoring of tolerance of enteral nutrition.
- Stop TPN, once 75% TE met with EN
- Ideally breastfeeds or specialised milks in those with SBS should continue for 1 year to allow for intestinal adaptation.
- Slowly progress to bolus oral feeding, by giving small 2 hourly feeds.
- Monitor tolerance of bolus feeds oral feeding, such as vomiting.
- Give bolus NGT feeds if there is poor oral skills.
- First attempt orally and rest passed through NGT.
- Refer to speech therapist if poor oral skills.
- Solids (lactose free diet) can be started at appropriate age.

Monitor tolerance of EN:
- *If Stool output : > 40 – 50 ml/kg* reduce rate and provide 8 hours of bowel rest.
- *Stool consistency & frequency:* watery, green, mucoid, turn nappy to plastic side if watery diarrhoea is suspected to be able to quantify consistency.
- *FOG (osmotic or secretory diarrhea);* secretory diarrhoea manage with octreotied, osmotic if on polymeric feed try semi elemental, if on semi elemental or elemental provide PN with 10 days of bowel rest. NB: Elemental feeds should not be given to manage diarrhoea as they have a high osmolality.
- *Low electrolytes:* replace with ORS
- *Daily weight:* >20 – 30g/day < 1 year and 10g/day in > 1 year.
- *Fat malabsorption:* send 3 day faecal fat
- Reducing substances: presence if on polymeric provide semi elemental, if on semi elemental or elemental provide 10 days bowel rest with PN
- *pH of stool:*
- Gastric aspirate: if more than 4 x previous hours infusion; withhold feeds for 12 hours

Follow up/Discharge
- Schedule a monthly follow up with dietitian
- Motivation to supply specialized feeds to local clinics or via medical scheme for private member.

Source: Adapted from Marino, L. Western Cape Guidelines for Management of short bowel syndrome.

Figure 71.1: Algorithm for the management of short bowel syndrome to ensure that each patient attains and maintains optimal nutrition.

Note: EN = enteral nutrition; FOG = faecal osmolar gap; LCT = long-chain triglycerides; MCT = medium chain triglycerides; MVT = multivitamins; NB = nota bene (note well); NGT = nasogastric tube; ORS =oral rehydration solution; PN = parenteral nutrition; TE = total energy (requirements); TPN = total parenteral nutrition.

Adaptation is driven by the increased load of fatty acids, carbohydrates, and proteins on the enteroglucagon-producing cells found in the ileum. Enteroglucagon stimulates ornithine decarboxylase, which in turn stimulates crypt cell proliferation. In animal models, other factors (e.g., glutamine, epidermal growth factor, cholecystokinin, and somatostatin) have also been shown to be involved in intestinal adaptation, although there is little evidence so far that their clinical use increases adaptation in humans.

The colon can become a digestive organ in patients with SBS. Bacteria in the colon can ferment undigested starch and fibres into short chain fatty acids, which are the preferred fuel for colonocytes. An intact colon will increase its energy absorption during the adaptive phase postoperatively by increasing the fermentation of carbohydrates.

The caloric requirement per kilogram also decreases with age, particularly after 1 year of age, which also contributes towards adapting to a shorter bowel length.

Management

The initial and primary consideration in the immediate period following extensive bowel resection[3] concerns fluid and electrolyte balance, even before calories. Gastric hypersecretion in the early period requires control with an H_2 receptor antagonist or proton pump inhibitor. Patients should be initially kept NPO (nothing by mouth) and have a nasogastric tube placed on free drainage, as well as a urinary catheter placed for monitoring fluid balance. All patients will require intravenous fluids to replace fluid losses.

Sodium and potassium chloride are the most important ions to closely monitor and replace. An infusion of normal saline (0.9%) with potassium chloride should be used to replace millilitre for millilitre measured enteral (stoma and nasogastric) fluid losses. Additional amounts of sodium and potassium may need to be given separately to avoid deficiency. Urine output should be monitored, and an adequate urine output maintained. Urinary sodium levels, where available can also be used to monitor sodium loss. A urine sodium level >30 mmol/l should be maintained.

Nutritional therapy should not be introduced until the patient is haemodynamically stable and fluid management is relatively stable, which is likely to be a few days after bowel resection.

Nearly all patients with SBS will require parenteral nutrition to survive the period while the bowel adapts. Avoidance of TPN depends on the anatomy of the remaining bowel; patients with an intact colon are the most likely to be able to survive without TPN.

Oral feeds can be started at the same time as parenteral feed and gradually increased as tolerated by the patient. Parenteral nutrition is then decreased as enteral feeding is increased.

In infants, breast milk with oral sodium and vitamin supplements can be used.

The initial oral treatment in older children should be with oral rehydration solution and a gradual introduction of carbohydrates. Children with SBS will require a diet high in calories from both fat and carbohydrates to provide sufficient calories despite malabsorption. They will also need supplements of potassium, sodium, magnesium, calcium, fat-soluble vitamins (large doses of vitamins A, D, and E), and zinc. Sodium is vital because it stimulates the bowel to absorb, promoting adaptation. Vitamin B_{12} injections are specifically required with the loss of the distal ileum.

Loperamide can be used to slow intestinal transit and decrease diarrhoea. In those patients with a stoma, effluent from the proximal bowel stoma can be introduced down the mucous fistula to promote bowel growth and adaptation of the distal bowel before stoma closure.

As feed is introduced, those patients who will tolerate enteral feeding and those who will be dependent on parenteral nutrition will become apparent. Bowel adaptation can take months or years, so survival of these patients will depend on funding for, and availability of, home parenteral nutrition.

Other medications used are cholestyramine to reduce the irritant effect of bile salts on the colon, ursodeoxycholic acid to reduce cholestasis, and intermittent use of oral antibiotics to reduce bacterial overgrowth (see algorithm in Figure 71.1).

Surgical Options

The main aims of surgery for SBS are to correct mechanical obstruction in order to decrease bacterial overgrowth, and to maximise bowel length. More recently, intestinal transplant has become a reality in selected centres worldwide. Stomas should be closed as early as possible so that all potentially functional bowel is used.

Tapering

Isolated dilated stagnant sections of bowel are a site for bacterial overgrowth. If symptoms of bacterial overgrowth are present, then dilated segments should be treated with tapering, especially in the duodenum and jejunum. This procedure involves excision of the antimesenteric border of the dilated portion of bowel. This enables more effective peristalsis, thus reducing stasis and bacterial overgrowth. Inversion placation has been used in an attempt to preserve mucosa but tends to unravel despite technical modifications such as seromuscular stripping of the inverted segment.

Bowel Lengthening

Bowel lengthening relies on the presence of dilated bowel resulting from intestinal adaptation and should therefore be reserved until 6 months to 1 year following initial bowel resection.

The two main bowel-lengthening procedures are Bianchi's longitudinal intestinal lengthening and tailoring (LILT)[4] and serial transverse entroplasty (STEP)[5].

Bianchi's LILT procedure (Figure 71.2) makes use of the bifurcation of the mesenteric vessels at the mesenteric border of the small bowel. The bowel is divided longitudinally between the mesenteric and antimesenteric borders along its dual blood supply, dividing the bowel into two limbs, each with a blood supply. These two limbs are then closed and anastomosed end to end, thus doubling that length of bowel.

In one series, 9 of 20 patients survived with this procedure, 7 of whom were able to wean off TPN. Factors associated with success were lack of liver failure and presence of at least 40 cm of intestine before the doubling procedure.

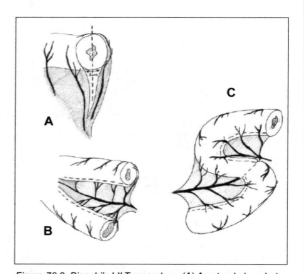

Figure 70.2: Bianchi's LILT procedure: (A) A natural plane between the leaves of the mesentery is found by dividing the bowel as shown (dotted line) and using upwards and outwards traction on the divided bowel. The bowel and mesentery are divided into two along the length so each hemisegment of bowel has a leaf of mesentery with blood supply. (B) The two hemisegments are then tubularised by using a continuous horizontal mattress 5/0 absorbable suture. (C) The opposite ends of the two new bowel segments are apposed and anastomosed in an S-shape with the bowel overlying the mesentery.

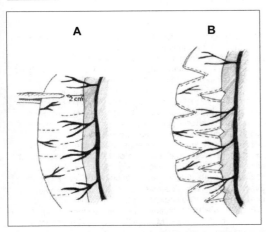

Figure 70.3: The STEP procedure: (A) A GIA stapler is used transversely across the dilated bowel from the antimesenteric border, leaving 2 cm of the bowel diameter uncut. The next cut is taken too distally this time from the antimesenteric border via a small gap created in the mesentery. (B) The GIA stapler is used down the bowel, alternating between the mesenteric and antimesenteric border as shown (dotted lines). Care is taken to keep the GIA stapler perpendicular to the mesentery to preserve the blood supply.

The STEP procedure is shown in Figure 71.3. STEP registry figures show a mean pre-STEP bowel length of 68 cm achieving a mean post-STEP bowel length of 115 cm. The percentage of enteral feeding increased from a mean of 33% preoperatively to a mean of 63% postoperatively.

Complications of bowel-lengthening procedures are high, including anastomotic and staple line leaks, bowel obstruction from adhesions or ischaemic strictures, bleeding, abscess formation, and death.

The limitations of bowel-lengthening procedures have led some authors to advocate that they should be reserved for those patients who, after 6 months of bowel adaptation, are tolerating more than half of their feeds enterally and would therefore have a greater chance of successfully becoming fully enterally fed following a lengthening procedure.

Intestinal Transplant

Intestinal transplant is offered in only a few centres worldwide. It is not an alternative to long-term TPN. It is reserved only for patients who are unable to have TPN, usually due to TPN-related liver disease or difficulty with venous access for TPN administration.

Intestinal transplant may involve (1) isolated bowel, for those with good liver function and normal motility; (2) bowel plus liver, for those with liver disease; or (3) multivisceral, which includes liver, bowel, stomach, and pancreas, for those with multiple abdominal organ failure and dysmotile bowel. The most frequent transplant performed for children with SBS is a liver plus bowel transplant. This procedure is currently limited to children weighing more than 5 kg due to the lack of size-matched donors.

Isolated liver transplants can be offered to some infants with early-onset liver failure but with sufficient bowel length such that adaptation could be expected.

The 5-year survival is approximately 70%; however, around 25% of patients die while on the waiting list for a transplant.

Prognosis and Outcomes of SBS

Long-term survival without TPN depends on the remaining bowel length. With TPN availability, survival is related to complications of TPN rather than to bowel length. The overall mortality of infants with SBS on TPN is 10–25%.

The two main causes of death and long-term morbidity in patients with short gut on TPN are liver failure and sepsis. In children, liver failure is secondary to intrahepatic cholestasis. This is most common in those who are entirely TPN dependent with no enteral feeding. It is also seen more frequently in neonates who are premature, have low birth weight, and have recurrent sepsis. The other main cause of death—septicaemia—arises because a complete lack of enteral nutrition results in bacterial overgrowth of the bowel and mucosal atrophy with impaired mucosal immunity, leading to an increased incidence of sepsis. Recurrent septicaemia is also related to central venous catheters. Early enteral feeding is therefore vital if these complications are to be reduced.

Even after discharge from hospital on full enteral feeds, infants are at risk during episodes of enteric infection, when rapid fluid and electrolyte loss may require emergency admission for intravenous rehydration. The management of a patient with SBS requires a multidisciplinary team, including paediatrician, surgeon, community nurse, dietitian, and pharmacist.

An audit of 63 patients with SBS seen at the Red Cross Children's Hospital between 1998 and 2006 revealed the following: The mean gestational age was 32 weeks (range 25–40 weeks). The most frequent causes were necrotising enterocolitis (NEC) (40%), along with intestinal atresia, midgut volvulus, intestinal aganglionosis, and gastroschisis. Overall, mortality was 36.5% (23/63). The mean number of days on parenteral nutrition was 95 (range 30–420 days).

Ethical Issues

The annual cost of care of a patient with SBS on parenteral nutrition has been estimated at between $100,000 and $150,000, making such care beyond the reach of all but a few. Treatment of patients with significant bowel loss in resource-poor settings is likely to be limited to those who attain enteral feeding quickly and have sufficient bowel function to require only increased oral calories and vitamin and mineral supplementation. There is therefore a need to counsel parents before surgery for bowel conditions that can potentially lead to short gut syndrome.

Evidence-Based Research

Table 71.2 presents a comparison of intestinal-lengthening procedures for patients with SBS.

Table 71.2: Evidence-based research.

Title	Comparison of intestinal lengthening procedures for patients with short bowel syndrome
Authors	Sudan D, Thompson J, Botha J, Grant W, Antonson D, Raynor S, Langnas A
Institution	Department of Surgery, Nebraska Medical Center, Omaha, Nebraska, USA
Reference	Ann Surg 2007; 246(4):593–601; discussion 601–604
Problem	Outcome of bowel-lengthening procedures.
Intervention	A review of the clinical results of 24 years of intestinal lengthening procedures at one institution.
Comparison/ control (quality of evidence)	A retrospective review of a single centre experience comparing the outcome of two intestinal-lengthening procedures (Bianchi and STEP) in terms of survival, total parenteral nutrition (TPN) weaning, and complications.
Outcome/ effect	This review involved 64 patients, including 14 adults, who underwent 43 Bianchi and 34 STEP procedures between 1982 and 2007. Three patients had prior isolated liver transplants. The median (range) remnant bowel length before first lengthening was 45 (11–150) cm overall (Bianchi = 44 cm; STEP = 45 cm); and 68 (20–250) cm after lengthening (Bianchi = 68 cm; STEP = 65 cm). Actual survival is 91% overall (Bianchi, 88%; STEP, 95%), with a median follow-up of 3.8 years (Bianchi = 5.9 years; STEP = 1.7 years). Average enteral caloric intake in paediatric patients was 15 kcal/kg before lengthening and 85 kcal/kg at 1 year after lengthening. Sixty-nine percent of patients were off TPN at the most recent follow-up, including 8 who were weaned from TPN after intestinal transplantation. Liver disease (when present) was reversed in 80%. Surgical complications occurred in 10%, more commonly requiring reoperation after Bianchi than STEP. Intestinal transplantation salvage was required in 14% at a median of 2.9 years (range = 8 months to 20.7 years) after lengthening.
Historical significance/ comments	Surgical lengthening with both Bianchi and STEP procedures results in improvement in enteral nutrition, reverses complications of TPN, and avoids intestinal transplantation in the majority, with few surgical complications. Intestinal transplantation can salvage most patients who later develop life-threatening complications or fail to wean TPN.

Key Summary Points

1. Short bowel syndrome may be congenital or acquired.

2. The effect of bowel resection depends on the site and length of bowel resected and the bowel remaining.

3. Intestinal adaptation takes place by means of bowel dilatation, lengthening, and thickening to increase the efficiency of absorption per unit of length.

4. Medical management is mainly supportive along with fluid and electrolyte balance, nutritional support with or without TPN, and infection control.

5. Surgical options include tapering, bowel lengthening using the Bianchi approach, the STEP procedure, or bowel transplant.

6. Long-term survival without TPN depends on the remaining bowel length. With TPN availability, survival is related to complications of TPN rather than to bowel length.

References

1. Gupte GL, Beath SV, Kelly DA, Millar AJW, Booth IW. Current issues in the management of intestinal failure. Arch Dis Child 2006; 91:259–264.

2. Duro D, Kamin D, Duggan C. Overview of pediatric short bowel syndrome. J Pediatr Gastroenterol Nutr 2008; 47(suppl 1):533–536.

3. Ching YA, Guruk K, Modi B, Jaksic T. Pediatric intestinal failure: nutrition, pharmacologic and surgical approaches. Nutr Clin Pract 2007; 22:653–663.

4. Goulet O. Short bowel syndrome in pediatric patients. Nutrition 1998; 14:784–787.

5. Bianchi A. Intestinal loop lengthening: a technique for increasing small intestinal length. J Pediatr Surg 1980;15:145–151.

6. Tannuri U. Serial transverse enteroplasty (STEP): a novel bowel lengthening procedure, and serial transverse enteroplasty for short bowel syndrome. J Pediatr Surg 2003; 38:1845–1846.

CHAPTER 72
GAASTROINTESTINAL STOMAS IN CHILDREN

Osarumwense David Osifo
Johanna R. Askegard-Giesmann
Benedict C. Nwomeh

Introduction

A stoma (or ostomy) is the deliberate creation of an opening that communicates between the GIT and the exterior. The purpose could be for feeding, drug administration, bowel decompression, protecting distal anastomosis or other gut lesions, controlling faecal effluent in some cases of incontinence, or a combination of these indications. The basic types of stomas derive their names from the gastointestinal segment in which they are sited. For example, gastrostomy is sited in the stomach, jejunostomy in the jejunum, ileostomy in the ileum, and colostomy in the colon. Stomas may be categorised on the basis of the purpose for their creation; specific examples of commonly used stomas in children are shown in Table 72.1.

The use and management of gastrointestinal stomas in children has evolved since the early success with colostomy formation in the 1800s. Improved surgical techniques, better understanding of the physiologic and psychological consequences of intestinal stomas, and advances in stoma care have contributed to a more rational use by paediatric surgeons and a wider acceptance in the medical and lay communities.[1,2].

Although creating a stoma may be life saving and necessary to maintain a child's health, the affected child and the child's family or caregivers need to understand why the surgeon is considering stoma creation and should have some input. They need to understand what a stoma is, why it is necessary, and how it will function.[3] It is also important that the child and the family understand the difficulties or complications that can be encountered. Discussions with the child's school during the planning phase can also be helpful, as this can ensure the child's smooth reintegration after surgery. The creation of a permanent stoma may need to be discussed openly, as some children and their families may believe that stoma creation is only a temporary measure.[3]

Common Types of Gastrointestinal Stomas

A good stoma is best obtained by careful preoperative planning, meticulous surgical technique, and detailed attention to skin care. Different types of stomas are created for a variety of clinical reasons. Colostomy, the most common enterostoma used in children in sub-Saharan Africa, is discussed in greater detail in this chapter.

Gastrostomy

Gastrostomy is the creation of an opening between the stomach and the skin for the purpose of feeding, drug administration, and proximal decompression of the GIT. Other clinical scenarios that may require a gastrostomy include oesophageal obstruction due to corrosive oesophageal stricture, severe maxillofacial trauma, achalasia of the cardia, and oesophageal carcinoma (in adults). A gastrostomy tube is most commonly placed by using the standard Stamm technique, but percutaneous endoscopic gastrostomy (PEG) and laparoscopic insertion are being introduced in a few centres.

Table 72.1: Categories of stomas with specific examples of common types in children.

Groups/purpose of enterostoma	Specific examples
Stomas created without entering through bowel wall	Nasogastric tube Nasogastrojejunal tube Nasojejunal tube Rectal tube Colonic tube
Minimally invasive stomas through bowel wall	Tunneled catheter Needle catheter T-tube Button, etc.
Isolated jejunal loop brought to abdominal wall	Roux-en-Y loop
Proximal decompression with distal loop for feeding	Nasogastric/nasojejunal tubes Double-barrel jejunostomy Double-barrel ileostomy
Antegrade irrigation and decompression	Caecostomy through appendix stump Catheter placement, T-tube, etc.
Colonic decompression, faecal/flatus diversion or evacuation	End stoma, single opening Double-barrel stomas End stoma with anastomosis below abdominal wall. Loop over a small rod or skin bridge. Open loop with occluding valve, T-tube device, etc. Catheterisable pouch

Jejunostomy/Ileostomy

Stomas of the small bowel are commonly used for feeding, bowel decompression, or diversion of distal disease. Specific indications include

- bypass of gastric outlet obstruction;

- protection of distal anastomosis;

- as a life-saving diversion procedure in clinically compromised children with obstructive distal bowel lesions; and

- to rest and/or decompress distal bowel in cases of perforation and severe enterocolitis with surgical complications.

Colostomy

Colostomy is a stoma of the colon with the aim of diverting faeces and flatus. It is the most common stoma used in children. Indications for creation of a colostomy may be either congenital or acquired.

Congenital indications are more common and include high anorectal anomalies and Hirschsprung's disease. More rare congenital indications are rectovesical/rectovaginal fistula, cloacal exstrophy, and severe spina bifida with incontinence. Colostomy may also be beneficial for faecal diversion prior to resection of large congenital intrapelvic masses.

Acquired indications include bowel perforation, high fissure-in-ano, severe perineal traumas, posttrauma paralysis, and to protect distal anastomoses (such as coloanal anastomosis of pull-through procedures).

Classifications of Stomas

Stomas may be classified by using temporal, anatomical, or constructional criteria.

Temporal Stomas

Temporal classification is based on the anticipated duration of the stoma and is either temporary or permanent. Most stomas in children are temporary and are reversed as soon as possible. Permanent stomas may be necessary for patients with spinal cord injury and resultant paralysis or severe spina bifida.

Anatomical Stomas

Anatomical classification is based on the anatomical portion of the colon in which the stoma is sited. Examples include sigmoid colostomy, when sited in the sigmoid colon; transverse colostomy, when sited in the transverse colon, which can be further subdivided into right-transverse, mid-transverse, and left-transverse colostomy; and caecostomy, when sited in the caecum.

Constructional Stomas

Constructional classification is based on how the stoma is constructed, and is of two major types: loop colostomy and divided colostomy.

Loop colostomy

An opening is made on the antimesenteric border of the colon without completely dividing it. A loop colostomy does not interrupt colon continuity and allows faecal material to pass beyond the stoma. Because some enteric material still enters the distal bowel, it is in essence a non-defunctioning stoma.[1] The stoma may be looped over a rod to prevent retraction. Loop colostomies are easy to create and are quite useful in clinically compromised children when prolonged anaesthesia is undesirable. Loop ostomies are associated with a higher rate of complications; therefore, most paediatric surgeons prefer divided stomas.[4]

Divided colostomy

In the divided stoma, the bowel is completely divided and the bowel continuity interrupted. Because intestinal content does not enter the distal bowel, divided stomas are also called defunctioning stomas. Divided stomas may be further subclassified based on what the surgeon does with the proximal and distal limbs. The most common variations are the double-barrel, Devine, and end stomas.

Stomas in which the distal limb is brought to the surface permit the release of secreted mucus, and provide access for contrast studies for the diagnosis of distal lesions and to assess the patency and integrity of the distal bowel before stoma closure. With end stomas, care must be taken to avoid leaving a Hartmann's pouch in which complete drainage through the anus is prevented by an obstructing lesion within the distal bowel. In such cases, mucous distention of bowel above the obstruction may lead to perforation of the Hartmann's pouch.

Double-barrel stoma

Both the proximal and distal limbs may or may not be plicated together but are brought out side-by-side through the same wound like a double-barrel gun. The proximal limb discharges faeces and flatus, and the distal limb discharges mucus. If the two ends are brought too close together, or are included in a single stoma pouch, enteric contents may pass into the distal bowel, and such a stoma may not be completely defunctioning.

Devine stoma

In a Devine stoma, both proximal and distal limbs are brought out separately, sometimes through different incisions, and are separated by a skin bridge. When complete diversion of stool from the distal bowel is desired, this type of stoma is preferred over the double-barrel variety.

End stoma

Here the proximal limb is brought out to evacuate faeces and flatus, and the distal limb is closed or oversewn and returned to the peritoneal cavity. The blind distal bowel, the Hartmann's pouch, opens distally into the anus.

Complications of Gastrointestinal Stomas

Major complications could occur in up to 75% of children following colostomy or ileostomy, with an overall revision rate of approximately 15% (Table 72.2). Skin complications, such as dermatitis, granuloma, and ulceration, are the most frequent problems with ostomies. Most surgeons in Africa will not have access to dedicated enterostomal therapists, and therefore they need to be knowledgeable in the care of stomas and in the prevention and management of skin problems and other complications.

Stomas made in the small intestine (enterostomas) are associated with more complications than colostomies. In addition, transverse colostomies cause more problems than sigmoid colostomies. With temporary stomas, the occurrence of complications should prompt consideration for closure of the ostomy, rather than revision.

Table 72.2: Stoma complications in children.

Complication	Incidence (%)
Ischaemia/necrosis	<1
Stenosis/stricture	3–6
Retraction	2–4
Prolapse	12–24
Parastomal hernia	1
Skin excoriation	20–30
Bleeding	1–10
Obstruction	1–6

Source: Nwomeh B. Reoperation for Stoma Complications. In: Teich S, Caniano DA, eds. Reoperative Pediatric Surgery. Humana Press, 2008, Pp 279–285.

Skin Excoriation

Skin excoriation is one of the most common complications following colostomy creation. It usually occurs due to (1) continuous wetting of the surrounding skin by effluent, which results in maceration; (2) allergic reaction to effluent; (3) enzymatic digestion of macerated tissues; and (4) bacterial and fungal growth on the macerated exposed tissues. It is graded from 1 to 4, depending on the depth of excoriation. Management includes using a properly fitted colostomy bag, applying zinc oxide paste to the skin (or petroleum jelly when zinc oxide paste is not available), and keeping the skin dry as much as possible. In severe cases, it may be necessary to revise or relocate the stoma.

Wound Infection

Wound infection is most common when the stoma is sited within the main incision. To reduce the incidence of postoperative infection, the stoma should be placed at a separate location. Treatment is usually with antibiotics and good peristomal skin care. Drainage may be necessary if an abscess develops.

Retraction

Retraction occurs when the stoma retracts back to the peritoneal cavity. It is important to identify the cause of stomal retraction. The most common problem is undue tension on the stoma because the proximal bowel and its mesentery had not been adequately mobilised. Anchoring the bowel to the fascia with sutures cannot be relied upon to prevent retraction of the stoma because it does not mitigate the tension in the bowel. A second cause is stomal necrosis. Also, retraction may be due to prolonged serositis with subsequent shortening of bowel when the stoma has not been matured. The retracted stoma causes leakage of intestinal contents, which may interfere with the secure application of the appliance.

Revision of the retracted stoma is usually required. The retracted stoma is often fixed in position and the goal is to mobilise sufficient length of bowel and mesentery so that maturation of the stoma can be accomplished without tension. Additional mobilisation of bowel often requires a laparotomy, and limited bowel resection is performed to remove an ischaemic or stenotic segment. If the retracted stoma is sufficiently mobile to allow the bowel to be everted, the bowel walls can be fixed together by inserting several interrupted absorbable sutures with full thickness bites. The new stoma should be matured at the same site, except when retraction has resulted in significant skin excoriation or abdominal wall sepsis; in these cases, a new ostomy site should be established.[4]

If available, several firings of a noncutting linear stapler (e.g., the GIA stapler without the blade) will simplify the procedure (Figure 72.1). Adhesion between the serosal surfaces of the everted stoma will usually have occurred before the sutures are absorbed. The stapling technique involves the following steps:

1. The stoma is retracted to its full extent by placing three pairs of Babcock's forceps (not shown in Figure 72.1).

2. A noncutting linear stapler (without the blade) is placed with the jaws toward the mucocutaneous junction between the Babcock forceps. Care is taken to avoid the mesentery before firing the stapler.

3. Three parallel rows of staples fix the two walls of the ileum together.

Prolapse

Stoma prolapse is a common and often frightening and distressing complication to the child and family. Loop stomas are more likely than end stomas to prolapse, and the distal segment of the loop stoma is most frequently affected. It often begins as a prolapse of the mucosa through the stoma, subsequently extending to the entire circumference of the bowel. Prolapse usually occurs when a skin opening is made to accommodate dilated bowel, which, upon shrinking, leaves a loose stoma. It may also be caused by inadequate fixation of the mesentery to the parietal peritoneum. A prolapsed stoma may be traumatised by desiccation or by an ill-fitting appliance, which may lead to mucosal ulceration and bleeding. In the early stage, spontaneous or manual reduction is usually possible, but in cases of persistent prolapse, intestinal obstruction, or strangulated bowel, surgical intervention is required.

For temporary relief, a nonabsorbable monofilament material (polypropylene or nylon) is used to place a simple purse-string suture, similar to the Thiersch technique for rectal prolapse (Figure 72.2). If this procedure is used in permanent stomas, however, the fixed ring may produce stenosis as the child grows. The procedure for the purse-string suture technique follows:

1. A 1-cm skin incision is made at the medial angle of the stoma down to the subcutaneous tissue (Figure 72.2(A)).

2. A finger is inserted into the stoma as a guide, and a 1-0 monofilament nonabsorbable suture with a round cutting needle is passed around the colostomy, staying within the subcutaneous layer (Figure 72.2(B)). The needle is placed as far as it can comfortably go, usually about a quarter of the circumference, then brought out through the skin.

3. The needle is passed again through the same skin exit site toward the lateral corner (Figure 72.2(C)).

4. One or two more passes of the needle are made as it marches circumferentially around the stoma until it is brought out through the medial incision. With a finger remaining in the lumen, the suture is tied, causing puckering of the stoma without completely occluding the lumen (Figure 72.2(D)).

Another technique for temporary control of prolapsed stoma, described by Gauderer,[5] involves the placement of a "U" stitch from the lumen of the reduced bowel through the abdominal wall with a double-armed needle (Figure 72.3). Before tying the suture ends, each needle is passed through a pledget, thus creating an internal and external bolster that attaches the bowel to the body wall and prevents the suture from cutting through. The pledget made from a rubber catheter may be used. This technique has the following steps:

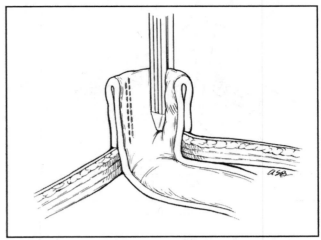

Source: Nwomeh BC. Reoperation for stoma complications. In: Teich S, Caniano DA, eds. Reoperative Pediatric Surgery. Humana Press, 2008. Reproduced with permission.

Figure 72.1: The stapling technique for fixation of a retracted stoma. See text for procedure.

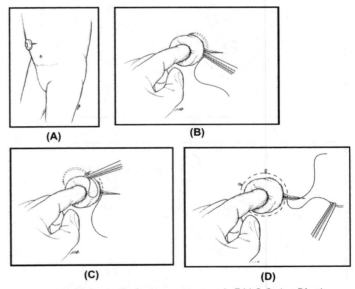

Source: Nwomeh BC. Reoperation for stoma complications. In: Teich S, Caniano DA, eds. Reoperative Pediatric Surgery. Humana Press, 2008. Reproduced with permission.

Figure 72.2: Purse-string suture technique for correcting prolapsed stoma. See text for procedure.

1. The prolapse is reduced with a gentle inward pressure (Figure 72.3(A)).

2. A double-armed 3-0 nonabsorbable monofilament suture is used. One needle is placed through a latex bolster (or pledget) and a second needle is passed 2–3 cm into the reduced limb of the stoma, then through the bowel wall and out the abdominal wall an equal distance from the stoma. The needle is then placed through a separate bolster (Figure 72.3(B)).

3. The suture is tied without undue tension, sandwiching the bowel and abdominal wall between the bolsters (Figure 72.3(C)). The inset in the figure shows the bowel adherent to the abdominal wall following removal of the bolsters 2 weeks later.

Definitive relief may require resection of the prolapsed bowel and fixation of the mesentery. This procedure usually requires reopening the main abdominal incision. A prolapsed loop ostomy may be divided with the closed distal end returned into the abdomen, thereby converting the loop to an end ostomy that is less likely to prolapse. When appropriate, closure of the ostomy is the best option.[4]

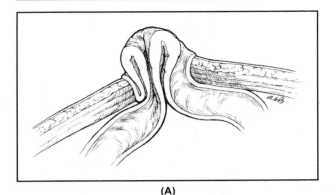

(A)

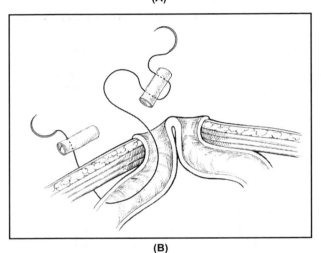

(B)

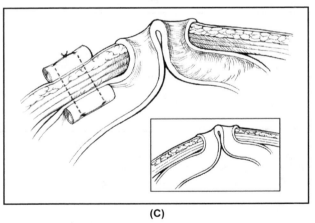

(C)

Source: Nwomeh BC. Reoperation for stoma complications. In: Teich S, Caniano DA, eds. Reoperative Pediatric Surgery. Humana Press, 2008. Reproduced with permission.

Figure 72.3: An alternative technique for temporary control of prolapse of one limb of a looped ostomy. See text for procedure.

Colostomy Dehiscence

When prolapse occurs before the colostomy is matured (a minimum of 2 weeks after formation), it may detach from the skin and allow evisceration of the intraabdominal content. This is a serious complication that requires emergency revision.

Ischaemia or Necrosis

The complication of significant ischaemia or frank necrosis is apparent early in the postoperative period. The cause is devascularisation from excessive stripping of the mesentery, venous congestion due to tension on the bowel, or a tight fascial opening. Some degree of oedema and venous congestion normally occurs with new stomas, especially if previously distended bowel is used, but this usually resolves within 48

hours. If mucosal necrosis is limited to the portion superficial to the fascia, an expectant approach may be employed, but the stoma should be monitored closely for progressive necrosis or subsequent development of stenosis, stricture, or retraction.[4]

Haemorrhage

Bleeding may occur from the mucosa or the stoma edge itself. Haemorrhage may occur postoperatively due to dislodgement of a clot or suture following crying or an increase in blood pressure when adequate haemostasis was not achieved in the operating room. Pressure with a gauze pad is usually sufficient to control the bleeding, but endoscopy or operative intervention may be necessary. Areas of the abdominal wall with major vessels, such as epigastric vessels, should be avoided when choosing the stoma site.

Stoma Stenosis or Stricture

Stenosis or stricture of the stoma may occur at the skin or fascial level and is clinically apparent as reduced stoma output or frank bowel obstruction. This may occur when the skin or fascial opening is tight, leading to ischaemia at the mucocutaneous junction. If the stoma had not been matured, prolonged serositis with subsequent fibrosis may also lead to stenosis. Serial dilatation with anal (or Hegar) dilators may resolve the obstruction, but this procedure carries the risk of bowel perforation. In many cases, a formal surgical revision is needed.

High Stoma Output

Excessive stoma output occurs in more proximal stomas. Stoma losses can cause profound fluid and electrolyte derangement. Adequate monitoring and replacement of losses are important.

Faecal Impaction

Faecal impaction should prompt the evaluation for stomal stenosis. It may be relieved with enemas administered through the stoma or by manual disimpaction, which should be done under sedation or general anaesthesia.

Parastomal Hernia

A parastomal hernia is a herniation that occurs at the site of the colostomy (Figure 72.4). Parastomal hernia appears to occur less frequently in children than in adult patients, with an incidence of less than 1%. The most likely cause is the creation of a fascial aperture relatively larger than the bowel used for the ostomy. Other factors predisposing to parastomal hernia include wound infection, malnutrition, and obesity. Fortunately, more serious complications, such as intestinal obstruction and strangulation, are rare. The stoma appliance is more difficult to retain, and persistent leakage may occur. In such cases, operative repair should be considered. The simplest procedure is to mobilise the stoma, repair the hernia snugly around the bowel, and then mature the ostomy at the same site. Alternatively, the hernia could be repaired and the stoma relocated to another site. It is often best to relocate or close the stoma because recurrence is frequent after local revision.[4]

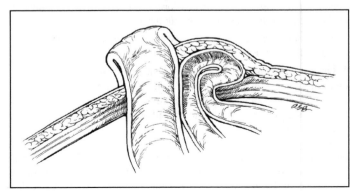

Source: Nwomeh BC. Reoperation for stoma complications. In: Teich S, Caniano DA, eds. Reoperative Pediatric Surgery. Humana Press, 2008. Reproduced with permission.

Figure 72.4: Parastomal hernia, with a bulge in the abdominal wall to one side of the stoma.

Other Complications

Peritonitis may be a caused by early stoma retraction or wound infection and may lead to intraperitoneal abscess, particularly in neonates. Antibiotic treatment or operative drainage may be indicated. Bowel obstruction may occur due to improper alignment and twisting at the time of stoma construction. This requires urgent surgical correction to prevent necrosis and resection and possible sepsis.

Exteriorisation of the wrong bowel segment may occur. For example, the small intestine may be mistakenly used instead of the colon, or the distal limb of the colon may be used as the stoma while the proximal limb is closed and returned to the peritoneal cavity as the Hartmann's pouch. When performing a left-sided colostomy, it is recommended to place a rectal tube to aid the identification of the colon. The problem usually manifests as a complete bowel obstruction and requires immediate surgical correction.

Other, less serious complications include granulation and/or polyp formation and ulceration. These are typically managed with local cauterisation therapies and observation. Psychological trauma, which may be a serious problem for families and school-age children, can be mitigated by adequate preoperative counselling and constant support.

Stoma Care

In most African hospitals, specialised nurses, such as enterostomal therapists, are not available. The paediatric surgeon is therefore the primary source of care and support for children with stomas and their families.

Management at Home

Children and their families adapt to stomas in various ways. Adequate planning by families is needed, and older children should be incorporated into care planning for their stomas. The use of an adequate size stoma bag is important to prevent the effluent from making contact with the skin. The nonavailability of stoma bags for children with colostomy is a major problem in this subregion. Some innovation may be needed, given the resources available locally. For example, a cut-off leg portion of a thick cotton pant slid over a soft napkin can be applied over the stoma.[6] This must be cleaned regularly to reduce offensive odour, and zinc oxide paste or petroleum jelly should be applied to protect the peristomal skin.

Management at School

The psychological effect on the school-age child is important. Some children will be open and discuss the stoma with their friends and classmates, but others may choose to conceal it. In some cases, however, the whole class and schoolmates may be told about the child's stoma so as to avoid subjecting the child to manual labour and overzealous play and physical contact in the playground. The child should be taught how to change the stoma bag and clean it regularly, even at school, to reduce offensive odour.

Stoma Closure

In temporary stomas, closure is imperative to restore bowel continuity as the last step in the treatment of the child. Provided there is no distal obstruction, the majority of tube stomas require no surgical closure. Removal of the tube (e.g., gastrostomy tube) with pressure dressing applied over the stoma results in spontaneous closure in most cases. However, if a persistent gastrocutaneous fistula develops, surgical closure is indicated.

Stomas should be closed when the underlying condition has resolved. Although there is no urgency to the timing of stoma closure, the psychological stress and cost of providing stoma care should be considered. A contrast study (distal loopogramme) and/or endoscopic assessment of the distal bowel may be done to ascertain normalcy (and patency) before closure. In cases of Hirschsprung's disease and anorectal anomalies, a stoma is usually in place at the time of definitive pull-through. After the anastomosis has healed, it is helpful to begin anal dilatation for up to a week before stoma closure. As mentioned previously, the occurrence of complications in temporary stomas should prompt consideration for closure of the ostomy rather than revision.

Complications of closure include:

1. wound infection;
2. anastomotic leak;
3. enterocutaneous fistula;
4. stenosis/stricture at the site of anastomosis;
5. intestinal obstruction; and
6. abdominal scars.

Evidence-Based Research

Table 72.3 presents a retrospective review of colostomy complications in children.

Table 72.3: Evidence-based research.

Title	Colostomy complications in children
Authors	Mollittt DL, Malangoni MA, Ballantine TV, Grosfeld JL
Institution	James Whitcomb Riley Hospital for Children, Indianapolis, Indiana, USA
Reference	Arch Surg 1980; 115:455–458
Problem	Intestinal stomas.
Comparison/ control (quality of evidence)	Single institution retrospective review.
Outcome/ effect	Analysis of 146 paediatric patients with colostomies, specifically related to formation, management, and subsequent closure of colostomies. The majority of the colostomies were performed for congenital diseases (Hirschsprung's and imperforate anus). There were more loop colostomies than divided colostomies, but also more complications noted with loop versus divided colostomies. No deaths were related to colostomy closure. Sigmoid colostomies were associated with the lowest rate of complications.
Historical significance/ comments	This study underscores the importance of location and type of colostomy (specifically sigmoid colostomy), attention to technical details, principles of stoma care, and proper instruction for parents in minimising complications from colostomies.

Key Summary Points

1. Gastrointestinal stomas are rare in children.

2. Stomas are typically created in emergency surgery situations, but may be necessary in the treatment of congenital abnormalities.

3. Stomas may be classified as temporary or permanent, as well as by where they occur in the intestinal tract.

4. Divided stomas are more common in paediatric patients and tend to have a lower risk of complications compared to loop ileostomies or colostomies.

5. The majority of complications from gastrointestinal stomas require some surgical intervention; however, initial nonoperative management is often appropriate.

6. Prolapse or retraction of temporary stomas may best be treated by restoring intestinal continuity, if possible, rather than revision of the stoma.

References

1. Gauderer MWL. Stomas of the small and large intestine. In: O'Neill JA, Rowe MI, Grosfeld JI, Fonkalsrud EW, Coran GA, eds. Pediatric Surgery, 5th ed. Mosby Year Book, 1998, Pp 1349–1359.

2. Minkes RK, Mazziotti MV, Langer JC. Stomas of the small and large intestine. eMedicine Specialties→Pediatrics: Surgery→General Surgery. Available at emedicine.medscape.com/article/939455-overview. Accessed 26 June 2009.

3. Sanders C, Bray L. Managing children with stomas. Charter Stoma Care. Hayward Medical Communications, 2007; 29:9–10.

4. Nwomeh B. Reoperation for Stoma Complications. In: Teich S, Caniano DA, eds. Reoperative Pediatric Surgery. Humana Press, 2008, Pp 279–285.

5. Gauderer MW, Izant Jr RJ. A technique for temporary control of colostomy prolapse in children. J Pediatr Surg 1985; 20(6):653–655.

6. Osifo OD, Osaigbovo EO, Obeta EC. Colostomy in children: indications and common problems in Benin City, Nigeria. Pak J Med Sci 2008; 24:199–203.

COLON, RECTUM, AND ANUS

CHAPTER 73
COLONIC ATRESIA

Alastair J. Millar
Sharon Cox
Kokila Lakhoo

Introduction

Atresia of the colon is an uncommon entity distinct from congenital pouch colon, which is a more frequent occurrence in India and Asia, and is associated with anorectal malformations. Although the underlying cause of colonic atresia may be vascular insufficiency, the association with Hirschsprung's disease, in particular, and the gross discrepancy between the proximal and distal bowel diameters militate against management strategies described for small bowel atresias.

Demographics

Atresia of the colon is a relatively rare form of intestinal atresia with an incidence of 1:40,000–60,000 live births, comprising less than 5% of the total number of gastrointestinal tract atresias. (In the Red Cross War Memorial Children's Hospital series of 316 bowel atresias distal to the duodenum, the incidence was 4.4%.) There is no gender or racial predilection for the abnormality. There is, however, an association with gastroschisis, malrotation/nonfixation of the bowel, a more proximal atresia of the small bowel and Hirschsprung's disease. The association with cloacal exstrophy is well known but will not be described here.

Aetiology/Pathophysiology

The association with gastroschisis and intestinal atresia is considered a result of a vascular accident in utero. It is not clear why aganglionosis is found in some. It may be that the dilated loop proximal to the transition to aganglionosis undergoes volvulus with bowel ischaemic injury and thus the development of atresia, or it may suggest an early event whereby migrating nerve cells are arrested in their progress to populate the distal gut. This implies an early gestational interruption.

Clinical Presentation

History

In the situation of an isolated atresia, patients present with neonatal intestinal obstruction and gross abdominal distention. A pitfall to be avoided is that with colonic atresia distal to a small bowel atresia, the colon in outward appearance may look normal. It is therefore essential for the colon to be evaluated in any small bowel atresia, preferably preoperatively, by contrast enema. The abdominal x-ray is typical in showing one or two very dilated gas- and fluid-filled loops.

Physical

Aspiration of gastric content of a volume >25 ml via orogastric or nasogastric tube, or emesis that is bile stained along with abdominal distention and failure to pass normal meconium are suggestive of a distal bowel obstruction.

Investigations

Abdominal x-ray is essential (Figure 73.1), and contrast enema (Figure 73.2) prior to surgery is advisable. Rectal suction biopsy to exclude Hirschsprung's disease is mandatory if primary anastomosis is contemplated.

Management

Management should include full investigation for associated anomalies, exclusion of Hirschsprung's disease and a second atresia or stenosis by biopsy of the bowel distal to the atresia, and contrast enema. The fashioning of a stoma at the level of the atresia is the preferred initial treatment rather than an attempt at primary anastomosis. The gross dilatation of the blind end (Figures 73.1 and 73.3) may need to be tapered or resected to assist in fashioning a manageable stoma.

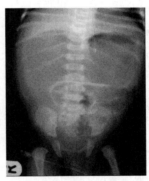

Figure 73.1: Anteroposterior abdominal radiograph showing disproportionately large loops of bowel.

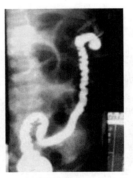

Figure 73.2: Barium enema of patient showing sigmoid atresia and distal microcolon.

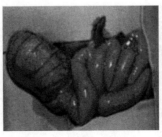

Figure 73.3: Operative photograph of patient with sigmoid atresia, showing dilated transverse colon.

Postoperative Complications

Missed diagnosis should not occur if the principles stated above are followed. In our series of 14 cases, there was one mortality due to a second colonic atresia, which was missed in a patient presenting with a small bowel atresia, causing a leak from the more proximal anastomosis, peritonitis, and death.

Prognosis and Outcomes

Outcomes should be good but are limited by associated intestinal atresias with short gut and the extent of other anomalies. Mortality in various series ranges from 7% to 61%. The type of surgery as well as coexistent pathology are major determinants of outcome, with initial primary anastomosis frequently being associated with complications and a poor outcome.

As in any resource-poor environment, the need for parenteral nutrition may be the major determinant for survival.

Evidence-Based Research

Tables 73.1 and 73.2 present studies on intestinal atresias and atresias of the colon, respectively.

Table 73.1: Evidence-based research.

Title	Colonic atresia: spectrum of presentation and pitfalls in management: a review of 14 cases
Authors	Cox SG, Numanoglu A, Millar AJW, Rode H
Institution	Department of Paediatric Surgery, Red Cross War Memorial Children's Hospital, Cape Town, South Africa
Reference	Ped Surg Int, 2005; 10:813–818
Problem	This study describes a case series of 14 patients with colonic atresia.
Intervention	This study seeks to identify predictors of untoward outcomes.
Comparison/ control (quality of evidence)	Fourteen cases of colonic atresia seen over a 38-year period are reviewed with particular reference to clinical presentation and pitfalls in management. Seven had Type I atresia, two had Type II and five had Type IIIa. Ten had associated gastrointestinal anomalies. Management varied considerably. Six had primary colonic anastomosis. Two of these developed complications due to unrecognized distal hypoganglionosis, two had associated jejunal atresias resulting in short bowel syndrome, and two had primary anastomosis protected by proximal ileostomies. Seven had a staged repair with initial defunctioning enterostomy, with only one complication, an unfixed mesentery that later resulted in midgut volvulus. The only mortality was a patient in which a jejunal atresia repair leaked as a result of a missed colonic atresia. Operative strategy should depend on the clinical state of the patients, the level of atresia, associated small bowel pathology and exclusion of distal pathology.
Outcome/ effect	Primary anastomosis would only rarely be advised with a circumspect approach. Long-term outlook, as in small bowel atresia, is generally excellent.

Table 73.2: Evidence-based research.

Title	Atresia of the colon
Authors	Etensel B, Temir G, Karkiner A, Melek M, Edirne Y, Karaca I, Mir E
Institution	Department of Pediatric Surgery, Adnan Menderes University, Aydin, Turkey
Reference	J Pediatr Surg 2005; 40(8):1258–1268
Historical significance/ comments	Colonic atresia (CA) is one of the rarest causes of neonatal intestinal obstructions, and no large series can be reported. Therefore, a retrospective clinical trial was performed to delineate our CA cases and carry out a literature survey. We reviewed the charts of CA cases treated in our center between 1992 and 2002. We aimed to collect all reported cases in Medline, and personal communications with the authors of published series were used to reach the missing data.

The chart review revealed 9 newborns with CA treated in our center (6 cases of type III, 2 cases of type II, and 1 case of type IV). These accounted for 3.7% of all gastrointestinal atresias managed in our center. Of the CA cases, 3 were isolated and 6 had at least one or more associated congenital anomalies. The preferred surgical technique at the initial treatment of CA was performing a proximal stoma and distal mucous fistula in an average of 59.4 hours postnatal. The literature survey enabled us to reach 224 cases of CA, including our cases.

Because of the low incidence of CA generally, delay in diagnosis and treatment may occur. The mortality is statistically higher when the surgical management is performed after 72 hours of age. However, the prognosis of CA is satisfactory if diagnosis and surgical management can be made promptly and properly. |

Key Summary Points

1. A very large dilated loop with a fluid level on abdominal x-ray is suspicious.

2. Beware the second atresia in the colon of a patient with a small bowel atresia and perform a preoperative contrast enema to rule this out.

3. Exclude Hirschprung's disease distal to the atresia.

4. Avoid primary anastomosis.

5. Note the association with nonrotation of the midgut.

Suggested Reading

Akgur FM, Cahit T. Colonic atresia and Hirschsprung's disease association shows further evidence for migration of the enteric neurons. J Pediatr Surg 1993; 26(4):635–636.

Benson CD, Lotf MW, et al. Congenital atresia and stenosis of the colon. J Pediatr Surg 1968; 3(2):253–257.

Boles ET, Vassy LE, et al. Atresia of the colon. J Pediat Surg 1976; 11(1): 69–75.

Cox S, Numanoglu A, Millar AJW, Rode H. Colonic atresia: spectrum of presentation and pitfalls in management: a review of 14 cases. Ped Surg Int 2005; 10:813–818.

Davenport M, Bianchi A, et al. Colonic atresia: current results of treatment. J R Coll Surg Edin 1990; 35(1):25–28.

Erskine JM. Colonic stenosis in the newborn: the possible thromboembolic aetiology of intestinal stenosis and atresia. J Pediatr Surg 1970; 5(3):321–333.

Fishman SJ, Islam S, et al. Non-fixation of an atresic colon predicts Hirschsprung's disease. J Pediatr Surg 2001; 36(1):202–204.

Harbour MJ, Donald MD, et al. Congenital atresia of the colon. Radiol 1965; 84:19–23.

Harris J, Kallen B, et al. Descriptive epidemiology of alimentary tract atresia. Teratology 1995; 52:15–29.

Landes A, Schuckett B, et al. Non-fixation of the colon in colonic atresia: a new finding. Pediatr Radiol 1994; 24:167–169.

Louw JH, Barnard CN. Congenital intestinal atresia: observations on its origin. Lancet 1955; ii:1065–1067.

Millar AJW, Rode H, Cywes S. Intestinal atresia and stenosis, 3rd ed. Pediatr Surg Ashcraft 2000; 30:406–424.

Moore SW, Rode H, et al. Intestinal atresia and Hirschsprung's disease. Pediatr Surg Int 1990; 5:182–184.

Peter CW, Riccardo A, et al. Colonic atresia combined with Hirschsprung's disease: a diagnostic and therapeutic challenge. J Pediatr Surg 1995; 30(8):1216–1217.

Pohlson EC, Hatch EI, et al. Individualized management of colonic atresia. Amer J Surg 1988; 155:690–692.

CHAPTER 74
APPENDICITIS

Behrouz Banieghbal
Kokila Lakhoo

Introduction

Acute appendicitis is the commonest and one of the most important causes of intraabdominal surgical conditions in children, particularly in adolescents. The time-honoured tradition of appendectomy through a midline or Lanz incision is considered to be the one basic requirement for trainee surgeons in both adult and paediatric surgical practice. Depending on the pathology of the appendix, acute appendicitis is divided into either simple or complicated appendicitis, with perforation and/or abscess formation occurring in the latter.

Demographics

In most First World countries, the lifetime incidence of appendicitis is considered to be around 7%, with a slightly higher incidence in males, and more than half occurring in childhood. In Africa, the incidence of appendicitis is much less, with a reported lifetime incidence rate of <1%.[1,2] This is probably due to the higher amount of fibre in the African diet compared to the refined food diet of Western Europe and North America.[3]

Although the condition is relatively uncommon during infancy and early childhood, a disproportionately higher incidence of complicated appendicitis occurs in children <5 years of age, potentially due to late presentation and difficulties in establishing an early diagnosis.

Pathophysiology

Most authors believe that the cause of appendicitis is intraluminal obstruction caused by lymphoid hyperplasia, parasite-infected faecal matter and ingested foreign bodies.[4] This may explain the increased rate in teenagers, as the submucosal lymphoid tissue reaches its peak number in adolescence followed by a gradual decrease after age of 30 years. Once the lumen is obstructed, mucus and bacterial proliferation result in venous congestion, which in turn will cause arterial flow obstruction, ischaemia, necrosis, and free perforation into the peritoneal cavity. The human defense system of omentum often wraps itself around the organ and limits the free perforation and result in appendix mass formation.

Clinical Presentation

Just as for most human diseases, the diagnosis of acute appendicitis can usually be made on careful history and clinical evaluation. The need for an appendectomy is usually based on the diagnosis of acute appendicitis, which is made on clinical grounds in most cases. Medical students are taught to look for a history that classically includes anorexia without vomiting, and umbilical pain that then moves to the right iliac fossa.

Once localized, any movement causes exacerbation of the pain, which is described as sharp in nature. Fever is usually low grade unless perforation has occurred, in which case there is generalized peritonitis and high fever. Other classic signs are that of rebound tenderness, which is best elicited with gentle "tapping" over the right iliac fossa. However, in obese children and patients with retrocaecal appendicitis, the signs are often absent or equivocal in nature.

Complicated appendicitis occurs as a result of perforated appendix with or without abscess formation. Physical findings may reveal diffuse peritonitis or a tender right lower quadrant mass, which is due to an organized abscess. It is more common to have diffuse peritonitis in young children because they have less omental fat to isolate the infection. Older children are more likely to have an appendiceal abscess. However, simple appendicitis may not always be differentiated from complicated cases prior to surgery. Diagnostic laparoscopy and appendectomy can be employed when the preoperative diagnosis of appendicitis is uncertain.[5]

Investigation

Most surgeons request blood tests and expect to find an elevated white cell count, with a disproportionately elevated neutrophil percentage and a high C-reactive protein. A urine dipstick is also done, which, in the case of appendicitis, should show no or a few red cells and white cells.

Plain abdominal x-ray is usually not helpful but may show a faecolith (Figure 74.1), dilated sentinel small loop, relative absence of bowel gas in the right iliac fossa, mild scoliosis, and even free air under the right subdiaphragm.

Sonar and computed tomography (CT) scans are done more frequently than x-rays, especially in academic and private hospitals worldwide to identify and decrease the rate of negative appendectomies. Shortcomings are due to lack of expertise and experience of the radiologists performing the sonar and the expense and radiation concern (and safety consideration for intravenous contrast material) used for CT scans. However, a good-quality CT scan has a very high sensitivity and specificity in children (>95%)[6] (see Figure 74.2).

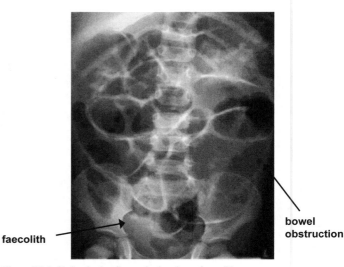

faecolith

bowel obstruction

Figure 74.1: Abdominal radiograph showing a faecolith.

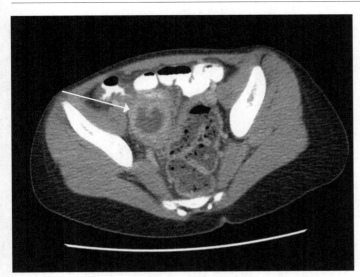

Figure 74.2: CT scan showing perforated appendix with collection (arrow).

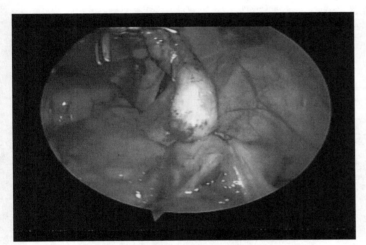

Figure 74.3: Laparoscopic interval appendectomy for a 15-year-old girl.

Management

Nonoperative Treatment

Occasionally, a child is admitted with a palpable right iliac fossa mass and low-grade fever but is otherwise well and can tolerate oral fluid. The current management for this subgroup of patients is to treat them as having an "appendix mass". Intravenous antibiotics alone usually resolve this mass, and the child can be discharged 7–10 days later. Most, but not all, surgeons normally readmit the child 6–8 weeks later and perform an interval appendectomy, which can be done open or laparoscopically (Figure 74.3).

Open Surgery

Even though surgery remains the most generally accepted treatment for simple acute appendicitis, the management for complicated disease—namely, perforated appendicitis and appendiceal mass—has been controversial for decades. The surgical treatment of acute appendicitis has evolved over the past few decades.

Appendectomy can be simply defined as surgical resection of the appendix. Although it is usually done in an urgent setting for a patient with acute appendicitis, a number of studies have demonstrated no deleterious effect from a period of hydration and antibiotics of up to 24 hours prior to appendectomy.[7,8]

Right lower quadrant abdominal incisions for simple appendicitis and extended incision for delayed presentation of perforated appendicitis

have stood as the gold standard approach for appendectomy for more than a century. Ever since the classic description by McBurney in 1889, surgeons have largely employed a transverse right lower quadrant (Lanz) incision for simple appendectomy. Abdominal muscles are split in the direction of the fibres. After locating the appendix, the mesoappendix is divided before the appendix is excised close to its base. Management of the appendiceal stump varies from simple ligation, to ligation with inversion using a purse string, to inversion without ligature, depending on the surgeon's preference. In cases of retrocaecal appendicitis, the base is tied first and the appendix is delivered in an antegrade manner; alternatively, the incision is extended laterally and the caecum is mobilized medially and eviscerated, revealing the entire appendix.

In cases of perforation, a methodical abdominal washout with warm water is completed by most surgeons. Closure is accomplished with continuous suturing, and drains are used based on the pathology and surgeon's preferences. The skin may be closed with interrupted nonabsorbable sutures.

Intravenous antibiotics such as ampicillin, cephalosporins, aminoglycosides, and metronidazole are given before surgery. The choice and duration of antibiotic therapy is determined by the operating surgeon based on the severity of the disease and perforation, and can last from 1 to 10 days.

Laparoscopic Appendectomy

In recent years, laparoscopic appendectomy has gained wide popularity. It seems reasonable to state that laparoscopic appendectomy, performed by an experienced laparoscopist, is considered to be at least equivalent to open surgery.[9]

Laparoscopic appendectomy usually involves a 3-trocar technique. A 5- or 10-mm cannula is usually placed in the umbilicus to allow the passage of the telescope and the retrieval of the appendix. One 5-mm cannula is placed below the bikini line in the left lower quadrant and in the right upper quadrant. Uni- or bipolar diathermy is used for division of the mesoappendix, but close to the appendix because these vessels are small in caliber and will not re-bleed with coagulation. The base of the appendix can be ligated inside the abdomen with endoloops, suture ligated, or simply secured extracorporeally with the appendix drawn out through a skin stab incision at the right lower quadrant. If possible, the appendix should be extracted through the umbilical cannula to avoid direct contact with the wound. If the appendix is too thick, it should then be placed in a retrieval bag, which is withdrawn through the port site. A cheap sterile retrieval bag can be made by cutting one of the "fingers" of a surgical glove.

Prognosis and Outcomes

Appendectomy is one of the safest surgical procedures, with minimum mortality. Morbidity after surgery for acute nonperforated appendicitis is confined to superficial wound sepsis, which often requires reopening the skin and releasing the pus. Secondary suturing may be required if the wound is extensively dehisced. In contrast, perforated appendicitis is known to have an increased risk of intraabdominal abscess (5–10% in most reports), frequently requiring relook laparotomy and per rectal draining of the collection.[10,11] Mortality is limited to the patients who are admitted with a prolonged delay and often a misdiagnosis of appendicitis. Many of these patients are in a moribund state on admission and succumb to multiorgan failure secondary to gram-negative septic shock.

Prevention

Currently, there are no known dietary measures to decrease the risk of appendicitis; however, a high-fibre diet is possibly associated with a decreased incidence.

Ethical Issues

In Africa, many patients with appendicitis are taken to traditional healers or so-called "witch doctors", who give affected children herbal medication and herbal laxative enemas. The content of these enemas can be quite toxic and result in renal or liver failure in an already compromised child, further delaying definitive surgical treatment. This group of children is at highest risk for multiple organ failure and death. Marks on the body made by traditional healers may identify the area of the pathology in a patient with communication difficulties.

Evidence-Based Research

Table 74.1 presents an analysis of the diagnostic accuracy of appendicitis.

Table 74.1: Evidence-based research.

Title	Acute appendicitis in children: emergency department diagnosis and management
Authors	Rothrock SG, Pagane J
Institution	Department of Emergency Medicine, Orlando Regional Medical Center, Orlando, Florida, USA
Reference	Ann Emerg Med 2000; 36:39–51
Problem	Despite considerable recent expansion of knowledge concerning appendicitis, accurate diagnosis remains suboptimal.
Intervention	Analysis of diagnostic accuracy of appendicitis.
Comparison/ control (quality of evidence)	State-of-the-art lecture.
Outcome/effect	Despite modern laboratory tests and imaging, the diagnosis is essentially clinical.

Key Summary Points

1. Appendicitis is rare in the African population.

2. Adolescence is the common age group for appendicitis.

3. Diagnosis is usually made based on a clinical evaluation.

4. Imaging usually is helpful in assessing complicated appendicitis.

5. The outcome is the same for open and laparoscopic appendectomy.

References

1. Rogers AD, Hampto MI, Bunting M, Atherstone AK. Audit of appendicectomies at Frere Hospital, Eastern Cape. S Afr J Surg 2008: 46(3):74–77.

2. Madiba TE, Haffejee AA, Mbete DL, Chaithram H, John J. Appendicitis among African patients at King Edward III Hospital, Durban, South Africa. East Afr Med J 1998; 75(2):81–84.

3. Jones BA, Demetriades D, Segal I. The prevalence of appendical faecolith in patients with and without appendicitis: a comparative study from Canada and South Africa. Ann Surg 1985, 202:80–82.

4. Anderson KD, Parry RL. Appendicitis. In O'Neill JA, Rowe MI, Grosfeld JL (eds). Pediatric Surgery, 5th ed. Mosby-Year Book Inc, 1998, Pp 130–136.

5. Morrow SE, Newman KD. Appendicitis. In Ashcraft KW, Holcomb G, Murphy JP (eds). Pediatric Surgery, 4th ed. Elsevier-Saunders, 2005, Pp 577–585.

6. Civit CJ, Applegate KE, Stallion A. Imagining evaluation of suspected appendicitis in a pediatric population: effectiveness of sonography versus CT. Am J Roentgeno 2000; 175:977–980.

7. Omundsen M, Dennet E. Delay to appendectomy and associated morbidity: a retrospective review. ANZ J Surg 2006; 76(3):153–155.

8. Yardeni D, Hirschl RB, Drongowaski RA. Delayed versus immediate surgery in acute appendicitis: do we need to operate during the night? J Pediatr Surg 2004; 39:464–469.

9. Lintula H, Kokki H, Vanamo K. Single-blind randomized clinical trial of laparoscopic versus open appendectomy in children. Br J Surg 2001; 88(4):510–514.

10. Fishman SJ, Pelosi L, Klavon SL. Perforated appendicitis: prospective outcome analysis for 150 children. J Pediatr Surg 2000; 35(6):923–926.

11. Lund DP, Murphy EU. Management of perforated appendicitis in children: a decade of aggressive treatment. J Pediatr Surg 1994; 29(8):1130–1134.

CHAPTER 75
INFLAMMATORY BOWEL DISEASE

Hugh W. Grant
Atonasio Taela

Introduction

Inflammatory bowel disease (IBD) refers to a group of disorders that causes intestinal inflammation. The commonest types of IBD are ulcerative colitis (UC) and Crohn's disease (CD). Other, rare forms of IBD include collagenous colitis, lymphocytic colitis, ischaemic colitis, and diversion colitis. Diagnosis is based on clinical symptoms and signs, upper endoscopy with biopsies, colonoscopy with biopsies (including terminal ileum), and radiological examination (contrast follow-through or enema).

Overall, 25–30% of patients with IBD present in childhood or adolescence. The overall incidence of IBD in children in Africa is unknown, but it is thought to be lower than in Europe and the United States, where it has an incidence of 7 per 100,000 children.[1] In the United Kingdom, approximately 18% of children with IBD are non-Caucasian—mainly Afro-Caribbean or Asian.[2] The literature contains reports of IBD from all over Africa: Tunisia, Egypt, Sudan, Senegal, Côte d'Ivoire, Nigeria, Ethiopia, Zimbabwe, and South Africa. IBD has been reported in all population groups in South Africa—Caucasians, Jews, Africans,[3] and Asians.[4]

Inflammatory bowel disease is thought to be uncommon in Africa—this may be due to underdiagnosis because infectious diseases of the gastrointestinal (GI) tract are very common. Infectious diseases may mimic the signs and symptoms of IBD, so it is highly likely that some cases of chronic diarrhoea in children are misdiagnosed.

Aetiology and Pathophysiology

Genetics, immunity, environment, and diet all play a part in the aetiology and pathogenesis of IBD. The basic problem in Crohn's disease is a breakdown in the immune tolerance of the gut to intraluminal flora.

Genetics

The genetics of IBD have not been fully delineated. In Crohn's disease, monozygotic twins have 44–55% disease concordance.[5] The lifetime risk for CD for first-degree relatives is 7% in Caucasians, but 16.8% in Jewish families.[6] Thirty percent of children presenting before 20 years of age have a family history of IBD. A number of IBD-susceptibility genes have been identified (e.g., CARD15 on chromosome 16q).

Immunity

Patients with IBD demonstrate an abnormal immune response within their own GI tract. There are features of autoimmunity, and the disease can affect other organs outside the gut, such as eyes, skin, and joints. Inflammatory mediators (e.g., Interleukin 23) are overexpressed in IBD, and lymphocyte subsets (CD4) have been implicated in the pathogenesis of the inflammatory response. A recent hypothesis postulates that IBD is caused by an overactive immune system that attacks the digestive tract in the absence of such traditional targets as parasites and worms. This is similar to the hygiene hypothesis of many allergic conditions, and might explain the low incidence of IBD in Africa, where helminthic and parasitic infestations are endemic.

Environment

Smoking exacerbates CD in adults and children. Diet may be important—serum antibodies to cow's milk protein are elevated in many patients with CD.

Infection

The pathological processes seen in CD have similarities to tuberculosis (TB), but no specific organism has ever been identified as an aetiological agent.

Pathology

Ulcerative Colitis

UC is a disease that affects the colon. It primarily affects the rectum and a variable extent of more proximal colon. The disease is generally confluent with no skip lesions (unless the patient has undergone treatment). Macroscopically, it can appear as a granular proctitis with superficial ulcers, slough, and contact bleeding (Figure 75.1).

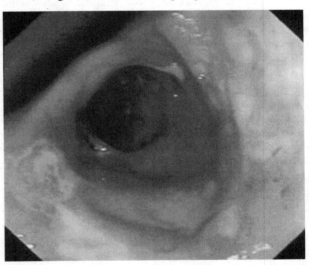

Source: Courtesy of Dr Peter Sullivan, Paediatric Gastroenterologist, John Radcliffe Hospital, Oxford, UK.

Figure 75.1: Macroscopic appearance of ulcerative colitis at colonoscopy.

Microscopically, the disease is limited to the mucosa. Inflammation starts at the base of the crypts with acute and chronic inflammatory cell infiltration. Crypt abscesses may be seen well as Goblet cell depletion. There is compensatory cell proliferation. Pseudopolyps are seen when islands of preserved mucosa are surrounded by superficial ulcers (Figure 75.2).

Ulcerative colitis is also associated with extragut manifestations such as arthropathy, uveitis, and skin lesions (pyoderma gangrenosum).

Crohn's Disease

Crohn's disease can affect any part of the GI tract from mouth to anus. In children, it manifests mainly as terminal ileal disease, colitis, or perianal disease. The lesions can be skip lesions. Macroscopically, CD can appear as patchy or confluent inflamed areas with a cobblestone appearance and apthous ulceration (Figure 75.3). At operation, there may be fat wrapping around the bowel wall.

Microscopically, CD affects all the layers of the bowel wall, with chronic inflammatory cell infiltrate, deep ulceration, granulomas, a thickened mesentery, and lymphadenopathy (Figure 75.4).

The features of CD can mimic tuberculosis. It is also associated with extragut manifestations, such as erythema nodosum, pyoderma gangrenosum, arthropathy, and uveitis.

When the pathologist cannot determine whether the problem is UC or CD, it may be labelled as "indeterminate colitis" or "IBD (not otherwise specified)". It is generally best treated as ulcerative colitis until the clinical picture becomes clear.

Clinical Presentation

History

Differences exist in the way IBD presents in children and adults. Abdominal pain is the most frequent symptom in children with IBD,[7] whereas adults tend to present with rectal bleeding in UC and with diarrhoea in CD. Forty percent of children have growth failure at the time of diagnosis[8]—however, this is not an issue with adults.

In ulcerative colitis, the commonest features in children are diarrhoea, abdominal pain, and blood per rectum.[9] UC is predominantly confined to the rectum and left colon in adults, whereas children tend to have pancolitis.[9]

In Crohn's disease, the classic adult triad of abdominal pain, diarrhoea, and weight loss was present in only 25% of children.[7] Many young CD patients present with vague complaints of nausea, vomiting, fever, growth retardation, malnutrition, or extra intestinal manifestations.[1] This clearly makes diagnosis very difficult in Africa, where anaemia, fever, weight loss, malaise, and diarrhoea are very common. For these reasons, the Porto criteria[1] for diagnosis are largely unworkable in Africa.

Physical Examination

In ulcerative colitis, external physical examination is often unremarkable; there may be some abdominal discomfort. It is important to look for extragut manifestations—pallor, arthropathy, and skin changes.

In Crohn's disease, physical examination may demonstrate identifiable disease. There may be mouth ulcers (Figure 75.5); abdominal tenderness; an inflammatory mass; or perianal tags, fissures, and abscesses (Figure 75.6). Check for extragut manifestations.

Investigations

For general testing, send the stool to the lab to exclude infective causes. Perform baseline blood tests: a full blood count (FBC) (looking for anaemia, high white blood count, raised platelets); inflammatory markers (raised erythrocyte sedimentation rate (ESR) or C-reactive protein (CRP)); electrolytes (for dehydration); and albumin.

Specific tests depend on their availability.

• *Upper endoscopy and colonoscopy* (with ileal intubation) should be performed if possible. Multiple biopsies should be taken along the length of GI tract.

• *Sigmoidoscopy and proctoscopy* can usually be performed if colonoscopy is not available.

• *Double contrast enema* should be performed if the colon is largely affected, and small bowel follow-through (or enema) if Crohn's disease is suspected (Figure 75.7).

• *Ultrasound scan* can be helpful for an inflammatory mass in Crohn's disease.

Differential diagnoses in children presenting with IBD include infective diarrhoea (viral and bacterial, especially *Yersinia enterocolitica* and *Entamoeba histolytica*); enteropathies; malnutrition from dietary deprivation; worm infestations; and tuberculosis. A wise approach is to investigate and treat the common causes of these symptoms but to consider IBD in chronic cases that do not respond to the usual treatments. In CD, tuberculosis must always be excluded before major surgery is undertaken.

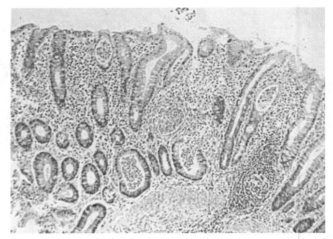

Source: Courtesy of Dr Peter Sullivan, Paediatric Gastroenterologist, John Radcliffe Hospital, Oxford, UK.

Figure 75.2: Microscopic appearance of ulcerative colitis.

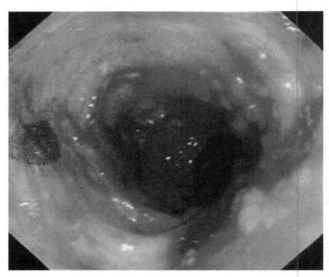

Source: Courtesy of Dr Peter Sullivan, Paediatric Gastroenterologist, John Radcliffe Hospital, Oxford, UK.

Figure 75.3: Macroscopic appearance of Crohn's disease affecting the terminal ileum.

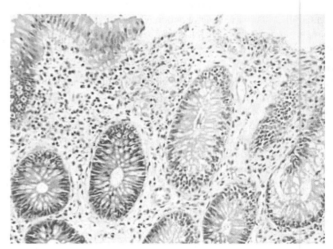

Source: Courtesy of Dr Peter Sullivan, Paediatric Gastroenterologist, John Radcliffe Hospital, Oxford, UK.

Figure 75.4: Microscopic appearance of Crohn's disease.

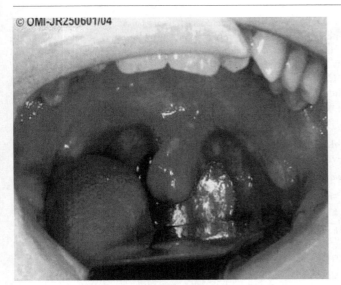

Source: Courtesy of Dr Peter Sullivan, Paediatric Gastroenterologist, John Radcliffe Hospital, Oxford, UK.

Figure 75.5: Mouth ulcers in Crohn's disease.

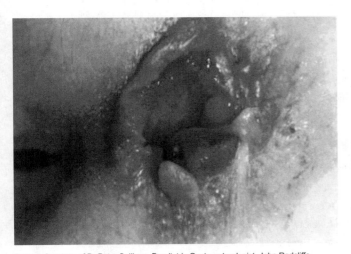

Source: Courtesy of Dr Peter Sullivan, Paediatric Gastroenterologist, John Radcliffe Hospital, Oxford, UK.

Figure 75.6: Perianal tags and fistula in Crohn's disease.

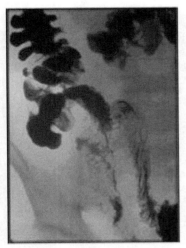

Source: Courtesy of Dr Peter Sullivan, Paediatric Gastroenterologist, John Radcliffe Hospital, Oxford, UK.

Figure 75.7: Contrast follow-through demonstrating stricture in terminal ileum.

Management

Medical Management

In ulcerative colitis, management is primarily medical and depends on the severity and extent of the disease.[2] For mild disease (i.e., fewer than four motions per day), oral aminosalicylates and corticosteroids are prescribed for 2 weeks. Mesalazine enemas are given daily until the bleeding stops, and then on alternate days for one week. For moderate disease (i.e., four to six motions per day, anaemia, slight toxicity), treat as above with oral steroids in a higher dose (2 mg/kg; maximum 40 mg) for 1 month and then reduce slowly over the following weeks. If there is a poor response, treat as for severe disease. For severe disease (i.e., more than six motions per day, toxicity, fever, anaemia), intravenous methylprednisolone or hydrocortisone are given for 3 days, and rectal hydrocortisone or prednisolone enemas are given twice daily. Intravenous fluids, blood transfusion, and total parenteral nutrition may also be required. If a relapse occurs, the patient should go back on rectal corticosteroids and a course of oral corticosteroids. Salicylates are generally lifelong for maintenance. If relapses occur, steroids or azathioprine (in order to limit the dose and complications of steroids) can be given. Other immunomodulating drugs include ciclosporin, methotrexate, and inflixamab.

In Crohn's disease, management is also primarily medical. Relapses can be expected, and many patients will require surgery. An elemental or polymeric diet for 6 weeks can produce remission in small bowel disease, but relapse is frequent. This diet has the advantage of having few side effects, but is poorly tolerated (due to its awful taste). It can be given either orally, through a nasogastric tube, or via a gastrostomy. For acute flare-ups, prednisolone should be given until remission occurs (2 mg/kg; maximum 40 mg) and then slowly reduced (by 5 mg per week). Mesalazine appears to be effective for treatment of small bowel and colonic disease. Azathioprine is effective for long-term maintenance and has steroid-sparing effects. Metronidazole can be helpful in controlling perianal disease with fistulas. Tumour necrosis factor (TNF) antagonists (inflixamab) are increasingly used but are not generally available in Africa.

Surgical Management

In ulcerative colitis, the indications for surgery are acute toxic mega-colon, intractable disease with ongoing symptoms and multiple frequent relapses despite maximum medical therapy, and growth failure. There is a risk of cancer in patients who have had pancolitis for more than 10 years. In ulcerative colitis, the disease affects the colon and can therefore be "cured" by removing the colon. The underlying principle is to remove all the mucosal disease (from the appendix and caecum to the anal margin). Surgery is usually performed in unwell children and it is safest to do this as a staged procedure.

An upper transverse incision should be performed in small children, and a midline for adolescents. A subtotal colectomy (leaving a rectal stump at the pelvic brim) and formation of an ileostomy (spouted) will remove the vast amount of the disease in the affected child. This is increasingly being done laparoscopically. If proctitis is a major problem, the rectal stump can be short. At a later date (usually around 6 months) when the child is off all immunosuppressive medications and when the ileostomy effluent is thicker and of less volume, the standard operative procedure is a restorative proctocolectomy (ileo-anal "J" pouch, with covering loop ileostomy). Six weeks later, a distal loopogram is performed, an examination under anaesthetic is performed (to check on possible stenosis and the condition of the pouch), and—if all is well—the covering ileostomy is closed. In Africa, a simple ileo-anal anastomosis is more appropriate. The eventual endpoint is the same (5-10 stools per day) but takes longer. It avoids any problems relating to the pouch (e.g., pouchitis). When performing an ileo-anal anastomosis, approach from below and start the dissection 1 cm above the dentate line, strip the mucosa for 3–4 cm (keeping very superficial), and then excise the entire rectal stump (like an endorectal pull-through). Anastomosis is best performed by using interrupted absorbable sutures.

In Crohn's disease, the indications for surgery are intestinal obstruction (due to stricture or inflammatory mass), failure of medical management with relapses, growth failure, fistulas, and perforation. The type of surgery depends on the location and extent of disease: For local small bowel disease, consider stricturoplasty, take out as little bowel as necessary, and avoid stomas if possible. For colonic disease, partial colectomy (preserve unaffected colon) may be required. For perianal disease, drain abscesses, use seton if indicated for fistulas, and avoid sphincter-damaging procedures.

Postoperative Complications

Complications are common after surgery for IBD.[10,11] The patients are often unwell, malnourished, have depressed immunity (e.g., steroids, failure to thrive), and are generally in poor condition. Specific short-term surgical complications include postoperative bleeding (salicylates), anastomotic leakage (impaired wound healing), fistula formation (part of CD), fluid and electrolyte imbalance, and short-gut syndrome. Medium- to long-term problems include recurrent disease in 10–40% of patients with CD,[12] small bowel obstruction due to adhesions in up to 25%,[10] and reduced fertility in girls following pouch surgery.[13] There is some evidence that continuing immunosuppressive therapy with azathioprine after surgery can reduce the reoperation rate in Crohn's disease.

Prognosis

Ulcerative colitis can generally be "cured" by colectomy and ileo-anal anastomosis, and patients can come off their medications. In Africa, colectomy carries the hazard of removing the vital absorptive capacity of the colon and may predispose patients to dehydration if they were to pick up infective diarrhoea. Long-term function is generally good, but may take up to 18 months to achieve acceptable bowel control and bowel frequency.

Crohn's disease is not curable; it follows a relapsing and remission pattern.[12] Previously indolent disease can flare up, and previously uninvolved areas can become diseased.

Evidence-Based Research

Table 75.1 presents a study that is an overview of inflammatory bowel disease.

Table 75.1: Evidence-based research.

Title	Inflammatory bowel disease
Authors	Baillie RM, Croft NM, Fell JM, Afzal NA, Heuschkel RB
Institution	Paediatric Medical Unit, Southampton General Hospital, Southampton, UK
Reference	Arch Dis Child 2006; 91:426–532
Outcome/ effect	Twenty-five percent of inflammatory bowel disease presents in childhood. Growth and nutrition are key issues in the management, with the aim of treatment being to induce and then maintain disease remission with minimal side effects. Only 25% of Crohn's disease presents with the classic triad of abdominal pain, weight loss, and diarrhoea. Most children with ulcerative colitis have blood in the stool at presentation. Inflammatory markers are usually, although not invariably, raised at presentation (particularly in Crohn's disease). Full investigation includes upper gastrointestinal endoscopy and ileocolonoscopy. Treatment requires multidisciplinary input as part of a clinical network led by a paediatrician with special expertise in the management of the condition.

Key Summary Points

Ulcerative Colitis

1. Surgery is indicated for complications.
2. Staged procedures should be considered in unwell children.
3. Remove all colon down to anal verge (anal transition zone).
4. Standard operative procedure is ileo-anal anastomosis or ileo-anal J pouch (restorative proctocolectomy).

Crohn's Disease

5. Surgery will never cure the disease.
6. Keep surgery simple (consider stricturoplasty).
7. Take out as little bowel as necessary.
8. Avoid stomas, if possible.
9. Drain perianal disease (use seton if indicated) and avoid sphincter-damaging procedures.

References

1. Medical Position Paper ESPGHAN, IBD Working group. Inflammatory bowel disease in children and adolescents, recommendations for diagnosis—the Porto criteria. J Pediatr Gastroenterol Nutr 2005; 41:1–7.

2. Coulter B. Inflammatory bowel disease. In: Southall D, Coulter B, Ronald C, Nicholson S, Parke S (eds). Intestinal Child Health Care. A Practical Manual for Hospitals Worldwide. BMJ Books London, 2002, Pp 289–293.

3. Segal I. Ulcerative colitis in a developing country of Africa. The Baragwanath experience of the first 46 patients. Int J Colorectal Dis 1988; 3(4):222–225.

4. Rajput HL, Seebaran A, Desai Y. Ulcerative colitis in the Indian population in Durban. S Afr Med J 1992; 81(5):245–248.

5. Tysk C, Lindberg E, Jarnerot G, Floderus-Myrhed B. Ulcerative colitis and Crohn's disease in an unselected population of monozygotic and dizygotic twins. A study of heritability and the influence of smoking. Gut 1988; 29:990–996.

6. Yang H, McElree C, Roth MP, Shanahan F, Targan SR, Rotter JI. Familial empirical risks for IBD: differences between Jews and non Jews. Gut 1993; 34:517–524.

7. Sawczenko A, Sandhu BK. Presenting features of inflammatory bowel disease in Great Britain and Ireland. Arch Dis Child 2003; 88:995–1000.

8. Motil KJ, Grand RJ, Davis-Kraft L, Ferlic LL, Smith EO. Growth failure in children with inflammatory bowel disease: a prospective study. Gastroenterol 1993; 105(3):681–691.

9. Baillie RM, Croft NM, Fell JM, Afzal NA, Heuschkel RB. Inflammatory bowel disease. Arch Dis Child 2006; 91:426–532.

10. Rintala RJ, Lindahl HG. Proctocolectomy and J-pouch ileo-anal anastomosis in children. J Pediatr Surg 2002; 37(1)66–70.

11. Romanos J, Stebbings JF, Mortensen NJ, Kettlewell HG. Restorative proctocolectomy in children and adolescents. J Pediatr Surg 1996; 31(12):1655–1658.

12. Lock MR, Farmer RG, Fazio VW, Jagelman DG, Lavery IC, Weakley FC. Recurrence of reoperation for Crohn's disease: the role of disease location in prognosis. N Engl J Med 1981; 304(26):1586–1588.

13. Waljee A, Waljee J, Morris AM, Higgins PD. Threefold risk of infertility: a meta-analysis of infertility after ileal pouch anal anastomoses in UC. Gut 2006; 55(11):1575–1580.

CHAPTER 76
HIRSCHSPRUNG'S DISEASE

Sam W. Moore   Paul T. Nmadu
N. Tsifularo   John R. Gosche

Introduction

Hirschsprung's disease (HSCR or HD) may be defined as a functional intestinal obstruction resulting from the congenital absence of para-sympathetic ganglion cells in the myenteric plexus of the distal bowel.

The initial description of congenital aganglionosis (Hirschsprung's disease) by Harald Hirschsprung, heralded as the Father of Danish Paediatrics, in 1886,[1] could not have anticipated the worldwide interest it would evoke. Successful treatment of the condition had to wait for 50 years until the pivotal role of the distal aganglionic segment and its vital role in the pathophysiology of Hirschsprung's disease was identified.[2,3] The development of successful surgical management in the same year[4] has made HSCR one of the success stories of paediatric surgery in the modern era.

Demographics

Hirschsprung's disease is a congenital cause of functional intestinal obstruction mostly diagnosable at birth but often presenting late in resource-poor environments.[5] It has long been regarded as a special condition in Africa, often presenting with advanced disease and malnutrition (the oldest patient we have encountered is 21 years of age). In Africa, patients often present following failure of traditional herbal enemas to afford relief. It may be difficult to separate from other conditions of megacolon, particularly in Africa where it may present in a way similar to other conditions, such as degenerative leiomyopathy. As a result, many believe that there is a special phenotypic expression in Africa. Although difficult to prove, there is a suspected interethnic variation in terms of genetic haplotypes within the promoter region of the REarranged during Transfection (RET) proto-oncogene in African patients. This is based on extrapolated data and has yet to be substantiated in Africa itself.

The HSCR incidence worldwide is approximately 1 in 5,000 live births. This has been substantiated in South Africa, where large series have reported a frequency of approximately 1 patient in every 5,726 live births, with all ethnic groups being affected.[6,7] The male-to-female ratio is approximately 4:1 overall worldwide, but appears to vary between the various ethnic groups represented in South Africa.[6] This ratio was 3.6:1 in caucasians and 3.9:1 in black African patients, but dropped to 2.5:1 in those of mixed descent, where a greater proportion of females were observed. The male-to-female ratio is also affected by the length of the aganglionic segment, which approaches 1:1 in total colonic aganglionosis (TCA). An overall male predominance is apparent, with incomplete gene penetrance and a variable phenotype.

Most babies with HSCR are born to mothers with a normal antenatal history (92%) with the majority having good Apgar scores. HSCR is mostly associated with big babies (average birth weight of 3,129 gm), and has been generally thought to be rare or absent in premature babies. This widely held belief has not been substantiated in recent studies, although our series had 12.2% who weighed less than 2.5 kg at birth, but in only 3 (1.9%) could a gestational age <37 weeks (28, 32, 33 weeks) be documented.

Hirschsprung's disease has been described as a sex-linked heterogonous disorder with various degrees of severity. It has a variable pattern of inheritance, which includes dominant, recessive, and multigenic patterns of transmission.

Associated Anomalies

The reported incidence of HSCR-associated anomalies varies between 5% and 32%, with a mean of 21.1%; no associated link between associated anomalies and familial HSCR transmission has been observed. Twelve percent are associated with chromosomal anomalies; Down syndrome is one of the most frequent (5.82% on average). These genetic variations account for more than 50% of the observed abnormalities associated with HSCR. Other associated anomalies include congenital eye problems and other associated syndromes (e.g., Waardenburg syndrome, sensorineural deafness, neurofibromatosis).

Associated anomalies (see Figure 76.1 for relative frequencies) include gastrointestinal (GIT), central nervous system (CNS), genito-urinary (G-U), musculo-skeletal, cardiovascular system (CVS), craniofacial, and skin.

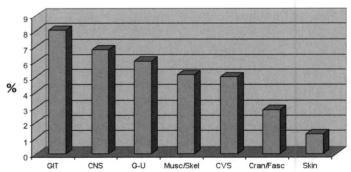

Figure 76.1: Hirschsprung's-associated abnormalities.

Although Hirschsprung's disease is described in association with several congenital abnormalities, there are two main reasons for their significance:

1. The majority may be attributed to abnormal genetic development signalling, yielding clues as to the genetic background of HSCR and its pathogenesis.

2. The influence of these associated anomalies on prognosis.

Familial Transmission

HSCR has a well-documented inherited familial predisposition (2.4–9%) and has also been reported in mono- and dizygotic twins. Affected families are known to carry an approximately 200 times higher risk of recurrence.[8] No significant difference is noted between male and female probands, but in our series, 50% of male TCA patients had a family history, transmitted through a female sibling in only two cases.

An association also exists between aganglionosis extending beyond the rectosigmoid and a family history (59% of familial versus 26% of the nonfamilial), with the frequency of TCA being significantly higher (P< 0.01) in the familial group. In addition, HSCR may recur in 15–21% of families with long-segment aganglionosis (L-HSCR), and as high as 50% in patients with ultra-long-segment aganglionosis (Zuelzer's disease). In our series, a progression of the length of segment was also observed in succeeding generations in two families.

The pattern of inheritance appears to vary in terms of the length of the affected segment, long-segment Hirschsprung's disease being considered to have an autosomal dominant inheritance pattern with incomplete penetrance (mostly RET; see nest section), whereas short-segment Hirschsprung's disease appears to be transmitted in an autosomal recessive manner or due to multiplicative effects of a number of involved genes.[9] In addition, several known associated syndromes are also inherited in an autosomal dominant manner.

Aetiology/Pathophysiology

The normal migration of neuroblasts in a cephalo-caudal direction within the bowel reaches the rectum by 12 weeks. Should the normal development be disturbed, a part of the colon will lack the normal ganglion cells and result in a functional loss of coordinated peristalsis, as occurs in HSCR.

At a molecular level, HSCR essentially appears to result from disruption of normal signalling during development. As a result, the cues controlling the migration of the neural crest cells go awry, resulting in aganglionosis of the distal bowel.

Current evidence would appear to support a large genetic component in HSCR aetiology. The patterns of conditions associated with HSCR have already been of great value in revealing many of the genetic components of the condition. Known genetic variations have been identified in at least 12% of HSCR cases which is higher than the expected in the normal population. Although much progress has been made in assessing possible mechanisms by which this gene malfunction may be involved in the pathogenesis of HSCR, the aetiology of HSCR is complex probably involving both genetic and microenvironmental influences in the development of the clinical phenotype. The extent of the complexity is shown by the number of genes implicated in its pathogenesis (at least nine). This is hardly surprising, as the signals governing cell migration and development in the embryo are extraordinarily complicated, and signalling molecules are notorious for crosstalk and redundancy.

Although the reason for the incomplete migration and development of ganglion cells is as yet not completely clear, the identification of major susceptibility genes (namely, the REarranged during Transfection (RET) gene and the Endothelin B receptor gene (EDNRB) and other genetic variations) have helped in understanding the aetiology of the condition. Ongoing research has identified a number additional HSCR susceptability genes (the EDNRB ligand EDN 3, the glial cell line derived neurotrophic factor (GDNF) situated at chromosome 5p12-13, and its related GFRα). In addition, the recently described association with PHOX2B and the SOX-10 gene on chromosome 22q13 and appears to synergise with the endothelin system in very long aganglionic segments.

Pathology

Hirschsprung's disease results in a functional obstruction of the bowel with dilatation of the proximal colon and hypertrophy of the muscles (i.e., megacolon).

Macroscopically, HSCR features a narrow aganglionic segment and a transitional zone, and then the dilated proximal portion with a thickened bowel wall as a result of hypertrophy of the muscular wall of the intestine.

HD classically affects the rectum and sigmoid (70%), but can also involve a long portion of colon and can affect the entire large bowel. In 20% of cases, a long segment of colon is affected, with the total colon being aganglionic in 8–10%.

Extensive ultra-long aganglionosis with extensive small bowel involvement is uncommon, occurring in <2%.

The functional abnormality always includes the internal anal sphincter and extends proximally for short or long distances, depending on the type.

HSCR, although regarded at one stage as a relatively easy diagnosis, has on occasion become "one of the most difficult diagnoses in Paediatric Surgery",[10] mainly due to difficulties in interpreting the histological, clinical, and radiological findings.

Histologic Diagnosis

The classic histological picture of Hirschsprung's disease is the absence of ganglion cells in intramuscular myenteric (Auerbach's) plexus and the submucosal Meissner's plexus. In addition, proliferation of peripheral nerves may also be seen in the affected bowel.

The method of suction biopsy initially described by Helen Noblett[11] allows specimens of the submucosal and mucosal layers to be obtained with minimal discomfort and without anaesthesia. A number of innovations to the biopsy forceps over the years have culminated in the availability of a superior tool with disposable capsules for specimen taking. This method, although reliable, is underutilized due to the expense of the disposable capsules. A more durable tool of the old-fashioned type is still manufactured, but can be difficult to locate (one possible source can be found at http://www.Trewavis.com.au/).

Biopsy specimens are taken at 2 and 4 cm (3 and 5 cm in older children). Failure to obtain adequate diagnostic yield on rectal suction biopsy will necessitate a full thickness biopsy, which causes problems during surgical procedures that require mucosal stripping (e.g., endorectal pull-through procedures). The biopsy specimens are then snap frozen and sectioned into slices ±15 μm thick.

Acetylcholinesterase Increase

Acetylcholinesterase (AChE) staining techniques remain the investigation of choice to evaluate suction biopsies to show an increased activity in the parasympathetic nerves of the affected zone as well as neurofibrils within the lamina propria and muscularis mucosa (Figure 76.1). This technique remains the gold standard on rectal suction biopsies in Europe and many parts of the world.

Because AChE staining techniques are mostly confined to specialized centres, many pathology units in Africa have a problem in obtaining access and rely on H&E (hematoxylin and eosin) staining, which may present difficulties in identifying immature ganglion cells from plasma cells or lymphocytes.

Interpretation of AChE staining may be influenced by the different patterns of AChE seen (particularly in neonates). The classic type A staining shows prominent AChE positive nerve fibrils throughout the lamina propria. The type B pattern shows similar AChE neurofibrils in the muscularis mucosa and neighbouring lamina propria.[12] Patients demonstrating the type B histochemical pattern may go on to display typical type A patterns after a few weeks.

Other immunohistochemical staining methods abound. NADPH-d immunocytochemistry yields a blue identification of both submucosal and myenteric ganglia.

The morphologic diagnosis of HSCR therefore rests on the following:

• Absence of ganglion cells in the submucosal layer (and/or intermyenteric (Auerbach's) plexus)

• Presence of the enlarged peripheral nerve trunks in the submucosa

• Increased AChE staining—proliferation of neurofibrils in the lamina propria and the muscularis mucosa (absent in normally innervated intestine; see Figure 76.2)

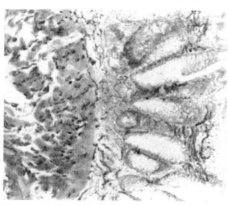

Figure 76.2: Acetylcholinesterase stain (Meier-Rüge), showing neurofibrils within the lamina propria in Hirschsprung's disease.

Clinical Features

The clinical evaluation of the patient remains the most important diagnostic step in the diagnosis of HSCR.

History

A delay in passage of meconium is the most important neonatal observation. Normal babies pass meconium within 24 hours, and a small percentage will also pass meconium by 48 hours. A significant delay in the passage of meconium after birth indicates a congenital cause. Any baby who has a delay in the passage of meconium of more than 24 hours or who passes little meconium should be investigated for HSCR.

Other signs in the neonate are a functional intestinal obstruction and bile-stained vomiting, often from day 2. In the older child in Africa, the main complaints are abdominal distention, constipation, wasting, diarrhoea, and retardation in growth.

A family history of HSCR or severe constipation are other significant factors. A family history is present in 4%, with a 61% possibility of a long segment. Other associated anomalies account for 16% of the cases of HSCR.

Physical Presentation

The clinical presentation depends not only on the length of the aganglionosis but also the age of the patient.

Neonate (50–80%)

- Most cases (>90%) present with signs in the neonatal period but are sometimes overlooked in poorly resourced health situations.

- In Africa, the number of neonatal diagnoses made may be as low as 10%.

- Intestinal obstruction presents with bile-stained vomiting and abdominal distention (often by day 2).

- Delayed passage of meconium is a presenting feature in more than 80% of patients with Hirschsprung's disease.

- Hirschsprung's-associated enterocolitis (HAEC) (16%) presents with bloody diarrhoea and mucus associated with abdominal distention and vomiting. The majority of cases of enterocolitis present during 2–4 weeks after birth. This is an important diagnosis because it accounts for 53% of the mortality arising from Hirschsprung's disease.

Older child (+10–50%)

- Some patients have early onset of mild constipation followed by acute low intestinal obstruction. The early onset of chronic constipation (often since birth) is an indication to exclude HSCR. Stools when passed are irregular and passed with great difficulty.

- Abdominal distention occurs in almost 100% (may be marked).

- Megacolon of the proximal colon is a classic sign of HSCR.

- The child does not develop normally and is often thin and malnourished.

- In contrast to the rectal findings in chronic constipation, the rectum is often empty on examination in HSCR and should the examining finger push beyond the aganglionic zone, there is an explosive evacuation of soft stool.

- Hirschsprung's-associated enterocolitis can also occur in the older patient or after surgery. This may lead to toxic megacolon.

- Secondary urogenital problems may occur in patients as a result of the chronic obstruction (e.g., vesicoureteric reflux, hydronephrosis).

Diagnostic Investigations

History and Examination
Look for clinical features of HSCR.

Abdominal X-rays
The diagnostic accuracy of abdominal x-rays is 52%.

- Look for signs of low intestinal obstruction and distended bowel loops of different calibres (Figure 76.3).

- Erect plates can demonstrate in fluid levels.

- A lateral view may demonstrate the narrow rectum.

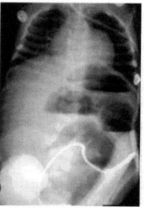

Figure 76.3: Abdominal radiograph showing a low intestinal obstruction and varying distended bowel loops.

Contrast Enema

- A contrast enema is diagnostic in two-thirds of patients if low pressures are used. Irrigation of the colon before the contrast must not be performed as it may result in possible decompression of the megacolon or the distended bowel.

- The narrow aganglionic segment is shown with a dilated proximal bowel segment, and a transitional zone is diagnostic.

- Care must be taken not to apply pressure in neonates, as the bowel can easily be distended (Figure 76.4).

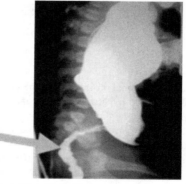

Figure 76.4: Underfilled contrast enema showing a narrow distal segment and distended proximal bowel (right).

• The aganglionic segment may be irregular, demonstrating a saw-tooth appearance, probably as a result of muscular fasciculations.

• A delay in the clearing of contrast (barium sulphate) within 24 hours is also a reliable sign, and a follow-up x-ray should be performed the following day.

Manometry

In normal people, distention of the rectum results in the reflex relaxation of the internal sphincter (rectosphincteric reflex; see Figure 76.5). This is absent on manometry in patients with Hirschsprung's disease.

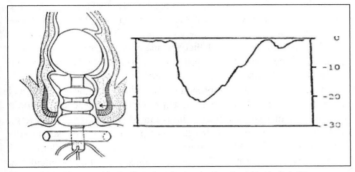

Figure 76.5: Manometric tracing showing normal rectosphincteric reflex.

Rectal Biopsy

See the section in this chapter on Pathology.

Differential Diagnosis

Differential diagnosis includes the following:

• Small left colon syndrome, particularly in diabetic mothers

• Meconium plug syndrome in neonates.

• Chronic idiopathic intestinal pseudo-obstruction (CIIP, or CHIPS)

• Other dysganglionosis of the gastrointestinal tract

• African degenerative leiomyopathy (ADL)[13]

• Acquired megacolon (generally at >1 year of age), resulting from anal fissure, anal or rectal stricture, anorectal malformations, tumour, or psychogenic reasons

Management

The standard surgical management of Hirschsprung's disease varies among centres.

The initial aim of management is to confirm the diagnosis. The patient is resuscitated and antibiotics are given (some children with enterocolitis have clostridium difficile infection).

The second aim is to correct the problem (i.e., relieve the intestinal obstruction) by means of definitive surgery. The aim of definitive surgery is to resect the abnormal aganglionic bowel and to anastomose normally ganglionated bowel to the rectum without affecting continence. Fluid and electrolyte losses are corrected and antibiotics commenced, if required.

Principles of Surgical Management and Results

A defunctioning colostomy (colostomy located at site of normal ganglionated bowel as determined by the presence of ganglion cells on frozen section) is the traditional way of relieving obstruction. This is then followed by a definitive pull-through procedure 3 to 9 months later.

Although a covering colostomy appears to decrease the incidence of infection, complications from the colostomy are not uncommon, including skin excoriation and bleeding from the stoma and prolapse.

In modern practice, temporary decompression is first attempted by means of washouts with warm saline. Should this be successful, it can be continued until definitive surgery can be performed. The recent swing to management by bowel irrigation techniques allows for early one-age surgery to be performed at a much earlier stage (mostly still within the neonatal period). Colostomy may still be necessary in resistant cases or if nursing care is unreliable.

Definitive pull-through surgical procedures have undergone numerous modifications since the original description by Swenson. Most of these modifications are based on the original concept described in 1948 by Swenson and Bill[4] and adhere to the principle of removing the functionally obstructive segment of aganglionic bowel and reanastomosis. In recent years, the endorectal pull-through (ERP) described by Soave[14] has gained popularity.

Neonatal Pull-Through

The current trend is for primary anal ERP either as a primary procedure or as a laparoscopically assisted pull-through procedure once the patient has been stabilized. Many argue for the latter because the laparoscope allows for histological mapping to identify the level of the transitional zone by biopsy It appears to make the procedure considerably easier in the neonate.

It would appear that neonatal pull-through is a safe and feasible method of treatment of Hirschsprung's disease and is suitable for those patients diagnosed in the neonatal period. Unfortunately, this applies to fewer HSCR cases in much of Africa. The remainder, who present with grossly distended megacolon, are probably best managed by surgical diversion of the faecal stream, allowing the chronically distended bowel to return to a normal calibre lumen before definitive surgical correction.

The major disadvantage of the one-stage neonatal pull-through procedure is that the determination of normal bowel is entirely dependant on frozen section histopathological evaluation. An expert pathological service is essential for this procedure to be carried out safely; the time taken for this procedure may vary but may add considerable delay. In addition, longer aganglionic segments present certain technical difficulties, resulting in a significant number of conversions to standard operative procedures.

Definitive Surgical Procedures

Five surgical procedures have received reasonably wide acceptance.

Swenson Procedure

This was the original operation described by Swenson in 1948. It involves resection of the aganglionic segment deep into the pelvis and direct end-to-end anastomosis of the proximal colon to the anorectal canal.

Duhamel Procedure

In the Duhamel procedure (retrorectal pull-through), the lower but aganglionic rectum is retained and the ganglionated bowel brought posteriorly and anastomosed to the aganglionic remnant in a side-to-side anastomosis.

Soave Procedure

The Soave procedure (extramucosal endorectal pull-through), along with its variations, is the most frequently performed procedure in the world for short-segment Hirschsprung's disease. See Figure 76.6. It has more recently been popularized as a laparoscopic-assisted or anal approach.

The procedure involves an extramucosal resection of a retained aganglionic rectal segment. The rectal mucosa is removed and a muscular cuff retained. The ganglionated colon is brought through this cuff and anastomosed to the dentate line in the rectum, thus forming an endorectal pull-through.

Rehbein Procedure

Largely abandoned, the Rehbein procedure (deep anterior resection) involves bringing the proximal ganglionic colon into the pelvis and anastomosed to the rectal stump by means of an end-to-end anastomosis higher than in the other operations (i.e., at the level of the levator ani muscle). It is very similar to the low anterior resection performed in adults.

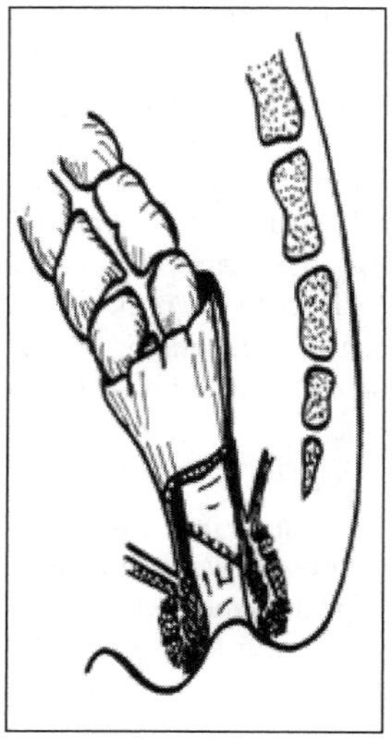

Figure 76.6: Soave procedure.

Transanal Pull-Through

The transanal pull-through approach is through the anus, thus avoiding abdominal scars. It is currently in vogue in many parts of the world, being mostly suited to a short aganglionic segment. It is similar to the Soave procedure, but is performed in reverse through the anus.

The technique involves the patient being placed in lithotomy and the rectum irrigated until clean. Retraction sutures are placed to expose the rectal mucosa and open the anus. Submucosal dissection is commenced 3–5 mm from the dentate line and the cut line controlled by multiple fine traction sutures. Following the completion of the submucosal dissection, the rectum is transected. The dissection is continued proximally until the peritoneal reflection where the sigmoid colon is mobilized and delivered. Following histological confirmation of ganglion cells in the proximal bowel, the aganglionic segment is resected, and a sutured anastomosis is performed. Many recommend a laparoscopic first stage to mobilize the bowel and perform biopsies to facilitate the resection margins.

Postoperative Complications of Hirschsprung's Surgery

Early postoperative complications appear to occur at a similar rate regardless of the age at surgery. The majority of reports of neonatal correction of Hirschsprung's disease describe initial experiences, and a paucity of long term-data exists. The Toronto group[15] have shown that the complication rate of single-stage repair was unaffected by whether the repair was performed prior to or later than the neonatal period, and the short-term outcome was similar for those weighing less than 4 kg.

There is a paucity of long-term evaluations, although one large study[16] reported a 6% incidence of postoperative enterocolitis and a 4% stricture rate. The overall long-term development of function (continence, sexual, and psychological) remains largely unevaluated.

Early Complications

Early postoperative complications include anastomotic insufficiency, stenosis, prolonged ileus, adhesive obstruction, intestinal obstruction, and retraction of the neorectum. Wound sepsis may be present to varying degrees, and other complications of sepsis or pelvic or presacral abscesses may be evident. Acidosis may be associated with excessive fluid and electrolyte losses in long-segment disease, and enterocolitis associated with Hirschsprung's disease may be present. Early complications following the Soave procedure are a reported higher rate of anastomotic leakage (4–7.7%) and stenosis (9.4–23.7%) compared with other procedures.

Late Complications

It is essential that the operative details are available in the assessment of long-term complications, so that like can be compared with like. The evolving nature of the surgery of Hirschsprung's disease should be borne in mind, as it has evolved from the original three-stage procedure to a two-stage and now one-stage (mostly neonatal) pull-through (often laparoscopic assisted). These technical advances have largely altered the nature and frequency of early complications, and it would appear from available evidence that the newer modifications give a lower incidence of enterocolitis and stricture formation. Reliable data and evaluation of late complications are largely unavailable regarding constipation incidence, continence, social integration, and sexual function, among others.

It is generally recognised that the major long-term complications in the postoperative period following Hirschsprung's surgery are constipation and Hirschsprung's-associated enterocolitis. The long-term incidence of constipation approaches 9% following almost all surgical procedures, but this figure may be considerably influenced by certain procedures with a well-established higher incidence of constipation (e.g., the Rehbein procedure). The incidence of postoperative constipation is one of the most practical methods of measuring successful therapy, although its assessment is often highly subjective. The true incidence may, in fact, be hidden, due the fact that many patients receive some form of treatment (e.g., stool softeners, etc.). Postsurgical obstructive symptoms must be separated from HAEC because diarrhoea and enterocolitis may persist into the postoperative period (especially following extensive gastrointestinal (GI) involvement such as TCA). The incidence of HAEC may also be influenced by obstruction due to the presence of stenosis or cuff strictures.

Constipation and obstructive symptoms may be related to a number of possible causes, which include a residual aganglionic segment, sphincter achalasia, associated dysganglionosis of the enteric nervous system, strictures, restrictive cuff following ERP, retained spur following Duhamel procedures, "acquired" aganglionosis, and other functional causes. Most large series include a small number of patients with incomplete resection of the aganglionic segment (namely, 2.2% for the Soave procedure; 3.6% and 3.8% for the Swenson and Rehbein techniques, respectively; and 1.2% following the Duhamel procedure), and repeat biopsies may be required to ascertain the status of the pull-through segment.

In many cases of postsurgical obstructive symptoms, failure to identify a cause on routine clinical and pathologic investigations suggests some degree of sphincter achalasia due to the failure of the internal sphincter to relax. Sphincter achalasia may be difficult to treat, and previous attempts at repeated anal dilatation have had mixed success. We have found the topical application of a glyceryltrinitrate paste to be fairly effective, and it is a cheap alternative to the injection of botulin toxin advocated by some.

Although the majority of patients do well following the modified surgical techniques currently employed for treating HSCR, some patients experience some degree of lack of control on follow-up. The incidence of incontinence following the ERP technique appears to be low, although sufficient long-term follow-up is as yet not available to assess the long-term outcome of neonatal or the transanal ERP techniques. Intermittent soiling may be associated with constipation, diarrhea, and a faeculoma, thus appearing to be related to overflow rather than inadequate sphincters. Some may be attributed to ill-advised sphincterotomy (largely historical).

There is a reported incidence of 0–9.7% of patients with genitourinary symptoms such as enuresis, incontinence of urine, dysuria, and impotence. The possibility that this could have resulted from damage to pelvic nerves (especially with techniques involving extensive pelvic dissection) has largely been confined to historical series. It has also been suggested that these symptoms may be related to psychological disturbances associated with long periods of hospitalization and trauma.

A relationship with perirectal abscess formation has been reported, and postoperative septic complications resulting in subsequent perianal fistulas appear to be uncommon, although they have been reported in isolated cases following the Swenson, Duhamel, and Soave procedures.[17]

Mortality, although uncommon, has been reported in 1.5–2.8%, depending on the surgical procedure employed. This can be partly influenced by HAEC and Down syndrome (where the mortality rate approaches 26%).[18,19]

Management of Special Problems

Enterocolitis management

Avoid surgery in the acute stage of HAEC because it may result in an increased incidence of complications. Management of HAEC includes resuscitation, antibiotics, decompression (6-hourly), and colostomy when stabilized.

Total colonic aganglionosis

Total colonic aganglionosis poses special problems due to the length of the bowel involved. It is usually treated by means of an ileostomy, a subsequent anal pull-through procedure with preservation of some aganglionic bowel, and anastomosis by means of a long side-to-side anastomosis.

Other

Obstructive symptoms may occur in the postoperative phase with recurrent episodes of abdominal distention associated with watery diarrhea.

Prognosis and Outcome

Ethical Issues

- Hirschsprung's disease is surgically correctable, and the majority of patients with the disease can live productive, satisfying lives.

- Physical growth and development generally approximate normal.

- Intellectual function is mostly good.

- Most HSCR patients (93%) achieve acceptable anorectal function, given sufficient time to adjust.

- Long-term functional results are excellent in some, good in the majority, and poor in approximately 15–30%.

- Functional results depend on the length of aganglionosis, procedure performed, surgical complications, social circumstances, family support, and associated anomalies, among other factors.

- Psychological problems may be magnified in those with poor support systems.

- Ethical issues do arise in cases of very long aganglionic segments, leading to intestinal failure.

- Ethical issues may be pertinent in certain disabling associated anomalies.

- Genetic counselling (if not handled correctly) also has the potential for giving rise to ethical issues, but should not be handled in isolation.

Genetic Counselling and Prevention

Although genetic factors are clearly implicated in the aetiology of HSCR, no clear pattern of inheritance exists, and autosomal dominant, recessive, and multigenic patterns have all been reported. This all strongly suggests a multifactorial and multigenic HSCR aetiology, and the majority of HSCR cases can be classified as complex genetic disorders for which familial aggregation is observed with variable Mendelian inheritance. Genetic counselling via pedigree analysis alone is particularly difficult in such a multifactorial condition, as it may be affected by a number of other unrelated factors (e.g., small family size, poor history, and adoption, as well as the lack of an identifiable genetic mutation). As a result, practical therapeutic interventions still appear to be mostly unattainable.

Nevertheless, apart from being an integral part of the ethics surrounding DNA testing, genetic counselling has become highly sought by families at risk. It is currently mostly carried out on empiric grounds. This will help to drive the process forward and DNA analysis of at least the major susceptibility genes in the family is an achievable goal. Should a major genetic defect be detected in this manner, the door is open for foetal genetic testing and evaluation of risk.

Key Summary Points

1. Hirschsprung's disease (HSCR) occurs in 1 out of every 5,000 live births worldwide.

2. HSCR is a functional intestinal obstruction occurring most frequently in large, term babies.

3. The male-to-female ratio is approximately 4:1 overall, but approaches 1:1 in long-segment Hirschsprung's disease (L-HSCR).

4. The aetiology is multifactorial, with genetics playing a major role.

5. The family recurrence varies between 4% and 9%.

6. The main susceptability gene is the REarranged during Transfection (RET) gene on chromosome 10 (10q22), but at least nine other genes have been implicated (including the Endothelin B receptor (EDNRB)).

7. The disease is caused by the congenital absence of ganglion cells (aganglionosis) in the distal bowel (histopathologically).

8. Aganglionosis may be confined to the rectosigmoid area in >70% (short-segment; S-HSCR).

9. Aganglionosis may extend up the large bowel for varying lengths (long-segment; L-HSCR) and may involve the entire colon (total colonic aganglionosis, or TCA), and even up the small bowel.

10. The majority of affected patients present with delay in the passage of meconium after birth, constipation, and abdominal distention.

11. Hirschsprung's-associated enterocolitis (HAEC) is a serious complication that contributes to morbidity and mortality.

12. Surgery involves relief of intestinal obstruction, confirming the diagnosis, and a corrective pull-through surgical procedure.

13. The majority of patients with Hirschsprung's disease are surgically correctable and can live productive, satisfying lives.

14. Most HSCR patients (93%) achieve acceptable anorectal function, given sufficient time to adjust.

References

1. Hirschsprung H. Stulträgheit Neugeborener in Folge von Dilatation und Hypertrophie des Colons. Jb Kinderheilk 1887; 27:1–7.

2. Zuelzer WW, Wilson JL. Functional intestinal obstruction on a congenital neurogenic basis in infancy. Am J Dis Child 1948; 75:40–64..

3. Whitehouse FR, Kernohan JW. Myenteric plexus in congenital megacolon. Study of eleven cases. Arch Int Med 1948; 82:75–111..

4. Swenson O, Bill AH. Resection of rectum and rectosigmoid with preservation of sphincter for benign spastic lesions producing megacolon. Surgery 1948; 24:212–220.

5. Nmadu PT. Hirschprung's disease in Zaria Nigeria: comparison of 2 consecutive decades. Ann Trop Paediatr 1994; 14:65–69..

6. Moore SW. The study of the etiology of post-surgical obstruction in patients with Hirschsprung's disease, MD thesis, University of Cape Town 1993.

7. Gordon H, Torrington M, Louw JH, Cywes S. A genetical study of Hirschsprungs disease. S Afr Med J 1966; 40:720–721.

8. Amiel J, Lyonnet S. Hirschsprung's disease, associated syndromes and genetics, a review. J Med Genet 2001; 38:729–739.

9. Carrasquillo MM, McCallion AS, Puffenberger EG, Kaschuk CS, No N, Chakravarti A. Genome-wide association study as well as the study of mouse models help to identify the interaction between RET and EDNRB pathways in Hirschsprung disease. Nature Genet 2002; 32:237–244.

10. Martucciello G. Hirschsprung's disease, one of the most difficult diagnoses in pediatric surgery: a review of the problems from clinical practice to the bench. Eur J Pediatr Surg 2008; 18(3):140–149.

11. Noblett HR. A rectal biopsy tube for the diagnosis of Hirschsprung's disease. J Pediatr Surg 1969; 4:406–409.

12. Huntley CC, Shaffner LD, Challa VR, Lyerly AD. Histochemical diagnosis of Hirschsprung disease. Pediatrics 1982; 69(6):755–761.

13. Moore SW, Schneider JW, Kaschula ROC. Non familial visceral myopathy clinical and pathologic features of African degenerative leiomyopathy. Pediatr Surg Inter 2002; 18(1):6–12.

14. Soave F. A new surgical technique for the treatment of Hirschsprung's disease. Surgery 1960; 56:1007–1014.

15. Hackam DJ, Superina RA, Pearl RH. Single-stage repair of Hirschsprung's disease: a comparison of 109 patients over 5 years. J Pediatr Surg 1997; 32(7):1028–1031.

16. Langer JC, Durrant AC, de la Torre L, Teitelbaum DH, Minkes RK, Caty MG, et al. One-stage transanal Soave pullthrough for Hirschsprung disease: a multicenter experience with 141 children. Ann Surg 2003; 238(4):569–583.

17. Kleinhaus S, Boley SJ, Sheran M, Sieber WK. Hirschsprung's disease—a survey of the members of the Surgical Section of the American Academy of Pediatrics. J Pediatr Surg 1979; 14(5):588–597.

18. Caniano DA, Teitelbaum DH, Qualman SJ. Management of Hirschsprung's disease in children with trisomy 21. Am J Surg 1990; 159(4):402–404.

19. Moore SW, Johnson GA. Hirschsprung's disease: genetic and functional associations of Downs and Waardenburghs syndromes. Sem Paediatr Surg (USA) 1998; 7(3):156–161.

CHAPTER 77
ANORECTAL MALFORMATIONS

Donald E. Meier
Afua A. J. Hesse

Introduction

Anorectal malformations (ARMs) occur commonly throughout the African continent.[1] Even under the best of circumstances, children undergoing operative treatment for ARMs may have lifelong bowel management problems of constipation, incontinence, and encopresis. In some areas of Africa with severely limited resources, few surgeons have expertise in the definitive management of these malformations. Operations are often performed out of desperation by doctors with minimal experience using inadequate equipment. Many of the affected children, not unexpectedly, suffer a lifetime of misery from bowel management problems. Other children undergo a colostomy in the newborn period, and definitive treatment is delayed until a surgeon with appropriate expertise is available. Due to the paucity of trained paediatric surgeons in most of Africa, many children throughout Africa may be living with a colostomy and hoping that someone with expertise will come along to help them achieve a more normal life. In some instances, particularly in rural areas, neonates identified with ARMs at birth are abandoned or euthanized because they are considered "nonviable" due to their abnormality. Some females with rectovestibular fistulas large enough for adequate defecation are not brought for operative correction until it is time for marriage (Figure 77.1).

Pathophysiology

A description of the embryological events resulting in ARMs is beyond the scope of this chapter. It is much more important that the African paediatric surgeon concentrate on understanding the various types of ARMs and how to best manage them. ARMs occur in an estimated 1 in 4,000 births worldwide, but this estimate is based on data from more developed countries where accurate birth records are available. To the paediatric surgeon sitting in a grossly overcrowded surgery clinic in a major African teaching hospital, the incidence of ARMs appears much higher. This, however, may be an artifactual observation because most children with ARMs are referred to these tertiary referral centres, whereas children with other less complicated operative problems are managed locally without referral. An impressive multicentre African study[1] demonstrated that ARMs are at least as common in Africa as in other parts of the world. ARMs in children are among the most common and most complex problems that the African paediatric surgeon will confront.

The term "imperforate anus" has traditionally been used to describe all anorectal abnormalities in females and males. Although imperforate anus implies that the anus never opened anywhere, a purely blind anal pouch is actually rare. Usually the rectum has opened either onto the perineum or into the genitourinary tract. The spectrum of abnormalities is quite broad, and therefore this chapter uses the term "anorectal malformations" for all of these abnormalities with further clarification to describe the specific malformation. "Imperforate anus" then refers to the specific portion of any anomaly where the rectum does not open properly through the anal musculature.

The most common ARM defect in males is imperforate anus with a rectourinary tract (usually urethral) fistula (Figure 77.2(A)). The next

most common ARM defect for males is a fistula into the perineum, a bucket-handle abnormality, or the presence of meconium in a midline perineal, scrotal, or penile raphe.

In females, the most common defect is imperforate anus with a rectal fistula into the vestibule of the vagina (Figure 77.2(B)). Perineal fistulas and bucket-handle deformities also occur occasionally in females. An uncommon but very complicated female defect is persistent cloaca, in which the urethra, vagina, and rectum empty into a single common perineal opening (Figure 77.2(C)).

Diagnosis

The diagnosis of ARM should be made during the newborn physical examination. Many children in Africa are not born in health care facilities, however, and the absence of an anus may not be appreciated by the family until hours or days after birth,[2,3] when it is noted that the child's abdomen is distending and the infant has not passed meconium (Figure 77.3).

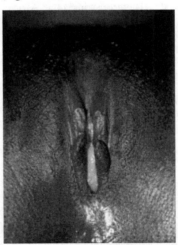

Figure 77.1: Previously untreated congenital ARM (rectovestibular fistula) in a 22-year-old female. The patient was brought for operative correction by her father, who hoped to increase her bride price. Note previous female circumcision.

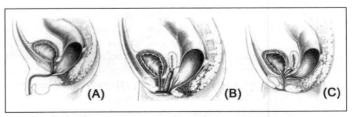

Source: ©1990, Springer-Verlag New York, Inc. From Peña A, Atlas of Surgical Management of Anorectal Malformations, Springer-Verlag, 1990, Figures 3.1, 4.1, and 4.12. Reproduced with kind permission of Springer Science+Business Media.

Figure 77.2: Three types of anorectal malformations: (A) male rectourethral fistula, (B) female rectovestibular fistula, (C) female persistent cloaca.

When consulted for a newborn with ARM, the African surgeon should initially note the child's gender and examine the perineum carefully to see whether there is any evidence of meconium from a perineal fistula (Figure 77.4) or along a midline raphe (Figure 77.5) or whether the child has a true bucket-handle deformity (Figure 77.6). If the child is male and there is no initial evidence of visible meconium, the child should be observed for 12 hours or more to see whether meconium appears in the perineum. During this time, gauze is placed over the penis so that the urine can be examined for evidence of meconium. If there is meconium in the urine, the diagnosis of a rectourinary tract fistula is made, and no further diagnostic procedures are indicated.

If, however, there is no meconium identifiable in the urine or on the perineum, an invertogram is performed because a very small percentage of children (more common in children with Down syndrome) will have a blind pouch without a fistula. The child is placed in a prone jackknife position with the buttocks higher than the rest of the body for at least 30 minutes. After that time, a radio-opaque object (drop of barium or coin) is placed on the anal dimple, a cross-table lateral x-ray is performed, and the distance between the rectal air bubble and the perineal skin is measured (Figure 77.7). If the distance is less than 1 cm, the lesion can be treated as a low lesion (see next section), but any distance greater than 1 cm should be managed as a high lesion. In females, the labia should be grasped for traction and the posterior portion of the vestibule (just external to the hymen) examined for a rectovestibular fistula (Figure 77.8). In persistent cloaca, there is only one perineal opening, and therefore the separate openings for urethra, vagina, and rectum are not visible.

When the diagnosis of ARM is made, the child should be examined for other components of the VACTERL (Vertebral and spinal cord, Anorectal, Cardiac, TracheoEsophageal, Renal and other urinary tract, Limb) complex of anomalies. Diagnostic modalities must be appropriate for the particular locale. Therefore, in some African locales an echocardiogram may be utilized, whereas in others a stethoscope may be the only cardiac diagnostic modality available. An orogastric tube is used to test for patency of the esophagus. An ultrasound, if available, is the best way to initially assess the urinary tract for abnormalities.

Treatment

Initial determination of the particular type of ARM will determine the proper initial treatment for the newborn. For many years, defects were classified as high, mid, or low. For the purpose of simplifying the treatment protocol for African paediatric surgeons, lesions in this chapter will be classified only as high or low. A colostomy is recommended as the initial treatment for high lesions, whereas low lesions can be treated primarily with an anoplasty. Low lesions that can be treated without a colostomy include those with evidence of meconium in the perineum or a bucket-handle lesion and those with a blind pouch less than 1 cm from the anal dimple, as demonstrated on invertogram. The most common lesions, including rectourinary tract fistulas in males and rectovestibular fistulas in females, should be treated as high lesions with an initial colostomy.

Creation of a proper colostomy is a difficult operation; it should *not* be assigned by default to the lowest-ranking physician who happens to be taking call after a long day in the operating theatre. The most common colostomy performed in African hospitals is a right transverse loop colostomy because it can be done quickly by simply pulling the colon out through a small incision and keeping it from returning to the abdomen by placing a rubber catheter beneath the protruding colon. Without adequate fixation, however, prolapse often occurs[4] (Figure 77.9), which can reach gigantic proportions. Death has even been reported from complications of a colostomy.[5] Children in Africa often have to live with their colostomies for months or years, and mistakes made at the initial colostomy creation result in long-term misery for the patient and the family (Figure 77.10).

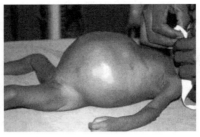

Figure 77.3: Four-day-old male with ARM brought to hospital moribund with a history of abdominal distention and no meconium since birth.

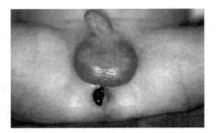

Figure 77.4: Perineal fistula in male newborn.

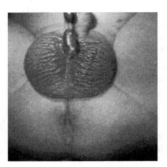

Figure 77.5: Newborn male with peno-scrotal midline raphe meconium.

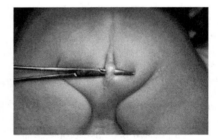

Figure 77.6: Bucket-handle deformity.

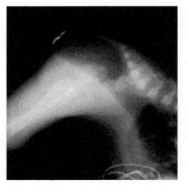

Figure 77.7: Invertogram demonstrating a low (<1 cm) blind pouch.

Alberto Peña has repeatedly emphasized the importance of a double-barrel colostomy to achieve total diversion of faeces.[6] This is particularly important in males because there is usually a fistula between the distal colon and the urinary tract, and undiverted stool in the distal colon may cause repeated urinary tract infections (UTIs). It is best to place the colostomy in the distal descending or proximal sigmoid colon to make the distal limb shorter than it would be in a transverse colostomy. Many male children with ARMs have urine flow from the urethra into the distal colon and then out the mucous fistula (distal stoma), and if urine stays in the colon for long periods of time, it can cause a significant metabolic acidosis. However, if the distal sigmoid is mistakenly selected for the colostomy, the distal colon may be too tethered to properly come down to the perineum and may require taking down the colostomy at the time of anorectoplasty.

A recommended method for creation of a colostomy is to make a transverse muscle transecting incision in the left abdomen just below the level of the umbilicus. The sigmoid colon is identified and traced proximally and distally to be sure that it is truly the sigmoid and not the transverse colon. A point is selected in the *proximal* sigmoid area, and the colon is transected at this point. The proximal sigmoid is less likely to prolapse because the distal descending colon is fixed to the left lateral peritoneal reflection. After transecting the colon, it is quite important to irrigate the distal colon with warm normal saline to remove all meconium, taking care that the effluent does not get into the peritoneal cavity. If this meconium is not properly removed at the time of colostomy, the meconium will desiccate and form large impacted faecal rocks, which complicate subsequent anorectoplasty. In order to prevent prolapse, the two stomas are secured to the peritoneum and fascia at opposite ends of the wound by using a minimum of six small absorbable sutures (3/0-5/0 vicryl) for each stoma. Approximately 2 cm of each stoma should protrude past the skin level. There is no need to mature these small stomas because they will spontaneously mature, and attempts at operative maturation may occlude the lumen. One or two sutures (3-0 vicryl, polydiaxanone, nylon, silk) are used to approximate the peritoneum, fascia, and muscle between the stomas to minimize parastomal herniation.

A skin bridge is created between the stomas by using interrupted, rapidly absorbable small sutures. The bridge must be wide enough to totally separate the stomas (Figure 77.11). When the child reaches approximately 2–3 months of age, and if the child appears in very good nutritional status as evidenced by a weight of 8–10 kg, a definitive posterior sagittal anorectoplasty (PSARP) can be considered. In males, a distal colostogram should be performed prior to operation to determine the site of the fistula. This is performed by inserting a Foley catheter into the mucous fistula and inflating the balloon enough to occlude the colon lumen. The child is placed in a lateral position on the x-ray table with the hips flexed. Under fluoroscopy, if available, a water-soluble contrast medium is injected to fill the distal rectum and adequately identify the place of entry into the urinary tract (Figure 77.12). If fluoroscopy is not available, proper timing of injection with a plain film x-ray can usually adequately define the fistula.

Posterior Sagittal Anorectoplasty Technique

The technique of PSARP, popularized by Alberto Peña in the 1980s,[7] is currently the most commonly utilized procedure for repairing ARMs. This is the procedure, with a few modifications for African practitioners, that is described in this chapter. PSARP in a male with a urethral fistula is described first because this is a commonly encountered lesion and is the most difficult to repair. A urinary catheter is inserted before definitively positioning the patient. Sometimes the catheter goes through the fistula and into the rectum instead of into the urinary tract. If no urine is obtained from the catheter, the balloon should not be inflated in case it has curled up in the urethra. If the catheter is in the rectum, it can later

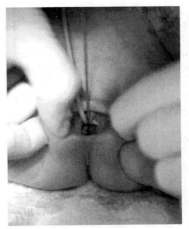

Figure 77.8: Most common female ARM. Catheter is in urethra; probe is in rectovestibular fistula.

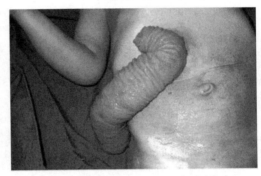

Figure 77.9: Prolapsed right transverse loop colostomy.

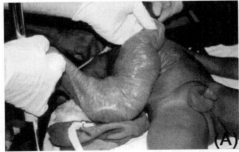

Source: Meier, DE, Opportunities and improvisions--suggestions for successful short-term pediatric surgical volunteer work in resource-poor areas. World J Surg 2010; 34(5): fig 1. Reproduced with permission from Springer Science+Business Media.

Figure 77.10: This three-year-old child with Hirschsprung's disease underwent a colostomy at three months of age. Now he is awaiting someone to perform a definitive procedure. (A) Tremendous prolapse. (B) Colostomy bag improvised by the mother to keep child from stepping on his colostomy.

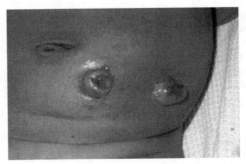

Figure 77.11: Double-barrel colostomy with intervening skin bridge.

be manipulated into the bladder. PSARP is performed with the child in a prone, jackknife position with all pressure points properly padded (Figure 77.13).

A Peña muscle stimulator is the best method for visualizing the perineal musculature, but these stimulators are quite expensive (>US$3000), so they are economically inaccessible for most African paediatric surgeons. As a result, many African surgeons use an electrocautery to identify the musculature, but this may cause damage to precious tissues, even on a low setting. The risk is decreased if a needle-point diathermy is used for all incisions. A much less expensive (US$50) and more appropriate stimulator can be improvised by using an anaesthesia nerve stimulator and a piece of solid, double-pronged, insulated wire, available in hardware stores around the world (Figure 77.14).

The insulation is removed for a distance of 1 cm from both ends of both pieces of the wire. The wire itself can be sterilized by soaking in an appropriate sterilizing solution. One end of both wires is connected to the stimulator. The other ends of the wire are left close to, but not touching, each other. This then serves as the handpiece used to touch the patient. Nonsterile personnel push the "continuous tetany" button on the stimulator whenever the surgeon wants to stimulate the patient with the handpiece to assess muscle contraction.

It is important during PSARP operations that anaesthesia personnel not administer a muscle relaxant because this impairs the use of any muscle or nerve stimulator. If a muscle relaxant is absolutely necessary for intubation, it must be a very short-acting one because the muscle/ nerve stimulator should be used early in the operation to define the musculature before any incision is made.

After mapping out the perineal musculature with a stimulator, temporary stay sutures are placed on either side of the midline at the anterior and posterior limits of the anal muscle complex (sphincter muscle) to identify the limits of the complex later in the operation if needed. A posterior sagittal incision is performed from the coccyx to the perineal body area, preferably with a needle-tip electrocautery placed on "cutting" current. After incising the skin, the deeper tissues can be incised by using the "coagulation" setting. The stimulator is used frequently to ensure that a true midline incision is being performed with equal musculature on either side. The incision is carried in the midline through the parasagittal fibres, the muscle complex, and the levator muscle (Figure 77.15(A)).

Deep to the levator, the white appearance of the rectum should be visualized. Attempts at dissecting around the rectum at this time should be avoided. Distally, the rectum is opened longitudinally to view the inside of the rectal lumen (Figure 77.15(B)). Anteriorly, the small fistula into the urinary tract is seen. Traction sutures are placed, and the anterior rectal wall is very carefully dissected from the posterior urethral wall (Figure 77.15(C)). This is the most difficult part of the operation.

After the initial dissection from the urethral wall itself, the dissection becomes easier above the prostate at the level of the bladder itself. The urinary fistula site should be carefully closed with an absorbable, fine suture. The rectum is then dissected circumferentially, staying close to the rectum itself so as to avoid damage to surrounding nerves, muscle, and urinary tract structures (Figure 77.15(D)). Fibrotic neurovascular bands are taken down to further free the rectum (Figure 77.15(E)). When the rectum is freed enough to come to the perianal skin without significant tension, the closure is performed. Significant tension will cause the neoanus to retract, resulting in lack of epithelial continuity with subsequent scarring and the need for another operation. The muscle anterior to the neoanus, including the perineal body, is closed with fine (4/0, 5/0 vicryl), absorbable suture (Figure 77.15(F)). The colon is placed deep to the levator muscle, and the levator approximated in the midline, taking a bite of the posterior colon wall also. The closure continues along the posterior portion of the muscle complex (sphincter muscle) out to the skin (Figure 77.15(G)). This closure should be close to the previously placed stay sutures marking the posterior limits

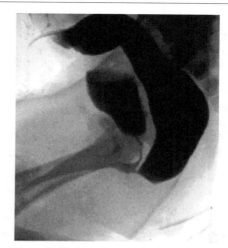

Figure 77.12: Colostogram showing fistula of rectum into bulbous urethra.

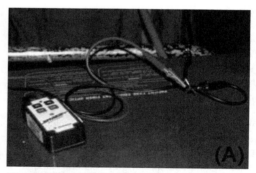

Figure 77.13: Positioning of patient for PSARP.

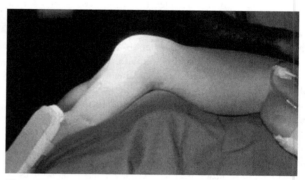

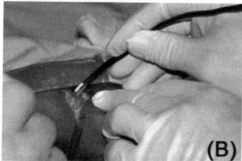

Source: Meier, DE, Opportunities and improvisions--suggestions for successful short-term pediatric surgical volunteer work in resource-poor areas. World J Surg 2010; 34(5): fig 2. Reproduced with permission from Springer Science+Business Media.

Figure 77.14: Improvised anal stimulator: (A) anaesthesia nerve stimulator; (B) handpiece made from solid, double-pronged, insulated wire.

of the muscle complex. Any protruding rectum is debrided, but care is taken to avoid excess tension on the subsequent anastomosis. A 16-suture anoplasty is performed by suturing the full thickness of the colon (neoanus) to the full thickness of the skin (Figure 77.15(H)). A dilator is placed to be sure that the lumen has not been occluded. The rest of the closure is performed, including the parasagittal muscles and subcutaneous tissue. The skin is closed with interrupted full-thickness rapidly absorbing suture (gut) or with a removable running subcuticular suture. There is no good way to secure a dressing to the area, so it is either left open to the air or covered with an antibiotic ointment.

When the rectal fistula goes into the urinary bladder instead of the urethra, a combined abdominal and perineal approach is utilized. The urethral catheter is left in situ for 5–7 days after a male PSARP, and the urine is cultured on its removal. If the patient is nursed prone postoperatively, there is less likelihood of contamination of the wound.

The most common female lesion, a rectovestibular fistula, is also repaired by using PSARP, as described for male lesions. Stay sutures are placed around the vestibular fistula site, and the rectum is carefully dissected from the posterior vaginal wall. This part of the dissection is the most difficult part of the female operation. The rest of the female operation is almost identical with that described above for males.

Females with a persistent cloaca defect present a very difficult challenge. These children should undergo initial decompression with a divided colostomy and a vesicostomy or vaginostomy, as needed to adequately provide urinary drainage. The definitive operation for repair of a persistent cloaca with an anorectoplasty and urogenital mobilization[8] should be delayed until a surgeon with proper expertise can undertake this difficult procedure in an appropriate referral centre.

Dilatation of the neoanus should begin 2–3 weeks postoperatively if the perineal wound has healed well. Ideally, plastic-graded dilators (commercially available for approximately US$10 each) can be provided for the mother to use at home. When such dilators are not available (the usual scenario), the mother can be taught to use her gloved fingers, progressing from the distal phalanx of the little finger to the proximal phalanx of the long finger over a few weeks. Another alternative is the use of an appropriately sized candle for the dilatations. The first dilatation should be performed by the surgeon in the clinic or ward. Starting with an 8-mm size, the surgeon sequentially passes dilators until there is slight resistance. The mother is sent home with this minimally snug dilators and the next larger one. She dilates the anus twice a day for a week and then moves to the next larger size for twice per day dilatations for the next week. After 2 weeks, she is seen in the clinic again, and the next two larger dilators are utilized for the next 2 weeks. When the target size (12 or 13 mm) is reached, and if the perineum has totally healed, the colostomy can be closed, but the dilatations must be continued for at least a year postoperatively.

Anorectoplasties performed by surgeons without proper expertise or equipment can result in a grossly misplaced anus (see Figure 77.16(A)) and a potential lifetime of misery for the child. A secondary operation by a surgeon with both expertise and equipment, although not as successful as a primary operation, is highly recommended *before* closure of the colostomy (Figure 77.16(B)).

Bowel Management Programs

Even under the best of circumstances, some children—particularly those with high ARMs—suffer from constipation or faecal incontinence caused by encopresis (escape of liquid stool around a large, hard faecal impaction). Bowel management programs have been initiated by hospitals in the United States to help children with these problems.[9]

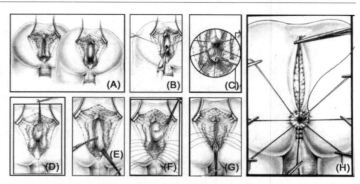

Source: ©1990, Springer-Verlag New York, Inc. From Peña A, Atlas of Surgical Management of Anorectal Malformations, Springer-Verlag, 1990, Figures 3.8–3.14. Reproduced with kind permission of Springer Science+Business Media.

Figure 77.15: The Peña technique for posterior sagittal anorectoplasty: (A) posterior sagittal incision through parasagittal fibres, muscle complex, and levator muscle; (B) distal rectum opened longitudinally; (C) dissection of rectum from fistula and posterior urethra; (D) circumferential dissection of rectum; (E) incision of neurovascular bands; (F) closure of muscle, including perineal body, anterior to rectum; (G) closure of levator muscle and posterior muscle complex; (H) 16-suture anoplasty.

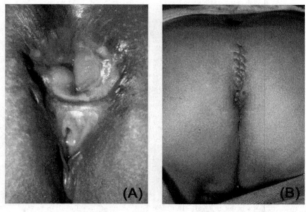

Source: Meier, DE, Opportunities and improvisions–suggestions for successful short-term pediatric surgical volunteer work in resource-poor areas. World J Surg 2010; 34(5): fig 4. Reproduced with permission from Springer Science+Business Media.

Figure 77.16: (A) Misplaced anorectoplasty. (B) Better placement after a secondary salvage operation.

The aim of these programs is to return children to normal lives at school in unsoiled underwear. The overriding principle behind bowel management is that the child learns to evacuate in a socially acceptable place (home) at a socially acceptable time (before or after school). The primary technique used to achieve continence is an enema regimen. The child is given enemas each night or early in the morning at home to completely evacuate the colon. The child can then go to school with confidence, knowing that there will be no stool accidents. After a successful enema regimen has been established, an antegrade continent enema (ACE) operation (known also as an ACE procedure) can be considered.[10] This procedure uses an appendicostomy as a conduit for administering antegrade enemas for evacuating the colon. This technique has been utilized with great success in achieving continence in children who were previously social recluses due to their bowel management problems.[11]

Key Summary Points

1. Anorectal malformations (ARMs) occur commonly and are a cause of significant morbidity for African children.

2. The most common ARM in males is a fistula of the rectum into the urinary tract (usually urethra); in females, it is a fistula into the vestibule of the vagina.

3. ARMs are one component of the VACTERL complex, and diagnostic techniques appropriate for a particular locale should be used to look for the other components of this complex.

4. The specific type of ARM is diagnosed on the basis of the newborn physical examination and a few technologically easy techniques.

5. Low lesions, which unfortunately constitute the minority of lesions, can be treated by a primary anoplasty without a colostomy.

6. Most ARMs are high lesions and should be treated initially with a sigmoid colostomy.

7. Improperly constructed colostomies can be a source of great morbidity for children.

8. The recommended definitive treatment for ARMs is a posterior sagittal anorectoplasty.

9. Even after the best of operations, children with ARMs can suffer from bowel management problems. A proper bowel management program can make a significant positive change in the life of a previously miserable child with faecal incontinence.

References

1. Moore SW, Alexander A, Sidler D, Alves J, Hadley GP, Numanoglu A, Banieghbal B, Chitnis M, Birabwa-Male D, Mbuwayesango B, Hesse A, Lakhoo K. The spectrum of anorectal malformations in Africa. Pediatr Surg Int 2008; 24:677–683.

2. Uba AF, Chirdan LB, Ardill W, Edino ST. Anorectal anomaly: a review of 82 cases seen at JUTH, Nigeria. Niger Postgrad Med J 2006;13(1):61–65.

3. Adejuyigbe O, Abubakar AM, Sowande OA, Olayinka OS, Uba AF. Experience with anorectal malformations in Ile-Ife, Nigeria. Pediatr Surg Int 2004; 20:855–858.

4. Archibong AE, Idika IM. Results of treatment in children with anorectal malformations in Calabar, Nigeria. S Afr J Surg 2004; 42(3):88–90.

5. Johnson O, Ghidey Y, Habte D. Congenital malformation of anus and rectum in Ethiopian children. Ethiop Med J 1981; 19(1):9–15.

6. Peña A. Anorectal malformations. In: Ziegler M, Azizkhan R, Weber T, eds. Operative Pediatric Surgery. McGraw Hill Publishers, 2003, Pp 739–761.

7. Peña A. Atlas of Surgical Management of Anorectal Malformations. Springer-Verlag, 1989.

8. Peña A. Total urogenital mobilization: an easier way to repair cloacas. J Pediatr Surg 1997; 32:263–268.

9. Peña A, Guardino K, Tovilla JM. Bowel management for fecal incontinence in patients with anorectal malformations. J Pediatr Surg 1998; 33:133–137.

10. Malone PS, Ransley PG, Kiely EM. Preliminary report: the antegrade continence enema. Lancet 1990; 336:1217–1218.

11. Meier DE, Foster E, Guzzetta PC, Coln D. Antegrade continent enema management of chronic fecal incontinence in children. J Pediatr Surg 1998; 33(7):1149–1152.

CHAPTER 78
POLYPS

Behrouz Banieghbal
Kokila Lakhoo

Introduction

Polyps and polypoid disorders in children, unlike those in adults, are relatively rare and are mostly benign. A complete understanding of these conditions is required for correct treatment and follow-up of these children. Polypoid disorder of the gastrointestinal (GI) tract include true polyps (juvenile and adenomatous), a variety of uncommon polyp syndromes, and a number of miscellaneous diseases of the intestinal tract that may present polypoid masses in the lumen of the intestine.

Demographics

Most reports of large series estimate that close to 1% of the population have polyps sometime during their childhood. Juvenile polyps are the most common type of lesion found in the GI tract in children, accounting for more than 80% of juvenile polyps. They are slightly more common in boys than in girls. The reported incidence of juvenile polyposis syndrome is 1:100,000.

Other polyposis syndromes, such as Peutz-Jeghers syndrome and familial adenatomoid polyposis (FAP) with its many variants, are reported to have an incidence of 1:200,000 and 1:35,000, respectively, with no racial variation.[1]

Juvenile Polyps

Juvenile polyps are the most common type of polyp in the gastrointestinal tract accounting for more than 80% of polyps in children. The affected age group is between 2 and 5 years. Macroscopically, these lesions appear as beefy red and range from several millimeters to several centimeters in size. Microscopically, they represent benign harmatomas with no malignant potential (Figures 78.1 & 78.2). The most common presentation of these polyps is painless bleeding, which is caused by inflammation and mucosal ulceration of the polyp. They may be asymptomatic and occasionally present with abdominal pain (10%) or prolapse (4%) if located low in the rectum. Diagnosis is made through history, rectal examination, sigmoidoscopy, colonoscopy, and / or air contrast enema. Histological examination of the polyp is vital to the management of the patient.

Many polyps are located in the rectum and lower sigmoid colon and can be snared and removed through a flexible sigmoidoscope. Some of these lesions can be prolapsed through the anus and removed by suture ligation of the pedicle (see Figure 78.1). For higher lesions, a snare and cautery through a colonoscopy may be performed. It is rarely necessary to perform a laparotomy with colostomy for removal of a juvenile polyp. If more than five polyps are identified, a colonoscopic excision of the polyps should be performed. This latter clinical scenario of more than five polyps may indicate juvenile polyposis syndrome (see next section) and would place the child at risk for future colorectal malignancies. Complications after endoscopic removal of juvenile polyps have been rare. Perforation and subsequent bleeding from additional or recurrent juvenile polyps is believed to be approximately 5%. The natural history of juvenile polyps is that they are self-limited and seem to disappear, presumably by auto amputation.

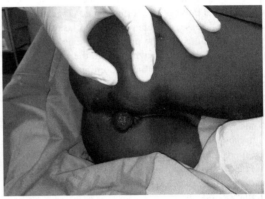

Figure 78.1: A prolapsed juvenile polyp prior to surgical excision in a 3-year-old girl.

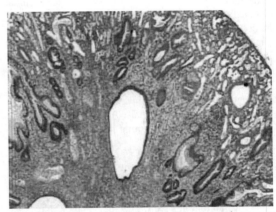

Figure 78.2: Cystic hamartomatous appearance on microscopy of a juvenile polyp.

Juvenile Polyposis Syndrome

Juvenile polyposis syndrome is a dominant inherited disorder that can present as diffuse juvenile polyposis of infancy (age 0–3 months), diffuse juvenile polyposis (age 6 months–5 years) and juvenile polyposis coli (age 5–15 years). Diarrhoea, rectal bleeding, intussusception, anaemia, prolapse, and failure to thrive are common presenting signs. The diagnosis is made as per juvenile polyps (see preceding section), and the presence of more than five polyps in sporadic cases and one polyp in cases with a family history confirms the diagnosis. Although polyps in this disorder are benign, patients have a 17% risk of developing cancer (significantly less than patients with a family history of FAP). The average age for the diagnosis of cancer is 30 years and older. Additionally, gastric duodenal and pancreatic cancers have been reported. In contrast to sporadic juvenile polyps, new polyps almost always form after a polyp is removed, and polyps continue into adulthood. Surveillance colonoscopy every 3 years should begin in the early teens, even in asymptomatic cases. Many surgeons recommend prophylactic colectomy and rectal mucosectomy with endorectal pull-through as the primary treatment for the disease as soon as the diagnosis is established.

Juvenile polyposis syndrome is a genetic disease linked to a number of mutations on mothers against decapentaplegic homolog 4 gene and SMA protein (collectively called SMAD4 on chromosome 18q21.2), which is a transforming growth factor intracellular protein; bone morphogenetic protein receptor type IA (BMPR1A on chromosome 10p22.3), an important protein in cell differentiation; and finally phosphatase/tensin homolog (PTEN) oncogene, which is a tumour suppressor gene on chromosome 19q32.[2]

Peutz-Jeghers Syndrome

Peutz-Jeghers syndrome is characterized by the presence of intestinal polyps with mucocutaneous pigmentation of the mouth, hands, and feet (Figure 78.3). The relationship of mucocutaneous pigmentation to polyposis is unknown; intestinal polyps are not pigmented (Figure 78.4). It is an autosomal dominant disease, and the polyps are classified as harmatomas of the muscularis mucosa. The polyps are mainly located in the small intestine but may be found anywhere from the stomach to the rectum. Patients often present with cramping abdominal pain and bowel obstruction secondary to intussusception of a polyp. These patients have an increased risk of cancer with transformation of hamartomas into carcinomas. Whether the carcinoma develops in these polyps or elsewhere in the mucosa is unknown. Patients are at an increased risk of developing malignancies in epithelial tissues; for example, it has been estimated that there is an 84-, 213-, and 520-fold increased risk of developing colon, gastric, and small intestinal cancers, respectively. A further 10% of patients with Peutz-Jeghers syndrome develop ovarian, cervical, and testicular neoplasms.

Diagnosis is made by family history, pigmented lesions, and cramping abdominal pain. Current recommendations for treatment include annual physical examinations, full blood count, breast and pelvic examinations, testicular examinations with ultrasound, and pancreatic examination with ultrasound. Oesophagogastroduodenoscopy and colonoscopy are recommended annually. Polyps larger than 5 mm are removed.

Peutz-Jeghers polyps arise from mutations in the serine/threonine kinase 11 (STK11/LKB1) tumour suppression gene (chromosome 19p13.3) in 70% of patients.[3] This is an important kinase protein that is involved with intracellular growth signals. A different and as yet unrecognized gene is involved in the remaining patients.

Familial Adenomatous Polyposis

Familial adenomatous polyposis is an autosomal dominant syndrome with a 100% risk of developing cancer. It is caused by germ-line mutations in the adenomatous polyposis coli (APC) gene. Presentation includes rectal bleeding, abdominal pain, anaemia, and/or diarrhoea. Diagnosis is usually made during screening of children from affected families and screening for the APC gene. Diagnosis is established by sigmoidoscopy, which reveals a colon carpeted with polyps. Polyps can also occur in other parts of the gastrointestinal tract.

In patients with FAP and its variants, the risk of malignancy in adulthood is so high that prophylactic colectomy is recommended for most cases (Figure 78.5). This is usually delayed until the midteen years.[4] The surgical options include: total colectomy with mucosal proctectomy and the endorectal ileal-pouch anal anastomosis (IPAA); or subtotal colectomy and ileorectal anastomosis (IRA).

IPAA is a more extensive procedure with a higher complication rate but a lesser incidence of rectal cancer in the follow-up period. It is therefore the recommended procedure for patients with >1,000 polyps or if available in FAP with known genetic mutations at condons 1250–1464. Lesser surgery such as IRA is thus reserved for "attenuated" FAP patients or those who have 50–100 polyps on endoscopy.[5]

Oral use of nonsteriodal anti-inflammatory drugs (NSAIDs, especially sulindac) has remained controversial, but it has been shown to cause regression of polyps in patients, especially if used after rectum-sparing surgery. Lifetime surveillance is still needed, however,

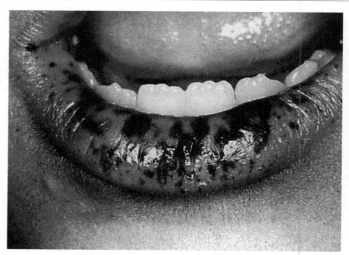

Figure 78.3: Oral pigmentation in an adult with Puetz-Jeghers syndrome.

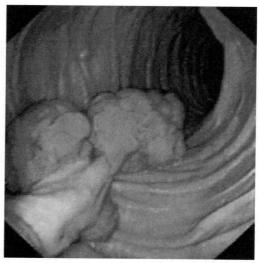

Figure 78.4: Duodenal polyp in a patient with Peutz-Jeghers syndrome.

as rectal carcinoma has been reported in these patients. The rare cases with MAP-type attenuated FAP can be spare surgery and instead have colonoscopic surveillance and regular snare polypectomies.

Mutations within the loci of the tumour suppressor APC gene across the band 5q21-22 result in the multitude of clinical manifestations of this condition. The APC gene encodes a 2843 amino acid protein involved in cell adhesion and signal transduction, the failure of which sets the stage for epithelial tumours. Proximal APC mutations (i.e., proximal to codon 1249) produce a milder FAP syndrome with sparse polyposis, otherwise known as attenuated FAP. However, APC mutations between codons 1250 and 1330 present with tremendous degrees of polyposis (>5,000 adenomas) and intracerebral malignancy (Turcot syndrome), hepatoblastoma, or intraabdominal desmoid tumours (Gardner's syndrome).

FAP is an autosomal dominant disorder, and registries are in place in most First World countries to monitor families with this disorder, which account for 80% of the cases. Recently, another type of attenuated FAP, termed mutYH-associated-polyposis (MAP), was described in the remaining 20% of the cases; these cases are all attenuated FAPs that— unlike classic FAP—are autosomal recessive in nature and not related to mutation on the APC gene. Rather, mutation is reported to occur on mutY homolog gene on chromosome 1p34.3.[6]

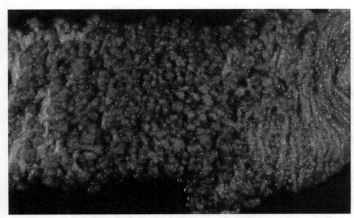

Figure 78.5: Colectomy specimen of a teenager with FAP.

Other Syndromes

Gardner's syndrome is an autosomal dominant disorder described as the association between colonic familial adenomatous polyposis and multiple osteomas, fibromas, and epidermoid cysts. The natural history and treatment of the colonic polyps is the same as for FAP. Turcot syndrome is the association of colonic FAP and brain tumours.

Pseudopolyps

Pseudopolyps consist of submucosal intestinal lymphatic tissue secondary to hyperplasia due to nonspecific infectious causes. Ulceration of these lesions may cause bleeding and anaemia. Diagnosis is confirmed at colonoscopy. Treatment is directed toward eradicating the underlying infectious process.

Differential Diagnosis

The differential diagnosis for rectal bleeding includes the common causes such as anal fissures, which generally can be visualized externally; and acute and chronic inflammatory bowel disease, which usually is accompanied by diarrhoea and blood dyscrasias, such as Henoch-Schönlein purpura. Bleeding from Meckel's diverticulum, duplication cysts of the intestine, and terminal ileal tuberculosis is usually of greater magnitude, dark, and mixed with stool. Bleeding from intussusception is usually accompanied by severe cramping abdominal pain and bilious vomiting.

Prognosis and Outcomes

Polypoid syndromes with known genetic anomalies have significant carcinoma risks; in FAP, surgical strategies as described above minimize these. A close follow-up is needed to detect and deal with other concurrent tumours with these genetic disorders. Counselling of the patients and their immediate relatives should be conducted.[7]

Ethical Issues

All children with polyps must have an expert histological examination of the excised polyp. If this proves to be an adult-type adenomatous polyp, then long-term surveillance with colonoscopies every 2 to 3 years is warranted. All close relatives must also undergo colonoscopies to exclude FAP in the family.

Evidence-Based Research

Table 78.1 presents a review article colonic polyps in children and adolescents.

Table 78.1: Evidence-based research.

Title	Colonic polyps in children and adolescents
Authors	Durno CA
Institution	The Hospital for Sick Children, Division of gastroenterology and Nutrition, University of Toronto, Canada
Reference	Can J Gastroenterol 2007; 21(4):233–239
Problem	The challenge is determining the precise risk of colorectal cancer in polyposis disease of childhood and adolescence.
Intervention	Debate on timing and type of surgery for colonic polyps with malignant potential.
Comparison/ control (quality of evidence)	Review article.
Outcome/ effect	Juvenile polyps are a common and benign disease. Other polyps require genetic screening and surveillance, and have high degree of malignant transformation.

Key Summary Points

1. Polyps and polypoid disorders in children are mostly benign.

2. Polypoid disorder of the GI tract includes true polyps (juvenile and adenomatous), a variety of uncommon polyp syndromes, and a number of miscellaneous diseases.

3. Juvenile polyps are benign, whereas adenomatous polyps have 100% malignant transformation.

4. Syndromic polyposis diseases also have malignant potential.

5. Presentation may be rectal bleeding, diarrhoea, abdominal pain, intussusceptions, and/or bowel obstruction.

6. Diagnosis is made through history, rectal examination, sigmoidoscopy, colonoscopy, and/or air contrast enema.

7. Treatment is dictated by the histology of the polyp, which includes simple excision or total colectomy.

8. Surveillance is highly recommended for any polyp with malignant potential.

References

1. Tietelbaum DH. Polypoid diseases of the gastrointestinal tract. In: O'Niell JA, Grosfeld JL, Fonkalsrud EW, Coran AG, Caldamone AA (eds). Principles of Pediatric Surgery, 2nd ed, Mosby-Year Book Inc. 2004, Pp 547–556.

2. van Hattem WA, Brosen LA, De Lang WW, Morsink FH, et al. Large genomic deletions of SMAD4, BMPR1A and PTEN in juvenile polyposis. Gut 2008; 57(5):623–627.

3. Durno CA. Colonic polyps in children and adolescents. Can J Gastroenterol 2007; 21(4):233–239.

4. Vasen HFA, Moslein G, Alonso A, Aretz S, et al. Guidelines for the clinical management for familial adenomatous polyposis. Gut 2008; 57(5):704–713.

5. Burt RW, Jacoby RE. Polyposis syndromes. In: Yamada T (ed). Textbook of Gasteroenterology, 4th ed. Lippincott Williams & Wilkins. 2003, Pp 1914–1939.

6. Al-Tassan N, Chmiel NH, Maynard J. Inherited variants of MYH associated with somatic G:C-T:A: mutations in colorectal tumours. Nat Genet 2002; 30(4):227–232.

7. Petersen GM, Boyd PA. Gene testing and counseling for colorectal cancer risk; lessons from familial polyposis. J Natl Cancer Inst Monogr 1995; 17:67–71.

CHAPTER 79
OTHER ANORECTAL CONDITIONS

John Chinda

Emmanuel A. Ameh

Kokila Lakhoo

Introduction

Children have a variety of anorectal problems that cause considerable distress to the patients and challenges to the surgeons. The presentation of these conditions may be age specific. Abscesses, fistulas, and fissures appear more commonly in infants and young children, whereas hemorrhoidal diseases are more common in older children and teenagers. The anorectal conditions discussed in this chapter include:

• Anorectal abscess and fistula-in-ano

• Fissure-in-ano

• Rectal prolapse

• Haemorrhoids

•Condylomata accuminatum

• Acquired rectovaginal fistula

Anorectal Abscess and Fistula-in-Ano

An anorectal abscess is essentially a "boil" of the perianal region. The abscess and the fistula are usually part of a continuum, the latter presenting as a progression of the former. Up to 85% of children with perianal abscess (PAA) may progress to form a fistula-in-ano (FIA).[1]

Demographics

Perianal abscess is relatively common in infants.[2] The true incidence is not known, but in some large series of patients with perianal fistula (adults and children),[3–5] 0.5% to 4.3% are children. The disease presents before the age of 1 year in 57%–86% of affected children,[6,7] mostly in males.

In reports of small numbers of patients from parts of sub-Saharan Africa, the median age of children with PAA and FIA was 3 years, again mostly in boys.[8]

Aetiology/Pathogenesis

The aetiology in infants has been a subject of controversy. The derivation of FIA from PAA has long been accepted.[9] Infection within the crypts of Morgagni at the dentate line gives rise to an abscess and triggers an inflammatory response that may result in a fistula.

Dermal infections, especially diaper dermatitis, might be a cause of PAA that may not necessarily develop into FIA after drainage.[10]

An androgen imbalance (androgen excess or imbalance in the androgen-estrogen ratio) has been incriminated as a congenital aetiology. This is thought to create abnormal anal glands that favour the formation of fistulas.[6] These abnormal crypts were noted in continuity to the fistula in 33 consecutive patients, and opening these crypts reduced their recurrence. Others have disputed the crypts' role in the aetiology of FIA.[11] Some have described irregular thickened tissue at the dentate line that predisposes to cryptis by trapping bacteria,[12] whereas others have suggested that aberrant migration of the urogenital sinus or hindgut could give rise to fistulous tracts.[13] In addition, entrapped migratory ectopic transitional cells have been demonstrated in the histology of excised fistulous tracts and have been suggested as

the cause of the fistula,[13] although inflammatory metaplasia can also explain the cellular ectopia. In some cases, FIA may be a complication of an anorectal surgery.[8]

Clinical Evaluation

Perianal abscess is often a very painful swelling in the perianal region. There may be associated pyrexia and passage of loose stools, particularly in ischiorectal and supralevator abscess. In sub-Saharan Africa, the abscess may burst spontaneously before presentation, and this may progress to rapidly developing necrotising fasciitis of the perineum.[8,14]

Fistula-in-ano frequently follows a spontaneously discharged or surgically drained PAA.

Digital rectal examination and anoscopy should be performed. In PAA, severe tenderness may preclude this, and a general anaesthetic may be required, especially in younger patients. The internal opening of the fistula should be identified; the opening is usually a small area of heaped up granulation tissue with pus in the punctate opening, often located at the dentate line. The tract is a cord-like structure leading to the anal sphincter.

Duhamel noted that FIA in infants and children have certain characteristics that seem to separate them from adult cases.[7] The characteristics of FIA in children can be summarized as follows:

• FIA mostly occurs in males.

• FIA mostly occurs in infants <1 year of age.

• All fistulas appear to be contiguous with the closest crypt.

• Multiple but separate tracts are fairly frequent (17–20%).

• Complex ramifying tracts are rare.

• Recurrence is not uncommon.

Investigations

Microbiology and serology

Any discharging fluid or pus should be cultured and antibiotic sensitivity obtained. Staining for acid-fast bacilli is necessary if tuberculosis (TB) is suspected in FIA.

Human immunodeficiency virus (HIV) serology should be done in cases that are recurrent or difficult to treat, after appropriate counselling.

Haematological

A complete blood count should be done. In PAA, leucocytosis is usually present.

Biochemical

If diabetes mellitus is suspected as an underlying condition, this should be ascertained by doing a urine and blood sugar assay.

Histopathology

Any tissue obtained at surgical treatment should be subjected to histopathology, particularly in the African setting, to exclude chronic granulomatous disease, including tuberculosis.

Radiology

If TB is suspected, a chest radiograph should be done to identify any evidence of the disease.

Management

General measures

Appropriate broad-spectrum antibiotics, effective against gram-negative enteric bacilli, gram-positives, and anaerobes is given. In early stages of PAA, this may be enough to control the infection and prevent progression.

Analgesics are given in PAA after establishing a diagnosis, as the condition is quite painful.

Specific measures

• *PAA.* Once an abscess is fully formed, adequate incision and drainage is done under general anaesthetic. It is important that appropriate antibiotics be started before the abscess drainage to prevent dissemination of the infection, which may cause portal pyaemia. Following drainage, the abscess cavity is lightly packed with gauze soaked in EUSOL (Edinburgh University solution) or native honey. The cavity is cleaned and lightly packed daily to allow gradual filling of the cavity by granulation tissue.

• *FIA.* The use of appropriate antibiotics and a sitz bath is done initially to control infection. Most FIA in children is of the intershincteric type, and the aim of treatment is to completely lay open the fistulous tract. The definitive treatment of these fistulas is fistulotomy or fistulectomy.[1] If the corresponding anal crypt can be identified, it should be included in the fistulotomy or fistulectomy. If fistulotomy is done, a biopsy is taken from the tract and sent for histopathology. Following fistulectomy, the entire specimen is sent for histopathology. Any primary underlying condition, such as tuberculosis and immunosuppresion, should be appropriately treated.

Outcome

After incision and drainage or spontaneous drainage of PAA, up to 35% develop a FIA. Following fistulotomy or fistulectomy for FIA, a recurrence rate of up to 68% has been reported.[1,15–17] Figures 79.1 and 79.2 illustrate the result in one large series.[1] Most recurrences follow shortly after treatment, and late recurrences are uncommon.[1] In a few instances, poor healing may result in perianal scarring, which may interfere with proper cleaning. Although some mild faecal soilage may occur initially, this would usually resolve and rarely causes any functional problems.

Fissure-in-Ano

Anal fissure (AF) is a tear in the anal mucosa that extends distally from the dentate line to the anal verge. With each bowel movement, the anal mucosa is stretched and the fissure reopened. Most acute fissures heal spontaneously within a few weeks, but some become chronic. AF is a common cause of haematochezia and anal pain in children.

Aetiology/Pathogenesis

The aetiology for anal fissure is still largely obscure. Initial trauma occurs with subsequent failure of healing. This initial trauma is usually caused by hard stools following constipation, although diarrhea can also be associated with the condition. Other diseases, such as HIV infections and Crohn's disease, or previous surgery can also be responsible. Repeated sexual abuse[17] (Figure 79.3) can also cause AF.

Fear of painful defaecation may lead to faecal retention and rectal distention, resulting in decreased rectal sensation. This may result in frequent bulky and hard stools that prevent healing of the fissure, creating a vicious circle.[18] The failure of healing can also be attributed to ischemia, which usually results from intense associated muscle spasm and sphincteric hypertonicity.[19]

Clinical Evaluation

The classic presentation of AF is that of a child crying with each bowel motion and the presence of bright red blood streaks in stools. The pre-

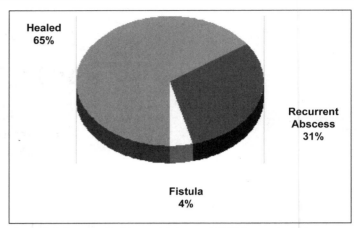

Figure 79.1: Results of incision and drainage of 26 PAA cases in children.

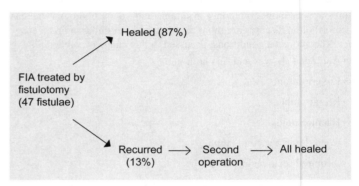

Figure 79.2: Results of treatment of 47 FIA cases in children.

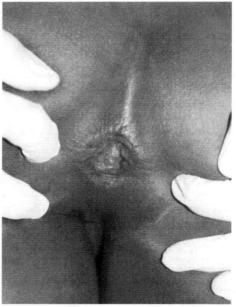

Figure 79.3: Fissure-in-ano resulting from repeated anal sexual abuse in a boy.

sentation is often associated with constipation.

Firm faecal masses may be palpated on the left side at abdominal examination, usually the result of faecal retention from the severe anal pain.

The diagnosis is made on anal inspection. AF is usually identified as a posterior midline longitudinal mucosal tear distal to the dentate, but it may be found anywhere along the anal circumference. Chronic fissures can be associated with a finding of hypertrophied anal papillae, sentinel tags, polyps, or haemorrhoids.

The fissures from chronic anal sexual abuse may be multiple, and the anus may appear rather patulous.

Digital rectal examination is best avoided, as this may produce severe pain.

Management

The goal of treatment for anal fissure is to relieve pain, aid normal defaecation, and achieve and maintain healing of the fissure. The majority of anal fissures will heal on medical treatment, but surgery may be needed if medical measures fail.

Medical treatment

Control of pain helps to relieve sphincter spasm and encourage defaecation. Oral analgesics can achieve this. If the pain is acutely severe, topical analgesics/anaesthetics using lignocaine gel (or another appropriate topical agent) help to produce quick relief of pain.

To aid normal defaecation, treatment should include the following measures:

- Encourage a high-fibre diet to help avoid constipation and the formation of hard stools.

- The use of stool softeners in addition to analgesia helps to establish normal defaecation and interrupts the vicious process created by fissure and hard stools.

- The use of topical 0.2% glyceryl trinitrate *cream* has been found to be effective in healing fissures in children.[20,21] However, one randomized control study concluded that topical 0.2% glyceryl-trinitrate *paste* is not beneficial in relieving pain in acute fissures.[22]

- Injection of botulinum toxin into the internal anal sphincters has been used to reduce internal sphincter spasm. This enhances defaecation as well as relieving pain.

With medical treatment, most fissures should heal. In a minority of patients, medical treatment may fail and surgical measures may become necessary.

Surgical treatments

Anal dilatation under general anaesthetic helps to interrupt sphincter spasm. This would aid defaecation and allow the fissure to heal. Anal dilatation should be combined with medical measures to achieve maximal benefits. Anal dilatation should be used with caution in children, however, as overenthusiastic dilatation may result in faecal incontinence.

Lateral internal anal sphincterotomy[23,24] is a surgical disruption of the internal anal sphincter aimed at relieving spasm and enhancing defaecation. It produces symptom relief in up to 98% of patients.[23] After sphincterotomy, the fissure usually heals in about 10–14 days. Continue medical measures for about 2 weeks after fissure healing to avoid recurrence.

Fissurectomy entails complete excision of the fissure, and should be reserved for the occasional nonhealing fissure or those with troublesome recurrence.

Rectal Prolapse

Rectal prolapse is a relatively common, self-limiting condition in children between 1 and 3 years of age.

Aetiology

Rectal prolapse occurs frequently as a result of diarrheal illness, constipation, weight loss or malnutrition, recurrent straining, and prolonged sitting on the toilet (usually due to tenesmus from parasitic infestation). Commonly implicated parasites include *Enterobius vermicularis, Trichuris trichuria*, and *Entamoeba histolytica*.

Pathology

Dilatation of the levator mechanism results in herniation of the rectum, causing prolapse. Due to persistent straining, the pelvic peritoneum is stretched and so are the suspensory vessels and adjacent structures,

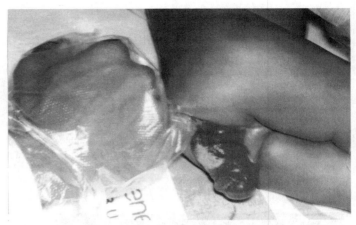

Figure 79.4: Differentiating between rectal prolapse and intussusceptions protruding through the anus (note the extent of insinuated finger into the sulcus between bowel loop and anal wall).

resulting in a prolapse. Other contributing factors are a short, straight sacrum and a redundant sigmoid colon.

In some congenital conditions, such as bladder exstrophy and myelomeningocele, rectal prolapse is one of the symptoms and is the result of true weakness of rectal supports. Nonoperative management is rarely successful in these situations.

Evaluation

Diagnosis is usually based on a history of a protruding mass and discomfort in the anus during defaecation, which either reduces spontaneously or is returned manually. The rosette rectal mucosa is usually noted. This can be differentiated from intussusception by insinuating a finger in the sulcus between the mass and perianal skin; the sulcus is endless in the latter, but blind-ended in the former (Figure 79.4). Confusing a rectal prolapse with intussusception is known to cause delays in referral for intussusceptions in parts of sub-Saharan Africa.[25]

Rectal examination is indicated to exclude polyps and lead points.

Stool microscopy

Microscopic examination of the stool is necessary to identify any parasite ova or trophozoites of *Entamoeba hystolytica*.

Barium enema

In recurrent cases, a barium enema may be needed to exclude other rectal pathology as well as elongated and redundant rectum.

Colonoscopy

Colonoscopy is helpful in difficult recurrent cases to help identify any rectal pathology that may be preventing resolution of the prolapse.

Management

Nonoperative treatment

In most cases, the condition is self-limiting, so nonoperative treatment should be employed at the outset. This consists of prompt reduction of the prolapse and teaching the parents how to reduce it. This reduction should be done each time the rectum prolapses.

The cause of any diarrhoea or constipation should be treated. Anhelminthics should be given for parasites identified at stool microscopy.

Nutritional rehabilitation should be instituted for those who are malnourished.

In symptomatic prolapse, the treatment should be nonoperative. In exstrophy, the prolapse usually disappears after correction of the primary cause. In myelomeningocele, the success of treatment depends on the severity of the condition.

Operative treatment

Surgery is indicated in cases with intractable prolapse after 6 months of nonoperative management.

A Thiersch suture may be applied to keep the prolapse reduced while treating the precipitating cause.

More radical surgical options include excision of redundant rectal mucosa and plication of the rectum. More extensive procedures, such as rectopexy, are rarely required and should be reserved for troublesome recurrent cases.

Occasionally, the prolapsed rectum undergoes dessication, ulceration, and may become infected. A few may develop necrosis of the prolapsed rectum (Figure 79.5). These complications put the patient at risk of pyelephlebitis. The patient should be quickly resuscitated and any gangreneous or compromised rectum resected transanally. If the rectum is only infected or ulcerated, control of infection and nonoperative measures are usually successful.

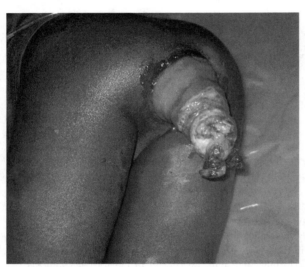

Figure 79.5: Rectal prolapse with oedema, ulceration, and necrosis in a 2-year-old boy following acute diarrhea.

Outcome
Rectal prolapse is usually self-limiting in a vast majority of patients and should resolve after appropriate treatment of the precipitating cause. Even in those requiring surgery, recurrence is unusual.

Haemorrhoids
Haemorrhoids are an uncommon condition in the paediatric population. Aetiology is mainly related to other conditions such as portal hypertension or cystic fibrosis and rarely is a result of straining at stool. Presentation includes painless bleeding and perianal pruritus. On examination, bluish discoloration or a prolapsed haemorrhoid may be noticed in the perianal area. Treatment is mainly conservative with local hygiene and cold packs. If conservative management fails, injection schlerotherapy with phenol in almond oil is a safe option in children.

Acquired Rectal Fistula
With the surge of HIV infection especially in sub-Saharan Africa, acquired rectal fistula has become one of the commonest surgical pathologies seen among children with HIV.[26-30] It is more common in girls,[27] but boys can also be affected.

Aetiology/Pathogensis
The pathophysiology of acquired rectal fistulas is largely unknown. Such fistulas have been noted to arise from the dentate line, and anal gland infections are proposed as the initiating factors.[28] There is, however, a recognized clinical pattern in these patients, in which HIV-related rectal fistula follows a diarrhea infection, and crypt abscess and fistulation into the vagina in girls and the urethra in boys. However, the exact mechanism of this process remains unknown.

Pathologically, the fistula is usually located at the dentate line. There is nonspecific inflammatory ulceration and acute chronic procititis.[27] One postmortem examination of the fistula edge showed a nonspecific ulcer.[31] Cytomegalovirus (CMV) has been noted in the rectal mucosa in a small minority of patients.[27]

Management
In patients not already known to have HIV infection, the serum should be tested for HIV to confirm diagnosis. In boys, a voiding cystourethrogram is helpful in identifying the urethral site of the fistula.

The main focus of initial treatment should be the administration of appropriate antiretroviral drugs. Appropriate antibiotics should be given if there are superimposed infections, and the nutritional status of the child should be significantly improved.

Once the CD4 count has improved to adequate levels, the fistula can be excised and the wound repaired, preferably under a protective diversion colostomy.

Initial surgical excision of the fistula should be avoided as much as possible because wound healing is not so good in these patients, and such wounds would break down with recurrence of the fistula.

Condylomata Accuminatum
Condylomata acuminatum (CA) is an infection caused by the human papillomavirus. It is normally a sexually transmitted disease in adults, but may occasionally be found in children of affected mothers. Sexual abuse should always be excluded.[32,33]

CA presents as a warty or verrucous growth in the perineal and anal region. It may be only a few growths, but it could be extensive. Diagnosis is confirmed at the histology of the biopsied growth.

The treatment may be medical, using such local agents as podophyllin, but this needs to be applied for several weeks, and recurrence may be a problem.

Fulguration or surgical excision is effective. Cryosurgery has also been found to be effective.

Evidence-Based Research
Table 79.1 presents evidence-based research for HIV-positive African children with rectal fistulas.

Table 79.1: Evidence-based research.

Title	HIV positive African children with rectal fistulae
Authors	Wiersma R
Institution	Department of Paediatric Surgery, Nelson R. Mandela School of Medicine, University of Natal, Durban, South Africa
Reference	J Pediatr Surg 2003; 38:62–64
Problem	Occurrence and treatment of HIV-related rectal fistulae in children.
Intervention	Fistula closure/repair.
Comparison/ control (quality of evidence)	A 6-year (1996 through 2001) retrospective study found 39 children presenting with HIV-related rectal fistulae. Thirty-seven girls were seen with rectovaginal fistulae (RVF), and supportive documentation shows an increase in this condition throughout Southern Africa. Until now, boys have not been described with this condition. Two boys who complete this spectrum of HIV-related acquired rectal fistulae are presented.
Outcome/ effect	All patients were found to have rectal fistulae at the dentate line. In girls, they varied in size from pinpoint to 5 mm in diameter, tracking anteriorly into the vagina. When closure of the fistula was attempted, it broke down. The two boys had large fistulae, which tracked to the prostatic urethra on the right of the verumontanum. The first patient underwent a successful repair. The second patient had a Y-shaped fistula based at the dentate line, with the second limb passing into the bladder. The parents refused further treatment and took the child home.
Historical significance/ comments	HIV disease affects increasing numbers of children. A spectrum of rectal fistulae now has been seen in both girls and boys. These acquired rectal fistulae arise at the dentate line in both genders. Girls with these fistulae are seen more commonly, presenting with RVF. The closure of a fistula has been successful in only one boy.

Key Summary Points

1. Noncongenital anorectal conditions affect children and are commonly infective in nature.

2. Some rectal fistula diseases may be the result of sexual abuse, and these children should be evaluated for abuse when relevant.

3. Rectal fistula is now a common presentation in HIV-infected children, and HIV infection should be excluded in children presenting with noncongenital rectal fistula.

4. Most of these anorectal conditions can be treated by simple measures, and several are self-limiting.

5. Radical or extensive surgical treatment should be avoided as much as possible, except in difficult recurrent cases.

References

1. Festen C, Van Harten H. Perianal abscess and fistula-in-ano in infants. J Pediatr Surg 1998; 33:711–713.

2. Rosen NG, Gibbs DL, Soffer SZ, Hong H, Sher M, Pena A. The non-operative management of fistula-in-ano. J Pediatr Surg 2000; 35:938–939.

3. Hill JR. Fistulas and fistulous abscesses in the anorectal region. Personal experience in management. Dis Colon Rectum 1967; 10:421–434.

4. Matt JG. Anal fistula in infants and children. Dis Colon Rectum 1960; 3: 258–261.

5. Mazier WP. The treatment and care of anal fistulas: a study of 1000 patients. Dis Colon Rectum 1971; 14:134–144.

6. Fitzgerald RJ, Harding B, Ryan W. Fistula in childhood: a congenital aetiology. J Pediatr Surg 1985; 20:80–81.

7. Duhamel J. Anal fistulae in childhood. Am J Proctol 1975; 26:40–43.

8. Ameh EA. Perianal abscess and fistula in children in Zaria. Niger Postgrad Med J. 2003; 10:107–109.

9. Poenaru D, Yazbeck S. Anal fistula in infants: etiology, features, management. J Pediatr Surg 1993; 28:1194–1195.

10. Eisenhammers S. The internal anal sphincter and the anorectal abscess. Surg Gynecol Obstet 1956; 103:501–506.

11. Takatsuki S. An aetiology of anal fistula in infants. Keio J Med 1976; 25:1–4.

12. al Salem AH, Qureshi SS. Perianal abscess and fistula-in-ano in infancy and childhood: a clinico pathological study. Pediatr Pathol Lab Med 1996, 16:755–764.

13. Shafer AD, Glone TP, Flanagen RA. Abnormal crypts of Morgagni, the cause of perianal abscess and fistula in ano. J Pediatr Surg 1987; 22:203–204.

14. Pople IK, Ralps DN. An aetiology for fistula-in-ano. Br J Surg 1988; 75:904–905.

15. Mshelbwala PM, Sabiu L, Ameh EA. Necrotising fasciitis of the perineum complicating ischiorectal abscess in childhood. Ann Trop Paediatr 2003; 23:227–228.

16. al Salem AH, Laing W, Talwalker V. Fistula-in-ano in infancy and childhood. J Pediatr Surg 1994; 29:436–438.

17. Watanabe Y, Todeni T, Yamamoto S. Conservative management of fistula-in-ano in infants. J Pediatr Surg 1998; 13:274–276.

18. Ameh EA. Anal injury and fissure-in-ano from sexual abuse in children. Ann Trop Paediatr 2001; 21:273–275.

19. Lund JN, Scholefield JH. Aetiology and treatment of anal fissure. Br J Surg 1996; 83:1335–1344.

20. Demirbag S, Tander B, Atabek C, Surer I, Ozturk H, Cetinkursun S. Long-term results of topical glyceryl trinitrate ointment in children with anal fissure. Ann Trop Paediatr 2005; 25:135–137.

21. Tander B, Geven A, Demirbag S, Ozkan Y, Ozturk H, Cetinkursun S. A prospective, randomized, double-blind, placebo-controlled trial of glyceryl-trinitrate ointment in the treatment of children with anal fissure. J Pediatr Surg 1999; 34:810–812.

22. Kenny SB, Irvine T, Driver CP, et al. Double-blind, randomized, controlled trial of topical glyceryl trinitrate in anal fissure. Arch Dis Child 2001; 85:404–407.

23. Argor S, Levandovsky O. Open lateral sphinctomy is still the best treatment for chronic anal fissure. Am J Surg 2000; 179:201–202.

24. Cohen A, Dehn TCB. Lateral subcutaneous sphincterotomy for treatment of anal fissure in children. Br J Surg 1995; 82:1341–1342.

25. Ameh EA, Mshelbwala PM. Transanal protrusion of intussusception in infants is associated with high morbidity and mortality. Ann Trop Paediatr 2008; 28(4):287–292.

26. Botgstein ES, Broadhead RE. Acquired recto vaginal fistula. Arch Dis Child 1991; 71:165–166.

27. Oliver ME. Spontaneous occurring rectovaginal fistula in children and adults with HIV infection. East Central Afric J Surg 1995; 1:23–25.

28. Wiersma R. HIV positive African children with rectal fistulae. J Pediatr Surg 2003, 38:62–64.

29. Banieghbal B, Fonseca J. Acquired vaginal fistula in South Africa. Arch Dis Child 1997; 77:94.

30. Uba AF, Chirdan LB, Ardill W, Ramyil VM, Kidmas AT. Acquired rectal fistula in human immunodeficiency virus-positive children: a causal or casual relationship? Pediatr Surg Int 2004; 20:898–901.

31. Hyde, Jr GA, Sarbah S. Acquired rectovaginal fistula in human immunodeficiency virus-positive children. Pediatrics 1994; 94:940–941.

32. Teran CG, Villarroel P, Teran-Escalera CN. Severe genital human papillomavirus infection in a sexually abused child. Int J Infect Dis 2009; 13:e137–e138.

33. Culton DA, Morrell DS, Burkhart CN. The management of condyloma acuminata in the pediatric population. Pediatr Ann 2009; 38:368–372.

Hepatobiliary System, Pancreas, and Spleen

CHAPTER 80
OBSTRUCTIVE JAUNDICE

Francis Aba Uba
Mohammed A. Latif Ayad
Alaa F. Hamza

Introduction

Neonatal cholestasis is defined as prolonged elevation of serum levels of conjugated bilirubin beyond the first 14 days of life. Neonatal hyper-bilirubinaemia is usually physiologic, unconjugated, and self-limited. Only 2–15% of neonates remain jaundiced past 2 weeks of life, and just 0.2–0.4% have cholestatic jaundice from either intrahepatic cholestasis or structural abnormalities that cause biliary obstruction. Intrahepatic cholestasis may result from numerous infectious or inflammatory causes, as well as from inherited metabolic defects. The major structural diseases include biliary atresia and choledochal cyst. A variable element of hepato-cellular dysfunction is common to all of these, thus rendering initial dis-crimination between medical and surgical cholestatic disease challenging.

Obstructive jaundice in infancy presents a surgical challenge, not only because of the difficulty in differentiating those cases that are amenable to surgical correction from those that are not, but also because of the desire to improve the persistently low salvage rate obtained even for correctable cases. Only if surgery is undertaken before 3 months of age, and preferably by 2 months of age, can the ravages caused by prolonged obstruction—namely, cirrhosis, portal hypertension, liver failure, and death—be prevented. Survival of patients whose obstruction is surgically relieved after 3 months of age is rare, and when they do survive, many of them (even those operated on before this time) have a severe morbidity or even mortality caused by cirrhosis and, later, portal hypertension. Thus there is only a short time between the appearance of the jaundice (usually between the ages of 4 and 6 weeks) and the optimal time for surgical intervention.

Aetiology/Pathophysiology

Biliary atresia is the most common cause of obstructive jaundice requiring operation in children, followed by choledochal cyst, choleli-thiasis, and spontaneous perforation of the bile ducts. Other causes of obstructive jaundice in infants are infantile obstructive cholangiopathy (biliary hypoplasia or hepatitis syndrome of infants), inspissated bile syndrome, extrinsic compression of the bile duct (e.g., pressure from huge intraabdominal masses), and cholestasis associated with intrave-nous feeding and gallstones in older children (Table 80.1).

Several hypotheses have attempt to explain the aetiology/pathophysiology of obstructive jaundice in the newborn infant. Biliary atresia and choledochal cyst belong to the same spectrum; they result from a single inflammatory process, probably viral, which leads to progressive destruction of liver parenchymal cells and desquamation of the epithelial lining of incompletely formed extrahepatic ducts late in gestation. Some of the other hypotheses include ischaemic or toxic injury in case of biliary atresia; abnormally long union of the pancreatic and common bile ducts (which permits the reflux of pancreatic secretions in the biliary tree, inducing inflammatory reactions that lead to progressive destruction, obliteration, or local weakening of the ductal walls); and a fault of ductal embryogenesis resulting from failure of the extrahepatic biliary system to develop patency.

At the moment, all of the proposed aetiological factors remain speculative because none of them fully explains the associated

Table 80.1: Most likely causes of cholestasis in infants younger than 2 months of age

Disease	Causes
Obstructive cholestasis	Biliary atresia Choledochal cyst Gallstones or biliary sludge Alagille syndrome Inspissated bile Cystic fibrosis Neonatal sclerosing cholangitis Congenital hepatic fibrosis/Caroli's disease
Hepatocellular cholestasis	Idiopathic neonatal hepatitis Viral infection Cytomegalovirus Human immunodeficiency virus (HIV)
Bacterial infection	Urinary tract infection Sepsis Syphilis
Genetic/metabolic disorders	α_1-antitrypsin deficiency Tyrosinaemia Galactosaemia Hypothyroidism Progressive familial intrahepatic cholestasis (PFIC) Cystic fibrosis Panhypopituitarism
Toxic/secondary	Parenteral nutrition–associated cholestasis

polysplenia syndrome, the frequent postnatal onset of jaundice and pale-coloured stools, and the discordance in twins.

Evaluation

The evaluation of the infant with jaundice should follow a logical, cost-effective sequence in a multistep process. Although cholestasis in the neonate may be the initial manifestation of numerous disorders, the clinical manifestations are usually similar and provide very few clues about aetiology. Affected infants have icterus, dark urine, light or acholic stools, and hepatomegaly, all resulting from decreased bile flow due to either hepatocyte injury or bile duct obstruction. Hepatic synthetic dysfunction may lead to hypoprothrombinaemia and a bleeding disorder. Therefore, administration of vitamin K should be the initial treatment of cholestatic infants to prevent haemorrhage.

Most newborn infants whose jaundice is of medical origin tend to be of low birth weight, and most often the jaundice is present at birth. This contrasts with jaundice caused by biliary atresia in the well-fed, healthy-looking newborn, who may have had normal stools at birth with minimal jaundice, but in whom jaundice usually becomes apparent in the first few days and certainly within the first 4 weeks after birth. Most infants with choledochal cyst present with mild intermittent jaundice, which might have been taken for granted for months or years. One-third of patients present with a classic triad of abdominal pain, jaundice, and abdominal mass, primarily in older children. Other early manifestations are pancreatitis and cholangitis.

The initial step in identification of cholestasis is the finding that more than 20% of the hyperbilirubinaemia is conjugated bilirubin. The next step is to recognize conditions that cause cholestasis and for which specific therapy is available to prevent further damage and avoid long-term complications such as sepsis, an endocrinopathy (hypothyroidism or panhypopituitarism), nutritional hepatotoxicity caused by a specific metabolic illness (galactosaemia), or other metabolic diseases (e.g., tyrosinaemia).

Hepatobiliary disease may be the initial manifestation of homozygous α_1-antitrypsin deficiency or of cystic fibrosis. Neonatal liver disease may also be associated with congenital syphilis and specific viral infections, notably echo virus and herpes viruses, including cytomegalovirus (CMV). The hepatitis viruses (A, B, C) rarely cause neonatal cholestasis. The final step in evaluating neonates with cholestasis is to differentiate extrahepatic biliary atresia from neonatal hepatitis.

Urgent diagnosis must be accomplished by radiologic examination of the extrahepatic biliary system because the assistance from the laboratory data is inconclusive. The value of ultrasonography (US) as a rapid, safe, noninvasive means of evaluating the jaundiced infant has been enhanced by the development of high-resolution real-time imaging.

The distinction between jaundice of parenchymal origin and biliary atresia or choledochal cyst can be accomplished by hepatobiliary imaging by using technetium-99m iminodiacetic acid (IDA). If the nucleotide uptake by the hepatocytes is rapid but excretion into the bowel is absent (even on delayed films), the jaundice is most likely to be due to biliary atresia; when the uptake is delayed by the diseased hepatocytes with poor or nonexcretion into the intestine, the jaundice is likely to be of hepatocellular (parenchymal) origin.

Operative cholangiography is preferred because it helps in proper surgical management decisions, but one-fifth of the interpretations of the cholangiographic films have suggested a diagnosis ultimately found to be incorrect. Other imaging approaches, such as computed tomography (CT), endoscopic retrograde cholangiopancreatography (ERCP), and magnetic resonance cholangiopancreatogram (MRCP), are also useful studies that can contribute to the diagnosis.

Liver biopsy, either percutaneous or open, is both safe and useful as a diagnostic modality. In approximately one-third of the specimens obtained by either method, the histological findings are not clear-cut, so further evaluation is necessary; for example, α_1-antitrypsin deficiency can be definitely differentiated from biliary atresia only by determining the α_1-antitrypsin level. A combination of open biopsy (with a guaranteed adequacy of size of specimen) and operative cholangiography is recommended as the ideal approach to the obstructed child.

Choledocholithiasis

Common bile duct stones are rare, but are relatively more frequent in infants and children with sickle cell disease. Obstructive jaundice, cholangitis, and/or pancreatitis are typical presenting features in symptomatic cases. Although US (conventional or endoscopic), MRCP, and CT may be helpful in diagnosis, ERCP offers the possibility of both diagnosis and treatment. ERCP and sphincterotomy with stone retrieval can be performed before or after laparoscopic cholecystectomy. Early ERCP is recommended for common duct stones associated with obstructive jaundice (bilirubin >100 μmol/L) and/or cholangitis, but not for most cases of gallstone pancreatitis because the stone usually passes spontaneously. Laparoscopic cholecystectomy with intraoperative cholangiography is usually undertaken a few weeks after the episode of gallstone pancreatitis.

Choledocholithiasis can be treated by open exploration of the common bile duct; laparoscopic common duct exploration; or ERCP, sphincterotomy, and stone extraction. In some centers, percutaneous

techniques are used. In small infants, cholecystotomy and irrigation may be successful. An initial short period of observation may be worthwhile if the infant is well without evidence of sepsis or progressive obstruction because some stones will pass spontaneously.

Idiopathic Perforation of Extrahepatic Bile Ducts

Spontaneous perforation of the extrahepatic bile ducts should always be considered in a young infant who develops obstructive jaundice after an initial period of good health or who presents with progressive ascites. The majority of infants present subacutely within 3 months of birth with mild, fluctuating, obstructive jaundice and slowly progressive biliary ascites. An acute presentation with abdominal distention and tenderness is rare.

The typical site of bile duct perforation is at the junction of the cystic and common bile ducts. The cause is unknown, but biliary obstruction from inspissated bile in the distal common bile duct or from ampullary stenosis may account for some cases. The differential diagnosis includes bile duct perforation secondary to trauma, choledochal cyst, or necrotising enterocolitis.

Abdominal US may show a complex loculated collection of bile around the common bile duct (which may be mistaken for a choledochal cyst) and within the lesser sac and/or generalized ascites. A hepatobiliary radionuclide scan confirms intraabdominal extravasation of bile.

Operative cholangiography via the gallbladder will confirm the site of perforation and assess the patency of the common bile duct. Definitive treatment is dictated by the findings. Cholecystectomy is sufficient for rare instances of cystic duct perforation, but for the usual site of perforation, tube cholecystostomy and simple drainage are appropriate if there is free flow of contrast into the duodenum. If there is distal common bile duct obstruction, catheter irrigation may clear inspissated bile, but drainage should be combined with cholecystostomy. If a distal bile duct stricture is demonstrated, hepaticojejunostomy is indicated.

Inspissated Bile Syndrome

Inspissated bile within the distal common bile duct may cause obstructive jaundice in newborns. It can be due to haemolysis, diuretic therapy, parenteral nutrition, prematurity, or cystic fibrosis. Inspissated bile plug syndrome may be difficult to distinguish from biliary atresia. In both conditions, there may be jaundice and acholic stools, conjugated hyperbilirubinaemia, and no biliary excretion on a radionuclide scan. However, US usually reveals dilated proximal bile ducts and inspissated bile.

Spontaneous resolution may occur. Treatment with ursodeoxycholic acid may help. More persistent obstruction can be cleared by percutaneous, transhepatic irrigation of the bile ducts, ERCP and retrograde irrigation, or cholecystectomy and bile duct irrigation. Occasionally, transduodenal sphincteroplasty may be required to remove an impacted mass of material or stones.

Biliary Hypoplasia

Biliary hypoplasia is a unique classification within the cholestatic spectrum. The liver histology is characterized by a paucity of intrahepatic ducts (i.e., a significantly decreased ratio of the number of interlobular bile ducts to the number of portal tracts). Biliary hypoplasia is best regarded as a condition secondary to decreased bile flow from the liver rather than a primary structural abnormality of the ducts. Biliary hypoplasia is either syndromic (Alagille syndrome) or nonsyndromic.

Alagille syndrome

Alagille syndrome is a genetic disorder that affects the liver, heart, and other systems of the body. Problems associated with the disorder generally become evident in infancy or early childhood. The disorder is inherited in an autosomal dominant pattern, and its estimated prevalence is 1 in every 100,000 live births. The severity of the disorder can vary within the same family, with symptoms ranging from being so mild as to go unnoticed to severe heart and/or liver disease requiring transplantation. Signs and symptoms arise from liver damage, cholestasis, and deposits of cholesterol in the skin xanthomas. Other signs of Alagille syndrome include congenital heart problems, tetralogy of Fallot, and vertebral arch defects with failure of anterior vertebral arch fusion (butterfly vertebrae). Many people with Alagille syndrome have similar facial features, including a broad prominent forehead; deep-set, widely spaced eyes; a long straight nose; and a small pointed chin with underdeveloped mandible. The kidneys and central nervous system may also be affected.

Nonsyndromic biliary hypoplasia

Nonsyndromic patients may initially be confused with those who have biliary atresia. Differentiation is crucial because transplantation is the only appropriate therapy for the end-stage liver disease in biliary hypoplasia. Percutaneous liver biopsy samples from affected infants lack the hepatic fibrosis and ductal proliferation characteristic of biliary atresia. The liver is smooth and often chocolate brown. Cholangiography demonstrates a diminutive biliary tree. Outcomes range from clinical improvement with resolution of cholestasis to end-stage liver disease with progressive cirrhosis.

Evidence-Based Research

Endoscopic ultrasonography (EUS) is a major advance in gastrointestinal imaging. It is used to image suspected pathology in the gastrointestinal tract and in the adjacent organs. It is a less invasive modality and may be equal or superior to ERCP in visualising the biliary tree. Its diagnostic accuracy in the evaluation of pancreatico-biliary diseases exceeds 90%. Its role and feasibility in children need to be accurately defined. Table 80.2 presents a study comparing EUS and ERCP in children with chronic liver disease.

Table 80.2: Evidence-based surgery.

Title	A comparative study of EUS versus ERCP in children with chronic liver disease (CLD)
Authors	El-Karaksy HM, El-Koofy NM, Okasha H, Kamal NM, Naga M
Institution	Department of Pediatrics and Department of Internal Medicine, Cairo University, Cairo, Egypt
Reference	Ind J Med Sci 2008; 62:345–351
Problem	The primary aim is to evaluate the role of EUS in comparison to ERCP in the pancreatico-biliary assessment of children with CLD. The secondary aim is to compare the findings obtained by EUS with those obtained by conventional abdominal ultrasound.
Intervention	Children with sonographic or histopathological evidence of biliary pathology, autoimmune hepatitis, cryptogenic CLD, and neonatal cholestasis underwent EUS and ERCP.
Comparison/ control (quality of evidence)	A descriptive comparative study carried out on 40 children older than 4 years of age suffering from CLD. All patients were subjected to EUS, ERCP, and abdominal ultrasound.
Outcome/ effect	EUS was equal to ERCP in diagnosis of biliary pathology. However, one false positive case was described to have dilatation and tortuosity of the pancreatic duct by EUS as compared to ERCP. EUS could detect early pancreatitis in five cases. One case with cryptogenic liver disease proved to have sclerosing cholangitis diagnosed by both EUS and ERCP.
Historical significance/ comments	In this study, EUS proved to be superior in detecting the cause of common bile duct (CBD) dilatation in patients in whom US could not demonstrate the cause of dilatation or in whom US revealed equivocal results. EUS was superior to ERCP in diagnosing chronic pancreatitis. In addition, negative cases should not be subjected to further evaluation by ERCP. ERCP should be performed if pancreatic duct pathology needs further assessment or if intervention is planned. More studies are needed to justify accurately the role of EUS in children with CLD and to highlight the feasibility of its usage for young ages.

Key Summary Points

1. Neonatal cholestasis is a prolonged elevation of serum levels of conjugated bilirubin beyond the first 14 days of life.

2. From 0.2% to 0.4% of neonates have cholestatic jaundice from either intrahepatic cholestasis or structural abnormalities that cause biliary obstruction.

3. Obstructive jaundice in infancy presents a surgical challenge; differentiation and surgical correction should be done by the age of 2 months.

4. Biliary atresia is the most common cause of obstructive jaundice requiring operation in children.

5. Evaluation of the jaundiced infant should follow a logical, cost-effective sequence in a multistep process.

Suggested Reading

A-Kader HH, Balistreri WF. Cholestasis. In: Behrman RE, Kliegman RM, Jenson HB (eds). Nelson Textbook of Pediatrics, 17th ed. W B Saunders, 2003, Pp 1314–1319.

Alagille D, Estrada A, Hadchouel M, et al. Syndromic paucity of interlobular bile ducts (Alagille syndrome or arteriohepatic dysplasia): review of 80 cases. J Pediatr 1987; 110:195–200.

Altman RP, Buchmiller TL. The jaundiced infant: biliary atresia. In: Grosfold JL, O'Neill JA Jr, Fonkalsrud EW, Coran AG (eds). Pediatric Surgery, 6th ed. Mosby, 2006, Pp 1603–1619.

Davenport M, Betalli P, D'Antiga L, et al. The spectrum of surgical jaundice in infancy. J Pediatr Surg 2003; 38:1471–1479.

Heaton ND, Davenport M, Howard ER. Intraluminal biliary obstruction. Arch Dis Child 1991; 66:1395–1398.

Hoffenberg EJ, Narkewicz MR, Sondheimer JM, et al. Outcome of syndromic paucity of interlobular bile ducts (Alagille syndrome) with onset of cholestasis in infancy. J Pediatr 1995; 127:220–224.

Holcomb GW, Morgan WM, Neblett WW, et al. Laparoscopic cholecystectomy in children: lessons learned from the first 100 patients. J Pediatr Surg 1999; 34:1236–1240.

Howard ER. Spontaneous biliary perforation. In: Howard ER, Stringer MD, Colombani PM (eds). Surgery of the liver, bile ducts and pancreas in children, 2nd ed. Arnold, 2002, Pp 169–174.

Ibanez DV, Vila JJ, Fernandez MS, et al. Spontaneous biliary perforation and necrotizing enterocolitis. Pediatr Surg Int 1999; 15:401–402.

Jonas A, Yahav J, Fradkin A, et al. Choledocholithiasis in infants: diagnostic and therapeutic problems. J Pediatr Gastroenterol Nutr 1990; 11:513–517.

Kumar R, Nguyen K, Shun A. Gallstones and common bile duct calculi in infancy and childhood. Aust NZ J Surg 2000; 70:188–191.

Mishra A, Pant N, Chadha R, Choudhury SR. Choledochal cysts in infancy and childhood. Indian J Pediatr 2007; 74:937–943.

Stringer MD. Disorders of the gallbladder and biliary tract. In: Oldham KT, Colombani PM, Foglia RP, Skinner MA (eds). Principles and Practice of Pediatric Surgery, 4th ed. Lippincott, Williams & Wilkins, 2005, Pp 1496–1509.

CHAPTER 81
BILIARY ATRESIA

Sanjay Krishnaswami
Richa Lal
Katrine Lofberg
Alaa Fayez Hamza

Introduction

Biliary atresia (BA) is a neonatal disease characterised by the inflammatory and sclerotic obliteration of part or all of the extrahepatic biliary tree, with varying involvement of the intrahepatic bile ducts. Although seen in only a small percentage of jaundiced neonates, this disorder is one of the more common structural causes of neonatal cholestatic jaundice.

If left untreated, biliary atresia is almost uniformly fatal. Hepatic failure, infection, or bleeding secondary to portal hypertension causes death by the age of 1 to 2 years in the vast majority of patients.[1,2] In the current era, despite the diagnostic difficulties and technical challenges that BA poses, early recognition and the proper performance of a Kasai portoenterostomy procedure can be life saving. When available, liver transplantation can serve as the ultimate therapy for those who have end-stage disease.

Demographics

Based mostly on Western series, the incidence of biliary atresia is between 1:8,000 and 1:17,000 live births, with an overall female preponderance of up to 1.7:1.[3] In most of Africa, incidence data are not available, but individual institutional reports suggest that up to five children with this disorder are encountered yearly in many centres.[4–6] Therefore, although cholestasis secondary to infectious causes is more common, BA is encountered fairly frequently in Africa.[4,7,8] No specific genetic factors are associated with the disease, but associated congenital malformations occur in 11–20% of the cases.[3] The most commonly associated anomaly is polysplenia; other associated anomalies include intestinal atresias, abdominal situs inversus, malrotation, and genitourinary and cardiac anomalies.

Aetiology/Pathology and Classification

Many aetiologies for the disease have been proposed, including genetic factors, congenital developmental causes such as a failure of recanalisation or antenatal ischaemia, and viral or other infectious causes. None have been proven, however, and the pathogenesis remains unknown. Because two groups of patients are affected—those with other congenital anomalies and those with a late foetal or perinatal anomaly that appears to occur in isolation—there may in fact be an interplay of these various aetiologies in the development of BA in any individual patient.

Microscopic examination of the biliary system reveals fibrosis of the ductules with varying degrees of inflammation. Early in the disease, bile duct proliferation, biliary plugs, and mild portal fibrosis are present. Later in the disease, this fibrosis extends intrahepatically and will manifest as bridging fibrosis of the biliary structures.

Classification of biliary atresia is generally based upon the macroscopic location of the fibrotic biliary cord remnants (Figure 81.1). The most common type is complete fibrosis of the entire extrahepatic biliary system, seen in up to 70–80% of cases. Gallbladder and common bile duct patency with obliteration of the porta and hepatic duct is the next most frequent (12–20%). Absence of portions of the biliary system with fibrosis of the remaining portions as well as distal fibrosis with proximal hilar cyst variants can also be seen. Macroscopically, these

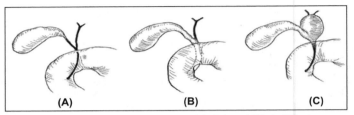

Source: Karrer FM, Pence JC. Biliary atresia and choledochal cyst. In: Ziegler MM, ed. Operative Pediatric Surgery. McGraw-Hill, 2003. Reproduced with permission from the McGraw-Hill Companies.

Figure 81.1: Illustration of common types of biliary atresia: (A) complete extrahepatic biliary obliteration (most common, affecting about 80%); (B) proximal obliteration, distal patency; and (C) common hepatic duct cystic dilatation with portal and distal common bile duct obliteration.

mucus-containing cyst variants can be confused for a fibrotic hilar cone or for a choledochal cyst. As these cysts do not communicate with the biliary tree, all such structures need to be resected. Failure to recognise this variant can lead to a nonfunctional anastomosis with the sequestered cyst.[3]

Clinical Presentation

Most children with biliary atresia appear normal at birth but become increasingly jaundiced after 3 to 6 weeks of age. Additionally, in those children with physiologic jaundice from birth that does not resolve spontaneously, BA should be suspected because persistence of jaundice after 2 to 3 weeks of life should always be considered pathologic until proven otherwise. This sign, coupled with the findings of progressively acholic stools and dark urine, is suggestive of BA.

As the liver becomes progressively obstructed, it grows in size and firmness. Malabsorption of fat-soluble vitamins resulting from hepatic obstruction and failure can lead to diarrhoea, anaemia, and malnutrition. Overall growth of the infant may therefore appear normal in the first few weeks or months after birth, but most patients develop failure to thrive once liver failure is more significant. Prolonged bleeding can be seen from the umbilical stump in such cases. Finally, splenomegaly, bleeding oesophageal varices, and other signs of portal hypertension can also be significant parts of the examination in patients who present with advanced illness.[9] By recent African reports, up to two-thirds of patients present late in the illness after advanced signs of liver failure are present.[10]

The value of the experienced paediatrician in recognising the jaundiced baby with persistently acholic stools cannot be overstated. It is important to recognise these and other physical findings early because successful outcomes after surgery for biliary atresia are tied closely to age at performance of Kasai portoenterostomy.[11] Note, however, that the physical signs and symptoms of BA described above overlap with myriad other causes of jaundice in infancy (discussed in the next section), and none of these findings should be considered as conclusive for BA. Rather, early recognition of signs of persistant jaundice should prompt swift referral to centres capable of completing the diagnosis and instituting definitive surgical intervention, if warranted.

Investigation

The differential diagnosis of neonatal jaundice is prodigious and includes such surgically correctable obstructive lesions as biliary atresia and choledochal cyst as well as inborn metabolic errors, congenital infectious causes, and other causes, as listed here:

- *physiologic:* immaturity of glucuronyl transferase (resolves quickly);

- *breast milk feeding;*

- *hematologic:* Rh/ABO blood group incompatibility, hemolytic diseases (spherocytosis);

- *infectious:* the TORCH (TOxoplasmosis, Rubella, Cytomegalovirus (CMV), Herpes) complex; syphillis, hepatitis, and others;

- *genetic/metabolic:* α1-antitrypsin deficiency, galactosaemia, tyrosinaemia, cystic fibrosis (CF), hypothyroidism, Gaucher's disease, iron storage disease;

- *hepatocellular dysfunction:* Gilbert's disease, Crigler-Najjar syndrome;

- *neonatal hepatitis;*

- *total parenteral nutrition (TPN)-related cholestasis;* and

- *extrahepatic processes:* BA, choledochal cyst, Alagille syndrome (arteriohepatic dysplasia), inspissated bile plug syndrome, bile duct stenosis or stricture, spontaneous perforation of the bile duct.

Testing

The main goal of early testing is to rapidly differentiate jaundice due to obstruction from that due to other causes. A proper combination of serology testing, imaging, and biopsy prior to or during an operative cholangiogram leads to an accurate diagnosis in >95% of patients.[12] Conventional serum liver function tests are nonspecific. Hyperbilirubinaemia, usually in the 5–12 μg/L range, is typical of the early stage of the disease. However, bilirubin fractionation is not useful in distinguishing obstructive jaundice due to BA from the more common intrahepatic cholestatic diseases (e.g., neonatal hepatitis) because there is elevation of indirect, unconjugated as well as direct, conjugated bilirubin in both diseases. Similarly, alanine transaminase (AST) and aspartate transaminase (ALT) are also often elevated in both cases, although extreme elevations of these are unusual in BA. In contradistinction to this, alkaline phosphatase and gamma-glutamyl transpaptidase (GGT) are often very elevated, and low levels of these may suggest an alternate diagnosis. Alterations in hepatic function tests, such as prothrombin time, partial thromboplastin time, and albumin, are typically seen only in advanced cases of BA. Serum testing should also be done to screen for both inborn metabolic errors and classic infectious causes such as TORCH and syphilis, among others. An exhaustive hunt to rule out all these possibilities can take many weeks, so one should not wait for the results of testing prior to imaging, which may help confirm or eliminate the possibility of an obstructive, mechanical cause of jaundice.[1,9]

Imaging

The two most useful imaging modalities in further differentiating surgically amenable causes from other causes of cholestasis are ultrasound (US) and nuclear hepatobiliary imaging. Although operator-dependant, US is available in many African centres and offers a safe and noninvasive way to evaluate the jaundiced neonate. It can be used to assess the size of the gallbladder and intra- and extrahepatic biliary ducts and to visualise gallstones. Although the presence of a cystic extrahepatic or intrahepatic ductal dilatation typically rules out BA, the disease is suspected if there is a very small or absent gallbladder, extrahepatic ducts are not at all visualised, or the cone-shaped fibrotic portal plate is seen.[13] The presence of polysplenia or pre-duodenal portal vein lends further support to a diagnosis of biliary atresia. Doppler use helps to correctly interpret the adjacent hepatic artery as a vascular rather than a biliary duct structure.

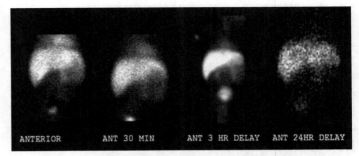

Figure 81.2: Nuclear hepatobiliary scan demonstrating prompt uptake of technecium tracer with no excretion into the gut after 24 hours. This image is suspicious for biliary atresia, but could still be consistent with neonatal hepatitis. Excretion into the gut at any time rules out biliary atresia.

Nuclear imaging is performed with intravenous administration of technecium-99m, which is taken up by the liver. In neonatal hepatitis, there is delayed technecium uptake due to hepatocellular dysfunction and delayed or absent excretion into the gut. In BA, uptake is usually prompt (especially early in the disease) but there is no gut excretion (Figure 81.2). Therefore, visualisation of tracer in the intestine rules out BA, whereas absence of tracer visualisation in the intestine could be due to either process. In resource-poor locations without nuclear imaging techniques, it may be judicious to proceed straight to either percutaneous biopsy or operative biopsy and cholangiogram via a laparoscopic or open technique.

Management

If, after initial investigation, the diagnosis of BA is still suspected, prompt operative intervention is warranted to definitively determine whether the patient has BA and, if so, to perform a Kasai portoenterostomy procedure.

Preoperative Considerations

In addition to routine preoperative care for any abdominal procedure, a dose of vitamin K (1 mg/kg) can be given several days prior to surgery. Coagulation factors (prothrombin time/international normalization ratio/partial thromboplastin time, or PT/INR/PTT) should be checked to ensure suitability for operation, and type-specific blood should be available. Routine bowel preparation is not necessary, but a dose of preoperative broad-spectrum antibiotic is given prior to incision.

Initial Intraoperative Considerations: Cholangiogram and Liver Biopsy

Traditionally, the operation commences with a small right upper quadrant transverse or oblique incision. However, if available, laparoscopy can also be utilised for the initial portion of the procedure. If a gallbladder is visualised and is patent, an operative cholangiogram is the next manoeuvre, wherein the tip of the gallbladder is cannulated with an angiocatheter and contrast is instilled under fluoroscopy. Contrast in the duodenum and continuity with the intrahepatic ducts rules out BA (Figure 81.3)

If biliary atresia is ruled out and a biopsy has not previously been done, a generous wedge biopsy of the liver is performed and the incision(s) is (are) closed. An "adequate" liver biopsy specimen that has at least five portal tracts, reported by an experienced pathologist done after 4–6 weeks of age, should have an overall accuracy of 96%. The biopsy not only helps to differentiate BA from neonatal hepatitis, but also points towards specific aetiologies of neonatal hepatitis as well as α_1-antitrypsin deficiency and storage disorders such as Niemann-Pick disease. In addition to being sent for pathologic exam, a portion of the biopsy specimen should be sent for viral and bacterial cultures.

If no gallbladder or a fibrotic gallbladder is present, or if cholangiogram reveals a lack of either the proximal or distal extrahepatic ducts (Figure 81.4), the right upper quadrant incision should be widened or the procedure converted to open from laparoscopic in preparation for hepatic portal exploration and the Kasai procedure.

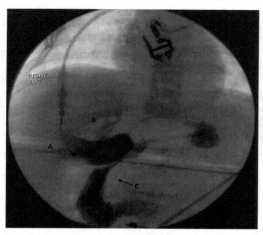

Figure 81.3: Intraoperative cholangiogram with contrast filling hypoplastic proximal and distal duct system with emptying into duodenum: (A) contrast-filled catheter within gallbladder; (B) left and right hepatic ducts; (C) intrapancreatic common bile duct. Patient had Allagille syndrome, not biliary atresia.

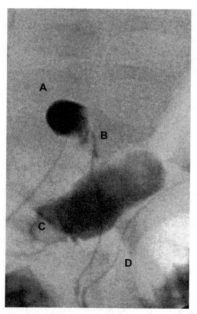

Figure 81.4 : Intraoperative cholangiogram demonstrating emptying of contrast into the duodenum with no proximal duct filling (proximal biliary atresia): (A) contrast being administered through a small but patent gallbladder; (B) stenotic but patent common bile duct passing intrapancreatic and emptying into the duodenum; (C) contrast in the duodenum; (D) retrograde filling of the pancreatic duct.

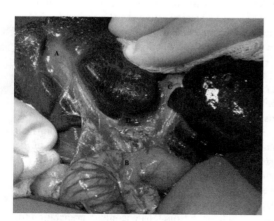

Figure 81.5. Biliary atresia: view of porta hepatis and hepatoduodenal ligament prior to dissection: (A) fibrotic gallbladder; (B) duodenum; (C) falciform ligament; (D) approximate location of fibrotic endplate.

Kasai Roux-en-Y Portoenterostomy

The portoenterostomy procedure, first described by Kasai and Suzuki in 1959,[14] uncovers patent biliary microductules proximal to the level of extrahepatic biliary fibrosis and allows these structures to drain directly into a segment of defunctionalised intestine.

The procedure begins with separation of the gallbladder from its liver bed down to the junction of the cystic and common bile ducts.

1. The peritoneum over the hepatoduodenal ligament is opened, exposing the biliary and hepatic arterial structures (Figure 81.5). The fibrous common duct is dissected and transected at its margin with the duodenum.

2. The entire gallbladder and fibrous common duct is placed on traction in a superior direction. The cystic artery is ligated, being careful to definitively identify it from the right hepatic artery.

3. The ductal remnants are then dissected from the adjacent hepatic artery and portal vein until the right and left branches of the portal vein are identified (Figure 81.6).

4. Further dissection reveals the widening of the fibrotic duct into a cone-shaped mass entering the liver superiorly. This fibrotic hepatic endplate is then transected at the point at which it is flush with the liver edge. In order to identify this level, small branches of the portal vein to the central portion of the fibrotic endplate must often be divided such that the most superior dissection is actually behind the portal vein. (Figure 81.7).

5. If there is discontinuity of the proximal biliary tree, meticulous exploration over the bifurcation of the portal vein will lead to identification of the fibrotic cone. Once the endplate is divided, cautery on this portion of the liver should be avoided, and a moist gauze should be placed here while attention is turned to the construction of a Roux-en-Y intestinal limb. The completed portal dissection is shown in Figure 81.8.

6. A 40-cm Roux-en-Y limb is constructed by dividing the bowel 10–15 cm after the ligament of Treitz. The distal cut edge is advanced in a retrocolic fashion up to the level of the liver. A handsewn end-to-end or side-to-side jejunojejunostomy re-establishes intestinal continuity. The mesenteric defect at the jejunojejunostomy is closed, and the Roux limb is tacked to the colonic mesentery at its retrocolic window to prevent internal hernia and excessive tension on the portoenterostomy (Figure 81.9).

7. The portoenterostomy is performed in a single layer, end-to-side or end-to-end fashion, using long-term absorbable sutures in an interrupted or running fashion, being careful to take meticulous full thickness bites of only the periphery of the porta hepatis (Figures 81.10 and 81.11). This ensures that the portoenterostomy incorporates the entire portion of tissue that may contain biliary channels and that risk of microductular structure compromise is minimised.

8. The completed portoenterostomy is shown in Figures 81.12 and 81.13. A closed-suction drain can be placed posterior to the portoenterostomy, and the abdomen is closed in layers.

To limit potential postoperative cholangitis, many modifications of the original portoenterostomy have been proposed over the years since Kasai first described the technique. These have included initial externalisation of the biliary conduit via a stoma and an antireflux intussusception valve within the Roux limb, among others. However, as none of these have been successful in preventing cholangitis, and in fact have been associated with unique complications of their own, their use should be discouraged.

Postoperative Considerations

Nasogastric drainage is continued for several days after the operation until gut function resumes. At that time, an oral diet is given as tolerated. Perioperative intravenous antibiotics, such as a cephalosporin, are administered by most surgeons for at least the first 12–24 hours. Many surgeons administer long-term oral antibiotics (e.g., trimethoprim/sulfa, 2 mg/kg per day) as well as choleretic agents, such as ursodeoxycholic acid (10–15 mg/kg per day) upon discharge in the hope of lessening the incidence of cholangitis following a Kasai procedure.[11]

Steroids are purported to benefit biliary function after a Kasai procedure through stimulation of salt-independent bile flow in addition to their marked anti-inflammatory, immunosuppressive, and scar-limiting properties. They were originally proposed for use along with broad-spectrum antibiotics in cases of postoperative cholangitis and in cases of sudden cessation of bile flow in a previously well-functioning portoenterostomy.[1,14] More recently, the routine use of steroids in the postoperative period has become standard for some surgeons. Although its use remains controversial, especially in light of reports showing equivocal benefits, this practice is widespread. The evidence for steroids comes from multiple studies reporting improved short- and long-term outcomes after standard postoperative steroid use as reflected by decreased bilirubin level several months after the Kasai procedure, decreased mortality at one year postoperatively, and improved jaundice-free survival with native liver at four- to five-year follow-up.[15–17] Although many of these studies involved small numbers of patients and many potentially confounding variables exist, none of the studies noted significant adverse reactions from steroid use, such as infectious complications or wound issues. The optimal dose and length of steroid treatment to achieve positive effects is unknown and varied across the studies cited. One author of this chapter prefers a three-week tapering course of oral prednisone (2 mg/kg per day) beginning at hospital discharge.

Complications

Although the usual operative complications, such as severe bleeding and anastomotic leak, can occur, these are rare—even in patients with fairly advanced disease. The most common issues postoperatively are cholangitis, nutritional deficiencies, and portal hypertension.

Cholangitis occurs in one-third to two-thirds of patients; its incidence is highest within the first several years after a Kasai procedure. It is thought that bacteria in the Roux-en-Y conduit and bile stasis combine to cause this problem. The onset of cholangitis is heralded by fever, leukocytosis, and an increase in bilirubin. Most cases are responsive to supportive treatment with fluids and early institution of broad-spectrum antibiotics covering intestinal flora. In refractory cases, one can consider a short burst of intravenous corticosteroids, as previously described. If not already being used prior to the first episode of cholangitis, chronic oral suppressive antibiotics, ursodeoxycholic acid, or oral steroids may be of benefit to prevent recurrent episodes.[18] Reoperation to prevent cholangitis (by creation of an antireflux valve or lengthening of the Roux limb) is generally unsuccessful.[3]

Portal hypertension is the most serious delayed complication, seen in up to 50–70% of long-term survivors.[19] It can occur even in patients who initially had a successful Kasai procedure and usually manifests as ascites, variceal bleeding, or hypersplenism. Treatment with diuretics, beta blockers, or variceal banding and splenectomy or splenic embolisation can be successful. However, without the possibility of liver transplantation, many of these patients will succumb to this portal hypertension.

Severe nutritional deficiency can accompany liver disease secondary to BA. Without adequate bile flow for intestinal fat absorption, children can develop essential fatty acid deficiency. Until adequate bile flow is achieved, it is prudent to administer formula feeds with a high percentage of medium-chained triglycerides that can be absorbed directly without the assistance of bile salts. Additionally, affected neonates can develop deficiencies of the fat-soluble vitamins (K, E, A, and D), which can result in diseases such as rickets (vitamin D deficiency) or severe coagulopathy (vitamin K deficiency). Monitoring vitamin levels and/or supplementation of these vitamins as available can prevent significant morbidity.

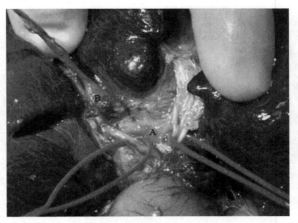

Figure 81.6: Porta after isolation of hepatic arteries and partial dissection of fibrotic endplate vessel loops around hepatic arteries: (A) portal venous confluence; (B) fibrotic ductal structures (medial portion of fibrous endcone already divided and reflected laterally).

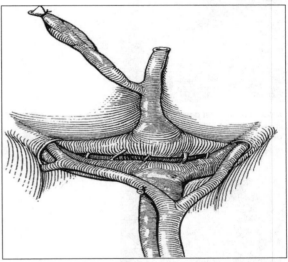

Source: Karrer FM, Pence JC. Biliary atresia and choledochal cyst. In: Ziegler MM, ed. Operative Pediatric Surgery. McGraw-Hill, 2003. Reproduced with permission from the McGraw-Hill Companies.

Figure 81.7: Fibrotic extrahepatic bile ducts with branches of portal vein to endplate.

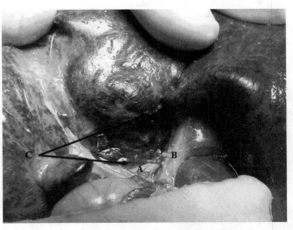

Figure 81.8: Intraoperative photo of completed dissection of porta prior to portoenterostomy in another patient: (A) portal vein confluence; (B) right hepatic artery; (C) portal plate after resection of fibrous cone; arrows mark anterior and posterior edges.

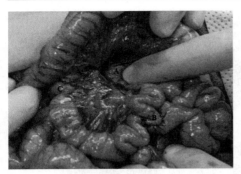

Figure 81.9: Completed jejunojejunostomy of Roux limb: (A) proximal jejunum at ligament of Treitz; (B) end-to-side jejunojejunostomy; (C) Roux limb to liver passing retrocolic, secured to transverse colon mesentery.

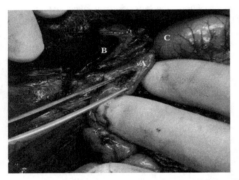

Figure 81.10: Distal Roux limb (superior to its retrocolic passage) being opened on its antimesenteric aspect in preparation for end-to-side anastomosis with porta: (A) side of Roux limb; (B) portal endplate; (C) pylorus posterior and adjacent to tip of Roux limb.

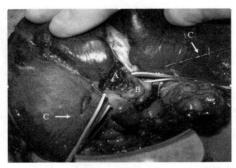

Figure 81.11: Posterior row of portoenterostomy anastomosis complete. Vessel loops around portal venous and hepatic arterial branches posterior to Roux limb: (A) inferior border of portal plate; (B) mucosal edge of jejunum ready for anterior row sutures; (C) lateral sutures leading to edge of posterior portion of anastomosis.

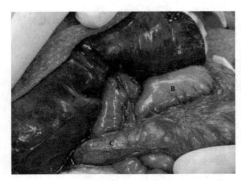

Figure 81.12 : Completed Kasai procedure: (A) Roux-en-Y end-to-side portoenterostomy anastomosis; (B) stomach and pylorus; (C) transverse colon with retrocolic Roux limb behind it.

Outcomes

Given that biliary atresia was previously a uniformly fatal disease, the Kasai operation has dramatically improved the survival rates of infants with this disease. However, the results are far from perfect. In general, by Japanese and Western reports, 60–80% of patients will achieve initial improvement in jaundice and early success with portoenterostomy, defined by some as normalisation of serum bilirubin to less than 2 mg% at 3 months following the procedure. Of these, one-half will have permanent relief and the other one-half will have progressive liver failure. The patients who never achieved initial improvement go on to experience progressive liver failure. The best five-year survival (up to 60%) has been reported by the Japanese Biliary Atresia Registry. Rates in most African reports are significantly lower, likely due to the patient's advanced age at the time of diagnosis and morbidities of advanced disease.[6,10]

Prognostic Factors

The most important long-term prognostic factors in predicting outcome after the Kasai procedure appear to be age at presentation, achievement of primary biliary drainage, experience of the centre, and occurrence of cholangitis.

Age at the time of the Kasai procedure is perhaps the most important prognostic indicator. Most reports state that the best outcomes, in both initial success and long-term survival, occur in patients younger than age 60–70 days at the time of operation (68% 10-year survival). The Japanese Biliary Atresia Registry extends such rates to patients up to 90 days of age, with a precipitous drop in success after that point.[3,11,20] Most series report performance of a Kasai procedure in infants after 70 days of age as a risk factor for failure; however, some do not agree with this.[21–23]

Although it is a very important postoperative prognostic factor, primary biliary drainage is not a guarantee of the long-term success of a portoenterostomy. Rather, it is a *requirement* for success in that nearly all patients who do not achieve primary biliary drainage will never do so. Surgical treatment via a second (redo) Kasai procedure for patients who did not achieve primary drainage as well as for those who had initial drainage but subsequent cessation, was met with initial interest secondary to case reports and small series of successes. Recent reports, however, suggest that redo portoenterostomy is not a useful strategy in the vast majority of patients.[24]

Role of Liver Transplantation

Liver transplantation, where available, is principally useful in cases of inadequate biliary drainage after portoenterostomy and in cases of progressive hepatic dysfunction or refractory portal hypertension despite initial portoenterostomy. Liver transplantation centres in North America, Europe, and Japan now report up to 85% 5-year survival after transplant for biliary atresia.[25] Given these excellent results, some in the West have advocated for primary liver transplantation in the neonate with BA. However, the long-term success of portoenterostomy in a significant percentage of patients, combined with the risks of long-term immunosupression beginning early in life (infectious and malignant), the expense of liver transplant, the shortage of donors, and the need for intense follow-up, make this a less attractive initial option in these patients. These issues are magnified in the African setting. In those regions where transplantation is an option, it should be noted that performance of an initial Kasai procedure has not been shown to affect the success of subsequent transplantation.[26]

Conclusion

The Kasai procedure remains the mainstay of initial treatment for biliary atresia throughout the world. In addition, it may offer the only hope for children with BA in most of Africa, where liver transplantation may not be available.

Despite the fact that many African reports state a poor outcome for even those BA patients who undergo portoenterostomy, likely due to the extremely late presentation of patients for the procedure, this should not discourage the use of the Kasai procedure in general.[6,10] It is therefore important for the surgeon to advocate to the community for early referral of patients with neonatal jaundice who may have biliary atresia. Time is of the essence, so accepting centres should have expertise in the rapid work-up of such patients. Subsequent thorough preoperative resuscitation and preparation and meticulous technique in the performance of Kasai portoenterostomy are crucial to the successful outcome of the patient who presents with potentially salvageable liver disease.

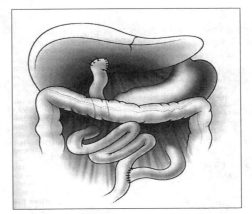

Source: Altman RP, Buchmiller TL. The jaundiced infant—biliary atresia. In: Grosfeld JL, O'Neill JA, Coran AG, Fonkalsrud EW (eds.). Pediatric Surgery, 6th ed., Vol. 2. 2006, Pp 1609.

Figure 81.13 : Illustration of completed Kasai procedure.

Key Summary Points

1. Although not as common as infectious aetiologies of neonatal cholestasis, biliary atresia is seen regularly in centres throughout Africa.

2. Persistent jaundice after 3 weeks of age is pathologic until proven otherwise.

3. The differential diagnoses for cholestasis in the newborn are large and include genetic/metabolic disorders, infectious agents, hepatocellular dysfunction, neonatal hepatitis, and extrahepatic obstructive disorders.

4. Early referral to a centre that can rule out extrahepatic biliary obstruction is vital to a successful outcome if biliary atresia is found.

5. A combination of ultrasound, nuclear imaging (if available), and operative cholangiogram with or without biopsy will definitively determine whether a patient has biliary atresia.

6. Kasai portoenterostomy is the cornerstone of therapy for biliary atresia.

7. Modifications of the Roux-en-Y portoenterostomy, such as externalisation of the biliary conduit and intussusception valves within the Roux limb, offer no benefit.

8. Cholangitis, the most frequent postoperative complication, is usually responsive to broad-spectrum antibiotics.

9. Advanced age at the time of the Kasai procedure is one of the most important indicators of poor outcome.

References

1. Karrer FM, Lilly JR. Corticosteroid therapy in biliary atresia. J Pediatr Surg 1977; 90:736.

2. Adelman S. Prognosis of uncorrected biliary atresia: an update. J Pediatr Surg 1978; 13:389–392.

3. Nio M, Ohio R, Miyano T, et al. Five- and 10-year survival rates after surgery for biliary atresia: a report from the Japanese Biliary Atresia Registry. J Pediatr Surg 2003; 38:997.

4. Obanafunwa JO, Elesha SO. Childhood liver diseases in Jos, Nigeria: a retrospective histopathological study. East Afr Med J 1991; 68:702–706.

5. Motala C, Ireland JD, Hill ID, Bowie MD. Cholestatic disorders of infancy—aetiology and outcome. J Trop Pediatr 1990; 36:218–222.

6. Mabogunje OA. Biliary atresia in Zaria, Nigeria: a review. Ann Trop Paediatr 1987; 7:200–204.

7. Muthuphei MN. Childhood liver diseases in Ga-Rankuwa Hospital, South Africa. East Afr Med J 2000; 77:508–509.

8. Akang EE, Osinusi KO, Pindiga HU, Okpala JU, Aghadiuno PU. Congenital malformations: a review of 672 autopsies in Ibadan, Nigeria. Pediatr Pathol 1993; 13:659–670.

9. O'Neill JA, Jr., Grosfeld JL, Fonkalsrud EW, Coran AG, Caldamone AA, eds. Principles of Pediatric Surgery. 2nd ed. Mosby, 2004.

10. Mshelbwala PM, Sabiu L, Lukong CS, Ameh EA. Management of biliary atresia in Nigeria: the ongoing challenge. Ann Trop Paediatr 2007; 27:69–73.

11. Altman RP, Lilly JF, Greenfeld J, et al. A multivariable risk factor analysis of the portoenterostomy (Kasai) procedure for biliary atresia: twenty-five years of experience from two centers. Ann Surg 1997; 226:348; discussion 353.

12. Zerbini MC, Gallucci SD, Maezono R, et al. Liver biopsy in neonatal cholestasis: a review on statistical grounds. Mod Pathol 1997; 10:793–799.

13. Sera Y, Ikeda S, Akagi M. Ultrasonographic studies for the diagnosis of infantile cholestatic disease. In: Ohi R, ed. Biliary Atresia. Professional Postgraduate Services, 1987.

14. Kasai M, Suzuki H, Ohashi E, et al. Technique and results of operative management of biliary atresia. World J Surg 1978; 2:571–580.

15. Dillon PW, Owings E, Cilley R, et al. Immunosuppression as adjuvant therapy for biliary atresia. J Pediatr Surg 2001; 361:80.

16. Meyers RL, Book LS, O'Gorman MA, et al. High-dose steroids, ursodeoxycholic acid, and chronic intravenous antibiotics improve bile flow after Kasai procedure in infants with biliary atresia. J Pediatr Surg 2003; 38:406.

17. Muraji T, Tusagawa C, Nishijima E, et al. Surgical management for intractable cholangitis in biliary atresia. J Pediatr Surg 1997; 32:1103; discussion 1106.

18. Bu LN, Chen HL, Chang CJ, et al. Prophylactic oral antibiotics in prevention of recurrent cholangitis after the Kasai portoenterostomy. J Pediatr Surg 2003; 38:509.

19. Lilly JR, Weintraub WH, Altman RP. Spontaneous perforation of the extrahepatic bile ducts and bile peritonitis in infancy. Surgery 1974; 75:664.

20. Grosfeld JL, Fitzgerald JF, Predaina R, et al. The efficacy of hepatoportoenterostomy in biliary atresia. Surgery 1989; 106:692; discussion 700.

21. Davenport M, Kerkar N, Mieli-Vergani G, et al. Biliary atresia: the King's College Hospital experience (1974–1995). J Pediatr Surg 1997; 32:479.

22. Maksoud JG, Fauza DO, Silva MM, et al. Management of biliary atresia in the liver transplantation era: A 15-year, single-center experience. J Pediatr Surg 1998; 33:115.

23. van Heurn LW, Saing H, Tam PK: Portoenterostomy for biliary atresia: Long-term survival and prognosis after esophogeal variceal bleeding. J Pediatr Surg 2004; 39:6.

24. Hasegawa T, Kimura T, Sasaki T, et al. Indication for redo hepatic portoenterostomy for insufficient bile drainage in biliary atresia: Re-evaluation in the era of liver transplantation. Pediatr Surg Int 2003; 19:256.

25. McDiarmid SV. Current status of liver transplantation in children. Pediatr Clin North Am 2003; 50:1335.

26. Vacanti JP, Shamberger RC, Eraklis A, Lillehei CW. The therapy of biliary atresia combining the Kasai portoenterostomy with liver transplantation: a single center experience. J Pediatr Surg 1990; 25:149.

CHAPTER 82
CHOLEDOCHAL CYST

Mohammed A. Latif Ayad   Alaa F. Hamza

Hesham M. Abdelkader   Donald E. Meier

Introduction

Congenital bile duct dilatation is a better term for the spectrum of anomalies known traditionally as choledochal cysts. Choledochal cysts may cause symptoms at any age, but typically present with obstructive jaundice and/or abdominal pain in infants and children. Although rare, they are more common in females (female-to-male ratio of about 3–4:1) and in some Asian races.

Anatomic Classification

Type I, II, and III forms of choledochal cysts were originally described by Alonso-Lej and colleagues. Subsequently, Todani and associates and others have further classified this anomaly into five main types and additional subtypes, based on analyses of cholangiograms. The two relatively common categories of cyst are types I and IV-A. The common varieties are as follows (see Figure 82.1):

- *Type I* consists of dilatation of the common bile duct, which may be cystic, focal, or fusiform (subtypes A, B, and C, respectively) (90–95% of cases).

- *Type II* is diverticulum of the extrahepatic bile duct.

- *Type III* involves choledochoceles.

- *Types IV:* Type IV-A, the second most common type, is defined as both intrahepatic and extrahepatic dilatation of the biliary tree. The rare malformation of multiple extrahepatic cysts is designated as type IV-B.

- *Type V* comprises single or multiple intrahepatic cysts. This type has been referred to as Caroli's disease when associated with hepatic fibrosis.

Pancreaticobiliary malunion may occur without choledochal dilatation, and this has been termed a forme fruste choledochal cyst.

Pathology

Histologic sections of the wall of extrahepatic choledochal cysts have demonstrated a thick-walled structure of dense connective tissue interlaced with strands of smooth muscle. In most instances, some degree of inflammatory reaction is noted; it is minimal in infants and gradually becomes more marked as patients get older. The histologic appearance of other forms of choledochal cysts is similar, with the exception of choledochocele. In these cysts, the lining is most commonly duodenal mucosa and only occasionally resembles the lining of the bile duct.

The findings on liver biopsy also vary with the age of the patient. In a newborn, the histologic appearance of the liver is usually interpreted as normal or having mild bile duct proliferation consistent with chronic biliary obstruction. Occasionally, in older patients, mild periportal fibrosis is noted. Although the bile duct is usually normal in appearance on histologic section, inflammation may be present, and stones and sludge may be seen in the common bile duct and occasionally in the intrahepatic ducts of older patients. Most patients with choledochal cysts have an anomalous pancreaticobiliary junction.

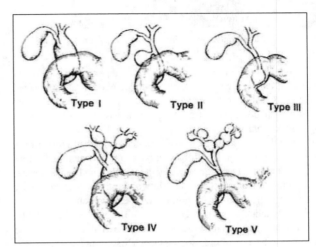

Figure 82.1: Classification of choledochal cysts.

Carcinomas arising in the wall of choledochal cysts are well recognized and believed to be the result of chronic inflammation. Biliary carcinoma has been noted in patients with an anomalous pancreaticobiliary junction even without a choledochal cyst. Carcinoma in the wall of a choledochal cyst has rarely been reported in a child, being primarily a problem of adults. Although the majority of these malignancies occur in the wall of choledochal cysts, other sites have included the gallbladder and the head of the pancreas in the region of the pancreaticobiliary junction. Because of the long interval over which these lesions seem to develop, it is presumed that they are the result of chronic inflammation from cholangitis. Inflammation is not a prominent feature in patients who have choledochoceles, although mild inflammation may lead to stenosis of the common bile duct and the pancreatic duct.

Aetiology

Choledochal cysts are congenital. Two main aetiologic theories have been proposed: (1) weakness of the wall of the bile duct due to pancreaticobiliary malunion (PBM), and (2) obstruction of the distal part of the bile duct.

In more than 75% of patients with a choledochal cyst (particularly type I and IV cysts), there is an anomalous junction between the distal common bile duct and the pancreatic duct; the ducts unite outside the duodenal wall some distance proximal to the ampulla of Vater. This common channel often exceeds 5–10 mm in length (Figure 82.2), and it is not surrounded by the normal sphincter mechanism. Consequently, pancreatic juice refluxes into the biliary tree. Isolated PBM without choledochal dilatation has been implicated in the pathogenesis of gallbladder cancer in adults. A common channel also predisposes to reflux of bile into the pancreatic duct, which may precipitate pancreatitis.

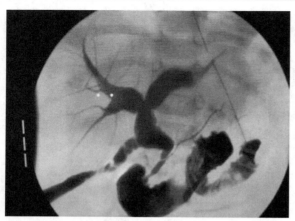

Figure 82.2: Intraoperative cholangiography showing a long common channel.

PBM is not found in all patients with congenital choledochal dilatation, and it can occur with a normal caliber bile duct. In addition, choledochal cysts have been detected as early as at 15 weeks gestation, a time when acinar development of the pancreas is rudimentary, which argues against a significant role for pancreaticobiliary reflux in such cases. An alternative and more plausible explanation is obstruction of the distal common bile duct. A distal obstruction could be functional rather than mechanical, and can occur as a result of PBM and an abnormal sphincter of Oddi. Kusunoki et al. have shown that there are abnormally few ganglion cells in the narrow portion of the common bile duct in patients with a choledochal cyst, as compared with controls. Presumably, this would result in functional obstruction and proximal dilatation in the same manner as achalasia of the esophagus or Hirschprung's disease.

Presentation

Patients with choledochal cysts usually present in one of two ways, which has led to them being classified as infantile or adult in nature. In the infantile form, patients ranging from 1 to 3 months of age present with obstructive jaundice, acholic stools, and hepatomegaly with a clinical picture indistinguishable from that of biliary atresia. Occasionally, signs of hepatic fibrosis are present, even in young patients, which is a strong argument for early treatment. Patients with the infantile form of this anomaly tend not to have abdominal pain or a palpable mass. Infants who have been diagnosed with a choledochal cyst prenatally do not ordinarily become jaundiced until 1 to 3 weeks after birth.

In the so-called adult form of choledochal cyst, clinical manifestations do not generally become evident until after the patient is 2 years of age; and most of these patients have fusiform deformities of the common duct without high-grade or complete obstruction. In this group of patients, the classic triad of abdominal pain, a palpable abdominal mass, and jaundice originally described by Alonso-Lej and colleagues may be noted. At least two features of the triad are found in 85% of children at presentation. Among the more commonly reported presenting features are cholangitis, pancreatitis, and biliary peritonitis from cyst rupture. However, it is important to emphasize that symptoms in older patients tend to be very subtle and intermittent, so the diagnosis frequently goes unrecognized. Because liver damage is progressive, these patients may present initially with cirrhosis and manifestations of portal hypertension.

Rare presentations include gastric outlet obstruction, neonatal bleeding tendency, duodenal intussusecption, and portal hypertension.

A choledochal cyst should always be considered in the differential diagnosis of obstructive jaundice or pancreatitis. Differential diagnosis includes duodenal atresia, an ovarian cyst, a duplication cyst, and cystic biliary atresia. Progressive enlargement of the cyst during gestation and the presence of dilated intrahepatic ducts on postnatal scan are indicative of a choledochal cyst rather than biliary atresia, but it may be difficult to distinguish between these two conditions.

Investigations

Ultrasound Scanning

Ultrasound scanning (US) can diagnose choledochal cysts with a specificity of 97% in children. Ultrasound is therefore an excellent first-line investigation of neonatal jaundice persisting more than 2 weeks after birth, and may help to differentiate choledochal cysts from biliary atresia. Antenatal diagnoses can be made on ultrasound, although diagnostic accuracy from this technique has been reported to be as low as 15%; also, it is not possible to differentiate between biliary atresia and choledochal cysts with antenatal ultrasound.

Radionucleotide Scintigraphy

Scintigraphy is safe and atraumatic, and has been used for a long time in the diagnosis of choledochal cysts. Scintigraphy follows the progression of an isotope from the biliary tract into the small intestine, and is reported to distinguish with 100% accuracy between choledochal cysts and biliary atresia. Type I cysts may be diagnosed with a sensitivity of 100%, but only two-thirds of type IV disease is detected, and the extent of the intrahepatic disease may be underestimated on scintigraphy.

Computed Tomographic Scan

Although there are reports of computed tomographic (CT) scans diagnosing choledochal cysts, others have found that cysts are missed on CT scans (especially in small size cysts or choledochocele), but picked up on magnetic resonance cholangiopancreatography (MRCP). A comparative study of 14 patients with choledochal cysts was performed, in which each patient had both CT cholangiography and MRCP performed. The MRCP investigation was superior at detecting and defining lesions. A better role for CT scanning may be in the postoperative period, where it has been shown to be superior to MRCP in locating the biliary-enteric anastomosis and in defining any stenosis thereof.

Magnetic Resonance Cholangiopancreatography

For the reasons outlined above, MRCP represents the current gold standard in the imaging of choledochal cysts. There are a few caveats to this, however. Although the technique is excellent for diagnosing and characterizing the cysts themselves, it is not so good at detecting anomalous pancreaticobiliary union, but this is probably not that important in determining patient management. Also, MRCP may not be as sensitive a tool in pediatric cases as it is in adults, where ultrasound has a preeminent role.

Endoscopic Retrograde Cholangiopancreatography

Investigation with endoscopic retrograde cholangiopancreatography (ERCP) is excellent for defining biliary anatomy, and as such has been used to diagnose cholodochal cysts. MRCP has been shown to be just as good if not better than ERCP, however, without the potential complications of the ERCP invasive technique.

Preoperative Preparation

Preoperative correction of any bleeding tendency with either parenteral vitamin K administration or even fresh frozen plasma is a must. Intravenous (IV) antibiotics are given to treat any attack of cholangitis.

Surgical Management

Historically, a cyst-enterostomy internal drainage procedure, either cyst-duodenostomy or cyst-jejunostomy, was considered the surgical management option for choledochal cysts. These approaches were abandoned due to complications, including malignancy in the remaining cyst, pancreatitis, and cholangitis.

The procedure currently recommended is cyst excision followed by Roux-en-Y hepaticojejunostomy or choledochojejunostomy, with the former thought to reduce the incidence of stricture formation postoperatively. Alternatives that have been suggested include hepaticoduodenostomy so that the anastomosis is accessible to ERCP in the event of postoperative complications. Hepaticoduodenostomy has not been widely adopted due to the potential for biliary reflux and cholangitis. The technique of appendix or free jejunal interposition hepaticoenterostomy similarly failed to gain widespread acclaim, as these grafts underwent stenosis with resultant hepatic fibrosis.

After excision of the cyst, the intrahepatic ducts should be probed and lavaged with saline to rid the ductal system of sludge and possible stones. Additionally, on occasion, obstruction may be found in the proximal biliary system, which can be dilatated. Therefore, intraoperative cholangiography before cyst excision is a must.

For many patients, particularly older ones who have had recurrent bouts of cholangitis, pericystic inflammation, and adherence to adjacent vascular structures, cyst excision is accomplished by using a plane of dissection between the inner and outer layers of the cyst (mucosectomy). The portion of the cyst wall that is adherent to the portal vein and hepatic artery are left undisturbed.

Patients with choledochoceles are not usually diagnosed until they are at least 5 years of age because the characteristic clinical symptom is abdominal pain of an intermittent nature that is not specific. A longitudinal duodenotomy permits complete exposure of an intraduodenal choledochocele. Once the choledochocele is exposed, it should be unroofed, and then the mucosa is reapproximated with multiple interrupted absorbable sutures. It is important to identify and calibrate the entry points of the common bile duct and the pancreatic duct to determine whether a sphincteroplasty of these ducts will be needed.

Patients with intrahepatic cysts or Caroli's disease are difficult to manage because they tend to develop severe recurrent bouts of cholangitis, subsequent biliary cirrhosis, and progressive segmental ductal ectasia. For this reason, these patients require frequent follow-up with US over a period of many years. A variety of techniques may be needed for management of intrahepatic cysts. Partial hepatic lobectomy may be done when the disease is localized and amenable to resection, but unroofing with drainage into a Roux limb of jejunum may be needed when proximal ductal obstruction is encountered. Otherwise, multiple cysts and Caroli's disease that are not amenable to localized resection or drainage may be an indication for liver transplantation.

Timing of Surgery

The timing of surgery should be early after diagnosis, even in asymptomatic prenatally diagnosed neonates (within the first 1–3 months of age), to reduce the incidence of complications, and particularly to prevent liver fibrosis in neonates.

Postoperative Complications

Intrahepatic Cholelithiasis

Intrahepatic stones are a particular problem in cases of type IV disease with residual intrahepatic cysts. Choledochoscopy is used at the time of surgery to detect and remove intrahepatic stones at operation. Intraoperative cholangiography with ductal probing and washout of debris reduces postoperative complications of stones retained in the biliary radicals.

Malignant Change after Cyst Excision

Even after cyst excision, there are reports of malignancy, usually from incomplete cyst excision. However, in a comprehensive review, the incidence of post-excision malignancy has been estimated at only 0.7%. Since malignancy may occur in the residual intrapancreatic portion of the choledochal cyst, close long-term follow-up for those patients with intra-pancreatic extension is recommended, with resection if needed.

The extent of the resection in type IV-A cysts is controversial. Several authors advocate management by excision of the extrahepatic component only, with hepaticoenterostomy. However, malignancy has been reported to arise in the intrahepatic cysts, as described above, and it has also been reported to occur after resection of the extrahepatic cyst with hepaticojejunostomy. Clearly, when the intrahepatic cysts are widespread, they cannot be excised; however, when the intrahepatic disease is localized, it is reasonable to perform a partial hepatectomy. Similarly, partial hepatectomy has been practiced for Caroli's disease.

Cholangitis

Patients who have had cyst excision with internal drainage have a lower incidence of postoperative cholangitis than do patients with biliary atresia who have had a similar type of drainage procedure. Hepaticoduodenostomy after cyst excision has long been claimed to be associated with a higher incidence of cholangitis and biliary reflux; however, our group (Ain Shams University in Cairo) has been using this type of biliary reconstruction after cyst excision for more than 50 cases with a follow-up period now approaching 6 years, and preliminary data refute the claim of higher cholangitis and biliary reflux rates with hepaticoduodenostomy.

Stricture Formation

Performing a higher anastomosis at the level of the confluence, as proposed by Todani and co-workers, may reduce the incidence of anastomotic stricture formation. Other investigators disagree and believe that conventional drainage at the level of the hepatic hilum is sufficient. We agree that an anastomosis to the common hepatic duct is sufficient, provided that a stricture of the right or left hepatic duct is not left in place.

Pancreatitis

Rarely, patients may develop pancreatitis after cyst excision and internal drainage. Acute pancreatitis due to protein plug formation is observed in more than 20% of patients followed long term. The morphology of the pancreatic duct and ductal dilatation, possibly caused by long-standing stagnation of pancreatic juice, may be associated with postoperative pancreatitis in choledochal cyst patients. Overall, however, pancreatitis is an uncommon event after excision and internal drainage of a choledochal cyst.

Laparoscopic Excision

Recently, laparoscopic cyst excision and hepaticojejunostomy have been described. It is too early to assess the long-term results of this approach in terms of anastomotic strictures and malignancy arising in residual cyst tissue. The principle of laparoscopic surgery for choledochal cysts is similar to that of open surgery, although it is much more technically demanding, especially in small children in whom the peritoneal space is very limited. The magnification of the laparoscope allows excellent visualization of the anatomy and, in turn, facilitates meticulous mobilization of the cyst from surrounding structures. Fashioning of the jejunal Roux loop can be performed through the enlarged umbilical wound. This enables meticulous bowel anastomosis, just like open surgery, and also avoids intraabdominal contamination.

Postoperative Follow-Up

Our routine is to keep the patients on low doses of ampicillin or trimethoprim-sulfamethoxazole for approximately 6 weeks postoperation to protect against cholangitis, after which the potential for this complication appears to diminish. Postoperative follow-up should be every 3 months for the first year and annually thereafter in asymptomatic patients. At each visit, liver function studies and serum amylase levels should be determined. Ultrasound of the liver and pancreas is done annually or when necessary if patients become symptomatic. US of the liver is particularly important in patients who are found to have intrahepatic ductal dilatation preoperatively. US is also helpful for long-term evaluation of the Roux-en-Y ductal anastomosis because occasional patients will develop late anastomotic strictures or stones. Patients who had hepaticoduedenostomy with a hepatobiliary iminodiacetic acid (HIDA) scan and barium meal and follow-through in the Trendelenberg position were investigated for biliary alkaline reflux; findings proved to be of no significance.

Evidence-Based Research

Table 82.1 presents a study of differences in characteristics between newborns and infants with choledochal cysts.

Table 82.1: Evidence-based research.

Title	The different clinical and liver pathological characteristics between newborns and infants with choledochal cysts
Authors	Hua MC, Chao HC, Lien R, Lai JY, et al.
Institution	Department of Pediatric Surgery, Chang Gung Memorial Hospital, Chang Gung University, Taoyuan, Taiwan.
Reference	Chang Gung Med J 2009; 32:198–202
Problem	Comparison of choledochal cysts presenting in the neonatal period with those presenting in older age groups, assuming there is a difference in the clinical and liver pathological aspects.
Intervention	Cyst excision and Roux-en-Y hepaticojejunostomy.
Comparison/ control (quality of evidence)	The patients were divided into two age groups: the newborn group comprised those who presented within 1 month of birth and the antenatally diagnosed patients; the infant group comprised those who presented between 1 and 12 months of age. All medical records of those patients who presented to the institution between March 1991 and November 2006 were retrospectively reviewed.
Outcome/ effect	Sixteen patients (45.7%) were categorized into the newborn group, including 12 patients in whom the cysts were detected by using antenatal ultrasound. Nineteen patients (54.3%) were in the infant group. According to Todani's classification, 74.2% of choledochal cysts were type I. Using chi-square and Student's t-tests, the infant group had significantly higher preoperative morbidity, abnormal levels of serum transaminase, gamma trans-peptide (γ-GT), and grade of liver fibrosis (≥ grade 2) (p < 0.05). The postoperative complications were not statistically significant between newborn and infant groups.
Historical significance/ comments	This report comparing the differences in clinical and pathological characteristics between newborns and infants presenting with choledochal cysts highlights the importance of such differentiation and its impact on management. Twelve patients had preoperative morbidities, including pseudopancreatitis, hypoalbuminemia, gallstone, poor body weight gain, cholangitis, cyst perforation with peritonitis, and inferior vena cava thrombus formation. These morbidities were more common in the infant group than in the newborn group. A liver biopsy specimen was obtained during the operations. The results of liver fibrosis based on Ohkuma's classification were consistent with a higher incidence of liver fibrosis in older infants.

The paper concludes that the favorable results of early surgical intervention for infants with choledochal cysts and the evidence of liver fibrosis in the older infants suggest that early surgery, even in asymptomatic patients, may be justified. |

Key Summary Points

1. Choledochal cysts are uncommon, but when encountered, they may appear nonspecifically rather than classically. A high index of suspicion will avoid a delay in diagnosis.

2. The imaging modality of choice for diagnosing and characterizing choledochal cysts is magnetic resonance cholangiopancreatography (MRCP).

3. Delayed diagnosis may have a variety of undesirable sequelae, including biliary cirrhosis, cholangiocarcinoma, pancreatitis, and cholangitis.

4. To avoid these complications, choledochal cysts should be treated by complete excision, whenever possible, with reconstruction using internal drainage.

5. Follow-up is essential to detect development of any complications, such as cholangitis, anastomotic stricture, or intrahepatic cholelithiasis.

Suggested Reading

Alonso-Lej F, Rever WB Jr, Pessagno DJ. Congenital choledochal cyst, with a report of 2, and an analysis of 94, cases. Int Abstr Surg 1959; 108(1):1–30.

Blankensteijn JD, Terpstra OT. Early and late results following choledechoduodenostomy and choledechojejunostomy. HPB Surg 1990; 2:151–158.

Iwai N, Yanagihara J, Tokiwa K, Shimotake T, Nakamura K. Congenital choledochal dilatation with emphasis on pathophysiology of the biliary tract. Ann Surg 1992; 215:27–30.

Kaneko K, Ando H, Watanabe Y, et al. Secondary excision of choledochal cysts after previous cyst-enterostomies. Hepatogastroenterology 1999; 46:2772–2775.

Kobayashi S, Asano T, Yamasaki M, Kenmochi T, Nakagohri T, Ochiai T. Risk of bile duct carcinogenesis after excision of extrahepatic bile ducts in pancreaticobiliary maljunction. Surgery 1999; 126:939–944.

Kusunoki M, Saitoh N, Yamamura T, Fujita S, Takahashi T, Utsunomiya J. Choledochal cysts: oligoganglionosis in the narrow portion of the choledochus. Arch Surg 1988; 123:984–986.

Metcalfe MS, Wemyss-Holden SA, Maddern GJ, et al. Management dilemmas with choledochal cysts. Arch Surg 2003; 138:333–339.

Miyano T, Yamataka A, Kato Y, et al. Hepaticoenterostomy after excision of choledochal cyst in children: a 30-year experience with 180 cases. J Pediatr Surg 1996; 31:417–421.

O'Neill JA Jr. Choledochal cyst. In: Grosfold JL, O'Neill JA Jr, Fonkalsrud EW, Coran AG. Pediatric Surgery, sixth ed. Mosby, 2006; Pp 1620–1634.

Todani T, Watanabe Y, Narusue M, et al. Congenital bile duct cysts: classification, operative procedure and review of thirty seven cases including cancer arising from choledochal cyst. Am J Surg 1977; 134:263–269.

Uno K, Isuchida Y, Kawarasaki H, et al. Development of intrahepatic cholelithiasis long after primary excision of choledochal cyst. J Am Coll Surg 1996; 183:583–588.

Yamataka A, Ohshiro K, Okada Y, et al. Complications after cyst excision with hepaticoenterostomy for choledochal cysts and their surgical management in children versus adults. J Pediatr Surg 1997; 32:1097–1102.

CHAPTER 83
CHOLELITHIASIS (GALLSTONES)

Bankole S. Rouma
Donald E. Meier

Introduction

Cholelithiasis (gallstones) in children is being diagnosed with increasing frequency in developed countries. This is related to an increase in recognition due to the widespread use of ultrasound (US) scans for abdominal complaints and an increase in the frequency of the disease secondary to some predisposing factors. These factors include an increase in childhood obesity, common use of total parenteral nutrition in fasting premature infants, an increase in the incidence of necrotising enterocolitis requiring ileal resection, more frequent use of lithogenic medications (e.g., ceftriaxone), improved medical treatment, longer survival of patients with haemolytic disease, and an increase in adolescent pregnancy. In Africa, children with sickle cell disease are more affected by cholelithiasis, and the incidence increases with age.

Demographics

The incidence of cholelithiasis in children is reported to be 0.15–0.22%, whereas the incidence in adults is approximately 10%.[1] The incidence of cholelithiasis in patients with sickle cell disease has been reported to be 10–70% in the United States.[1] In Nigeria, the prevalence of gallstones diagnosed in a predominantly teenage population of children with SS haemoglobin was found to be 9%, but there was a higher prevalence of 24.1% in older sickle cell patients.[2] A prevalence of 4% was found in Ghanaian children with sickle cell disease[3] and 9.4% in Senegalian sickle cell children.[4]

Embryology of the Bile Ducts

The liver develops from an endodermal bud in the ventral floor of the foregut at about 22 days gestation. The cells of the cranial portion give rise to the mature hepatocytes, intrahepatic bile ducts, proximal extrahepatic bile ducts, and gallbladder. The distal extrahepatic bile ducts are derived from cells in the caudal portion.

Physiologic Maturation of the Biliary System

Hepatocytes perform a wide variety of essential physiologic tasks, including production of plasma proteins, gluconeogenesis, glycogenolysis, biotransformation of toxins and chemicals, bile acid metabolism, cholesterol regulation, and bilirubin excretion. During gestation, many of these functions are performed for the foetus through placental transport and maternal hepatic function. Many of the excretory functions of the foetal liver mature only after birth. The physiologic immaturity of the premature liver plays a role in the pathophysiology of a variety of neonatal diseases characterised by abnormal bile composition or flow.

Maturation of Bile Acid Metabolism and the Enterohepatic Circulation

Bile acids are amphipathic sterols formed in the liver by stereospecific additions and modifications of cholesterol. Bile acid metabolism is a critical determinant of cholesterol regulation. The interaction of bile acids, phospholipids, and cholesterol leads to mixed micelle formation, allowing biliary excretion of these lipids and other compounds, and facilitating intestinal absorption of dietary fat.

The enterohepatic circulation maintains the bile acid pool by recycling 90% of the excreted bile acid. This occurs through a sodium-bile acid transport system, present on the ileal brush border that absorbs bile acid against a concentration gradient. The bile acids return to the liver through the portal circulation, where they are actively secreted by a second sodium-bile acid cotransporter across the hepatocyte canalicular basolateral membrane. Bacteria present in the jejunum and ileum metabolise a portion of the primary bile acids to secondary bile acids, which are passively absorbed in the colon and re-enter the hepatic circulation. Maturation of hepatic and ileal bile acid transport does not begin until around the time of birth.

Foetuses and newborns have qualitative differences from adults in bile acid composition. Foetal bile contains an increased chenodeoxycholic/cholic acid ratio, a predominance of taurine conjugates, and the presence of unusual bile acids with specific hydroxylations seen in adults with cholestasis. Therefore, the preterm or term infant has several predispositions to cholestasis. The diminished bile acid pool and decreased intraluminal concentration of bile acid result in decreased bile acid flow, which favours the development of sludge or cholelithiasis.

Maturation of Bile Pigment Excretion

Most bilirubin is the end product of the degradation of haem derived from erythrocytes normally removed from the circulation and destroyed in the reticuloendothelial system.

Erythrocyte half-life is shorter in the foetus and neonate, and therefore production of unconjugated bilirubin is greater than in an adult. Bilirubin UDP-glucuonyl tranferase activity, which conjugates bilirubin, is first detected at about 20 weeks gestation and remains low until after birth. The reabsorption of unconjugated bilurubin from the intestine may also contribute to the increased bilirubin load after birth. Conjugated bilirubin gradually accumulates in meconium during foetal life. Bacterial flora responsible for the conversion of conjugated bilirubin to urobilin are absent or reduced in the gut of the newborn infant, which allows the enzyme B glucuronidase to deconjugate the accumulated bilirubin. This process results in the absorption of a significant load of unconjugated bilirubin from the newborn intestine.

Pathogenesis

The pathogenesis of cholelithiasis in children is multifactorial and differs according to age at presentation. In infants, the normal immaturity of the hepatic excretory function and the enterohepatic circulation lower the threshold for stone formation when combined with lithogenic factors (parenteral alimentation, fasting, dehydration, furosemide treatment, ileal resection related to necrotising enterocolitis or volvulus, biliary tract anomalies, and polycythaemia). In this age group, cholestasis can manifest as liver functional abnormality, as biliary sludge, or as true cholelithiasis directly related to the duration of fasting.

In the prepubertal child, stones are more likely to be idiopathic or related to chronic haemolysis, cystic fibrosis, ileal resection, or ceftriaxone therapy. In this age group, stone composition is predominantly calcium bilirubinate or calcium carbonate, and the gender incidence is equal.

After puberty and in the adult population, stones are more likely to be predominantly cholesterol. The solubility of cholesterol depends on the concentration of lecithin, bile salts, and cholesterol within bile. Any disturbance in the concentration of these three substances may leave the bile lithogenic and predisposed to formation of cholesterol stones. These stones result when the bile cannot solubilise all the cholesterol. In this age group, there is an increased female-to-male ratio. Racial and genetic influences, obesity, oral contraceptives, and pregnancy are also predisposing factors.

Haemolytic Disease

Pigmented stones can be black or earthy brown (calcium bilirubinate). Black-pigmented stones usually are associated with a haemolytic process such as sickle cell disease, thalassaemia major, hereditary spherocytosis, pyruvate kinase deficiency, autoimmune haemolytic anaemia, or other haemolytic processes. Calcium bilirubinate stones are found in patients with infected bile or biliary structures. Although the exact cause of the development of pigmented stones is unclear, the bile in these patients contains an excess amount of unconjugated bilirubin and beta-glucuronidase, an enzyme produced by bacteria that may hydrolyze soluble bilirubin glucuronide to insoluble unconjugated bilirubin and glucuronic acid. Unconjugated bilirubin may form calcium bilirubinate. Stasis and nucleating factors also may play roles in the development of these stones. Jaundice also may occur intermittently because of haemolysis; therefore, jaundice does not necessarily mean that common duct calculi are present.

Sickle Cell Anaemia

The incidence of gallstones increases with age in children with sickle cell anaemia: 12% are affected in the 2–4 year age group and 42% in the 15–18 year group.[2] It can be difficult to differentiate symptoms of biliary colic from an abdominal crisis in the sickle cell patient. Utrasound should be performed in all children with sickle cell disease and abdominal pain, as there is an increased risk of complications related to cholelithiasis in patients with sickle cell disease. Careful preoperative preparation of a child with sickle cell anaemia is essential to avoid perioperative sickling of the abnormal red blood cells. This sickling may be precipitated by hypoxia, hypovolaemia, acidosis, hypothermia, and a high level of haemoglobin S. Cholecystectomy is currently not recommended for children with sickle cell disease unless symptomatic. Cholecystectomy should be performed electively rather than as an emergency procedure during a haemolytic crisis. Partial exchange transfusion is necessary before operation to reduce the haemoglobin S level to less than 40%.

Thalassaemia Major

The incidence of gallstones varies from 2.3% to 23% and increases with age.[1] The risk of cholelithiasis in the patient population with thalassaemia major is decreasing because of hypertransfusion therapy that blocks the bone marrow so that the fragile cells of thalassaemia major are no longer produced. For all symptomatic patients and for patients undergoing splenectomy in whom preoperative ultrasound shows the presence of gallstones, cholecystectomy is recommended.

Hereditary Spherocytosis

Hereditary spherocytosis is rare in the Africa population.[5] The incidence of cholelithiasis in this disease is 43–63% and is slightly more common in girls than boys. Abdominal ultrasound should be performed before elective splenectomy to detect the presence of gallstones. Demonstration of stones dictates that a simultaneous cholecystectomy should be performed.

Congenital Deformities of the Gallbladder

Agenesis, duplication, bilobation, floating gallbladder, diverticula, and ectopia are usually of no real clinical relevance unless they impair gallbladder emptying; calculi are frequent in such cases.

Clinical Presentation

Clinical presentation depends on age. Gallstones are frequently asymptomatic in all age groups and detected on evaluation for other problems. Diagnosis in infancy requires clinical suspicion because the presentation is nonspecific. Persistent direct hyperbilirubinaemia should lead to an evaluation of the biliary tract, including evaluation for cholelithiasis. Jaundice and fever in an infant with any predisposing factors should lead to prompt evaluation for stones.

In older children, the presenting complaint is almost always abdominal pain. Younger children may not be able to localise abdominal pain, whereas older children have more typical right upper quadrant or subscapular pain. Diagnosis is often delayed due to a lack of suspicion in children and an absence of predisposing conditions. Evaluation of children with recurrent unexplained abdominal pain should include an evaluation for biliary disease. Abdominal pain in patients with chronic haemolysis or other predisposing factors should prompt immediate biliary evaluation.

Presentation in the postpubertal population is similar to that in adults. Pain is usually dull and subcostal in location and may radiate to the subscapular region. Fatty food intolerance with associated nausea and vomiting may be present.

In children with chronic cholecystitis and cholelithiasis, the physical examination is often normal. Patients with acute cholecystitis may show elevated temperature, signs of dehydration, nausea, and right upper abdominal tenderness and muscle guarding. Some patients may have a tender, palpable mass (Murphy's sign). Laboratory findings include leukocytosis and elevated serum direct bilirubin, alkaline phosphatase, and glutamyl transferase levels. Because pancreatitis can occur in 10% of such patients, serum amylase and lipase level should be monitored as well.

Diagnosis

Most gallstones in children are radiolucent, and US is the diagnostic modality of choice. Ultrasound diagnosis (Figure 83.1) of stones requires the presence of moveable, echogenic structures within the gallbladder, with associated shadowing. Sludge is a fluid substance that on US examination can be seen layering out in the dependent portion of the gallbladder. An US finding of an impacted stone at the ampulla, associated gallbladder wall thickening, or localised pericholecystic fluid support the clinical diagnosis of acute cholecystitis.

Common bile duct dilatation suggests choledocholithiasis, and confirmatory endoscopic retrograde cholangiopancreatography (ERCP) or operative or transhepatic cholangiography may be required.

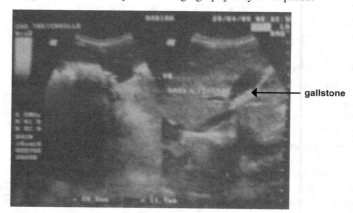

gallstone

Figure 83.1: Ultrasound of an 8-year-old sickle cell disease girl with gallstone.

Differential Diagnosis

Hydrops of the Gallbladder

Acute distention of the gallbladder with oedema of the gallbladder wall has been reported in association with septic or shocklike states, severe diarrhoea with dehydration, hepatitis, scarlet fever, Kawasaki disease, leptospiroses, and mesenteric adenitis. Hydrops is suspected if a palpable mass of the gallbladder is confirmed by US. Generally, hydrops resolves spontaneously. If symptoms intensify, cholecystectomy may be necessary.

Acalculous Cholecystitis

Acalculous cholecystitis may occur as a complication during treatment of various disease states. This condition may occur in newborns, but it is more common in older children. Patients are often severely ill and sometimes intubated in an intensive care unit, so early manifestations of the disease are not evident. The most common presentation is deterioration and signs of sepsis in a previously stable patient. The diagnosis is confirmed by US, which demonstrates gallbladder distention and intraluminal echogenic debris. Treatment in mild cases can be conservative with antibiotics, but if the patient's condition deteriorates, cholecystectomy should be performed. If the patient is very ill, percutaneous or open cholecystostomy may be useful as a temporary measure.

Biliary Dyskinesia

Biliary dyskinesia is a distinct clinical entity that occurs primarily in older children and adults. It is characterised by poor gallbladder contractility and the presence of cholesterol crystals in the gallbladder bile. There is often a delay in diagnosis in patients with this condition because US does not show cholelithiasis. Biliary dyskinesia is diagnosed with a cholecystokinin-stimulated hepato-iminodiacetic acid (HIDA) scan that shows poor biliary excretion.

Other differential diagnoses of right upper quadrant pain are acute appendicitis, peptic ulcer disease, inflammatory bowel disease, hepatitis, pancreatitis, intussusception, acute sequestration crisis, and malaria fever.

Treatment

Numerous nonoperative therapies were introduced for the management of gallstones, including dissolution of cholesterol gallstones with oral administration of chenodeoxycholic acid, the use of extracorporeal shock-wave lithotripsy, and percutaneous endoscopic cholecystolithotomy. These therapies have been all but abandoned. In developed countries and in some developing countries, laparoscopic cholecystectomy has become the preferred standard for the management of symptomatic children with cholelithiasis.[1,4,6,7]

Preoperative ultrasound is performed on each patient to confirm the diagnosis of cholelithiasis and to evaluate the presence or absence of common duct involvement. In developed countries, if choledocholithiasis is suspected on initial evaluation, ERCP and sphincterotomy are recommended before laparoscopic cholecystectomy. The expertise to remove the stones endoscopically is not available in all children's hospitals, however. If choledocholithiasis is documented and the stones cannot be removed endoscopically, the surgeon must decide whether to proceed with laparoscopic cholecystectomy and laparoscopic choledochal exploration or to perform an open operation.

Laparoscopic Cholecystectomy

Laparoscopic cholecystectomy is now the standard method for cholecystectomy for children in more developed locations. Since the technique is so technologically dependent, however, it is not appropriate for resource-poor locations that do not have a dependable supply of electricity or the money to purchase enough equipment to have reserve supplies whenever there is a malfunction of the primary equipment (a frequent occurrence, even in developed locations). There is a very steep learning curve for this procedure, and the complications of injury or ligation of the common bile duct are often catastrophic. Therefore laparoscopic cholecystectomy is recommended only for the most advanced African hospitals with excellent equipment and supplies. It is quite important that all surgeons undertaking laparoscopic cholecystectomy know how to expertly perform open cholecystectomies and common bile duct explorations.

Procedure

General endotracheal anaesthesia is administered with a muscle relaxant to assist with the pneumoperitoneum. The abdomen is prepared and draped in a sterile fashion.

1. A 10-mm incision is made in a vertical direction through the umbilical skin and carried down through the umbilical fascia with a cautery.

2. A 10-mm port is introduced directly into the abdominal cavity.

3. A pneumoperitoneum is created with insufflation of CO_2 up to a maximum pressure of 15 mm Hg.

4. The other ports are introduced under telescopic vision after creation of the pneumoperitoneum. The position of the other incisions and ports varies according to the patient's size. It is important to place these ports widely in the younger patient because the intraabdominal working space is reduced. Two 3- or 5-mm ports are placed on the right side of the abdomen, one below the right costal margin and one in the right mid to lower abdomen.

5. The fourth incision is 5 mm (or 10 mm if a 10-mm endoscopic clip applier is required), and it is situated in the epigastric region in the older child or to the left of the midline in the younger child.

6. The fundus of the gallbladder is grasped with a grasping forceps that has been introduced through the lower, lateral cannula, and the gallbladder is retracted superiorly and ventrally over the liver.

7. The infundibulum is retracted to the patient's right using the right upper port for access. This allows the cystic duct to enter the common duct as close to a 90° angle as possible. If the infundibulum is retracted cephalad instead, the cystic duct approaches the common duct, and injury or ligation of the common duct is more likely to occur.

8. The cystic duct is skeletonised. Cholangiography often is not necessary, but if it is, it can be performed at this point by making an incision in the cystic duct and introducing a cholangiogram catheter.

9. If a cholangiogram is not performed, or after it is performed, the cystic duct is triply clipped and divided between the proximal clips and the distal third clip, leaving two clips on the cystic duct stump and one clip on the duct next to the gallbladder so that bile will not be leaking during the rest of the case.

10. The cystic artery is triply clipped and divided in a similar fashion in Calot's triangle.

11. The gallbladder is dissected from its liver bed in a retrograde fashion with a hook or spatula cautery. Before complete detachment of the gallbladder from the liver, the area of the dissection is inspected carefully and haemostasis is achieved. The gallbladder is detached completely from its liver bed.

12. The telescope is moved from the umbilical port to the cannula of the epigastric port.

13. The gallbladder is removed through the umbilical cannula or through the fascial defect if it is necessary to remove the cannula.

14. The dissected area is inspected again and haemostasis assured. Ports and instruments are removed, and the incisions are closed.

Advantages

The advantages of the laparoscopic approach include less operative discomfort, reduced hospitalisation, and early return to full activity.[7,8] Laparoscopic cholecystectomy decreases the chance for wound infection, a common complication following open cholecystectomy in developing countries. Even sickle cell disease children can benefit from laparoscopic cholecystectomy if the following rules of general anesthesia are respected: preoperative transfusion or blood exchange and the prevention of pain, hypovolaemia, hypothermia, and acidosis during the perioperative period.

Open Surgery

Using a right subcostal incision, the same steps as for the laparoscopic cholecystectomy can be performed. In cases of acute cholecystitis, the cystic duct may be difficult to visualise. In these instances, the gallbladder can be taken down in a prograde direction (from fundus to ampulla) before ligating the cystic duct and artery. This more safely identifies the junction of the gallbladder and cystic duct and minimises the chance of damage to the common bile duct.

Complications

Significant complications have been reported in laparoscopic cholecystectomies. There is a definitive learning curve with a significant decrease in complications with increased operator experience. Bile duct injuries have been reported in 0.1–2.3% of patients, and bile leak in 1.5–2.0% of patients.[1]

In sickle cell disease children, postoperative complications include acute chest syndrome, haemolysis, and vaso-occlusive crisis.[6]

Key Summary Points

1. Jaundice may occur intermittently in haemolytic cholelithiasis (sickle cell disease) children because of haemolysis; therefore, common bile duct calculi are not necessarily present.

2. Jaundice and fever in infants with any other disposing factor (ileal resection, fasting, dehydration, parenteral nutrition, necrotising enterocolitis, biliary tract anomalies, polycythaemia) should prompt evaluation for stones.

3. It is important before surgery to rule out choledocholithiasis by ultrasound.

4. In sickle cell disease, cholecystectomy is currently not recommended unless symptomatic, and cholecystectomy should be performed electively rather than as an emergency procedure during a haemolytic crisis.

5. Partial exchange transfusion is necessary before operation to reduce the haemoglobin S level in sickle cell disease children.

6. In patients with spherocytosis, ultrasound is recommended before splenectomy; demonstration of a stone dictates that a simultaneous cholecystectomy should be performed.

7. African paediatric surgeons must have training in laparoscopic surgery and be able to do laparoscopic cholecystectomy safely because the advantages are important in developing countries.

8. During laparoscopic cholecystectomy, it is important to retract the infundibulum laterally, which orients the cystic duct at a right angle to the common bile duct.

References

1. Holocomb GW III. Gallbladder disease. In: O'Neill JA Jr., Grosfeld JL, Fonkalsrud EW, Coran AG, Caldamone AA (eds). Principles of Pediatric Surgery. Mosby, 2004, Pp 645–651.

2. Akamaguna AI, Odita JC, Ugbodaga I, Okafor LA. Cholelithiasis in sickle cell disease: a cholecystographic and ultrasonographic evaluation in Nigerians. Europ J Radiol 1985; 5:271–272.

3. Darko R, Rodrigues OP, Olivier Commey JO. Gallstones in Ghanaian children with sickle cell disease. West Afr J Med 2005; 24:295–298.

4. Fall B, Saga A, Diop PS, Faye EAB, Diagnel, Dia A. Laparoscopic cholecystectomy in sickle cell disease. Annales de Chirurgie 2003; 128:702–705.

5. Olubode OA, Esan GJ, Isaac-Sodeye WA, Ukaejiofo EO. Hereditary spherocytosis in Nigeria. Niger Med J. 1976; 6:44-48.

6. Diop Ndoye M, Diao Bah M, Ndiaye Pape I, Diouf E, Kane O, Bèye M, Fall B, Ka-Sall B. Perioperative management of laparoscopic cholecystectomy in children with homozygous sickle cell disease. Archives de Pédiatrie 2008; 15:1393–1397.

7. Bankolé R, Kirioua B, Guemaleu P. Pediatric laparoscopic surgery in Abidjan (Côte d'Ivoire). J Laparoendosc Adv Surg Tech 2008; 18:537.

8. Holocomb GW III, Morgan WM III, Neblett WW III, et al. Laparoscopic cholecystectomy in children: lessons learned from the first 100 patients. J Pediatr Surg 1999; 34:1236–1240.

CHAPTER 84
ANNULAR PANCREAS

Ashley Ridout

Kokila Lakhoo

Introduction

Annular pancreas (from the Latin annularis, meaning ring-shaped) is a rare congenital disorder of the pancreas first recognised by Tiedeman in 1818. This abnormality, although at times clinically silent, may be the cause of a broad spectrum of disease. Complications range from neonatal intestinal obstruction to more complex pathologies in the adult. In cases of neonatal obstruction, annular pancreas is an important structural and anatomical cause that must be identified and treated appropriately. Currently, the majority of cases are diagnosed early in life, and prenatal diagnosis is becoming increasingly important.

Demographics

The incidence of this congenital anomaly is reported as 1–3 in 20,000,[1,2] and some studies have shown that it is more common in males. Detection of the condition is variable, as it may be asymptomatic and therefore detected only incidentally or at postmortem. However, the vast majority of cases are diagnosed either prenatally or in the first few days of life. If the condition is not diagnosed prenatally or does not present with complications in early life, it may be undetected until adulthood. The detection of an annular pancreas may occur at any time during adulthood (presentation age shows a bell-shaped distribution[1]), and may be discovered either incidentally or after presentation due to a complication such as pancreatitis.

There is a strong association between annular pancreas and other congenital abnormalities—up to 71% of cases have coexisting congenital anomalies.[1] The most common association is with Down syndrome. However, there may be a wide range of associated cardiac and gastrointestinal anomalies (including Hirschsprung's disease and imperforate anus), as well as tracheo-oesophageal fistula and oesophageal atresia.[3]

Aetiology and Pathophysiology

Annular pancreas is an embryological defect of the foregut. Development of the pancreas begins during week 5 of gestation. One dorsal and two ventral buds develop from the primitive foregut. By week 7, the ventral bud rotates with the gut to fuse with the dorsal bud, after passing behind the duodenum. The dorsal bud forms the body and tail of the pancreas, and the ventral bud forms the inferior part of the pancreatic head and the uncinate process. Fusion of the buds forms the main pancreatic duct.

Several theories have been proposed to explain the development of annular pancreas. One theory suggests that the tip of the ventral bud fuses abnormally to the duodenum, therefore rotating incorrectly around the duodenum and resulting in a band of fibrous or pancreatic parenchymal tissue around the second part of the duodenum.[1] An alternative theory posits that hypertrophy of the dorsal and ventral buds results in a complete band of pancreatic tissue around the duodenum (a complete ring is found in approximately 25% of the cases[4]).

Clinical Presentation

History

The diagnosis of annular pancreas may be made prenatally, upon emergency presentation, or incidentally after imaging, at operation, or postmortem. If the band of pancreatic tissue causes a duodenal obstruction, symptoms may appear within the first few hours of life. Signs of neonatal intestinal obstruction may initially be nonspecific, including poor feeding, vomiting, and irritability. If proximal to the ampulla of Vater, vomiting may be nonbilious, and therefore could be confused with less severe, non–life-threatening conditions.

The nature of presentation differs according to patient age, although most presentation occurs most commonly in infancy or early childhood. Children frequently present with gastrointestinal (GI) symptoms, including poor feeding, vomiting, and abdominal distention. In Africa, most patients present late, with malnutrition, failure to thrive, bile-stained vomiting, and—less frequently—abdominal cramps.

Of note is the fact that adults are much more likely to describe upper abdominal pain or present acutely with pancreatitis.[1] Complications arising due to the presence of an annular pancreas are a rare cause of neonatal or childhood presentation, but must be kept in mind, as cure requires identification and treatment of the abnormality.

Physical

Clinical examination findings will vary according to the age at presentation and the extent of systemic upset. For some patients, access to a hospital may be difficult—this includes patients whose presentation is delayed by parents and those who have to travel long distances to reach the hospital. These patients will likely be more unwell at presentation and may even die before they reach the hospital.

When presenting as intestinal obstruction, the abdomen will be distended (before decompression), and there may be palpable peristalsis. Bowel sounds are variable. If presentation is delayed, there may be clinical signs of hypovolaemic shock, including pallor, poor capillary refill, and drowsiness or lethargy.

Investigations

Prenatal diagnosis

It is becoming increasingly possible to detect the presence of annular pancreas in foetal life (2nd trimester). A nonspecific diagnosis of duodenal obstruction can be made prenatally with identification of simultaneous dilatation of the stomach and duodenum—the "double bubble" sign.[4] This does not predict the specific cause of the duodenal obstruction, and certainly is not specific to the diagnosis of annular pancreas. Indeed, presence of an annular pancreas is the cause in only 1% of cases of neonatal duodenal obstruction.[5] Therefore, there is a search for more specific prenatal markers of annular pancreas. Several groups have shown that the presence of hyperechogenic bands around the duodenum specifically indicates the presence of an annular pancreas.[4] This finding can now be used to specifically detect the presence of annular pancreas during foetal life.

Imaging modalities

Abdominal radiography

The plain abdominal radiograph will not provide diagnostic structural information about the pancreas, in part due to the lack of tissue contrast. Cross-sectional imaging modalities are much more useful in delineating the precise anatomy of this area. However, if obstruction is complete, duodenal obstruction classically appears as a double bubble on abdominal radiograph. This represents dilatation of the stomach (seen in the left upper quadrant) and proximal duodenum (seen in the right upper quadrant). A double bubble on abdominal radiograph is sufficient to diagnose a complete duodenal obstruction. However, an upper gastrointestinal contrast radiograph is helpful for diagnosing a partial duodenal obstruction.

Ultrasonography

The use of ultrasonography (US) allows a real-time evaluation of the paediatric pancreas, without the use of ionising radiation and usually without the need for sedation. This modality provides a safe, relatively cheap, and often readily available technique for imaging the paediatric pancreas. The reduced body wall thickness of the child, in combination with the anatomical "window" provided by the liver, ensures that a better quality of pancreatic image is obtained in the child, as compared to the adult.[3]

Computed tomography

The lack of intraabdominal fat in children, combined with the often thin band of pancreatic tissue around the duodenum, may make identification of the annular pancreas with computed tomography (CT) difficult. Despite this, detection rates can be greatly improved with a specific, intravenous (IV)-contrast-enhanced, pancreatic study.[3,6] CT may also highlight extrinsic compression of the duodenum, which must be differentiated from thickening of the wall of the duodenum. CT may be used for further investigation of abnormalities detected with ultrasound imaging.

Magnetic resonance imaging

Magnetic resonance imaging (MRI) is an alternative to CT imaging for evaluation of the pancreas. Combined with magnetic resonance cholangiopancreatography (MRCP), it allows detailed imaging of the biliary system.[3]

Typically, the exact cause of the duodenal obstruction is not known until surgical exploration.

Management

In clinically silent cases of annular pancreas, no specific intervention is required. Specific management will depend upon the nature of the complication or symptoms caused by the annular pancreas.

Duodenal Obstruction

Ultimately, urgent surgical intervention is required in cases of duodenal obstruction, even if the precise cause of the obstruction is unclear. Initially, however, management must include decompression with a nasogastric tube and fluid resuscitation. It is appropriate for patients to be transferred to a special care/high dependency unit, if available, where appropriate monitoring and interventions can be instigated. Delayed presentation may result in significant systemic upset, and it is vital that adequate resuscitation be carried out before surgery. Prior to surgery, fluid and electrolyte resuscitation is an absolute requirement.

The management of duodenal obstruction in the presence of annular pancreas requires surgical bypass of the obstruction with duodenoduodenostomy, or duodenojejunostomy. Laparotomy may be required to determine the cause of obstruction if this is not specifically identified on preoperative imaging. Tapering of the bowel is not necessary, even if the proximal segment is grossly dilatated. Transanastamotic nasogastric tubes may be necessary in centers where parenteral nutrition is not available, due to the delay in enteral feeding as a result of the dilatated proximal segment.

Prognosis and Outcomes

Successful treatment of neonatal intestinal obstruction requires rapid identification, resuscitation, and definitive management. In addition to the technical skill required to bypass the obstruction caused by aberrant pancreatic tissue, appropriate perioperative care is required to ensure a successful outcome after surgery. Surgical treatment of annular pancreas has an excellent prognosis,[7] as long as there is sufficient appropriate perioperative and postoperative care. This includes appropriately trained anaesthetic staff, ventilatory support, and the facility for parenteral nutrition.[8]

Ultimately, and despite appropriate surgical intervention to relieve duodenal obstruction if present, the outcome may be affected by the presence of severe associated congenital abnormalities.

Prevention

With the improvement in prenatal diagnosis—in particular, the identification of specific markers for annular pancreas—detection of this congenital abnormality can be optimised. Although it cannot be prevented, earlier identification of complications—in particular, intestinal obstruction—will help to ensure that appropriate treatment can be instigated as soon as possible.

Evidence-Based Research

Table 84.1 presents a retrospective review of cases of annular pancreas for a period of 10 years.

Table 84.1: Evidence-based research.

Title	Annular pancreas in children: a recent decade's experience
Authors	Jimenez JC, Emil S, Podnos Y, Nguyen N
Institution	Division of Pediatric Surgery, Irvine Medical Centre, Orange, California, USA; Department of Surgery, Miller Children's Hospital, Long Beach, California, USA
Reference	J Pediatr Surg 2004; 39(11):1654–1657
Problem	A 10-year review of clinical, radiological, and prognostic findings in patients with annular pancreas.
Intervention	Retrospective review of all cases of annular pancreas between 1993 and 2002
Outcome/effect	All patients required surgical intervention, and all patients survived to be discharged from hospital (mean stay, 24 days).
Historical significance/ comments	This paper highlights the rarity of this condition and its association with other congenital abnormalities. Despite the high percentage of concurrent abnormalities, all patients survived and were discharged from the hospital.

Key Summary Points

1. Annular pancreas is a rare congenital structural abnormality of the primitive foregut.

2. There is a strong association between annular pancreas and other congenital abnormalities, particularly Down syndrome.

3. The spectrum of disease that may be caused by annular pancreas is broad.

4. Diagnosis may be made prenatally with evidence of duodenal obstruction. More specific markers for prenatal detection of annular pancreas are currently under investigation.

5. A plain abdominal radiograph will show evidence of duodenal obstruction, but ultrasound or cross-sectional imaging techniques are required to specifically identify annular pancreas.

6. Urgent surgical intervention is required in cases of duodenal obstruction caused by annular pancreas. Surgery is not required to correct annular pancreas if there are no complications caused by its presence.

7. Prognosis after surgery for duodenal obstruction is good; however, overall outcome will also be affected by the severity of associated congenital anomalies.

References

1. Zyromski N, Sandoval J, Pitt H, et al. Annular pancreas: dramatic differences between children and adults. J Am Coll Surg 2008; 206:1019–1025.

2. Ohno Y, Kanematsu T. Annular pancreas causing localized recurrent pancreatitis in a child: report of a case. Surg Today 2008; 38:1052–1055.

3. Nijs E, Callahan M, Taylor G. Disorders of the pediatric pancreas: imaging features. Pediatr Radiol 2005; 35:358–373.

4. Dankovcik R, Jirasek J, Kucera E, Feyereisl J, Radonak J, Dudas M. Prenatal diagnosis of annular pancreas: reliability of the double bubble sign with periduodenal hyperechogenic band. Fetal Diagn Ther 2008; 24:483–490.

5. Lohr C, Emch T, Patton H, et al. Annular pancreas. Applied Radiology 2007; 36(4).

6. McCollum M, Jamieson D, Webber E. Annular pancreas and duodenal stenosis. J Pediatr Surg. 2002; 37:1776–1777.

7. Jimenez JC, Emil S, Podnos Y, Nguyen N. Annular pancreas in children: a recent decade's experience. J Pediatr Surg 2004; 39:1654–1657.

8. Chirdan L, Uba A, Pam S. Intestinal atresia: management problems in a developing country. Pediatr Surg Int 2004; 20:834–837.

CHAPTER 85
PANCREATITIS

Ashley Ridout
Kokila Lakhoo

Introduction

Pancreatitis is defined as inflammation of the pancreas (Figure 85.1). It is a rare, but significant, cause of disease in children. This relative rarity in childhood, compared to that in adulthood, may have previously resulted in the underestimation of its significance, and, indeed, to underestimation and underreporting of its true incidence.

The disease is divided into acute and chronic pancreatitis, conditions that show contrasting patterns of aetiology, clinical presentation, and outcome. Acute pancreatitis is defined as sudden, reversible inflammation of the pancreas. Chronic pancreatitis is the irreversible result of persistent inflammation and is associated with destruction and infiltration of normal pancreatic tissues.

Despite its relative rarity, pancreatitis continues to cause significant morbidity and mortality throughout the world. Prognosis is variable, according to the severity of the disease, but episodes of acute pancreatitis in children are usually mild and associated with a good prognosis. Research continues into the precise pathogenesis of this disease. However, it is most important that this condition be considered and excluded when appropriate.

Demographics

The incidence of both acute and chronic pancreatitis in childhood is low. Recent studies have reported the incidence of acute pancreatitis as approximately 1 in 50,000 in the United States.[1] An apparent increase in incidence over the past few decades may reflect either a true increase in disease prevalence or increased awareness and diagnosis of the disease.

Aetiology/Pathophysiology

The aetiology of pancreatitis in childhood is diverse. There is a definite contrast between the most common causes of pancreatitis in adults (namely, gallstones, alcohol, and—increasingly —hypertriglyceridaemia) and the causes of pancreatitis in children.

Acute Pancreatitis

Two of the most common causes of acute pancreatitis in children are blunt abdominal trauma and multisystem disease.[2] Other causes include drugs and toxins (including alcohol), infections, idiopathic causes, and congenital abnormalities. It has previously been reported that acute pancreatitis diagnosed in children under the age of 3 years is always associated with a concurrent systemic disease process.[3] In cases of trauma, it is important to also consider nonaccidental injury. Goh et al.[4] reported 12 cases of acute pancreatitis seen in their institution over a 4-year period. Two of the 5 cases attributable to trauma were a result of nonaccidental injury.[4]

More than 85 drugs have been reported to cause acute pancreatitis.[5] Important examples include the nucleoside analogues didanosine (up to 23% of cases[5]) and zalcitabine, used in the treatment of human immunodeficiency virus (HIV); cytotoxic drugs, such as L-asparaginase; and immunosuppressive drugs, such as azathioprine and mercaptopurine (3–5% of cases[5]). Other drugs associated with acute pancreatitis include analgesics (paracetamol, salicylates); thiazides; sodium valproate; corticosteroids; and antibiotics (tetracyclines and erythromycin).

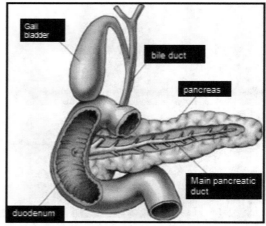

Figure 85.1: Normal anatomy of the pancreas.

A wide variety of infections (bacterial, viral, and parasitic) also have been associated with acute pancreatitis. These include mycoplasma, Epstein-Barr virus (EBV), cytomegalovirus (CMV), influenza A, mumps, measles, rubella, malaria, ascariasis, cryptosporidium, and leptospirosis. Multisystem diseases implicated with acute pancreatitis include systemic lupus erythematosus (SLE), Henoch-Schönlein purpura (HSP), Kawasaki disease, Reye's syndrome, and haemolytic-uraemic syndrome.

Congenital abnormalities of the pancreas, biliary tree, or alimentary system (including pancreas divisum, annular pancreas, pancreatic duct obstruction, choledochal cysts, and enteric duplication cysts) lead to periampullary obstruction and therefore may contribute to the development of acute pancreatitis.[6]

The process of inflammation within the pancreas involves both pancreatic acinar cell injury and premature conversion of trypsinogen to trypsin in the pancreas. This proenzyme is normally activated in the duodenum by enterokinase or trypsin. However, autodigestion and pancreatic cell damage will occur if autoactivation takes place within the pancreas. Pancreatic trypsinogen is stored in close association with other proenzymes, and its untimely activation may result in an uncontrolled production of other digestive enzymes.[2]

Chronic Pancreatitis

Chronic pancreatitis is more commonly seen in adults, particularly those with a history of alcohol misuse. However, this disease also occurs in childhood, and one of the most common causes of chronic pancreatitis in children—tropical calcific pancreatitis—occurs in the developing world. This is also known as tropical pancreatitis, juvenile tropical pancreatitis syndrome, tropical calculous pancreatopathy, or nutritional pancreatitis.[7] Other causes of chronic pancreatitis include cystic fibrosis, fibrosing pancreatitis, hereditary chronic pancreatitis, and inborn errors of metabolism.

Several hypotheses have been proposed to explain the pathophysiology of chronic pancreatitis. The necrosis-fibrosis hypothesis[8] suggests that repeated episodes of acute inflammation lead to fibrosis of pancreatic tissues. Another theory suggests that a single, severe, pathological incident is the critical factor for development of chronic pancreatitis. This event is significant enough to result in attraction of monocytes and subsequent infiltration, differentiation, and proliferation of pancreatic stellate cells.[9] Fibrosis is associated with chemokine and cytokine release, caused by recurrent cell injury.

Furthermore, work is currently under way to investigate the role of genetic mutations in the development of chronic pancreatitis. Mutations in the cationic trypsinogen gene, cystic fibrosis transmembrane conductance regulator (CFTR), and serine protease inhibitor Kazal type 1 (SPINK1) are all currently under investigation.[2]

The most common mutations in the cationic trypsinogen gene are mutations R122H and N291. These cause hereditary pancreatitis, and most patients develop chronic pancreatitis within 10 years of the onset of the initial disease. Both CFTR and SPINK1 mutations act in combination with other mutations and environmental factors to predispose individuals to development of pancreatitis. There are more than 1200 known mutations in the CFTR gene, which encodes a protein found in the apical membrane of pancreatic duct cells. This gives rise to a spectrum of disease from mild to severe, and a number of different mutation combinations predispose to development of pancreatitis. The SPINK1 mutation predisposes to idiopathic chronic pancreatitis. Ninety percent of individuals with this mutation will develop pancreatitis before the age of 20 years.[2] This mutation is thought to increase susceptibility to recurrent acute and chronic pancreatitis, especially in patients with multiple genetic mutations and exposure to environmental risk factors.[6]

Clinical Presentation

The diagnosis of pancreatitis relies upon clinical suspicion, laboratory results, and radiographic evidence. However, in the initial stages of the disease, the clinical presentation may provide important clues as to the nature of the disease. Correct interpretation of relevant features in the history and clinical findings will allow more rapid diagnosis and instigation of resuscitation and therapeutic measures.

History

There may be great variety in clinical presentation. If able, the patient with acute pancreatitis may describe increasingly severe abdominal pain (usually, but not exclusively, in the epigastrium and upper abdomen) of either sudden or gradual onset. This may radiate to the left or right upper quadrants, and is exacerbated by foods (particularly high-fat foods) and movement. Classically, in adults the pain radiates to the back; however, this is rare in children, and has not been reported in 60–90% of childhood cases.[10,11] There is often a history of nausea and vomiting. Behavioural clues may include the child who lays very still, or who positions himself on hands and knees to relieve pain.[6]

The patient with chronic pancreatitis may describe a severe, constant, epigastric pain, radiating to the back. This may be relieved by sitting forward and worsened by eating. The pain is often associated with nausea and vomiting. As the disease progresses, pain may decrease. The patient may also describe greasy, bulky stools and weight loss. With loss of pancreatic endocrine function, patients develop diabetes, which is notoriously difficult to control.

Physical Examination

At acute presentation, patients may be dehydrated, and there may be an element of systemic upset with tachycardia, hypotension, and pyrexia. Severe cases with respiratory compromise may show reduced oxygen saturations. The abdomen may be distended, and there may be abdominal tenderness (particularly in the upper abdomen) and guarding. There may also be rebound tenderness, and bowel sounds may be reduced.

Patients with chronic pancreatitis may show evidence of other multisystem or genetic diseases, such as cystic fibrosis.

Investigations

Simple laboratory investigations can help in the diagnosis of acute pancreatitis:

- Serum amylase levels increase within 12 hours of onset of inflammation, and this elevation may persist for up to 5 days.[6] Prolonged elevation may suggest the presence of a pancreatic pseudocyst or other complication.

- Elevation of serum lipase also indicates acute pancreatitis.

Serum levels may remain elevated for longer than serum amylase. It is considered diagnostic when levels of amylase or lipase are raised three times above normal; however, these markers are not specific. In addition, the destruction of pancreatic tissue in chronic pancreatitis may result in a normal amylase level despite the presence of disease. In children, serum amylase is less sensitive and specific for pancreatitis than it is in adults. In one study, 40% of children with proven pancreatitis had a normal serum amylase.[12] Indeed, many other conditions may cause a raised serum amylase, including appendicitis, intestinal obstruction, disorders of the salivary glands, and renal failure.[6] If possible, it may also be helpful to determine the specific isoenzyme of amylase that is present in order to precisely identify its source.

Patients may also develop hypocalcaemia or hyperglycaemia, occasionally severe and symptomatic.

Imaging

Imaging is important in pancreatitis for initial diagnosis, identification of complications, and subsequent follow-up.

Plain Film Radiography

Abdominal x-ray (AXR; see Figure 85.2) may show a sentinel loop (single dilated loop of bowel), dilated loops of duodenum, or loss of the psoas muscle shadow. In up to 20% of cases, chest x-ray (CXR) may show unilateral or bilateral pleural effusions.[13]

Ultrasonography

Ultrasonography (US) is an inexpensive and often readily available imaging modality that may be useful in establishing the diagnosis of pancreatitis without exposing the child to ionising radiation. It also allows evaluation of other abdominal organs in a patient who presents with acute abdominal pain of unknown aetiology. US imaging may be extremely useful in combination with clinical examination and simple laboratory tests. In the case of pancreatitis, the pancreas may be enlarged and oedematous, with altered echogenicity. There may be biliary sludge, gallstones, or dilated common bile duct or intrahepatic ducts, suggesting an obstructive cause.[2] The presence of calcification may suggest chronic pancreatitis. US may also reveal structural abnormalities, such as pancreas divisum, annular pancreas, or a choledochal cyst.

Computed Tomography

Computed tomography (CT) scans can be useful in both confirmation of the diagnosis of pancreatitis and identification of subsequent complications. In addition, it can exclude other serious intraabdominal causes of pain that may be confused with pancreatitis, including damage caused by trauma and mesenteric infarction. In acute pancreatitis (Figure 85.3), the pancreas may be enlarged, with decreased echogenicity. Chronic pancreatitis shows calcification (see Figure 85.4).

Endoscopic Retrograde Cholangiopancreatography

Although rarely used during an acute episode of pancreatitis, endoscopic retrograde cholangiopancreatography (ERCP) may identify structural causes of recurrent pancreatitis and allow for therapeutic intervention at the time of diagnosis.

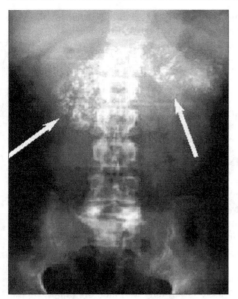

Figure 8.2: Abdominal x-ray showing pancreatic calcification.

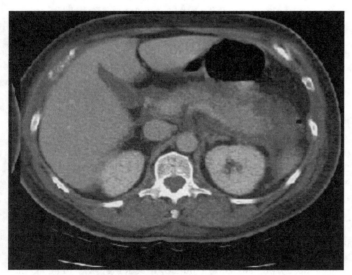

Figure 85.3: CT scan showing acute pancreatitis.

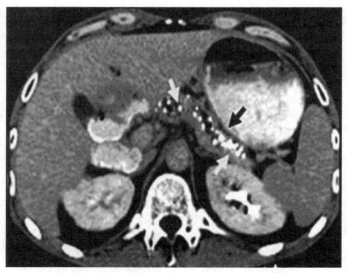

Figure 85.4: CT scan showing chronic pancreatitis with calcification (arrows).

Magnetic Resonance Cholangiopancreatography

Magnetic resonance cholangiopancreatography (MRCP) provides detailed imaging of the biliary tract without the need for an invasive procedure or exposure to ionising radiation. MRCP is frequently carried out in adults and has great potential for use in children.

Management

Acute Pancreatitis

Initially, management of acute pancreatitis must be supportive and symptomatic. This disease is commonly divided into mild and severe forms. Close monitoring is essential, as patients may deteriorate rapidly. This includes a strict fluid balance—patients may require considerable fluid resuscitation to counteract fluid losses into the "third space". Adequate analgesia is also essential. If the patient is vomiting, insertion of a nasogastric tube may increase patient comfort and significantly reduce the risk of such complications as aspiration.

In addition to these measures, resting the gut by making the patient nil by mouth for several days may promote recovery in mild cases of acute pancreatitis. These patients will require appropriate fluid management, with maintenance fluids in addition to resuscitation fluids. If recovery is prolonged, patients may require parenteral or jejunal nutrition. Unless pancreatic infection is suspected, it is not necessary to administer antibiotics.

In severe cases, patients may require much more intensive management, including high-dependency or intensive care.

Surgical intervention is required only in cases of acute pancreatitis that have become complicated by pancreatic necrosis. These cases require debridement of the necrotic tissue in an attempt to prevent secondary infection.

Chronic Pancreatitis

The management of chronic pancreatitis, once initial resuscitation and appropriate analgesia have been implemented, must focus on determining the aetiology and monitoring the disease consequences and complications. Pathological conditions, such as cystic fibrosis, other genetic mutations, and autoimmune diseases, must be excluded with genetic testing, if appropriate. Pancreatic imaging must be used to exclude structural abnormalities.

There may be functional implications of chronic pancreatitis. When pancreatic cell damage is sufficiently extensive, there will be a loss of endocrine (leading to diabetes mellitus) and exocrine (resulting in malabsorption) functions. These patients must be installed in a programme of follow-up, and they or their caregivers must receive appropriate education about their disease and its consequences.

Surgical intervention is usually indicated in chronic pancreatitis only for the relief of severe, persistent pain. These procedures aim to improve drainage of the pancreatic ducts and may also prevent disease recurrence in children.[1] This may be approached either endoscopically, with stent placement, or at open operations, such as lateral pancreaticojejunostomy.

Severity Scoring

In adults, a number of different scoring systems are used to assess the severity of acute pancreatitis. These scores are not absolutely transferable to children, but one group has compared a scoring system designed specifically to paediatric patients with these adult scoring systems.[14] This system compares eight variables to predict severe outcome and mortality during an episode of acute pancreatitis, and has been shown to have greater sensitivity and negative predictive value compared to the Ranson and Glasgow scoring systems. The factors considered were age (<7 years), weight (23 kg), admission white blood cell count (>18.5 × 10^9/L), admission LDH (>2000 IU/L), 48-hour trough albumin, 48-hour fluid sequestration, and 48-hour rise in blood urea nitrogen. Each factor is allocated a score of 1 point, and higher total scores are associated with an increased chance of severe pancreatitis and mortality. Scores of

5–7 points showed 80% severe outcome and 10% mortality; 2–4 points showed 38.5% severe outcome and 5.8% mortality; and 0–2 points showed 8.6% severe outcome and 1.4% mortality.

Complications

It is very important that patients be monitored for signs of complications of pancreatitis. Pancreatic imaging must be considered in patients whose symptoms do not improve or get worse.

Acute Pancreatitis

Most reports of acute pancreatitis suggest that the disease is mild and has a good prognosis. Goh et al.[4] reported that of a group of 12 patients, 5 had radiological evidence of pseudocyst formation (4 of which had acute pancreatitis attributed to trauma). This is in agreement with other reports that suggest that pancreatic pseudocyst development occurs most commonly in children who have trauma-induced pancreatitis.

In children, pseudocysts do not usually require surgical intervention and often resolve spontaneously. In the study by Goh et al.,[4] 2 patients developed pleural effusion, one of whom also developed pulmonary consolidation and coagulopathy, requiring administration of fresh frozen plasma. Pancreatic necrosis is rare in children; however, there have been reports of severe, haemorrhagic necrotic pancreatitis associated with very poor prognosis.

Recurrent episodes of acute pancreatitis may result in chronic pancreatitis, which has considerable implications for long-term morbidity and mortality.

Chronic Pancreatitis

Both local and systemic complications occur in chronic pancreatitis (Figure 85.5). Local complications include pseudocyst formation, splenic vein thrombosis, pseudoaneurysm, duodenal or common bile duct obstruction, pancreatic fistula, and the long-term complication of pancreatic adenocarcinoma.[6] Systemic complications, as previously mentioned, include malabsorption and development of diabetes mellitus.

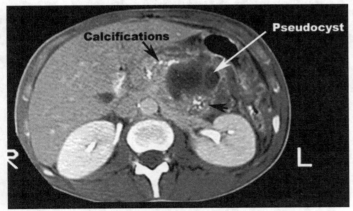

Figure 85.5: CT scan showing chronic pancreatitis with complications.

Prognosis and Outcomes

Acute Pancreatitis

In uncomplicated episodes of acute pancreatitis, prognosis is very good and symptoms may settle within days. However, the prognosis varies considerably between mild and severe forms. Mortality in mild disease is approximately 10%, compared with up to 90% in severe necrotizing or haemorrhagic disease. It has been shown that recurrent acute pancreatitis occurs in up to 10% of children after an episode of acute pancreatitis. This is more likely to occur in children with other predisposing risk factors, however.[14]

Chronic Pancreatitis

The systemic implications of chronic pancreatitis may have a significant impact upon the patient. The effects of irreversible loss of exocrine and endocrine pancreatic function may result in considerable morbidity. It has been shown that chronic pancreatitis is a risk factor for pancreatic adenocarcinoma, and a cohort study of patients with hereditary pancreatitis has reported an estimated cumulative risk of pancreatic cancer in these patients of 40% up to age 70.[15]

Prevention

As the onset of pancreatitis cannot be prevented, it is vital that this condition be considered in all children with acute abdominal pain and vomiting, especially those who may be at higher risk of the disease. These children include those who have known congenital abnormalities of the pancreas, are taking relevant medications, and have a known congenital abnormality of the pancreas or predisposing genetic condition. Early diagnosis, close monitoring, and appropriate follow-up will help to ensure a favourable outcome.

Evidence-Based Research

Table 85.1 presents a retrospective review of children with acute pancreatitis in a 4-year period.

Figure 85.1: Evidence-based research.

Title	Childhood acute pancreatitis in a children's hospital
Authors	Goh S-K, Chui C, Jacobsen A
Institution	KK Women's and Children's Hospital, Singapore
Reference	Singapore Med J 2003; 44(9):453–456
Problem	Review of all cases of acute pancreatitis, including clinical and radiological findings and outcome.
Intervention	Retrospective review of patients presenting with acute pancreatitis between 1998 and 2002.
Comparison/control (quality of evidence)	Twelve cases were identified as having acute pancreatitis. Most presented with abdominal pain (n = 11) and vomiting (n = 7). The most common aetiological cause was trauma (n = 5).
Outcome/effect	There was no mortality. Recurrence occurred in two patients, and one patient required surgical intervention. Mean hospital stay was 12.41 ± 4.54 days.
Historical significance/comments	This paper describes the rarity of acute pancreatitis, but highlights its clinical significance and excellent prognosis.

Key Summary Points

1. Pancreatitis (inflammation of the pancreas) is a rare but clinically significant cause of disease in children. It must be considered in all children presenting with abdominal pain and vomiting.

2. Acute pancreatitis is sudden, reversible inflammation of the pancreas.

3. Chronic pancreatitis is the irreversible result of persistent inflammation and is associated with destruction and infiltration of normal pancreatic tissues.

4. There is a broad spectrum of aetiology of pancreatitis; the aetiology is different in children and adults.

5. Imaging is important for initial diagnosis, identification of complications, and follow-up.

6. The management of acute pancreatitis is mainly supportive and symptomatic.

7. The management of chronic pancreatitis includes identification of causative factors, including cystic fibrosis, other genetic mutations, and autoimmune disease.

8. Episodes of acute pancreatitis are usually mild and associated with good prognosis. Complications such as pancreatic necrosis, however, are associated with high mortality (up to 90%).

9. Early diagnosis, close monitoring, and appropriate follow-up all contribute to a good prognosis.

References

1. Clifton MS, Pelayo JC, Cortes RA, et al. Surgical treatment of childhood recurrent pancreatitis. J Pediatr Surg 2007; 42:1203–1207.

2. Lowe ME. Pancreatitis in childhood. Curr Gastroenterol Rep 2004; 6:240–246.

3. Lopez MJ. The changing incidence of acute pancreatitis in children: a 10-year experience in Melbourne. J Pediatr Gastroenterol Nutr 2004; 39(Suppl.1): S167.

4. Goh S-K, Chui C, Jacobsen A. Childhood acute pancreatitis in a children's hospital. Singapore Med J 2003; 44(9):453–456.

5. Weizman Z. Acute pancreatitis in childhood: Research of pathogenesis and clinical implications. Can J Gastroenterol 1997; 11:249–253.

6. Nydegger A, Couper R, Oliver R. Childhood pancreatitis. J Gastroenterol Hepatol 2006; 21:499–509.

7. Kleinman R, Goulet O-J, Mieli-Vergani G, Sanderson I, Sherman P, Shneider B. Walker's Pediatric Gastrointestinal Disease, 5th ed. BC Decker, 2008.

8. Comfort MW, Gambrill EE, Baggenstoss AH. Chronic relapsing pancreatitis. A study of twenty-nine cases without associated disease of the biliary or gastro-intestinal tract. Gastroenterology 1968; 54(Suppl.):760–765.

9. Whitcomb DC. Hereditary pancreatitis: new insights into acute and chronic pancreatitis. Gut 1999; 45:317–322.

10. Haddock G, Coupar G, Youngson GG, MacKinlay GA, Raine PA. Acute pancreatitis in children: a 15-year review. J Pediatr Surg 1994; 29:719–722.

11. Weizman Z, Durie PR. Acute pancreatitis in childhood. J Pediatr 1988; 113(1 Part 1):24–29.

12. Cox KL, Ament ME, Sample WF, Sarti DA, O'Donnell M, Byrne WJ. The ultrasonic and biochemical diagnosis of pancreatitis in children. J Pediatr 1980; 96(3 Part 1):407–411.

13. Uretsky G, Goldschmiedt M, James K. Childhood pancreatitis. Am Fam Physician 1999; 59(9):2507–2512.

14. DeBanto JR, Goday PS, Pedroso MR, et al. Acute pancreatitis in children. Am J Gastroenterol 2002; 97:1726–1731.

15. Lowenfels AB, Maisonneuve P, DiMagno EP, Elisur Y, Gates LK Jr, Perrault J, et al. Hereditary pancreatitis and the risk of pancreatic cancer. J Natl Cancer Inst 1997; 89:442–446.

CHAPTER 86
SPLEEN

Johanna R. Askegard-Giesmann
Bankole S. Rouma
Brian D. Kenney

Introduction

The spleen, once thought to be a nonessential organ, has important functions in bacterial clearance, antibody formation, phagocystosis, and haematopoiesis. Aside from trauma, surgical intervention is mainly limited to haematologic diseases that affect the function of the spleen.

Demographics

The most common functional disease of the spleen is found in sickle cell disease and thalassaemic children in Africa. Splenomegaly is present in 21% of sickle cell disease patients in Nigeria.[1] Lebanese sickle cell disease children have a high prevalence (28.9%) of persistent splenomegaly.[2]

Aetiology/Pathophysiology

The spleen develops alongside the pancreas from mesenchyme of the dorsal pancreatic bud and the dorsal mesogastrium. The splenic primordium is first recognised at the 8–10 mm stage as a mesenchymal bulge in the left dorsal mesogastrium between the stomach and pancreas. By the fourth month of foetal life, the spleen produces both red and white cells, and it functions as a site of extramedullary haematopoiesis until approximately 1–2 months of age. This function gradually declines, as the spleen is rarely the site of clinically significant haematopoiesis in childhood.[3,4]

Anatomy and Function

Blood enters the spleen through segmental arteries that originate from the splenic artery and branch into trabecular arteries that eventually enter the white pulp. The white pulp consists of lymphocytes and macrophages arranged in germinal centers around a central artery. The white pulp is thought to function as an immune screening area that processes foreign antigen and antigen-antibody complexes. Approximately 20% of splenic volume is white pulp, with the remainder contributing to red pulp. The red pulp acts as a phagocytic filtration system that digests defective blood elements, foreign material, and bacteria. Encapsulated bacteria can be removed from the bloodstream by the spleen because of its variable antigenicity. The spleen functions in red blood cell maintenance, immune function, and as a reservoir.[3,4]

The spleen destroys red blood cells at the end of their life-span and repairs other damaged red cells. It selectively removes abnormal cells, such as spherocytes. As blood passes through the spleen, cellular and nuclear inclusion bodies are removed (i.e., Howell-Jolly bodies, Heinz bodies, and Pappenheimer bodies). After splenectomy, these inclusion bodies can be noted on peripheral blood smears.

The spleen's primary immune function is related to antigen processing of T cells. It also performs nonspecific immune functions by removing particulate matter from the bloodstream, primarily via macrophages. The spleen contains opsonins, which further activate the complement system and facilitate the destruction of organisms. The spleen functions as a biologic filter, which can assist in the clearance of bacteria. The spleen is a significant reservoir for platelets and factor VIII in the human body. The proportion of platelets within the spleen increases with splenomegaly and can occasionally lead to thrombocytopaenia.

Clinical Presentation

Aside from infections, injury, and trauma, splenic disorders can be classified into anatomic and functional abnormalities. Anatomic abnormalities are rarely the cause for surgical intervention, but may be associated with other surgical problems. Consequently, it is important for the paediatric surgeon to be aware of these conditions.

Congenital asplenia is usually associated with congenital heart disease, bilateral "right-sidedness" with bilateral three-lobed lungs, right-sided stomach, and a central liver. Patients with these disorders may have intestinal malrotation and are prone to overwhelming infections. Polysplenia, in which the spleen is divided into multiple splenic masses, may be associated with biliary atresia, preduodenal portal vein, situs inversus, cardiac defects, and malrotation.

Accessory Spleen

Accessory spleen is the most common anatomic abnormality, occurring in 13–30% of all children. Of those patients with accessory spleens, 80% have one, 11% have two, and 3% have three or more accessory spleens.[3,5,6] Nearly 75% of accessory spleens are located near the splenic hilum; the next location in terms of percentages is by the tail of the pancreas. Accessory spleens may also occur along the splenic artery, omentum, mesentery and retroperitoneum. When performing a splenectomy, it is important to routinely examine for accessory spleens because, if missed, they can account for recurrence of idiopathic thrombocytopaenic purpura (ITP) or hereditary spherocytosis.

Wandering Spleen

Wandering spleen is an anatomic abnormality characterised by the lack of ligamentous attachments to the diaphragm, colon, and retroperitoneum. The problem is related to a failure of development of the ligaments from the spleen to the dorsal mesentery. Children may present with episodic pain and abdominal mass from torsion and infarction of the spleen. Splenopexy is the preferred treatment; however, patients may require splenectomy for infarction. Among the variety of techniques of splenopexy are an extraperitoneal pocket, absorbable mesh bag or basket, or suture splenopexy. Laparoscopic techniques have also been described.

Splenogonadal Fusion

During embryologic development, early fusion between the spleen and the left gonad can occur, causing what is known as splenogonadal fusion. This developmental abnormality is often found with limb or anorectal abnormalities, indicative of some sort of embryonic event occurring between weeks 5 and 8 of development. Three types of fusion have been described: continuous, discontinuous, and combined. In the first type, a continuous cord consisting of splenic or fibrous tissue connects the spleen to the left gonad, typically originating from the upper pole of the spleen. The discontinuous type is characterised by ectopic splenic tissue fused to the left gonadal mesonephric structures, which are discrete from the spleen itself. The combined form is characterised by an extension of functioning splenic tissue without any actual connection to gonadal tissue. Male patients with this disorder may have an undescended testicle or may be presumed to have an inguinal hernia.

Splenic tissue may be mistaken for a tumour attached to the testicle and in most cases may be safely dissected off the testicle, thereby avoiding an unnecessary orchiectomy.

Splenic Cysts

Benign splenic cysts are rare. When they are asymptomatic, they are typically found incidentally during imaging for another reason. Splenic cysts can be classified by appearance as uni- or multilocular, or by origin: congenital, infectious (parasitic), or posttraumatic. Congenital cysts are typically unilocular with a squamous (epithelial) or endothelial cell lining filled with clear fluid. Infectious cysts are typically parasitic, originating from echinococcus (hytadid cysts). Echinoccocal cysts should be handled carefully during removal, and total splenectomy may be necessary in order to prevent rupture of the cyst. Posttraumatic cysts result from a resolving haematoma. Liquefaction of the haematoma forms a pseudocyst with a fibrous lining. Treatment for congenital or posttraumatic cysts is indicated only if they become symptomatic, which usually occurs at a size greater than 8 cm. Patients may present with pain, rupture, abscess of a previously uninfected cyst, or gastric compression. Treatment may consist of percutaneous drainage or sclerosis of the cyst cavity, but both congenital and posttraumatic cysts have a high rate of recurrence. Partial or total splenectomy may be necessary for primary treatment, or in treatment of recurrent symptomatic cysts.

Splenic Abscess

Splenic abscess is a rare occurrence in children, and usually is a result of secondarily infected haematoma, congenital or posttraumatic cysts, or an area of infarct. Patients with splenic abscess typically present with bacteraemia, fever, and left upper quadrant pleuritic pain, and they may be toxic. A computed tomography (CT) scan is usually diagnostic, and ultrasound may be useful as well. Unilocular abscesses can be drained percutaneously and combined with antibiotic therapy. Multilocular abscesses may respond to antibiotics alone. Patients with hemoglobinopathy and splenic infarct typically have infection with *Salmonella* species. Staphylococcus and streptococcus are more common in posttraumatic infections. Fungal infection may occur in immunosuppressed patients who have negative blood cultures. Empiric antibiotics should be started as soon as the diagnosis is suspected and can be tailored to blood culture and abscess drainage cultures as the results become available.

Hyperactive Malarial Splenomegaly

Hyperactive malarial splenomegaly (HMS) is thought to represent an immunological dysfunction of the spleen due to recurrent episodes of malaria. Specific criteria for the diagnosis are gross splenomegaly, high levels of antimalarial antibodies, IgM in serum at least two standard deviations above the local mean, and clinical and immunological response to antimalarial treatment. Detection of circulating malaria parasites by polymerase chain reaction (PCR) may represent a useful diagnostic tool.[7] In hospitals that do not have access to these laboratory tests, the diagnosis is made by exclusion or response to treatment.

Functional Abnormalities

Abnormalities in splenic function can be categorised broadly as hypersplenism or hyposplenism. Hypersplenism refers to the inappropriate sequestration of blood elements within the spleen and may be a primary or secondary occurrence. Primary hypersplenism is generally caused by hereditary spherocytosis, elliptocytosis, and idiopathic thrombocytopenic purpura. Secondary hypersplenism is most commonly caused by portal hypertension, but any cause of splenomegaly can result in hypersplenism. Treatment of secondary hypersplenism may consist of splenic artery embolisation or ligation, although if these options are not available, splenectomy may be necessary.

Hyposplenism occurs with splenectomy or sickle cell disease with splenic infarcts and eventual involution, and it has also been seen with ulcerative colitis. These patients are at risk of infection by encapsulated organisms. Hyposplenism may be detected by Howell-Jolly bodies

present in erythrocytes on peripheral blood smear, and patients may present with overwhelming sepsis. Early treatment with broad-spectrum antibiotics is essential in the face of sepsis if this diagnosis is suspected.

Hereditary Spherocytosis

Hereditary spherocytosis is an autosomal dominant hereditary disorder that is thought to be due to a spectrin deficiency. Spectrin is a cytoskeletal protein. The erythrocytes take on an abnormal spherical shape, have decreased cell wall flexibility, and are prematurely sequestered in the spleen. Index cases in a family may present with anaemia, jaundice, and splenomegaly; indirect hyperbilirubinaemia may occur in infants. The estimated incidence of spherocytosis in Algiers was reported as 1 in 1,000, with approximately the same features among Algerians as in people of European heritage.[8] It is very rare in sub-Saharan Africans and African Americans, with few literature reports.[9,10]

Diagnosis is made by demonstrating increased osmotic fragility of erythrocytes. Patients should also undergo a Coombs' test to rule out other immune causes of haemolytic anaemia. An aplastic crisis can occur in affected children from a parvovirus B19 infection, which results in suppression of erythrocyte production and severe anaemia due to ongoing erythrocyte destruction. Splenectomy is generally recommended for moderate to severe anaemia. Pigmented gallstones are a common occurrence in patients with hemolysis, so a preoperative ultrasound should be performed so that a concomitant cholecystectomy can be planned, if necessary. Hereditary elliptocytosis is a similar disorder, but most patients are asymptomatic and rarely require splenectomy.

Idiopathic Thrombocytopaenic Purpura

ITP is an autoimmune disorder of unknown aetiology. Antiplatelet autoantibodies, typically IgG, bind to platelet-associated antigens and cause destruction of platelets via phagocytosis within the spleen. Acute ITP occurs most commonly in children younger than 10 years of age after an acute viral illness. Symptoms are related to the severe thrombocytopaenia that results. The majority of patients have an acute form of ITP, which can generally be treated conservatively with restricted activity, corticosteroids, and intravenous immunoglobulin (IVIG). Medical treatment is indicated for platelet counts below 40,000/mm^3 or in older children with a higher risk of intracranial haemorrhage. Ten to twenty percent of patients with acute ITP will have persistence of their symptoms for more than 6 months, which is considered to represent chronic ITP. For patients who fail medical therapy, splenectomy may be an option, but failure to respond to either steroids or IVIG is also associated with a 70% chance of failure rate with splenectomy.[3,11] ITP in children is usually a self-limited disorder, and splenectomy should be considered only for chronic cases.

Sickle Cell Disease

Sickle cell disease occurs when valine is substituted for glutamic acid on the β-chain of hemoglobin A, resulting in hemoglobin S. The red cells are prone to become rigid and sickle in a hypoxic and acidic environment, such as in the spleen. The sickled cells block capillaries and can cause infarction distal to the obstruction, which can result in painful crises and, with regard to the spleen, areas of infarction. The spleen initially becomes large; then, with progressive infarction, slowly atrophies and produces a functional autosplenectomy. Persistent gross splenomegaly is found in patients with anaemic crises.[12] Acute splenic sequestration crisis (ASSC) can occur and is the most common indication for splenectomy. Classic presentation of patients with ASSC is a rapidly enlarging spleen with severe anaemia or hypotension and associated hypersplenism and thrombocytopaenia.[1] ASSC may be so severe that it causes circulatory collapse; it carries a high mortality rate.

Thalassaemia

Thalassaemia is a group of haemoglobinopathies related to abnormal production of α or β chains of haemoglobin that may be classified as of major (homozygous), minor (heterozygous), or intermediate form. Significant erythrocyte sequestration may occur within the spleen, and splenectomy has been utilised in an attempt to decrease transfusion requirements. Partial splenectomy may have benefit to these patients because postsplenectomy sepsis occurs in approximately 10% of these patients who have undergone total splenectomy.

Leukaemia and Lymphomas
The spleen is often involved in both leukaemia and lymphoma, and may lead to splenomegaly without hypersplenism. Splenectomy is typically not indicated in these patients and plays no therapeutic role. In chronic myelogenous leukaemia, patients may have pain, mass-related symptoms, and secondary hypersplenism, and splenectomy may be performed for palliation of symptoms. In acute myelogenous leukaemia (AML) and acute lymphocytic leukaemia (ALL), the degree of splenomegaly is much less. In these cases, splenectomy is rarely of benefit and may be detrimental in those in which the spleen has become an important site of extramedullary haematopoiesis.

Gaucher's Disease
Gaucher's disease is an autosomal recessive metabolic disorder caused by a deficiency of the enzyme β-glucocerebrosidase, which causes the body to accumulate glucosylceramide in the macrophages of the spleen, liver, lungs, and bone marrow. Patients may have massive splenomegaly that may cause hypersplenism. Splenectomy has been performed in these patients to improve erythrocyte, leukocyte, and platelet counts and to alleviate the hypersplenism. Partial splenectomy may help improve symptoms temporarily, but recurrence seems to be the rule.

Splenosis
Splenic trauma may result in fragmentation of the spleen with subsequent growth of splenic tissue within the abdominal cavity. This event is called splenosis. The splenic implants do not function in the same capacity as the entire spleen would, and specifically they do not clear encapsulated organisms. Consequently, patients with splenosis should be treated with immunisations and antibiotics as if they were asplenic.

Investigations
The spleen and splenic disorders can be visualised with many different imaging modalities. Ultrasound is often the easiest and safest way to visualise the spleen and can be useful for initial evaluation of abdominal masses. Cysts are well visualised with ultrasound. Splenic trauma, lacerations, or haematomas are not reliably diagnosed with ultrasound, and CT may be necessary. With limited resources, ultrasound would likely be the most beneficial imaging study for the paediatric surgeon and can be easily done at the bedside.

Management
Nonoperative management is the treatment of choice for a child with a blunt splenic injury who is hemodynamically stable. However, in areas of Africa where CT scans are not available, surgical management with splenorrhaphy or splenectomy predominates.[13,14] When elective splenectomy is planned, patients should receive three immunisations two weeks prior to surgery to provide adequate time for immunologic response. The immunisations include *Streptococcus pneumonia*, meningococcus, and *Haemophilus influenza B*. Preoperative transfusion may be necessary in sickle cell disease to improve anaemia and to reduce the hemoglobin S level to less than 30% to avoid complications related to bleeding or heart failure.

Open Splenectomy
The operative approach to splenectomy has recently become more variable, depending on the reason for surgery and the surgeon's operative experience.

1. The traditional open splenectomy is approached with the patient in the supine or right decubitus position with a midline, transverse, or left subcostal incision.

2. The short gastric vessels are divided (often with suture ligation to avoid the potential catastrophic event of a tie slipping off with haemorrhage) and the spleen mobilised by dividing the diaphragmatic, colic, and renal attachments. In cases of severe splenomegaly, it may be necessary to open the gastrocolic ligament laterally to expose and ligate the splenic artery at the superior aspect of the pancreas in order to decrease blood loss with further mobilisation.

3. The spleen, when fully mobilised, is lifted up into the wound to allow safe division of the splenic artery and vein at the hilum. The tail of the pancreas may extend into the splenic hilum. Care should be taken when dividing the hilar vessels to avoid injury to the pancreas.

4. Once the spleen has been removed, the splenic bed is inspected for hemostasis. A nasogastric tube is often left in the stomach to provide gastric decompression in an attempt to avoid bleeding from the short gastric vessels.

5. A careful search is made for any accessory spleens, especially if the indication for surgery is hemolytic anaemia or ITP.

Laparoscopic Splenectomy
The laparoscopic approach to splenectomy began in 1991 and has become the preferred method for many institutions for elective cases. Benefits include decreased pain, shorter hospital length of stay, and improved cosmesis. There is, however, a steep learning curve with this procedure, and the procedure can be quite challenging when splenomegaly is present.

1. A lateral approach is typically used, with the patient's left side up at approximately 45°. The table is rotated to the patient's left for trocar placement, then back to the right to achieve a right lateral decubitus position. Four ports are often used: three in the midline or just off to the right (upper, mid, and umbilicus) and one in the left midabdomen. Two grasping instruments are usually used in the upper ports to provide traction and elevate the spleen.

2. The harmonic scalpel is typically used to divide the short gastric vessels and other splenic attachments.

3. The endostapler is used to ligate the hilar vessels, and the spleen is placed in an endocatch bag and removed via morselisation through the largest port site, typically in the left midabdomen.[3]

The rate of conversion to open procedure has been reported up to nearly 3% in several large series,[3] with splenomegaly and bleeding as the most common reasons. It is imperative to search for accessory spleens, especially if the indication for splenectomy is ITP or hemolytic anaemia. Studies in paediatric patients have not detected a significant difference in the detection rate of accessory spleens in either open or laparoscopic procedures.[3] Patients may recover somewhat faster with less pain after laparoscopic splenectomy, but there is a steep learning curve, and operating room time is generally longer for the laparoscopic procedure. This may not be a feasible option for hospitals with limited resources and laparoscopic capabilities.

Partial Splenectomy
The segmental blood supply of the spleen allows for partial splenectomy along the lines of demarcation that are apparent after vessel ligation. The procedure has been done both open and laparoscopically, and has been primarily used for hemolytic anaemia. It has also been used for trauma, splenic cysts, haemangiomas, and hamartomas. Approximately 25% of the normal splenic remnant is left after successful partial splenectomy. If the spleen is totally mobilised, the remnant should be fixed to adjacent structures or the retroperitoneum to prevent torsion. Patients should receive preoperative immunisations and prophylactic antibiotics postoperatively until splenic immune competence is noted.

Postoperative Complications
Postoperative complications are rare after splenectomy, but thrombosis may occur in the splenic, portal, or mesenteric veins. This should be considered in the evaluation of postsplenectomy abdominal pain. Splenosis may occur after splenectomy if spillage of splenic contents occurred during the operation. This may simulate intraabdominal tumour implants and present as small bowel obstruction, haemorrhage, or relapse of haematologic disorder.[15]

Postsplenectomy sepsis (PSS) is the most worrisome complication of splenectomy and is thought to be due to decreased immunoglobulin levels as well as decreased clearance of encapsulated organisms. The overall incidence of PSS is 4%, with a higher incidence in patients with thalassaemia (nearly 10%), and mortality approaches 50%.[4,16] Patients typically have a fulminant infection caused by encapsulated bacteria (pneumococcus, *Haemophilus influenza B*, gonococcus, and *Escherichia coli*). Empiric antibiotics should be initiated as soon as possible in a patient with fever and illness after splenectomy.

Ideally, patients should receive immunisations prior to splenectomy, and booster immunisations are recommended every 5 to 10 years. Prophylactic antibiotics are recommended for patients after splenectomy, and the duration varies from 2 years to a lifetime. The risk of PSS declines significantly after 2 years from splenectomy.[17] There have also been case reports of severe malarial infections and fatality in patients after splenectomy such that lifelong prophylaxis is recommended for patients living in endemic areas.[14]

Prevention

There are no preventive measures to take regarding this disease process. Once a decision for elective splenectomy has been made, obtaining the immunisations preoperatively would be of highest importance in terms of reducing the risk of PSS as well as the availability of prophylactic postoperative antibiotics. Preoperative transfusion may be necessary in sickle cell disease, as previously mentioned.

Ethical Issues

The availability of postoperative health care may be of paramount concern in countries with decreased health resources. This extends to the availability of immunisations as well as antibiotics. Prophylactic antibiotic use after splenectomy may be problematic when both financial and pharmaceutical resources are scarce for the patients' families and their health care providers. Patients with symptomatic splenomegaly may have to wait until the severity of their symptoms outweighs the risks associated with asplenia.

Key Summary Points

1. The spleen is an important immunologic intraabdominal organ that functions in bacterial clearance, antibody formation, and phagocytosis.

2. Surgical splenectomy is mainly limited to haematologic diseases.

3. Both open and laparoscopic approaches are feasible for splenectomy, depending on the surgeon's experience and hospital resources.

4. Preoperative transfusion may be necessary in sickle cell disease to improve anaemia and to reduce the hemoglobin S level to less than 30% to avoid complications related to bleeding or heart failure.

5. Preoperative immunisations against *Streptococcus pneumonia*, meningococcus, and *Hemophilus influenza B* are of paramount importance to help reduce the risk of postsplenectomy sepsis.

6. Prophylactic antibiotics are recommended postsplenectomy for at least 2 years, and often for a lifetime, depending on the patient's clinical condition.

7. Postsplenectomy sepsis is the most feared complication, with an overall incidence of 1–4%; the risk decreases after 2 years from splenectomy.

8. Splenectomy may predispose to severe or even fatal malaria infestation, and lifelong prophylaxis is recommended for patients living in malaria endemic areas.

References

1. Olaniyi JA, Abjah UM. Frequency of hepatomegaly and splenomegaly in Nigerian patients with sickle cell disease. West Afr J Med 2007; 26:274–277.

2. Inati A, Jradi O, Tarabay H, et al. Sickle cell disease: the Lebanese experience. Int J Lab Hematol 2007; 29:399–408.

3. Rescorla FJ. The spleen. In: Grosfeld JL, O'Neill JA Jr, Fonkalsrud EW, Coran AG (eds): Pediatric Surgery. Mosby Elsevier, 2006, Pp 1691–1701.

4. Mehta SS, Gittes GK. Lesions of the pancreas and spleen. In: Ashcraft K, Holcomb GW III, Murphy JP (eds), Pediatric Surgery. Elsevier Saunders, 2005, Pp 639–658.

5. Halpert B, Alden ZA. Accessory spleens in or at the tail of the pancreas. Arch Pathol 1964; 77:652–654.

6. Halpert B, Gyorkey F. Lesions observed in accessory spleens of 311 patients. Am J Clin Pathol 1959; 32:165–168.

7. Puente A, Rubio JM, Subirats M, et al. The use of PCR in the diagnosis of hyper-reactive malarial splenomegaly (HMS). Ann Trop Med Parasitol 2000; 94:559–563.

8. Zerhouni F, Guetarni D, Henni T, et al. Occurrence and characteristics of hereditary spherocytosis in Algeria. Eur J Haematol 1991; 47(1):42–47.

9. Olubode OA, Esan GJ, Isaac-Sodeye WA, Ukaejiofo EO. Hereditary spherocytosis in Nigeria. Niger Med J 1976; 6:44–48.

10. Hassan A, Babadoko AA, Iser AH, Abunimye P. Hereditary spherocytosis in 27-year-old woman: case report. Ann Afric Med 2009; 8(1):61–63.

11. Davis PW, Williams DA, Shamberger RC. Immune thrombocytopenia: surgical therapy and predictors of response. J Pediatr Surg 1991; 26:407–413.

12. Adeodu OO, Adekile AD. Clinical and laboratory features associated with persistent gross splenomegaly in Nigerian children with sickle cell anaemia. Acta Paediatr Scand 1990; 79:686–690.

13. Ameh EA. Management of paediatric blunt splenic injury in Zaria, Nigeria. Injury: Int J Care Injured 1999; 30:399–401.

14. Ostrow B. Is splenic preservation after blunt splenic injury possible in Africa? Surgery in Africa—Monthly Review. Available at: http://www.ptolemy.ca/members/archives/2005/Splenic_Preservation_Africa_Sept_2005.pdf.

15. Zissin R, Osadchy A, Gayer G. Abdominal CT findings of delayed postoperative complications. Can Assoc Radiol J 2007; 58:200–211.

16. O'Sullivan ST, Reardon CM, O'Donnell JA, et al. How safe is splenectomy? Ir J Med Sci 1994; 163:374–378.

17. Price VE, Dutta S, Blanchette VS, et al. The prevention and treatment of bacterial infections in children with asplenia or hyposplenia: practice considerations at the Hospital for Sick Children, Toronto. Pediatr Blood Cancer 2006; 46:597–603.

CHAPTER 87
PORTAL HYPERTENSION

Alastair J. W. Millar

Introduction

Portal hypertension (PHT) may be caused by a wide variety of conditions, each with a different natural history. It frequently presents with bleeding from oesophageal varices, which is the commonest cause of serious upper gastrointestinal haemorrhage in children. Precise diagnosis, a sound understanding of the therapeutic options, and a multidisciplinary approach are essential for successful management.

Demographics

Portal hypertension is common in Africa and other developing regions, particularly as a result of endemic hepatitis B–related cirrhosis and, in affected areas, schistosomiasis and some particularly unique toxins that cause veno-occlusive disease.

Portal hypertension in children may be due to:

- primary venous obstruction at a prehepatic (e.g., portal vein obstruction); intrahepatic (e.g., hepatoportal sclerosis); or posthepatic (e.g., veno-occlusive disease and Budd-Chiari syndrome) level (rarely, an arterioportal venous fistula causes portal hypertension in an unobstructed system);

- intrinsic liver disease (e.g., cirrhosis, fibrosis, nodular hyperplasia);

- chronic liver disease, the commonest overall cause of PHT; or

- portal vein occlusion (PVO), the most frequent cause of extrahepatic PHT.

Occasionally, the picture is mixed, as in cirrhosis complicated by portal vein thrombosis.

Aetiology/Pathophysiology

Portal hypertension is defined by an increased hepatic venous pressure gradient (>5 mm Hg), which is the difference between wedged hepatic venous pressure (an indicator of portal venous pressure) and free hepatic venous pressure. A gradient of more than 12 mm Hg is necessary for the development of oesophageal varices. Although the relationship is not linear, the risk of variceal bleeding is increased in larger varices and in those with a higher internal pressure and wall tension. In established cirrhosis, the risk of variceal bleeding is related to the severity of the liver disease.

Portal venous pressure is the product of blood flow from the gut and spleen being increased in cirrhosis due to splanchnic vasodilatation, and vascular resistance. Within the liver, vascular resistance includes both fixed (fibrosis and architectural distortion) and dynamic (sinusoidal vascular tone) components.

A rise in portal pressure leads to splenomegaly and the development of portosystemic collaterals at various sites: the distal oesophagus and gastric cardia (oesophageal and gastric varices), the anal canal (anorectal varices), the falciform ligament (umbilical varices), and varices in the abdominal wall and retroperitoneum. The junction between mucosal and submucosal varices in the lower 2–5 cm of the oesophagus is the usual site of rupture leading to variceal bleeding.

Clinical Presentation

History

Presentation is typically with acute gastrointestinal haemorrhage (haematemesis and/or malaena) and/or splenomegaly, or as part of the manifestation of chronic liver disease with spider naevi, clubbing, varices, ascites, and bleeding in patients with cirrhosis.

Physical

Children with PVO present with variceal bleeding at a younger mean age than those with cirrhosis (5 years of age versus 8 years), but onset of haemorrhage may occur at any age. The risk of bleeding is often precipitated by an upper respiratory tract infection, but this may reduce with age and the spontaneous development of portosystemic collaterals.

Splenomegaly may be associated with evidence of hypersplenism. However, unlike cirrhotics, humoral immunity is preserved in those with PVO. Ascites usually denotes the presence of chronic liver disease but may occur transiently after a major variceal bleed in those with extrahepatic portal hypertension. Encephalopathy may complicate an episode of bleeding in cirrhotics but is rarely detectable in children with PVO.

Portal hypertension may cause mucosal oedema in the small intestine, leading to malabsorption, protein loss, and failure to thrive. Thus, growth failure is common in cirrhosis and may also be found in children with PVO. In established PHT, dilated cutaneous collateral veins carry blood away from the umbilicus towards the tributaries of the vena cava (caput medusae). In long-standing disease, varices around the common bile duct may cause bile duct dilatation and, rarely, obstructive jaundice. Also rarely, pulmonary hypertension may coexist with portal hypertension—more often in children with cirrhosis than those with PVO. In cirrhotics, 30–50% will have varices and nearly half will have a significant bleed. There is 5–20% mortality during the first bleed, and half of the survivors will bleed again. In PVO, the mortality from the first bleed is <3%, with a lifetime mortality from bleeding of 10–15%.

Investigations

A full blood count may show anaemia, leucopenia, and/or thrombocytopenia from hypersplenism. The prothrombin time is commonly prolonged in patients with intrinsic liver disease or Budd-Chiari syndrome. In PVO, the prothrombin time is often slightly prolonged in association with a reduced factor VII concentration. The presence of reduced procoagulant and anticoagulant protein concentrations in PVO is probably due to reduced portal blood flow and/or portosystemic shunting. In patients with Budd-Chiari syndrome, an underlying myeloproliferative disorder or thrombophilic state should be excluded by bone marrow aspirate, and estimation of protein C, S, factor V Lieden, and lupus anticoagulant.

Biochemical liver function tests are essentially normal in PVO but reflect the level of chronic disease in cirrhosis, particularly with low serum albumin. In Budd-Chiari syndrome, both liver and renal function may be disturbed.

Abdominal Ultrasound Scan

An abdominal ultrasound scan confirms nonspecific features of portal hypertension, such as large collateral veins and splenomegaly. Hepatic echotexture may indicate the presence of chronic liver disease. Colour Doppler flow studies provide information on the direction and velocity of flow in the portal vein, hepatic veins, and vena cava.

Gastrointestinal Endoscopy

Endoscopy can be used to evaluate gastro-oesophageal and anorectal varices and mucosal features of portal hypertension at all ages. Oesophageal varices are graded according to severity. Large varices may show "red signs" of recent or impending variceal haemorrhage; these stigmata include "cherry-red spots" and "varices on varices". Endoscopic ultrasound assessment of submucosal and para-oesophageal varices is a distinct advance with diagnostic accuracy. Portal gastropathy is characterized by mucosal hyperaemia and dilated submucosal veins.

Computed Tomography and Magnetic Resonance Imaging

Both computer tomography (CT) and magnetic resonance imaging (MRI) are useful in evaluating focal liver lesions associated with portal hypertension and in Budd-Chiari syndrome. In the latter, the findings depend on the duration and degree of venous obstruction; in chronic cases, there is splenomegaly and ascites, and the liver parenchyma shows patchy contrast enhancement and caudate lobe hypertrophy. In PVO, a variable degree of liver atrophy may be seen.

Angiography

Magnetic resonance angiography is being used increasingly as a noninvasive alternative to conventional angiography. It confirms the diagnosis of PVO and assesses the patency and calibre of veins throughout the portomesenteric system. Angiography is particularly important when considering portosystemic shunt surgery, including meso-Rex surgery, and when assessing patients with a thrombosed or abnormal portal vein before liver transplantation. Conventional angiography can be performed by several routes, but the commonest is by indirect portography. Direct splenoportography after percutaneous needle puncture of the spleen also enables the measurement of splenic pulp pressure (an index of portal hypertension), which may be of value in assessing anastomotic portal vein strictures posttransplant. Percutaneous transhepatic portography is occasionally used. Hepatic venography shows a typical "spider web" pattern of venous collaterals around hepatic vein thrombosis in Budd-Chiari syndrome. Inferior vena cavography or magnetic resonance venography may be necessary to determine the patency of the inferior vena cava (IVC) or the intrahepatic portal and Rex veins.

Liver Biopsy

If there are no contraindications (poor clotting not corrected by replacement therapy of vitamin K, fresh frozen plasma, or clotting factor concentrates), a biopsy is usually undertaken to diagnose any underlying liver disease. Open or laparoscopically observed biopsy may be a safer option, as postbiopsy bleeding is a real risk. In extrahepatic PVO, the liver architecture is normal, but mild periportal fibrosis may be seen. In hepatic vein obstruction, liver biopsy typically shows marked venous congestion around central venules with hepatocyte necrosis; in chronic cases, there is progression to hepatic fibrosis and cirrhosis.

Management

Primary Prophylaxis of Variceal Bleeding

Beta-blockers

Propranolol reduces portal pressure by causing splanchnic vasoconstriction and reducing cardiac output. If there are no contraindications to beta-blockers (e.g., asthma), primary prophylaxis may be worthwhile in children with PVO or cirrhosis and large varices. Therapy should aim to reduce the resting pulse rate by 25%.

Endoscopic therapy

Prophylactic use of injection sclerotherapy or banding is controversial. A small proportion of patients with PVO never bleed. At present, primary endoscopic prophylaxis cannot be recommended except for situations in which a child may be returning to an environment where treatment is limited.

Emergency Management of Variceal Bleeding

Bleeding from oesophageal varices is life threatening and requires hospital admission. Mortality is closely related to the severity of any underlying liver disease.

Octreotide, a long-acting analogue of somatostatin, with a plasma half-life of more than 1 hour, is given as an intravenous infusion and is effective in controlling acute variceal bleeding, particularly when used in combination with endoscopic therapy.

A balloon tamponade may be required to control active variceal bleeding. A Sengstaken-type tube can be inserted by an experienced clinician after securing the airway by endotracheal intubation. Only the gastric balloon need be inflated, and correct positioning must be verified by x-ray. Moderate traction is applied; excessive traction may cause mucosal ulceration or balloon displacement. The balloon is deflated after 12–24 hours at the time of endoscopy. Balloon deflation may be followed by severe bleeding, especially with gastric fundal varices.

Endoscopic Treatment of Oesophageal Varices

Injection sclerotherapy

Endoscopic injection sclerotherapy (EIS) has been a standard technique for inducing variceal thrombosis for many years but has largely been superseded by oesphageal banding in older children. EIS is applicable to all age groups and is best performed under general anaesthesia with an endotracheal tube in place. It is now used only in small infants, in whom it is not possible to pass the endoscope with the banding equipment, as well as where banding equipment is not available. A variety of injection techniques and sclerosants have been used, with 5% ethanolamine oleate being the most widely used. Between 1 and 3 ml of sclerosant are injected into each of the major variceal columns just above the gastro-oesophageal junction. Paravariceal injection or a combination of the two is equally efficacious.

Varices should be initially injected every 1 to 2 weeks and then at monthly intervals until sclerosis is complete. Patients are given oral sucralfate for 48 hours and ranitidine for 2 weeks after each injection session to reduce complications from ulceration. Endoscopic review is undertaken after 6 months and then annually, but only large recurrent varices require treatment.

Variceal ligation (banding)

In variceal ligation, the varix is aspirated into a transparent cylinder fitted to the end of a flexible endoscope and an elastic band is released by a trip wire passing through the biopsy channel, causing strangulation of the varix, which then thromboses and sloughs. Treatment begins with ligation of the most distal varix in the oesophagus, just above the cardia. Up to four bands can be applied to the varices at each session; the treatment is repeated after 1 to 2 weeks and then monthly until the varices have been obliterated. Multiband devices allow the application of several bands with one pass of the endoscope.

Gastric Varices

Many gastric varices are fundal and directly contiguous with lower oesophageal varices. Most are present at the initial endoscopy and are eradicated during treatment of oesophageal varices. However, 5–10% of patients develop significant gastric varices after treatment of oesophageal varices by EIS. Bleeding from gastric varices may respond to EIS, but this is much less likely if the gastric varices are isolated and not contiguous with oesophageal varices. Alternative sclerosants, such as bovine thrombin and cyanoacrylate, have been used successfully in adults but have not been evaluated in children. Banding of gastric varices is associated with a high rebleeding rate. If sclerotherapy is ineffective or inappropriate, then portosystemic shunting or a local devascularization procedure should be considered in those with satisfactory liver function.

Surgery for Portal Hypertension

Surgical shunts

Shunt surgery (see Figure 87.1) and endoscopic therapy are complementary procedures in the management of portal hypertension.

Indications for surgery include:

- uncontrolled bleeding from oesophageal varices (not responding to at least two sessions of banding or sclerotherapy) in children with PVO or those with chronic liver disease and reasonable liver function;

- bleeding gastric or ectopic varices that cannot be controlled endoscopically;

- massive splenomegaly, causing severe hypersplenism or abdominal pain; and

- lack of access to expert endoscopy.

A case can be made for mesoportal bypass surgery in children with extrahepatic PVO and cavernoma as prophylactic therapy because of the added benefit of not only relieving PHT but also redirecting portal venous blood into the liver.

Many types of portosystemic shunt have been described, but mesocaval and splenorenal shunts have been used most often in children. The distal splenorenal (Warren) shunt is considered to be a selective shunt in that it achieves gastrosplenic variceal decompression while maintaining portal perfusion.

Shunt patency is confirmed by improvement in hypersplenism, as evidenced by an increase in platelet counts, a reduction in splenomegaly, and regression of oesophageal varices observed endoscopically. Shunt thrombosis is a major complication and frequently manifests as recurrent variceal bleeding. It is more likely in children younger than 5 years of age. Shunt patency may be assessed directly by a variety of imaging modalities including colour Doppler ultrasound imaging of the shunt, magnetic resonance angiography, and conventional angiography, or indirectly by ultrasound examination of flow patterns in portomesenteric and systemic veins.

Encephalopathy is a well-recognized complication of portosystemic shunt surgery in cirrhotics but is very rare in children with PVO. Improvement in some areas of cognitive function has been documented after restoration of normal portal blood flow into the liver by means of the mesenterico-left portal (Rex) shunt (Figure 87.2).

The introduction of the Rex shunt has significantly broadened the indications for shunt surgery in PVO. In this shunt, a vein graft is interposed between the superior mesenteric vein and the (intrahepatic) left portal vein, which is located in the Rex recessus adjacent to the falciform ligament. The portal vein occlusion is bypassed, hepatic portal blood flow is restored, and portal hypertension is corrected. The operation demands the presence of an adequate calibre, patent intrahepatic left portal vein and patent splenic and mesenteric veins; this must be established preoperatively by angiography, ultrasound, and/or retrograde hepatic venography. This shunt is a valuable option for selected children with PVO because it restores normal physiology. However, it is not feasible in all cases. Shunt failure is a potential problem, but medium-term follow-up studies indicate that excellent results can be achieved with autologous vein grafts.

Mesocaval shunting has been a successful form of treatment in the past and may be preferred to selective or side-to-side splenorenal shunts because the vessels used are larger and more likely to remain patent. As with all nonselective shunts, there is the long-term risk of encephalopathy.

Nonshunt surgery

Other surgical techniques to control variceal bleeding have been disappointing in the long term because of a high rate of rebleeding.

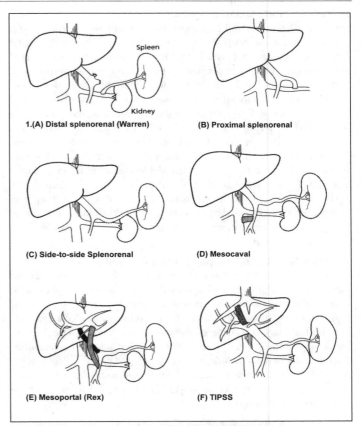

Figure 87.1: Diagrams showing the different types of shunt procedures: (A) distal splenorenal (Warren); (B) proximal splenorenal with splenectomy; (C) side-to-side splenorenal; (D) mesocaval interposition graft; (E) mesoportal (Rex); (F) transjugular intrahepatic portosystemic shunt (TIPSS).

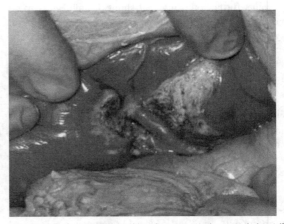

Figure 87.2: A patent internal jugular mesenterico-portal shunt (Rex) at surgery for extrahepatic portal hypertension.

Splenectomy alone, suture ligation of varices, and oesophago-gastric transection have generally yielded only short-term success, except in gastric variceal bleeding from isolated splenic vein thrombosis when splenectomy may be curative. Splenectomy is rarely indicated for massive splenomegaly causing severe hypersplenism or abdominal pain, but shunt surgery should be considered in such cases. Splenic embolisation is an alternative, but its effects may be temporary, and the procedure is not without morbidity.

Liver transplantation

Liver transplantation is the treatment of choice for most children with variceal bleeding complicating end-stage chronic liver disease.

Surgery for Budd-Chiari syndrome

Rarely, posthepatic portal hypertension has a radiologically or surgically treatable cause, such as a caval web. Many children with hepatic vein thrombosis are successfully managed by medical therapy directed at controlling ascites and preventing progressive venous thrombosis. Portal decompression is necessary for variceal bleeding, deteriorating liver function associated with zonal necrosis on liver biopsy, and intractable ascites. Portosystemic shunting converts the portal vein into a venous outflow tract. Occasionally, more complex shunts are needed in those with IVC obstruction. These procedures are potentially hazardous, and a transjugular intrahepatic stent is a less invasive alternative. In this procedure an expandable wire stent is placed in the hepatic vein after balloon dilatation. Prolonged anticoagulation with warfarin is required. Liver transplantation is indicated for fulminant liver failure or cirrhosis, but recurrence of Budd-Chiari syndrome in the graft is a risk, and patients with thrombophilia usually require long-term anticoagulation.

Transjugular intrahepatic portosystemic stent shunt

A transjugular intrahepatic portosystemic stent shunt (TIPSS) requires sophisticated technology and a skilled interventional endoscopist. It involves the percutaneous insertion of an expandable metal stent via the jugular vein into a hepatic vein and major portal vein. Selected patients with Budd-Chiari syndrome or intractable ascites may also benefit. Portal vein occlusion and uncorrected coagulopathy are contraindications. The major risks include stent occlusion and hepatic encephalopathy. The incidence of stent occlusion increases with time. These and other complications and the technical demands of the procedure have limited its role in children.

Postoperative Complications

Complications after EIS are those of rebleeding, oesophageal ulceration, and stricture. Perforation with mediastinitis has occurred only rarely. With occult bleeding (OB), the ulcers tend to be more superficial and the rebleeding rate less. Shunt surgery, if successful, reduces portal pressure and prevents further bleeding, but shunt thrombosis is more frequent in smaller children with a shunt diameter of less than 0.5 cm. Encephalopathy is a real concern, particularly in children shunted for cirrhosis. Selective distal splenorenal shunts generally have a better record. For PVO, the mesenteric left portal bypass is the treatment of choice, but may not be possible in up to 30% of cases.

Prognosis and Outcomes

Prognosis depends on shunt patency and on the severity of liver disease. Those with cirrhosis eventually require liver transplantation before the development of end stage disease. With complimentary medical therapy, endoscopic intervention, and shunt surgery, the ultimate prognosis is excellent.

Prevention

Control of hepatitis B, schistosomiasis, and toxins may prevent liver disease, which subsequently presents as portal hypertension.

Ethical Issues

Where follow-up is poor, early recourse to shunt surgery—if the skills are available—may be preferred to serial endoscopic injection sclerotherapy or banding. Liver transplantation should not be undertaken unless life-long supervision and immunosuppressive therapy are available.

Evidence-Based Research

Table 87.1 presents a study comparing sclerotherapy and ligation for treating bleeding eosophageal varices in children. Table 87.2 presents a study of endoscopic sclerotherapy for bleeding oesophageal varices in Sudan.

Table 87.1: Evidence-based research.

Title	Endoscopic ligation compared with sclerotherapy for bleeding esophageal varices in children with extrahepatic portal venous obstruction
Authors	Zargar SA, Javid G , Khan BA, et al.
Institution	Department of Gastroenterology, Sher-i-Kashmir Institute of Medical Sciences, Srinagar, Kashmir, India
Reference	Hepatology 2002; 36(3):666–672
Problem	Endoscopic sclerotherapy is an effective treatment for bleeding esophageal varices, but it is associated with significant complications. Endoscopic ligation, a new form of endoscopic treatment for bleeding varices, has been shown to be superior to sclerotherapy in adult patients with cirrhosis.
Intervention	To determine the efficacy and safety of endoscopic sclerotherapy and ligation, the two methods were compared in a randomized control trial in 49 children with extrahepatic portal venous obstruction who had proven bleeding from oesophageal varices.
Comparison/ control (quality of evidence)	Twenty-four patients were treated with sclerotherapy and 25 with band ligation. No significant differences were found between the sclerotherapy and ligation groups in arresting active index bleeding (100% each) and achieving variceal eradication (91.7% versus 96%, P = .61). Band ligation eradicated varices in fewer endoscopic sessions than did sclerotherapy (3.9 ± 1.1 versus 6.1 ± 1.7, respectively, P < .0001). The rebleeding rate was significantly higher in the sclerotherapy group (25% versus 4%, P = .049), as was the rate of major complications (25% versus 4%, P = .049). After eradication, esophageal variceal recurrence was not significantly different in patients treated by ligation than in those treated by sclerotherapy (17.4% versus 10%, P = .67).
Outcome/ effect	In conclusion, variceal band ligation in children is a safe and effective technique that achieves variceal eradication more quickly, with a lower rebleeding rate and fewer complications compared with sclerotherapy.

Table 87.2: Evidence-based research.

Title	Endoscopic sclerotherapy for bleeding oesophageal varices: experience in Sudan
Authors	Gasim B, Fedial SS, Musaad AM, Ahmed W, Salih SM, Ibn-Ouf M
Institution	National Centre for Gastrointestinal and Liver Disease, Ibn Sina Hospital Faculty of Medicine, University of Khartoum, Khartoum, Sudan
Reference	Tropical Gastroenterol 2002; 23(2)107–109
Problem	Bleeding due to oesophageal varices is the commonest cause of upper gastrointestinal tract haemorrhage in Sudan. Endoscopic injection sclerotherapy is a valuable therapeutic modality for the management of variceal bleeding. Other options for treatment, such as variceal banding, are either too expensive or unavailable.
Intervention	A retrospective study to evaluate the outcome of EST in the management of bleeding oesophageal varices due to portal hypertension in a developing country (Sudan).
Comparison/ control (quality of evidence)	A total of 1070 patients over a period of 10 years (1986–1996) were studied. The inclusion criterion was bleeding oesophageal varices consequent to portal hypertension. EIS was performed using a standard technique. Ethanolamine oleate 5% was the sclerosing agent. The procedure was done on a day-case basis. There were 904 males (84.5%) and 166 females (15.5%). The cause of portal hypertension was schistosomal periportal fibrosis (PPF) in 999 (93.3%) patients, liver cirrhosis in 59 (5.5%), mixed PPF and cirrhosis in 5 (0.46%), portal vein thrombosis in 6 (0.64%), and congenital hepatic fibrosis in 1 patient. A total of 100 (9.4%) patients presented with bleeding after surgery. Full obliteration of varices required a mean of 4 sessions with a range of 2–6. Follow-up of 462 patients (43.2%) continued until complete sclerosis of varices.
Historical significance/ comments	This study provides evidence that endoscopic injection sclerotherapy is an essential component in the management of bleeding oesophageal varices caused by portal hypertension. It is a feasible and cost-effective therapeutic strategy in developing countries.

Key Summary Points

1. Portal hypertension is common in developing regions, and variceal haemorrhage may be lethal.

2. Noncirrhotic portal hypertension can satisfactorily be treated with a combination of medical, endoscopic, and surgical treatment modalities.

3. Shunt surgery, particularly the mesenterico-portal bypass operation for PVO, has excellent long-term results and not only cures portal hypertension but also restores normal liver splanchnic blood flow.

4. Liver transplantation is the treatment of choice for cirrhosis but should be attempted only with lifelong supervision.

Suggested Reading

Abraldes JG, Bosch J. Somatostatin and analogues in portal hypertension. Hepatology 2002; 35(6):1305–1312.

Alagille D, et al. Long-term neuropsychological outcome in children undergoing portal-systemic shunts for portal vein obstruction without liver disease. J Pediatr Gastroenterol Nutr 1986; 5(6):861–866.

Arakawa M, Masuzaki T, Okuda K. Pathomorphology of esophageal and gastric varices. Semin Liver Dis 2002; 22(1):73–82.

Bismuth H, Franco D, Alagille D. Portal diversion for portal hypertension in children. The first ninety patients. Ann Surg 1980; 192(1):18–24.

Cauchi JA, et al. The Budd-Chiari syndrome in children: the spectrum of management. J Pediatr Surg 2006; 41(11):1919–1923.

Chopra R, et al. Defibrotide for the treatment of hepatic veno-occlusive disease: results of the European compassionate-use study. Br J Haematol 2000; 111(4):1122–1129.

de Ville de Goyet J, et al. Direct bypassing of extrahepatic portal venous obstruction in children: a new technique for combined hepatic portal revascularization and treatment of extrahepatic portal hypertension. J Pediatr Surg 1998; 33(4):597–601.

DeLeve LD, Shulman HM, McDonald GB. Toxic injury to hepatic sinusoids: sinusoidal obstruction syndrome (veno-occlusive disease). Semin Liver Dis 2002; 22(1):27–42.

Fox VL, et al. Endoscopic ligation of esophageal varices in children. J Pediatr Gastroenterol Nutr 1995; 20(2):202–208.

Goncalves ME, Cardoso SR, Maksoud JG. Prophylactic sclerotherapy in children with esophageal varices: long-term results of a controlled prospective randomized trial. J Pediatr Surg 2000; 35(3):401–405.

Hayes, PC, et al. Meta-analysis of value of propranolol in prevention of variceal haemorrhage. Lancet 1990; 336(8708):153–156.

Heyman MB, LaBerge JM. Role of transjugular intrahepatic portosystemic shunt in the treatment of portal hypertension in pediatric patients. J Pediatr Gastroenterol Nutr 1999; 29(3):240–249.

Howard ER, Stringer MD, Mowat AP, Assessment of injection sclerotherapy in the management of 152 children with oesophageal varices. Br J Surg 1988; 75(5):404–408.

Jalan R, et al. TIPSS 10 years on. Gut 2000; 46(4):578–581.

Kato T, et al. Portosystemic shunting in children during the era of endoscopic therapy: improved postoperative growth parameters. J Pediatr Gastroenterol Nutr 2000; 30(4):419–425.

Lay CS, et al. Endoscopic variceal ligation in prophylaxis of first variceal bleeding in cirrhotic patients with high-risk esophageal varices. Hepatology 1997; 25(6):1346–1350.

Lebrec D. Ectopic varices in patients with portal hypertension. Arch Surg 1980; 115(7):890.

Lykavieris P, et al. Risk of gastrointestinal bleeding during adolescence and early adulthood in children with portal vein obstruction. J Pediatr 2000; 136(6):805–808.

Mack CL, et al. Surgically restoring portal blood flow to the liver in children with primary extrahepatic portal vein thrombosis improves fluid neurocognitive ability. Pediatrics 2006; 117(3): e405–e412.

Maksoud JG, et al. The endoscopic and surgical management of portal hypertension in children: analysis of 123 cases. J Pediatr Surg 1991; 26(2):178–181.

Millar AJ, et al. The fundal pile: bleeding gastric varices. J Pediatr Surg 1991; 26(6):707–709.

Odell JA, et al. Surgical repair in children with the Budd-Chiari syndrome. J Thorac Cardiovasc Surg 1995; 110(4, Pt 1):916–923.

Okudaira M, Ohbu M, Okuda K. Idiopathic portal hypertension and its pathology. Semin Liver Dis 2002; 22(1):59–72.

Shashidhar H, Langhans N, Grand RJ, Propranolol in prevention of portal hypertensive hemorrhage in children: a pilot study. J Pediatr Gastroenterol Nutr 1999; 29(1):12–17.

Steenkamp V, Stewart MJ, Zuckerman, M. Clinical and analytical aspects of pyrrolizidine poisoning caused by South African traditional medicines. Ther Drug Monit 2000; 22(3):302–306.

Stringer MD, et al. Patterns of portal vein occlusion and their aetiological significance. Br J Surg 1994; 81(9):1328–1331.

Superina R, et al. Surgical guidelines for the management of extra-hepatic portal vein obstruction. Pediatr Transplant 2006; 10(8):908–913.

Valayer J, Branchereau S. Portal hypertension: portosystemic shunts. In: Stringer MD, Oldham KT, Mouriquand PDE, Howard ER (eds). Pediatric Surgery and Urology Long-Term Outcomes, Cambridge University Press, 1998, Pp. 439–446.

Valla DC. Hepatic vein thrombosis (Budd-Chiari syndrome). Semin Liver Dis 2002; 22(1):5–14.

Webb, LJ, Sherlock S. The aetiology, presentation and natural history of extra-hepatic portal venous obstruction. Q J Med 1979; 48(192):627–639.

Paediatric Urology

CHAPTER 88
CYSTIC DISEASES OF THE KIDNEY

Osarumwense David Osifo
Edward Hannon

Introduction

Cystic diseases of the kidney are common lesions worldwide.[1-5] They are broadly divided into genetic and nongenetic cysts. A renal cyst is a fluid-filled sac arising from dilatation in any part of the nephrons or collecting ducts. The cysts may eventually separate from the nephrons or ducts and continue to enlarge. Although most are simple cysts, about one-third of people older than 50 years of age are said to have renal cysts.[1-3] Depending on the type, symptoms can occur at any age, and many cases may manifest symptoms in utero. Undiagnosed or untreated cases ultimately progress to end-stage renal disease (ESRD) and death. The outcome of the disease varies between developed and developing countries, due mainly to late presentation, lack of facilities required for prompt diagnosis, and a lack of facilities and manpower required for intrauterine interventions in developing countries, especially in children who manifest symptoms in utero.[3] Table 88.1 shows the classifications of cystic diseases of the kidney. This chapter discusses the common types, which include:

- multicystic kidney or multicystic dysplastic kidney (MCDK);
- autosomal dominant polycystic kidney disease (ADPKD); and
- autosomal recessive polycystic kidney disease (ARPKD).

Table 88.1: Classification of cystic diseases of the kidney.

Nongenetic	Genetic
Acquired disorders	*Autosomal dominant*
Simple renal cysts (solitary or multiple)	Autosomal dominant polycystic kidney disease*
Cysts of the renal sinus (or peripelvic lymphagiectasis)	Tuberous sclerosis complex
	von Hippel-Lindau disease
Acquired cystic kidney disease (in patients with chronic renal impairment)	Medullary cystic disease
Multilocular cysts (or multilocular cystic nephroma)	Glomerulocystic disease
Hypokalemia-related cysts	*Autosomal recessive*
Developmental disorders	Autosomal recessive polycystic kidney disease*
Medullary sponge kidney	Nephronophthisis
Multicystic dysplastic or multicystic kidney*	*X-linked*
Pyelocalyceal cysts	Orofaciodigital syndrome type 1

*Common type of cystic disease of the kidney

Source: Pirson Y, Chauveau D, Grunfeld JP. Autosomal dominant polycystic kidney disease. In: Davison AM, Cameron JS, Grunfeld JP, eds. Oxford Textbook of Clinical Nephrology. Oxford University Press, 1998, Pp 2393-2415.

Demographics

Incidence

No conclusive African figures on cystic kidney disease are available due especially to a poor database. There is, however, geographical variation in incidence as well as variation in incidence among the subtypes.[2,3] Available literature[1-6] from more developed countries suggests that:

- Multicystic kidney or MCDK has an incidence of 1 per 1,000–4,000 live births.
- ADPKD has an incidence of 1 per 400–1,000 among whites and accounts for 8–10% of all cases of ESRD.
- ARPKD has an incidence of 1 per 6,000–55,000 live births, with a heterozygous carrier frequency of 1 per 70.

Race

ADPKD is found worldwide in all races and ethnic groups, whereas acquired cystic renal disease is reported to be most common in white and African American men.

Gender

MCDK is more common in males than females, and symptomatic progression of ADPKD appears to be more rapid in men.

Age

ADPKD has a bimodal distribution of onset. It usually presents in infancy or childhood and adulthood, with rare occurrence in middle age. ARPKD often presents in infancy, childhood, or adolescence. In contrast, simple cysts are very rare in children but increase in frequency with age.

Aetiology/Pathophysiology

Generally, cysts develop due to increased tubular epithelial proliferation.[1-3] Many of the cysts may detach from the parent tubule after growing to a few millimeters in size.

Multicystic kidney is usually a sporadic, nonsyndromal, congenital anomaly. It occurs as a result of ureteropelvic dysplasia or atresia that results in an enlarged kidney and the formation of cysts of varying sizes that do not communicate. There is no demonstrable pelvis and calyces, but microscopic examination shows rudimentary lobes with no corticomedullary differentiation.

ADPKD occurs due to mutations in the genes PKD1 and PKD2, which encode polycystin proteins. It may require a second "hit" to result in ADPKD later in life.[5]

ARPKD occurs following mutations in PKHD1, a large gene that encodes fibrocystin/polyductin, which plays a critical role in collecting-tubule and biliary development.

Clinical Presentation

Clinical presentation depends on the type of cystic disease.[1-3]

Multicystic kidney is the second most common cause of a flank mass in the newborn. The diagnosis may be made in utero by ultrasonography (US) or palpation of an abdominal mass during examination for other conditions in neonates. Clinical symptoms are rarely seen unless it is complicated by infection. The contralateral kidney is usually normal but may be absent, hydronephrotic, ectopic, refluxing, or dysplastic.

Patients with ADPKD usually present in the fourth decade of life with flank pain or intermittent haematuria. Renal size increases exponentially with an equal growth rate in both kidneys over time due to the increase in cyst volume. The disease course varies significantly among affected individuals. Hepatic cysts are the most common extrarenal manifestation that increases with age. Recent reports[1,2] revealed an incidence of 20% and 75%, respectively, at the third and sixth decades of life. Patients with PKD1 genoytpe appear to develop more rapid disease progression.

ARPKD affects renal and hepatic development with varying degrees of organ involvement with age. It may be a cause of neonatal death due to pulmonary disease resulting from nephromegaly and oligohydraminios. Symptoms in infants include hypertension, diminished urine concentrating ability, and renal insufficiency. Almost half of affected individuals develop ESRD in the first decade of life. Occurrences in children between 4 and 8 years of age are predominantly hepatic involvement with kidneys often less severely affected.

Investigation

Cystic diseases of the kidney are usually diagnosed by imaging investigations, such as the following:

- *Ultrasonography:* US is a common investigation with high diagnostic accuracy. It is used for both diagnosis and follow-up of the patient. A US scan shows the cystic nature of the mass, but critical for the diagnosis of a renal cyst is the loss of internal echoes; rounded outline; sharply demarcated, smooth walls; and bright posterior wall echo.[4,6] Multiple cysts show similar features that are separated by septa with a lobulated appearance (Figure 88.1).

- *Intravenous urography:* Intravenous urography may show a nonfunctioning kidney in ESRD, loss of tubular connection in MCDK, and multiple cystic collections in polycystic kidney disease.[3,5]

- *Computerised tomography (CT) scan:* A CT scan gives better resolution than US or intravenous urography, which is especially useful when the US finding is not conclusive.

- *Magnetic resonance imaging (MRI):* MRI has a very high diagnostic accuracy and is quite useful for follow-up, but its nonavailability is a major drawback to its use in developing countries.

- *Nonimaging investigations:* Other investigations include genetic testing for polycystic kidney disease, serum electrolytes, urea and creatinines, and urine for microscopy culture and sensitivity.

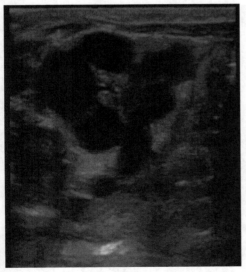

Figure 88.1: Ultrasound of a multicystic dysplastic kidney.

Management

The management of cystic disease of the kidney in the developed world, as in Africa, involves a multidisciplinary team approach involving paediatric urologists, paediatric nephrologists, and (as required and/or available) transplant surgeons and dialysis teams. The main differences in the management of these conditions is obviously influenced by the availability of resources in these locations, including antenatal scanning, availability of specialists, and, more specifically to renal disease, the availability of renal replacement therapy and transplantation. These key factors obviously play a role in the long-term outcomes of each of these conditions.

Multicystic Dysplastic Kidneys

The management of MCDK[7,8] in the developed world remains controversial, especially as the numbers of asymptomatic patients being picked up on routine antenatal screening increases. The most common presentation in developed countries is on antenatal US scan, with fewer cases now being picked up clinically. US scans remain the first-line investigation of choice and are usually diagnostic, but postnatal isotope scanning (dimercaptosuccinic acid (DMSA) or mercaptuacetyltriglycine (MAG3)) is being used increasingly to confirm a total absence in isotope uptake in the affected kidney and hence a diagnosis of MCDK. US also has a role in imaging the contralateral kidney, in which pelviureteric junction obstruction or vesicoureteric reflux may be demonstrated and may subsequently require investigation with a micturating cystourethrogram (MCUG) and/or MAG3 scanning.

Nephrectomy is the treatment of choice for large MCDK presenting clinically with a palpable mass in the neonatal period. Surgery is also indicated in those with smaller lesions and symptoms such as pain, haematuria, and hypertension. Management of asymptomatic patients is more controversial. Up to 50% of MCDK cases have been shown to involute by 5 years of age; however, for the remaining patients the role of "prophylactic" nephrectomy to minimise the risk of hypertension and malignancy is debatable. Hypertension is a rare but recognised complication of MCDK, and malignancy (Wilms' and renal cell carcinoma) is also documented; many authors and clinicians suggest the rarity of these complications makes prophylactic nephrectomy unnecessary in the asymptomatic patient, but opinion on this remains divided.

Autosomal Dominant Polycystic Kidney Disease

ADPKD is essentially a disease of adulthood but may be brought to the attention of the paediatric surgeon in developed countries, with occasional cases being picked up on antenatal scan or following US screening of family members of a patient. Management during childhood is typically expectant, managing any early complications of hypertension or infection as they occur. Rarely, nephrectomy may be required if these complications cannot be managed medically.

Autosomal Recessive Polycystic Kidney Disease

ARPKD,[7-9] in contrast to ADPKD, is a disease of childhood with a generally poor prognosis in both the developing and developed world due to the combination of end-stage renal failure and significant hepatic disease, which most patients experience. The mainstay of management is directed at treating the complications of renal and hepatic failure. The main difference in the developed world compared to developing countries is the wider availability of specialist medical care, dialysis, and transplantation; some studies suggest the prognosis may not be as poor as originally thought and that it is organ- and disease type-specific.[9] The survival rate therefore depends on many factors, including age of onset, presence of pulmonary disease, and relative degree of hepatic and renal involvement. Although severe perinatal disease has a universally poor prognosis, a survival rate of 46% at 15 years has been reported.[8]

Prognosis

The prognosis for cystic kidney diseases depends on the type of disease and age at presentation. Early diagnosis and surgical treatment of unilateral multicystic kidney disease is usually curative with an excellent outcome. The prognosis is good in patients with ADPKD, but those with PKD1 genoytpe appear to develop a more rapid disease progression, resulting in end-stage renal disease. The worst prognosis is in patients with ARPKD. Life expectancy is poor, as almost half of the affected individuals progress to ESRD and death in the first decade of life.

Prevention

There is no known preventive measure for cystic kidney diseases, but genetic counselling of couples intending to become parents may help in the prevention of polycystic kidney diseases.

Key Summary Points

1. Cystic disease of the kidneys is a common problem worldwide.

2. The three most common types of cystic kidney disease are:
   • multicystic kidney or multicystic dysplastic kidney (MCDK);
   • autosomal dominant polycystic kidney disease (ADPKD); and
   • autosomal recessive polycystic kidney disease (ARPKD).

3. MCDK is commonly sporadic and is usually diagnosed antenatally or neonatally on ultrasound. Nephrectomy may be required if patients are symptomatic; prognosis is excellent.

4. ADPKD is associated with the PKD1 and PKD2 genes, which encode for polycystin proteins. ADPKD usually presents in adulthood, but may be seen in the paediatric population antenatally or following screening of family members.

5. ARPKD is a disease of the liver and kidneys presenting in childhood. The prognosis of ARPKD is universally poor and depends on the disease type, organ involvement, and availability of renal replacement therapy.

6. Involvement of a multidisciplinary team with nephrologists is important for all cystic kidney lesions.

References

1. Grantham JJ, Nair V, Winklhoffer F. Cystic diseases of the kidney. In: Brenner BM, ed. Brenner and Rector's The Kidney, 6th ed. WB Saunders Company, 2000, Pp 1699–1730.

2. Trout AT, Siegal J. Cystic diseases of the kidney. Overview-eMedicine, updated 27 June 2006; accessed 25 May 2009. Available at: emedicine.medscape.com/article/453831-overview.

3. Kaplan BS, Mouriquand P, Ewalt DH, et al. Genitourinary and related disorders. In: O'Neill JA, Rowe MI, Grosfeld JI, Fonkalsrud EW, Coran GA, eds. Pediatric Surgery, 5th ed. Mosby Year Book Inc, 1998.

4. Pirson Y, Chauveau D, Grunfeld JP. Autosomal dominant polycystic kidney disease. In: Davison AM, Cameron JS, Grunfeld JP, eds. Oxford Textbook of Clinical Nephrology. Oxford University Press, 1998, Pp 2393–2415.

5. Germino CC. Autosomal dominant polycystic kidney disease: a two hit model. Hospital Pract 1997; 2:81–102.

6. Ravine D, Gibson RN, Walker RG. Evaluation of ultrasonographic diagnostic criteria for autosomal dominant polycystic kidney disease. Lancet 1994; 343:824–827.

7. Wu HY, Snyder HM III. Developmental and positional anomalies of the kidneys. In: Ashcraft KW, Holcomd GW, Murphy JP. Pediatric Surgery, 4th ed. Elsevier Saunders, 2005, Pp 723–731.

8. Thomas DFM. Cystic renal disease. In: Thomas DFM, Rickwood AMK, Duffy PG. Essentials of Paediatric Urology, 2nd ed. Informa UK Ltd, 2008, Pp 97–104.

CHAPTER 89
CONGENITAL URETEROPELVIC JUNCTION STENOSIS

Chris Heinick

John Lazarus

Introduction

Congenital ureteropelvic junction (UPJ) stenosis is a disturbance in the flow of urine at the crossover point from the kidney pelvis to the ureter, with a dilatated and obstructed renal-pelvic calyceal system (Figure 89.1). UPJ obstruction is the most frequent congenital malformation of the genitourinary system. Its incidence is around 1 out of 1,000 newborns.

The first sonographically demonstrable sign of URJ stenosis in early gestation is a dilatation of the renal-pelvic calyceal system. In part, this can be observed sonographically, in varying degrees, in the 18th to 20th week of gestation.

The outcome of a UPJ stenosis is quite good in general, given timely therapy, but the outcome often depends on whether there are concomitant malformations of the genitourinary system or other organ systems. The condition has been shown to be associated with congenital cardiac malformations, hydrocephalus, skeletal dysplasias, or trisomy 21. In the international literature, nonrenal concomitant malformations have been described in up to 12% of cases.

More frequent are further anomalies in the area of the urinary tract, for example, kidneys with two urinary track systems, horseshoe kidneys, mega-ureters, urethral valves, or contralateral multicystic renal dysplasia.

Demographics

The male-to-female ratio of congenital UPJ stenosis is 2:1. The left side is significantly more frequently affected in isolated cases than the right side. In 30% of the cases, both kidneys are affected. The literature does not indicate a racial predilection in UPJ stenosis.

Aetiology

At present, the cause of congenital UPJ stenosis has not been clearly determined. Extrinsic and intrinsic stenoses are distinguished. Extrinsic UPJ stenoses are caused, for example, by accessory polar vessels crossing the pelviureteric junction or by pressure exerted by an external tumour. The intrinsic form is characterised by an aetiologically unclear congenital disturbance in the texture of the ureter wall, which forms a stenotic fibrosis at the pelviureteric junction. This is regularly shown at histological investigation. A further cause of an intrinsic obstruction is a rare mucous membrane polyp at the pelviureteric junction.

Pathophysiology

The obstruction of the ureter results in a backflow of urine into the proximal urinary tract. When there is a functionally effective stenosis, it leads at first to a progressive dilatation of the renal pelvis and its calyxes. If this dilatation exerts a specific pressure on the renal parenchyma, the wall of the renal pelvis and the blood vessels for a certain amount of time, the result is, at first, a reversible but in time irreversible loss of kidney function due to renal atrophy. This process has been shown not to be pure pressure atrophy; the main cause of the hydronephrotic atrophy is circulatory disruption of the blood and lymph vessels due to increased tension in the renal pelvic wall. Many investigations have shown that the loss of kidney function after long-standing obstruction is irreversible, even after relief.

Prenatal Diagnosis

Prenatal ultrasound (US) can show reliably a dilatation of the renal pelvis at the 16th to 20th week of gestation (Figure 89.2), and can be used to follow the development of the dilatation during the course of pregnancy. The most frequent prenatal foetal abnormality is an isolated renal pelvis dilatation. Not every prenatal dilatation of the kidney results in a pathological condition, however. Many low-level prenatal dilatations of the renal pelvis can no longer be detected postnatally.

On the basis of many investigations, a prognostic limit for the prenatal renal pelvis width has been determined. The limit is around 10–11 mm for the posterior-anterior diameter of the renal pelvis. In general, prenatal dilatations below this value do not result in pathological conditions requiring postnatal treatment. Renal pelvis

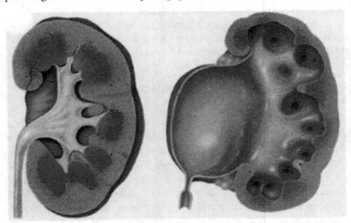

Normal renal pelvis   **UPJ stenosis**

Figure 89.1: Normal and stenosed ureteropelvic junction.

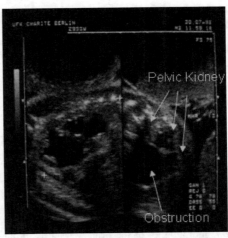

Figure 89.2: Prenatal ultrasound image of UPJ stenosis at the 16th (left) and 20th (right) week; renal pelvis diameter >10 mm.

dilatations during pregnancy that clearly exceed this limit and remain beyond it urgently require postnatal observation and treatment. In these cases, diagnosis frequently shows the presence of an UPJ stenosis requiring surgery.[1-4]

Clinical Symptomatology

The clinical symptoms of a congenital UPJ stenosis present a broad spectrum, depending upon the point in time of diagnosis. The majority of stenoses of the UPJ diagnosed prenatally by means of US show no symptoms either clinically or paraclinically. The newborns show no clinical signs of hydronephrosis. The diagnostic indication here is a conspicuous postnatal ultrasound image of the kidney associated with a prenatally determined dilatation of the renal pelvis.

In the age of prenatal diagnostics, general symptoms, such as poor growth, refusal to feed, recurring vomiting, and agitation, are usually not observed in connection with the stenosis because treatment begins early enough; these symptoms are often observed only in connection with an infection of the urinary tract. If US examination is not possible, infections of the urinary tract are usually indicative and should lead to further diagnostic procedures. Due to early diagnosis and the resulting possibility of timely treatment with antibiotics, the incidence of urinary tract infections has declined significantly.

In cases where a UPJ stenosis is not diagnosed prenatally or neonatally, symptoms other than the general one mentioned above arise during the course of the disease: characteristic pains in the area of the kidneys, haematuria (in 30% of late diagnoses), palpable intraabdominal masses, and infections of the urinary tract. In severe cases, the patient can have classic symptoms of urosepsis.

Untreated unilateral UPJ obstructions result in a nonfunctional, hydronephrotic, sacculated kidney; as the loss of kidney function progresses, children with untreated bilateral UPJ obstructions begin to show symptoms of renal insufficiency.[5,6]

Diagnostics

Clinical Diagnostics

As with all illnesses, prior to imaging diagnostics, a thorough medical history and physical examination of the child have to be undertaken. Particular attention should be paid here to the urination history and the family history. There is no known hereditary chromosomal influence in UPJ obstruction, although there is familial clustering. Furthermore, there are no typical physical malformations that accompany UPJ obstruction. Complete blood and urine tests have to be carried out to determine or exclude any accompanying nephrological or urological conditions or an infection.

Imaging Diagnostics

The goal of imaging diagnosis in children is to obtain reliable results while causing the least possible stress to the child. The following imaging procedures are available for routine diagnosis of a disturbance in the transport system for urine:

- ultrasound;

- voiding cystourethrography (VCUG);

- renal function scintigraphy; and

- uro-magnetic resonance imagery (uro-MRI).

In recent years, excretion urography has been used only for special examinations due to its high level of x-ray exposure.

Diagnostic Procedure

Generally, the following investigations provide a reliable basis for deciding how to proceed with treatment:

- *clinical and paraclinical examination:* medical history, current status, blood and urine tests;

- *ultrasound investigation:* morphology of the urinary tract as initial examination and as a basis for future observation;

- *VCUG:* to exclude a vesicoureteral reflux; and

- *renal function scintigraphy:* technetium-99m mercaptuacetlytri- glysine (T-99m MAG3) scintigraphy to evaluate functional processes such as renal perfusion and the renal function of both sides separately, as well as to evaluate an existing obstruction and use of a furosemide load; and dimercaptosuccinic acid (DMSA) scintigraphy to evaluate perfusion, especially after recurring kidney infections.[7-9]

A UPJ obstruction requiring surgery is present when US regularly shows a renal pelvis dilatation of more than 10–15 mm, with progressive dilatation. In general, infections of the urinary tract in cases of UPJ obstruction arise late, so they do not represent an isolated indication for surgery.

The decisive investigation is renal function scintigraphy, which not only shows the renal function for both sides, but is especially important for determining the flow relationships in the urinary tract collection system. In the case of an obstruction, Figure 89.3 shows a mounting curve on the affected side. It is important to carry out the T-99m MAG3 scintigraphy investigation together with a furosemide investigation.

The main reason for VCUG is to exclude a vesicoureteral reflux, which is associated with a significantly higher incidence of urinary tract infection (UTI). The US image can show a dilatation of the renal pelvis with a mega-ureter. The scintigram in Figure 89.3 shows no obstructive influence on the urinary flow.

There are, however, cases with combined malformations showing a UPJ obstruction and a vesicoureteral reflux on the ipsilateral side.

A UPJ obstruction requiring surgery shows a clear dilatation of the renal pelvis and an obstructive mounting curve with functional scintigraphy on an accompanying furosemide investigation. With timely diagnosis and treatment, the normal division of renal function can be maintained. When there is a clear obstruction, corrective surgery should be carried out; without waiting until there are possible signs of a loss of renal function in the affected kidney shown in a follow-up scintigram. Multiple studies have demonstrated that renal function does not improve, even after normal urinary flow conditions have been restored.

For any uncertain issues that still exist—for example, the presence of different simultaneous renal malformations or of a tumour—imaging procedures such as CT or uro-MRI can be employed.

Should the investigations show no flow obstruction of the urinary tract, despite sonographically detected dilatation, the child should undergo periodic examinations and, if the dilatation of the renal pelvis progresses or UTIs develop, the diagnostic procedure should be repeated, as shown in the algorithm in Figure 89.4.

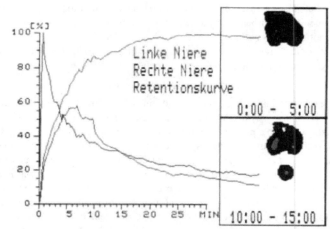

Figure 89.3: Renal function scintigraphy with a mounting curve for the left kidney, showing one obstructed curve (T-99m MAG3, furosemide investigation).

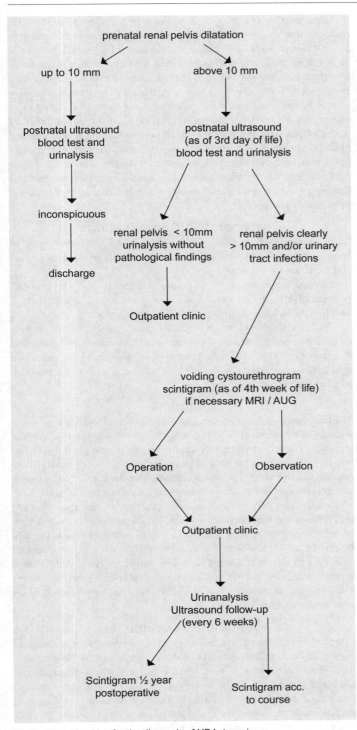

Figure 89.4. Algorithm for the diagnosis of UPJ stenosis.

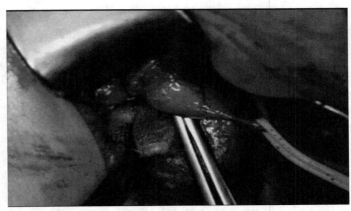

Figure 89.5: Surgical site intraoperative. The goal of all plastic-reconstructive surgical methods is the removal of the hindrance to the urinary flow with retention of the organ.

Treatment of a Congenital Ureteropelvic Junction Obstruction

The spectrum of treatment for a congenital UPJ obstruction reaches from conservative observation; to application of a temporary, percutaneous nephrostomy in acute emergency situations; to plastic reconstructive organ-preserving surgery methods; to the rare necessary excision of a nonfunctional organ.

All moderate renal pelvis dilatations for which the clinical, paraclinical, and imaging diagnoses have shown no further pathological condition beyond the dilatation—in particular, no obstruction with or without a loss of renal function—should be kept under regular US

observation in an outpatient clinic. In addition, regular urine and blood tests are necessary. Should UTIs occur, or should the US show an increase in the renal-pelvis calyceal system dilatation, a new series of urological imaging investigations should be carried out.

The goal of a temporary, percutaneous nephrostomy is immediate relief of the kidney, which is usually infected and painful due to the hydronephrosis. Normally, this is performed percutaneously under general anaesthesia, with US monitoring. This temporary drainage of urine results in a reduction in pain, allows an efficient antibiotic treatment of the infection, and enables an adequate diagnosis. The required surgical procedure can then be carried out on an organ that is not infected, and with the patient in the best possible general condition.

An indication for nephrectomy is given only when the renal parenchyma is so damaged by obstructive and/or infectious processes that the organ has become functionally worthless. The decision to perform a nephrectomy can be made only after thorough diagnostic evaluation and the reliable demonstration that the kidney is no longer functional. With acute hydronephrosis, especially in early infancy, it is advisable, after primary percutaneous relief of the kidney, to perform a renal function scintigraphy examination once again. In the literature, renal function below 10% is frequently given as an indication for nephrectomy.

Surgical techniques can be divided into those that involve resection and those that do not. Due to the relatively high rate of recurrence, the nonresectional flap techniques have not found acceptance internationally. In Figure 89.5, the stenotic region at the ureter junction is left in place and is extended by means of a folded-in ureteral flap.

In recent decades, resectional surgical techniques—in particular, that of Anderson-Hynes[10,11]—have gained acceptance. Common to all resectional methods is removal of the dysplastic portion of the ureter followed by a microsurgical anastomosis to connect the renal pelvis and the ureter. The Anderson-Hynes technique is seen today as standard. It can be carried out both in open surgery and—with older children, from around age 24 months—laparoscopically.[10,11] Once there is a surgical indication, the operation should be carried out regardless of the age of the child. Figures 89.6 to 89.8 show the essential steps in the Anderson-Hynes procedure.

Especially with small children, conventional open surgical retroperitoneal-dorsal access is usually preferred, for example, access according to the Bergmann-Israel procedure. After freeing the kidney, the renal pelvis, and the ureter, the dysplastic constriction at the ureter junction with the prestenotic dilated renal pelvis can be clearly seen. After placement of retention stitches, the resection of the ureter restriction is undertaken, together with a small part of the dilated renal pelvis, in order to avoid a Windkessel function postoperatively. Then the renal pelvis-ureter anatomosis is sutured continuously microsurgically by using thin, absorbable suture material corresponding to the age of the child (e.g., vicryl 6-0 or 7-0).

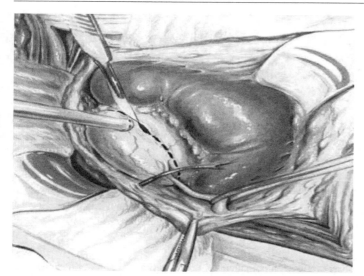

Figure 89.6: Resection line renal pelvis, ureter identified by ligature pelvic junction obstruction.

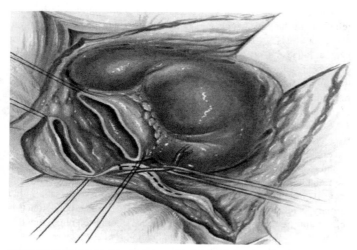

Figure 89.7: Resection line: ureter-renal pelvis cut through.

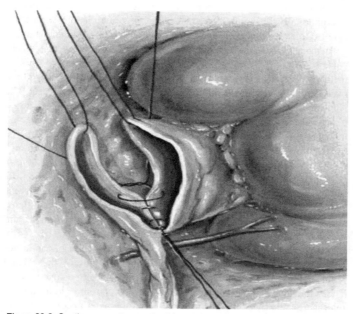

Figure 89.8: Continuous ureter-renal pelvis anastomosis with inserted pyelostomy.

Intraoperative insertion of a pyelostomy or a ureteral stent for postoperative securing and splinting of the anastomosis can be carried out in different ways. Both methods and whether they should be used at all are subjects of debate. If the surgeon decides to install a pyelostomy, it should be removed between the 7th and 10th postoperative day. Before its removal, the pyelostomy enables one to monitor the flow control of the anastomosis by means of x-ray contrast imaging or to influence the flow by a temporary "training" of the anastomosis by means of pinching it off for a time and then releasing it. For removal of an intraoperatively inserted, double-J ureteral stent about 3 months postoperative, a cystoscopy under general anaesthesia is required.

According to the international literature, a completely drainage-free surgery shows no inferior results—in particular, no higher rate of anastomosis leakage.[12,13]

Postoperative Complications

During the immediate postoperative phase, the focus with regard to complications is on anastomosis leakages, swelling of the anastomosis with resultant backflow of urine, and UTIs.

Intraoperative insertion of drain serves to reduce pressure postoperatively in the area of the anastomosis and can prevent a backflow or leakage of urine, which aids in recovery.

The patient should be protected against possible postoperative infections by perioperative and postoperative intravenous administration of antibiotics. This is carried out either on the basis of a antibiotic sensitivity or by using a wide-spectrum antibiotic such as cefuroxime, adapted for weight.

Outcome

The long-term results of the Anderson-Hynes procedure are very good, with the rate of recurrence of a stenosis being 3–5% in the international literature. The most frequent reason for a new operation is the development of a stenosis in the area of the anastomosis. In rare cases, suture granulomas or connective tissue accretions in the area of the surgery, which narrow or deform the pelviureteric junction, can be found.

Decisive for the success of the operation is not the complete reduction of the renal pelvis dilatation but the free, unobstructed flow of urine, as shown by scintigraphy. This follow-up investigation should be carried out 6 months to 1 year after surgery. All children operated on for a UPJ obstruction must remain in outpatient care. At the outset, regular urinalysis and US examinations should be carried out every 4 to 6 weeks. If no complications arise, the time between follow-up examinations can be extended.[14–19]

Concluding Comments

Congenital UPJ stenosis is a pathological condition of the genitourinary system that can be detected early on during pregnancy by US examination. These early prenatal signs make possible a timely diagnosis and treatment postnatally. Only in very severe cases does the condition result in a complete loss of the kidney and serious complications, despite timely treatment. As a rule, given timely diagnosis and the indicated treatment, it is possible to maintain kidney function at the level of the point in time of surgery without further complications.

Evidence-Based Research

Table 89.1 presents a landmark retrospective review of 1,000 children with hydronephrosis. Table 89.2 presents a natural history series of children with severe antenatal hydronephrosis managed nonoperatively.

Table 89.1: Evidence-based research.

Title	Prenatally diagnosed hydronephrosis: the Great Ormond Street experience
Authors	Dhillon HK
Institution	Great Ormond Street Hospital for Sick Children, London, United Kingdom
Reference	Br J Urol 1998; 81(suppl 2):39–44
Problem	Natural history series of 1,000 children with antenatal hydronephrosis.
Intervention	Anderson-Hynes pyeloplasty.
Comparison/ control (quality of evidence)	Retrospective review.
Outcome/ effect	Demonstrated the essentially benign nature of antenatally picked hydronephrosis. Only 5% of children with an AP measurement of <20 mm required pyeloplasty.
Historical significance/ comments	Landmark paper

Table 89.2: Evidence-based research.

Title	The long-term follow-up of newborns with severe unilateral hydronephrosis initially treated nonoperatively
Authors	Ulman I, Jayanthi VR, Koff SA
Institution	The Ohio State University, Columbus, Ohio, USA
Reference	J Urol 2000; 164:1101–1105
Problem	Natural history series of children with severe antenatal hydronephrosis managed nonoperatively.
Intervention	Nonoperative.
Comparison/ control (quality of evidence)	Retrospective review.
Outcome/ effect	Highlights the benign nature of most cases of antenatal hydronephrosis, but close follow-up is required to pick up children needing pyeloplasty.
Historical significance/ comments	Excellent natural history series.

Key Summary Points

1. Congenital hydronephrosis is the most common cause of a palpable neonatal abdominal mass, of which ureteropelvic junction obstruction is the most likely cause.

2. Not all dilatation seen on ultrasound and thought to be due to a ureteropelvic junction obstruction requires surgery.

3. True ureteropelvic junction obstruction must be attended by worsening dilatation on sonar and declining renal scan function.

4. An open dismembered pyeloplasty (Anderson-Hynes technique) offers excellent surgical outcomes.

References

1. Onen A, Jayanthi VR, Koff SA. Long-term follow-up of prenatally detected severe bilateral newborn hydronephrosis initially managed nonoperatively. J Urol 2002; 168:1118–1120.

2. Chertin B, Fridmans A, Knizhnik M, et al. Does early detecction of ureteropelvic junction obstruction improve surgical outcome in terms of renal function? J Urol 1999; 162:1037–1040.

3. Koff SA. The prenatal diagnosis of hydronephrosis: when and why not to operate? Arch Esp Urol 1998; 51:569–574.

4. Gonzalez FN, Lara DZ, Calleja LA. Fetal hydronephrosis. Case report and literature review. Glinecol Obstet Mex 2008; 76:487–492.

5. Rosen S, Peter CA, Chevalier RL, Huang WY. The kidney in congenital ureteropelvic junction obstruction: a spectrum from normal to nephrectomy. J Urol 2008; 179:1257–1263. Published online 20 February 2008.

6. Ulman I, Jayanthi VR, Koff SA. The long-term follow-up of newborns with severe unilateral hydronephrosis initially treated nonoperatively. J Urol 2000; 164:1101–1105.

7. Tan BJ, Smith AD. Ureteropelvic junction obstruction repair: when, how, what? Curr Opin Urol 2004; 14:55–59.

8. Tripathi M, Kumar R, Chandrashekar N, et al. Diuretic radionuclide renography in assessing Anderson-Hynes pyeloplasty in unilateral pelviureteric junction obstruction. Hell J Nucl Med 2005; 8:154–157.

9. Thomas DF. Prenatnatally diagnosed urinary tract abnormalities: long-term outcome. Semin Fetal Neonatal Ned 2008; 13:189–195. Published online 26 November 2007.

10. Lam PN, Wong C, Mulholland TL, et al. Pediatric laparoscopic pyeloplasty: 4-year experience. J Endourol 2007; 21:1467–1471.

11. Piaggio LA, Franc-Guimond J, Noh PH, et al. Transperitoneal laparoscopic pyeloplasty for primary repair of ureteropelvic junction obstruction in infants and children: comparison with open surgery. J Urol 2007;178:1579–1583. Published online 16 August 2007.

12. Elmalik K, Chowdhury MM, Capps SN. Ureteric stents in pyeloplasty: a help or a hindrance? J Pediatr Urol 2008; 4:275–279. Published online 7 March 2008.

13. Smith KE, Holmes N, Lieb JI, et al. Stented versus nonstented pediatric pyeloplasty: a modern series and review of the literature. J Urol 2002; 168:1127–1130.

14. Castagnetti M, Novara G, Beniamin F, et al. Scintigraphic renal function after unilateral pyeloplasty in children: a systematic review. BJU Int 2008; 102:862–868. Published online 11 March 2008.

15. McAleer IM, Kaplan GW. Renal function before and after pyeloplasty: does it improve? J Urol 1999; 162:1041–1044.

16. Zaffanello M, Ceccetto M, Brugnara M, et al. Pelvi-ureteric junction obstruction and renal function after pyeloplasty: a retrospective study in 29 children. Minerva Urol Nefrol 2008; 60:1–6.

17. Shokeir AA, El-Sherbiny MT, Gad HM, et al. Postnatal unilateral pelviureteral junction obstruction: impact of pyeloplasty and conservative management on renal function. Urology 2005; 65:980–985, discussion 985.

18. Boubaker A, Prior JO, Meyrat B, et al. Unilateral ureteropelvic junction obstruction in children: long-term follow-up after unilateral pyeloplasty. J Urol 2003; 170:575–579, discussion 579.

19. van den Hoek J, de Jong A, Scheepe J, et al. Prolonged follow-up after paediatric pyeloplasty: are repeat scans necessary? BJU Int 2007; 100 (5):1150–1152. Epub 29 May 2007.

CHAPTER 90
URETERIC DUPLICATIONS AND URETEROCOELES

V. T. Joseph

Introduction

Duplications of the ureter represent one of the most common anomalies of the urinary tract. Duplications may be complete or incomplete and can be associated with functioning renal moieties with orifices that open into the bladder. Duplications are often completely asymptomatic and often come to light only in the course of investigations for other reasons. Clinical problems are the result of obstruction, reflux, or ectopic openings, giving rise to hydronephrosis, infection, and incontinence. Antenatal diagnosis provides useful information for postnatal evaluation with a view to preserving renal function, when appropriate, or removing dysplastic components that potentially may cause infection and compromise the other elements of the renal tract.

Embryology

The ureteric bud develops from the wolffian (mesonephric) duct between 4 to 8 weeks in utero from a point just proximal to the junction with the cloaca. It elongates in a cranial direction to reach and penetrate the metanephric intermediate mesoderm to induce the formation of the kidney. The portion of the wolffian duct distal to the ureteric bud is called the common excretory duct. The common excretory duct is absorbed into the urogenital sinus to form the trigone, fusing with its component of the opposite side. The opening of the wolffian duct ends at the utricle, and the duct gives rise to the prostate, seminal vesicles, vas deferens, and epididymis. In females, the wolffian duct eventually undergoes involution but may persist as a Gartner's duct.

Abnormalities of Development

A large number of different types of anomalies of the ureteric bud exist. The ureteric bud may be atretic and fail to reach the metanephric mesoderm, giving rise to a multicystic dysplastic kidney. Or the ureteric bud may originate from a site other than its normal position on the mesonephric duct, giving rise to ectopia. The orifice may lie in the bladder but lateral or caudal to the normal site. The orifice may also lie outside the bladder, in the urethral, vestibular, vaginal, or vassal positions.

In males, ectopic ureters drain proximal to the urinary sphincter and hence wetting is not evident. In females, ectopic ureters discharge into the genital tract where they bypass the urinary sphincter, thus causing the classic pattern of wetting associated with normal voiding. Three circumstances associate ectopic ureters with wetting:

- The ectopic orifice is distal to the midpoint of the urethra (females only).

- The ectopic orifice is in the vagina (rare) or vestibule (common).

- The ectopic orifice is in the urethra but the hiatus where the ureter enters into the bladder wall is at the bladder neck and disrupts the sphincter, causing incontinence.

Ureteric Duplications

Ureteric duplications occur either due to bifurcation of a single ureter or when two ureteric buds arise from the wolffian duct. Single ureteric bifurcation may result in a whole spectrum of anomalies, ranging from bifid pelvis to almost complete duplication down to the intramural part of the ureter. Complete duplication occurs when two ureteric buds arise from the mesonephric duct and meet the metanephric mesoderm at separate points, thus giving rise to duplex kidneys.

In complete duplication, the cranially positioned bud reaches the upper portion of the mesoderm and the caudally positioned bud reaches the lower portion. However, at the bladder end, the relationships become more complex, owing to the tissue migration and incorporation into the outflow tract. When the buds are close to each other, the ureteric orifices are in the bladder in the normal position. When the buds are widely separated, the orifices may be ectopic. In such situations, the lower pole ureter (LPU) inserts normally and the upper pole ureter (UPU) crosses it anteriorly in the lower third and inserts ectopically (Weigert-Meyer law). The UPU is normally dilated and tortuous and is connected to dysplastic upper moiety. The lower end of the ureter is usually stenotic, causing obstruction, or may be associated with a ureterocoele. The LPU is usually of normal calibre but may be associated with vesicoureteric reflux.

Ureterocoeles

Ureterocoeles represent a cystic dilatation of the lower end of the ureter. The aetiology of ureterocoeles is not clear; it has been proposed that they result from the persistence of Chwalla's membrane or as a result of deficiency of the muscle in the distal ureter. They may be classified in several ways; the simplest system is to regard them as either intravesical or extravesical. In each category, additional features can be described as follows:

- *Stenotic:* The orifice is very tiny and difficult to identify.

- *Sphincteric:* The orifice is situated within the urethral sphincter zone.

- *Caecoureterocoele:* There is a caudal extension in the submucosal plane of the urethra.

- *Blind ureterocoele:* There is atrophy of the ureter distal to the ureterocoele.

Clinical Presentation

Routine antenatal maternal ultrasonography (US) can identify most urinary tract abnormalities. Currently, two-dimensional US is employed in routine screening with detection rates as high as 88%. The 20-week anomaly scan is designed to detect major foetal abnormalities as part of the foetal anatomical survey. US is highly observer-dependent, so the success of the screening program depends as much on the training of the professionals as on the quality of the equipment.

In ureteric duplications, the most common US findings are those of hydronephrosis and hydroureter. These findings are not specific and require postnatal evaluation to define the anomaly. Bladder outlet obstruction due to ureterocoeles presents with signs similar to posterior urethral valves and requires postnatal investigation with micturating cystourethrography to establish the cause.

Postnatal presentations are related to obstruction, infection, and urinary incontinence. Specifically:

- Acute obstruction occurs at the bladder outflow tract and is caused by ectopic ureterocoeles extending into the urethra. This represents the most common cause of bladder outlet obstruction in girls and is the second most common cause in boys after posterior urethral valves. The clinical presentation is that of a distended, palpable bladder with failure to pass urine.

- A prolapsing ureterocoele presents as a purplish mass protruding from the urethral orifice, showing congestion and oedema. The urethral opening can usually be identified and catheterised.

- Obstruction can also lead to hydronephrosis, which in severe cases presents with an abdominal mass.

- Urinary tract infection (UTI) occurs in 50% of cases. Patients present with flank pain and fever, indicating a pyelonephritis. This may also be associated with failure to thrive and nonspecific abdominal pain.

- Acute epididymo-orchitis in male infants may be the presentation of an ectopic ureter. Clinically, the child presents with an acute scrotum which is indistinguishable from torsion, and the diagnosis is made only on exploration.

- Incontinence in girls may be a manifestation of ectopic ureters opening outside the bladder. The typical history is that of voiding normally but wetting between voids. The degree of wetting may vary from slight dampness to significant leaks. Many cases are diagnosed as bladder dysfunction, and the true condition may remain undetected until later years, particularly after pregnancy.

Diagnosis

Ultrasound

The investigation of choice in the initial evaluation of ureteric duplications and ureterocoeles is the US scan, which includes complete evaluation of the kidneys, ureters, and bladder. The postnatal scan should be delayed for up to a week in the newborn because the relative state of dehydration at birth may mask some urinary tract abnormalities. However, in urgent situations, the scans should be conducted as soon as possible. Further investigations then can be used to follow up the findings. The kidney may show hydronephrosis of varying severity; in a duplex kidney, this may be confined to one moiety, thus making the diagnosis easy. In nondilated duplex systems, US scans do not show a clear demarcation of the two moieties, and thus other imaging techniques may be required.

Massive dilatation of the ureter is easily identified on US; it may be an obstructed ureter usually draining the upper moiety or a refluxing ureter to the lower moiety. Ectopic ureters can sometimes be identified passing behind and below the bladder, but it is not possible to determine the location of its opening with ultrasound.

US is the best modality for identifying ureterocoeles. These are visualised as cystic protrusions into the bladder; sometimes, urinary jets may be seen from their orifices.

Micturating Cystourethrogram

A micturating cystourethrogram (MCUG) involves filling the bladder with x-ray contrast media via a catheter under fluoroscopy. It is carried out in all cases where US has demonstrated a dilated upper tract or the presence of a ureterocoele (Figures 90.1 and 90.2). The MCUG may show reflux into the lower moiety of a duplex system and thus delineate the dilated ureter. However, where US shows a dilated ureter and MCUG shows either no reflux or reflux with a normal calibre ureter, the interpretation is that the dilated ureter is associated with the upper moiety. In this situation, further investigations are necessary.

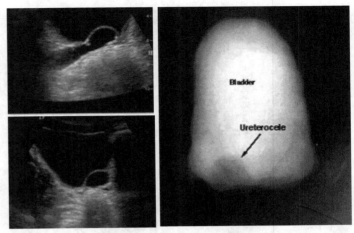

Figure 90.1: US scan (left) and MCUG (right), showing ureterocoele.

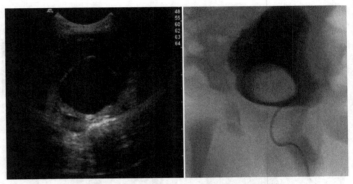

Figure 90.2: Large ureterocoele causing bladder outlet obstruction.

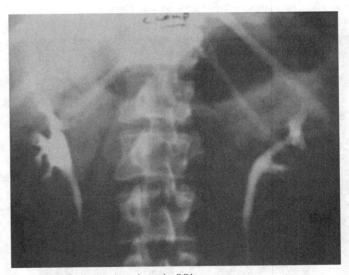

Figure 90.3: Duplex system shown by IVU.

Intravenous Urography and Magnetic Resonance Urography

Until recently, intravenous urography (IVU) was the only radiological method of demonstrating the renal elements in duplication anomalies (Figure 90.3). Because the upper moiety is frequently dysplastic with poor function it was not possible to visualise it with contrast. Instead, radiological signs such as the absent upper calyx, displacement of the lower moiety, and indentation of the lower moiety ureter were used to infer the presence of a dilated upper moiety.

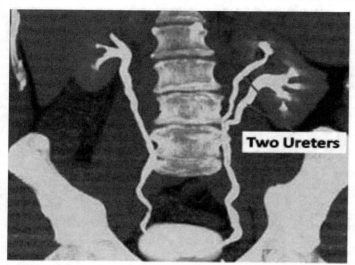

Figure 90.4: Bifid system on MRU.

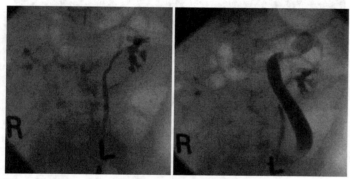

Figure 90.5: Retrograde pyelogram showing duplex system.

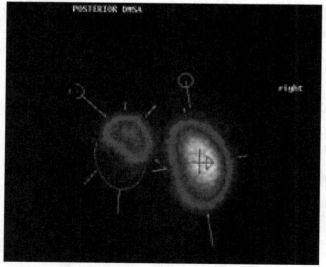

Figure 90.6: DMSA scan showing nonfunctioning lower moeity on the left.

The introduction of magnetic resonance urography (MRU; Figure 90.4) has made a dramatic difference in imaging the renal tract. It is now possible to sequentially image the entire upper tract and follow the ureter all the way down to the bladder and beyond. Even ectopic ureters can be traced down almost to where they actually open, thus providing vital information for the surgeon.

Cystoscopy

Cystoscopy is carried out in all cases of ueterocoeles and duplications presenting clinically with symptoms relating to obstruction, infection, and incontinence. A single ureteric orifice on the side of the duplication indicates the presence of an ectopic ureter. This can be further confirmed by doing a retrograde study (Figure 90.5) via the single opening to demonstrate that it is associated with one ureter going only to the lower pole. A careful search of the bladder neck area will usually reveal the ectopic ureteric opening. Careful examination of the vulva/ vestibule area in the female may occasionally show the ectopic opening and allow contrast examination to be performed.

Dimercaptosuccinic Acid Scan

The dimercaptosuccinic acid (DMSA) scan (Figure 90.6) is useful because the isotope is taken up only by functioning renal tissue. Thus, even a small dysplastic upper moiety may be visualised and the presence of renal scarring can also be assessed. This information is useful when a decision has to be made regarding nephroureterectomy in duplex systems.

Management

The principles of management in duplications of the upper urinary tract are based on a thorough evaluation of the symptoms and pathophysiological changes in the systems.

Each case has to be considered individually. Most duplications of the upper urinary tract are incomplete, and the majority are asymptomatic, being discovered only in the course of investigation for some other complaint. These cases do not need any further intervention. Complete duplications are often associated with clinical problems that require active intervention. The following guidelines are just a framework for detailed assessments.

Vesicoureteric Reflux

Urinary tract infections are often associated with vesicoureteric reflux into the lower moiety of a duplex system. (Vesicoureteric reflux is described in more detail in Chapter 91.) Rarely, reflux can also occur into the upper or both moieties. The clinical presentation is that of pyelonephritis with fever, loin pain and tenderness, dysuria, and a culture positive urine. Children with these symptoms can be very ill and need hospitalisation for administration of intravenous antibiotics and fluid resuscitation. A broad-spectrum antibiotic such as coamoxiclav is combined with one providing gram-negative cover, such as gentamycin, and treatment must be given until there is complete resolution of the UTI. The reflux needs to be treated, which can be done by cystoscopy—an on-table cystogram with endoscopic submucosal injection of Deflux®. If this technique fails to stop reflux, then reimplantation of the ureter will have to be done. This often means reimplantation of both ureters because they can be very close and even share a common sheath. In this situation, careful evaluation of the upper moiety function should be made preoperatively to decide whether preservation of this renal element is justifiable.

Obstruction

In some cases where infection occurs in an obstructed system, it is necessary to provide urgent drainage in addition to antibiotic therapy. This can be done by US-assisted percutaneous drainage if facilities are available, or by open nephrostomy. Following this, the anatomy and functional state of the affected moiety must be clearly assessed and a decision made as to the further surgical procedure that would be required. If sufficient renal function is present, the obstruction is dealt with by the appropriate method. This usually involves reimplantation of the lower end of the ureter into the bladder because most often that is the site of the obstruction. Difficulty may arise when a dilated, nonobstructed system is present. In this case, conservative treatment with stenting by using a double-J stent and prophylactic antibiotics would be an option. The stent is left in for a prolonged period of 3 to 6 months, and periodic assessments need to be made during this time, usually with US. This method has yielded remarkable results in a number of cases with significant reduction in upper tract dilatation. If conservative management fails and recurrent infections are a problem, the only definitive treatment is nephroureterectomy of the affected moiety.

Obstruction is usually associated with ureterocoeles and is considered next in that context.

Ureterocoeles

Single-system ureterocoeles are more common in boys than girls and are confined to within the bladder. They may obstruct the bladder outlet and can be confused with posterior urethral valves. They may also cause obstruction to the upper tract, although this is not common, and are known to be associated with recurrent UTIs. The treatment of choice is endoscopic incision, which is done with a fine electrode introduced through the cystoscope. The ureterocoele collapses and may not even be visible on subsequent imaging. Excision with reimplantation of the ureter is rarely indicated for this lesion.

Duplex-system ureterocoeles are associated with the upper moiety and can cause obstruction to the bladder outlet, the lower moiety ureter, and prolapse through the urethra in girls, sometimes appearing as a reddish-purple swelling at the urethral orifice. The initial management in all these cases is cystoscopy and incision of the ureterocoele. Subsequently, full investigations are carried out to determine renal tract anatomy and function.

A duplex-system ureterocoele associated with very poorly functioning upper moiety is best treated by upper pole nephroureterectomy, leaving the distal stump of ureter and ureterocoele behind. This usually does not cause any further problems.

When both upper and lower moieties have satisfactory renal function, the procedure of choice is excision of the ureterocoele and reimplantation of the ureters. With large ureterocoeles, the underlying bladder wall may be deficient and needs to be repaired to prevent diverticulum formation. Excision of the urethral lip of the ureterocoele has to be complete to avoid leaving a rim of tissue that can cause obstruction to outflow. At the same time, great care has to be taken to ensure that the sphincter musculature is not damaged. If both moieties have poor renal function, then nephrectomy and removal of as much of the ureters as possible is performed.

In some cases, it may be necessary to carry out complete excision of the upper moiety, its ureter, and the ureterocoele to achieve a satisfactory result. This operation also often requires reimplantation of the lower moiety ureter. Previously, this kind of surgery required the use of separate incisions for the kidney and bladder parts of the procedure. However, with technological advances in minimally invasive surgery, it is now possible to do this operation with suitably placed ports by using an intraperitoneal or retroperitoneal approach.

Evidence-Based Research

Table 90.1 presents a retrospective study of the long-term effectiveness of endoscopic puncture of a ureterocoele in children.

Table 90.1: Evidence-based research.

Title	Endoscopic puncture of ureterocele as a minimally invasive and effective long-term procedure in children
Authors	Chertin B, Fridmans A, Hadas-Halpren I, Farkas A
Institution	Department of Urology, Shaare Zedek Medical Center, Jerusalem, Israel
Reference	Eu Urol 2001; 39(3):332–336
Problem	Over a period of years, the surgical approach to ureterocele has evolved from complicated major surgery to minimally invasive endoscopic treatment. Because of the high rate of secondary surgery in some recently reported series, an upper pole partial nephrectomy is again recommended as the procedure of choice.
Intervention	A retrospective evaluation of the long-term results of endoscopic puncture of a ureterocele and its long-term effectiveness and applicability in children.
Comparison/ control (quality of evidence)	Over the past 8 years, 34 patients (20 female, 14 male) were treated with primary endoscopic puncture of a ureterocele. The mean age of the patients was 1.1 ± 4.3 (mean ± SD) years. Mean follow-up was 6.1 ± 2.4 years. Antenatal ultrasound detected the ureterocele in 5 (14%) patients, foetal hydronephrosis leading to the postnatal diagnosis in 13 (38%); 16 (48%) children presented with symptoms of urinary tract infection (UTI). The ureteroceles presented as part of renal duplication in 31 (91%) patients, 3 (9%) in a single system, and 1 had bilateral ureteroceles of a duplex system. Twenty (58%) children had intravesical ureteroceles, and the remaining 14 (42%) had ectopic ureteroceles. Very poorly functioning upper pole moiety presented in 26 (75%) of the cases, and nonfunctioning upper poles in 5 (14%). Twenty of 34 (58%) children had initial vesicoureteric reflux (VUR) to the lower moiety, either to the ipsi- (60%) or contralateral kidney (40%). A cold knife incision was carried out in 4 (11.7%), puncture by a 3-Fr Bugbee electrode in 20 (58%), and the stylet of a 3-Fr ureteral catheter was utilized to puncture the ureterocele in the remaining 10 patients (30.3%).
Outcome/ effect	Complete decompression of the ureterocele was observed in 32 of 34 (94%) children. Two patients required secondary puncture two years following the primary procedure and are doing well. Upper pole moiety function improved postoperatively in 2 infants and remained stable in all 32 patients; no patient presented with deterioration of the renal function. Six of 20 (30%) patients who had initial VUR to the lower pole, accompanied with recurrent UTI, required surgery. Three underwent ureteric reimplantation and another 3 submucosal polytetrafluoroethylene paste (Teflon®) injection. Eight (40%) patients presented with spontaneous resolution of VUR to the lower moiety following puncture of the ureterocele. An additional 6 (17.6%) patients developed VUR to the upper moiety following the puncture of the ureterocele, 3 after cold knife incision and 3 after simple puncture. In 2, submucosal Teflon injection solved the VUR; the remaining 4 patients were maintained on prophylactic antibiotics. In 1 child, the reflux resolved spontaneously, and no patient presented with UTI. In 2 cases with nonfunctional upper poles, partial nephrectomy was performed due to symptomatic UTI one and two years following the initial puncture, respectively, in spite of complete collapse of the ureterocele. No difference was observed in the reoperation rate between the patients with ectopic versus intravesical ureteroceles (p < 0.05).
Historical significance/ comments	Endoscopic puncture of a ureterocele presents an easily performed procedure that allows the release of obstructive ureters and avoids major surgery in the majority of cases, even after a long follow-up.

Key Summary Points

1. Duplications of the renal tract are often diagnosed on antenatal ultrasound scans.

2. Incomplete duplications rarely cause problems and do not require intervention.

3. Complete duplications may be associated with infection, obstruction, or incontinence.

4. Recurrent urinary tract infections associated with reflux into the lower moiety require an endoscopic antireflux procedure, which involves submucosal injection of Deflux® at the ureteric orifice.

5. Obstruction with very poor renal function is best treated by upper pole heminephroureterectomy.

6. Obstruction and infection presenting acutely with pyonephrosis is treated initially with drainage and subsequently according to the renal function present.

7. Ectopic ureters in the male are single system and open above the sphincteric zone. Hence, males do not experience the symptom of wetting but can present with epididymo-orchitis. Renal function is usually preserved, and the treatment is reimplantation of the ureter into the bladder.

8. Ectopic ureters in the female may open either above or below the sphincteric zone. They are often associated with duplex systems and can present with the symptom of wetting in spite of normal voiding. In most cases, the renal element has very poor function and the treatment is excision of the upper pole with its ureter.

9. Ureterocoeles are easily diagnosed on ultrasound and initially are best managed with endoscopic incision.

10. Surgical intervention is required if further problems relating to obstruction or infection continue to be present. In such cases, if renal function is preserved, the treatment of choice is excision of the ureterocoele and reimplantation of the ureter.

11. If the renal element has poor renal function, the treatment will be nephrectomy of the upper moiety and ureter, leaving the distal stump behind. In some cases, however, it will be necessary to carry out complete excision of the upper moiety, ureter, and ureterocoele.

Suggested Reading

Brueziere J. Ureteroceles. Ann Urol (Paris) 1992; 26:202–211.

Castagnetti M, El-Ghooeimi A. Management of duplex system ureteroceles in neonates and infants. Nat Rev Urol 2009; 6:307–315.

Chertin B, de Caluwe D, Puri P. Is primary endoscopic puncture of ureterocele a long-term effective procedure? J Pediatr Surg 2003; 38:116–119.

Merilini E, Lelli Chiesa P. Obstructive ureterocoele—an ongoing challenge. World J Urol 2004; 22:107–114.

CHAPTER 91
VESICOURETERIC REFLUX

Sarah Howles
Rowena Hitchcock

Introduction

Vesicoureteric reflux (VUR) is a common childhood condition that can be defined as the retrograde passage of urine from the bladder to the upper urinary tract due to the failure of the vesicoureteric junction (VUJ) to act as a one-way valve. This retrograde flow of urine predisposes sufferers to acute pyelonephritis by allowing bacteria to travel from the bladder to the usually sterile upper tracts. Pyelonephritis can lead to renal scarring (reflux nephropathy), which can progress to cause hypertension and renal impairment. In some cases, end-stage renal failure may ensue.

Demographics

Although VUR is common, its overall prevalence is difficult to quantify because many sufferers are asymptomatic, and invasive investigation leading to diagnosis is carried out only when clinically indicated. Studies carried out from the 1950s to the 1970s on healthy children suggest that up to 1.8% of newborns suffer from VUR.[1] More recently, it is has been shown that approximately one-third of children with urinary tract infection (UTI) will suffer from this condition.[2]

VUR has a well-recognised genetic component, although the mode of inheritance remains unclear. If a child suffers from VUR, there is a 34% chance that infant siblings will also have this condition. In addition, VUR has been shown to be present in 20–66% of the offspring of affected parents.[3]

VUR demonstrates important gender differences, with girls being more likely to suffer than boys. However, girls tend to present later than boys (2–7 years versus 0–2 years) with lower-grade reflux, often of a functional aetiology. Anatomical factors are more important in the aetiology of male disease.[4]

A study from the United States investigating the incidence of VUR in children with specific reference to age, gender, and race found that younger children are more likely to suffer from VUR than older children, that girls are twice as likely to be affected as boys, and that white children are three times more likely to have VUR than black children.[5]

Aetiologies

Vesicoureteric Reflux

VUR can be classified as being either primary or secondary in nature. Primary VUR is the product of an anatomical abnormality at the VUJ, and secondary VUR is due to abnormally high pressures within the bladder, causing an incompetent VUJ during voiding.

Note, however, that this traditional distinction between primary and secondary VUR may be an oversimplification. A proportion of patients will have a "borderline" incompetent VUJ with a degree of voiding dysfunction (such as detrusor-sphincter dyssynergia), and these two factors will act together to cause VUR. Additionally, in the first two years of life, intravesical voiding pressures are much higher than they are when the urinary system matures. These falling pressures will also contribute to the natural resolution of VUR that is seen in some cases.

Primary VUR

In the normal urinary system, a passive flap-valve mechanism prevents retrograde passage of urine from the bladder into the upper urinary tract, even at the increased pressures experienced during voiding. This valve mechanism is created by the terminal ureter travelling obliquely from the bladder wall to the trigone in an intramural and then submucosal tunnel. This enables the pressure of urine within the bladder to compress the distal ureter against the detrusor muscle and close the distal ureter as the bladder fills and then empties. The compliance of this valve depends on the length and angle of the intramural tunnel, the bladder wall thickness and tone and the site of the ureteric orifice.

In primary VUR, this valve mechanism fails with a ureter that is characteristically sited laterally and opens on the base of the bladder rather than the trigone. This shortens the intramural and submucosal portion of the distal ureter and alters the position of the ureteric orifice, resulting in reflux. Anatomical measurements suggest that the ratio of tunnel length to ureteral diameter must be at least 5:1 to prevent reflux. This observation is fundamental to almost all surgical procedures to correct the disorder. As a child grows, both the absolute and relative lengths of the submucosal tunnel increase, explaining the spontaneous resolution of VUR that is seen in some cases.

An inadequacy or absence of muscle support of the tunnel due to a local or generalised detrusor weakness, or an abnormal configuration of the ureteral orifice, can also cause primary VUR.

Secondary VUR

Secondary VUR is associated with such conditions as neuropathic bladder or posterior urethral valves, in which an elevated intravesical pressure causes retrograde passage of urine from the bladder to the upper urinary tract. Therefore, the initial management of VUR in these cases should always be to correct the underlying associated abnormality, for example, bladder augmentation to reduce pressures in the neuropathic bladder. If VUR still persists, specific surgical intervention to reduce VUR can then be carried out.

Reflux Nephropathy

Reflux nephropathy can be the result of (1) upper tract infections or (2) abnormal renal development associated with VUR. These two forms of renal injury are not mutually exclusive, however—for example, acquired renal scarring can be superimposed on congenital renal dysplasia. If a critical amount of renal parenchyma is affected, hypertension, renal insufficiency, and renal failure can result. Reflux nephropathy accounts for 5–12% of the cases of end-stage renal failure (ESRF) in North America, New Zealand, and Europe.[6] There are limited data regarding the causes of ESRF in the African setting.

Infection

In the presence of VUR, infective organisms from the lower urinary tract can be transported to the renal collecting system and parenchyma. This can lead to pyelonephritis and scarring, especially in the presence of intrarenal reflux—a phenomenon by which the anatomy of renal papillae allows backflow of urine into the collecting ducts. The cascade of inflammation resulting from this infective process can result in local tissue ischaemia and fibrosis. The kidneys of children younger than 3 years of age seem to be particularly susceptible to damage in this way, which may be the result of reduced levels of such antioxidants as renal superoxide dismutase.

Congenital

Many children with VUR are found to suffer from renal damage at presentation. This was previously thought to be due to a single episode of pyelonephritis causing significant renal scarring—a theory named the "big bang" effect by Ransley and Risdon.[7] It has since become clear, however, that much of this damage is due to abnormal renal development in association with VUR. This renal dysplasia can be severe and may be due to defective interactions between the ureteric bud and metanephric blastema. These abnormal interactions may also result in the failure of the ureteric bud to migrate to its normal position, causing an ectopic ureter or incompetent ureteric orifice. In congenital renal dysplasia, a global reduction in functioning renal tissue tends to be seen in contrast to the focal, polar scarring seen due to infection.

Classification

The severity of VUR historically has been classified by the International Reflux Grading System on the basis of the degree of retrograde filling and dilatation of the renal collecting system seen on a voiding cystogram. This classification is as follows:

• *Grade I:* Reflux fills the ureter only without dilatation.

• *Grade II:* Reflux fills the ureter and collecting system without dilatation.

• *Grade III:* Reflux fills and mildly dilates the ureter and collecting system. There is mild blunting of the calyces.

• *Grade IV:* Reflux fills and moderately dilates the ureter and collecting system. There is mild blunting of the calyces.

• *Grade V:* Reflux fills and grossly dilates the ureter and collecting system. The ureter appears tortuous and there is severe blunting of the calyces.

More recently, there has been a trend to describe VUR as either dilating or nondilating, with or without cortical scarring or dysplasia. This newer classification enables description of VUR from high-resolution ultrasound (US) images and also fits better with the natural history of the disease.

Presentation

Prenatal Presentation

Antenatal ultrasound will detect dilatation of the upper urinary tract. Antenatal US is undertaken routinely in the West, and primary VUR accounts for at least 12% of the prenatal uropathies that are detected.[8] Male children are much more likely to suffer from prenatally diagnosed VUR, with a male-to-female ratio of 3:1.[9] Children diagnosed prenatally will often progress through evaluation and treatment without clinically significant illness.

Postnatal Presentation

The most common presentation of VUR remains symptomatic UTI, with girls being twice as likely as boys to present in this way. Unfortunately, UTI can be difficult to diagnose in children because the signs and symptoms are often nonspecific. It is important to maintain a high index of suspicion and consider UTI in any child with an unexplained fever. Other possible features include vomiting, diarrhoea, anorexia, lethargy, failure to thrive in infants, voiding symptoms in the older child, and abdominal pain (particularly loin pain in pyelonephritis).

Occasionally, advanced nephropathy leading to renal failure may be the presenting feature, especially in the African setting. This nephropathy can be the result of recurrent untreated upper UTI or secondary to congenital nephropathy. Renal failure may manifest with the symptoms of uraemia such as lethargy, itching, or nausea, or those of untreated hypertension such as congestive cardiac failure or headaches.

A family history may be suggestive of VUR, but a definitive diagnosis is impossible in the absence of imaging investigations.

Investigation

Imaging studies form the basis of diagnosis of VUR. In the United Kingdom, it is recommended that all children who suffer from a proven UTI go on to have renal tract ultrasonography and those with severe or recurrent UTIs are evaluated for VUR with micturating cystourethrogram (MCUG) and dimercaptosuccinic acid (DMSA) scintigraphy. In Africa, the decision to investigate may be modified in UTI associated with kwashiorkor. Kala has shown the prevalence of UTI in kwashiorkor to be 42% and in these patients US scans did not reveal renal tract pathology.[10]

Ultrasound

US is a commonly used, noninvasive, and relatively inexpensive investigation. Renal US allows assessment of renal tract dilatation, renal size, renal parenchyma, and visualisation of the bladder (Figure 91.1).

It is important, however, to appreciate that renal US has a high false-negative rate when used to investigate VUR. Many children with a renal tract that appears normal on ultrasound can be shown to suffer from reflux with the use of an MCUG, but even an MCUG will miss VUR in 3–9% of the cases.

Hydronephrosis in the presence of a dilated ureter is consistent with VUR, whereas hydronephrosis with a nondilated ureter would imply ureteropelvic junction obstruction. Observation of changes in hydronephrosis and hydroureter during and after voiding can be used to identify VUR noninvasively.

Renal size can be measured and followed over time to assess growth. Abnormal or dysplastic kidneys will tend to be smaller and appear brighter. Measurements of bladder wall thickness can be taken; incomplete bladder emptying may be observed in bladder dysfunction.

High-resolution US allows accurate assessment of the renal cortex and cortical loss, and split renal function can be estimated from a three-dimensional calculation of total cortical volume.

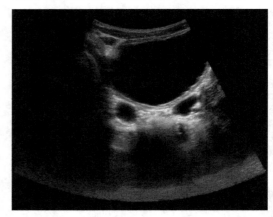

Figure 91.1: Transverse bladder view US scan showing thick-walled bladder with bilateral ureteric dilatation.

Micturating Cystourethrography

To perform an MCUG, the bladder is filled with contrast either urethrally or via suprapubic catheter. This allows the appearance of the ureters and urethra to be observed during voiding. This test also provides information regarding bladder capacity and emptying as well as revealing bladder trabeculation or diverticula, indicative of bladder outlet obstruction. Particular attention should be paid to the posterior urethra in boys to look for posterior urethral valves.

MCUG is the gold-standard investigation for the diagnosis of VUR and allows grading of the severity of disease (Figure 91.2). It is an invasive test, however, and should be performed only if the findings are likely to alter management. Additionally MCUG should be avoided during active UTI.

Dynamic Renography

A less invasive alternative to MCUG is dynamic renography using intra-venous radioactive mercaptoactyletrigylcerine (MAG3) or diethylene triamine pentaacetic acid (DTPA). However, to diagnose VUR, the child must be potty trained, and its use is therefore limited in the younger child, which is the age group most at risk of infective scarring. Dynamic renography is also less sensitive in diagnosing low-grade VUR and is therefore mainly used as a follow-up of VUR in the older child.

Dimercaptosuccinic Acid Scan

DMSA scintography is considered the best modality for assessing renal scarring and evaluating differential renal function (Figure 91.3). Persistent photopenic deficits, representing impaired tubular uptake of radionuclide isotope, correspond to renal scarring and irreversible renal damage. Diffuse decreased renal uptake may indicate renal dysplasia. This scan, however, does not provide any information regarding VUR itself.

Intravenous Urography

If DMSA is not available, intravenous urography (IVU) is an alternative method for assessing renal function, with a poorly functioning kidney showing reduced excretion of contrast.

Management

Medical Management

Many children with VUR are managed nonsurgically. The rationale for this is that in the absence of a UTI, there will be no further renal damage, and 50–85% of cases of mild to moderate VUR will spontaneously resolve.[11]

The initial treatment of UTI is discussed in all general paediatric care texts, such as the Nelson Textbook of Pediatrics,[12] but it should be noted that timely initiation of antibiotic therapy is crucial. Animal studies have suggested that permanent renal damage can occur in less than 72 hours.[13] Once this initial treatment has been completed, prophylactic antibiotics, such as trimethoprim (1–2 mg/kg per day), should be considered. Although prophylaxis is useful in some individual children, however, there is little evidence that it is effective in reducing infections or renal scarring, and prophylaxis is avoided in many countries.

Strategies to improve bladder dysfunction can also reduce VUR. Regular, timed voiding should be instituted and, in the presence of incomplete bladder emptying, double voiding should be encouraged. Anticholinergics may be a useful adjunct in bladder instability, but care should be taken not to compound problems of incomplete bladder emptying or constipation, which often coexists with bladder dysfunction.

Commitment from the medical team, child, and family are essential to the success of medical management. Arrangements need to be made to allow early treatment of breakthrough infections, and the family and child need to be motivated to correct voiding dysfunction. If the health care system does not allow for early and reliable treatment of breakthrough infection, there may be a role for primary surgical intervention.

Surgical Management

Indications for surgery are relative rather than absolute, and would include failure of medical management and reflux that is unlikely to spontaneously resolve. Dilating reflux with dysplasia or reflux associated with anatomical abnormalities, such as ureteric duplication, are unlikely to resolve spontaneously. Endoscopic treatment can be considered from the neonatal period onwards if a suitable cystoscope is available, but ureteric reimplantation will normally be delayed until the patient is older than 18 months of age unless UTIs are particularly severe.

Endoscopic intervention

The endoscopic subureteric injection of a bulking agent to prevent reflux was first popularised by O'Donnell and Puri in the 1980s.[14] The bulking agent elevates the ureteral orifice to narrow the ureteral

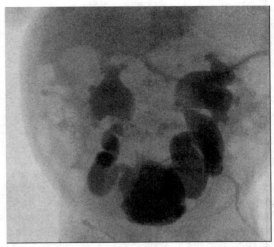

Figure 91.2: MCUG showing bilateral reflux with tortuous ureters. There is dilatation of the pelvicalyceal system with mild blunting of the calyces.

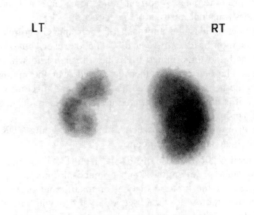

Figure 91.3: DMSA scan showing a small left kidney with cortical thinning and upper and lower pole scar. The right kidney is normal.

lumen, still allowing antegrade flow but preventing retrograde flow. A variety of inert bulking agents have been used, including Teflon®, a suspension of polytetrafluoroethylene (PTFE) in glycerine, dextrano-mer-hyaluronic acid copolymer (Deflux®), and polydimethylsiloxane (Macroplastique®). Teflon was the first substance used for this purpose, but it has recently fallen from favour because it has been shown to migrate to other organs, such as the lungs and brain. It is from this "subureteric Teflon injection" that the acronym STING was coined. Deflux is now the most commonly used bulking agent in Europe.

To allow endoscopic injection, a cystoscope with a working channel is introduced into the bladder under general anaesthetic. Through the working channel, a rigid or flexible needle is used to inject the bulking agent, bevel up, at the 6 o'clock position at the ureteric orifice. The needle should be withdrawn after the injection of 0.5–2.0 ml of material, at which point a mound should be seen. The ureteric orifice will now be elevated so that there is a slit-like opening at the top of the mound.

An alternative to this classic method is the hydrodistention-implantation technique (HIT). In this case, a pressurised stream of fluid is used to open the ureteric orifice so that a bulking agent can be injected directly into the submucosa within the ureteric tunnel. This procedure is useful when dealing with larger ureteric orifices.

Endoscopic correction is most useful for the correction of reflux that is complicated by breakthrough UTI. Injection may need to be repeated, particularly in higher grade reflux, where the HIT technique has improved success rates. However, in "golf hole" or abnormal ureteric orifices, it is less likely to be successful, and open surgery may need to be considered.

Ureteric reimplantation

Ureteric reimplantation is the definitive method for correcting primary VUR. A successful procedure relies on creating a submucosal channel for the affected ureter with a length-to-diameter ratio of 5:1 as well as on providing good detrusor muscle backing.

Cohen pioneered a technique that is now the favoured technique of most paediatric urologists, as it has a success rate of more than 95% and a low rate of postoperative complications.[15] In this technique, the bladder is opened, and the ureter is cannulated with a feeding tube and mobilised intravesically. A submucosal tunnel is made across the width of the trigone through which the ureter is then reimplanted. If the bladder is small and the ureter dilated, it can be difficult to achieve the required length-to-diameter ratio; in this case, the diameter of the distal ureter can be reduced by plication.

Postoperatively, the bladder should be drained for a short period either suprapubically or urethrally. The feeding tube used to cannulate the ureter may be left in place as a stent and brought out through the abdomen or the urethra in females. A current trend, however, is to leave no stent in situ unless transient obstruction is a concern.

An alternative operation is the approach of Lich and Gregoir, in which the ureter is mobilised extravesically. The detrusor, but not the mucosa, is opened and undermined to create a trough into which the ureter is placed. The detrusor can then be closed over the ureter. This technique has the benefits of reduced haematuria and discomfort postoperatively, but it is unsuitable for dilated ureters and is associated with postoperative voiding dysfunction.

Complications of reimplantation procedures include ongoing VUR, ureteric obstruction, haematuria, and infection:

- Persistent ipsilateral VUR will usually be the result of a technical problem, such as inadequate length of the submucosal tunnel, inappropriate placement of the ureteric orifice, or insufficient ureteral mobilisation, but may represent missed secondary reflux with underlying untreated bladder abnormality.

- Contralateral reflux may become apparent once the index side has been treated because it no longer acts as a pressure-relieving valve. The majority of these cases can be managed conservatively or with STING.

- Postoperative ureteric obstruction will often be secondary to oedema, blood or mucous clots, submucosal haematomas, or bladder spasm. Alternatively, ureteral angulation, ischaemia, or incorrect tunnel placement can cause chronic obstruction. Revision reimplantation can be undertaken if required, but the ureter should be transected outside the bladder before being reimplanted.

- Haematuria will usually be self-limiting.

- Infection should be treated with appropriate antibiotics.

Alternative operative procedures

Cutaneous vesicostomy or loop ureterostomy can be used to decompress the systems of young infants whose VUR is complicated by sepsis or impaired renal function. Vesicostomy will often fail to decompress the upper tracts of an infant with a particularly thick-walled bladder; in this situation, a loop ureterostomy may be more successful. Vesicostomies or ureterostomies can be reversed in the second or third year of life, when voiding pressures have fallen, and the bladder can be enlarged either as an isolated procedure or in combination with ureteric reimplantation.

Transuretoureterostomy can be used to manage recurrent VUR or ureteric obstruction complicating a reimplantation procedure.

Nephroureterectomy may need to be considered in the context of recurrent UTI and a poorly functioning kidney. Leaving the grossly scarred kidney in situ exposes the patient to the risk of hypertension and resultant systemic damage. If the differential function of the affected kidney is less than 10% and the contralateral kidney is normal, nephroureterectomy is reasonable. When removing the kidney, the ureter should also be resected in its entirety to prevent infection associated with a refluxing stump.

Prognosis and Outcomes

The outlook for children younger than 5 years of age with reflux of grades I–III is good, with more than 50% spontaneously resolving.[11] Even those with higher-grade reflux may resolve with time, but the rates are significantly lower.[16]

For those patients who do not improve with age, endoscopic subureteric injection with Deflux will cure 70% of patients with grade III reflux after only one injection.[17] For those patients who are not suitable for, or fail, endoscopic treatment, open reimplantation will definitively treat more than 95% of patients.[15,18]

Prevention

Although VUR itself cannot be prevented, once it is detected, steps can be taken to prevent renal damage. It is essential that UTI be treated quickly and effectively. Bladder function should be assessed, urolithiasis excluded, and factors such as constipation, poor voiding, and drinking patterns improved.

Evidence-Based Research

At present, there are no randomised control trials based in Africa regarding treatment of VUR. Therefore, decisions must be guided by studies carried out in the West. Table 9.1 presents the results of a clinical trial in New York that assesses whether surgical or medical management is better in preventing recurrent UTI.

Table 91.1: Evidence-based research.

Title	Results of a randomized clinical trial of medical versus surgical management of infants and children with grades III and IV primary vesicoureteral reflux.
Authors	Weiss R, Duckett J, Spitzer A
Institution	Albert Einstein College of Medicine, New York, New York, USA (coordinating centre)
Reference	J Urol 1992; 148:1667–1673
Problem	To determine, in children with primary VUR of grades III and IV, whether surgical management is better than medical management in preventing recurrent UTI and its complications.
Intervention	Ureteric reimplantation.
Comparison/ control (quality of evidence)	This study monitored 135 patients for new renal damage, kidney growth, changes in estimated glomerular filtration rate (eGFR), appearance of hypertension, and disappearance of VUR. These variables were assessed with urine cultures, blood pressure measurements, serum creatinine measurements, voiding cystogram, and intravenous pyelogram. Follow-up was for five years.
Outcome/ effect	Progression in renal scarring was found in a proportion of the patients, but there was no significant difference between the two groups (medical versus surgical). Similar rates of bacteriuria were found in both groups but medical patients were three times as likely to suffer from acute pyelonephritis. There were no significant differences between renal growth and eGFR between the two groups, and no new cases of hypertension. Grade IV reflux spontaneously resolved at a rate of 8% per year.
Historical significance/ comments	Rates of acute pyelonephritis are higher amongst patients managed with antibiotic prophylaxis than those undergoing surgical reimplantation. Despite this, both surgical correction and medical therapy are equally, but only partially, effective at protecting the kidney from new renal injury. Grade IV reflux will take 9 years to resolve in more than 50% of patients; therefore, prolonged medical therapy will be needed in this group.

Key Summary Points

1. Renal injury in VUR may be the result of congenital renal dysplasia associated with VUR, renal scarring secondary to infection, or a combination of these two factors.

2. Progressive renal damage may be prevented by the early treatment of UTI and not allowing a pattern of recurrent UTI to develop.

3. Taking steps to manage voiding dysfunction is crucial to effective medical treatment of VUR.

4. In the presence of mild to moderate reflux and breakthrough UTI, endoscopic treatment has an important role.

5. Open surgery should be undertaken only after considering medical and endoscopic management.

References

1. Sargent MA. What is the normal prevalence of vesicoureteral reflux? Pediatr Radiol 2000; 30:587–593.

2. Smellie JM, Norman ICS, Katz G. Children with urinary infection: a comparison of those with and those without vesicoureteric reflux. Kidney Int 1981; 20:717–722.

3. Boris C, Puri P. Familial vesicoureteral reflux. J Urol 2003; 169:1804–1808.

4. Rickwood AMK. Vesicoureteric reflux. In: Thomas DF, Rickwood AMK, Duffy PG. Essentials of Paediatric Urology. Martin Dunitz Ltd, 2002, Pp 45–46.

5. Chand DH, Rhoades T, Poe SA, Kraus S, Strife CF. Incidence and severity of vesicoureteral reflux in children related to age, gender, race and diagnosis. J Urol 2003;170: 1548–1550.

6. Ransley PG. Vesicoureteric reflux: continuing surgical dilemma. Urology 1978; 12:246–255.

7. Dillon MJ, Goonasekera CDA. Reflux nephropathy. J Am Soc Nephrol 1998; 9:2377–2383.

8. Malik M, Watson A. Antenatally detected urinary tract abnormalities: more detection but less action. Pediatr Nephrol 2008; 23:897–904.

9. Yeung CK, Godley ML, Dhillon HK, Gordon I, Duffy PG, Ransley PG. The characteristics of primary vesico-ureteric reflux in male and female infants with pre-natal hydronephrosis. BJU Int 1997; 80:319–327.

10. Kala UK, Jacobs WC. Evaluation of urinary tract infection in malnourished black children. Ann Trop Paediatr 1992; 12(1):75–81.

11. Keating MA. Role of periureteral injections in children with vesicoureteral reflux. Curr Opin Urol 2005; 15:369–373.

12. Elder JS. Urinary tract infections. In: Kleigman RM, et al. Nelson Textbook of Pediatrics, 18th ed. Saunders, 2007, Chap 538.

13. Roberts JA, Kaack MB, Baskin G. Treatment of experimental pyelonephritris in the monkey. J Urol 1990; 143:150–154.

14. O'Donnell B, Puri P. Treatment of vesicoureteric reflux by endoscopic injection of Teflon. BMJ 1984; 289:7–9.

15. Dewan PA. Ureteric reimplantation: a history of the development of surgical techniques. BJU Int 2000; 85:1000–1006.

16. Weiss R, Duckett J, Spitzer A. The International Reflux Study in Children. Results of a randomized clinical trial of medical versus surgical management of infants and children with grades III and IV: primary vesicoureteral reflux (United States). J Urol 1992; 148:1667–1673.

17. Lackgren G, Wahlin N, Skoldenberg E, Stenberg A. Long-term follow-up of children with dextranomer/hyaluronic acid copolymer for vesicoureteral reflux. J Urol 2001; 166:1887–1892.

18. Duckett, JW, Walker RD, Weiss R. Surgical results: International Reflux Study in Children–United States Branch. J Urol 1992; 148:1674–1675.

CHAPTER 92
BLADDER EXSTROPHY AND EPISPADIAS

William Appeadu-Mensah
Piet Hoebeke

Introduction

Exstrophy and epispadias are part of a spectrum of anomalies characterised by exposure of part or all of the mucosa of the lower urinary tract (bladder and urethra) to the external environment through a defect in the anterior abdominal wall. At one end of this spectrum is cloacal exstrophy, which is the most complex of these anomalies. It is characterised by exposure of the bladder mucosa together with the mucosa of the hind gut to the external environment through an anterior abdominal wall defect. At the other end of the spectrum is epispadias, which is characterised by a normal abdominal wall and bladder with a dorsal external urethral meatus, which may be anywhere from the base of the penis to the glans and may or may not be associated with an incompetent bladder neck and sphincter mechanism. Between these two extremes exist variations in pathology, with the most prevalent being classic bladder exstrophy. In most of the anomalies in this spectrum, there is concomitant bone involvement with diastasis of the symphysis pubis.

The most prevalent condition, classic bladder exstrophy, is characterised by exposure of the bladder and posterior urethral mucosa through a defect in the anterior abdominal wall. It is associated with a complete epispadias in boys and bifid clitoris in girls. At neonatal presentation, this anomaly results in the continuous dribbling of urine and exposure of bladder and urethral mucosa to the external environment. It leads to chronic irritation of this mucosa as well as social and emotional complications in Africa due to isolation of the affected person.

The medical literature on treatment of the epispadias-exstrophy complex presents many techniques. There is no ultimate excellent technique. Techniques used depend on various factors, such as extent of the abnormality, surgeon's experience, hospital staff and skills, and possibilities for follow-up, among many others.

This chapter presents examples of how to tackle the problem, specifically in the African situation. This chapter is not intended to be the final state-of-the-art approach to exstrophy; rather, the goal is to inspire those who are confronted with a child presenting with the epispadias exstrophy complex.

Demographics

The incidence of bladder exstrophy in Africa is not known, but various studies report it to be 3.3 per 100,000, with a male-to-female ratio of 2.3:1. In Africa, most children born with extreme congenital anomalies are neglected and allowed to die. It is therefore difficult to know the exact incidence. The incidence of epispadias is estimated to be 1 in 117,000 in males, with a male-to-female ratio of 3–4:1. The incidence of cloacal exstrophy is estimated to be 1 in 200,000 to 1 in 400,000. The risk of transmission from a patient with exstrophy to a child is about 1 in 70. The risk of recurrence in a particular family is estimated to be about 1 in 100. The worldwide incidence may be affected by antenatal diagnosis, which may increase the abortion rate.

Although rare anomalies, extrophy and epispadias are challenging conditions. These conditions are not life threatening if left untreated at birth, so the option of no treatment will not lead to death. Therefore, most children born with this devastating condition should be offered treatment even if they present late. In the African environment, these children sometimes present to hospital at age 6 to 9 years or even older.

Embryology

Due to the low prevalence of the condition, the exact aetiology of bladder exstrophy is not known. No genetic factors have been identified, but there is an increased risk among siblings, which indicates that a genetic origin is possible. It is also relatively more common among young mothers and multiparous mothers. Exstrophy is believed to result from a failure of incorporation of mesoderm into the cloacal membrane, leading eventually to rupture of this membrane. An overgrowth of the cloacal membrane as well as an abnormal insertion of the body stalk may contribute to this. The pathophysiology depends on the timing of this rupture. In cloacal exstrophy, the rupture occurs very early before the urogenital septum has divided the cloaca into the urogenital sinus and the anorectum. Other studies have shown later rupture of the cloacal membrane in cloacal exstrophy, suggesting that other factors, such as failure of embryogenesis, may contribute to this.

Epispadias is thought to be due to impaired migration of the genital tubercles to the midline.

Pathology

Classic Bladder Exstrophy

In classic bladder exstrophy (Figures 92.1 and 92.2), the pathological process affects the pelvic bones, anterior abdominal wall, pelvic diaphragm, urinary system (ureterovesical junction (UVJ), bladder, and urethra), the genitalia, and the anus.

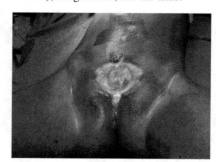

Figure 92.1: Classic bladder exstrophy in the female.

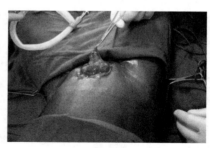

Figure 92.2: Classic bladder exstrophy in the male.

Boney Anomalies

The pubic bones are widely separated. There is a wider angle between the sacroiliac bones and the sagittal plane as well as between the sacrum and ilium and the ilium and pubis than in normal individuals. This can result in a waddling gait. Over time, however, this gait resolves with no obvious abnormality.

Muscular Anomalies

The rectus sheath is attached to the separated pubic bones. The pelvic diaphragm also inserts into the widely separated pubic bones and forms an intersymphyseal fibrotic band. The normal sphincteric function is therefore affected, leading to incontinence of urine, sometimes incontinence of stool, prolapse of the uterus, and sometimes prolapse of the rectum.

Anomalies of the urinary system

The exposed bladder surface is sometimes wide, elastic, and compliant, but may be small, fibrosed, and noncompliant. There exists a wide variation in the size of the bladder plate at birth. Some children have a large bladder plate, which can easily be closed, and others have, from birth, a small fibrotic plate that is difficult to close. If left unclosed, persistent trauma leads to inflammation, fibrosis, metaplasia, and possible carcinoma later in life. Long exposure to the open air can lead to progressive loss in elasticity and compliance. The UVJ is often incompetent, resulting in reflux in nearly all patients with exstrophy of the bladder.

Anomalies of the genitalia

In male children with classic bladder exstrophy, the penis is completely open dorsally as a complete epispadias. The penis has a dorsal chordee, which, together with the wide attachment of the corpora cavernosa to the separated pubis and short corpora, contributes to a short penis. There are, however, other anatomical variations in exstrophy (Figure 92.3), with the penis sometimes being completely bifid with each corpus attached separately to the pubic bones. The testes and vas deferens are usually normal, although there may be associated inguinal hernias. The prostate gland does not surround the urethra.

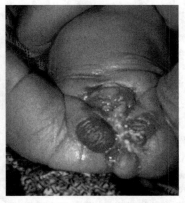

Figure 92.3: Bladder exstrophy, two hemiscrota, and abnormal perineum and anus.

In female children, there is a bifid clitoris and the labia are attached widely to the separated pubic bones. The vagina may be short but is otherwise normal, although it tends to be more anterior in position.

Anomalies of the anus

In both males and females, the anus tends to be placed more anteriorly; however, it most often functions normally.

Cloacal Exstrophy

Cloacal exstrophy is characterised by a defect in the anterior abdominal wall, exposing the mucosa of the caecum with bladder mucosa on both sides of it, and resulting in loss of the hindgut and no development of colon. In addition, a short remnant of the hindgut, the appendix, and the ileum open onto the exposed caecum. There are commonly associated spinal, boney, renal, gastrointestinal, and genital anomalies, such as bicornuate uterus.

Epispadias

In epispadias in the male, there is a dorsal penile opening of the urethral meatus with a dorsal penile curvature. In this anomaly, the spectrum is between a meatal anomaly alone and an abdominal wall abnormality with wide pubic symphysis and sphincteric incompetence. The exact position of the meatus on the dorsal surface of the penis varies and may be anywhere from the peno-pubic area to the glans. When in the peno-pubic region, the whole urethral mucosa is open dorsally. It is always associated with some degree of dorsal chordee and may or may not be associated with an incompetent sphincter. Vesicoureteric reflux (VUR) may also be present.

In the female, the urethral orifice may be lax and patulous in a normal position or be found anywhere from the bladder neck to the normal position. There may be an associated incompetent sphincter and VUR. There is usually associated diastasis of the pubic symphysis. The clitoris is usually bifid with an open attachment of the labia minora to the separated symphysis, but it may sometimes be normal.

Clinical Presentation

The presentation of bladder exstrophy can vary, depending on the type of anomaly.

Classic Bladder Exstrophy

In classic bladder exstrophy (see Figures 92.1 and 92.2), the newborn child may look well in all respects but for the abdomen, which shows a huge expanse of abdominal wall superiorly with a low-set umbilicus. There is an obvious defect in the lower abdomen, which reveals the bladder mucosa with urine dribbling continuously from the ureteric orifices. This is continuous with the urethral mucosa, which opens dorsally. Sometimes ectopic bowel mucosa is found in association with the bladder mucosa. There is a wide gap between the pubic bones with attached epispadiac penis in the male.

In the female, similar abdominal features are noted, but there is a bifid clitoris attached to the separated pubic bones. The vagina may be short and is relatively anteriorly placed. The labia are also attached widely to the pubic bones.

The anus is seen in the perineum in an anterior position. There may be associated inguinal hernias.

Cloacal Exstrophy

In cloacal exstrophy, the abdominal wall defect is occupied by two hemibladders laterally with caecal mucosa in the middle. The hemibladders may be joined together superiorly, laterally, or inferiorly. Three orifices are noted on the ceacal mucosa. These open into the ileum, appendix, and short hindgut. Arrangements of bladder and/or bowel mucosa can vary and may not have a classic pattern. Obvious inguinal swellings when the child strains demonstrate bilateral inguinal hernias.

The phallus in the male is obviously short and may have a varied presentation, being bifid, unilateral, or rudimentary. In the female, there is a bifid clitoris with separated labia. The vagina may be double or single.

There may be an imperforate anus with variations in anal pathology. There may be obvious spinal anomalies, such as myelomeningocoele, as well as limb anomalies. Associated anomalies are more common in patients with cloacal anomaly and involve practically all systems.

Epispadias

In males, epispadias presents with a dorsal penile meatus which opens anywhere from the penopubic region to the glans. There is an associated dorsal chordee. The prepuce may be noticed to be ventral and deficient dorsally.

In females, the urethral meatus may be at the normal site but lax and patulous with associated dribbling of urine or may be found anywhere from the bladder neck to the normal site with a dorsal open urethra distal to the orifice and a bifid clitoris. A definite gap may be palpated between the pubic bones. The labia minora may be seen attached to the separated pubic bones.

In both males and females, there can be associated incontinence of urine due to sphincteric incompetence.

Age at Presentation

In Africa, age at presentation tends to be late despite the obvious nature of this condition. Reasons for late presentation include cultural beliefs related to a child born with this condition, lack of finances to support the care of the child in a specialised hospital, long distance from specialist hospitals, and lack of available professionals able to manage this condition.

Exstrophy of the bladder may be diagnosed in utero and helps prepare the parents for birth in an appropriate child care centre with relevant expertise and equipment. It may, however, increase the abortion rate and anxiety of parents. Prenatal diagnosis is uncommon in Africa.

Investigations

The diagnosis is made basically by clinical examination, and investigations are done to rule out other anomalies. An abdominal ultrasound (US) examination helps to exclude associated renal anomalies. An x-ray of the abdomen and pelvis shows pubic diastasis and the wide angle between the pelvic bones.

Management

Exstrophy of the Bladder

Management of exstrophy of the bladder requires the involvement of a team of experts to help manage the various aspects of this complex anomaly. These include a counsellor, a neonatologist, and a team of paediatric surgeons, as well as nurses and anaesthesiologists.

Initial Management

Initial management involves counselling the parents to help them understand the pathological process, the management options, and the prognosis. They must be helped to appreciate that, with modern methods, the child will eventually be dry and continent. In addition, they must be helped to recognise the sex of the child in order to appropriately bring up the child. Gender assignment in typical exstrophy is easy. In boys, the scrotum is well developed and the testes are descended. Even in cloacal exstrophy, the scrotum is developed and the testes are descended despite the lack of penile development. In cloacal exstrophy, female gender assignment was readily done based on penile underdevelopment. Recent literature suggests that female-assigned cloacal exstrophy boys tend to have a higher prevalence of gender dysphoria.

In Africa, local beliefs must be taken into consideration and attempts made to diffuse the beliefs of parents that may result in neglecting the child. The financial burden on the parents must be recognised in the initial counselling and suggestions made as to how parents could be supported by available groups. In the absence of a team of experts, the available health attendant must initiate the counselling process.

As part of initial management, it is important that the bladder mucosa be protected from trauma from gauze, clothing, or the clip used on the umbilical cord. The umbilical cord should be ligated with a suture to avoid trauma from the clip. The mucosa may be protected by using plastic material to cover the mucosa. This is then removed and the surface irrigated with saline any time diapers are changed. If saline is not available, clean water may be used. The patient must then be referred to a tertiary centre where this condition can be managed. In most places in Africa, the parents need time to prepare financially and socially to move to a tertiary centre.

At the tertiary centre, the child is examined fully, and necessary investigations are done. The patient is cared for by a team of counsellors or social workers, neonatologists, paediatricians, anaesthetists, and paediatric surgeons, who may include a urologist and an orthopaedic surgeon. In some centres, a full team may not be available, and a surgeon with interest in managing this condition may be the only one to give all the necessary care. The surgeon helps the parents understand the various stages involved in the management of their child's condition, whereas the counsellor helps the parents accept the child and manage the social implications.

Definitive Treatment

Surgery should be done as soon as practicable to give the bladder the best chance of recovery after reconstruction. The timing of surgery depends, however, on the availability of personnel and facilities to manage a newborn undergoing an operation that may take several hours to complete. There must be a competent neonatal anaesthetist with relevant associated equipment, a surgeon or team of surgeons capable of performing an osteotomy and closure of the bladder, a neonatologist or paediatrician to assist with care after surgery, and a neonatal intensive care unit (NICU) with available equipment and personnel to handle the infant. In the absence of a well-equipped NICU, it might be necessary to delay the operation until the child is old enough to withstand a long operation. An appropriate age may be between 1 and 3 months of age in such patients, but surgery can be done from the first day of life. Once surgery is considered safe, initial surgery is done.

Surgical Procedures

Surgical options are staged reconstruction, complete primary reconstruction, or urinary diversion.

Indications for reconstruction include a bladder with a wide surface area, good elasticity, and compliance after assessment under anaesthesia. A small, fibrotic, inelastic bladder is not a candidate for reconstruction, and a form of diversion may be necessary. A bladder may be fibrotic at birth, but late presentation with long-term irritation tends to contribute to this. This is quite common in Africa. The procedures for reconstruction include bilateral osteotomies, bladder closure, posterior urethra and abdominal wall repair, epispadias repair, bladder neck reconstruction, and antireflux procedure. These can be done in one stage or as a staged procedure.

In staged repair, bilateral osteotomies, bladder closure, posterior urethra, and abdominal wall repair are done soon after birth. Repair of epispadias is performed between 6 months and 1 year of age. Finally, bladder neck reconstruction with an antireflux procedure is done when the bladder capacity is at least 85 ml.

In complete primary repair, a combination of bilateral osteotomies, bladder closure, posterior urethra, and epispadias repair may be done at any age in one stage. Bladder neck repair with antireflux surgery is then done when the child has an appropriate bladder volume. This approach is particularly useful in children who present at an older age, although it can be used instead of a staged repair in the neonatal period.

Osteotomies

Types of osteotomies include posterior iliac osteotomy, anterior pubic ramus osteotomy, anterior oblique innominate osteotomy, and combined transverse innominate and vertical iliac osteotomy. Osteotomies are necessary to ensure adequate repair of the anterior abdominal wall without tension, to place the bladder neck and posterior urethra deep in the pelvis, and to bring the pelvic muscles to the midline to aid eventual continence. In children less than 72 hours postnatal, this may not be necessary but should be done if there is any doubt about the ability to easily repair the abdominal wall without tension.

Combined vertical and transverse innominate osteotomies allow easy approximation of the pubic symphysis without the need to turn the baby during the procedure. Posterior iliac osteotomies are done in the prone position, after which the child is turned supine for the bladder repair. Anterior pubic osteotomy is not very effective. The anterior oblique osteotomy avoids the need to turn the patient. The type of osteotomy performed depends, among other things, on the expertise and training of the available surgeon. Results are usually acceptable in good hands.

After an osteotomy, immobilisation of the pelvis is necessary. The most popular means are mermaid casts; however, gallows traction and external fixators have been used. The availability of equipment such as external fixators in Africa may influence the type of fixation done postoperatively.

Technique of Anterior Oblique Osteotomy

1. After complete preparation of the child from the nipple to the leg, and with the child in a supine position, a skin incision is made along the iliac crest, beginning from the anterior superior iliac spine and extending posteriorly and deepened until the periosteum is reached.

2. An incision is then made in the periosteum along the iliac crest beginning 1 cm posterior to the anterior superior iliac spine.

3. The periosteum is elevated toward the sciatic notch. Both tables of ileum are divided down to the sciatic notch with the aid of an osteotome, reciprocating saw or Gigli saw, including cartilage at the level of the sciatic notch. This results in free movement of the anterior fragment.

4. The surgeon then proceeds to repair the bladder.

Technique of Repair of Bladder and Posterior Urethra

1. An incision is made just above the umbilicus and continues around the bladder mucosa to a point 1 cm away from the midline in the distal trigone on both sides (Figure 92.4(A,B)).

2. This incision is then continued in a parallel manner along the

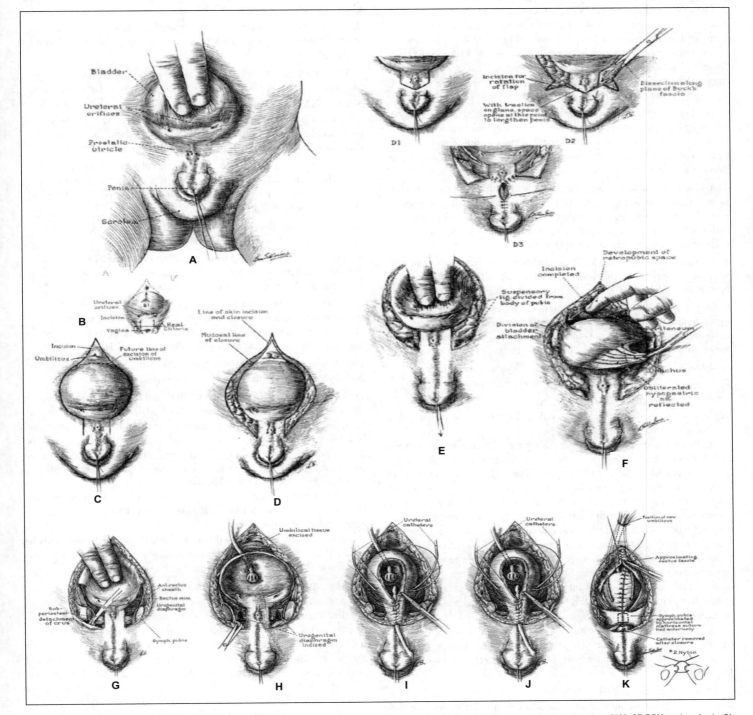

Source: Gearhart JP. Exstrophy, epispadias and other bladder anomalies. In: Walsh PC, Retik AB, Vaughan ED, et al., eds. Campbell's Urology, vol 3, 8th ed. Saunders, 2003, CD ROM version, chapter 61. Reproduced with kind permission of Elsevier Science.

Figure 92.4: Technique of repair of bladder and posterior urethra.

urethral plate distally (Figure 92.4(C,D)) to the region lateral to the verumontanum in boys and along the urethral plate in girls. No attempt is made to divide the urethra unless there are compelling reasons to believe the urethra needs to be lengthened

3. The incision is deepened in the region of the umbilicus and a plane developed between the rectus muscle and the bladder wall (Figure 92.4(D,E)).

4. The peritoneum is dissected off the bladder and dissection continued until the area lateral to the trigone is reached, where the urogenital diaphragm will be encountered (Figure 92.4(F)). Ureteric stents must be placed early to avoid inadvertently dividing the ureters.

5. The urogenital diaphragm is sharply dissected off the pubic bone deeply, parallel to the bladder and posterior urethra, until it is completely separated from the pubic bone (Figure 92.4(G,H)). Traction on the pubic bone using skin hooks or a stitch helps to accentuate the fibres and aid complete dissection of these fibres. This is a particularly important step because it ensures that the bladder neck is placed deeply at the end of the procedure and promotes continence later.

6. The bladder mucosa and posterior urethra are then closed in two layers by using long-term absorbable sutures well onto the urethra (Figure 92.4(I,J)). The final urethral orifice must be able to admit a 12 Fr to 14 Fr stent to allow adequate resistance for bladder growth while preventing outlet obstruction.

7. A suprapubic catheter and ureteric stents are left in situ, but no stent is left in the urethra (Figure 92.4(K)). Ideally, nonlatex silastic tubes should be used, but a Foley catheter may be used instead of a malecot catheter for suprapubic drainage, and feeding tubes may be used as ureteric stents in the absence of ideal tubes.

8. Care must be taken not to inflate the balloon of the catheter so much as to cause pressure on the thin mucosal wall; the tip of the Foley catheter beyond the balloon may need to be cut to avoid pressure in the urethra.

9. After bladder closure, the trochanters are brought together by the assistant and the pubic bones approximated with a #2 nylon stitch, ensuring that the knot remains outside the bone to avoid traumatising the urethra. A second stitch may be applied to reinforce the repair.

10. Finally, the abdominal wall is closed in layers. Antibiotics are given at induction to reduce the risk of septic complications.

Management after Primary Surgery
Postoperatively, gallows traction is applied for 3–6 weeks or an alternative method of fixation is used.

The child is observed to ensure adequate drainage of urine from both ureteric stents. The ureteric stents are left in situ for 10–14 days, and the suprapubic catheter for 4 weeks. The child is discharged, after urine examination has been done, abdominal US shows no upper tract dilatation, and there is no residual urine. If residual urine is observed, the urethral orifice can be calibrated to check for patency. Any infection noted on urine examination is treated and the patient placed on prophylactic antibiotics due to VUR. Abdominal US at 3 months and then at 6-month to yearly intervals is used to observe for any stasis in the urinary system. The presence of stasis may necessitate intervention in the form of dilatation, intermittent catheterisation, urethrotomy, refashioning of the bladder outlet, antireflux surgery, or urinary diversion.

Yearly calibration with the aid of cystoscopy and cystography helps to assess the bladder volume. At the age of about 1 year, epispadias repair is performed because this facilitates a gradual increase in bladder volume.

Technique of Epispadias Repair
There are various techniques of epispadias repair. These include the Cantwell-Ransley repair, the Modified Cantwell-Ransley repair, and Mitchell's total penile disassembly method. The aim is to obtain a functional, cosmetic penis by correcting dorsal chordee, urethroplasty, and glanduloplasty, and providing skin cover.

The Modified Cantwell-Ransley procedure, which achieves good results with a low complication rate, is described here (Figure 92.5). Testosterone may be given to increase the size of the penis. Repair may otherwise be done when the penis has an adequate size.

1. A stitch is placed in the glans for traction on the penis, and a longitudinal incision, made at the tip of the urethral mucosa, is closed transversely to widen the urethral mucosa at the distal end (Figure 92.5(A)).

2. The mucosa at the lateral ends of the glans is excised for glanduloplasty later (Figure 92.5(B)).

3. Parallel incisions are made over the urethral plate about 18 mm apart, from the prostatic urethral orifice to the tip of the penis (Figure 92.5(A,B,C)).

4. The skin at the base of the penis is incised with a Z-plasty incision to reduce the risk of later contracture, and all fibrotic tissue is excised.

5. The penile skin is dissected off the corpora ventrally from the corona to the base of the penis while leaving intact the mesentery to the urethral plate, which runs from ventral to dorsal between the corpora at the proximal part of the penis (Figure 92.5(C,D)).

6. The corpora are dissected off the urethral plate from the base to the tip of the penis while leaving intact the distal 1-cm attachment of the urethral mucosa to the glans. It is also dissected partially off the pubic ramus (Figure 92.5(E,F)).

7. The urethra is then tubularised with 6.0 polyglycolic acid sutures over a size 8 Fr stent (Figure 92.5(I)).

8. The corpora are rotated dorsally over the tubularised urethra and sutured together in two layers with 5.0 polyglycolic acid sutures to move the urethra ventrally (Figure 92.5(J,K)).

9. The neurovascular bundle may be dissected off the corpora only if chordee correction cannot easily be achieved and it is necessary to incise the corpora and suture the two defects in the corpora together in the middle to correct dorsal chordee (Figure 92.5(G,H)).

10. Glanduloplasty is done over the urethra with 5.0 and 6.0 polyglycolic acid sutures deeply and superficially.

11. The ventral skin is split in the midline and brought dorsally for skin cover in a bear-hug method (Figure 92.5(L,M)).

If dorsal chordee is too severe to be corrected this way, the urethra is considered too short, or skin cover is inadequate, skin graft on the dorsum of the corpora after incising the corpora may be used for correction of chordee, while skin flaps or grafts may be used to lengthen the urethra and for skin cover.

Many other techniques have been described, and some authors advocate that ventral rotation of the corpora results in a better bending penis and more penile length.

Whatever technique is used, any surgeon doing this repair must be aware of the lateral course of the neurovascular bundle, and must avoid damage to the neurovascular bundle.

Management after Epispadias Repair
Postoperatively, a urethral stent is left in place for 10 to 12 days. A Vaseline® gauze dressing may be applied directly to the wound followed by a dry roll of gauze held in place with adhesive plaster. The outer dressing may be changed any time it gets wet. After about a week, the wound may be exposed and allowed to stay dry. Dressings may be removed after 48 hours, and the wound allowed to remain exposed if the child is unlikely to handle the wound. The patient may be discharged soon after surgery if one can ensure a quick return to hospital if the need arises. Otherwise, the patient is kept in hospital until there is adequate healing. Analgesics, antispasmodics, and antibiotics are important adjuncts in the postoperative management to reduce pain, bladder spasm, and infection.

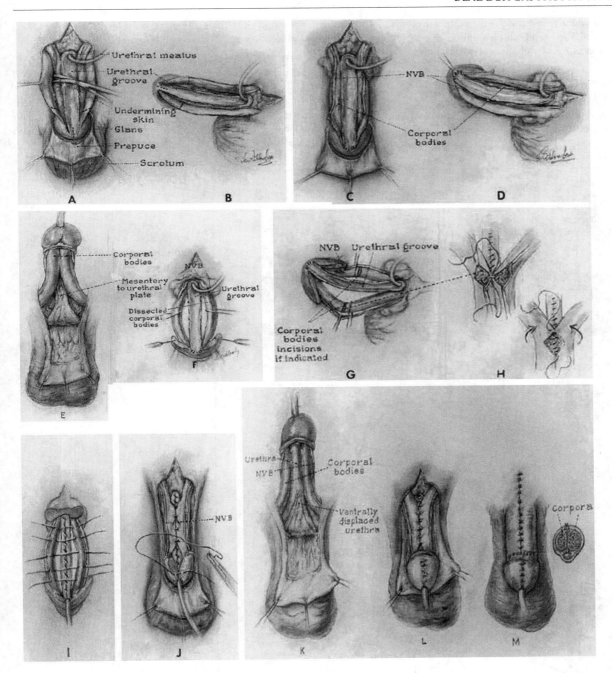

Source: Gearhart JP. Exstrophy, epispadias and other bladder anomalies. In: Walsh PC, Retik AB, Vaughan ED, et al., eds. Campbell's Urology, vol 3, 8th ed. Saunders, 2003, CD ROM version, chapter 61.. Reproduced with kind permission of Elsevier Science.

Figure 92.5: Technique of repair of epispadias.

Yearly assessment of bladder volume is done under anaesthesia. Assessment of bladder volume may be done with the aid of US, cystoscopy, cystography, or urodynamic studies. Urodynamic studies, which give added information on pressure in the bladder, are usually not available in most African countries. Once bladder volume is at least 85 ml, bladder neck reconstruction and antireflux surgery is done. This may take up to age of 4 years.

If bladder capacity is adequate for age but incontinence persists, which is usually the case, then bladder neck reconstruction should be considered. Outcome after primary closure tends to be better for girls than for boys.

Technique of Bladder Neck Repair

There are various techniques for bladder neck repair. The modified Young-Dees-Leadbetter repair gives good results and is described here (Figure 92.6).

1. A transverse incision is made at the bladder neck and extended vertically in a T-shape. Cohen transtrigonal reimplantation of the ureters is then done (Figure 92.6(A,B,C)).

2. A 15- to 18-mm wide and 30-mm long mucosal strip is chosen between the midtrigone and prostatic urethra. The bladder mucosa lateral to this is excised with the aid of gauze soaked in adrenaline for haemostasis (Figure 92.6(D)).

3. Multiple transverse incisions are made in the muscle edge lateral to this strip without making a transverse incision at the border with the bladder floor to reduce the risk of ischaemia (Figure 92.6(E)).

4. The strip of mucosa and underlying muscle is then tubularised with 4.0 polyglycolic acid sutures. The lateral muscle flaps are overlapped over the tubularised mucosa using 3.0 polyglyocolic acid sutures (Figure 92.6(F,G)).

5. The bladder neck is then suspended on the anterior rectus muscle (Figure 92.6(H)).

6. The bladder, bladder neck, and posterior urethra are completely dissected to ensure easy mobility and an adequate repair.

7. A size 8 urethral stent may be used to assist closure of the urethra, but this is not left in situ. Bilateral ureteral stents and a suprapubic catheter are placed for urinary diversion (Figure 92.6(I)).

Management after Bladder Neck Repair

The suprapubic tube is left for 3 weeks. Before removal, it is clamped for about 1 hour and then the child is observed for passage of urine. If this fails to occur, a size 8 Foley catheter is passed for 5 days and then another attempt made to void. These attempts are continued until the child is able to void. Some children, however, will be unable to pass urine and should be put on intermittent catheterisation. This can

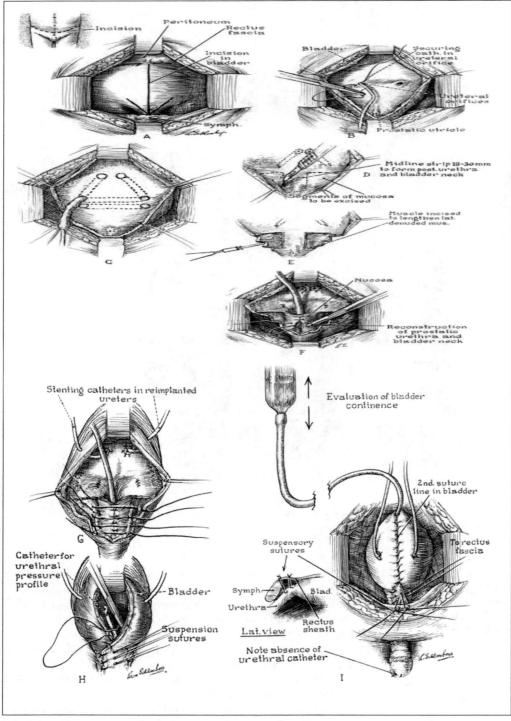

Source: Gearhart JP. Exstrophy, epispadias and other bladder anomalies. In: Walsh PC, Retik AB, Vaughan ED, et al., eds. Campbell's Urology, vol 3, 8th ed. Saunders, 2003, CD ROM version, chapter 61. Reproduced with kind permission of Elsevier Science.

Figure 92.6: Technique of repair of bladder neck.

be difficult after urethral reconstruction, and some children will need continent diversion (Mitrofanoff's technique) to be able to empty the bladder. The child is then discharged and followed up with regular US examinations to ensure adequate renal function. It is expected that within 1 to 2 years the child should achieve daytime dryness of 3 hours. Failure to achieve this is an indication to consider other methods of urinary control.

Other Techniques

Various forms of urinary diversion, bladder augmentation, the use of conduits, continent diversion, and artificial sphincters are necessary for various reasons in the management of bladder exstrophy. Indications include small contracted fibrotic bladder incapable of forming a bladder, failed repair of bladder, failure to achieve adequate bladder volume after primary repair, and failed bladder neck repair. Techniques include uretero-sigmoidostomy and modified forms of this, rectal bladders, ileocolonic bladders, ileal bladders, injection of bulking agents to augment sphincteric action, the use of conduits, and continent stomas. These methods may be important in Africa due to the late presentation of patients. However, the method chosen must require minimal follow-up and less cost because follow-up of patients is difficult in Africa.

Cloacal Exstrophy

Management of cloacal exstrophy is individualised due to the complex and varied nature of the anomalies present. Staged repair is particularly important here, although complete repairs may be done. Procedures that need to be done include repair of spinal defects; stomas for bowel management; osteotomies, and other diversions for urinary anomalies; and repair of genital anomalies.

Spinal and bowel anomalies must be dealt with first after the child is stable. Urinary and genital anomalies may then be managed later.

Gender assignment is another important part of the management of this condition because the male phallus may be so short that gender reassignment may be necessary at the onset.

Epispadias

Treatment of epispadias in the male follows principles similar to those used for exstrophy of the bladder. In those who are incontinent, which is usual in penopubic and penile epispadias, urethroplasty is done first and then bladder neck repair is done when the bladder volume is 85 ml. In the absence of incontinence, urethroplasty is done. The Modified Cantwell Ransley method and the Young-Dees-Leadbetter repair are adequate for urethroplasty and bladder neck repair, but many other techniques have been described.

Treatment of epispadias in the female follows the same principles as those used in the male with epispadias. Urethroplasty is done first, after which bladder neck repair is done.

1. For urethroplasty, the patient is placed in a lithotomy position, and a vertical skin incision is made on the mons and then extended laterally in a Y-shape from the apex of the urethral orifice distally to the open urethra between the 3 and 9 o'clock positions.

2. Parallel incisions are then made from this position proximally to the bladder neck.

3. The strip of urethra between these incisions is excised.

4. The urethra is tubularised around a size 10 or 12 Fr stent.

5. The mucosa on the medial aspect of the clitoris and labia minora on both sides is excised, and the clitoris and labia minora are repaired in the midline.

6. The skin is then closed in layers, ensuring that fat is brought together over the urethral repair.

Bladder neck repair is done when bladder volume is adequate and the Young-Dees-Leadbetter repair achieves good results. Reimplantatation of the ureters is necessary in many of these cases due to reflux and is done in addition.

If bladder volume is adequate at the onset, urethroplasty and bladder neck repair can be done in one stage.

Postoperative Complications

Table 92.1 outlines possible complications of surgery related to bladder exstrophy and epispadias.

Table 92.1: Complications of surgery.

Surgical procedure	Complication	Management
Primary bladder closure	Partial or complete wound, breakdown with wound dehiscence	Repeat reconstruction, diversion
	Bladder prolapse, inadequate bladder volume	Bladder augmentation
	Bladder outlet stenosis, infection, pyelonephritis	Urethral dilatation, urethrotomy, refashioning of bladder outlet, re-implantation of ureters
	Vesicoureteric reflux	Antibiotics
Osteotomies	Poor healing, nerve injury, osteomyelitis, diastasis	Good fixation, rest, antibiotics
Epispadias repair	Urethrocutaneous fistulas, stenosis, short penis, unpleasant scars, difficult catheterisation	Repair, further surgery
Bladder neck repair	Persistent incontinence	Diversion, bladder augmentation, artificial sphincters
Diversion	Metabolic acidosis, carcinoma, electrolyte imbalance, infection	Monitoring, antibiotics, alkaline drugs

Prognosis and Outcomes

The outcome of staged primary reconstruction and combined reconstruction has improved over the years. Continence, defined as daytime dryness of at least 3 hours, is obtained in 60–90% of patients. Success in becoming continent is related to the number of times surgery is done to close the bladder, the use of osteotomy after the age of 72 hours, and a bladder volume of at least 85 ml prior to bladder neck repair.

Urinary diversion has resulted in continence in up to 90% of patients whenever this has been necessary. This, however, may be associated with the risk of metabolic complications, infection, and carcinoma later in life.

Sexual function has been shown to be normal in most male and female patients with exstrophy. The male genitalia remains short, and further surgery may be needed to achieve better length and to excise unsightly scars later in adult life. Females may require vulvoplasty and/or vaginoplasty in adult life. Libido, erection, and orgasm occur successfully in both males and females.

Fertility is poor in males. It is poorer, however, after primary reconstruction than after urinary diversion due to malejaculation in the former procedure. Assisted reproductive techniques, such as gamete intrafallopian transfer, can be used successfully in these patients.

Females are fertile and have borne children successfully with this condition. Prolapse of the uterus is a common complication for which repair must be done.

For those with cloacal anomalies, modern techniques have made it possible for most to live independent lives. They may have to live with permanent stomas, but they remain socially continent.

Outcomes after surgery for epispadias are better than those for bladder exstrophy.

Ethical Issues

Exstrophy could be used as an example of the differences in approaches to congenital anomalies, depending on the place of birth. Whereas in most European and North American societies, children with exstrophy are transferred to referral centres within the first 48 hours of life, this is not the case in Africa. With neonatal referral, neonatal staged or complete repair is the first choice and offers the best chance of a final good outcome.

Even prenatal detection has changed the scene. In some European countries, early abortion after prenatal diagnosis is the rule.

Late referral, with children presenting as late as 6 or more years of age, is common in Africa, however. The bladder at this stage may be fibrotic and metaplastic, making urinary diversion a particularly important option for many in Africa. It is still possible, however, to find bladders that are compliant and elastic enough to allow primary reconstruction; combining bladder closure with epispadias repair may be the option of choice in such cases.

Next to late referral, other factors that contribute to prognosis in Africa include the cultural understanding of the condition, availability of experts to help manage this condition, and availability of resources. In a number of African communities, children born with such conditions are considered abnormal and may be neglected, with no attempt made to seek medical attention. The lack of financial resources and distance from a hospital with required expertise may contribute to this problem. Such children may therefore die or grow as social outcasts with possible psychological implications.

In Africa, where resources are scarce, it is important that a few centres be set up in each country or region in which resources and expertise are concentrated to help provide the best care to most of these children. Education about this condition should be instituted at the community level to help change concepts and make it possible for affected children to receive adequate care on time. Social groups with interest in such conditions need to be established to help provide financial and other social support so that parents do not abandon their children due to inability to bear the burden alone. Such groups may also help influence policy makers to ensure that policies are made to benefit these children.

Evidence-Based Research

Table 92.2 presents a retrospective study of a large number of patients that showed that bladder volume is an important determinant of continence after bladder neck repair.

Table 92.2: Evidence-based research.

Title	Modern staged repair of bladder exstrophy: a contemporary series
Authors	Baird AD, Nelson CP, Gearhart JP
Institution	Division of Pediatric Urology, Brady Urological Institute, The Johns Hopkins Hospital, Baltimore, Maryland, USA; Department of Urology, Royal Liverpool University Hospital, Merseyside, Liverpool, UK
Reference	J Pediatr Urol 2007; 3(4):311–315
Problem	Outcome after modern staged repair.
Intervention	Staged repair of exstrophy of the bladder.
Comparison/ control (quality of evidence)	Patients with bladder volume of at least 85 ml after repair of the bladder and compared with those who attained less bladder volume.
Outcome/ effect	Most patients who had a bladder volume of at least 85 ml after repair of the bladder were continent, compared with those who attained less bladder volume.
Historical significance/ comments	This study provides a guideline in decision making as to which patients should undergo bladder neck repair and the best stage at which bladder neck repair is likely to be successful. It also helps in the decision of when to divert urine rather than proceed to do a bladder neck repair that is likely to fail. Before proceeding to bladder neck repair, the patient should have a bladder volume of at least 85 ml.

Key Summary Points

1. Exstrophy of the bladder is part of a spectrum of diseases of varying severity.

2. Exstrophy of the bladder may result in carcinoma and social isolation.

3. Use plastic material to protect the bladder mucosa soon after birth.

4. Early surgery gives the best opportunity for reconstruction but must be done at an age when available support facilities can adequately maintain the child postoperatively.

5. Osteotomy is necessary after 72 hours of age.

6. Complete dissection of the urogenital diaphragm from the pubic bone is necessary for adequate closure of the bladder.

7. Bladder neck reconstruction gives the best results when bladder volume is at least 85 ml.

8. With modern reconstructive techniques, 80–90% achieve social continence.

9. Urinary diversion is important in the management of a number of patients and requires long-term follow-up.

Suggested Reading

Agwu KK. Imaging of the complicated bladder exstrophy presenting with ureteric duplication. West Afr J Radiol 2001; 8(1):29–32.

Attah CA, Enabulele UF, Ike CG, Chukwulebe AE. Exstrophy of the bladder—management options. Ebonyi Med J 2006; 5(1):1–6.

Baker LA, Gearhart JP. The staged approach to bladder exstrophy closure and the role of osteotomies. World J Urol 1998; 16(3):205–211.

Borzi PA, Thomas DF. Cantwell Ransley epispadias repair in male epispadias and bladder exstrophy. J Urol 1994; 151(2):457–459.

Catti M, Paccalin C, Rudigoz RC, Mouriquand C. Quality of life for adult women born with bladder and cloacal exstrophy: a long term follow-up. J Pediatr Urol 2006; 2(1):16–22.

Fahmy MA, Mansour AZ, Mazy A. Ureterorectostomy as continent urinary diversion. Int J Surg 2007; 5(6):394–398.

Gearhart JP. Exstrophy, epispadias and other bladder anomalies. In: Walsh PC, Retik AB, Vaughan ED, et al., eds. Campbell's Urology, vol 3, 8th ed. Saunders, 2003, CD ROM version, chapter 61.

Gearhart JP. Complete repair of bladder exstrophy in the newborn: complications and management. J Urol 2001; 165(6, pt 2):2431–2433.

Grady R, Mitchell ME. Complete repair of exstrophy. J Urol 1999; 162:1415.

Hafez AT, Elsherbiny MT, Ghoneim MT. Complete repair of bladder exstrophy: preliminary experience with neonates and children with failed initial closure. J Urol 2001; 165(6, pt 2):2428–2430.

Hernandez DJ, Purves T, Gearhart JP. Complications of surgical reconstruction of the exstrophy epispadias complex. J Pediat Urol 2008; 4(6):460–466.

Husmann DA, McLorie GA, Churchill BM. Closure of the exstrophic bladder: an evaluation of the factors leading to its success and its importance on urinary continence. J Urol 1989; 142:522.

Lowentritt BH, Van Zigl PS, Frimberger D, Baird A, Lakshmanan Y, Gearhart JP. Variants of the exstrophy complex: a single institution experience. J Urol 2005; 173(5):1732–1737.

Mteta KA, Mbwambo JS, Eshieman JL, Aboud MM, Oyieko W. Urinary diversion in children with mainly exstrophy and epispadias: alternative to primary bladder closure. Cent Afr J Med 2000; 46(12):318–320.

Njoku O, Wedderman K. Pregnancies following a treated ectopia vesicae. Port Harcourt Med J 2006; 1(1):62–64.

Schartz RB, King JA, Todd Purves J, Sponseller PD, Gearhart JP. Repeat pelvic osteotomy in cloacal exstrophy: applications and outcomes. J Pediatr Urol 2007; 3(5):398–403.

Sponseller PD, Bisson LJ, Gearhart JP, et al. The anatomy of the pelvis in the exstrophy complex. J Bone Joint Surg (AM) 1995; 77:177.

Youssif M, Badawy H, Saad A, Hanno A, Mokhless I. Single stage repair of bladder exstrophy in older children and children with failed previous repair. J. Paediatr Urol 2007; 3(5):391–394.

CHAPTER 93
URETHRAL VALVES

Stefan Wolke

Christopher C. Amah

Introduction

Posterior urethral valves (PUVs) are a rare malformation in the subcollicular region of the male urethra. They cause varying obstructions of the lower urinary tract. The resulting secondary pathological conditions extend from mild—in part, clinically unmanifested—urinary dysfunctions to severe, bilateral changes in the upper urinary tract and associated renal failure. The literature puts the incidence between 1 in 5,000 and 1 in 8,000 male births. No clear hereditary association has been demonstrated, although a certain hereditary aspect is probable.[1] An incidence in identical twins and, very rarely, a familial cluster have been described in the literature. There are usually no concomitant malformations outside the genitourinary tract.

The modern literature on PUVs had its origin in the publications of Young et al. in 1919.[2] Their differentiation of three types of valves is a subject of debate, but is still used regularly. From the perspective of paediatric surgery, type I and type III urethral valves are of particular significance. In these, the flow of urine is opposed either by mucous membrane folds projecting "backdrop-like" into the lumen in lithotomy position from 7 to 5 o'clock directly below the seminal colliculus (type I), or by an aperture-like stenosis (type III).

A more recent description of the valve structures with the designation COPUM (congenital obstructive posterior urethral membrane) subsumes Young et al.'s type I and II valves into one class. Endoscopic observations agree well with this classification, when it is taken together with the different structure known as "Cobb's collar", which is clearly distal of the seminal colliculus.[3]

Aetiology

The embryological aetiology of PUVs is not clear. The physiological and morphological changes do not fit easily into the accepted idea of the development of the urethra out of parts of the embryonic cloaca, the urogenital sinus, and parts of the wolffian duct. Further, dysplastic changes in the kidneys in severe cases of urethral valves suggest a dysontogenetic aspect in the development of the wolffian duct derivatives beyond the purely secondary changes resulting from the distal obstruction. Histologically, it is possible to find parallels here to findings obtained in cases of multicystic diseased kidney (MCDK).[4]

In addition to PUVs, so-called anterior urethral valves in the more distally located part of the male urinary tract occasionally have been described. These may represent a separate condition; they appear extremely rarely and have not been described uniformly in the literature. Therefore, they will not be covered in this chapter.

Pathological Features

In regions with a well-developed prenatal diagnostic infrastructure, suspicious findings pointing to urethral valves can be obtained early in pregnancy. Severe secondary changes, such as megacystis and bilateral hydronephrosis, are already visible in the 10th to 12th week of gestation.[5] For the most part, however, the pathological findings are obtained during the second trimester screening ultrasound (US) after the 20th week of pregnancy (Figure 93.1). At this point in utero, the kidneys are largely developed. As a result, intrauterine measures to protect the foetal kidneys are of doubtful value. The complete sonographic urethral valve picture with megacystis (keyhole bladder), bilateral hydronephrosis, and oligohydramnios need not be present, even in the case of a pronounced finding of urethral valves. More frequently, one finds—in addition to a conspicuously large, rarely emptying bladder (see Figure 93.1)—a single-sided hydronephrosis. In some cases, the subvesical obstruction causes a backup of urine that is relieved over a rupture, usually spreading out into the fornix area of the kidney, or more rarely of the urinary bladder. These cases become conspicuous because of an associated urinoma or an associated ascites.[6] This "pop-off" mechanism can bring about protection of the kidneys. If, as a result of the inadequate foetal excretion of urine, anhydramnios develops, the child shows the renofascial dysplasia known as Potter sequence. These children are not viable. In the case of oligohydramnios, as well, lung development and maturation of the foetus can be disturbed, which results in a disruption of postnatal adaptation.

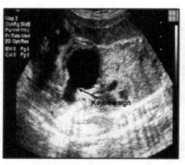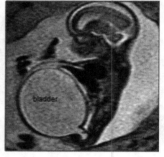

Source: Courtesy of Kokila Lakoo, Oxford Children's Hospital, Oxford, UK.

Figure 93.1: Foetal US (left) showing PUV and foetal magnetic resonance imaging (MRI; right) showing large bladder.

Neither the sonomorphology alone nor the point in time at which the secondary pathologies are determined are reliable predictors for the outcome of the patient. In addition, investigations of the foetal urine do not result in additional useful indications. The creatinine and urea of the foetus are excreted through the placenta through the mother's kidneys, so only after the first day of life can the retention parameters of the child be taken as an expression of the child's own renal functioning.

The natural course of the pregnancy when urethral valves are present does not result in a relevant premature delivery. In a case of megacystis or ascites causing displacement, foetoamniotic shunting or serial puncture can be considered. Experience with vesicoamniotic shunting has not been good due to frequent dislocation of the shunt. Serial amniotic fluid instillation also does not improve the prognosis. Because intrauterine interventions, including foetoscopic ablation of the valves, have to be carried out late in pregnancy, the prognostic advantage for the baby has to be questioned. In addition, as is often the case in prenatal therapy, we lack reliable prognostic factors for establishing reliable indication for therapy for individual cases. It is probable that prenatal diagnosis of PUV and the immediate postnatal therapy improve outcome only in cases with the most pronounced findings.

Given the situation of medical care in developing countries, both prenatal and, perhaps, postnatal sonographic diagnosis cannot be placed in the foreground.[7] In one reported series,[8] all diagnoses were based on postnatal US, micturiting cystourethrogram, and urethrocystoscopy in older children and adolescents. The great majority of patients become conspicuous due to the symptoms of urethral obstruction. These are mainly difficulty in urinating, recurring urinary tract infections (UTIs), or a palpable intraabdominal mass. This means that there can be a considerable delay in making a relevant diagnosis. The presence of associated urinomas or an associated ascites is possible. Special attention should be paid to urinary irregularities and to performing further diagnostic tests after recurring UTIs in boys.

Diagnostic Work-Up

Transperineal US can be used to detect urethral valves. However, the diagnosis of urethral valves is made on the basis of a voiding cysto-urethrography (VCUG) (Figure 93.2). This shows the dilated proximal urethra; the deformed, thick-walled urinary bladder with pseudodiverticuli; and (usually) the vesicoureteral reflux (VUR) (Figure 93.3). In cases of pronounced pathology of the upper urinary pathways involving disruption of urinary transport (grades IV–V), VUR can be absent. Even in the case of unclear findings with involvement of the upper urinary tract, diagnostic/therapeutic cystoscopy is recommended. Repeated determination of the retention parameters is necessary as a basis for estimating the global functioning of the kidneys. Initial pathologically raised retention parameters (serum creatinine > 1 mg/dl) and, more significantly, raised retention parameters later than two weeks after treatment are prognostically unfavorable results.[9] For the evaluation of single renal clearance and, if necessary, to determine the extent of the urinary transport disturbance, the authors perform, after therapy at no earlier than the age of 6 weeks (corrected for gestation age), a technetium-99m mercaptuacetyltriglycine (Tc-99m MAG3) scan with a furosemide (Lasix®) load (Figure 93.4).

Treatment Protocol

On suspicion of urethral valves, treatment of the symptoms is more important than diagnostics. Symptomatic therapy generally consists of insertion of a transurethral or vesical catheter to drain off the urine. Normally, there is no difficulty in overcoming retrograde entrance of the valve structures with a catheter. If urine drainage is expected to last longer than 2–4 weeks, surgical urine drainage such as vesicostomy is preferable.

At every age, treatment consists of endoscopic ablation of the urethral valves.

1. Incision of the valve structures using a neodymium:yttrium aluminium garnet (Nd:YAG) laser over a 6 Fr cystoscope can be carried out even with the majority of prematurely born children. Fundamentally, laser ablation using the Nd:YAG laser in contact procedure with the bare fibre is preferred.

2. With endoscopic monitoring employing very precisely dosed energy, the valve structures are incised at 12, 5, and 7 o'clock with the patient in the lithotomy position.

3. A bladder catheter is inserted for 1 week. Before the patient is discharged, the result of surgery is checked once again cystoscopically.

The alternative surgical option is cold incision of the structures by using the endoscopic resectoscope, which is larger in size. Electrocoagulation (fulguration) is not recommended for infants due to the risk of urethral strictures, which have not been observed after use of the laser. Technically simpler methods for destroying the valve structures are the use of a balloon catheter (either blind or with x-ray monitoring) or a transurethral incision by using the Mohan urethral valvotome.[10] In developing and resource-poor countries, catheter balloon avulsion, open

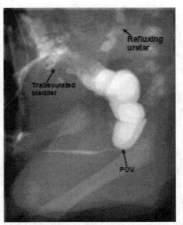

Source: Courtesy of Kokila Lakhoo, Oxford Children's Hospital, Oxford, UK.
Figure 93.2: Micturating cystourethrography (MCUG) showing PUV and sequel.

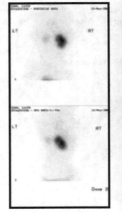

Source: Courtesy of Kokila Lakhoo, Oxford Children's Hospital, Oxford, UK.
Figure 93.3: Postnatal US showing thick bladder wall.

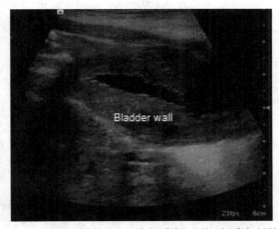

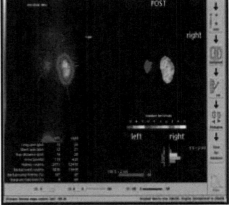

Source: Courtesy of Kokila Lakhoo, Oxford Children's Hospital, Oxford, UK.
Figure 93.4: MAG3 scan showing 4% function in the left kidney and 96% in the right kidney.

(suprapubic) excision, and endoscopic transurethral fulguration of the valves remain the main modalities of treatment.

Endoscopic treatment of the valves is the only causal therapy. Restoration of unimpeded flow in the urethra is the necessary precondition for the physiological and functional rehabilitation of the urinary bladder and the upper urinary tract. However, successful treatment does not ensure that the secondary pathologies will be cured.

Since the obstruction was present and active prenatally, it leads to functional and structural changes in the urinary bladder and the upper urinary tract known as the valve-bladder syndrome.

After successful treatment, the authors have observed both a complete restoration of urine flow as well as chronic functional disturbances of the urinary bladder and the kidneys. In the authors' patient population, all boys with a continued pathological increase in the retention parameters 2 weeks after successful surgery developed a terminal renal failure before reaching the age of 11 years.[9] The disorders in bladder function can be not only a lazy bladder, but also a hyperreflexive bladder of low capacity. The morphological correlates are a bladder with a large volume with high compliance and a significant amount of residual urine or a small bladder with a thick wall and low compliance. Urodynamic examinations of boys with a conspicuous pattern of excretion after the first year of life are conducted. An isolated enuresis nocturna as the sole symptom of a urethral valve disorder has not been observed. A subjective and objective reduced flow of urine requires clarification (sonography, VCUG, or possibly cystoscopy).[8]

If there is no possibility of a quick endoscopic treatment, surgical vesicostomy offers the possibility of an effective and technically simple temporary treatment.

From the perspective of maximal protection of the kidneys, a persistent restricted renal function can make introduction of a high diversion necessary. This can be achieved, for example, by means of a terminal cutaneous ureterostomy, loop ureterostomy, ureterostomy according to Sober, or pyelostomy. Catheter nephrostomy is suitable only for short-term relief due to the risk of infection. A vesicostomy *after* a successful treatment of the valves is not indicated and should be considered only in the case of nonrelevant, proximal disruption of urine transport.

Conclusion

In summary, in a case of conspicuous urethral valves—after immediate symptomatic treatment and carrying out the endoscopic procedure as quickly as possible following evaluation of the renal function—treatment of possible secondary pathologies such as VUR, renal flow obstruction, and voiding disorders should be undertaken in the first year of life, but as conservatively as possible. After the passage of a year, new examinations (sonography, VCUG, scintigraphy (if necessary), and urodynamics) are carried out to determine the course of the condition and whether there is need for a directed therapy. Any therapy here would focus on the individual primary conditions (ureteropelvic junction stenosis, ureteral orifice stenosis, severe vesicoureteral reflux, etc.) and be based on the criteria for their treatment. All children with initial restricted renal function—in particular, with persisting global renal restriction—have to be in nephrological/paediatric surgical (urological) outpatient care.

Studies have shown that, despite adequate surgical treatment, patients with an initial urethral valve symptomatology only rarely show no morphological or functional urinary tract pathologies on in-depth follow-up examinations. The prognosis of valve patients requiring transplants also depends on whether there are any persisting bladder dysfunctions. The bladder dysfunctions can be influenced therapeutically—for example, by medication. With this approach, it is possible to improve long-term prognosis in the treatment of posterior urethral valves.

References

1. Rajab A, Freeman NV, Patton M. The frequency of posterior urethral valves in Oman. Br J Urol 1996; 77(6):900–904.

2. Young HH, Frontz WA, Baldwin JC. Congenital obstruction of the posterior urethra. J Urol 1919; 3:289–365.

3. Dewan PA, Keenan RJ, Morris LL, Le Quesne GW. Congenital urethral obstruction: Cobb's collar or prolapsed congenital obstructive posterior urethral membrane (COPUM). Br J Urol 1994; 73(1):91–95.

4. Haecker FM, Wehrmann M, Hacker HW, Stuhldreier G, von Schweinitz D. Renal dysplasia in children with posterior urethral valves: a primary or secondary malformation? Pediatr Surg Int 2002; 18(2–3):119–122.

5. Dewan PA. Antenatal diagnosis of posterior urethral valves. Br J Urol 1994; 73(5):600–601.

6. Patil KK, Wilcox DT, Samuel M, Duffy PG, Ransley PG, González R. Management of urinary extravasation in 18 boys with posterior urethral valves. J Urol 2003; 169(4):1508–1511; discussion 1511.

7. Ikuerowo SO, Balogun BO, Akintomide TE, Ikuerowo AO, Akinola RA, Gbelee HO, Esho JO. Clinical and radiological characteristics of Nigerian boys with posterior urethral valves. Pediatr Surg Int 2008; 24(7):825–829. Epub 24 April 2008.

8. Aghaji AE, Amah CC. Posterior urethral valves. Nig J Surg Sci 1999; 9:18–22.

9. Eckoldt F, Heling KS, Woderich R, Wolke S. Posterior urethral valves: prenatal diagnostic signs and outcome. Urol Int 2004; 73(4):296–301.

10. Ikuerowo SO, Omisanjo OA, Balogun BO, Akinola RA, Alagbe-Briggs OT, Esho JO. Mohan's valvotome for the ablation of posterior urethral valves. J Pediatr Urol 2009; 5(4):279–282.

CHAPTER 94
HYPOSPADIAS

Ahmed T. Hadidi
Philemon E. Okoro

Introduction

Hypospadias is a wide spectrum of abnormalities involving the inferior surface of the penis and having in common a urethral opening that lies on the inferior surface of the penis, (*hypo* = under; *spadias* = opening or rent).

The spectrum of hypospadias anomalies includes an abnormal urethral opening, chordee (ventral curvature of the penis), an incomplete prepuce, rotation of the penis, abnormal raphe, and disorganised corpus spongiosum and penile fascia.

Worldwide, hypospadias surgery is known to be challenging and technically demanding. In some parts of Africa, this is complicated by unawareness and some deleterious cultural and religious beliefs. Hence, the majority of hypospadias patients in Africa are referred late, already circumcised or with signs of mutilation due to failed repair or cultural practices. In addition, suboptimal theatre conditions, lack of delicate instruments and suture materials, and high infection rates in some parts of Africa make hypospadias repair even more difficult.

Epidemiology

Hypospadias is the most frequent congenital urological anomaly, occurring in 1–3 per 1,000 live births. The incidence varies geographically from 0.26 per 1,000 live births in Mexico to 3.9 per 1,000 live births in the United States.[1]

Reports have suggested that the prevalence of hypospadias varies across different races, being highest among caucasians, less in Hispanics, and least in blacks.[2]

Embryology

During the 3rd week of gestation, mesenchymal cells migrate around the cloacal membrane to form slightly elevated cloacal folds. During the 4th week, the cloaca folds cranially to form the genital tubercle, and caudally to form the urethral folds anteriorly and the anal fold posteriorly. In the meantime, another pair of elevations, the genital swellings, become visible on each side of the urethral folds. These swellings later form the scrotal swellings in the male and the labia majora in the female. Until the end of the 6th week, it is impossible to differentiate between the two sexes.[3]

Development of the external genitalia in the male is under the influence of androgens secreted by the foetal testis and is characterised by rapid elongation of the genital tubercle, which is now called the phallus. During this elongation, the phallus pulls the urethral folds forward so that they form the urethral plate. This urethral plate extends along the undersurface of the elongated phallus into the glans (Figure 94.1).

The origin of the urethral mucosa has been variously described as endodermal,[4] ectodermal,[5] or mixed.[6] In the 1950s, Glenister proposed that the male urethra develops by fusion of the urethral folds over the urethral groove.[7] This fusion extends from the proximal to the distal end of the penis. The last part of the formation of the urethra is the canalisation of a cord of ectodermal cells extending from the apex of the glans to the distal end of the developing urethra. Thus,

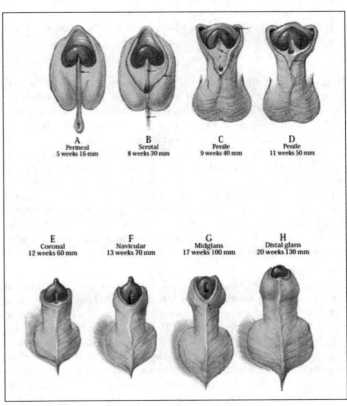

Source: Hadidi AT, Azmy AF, eds. Hypospadias Surgery: An Illustrated Guide, 1st ed. Springer Verlag, 2004. Reproduced with kind permission of Springer Verlag.

Figure 94.1: Normal urethral development. The urethral meatus shifts distally as the embryo gets older to reach the distal glans at about 20 weeks of gestation.

the distal urethra is the last to form and also the most common site of hypospadias.[8,9] The mesenchyme in the urethral folds subsequently becomes the corpus spongiosum. A ridge just proximal to the corona develops at about the 8th week of intrauterine life. This ridge is carried distally by active mesenchymal growth around the corona to form a cone-shaped prepuce. A defect of the urethra would, therefore, prevent the ventral aspect of the cone from developing. By the 12th week of intrauterine life, the labioscrotal folds fuse completely in the midline to form the scrotum.[10,11]

The formation of the urethra is still a matter of speculation. The long-accepted assumption that the urethra forms by fusion of the urethral folds in the midline—similar to closing a zipper—has been challenged in recent years. Van der Putte and Kluth failed to find any evidence of midline fusion.[12–15] Furthermore, the fusion theory cannot explain the wide spectrum of anomalies associated with hypospadias, such as chordee with or without hypospadias, torsion and different glans configuration, and meatus size commonly encountered in hypospadias.

Aetiology

A unifying aetiology for hypospadias remains elusive. Hypospadias probably results from multiple factors—namely, endocrine, genetic, and environmental.

- *Endocrine:* Hypospadias may result from disruption in the synthetic biopathway of androgens, defective local androgen receptors, or a subnormal testosterone response to human chorionic gonadotropin (hCG) stimulation.

- *Genetic:* Hypospadias may have a complex genetic background. The familial incidence of hypospadias is about 7%, which reflects a nonfamilial sporadic finding in most cases.[16]

- *Environmental:* The incidence of hypospadias is increasing world-wide. One possible explanation is environmental contamination. Insecticides, pharmaceuticals, plant estrogens—the so-called "endocrine disruptors"—have been incriminated.[17]

Morphology

Hypospadias presents in various ways. The abnormality usually affects more than one component of the male organ. It is very important for the surgeon operating on hypospadias to be aware of its different morphological features. Such variations influence dramatically the choice of the most suitable operation for an individual patient.

The task of the hypospadias surgeon is to try to correct all the different components of the hypospadias spectrum and not just bring the urethral meatus to the tip of the glans penis. The surgical technique that is suitable for a child with a cleft glans and wide, well-vascularised urethral plate is totally different from the technique suitable for a patient with flat glans and fibrotic, nonpliable, narrow urethral plate. For this reason, hypospadias surgery differs from surgery for most other anomalies of the human body.

The Meatus

The common shape of meatus in hypospadias is the transverse form. In some patients, the meatus may look like a longitudinal fissure, but in fact it is circular at the proximal end of the fissure. The other common type is the pinpoint type of meatus. The pinpoint opening may be surrounded by a soft yielding tissue that dilates during micturition or may be surrounded by a fibrous ring that may cause difficulty to pass urine. In glanular hypospadias, there may be an elevation (bridge) distal to the meatus. This usually suggests that the urethra is mobile and can be stretched to the tip of the glans. The double-Y glanuloplasty (DYG) or *M*eatal *A*dvancement and *G*lanulo*p*lasty *I*ncorporated (MAGPI) technique is suitable for such cases.

There may be several openings, which represent openings of paraurethral canals or lacula of Morgagni. The presence of a distal opening may lead the parents and the inexperienced practitioner to think that the hypospadias is more distal that it really is. As a general rule, *the most proximal orifice is the actual urethral orifice connected to the bladder.*[18]

The Glans

Patients with hypospadias have an abnormal-looking globular glans. The glans is classified into three categories based on the degree of clefting and urethral plate projection.[19]

1. Cleft glans (Figure 94.2(A)): There is a deep groove in the middle of the glans with proper clefting; the urethral plate is narrow and projects to the tip of the glans. An example is the "hidden hypospadias" (megameatus-intact prepuce). Tubularisation of the urethral plate without incision or pyramid repair gives good results.

2. Incomplete cleft glans (Figure 94.2(B)): There is a variable degree of glans split, a shallow glanular groove, and a variable degree of urethral plate projection. An inverted-Y tubularised plate (YTP) or inverted-Y meatoglanuloplasty usually gives good results.

3. Flat glans (Figure 94.2(C)): The urethral plate ends short of the

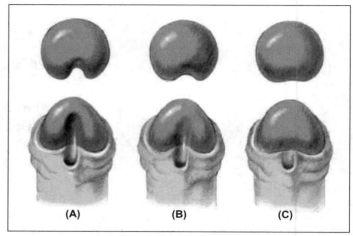

Source: Hadidi AT, Azmy AF, eds. Hypospadias Surgery: An Illustrated Guide, 1st ed. Springer Verlag, 2004. Reproduced with kind permission of Springer Verlag.

Figure 94.2: Different glans configurations.

glans penis; there is no glanular groove. Generous glans splitting is required to achieve good cosmetic and functional results. The new urethra has to be embedded deep into the glans to have a satisfactory cosmetic appearance and maintain a wide meatus.

Chordee

The term "chordee" was introduced into medical literature in the 17th century from the French in relation to gonorrhea. It was defined as a "painful downward curvature of the penis due to inflammation".[20] Most hypospadias pioneers in the 19th century used terms such as incurvation, curvature, or bending. Clinton Smith, in the 1930s, was probably the first to use the term chordee to describe congenital curvature associated with hypospadias.[21] Some publications mention that the word chordee comes from the Greek word *chorde* and means cord[22] and define chordee as a congenital defect of the genitourinary tract resulting in a ventral curvature of the penis, caused by presence of a fibrous band of tissue instead of normal skin along the corpus spongiosum.[22] This definition is inaccurate and may be misleading.

Chordee has a wide spectrum and may be due to disproportionate growth of one of the fascial coverings or skin. It may be classified into one of the following categories:

- *Chordee without hypospadias:* This occurs when there is deficiency or disproportionate growth of skin and/or dartos fascia, Buck's fascia, or corpus spongiosum. The urethra is normal, although it may be very thin, and it lies directly under the skin when the corpus spongiosum is also deficient.

- *Hypospadias with superficial chordee* (Figure 94.3): This condition is present when there is disproportionate growth of the urethra as well. In this situation, the disproportionate growth involves the fascial structures and skin superficial to the urethra. This may be encountered in some distal forms of hypospadias, and incision proximal to the meatus and mobilisation of the skin from the underlying urethra usually corrects this form of chordee.

- *Hypospadias with deep chordee* (Figure 94.4): This type of hypospadias is encountered when the Buck's fascia deeper to the urethra is also involved. The disorganised tissue is mainly distal to the meatus. This form of deep chordee is encountered in about 50% of proximal hypospadias. Incision of the urethral plate is needed to correct the curvature of the penis.

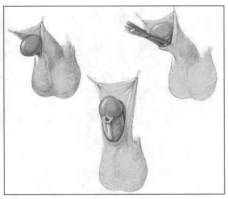

Figure 94.3: Superficial chordee.

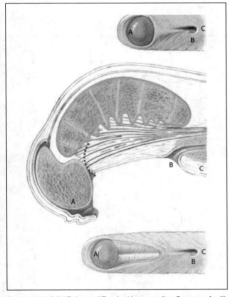

Figure 94.4: Deep chordee. Deep chordee is usually associated with proximal hypospadias. Incision of the urethral plate at the coronal sulcus will increase the distance between the tip of the penis (A) and the urethral meatus (B). The distance between the urethral meatus (B) and the penoscrotal junction (C) remains constant.

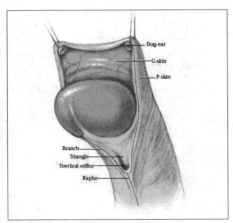

Figure 94.5: Prepuce in hypospadias.

• *Hypospadias with corporeal disproportion:* This condition is rather rare. The situation is encountered when the ventral tunica albuginea surrounding the corpora cavernosa is also contracted. Excision of the disorganised fascial tissue distal to the meatus is not enough to achieve a straight penis. This condition is thought to be encountered mainly in older children with long-standing uncorrected proximal hypospadias.

The Prepuce

The prepuce presents in several variations in hypospadias. In the majority of patients, the prepuce is longer than normal dorsally but absent ventrally. There are two lateral edges that are fixed at the lateral borders of the ventral aspect of the prepuce. Thus, the prepuce is deficient ventrally. To get an idea about the area of underdevelopment of the urethra and corpus spongiosum , draw two lines along the two lateral edges of the prepuce.

A common finding in many hypospadias patients is two rounded knobs laterally on the dorsum of the prepuce (like two little eyes, whirls, or dog-ears) (Figure 94.5). The significance of these two knobs is still unclear. These two little knobs are visible on the prepuce after preputial reconstruction following hypospadias repair. Attempts to excise the two knobs during the prepuce reconstruction usually results in a very short prepuce, and it is important to inform the parents of this beforehand.

The prepuce itself may accentuate the degree of penile chordee. In many cases, the family doctor reports the presence of penile chordee because of the hooded appearance of the prepuce and the presence of a peculiar line of cleavage.

In less than 5% of hypospadias patients, the prepuce is complete, covers the whole glans and is longer than normal. This may result in late diagnosis of hypospadias and excision of the prepuce wrongly in routine circumcision. This is considered as a separate entitiy and is called "hidden hypospadias" or mega-meatus intact prepuce (MIP) hypospadias.

The Urethral Plate

The urethral plate is a pink gutter of mucous membrane with a well-defined mucocutaneous line. This gutter may extend from the hypospadiac urethral orifice to the base of the glans penis. Rarely, it may extend well into the glans.

Paul and Kanagasuntheram have described the histological sections of this gutter to be stratified squamous epithelium with pigment in the malpighian layer.[23] These sections show no underlying layer of erectile tissue. In patients with perineal hypospadias, histology of sections within the scrotum showed pseudostratified columner epithelium rather than transitional epithelium. There is no erectile tissue.

The Penile Raphe

The penile raphe is normally situated in the ventral midline. In hypospadias, it is usually present (85%) and bifurcates proximal to the hypospadiac meatus into two branches that end distally into what is called eyes, whirls, or dog-ears (Figure 94.5). The area between the two branches of the raphe gives an idea of the extent of the developmental defect of the corpus spongiosum and ventral fascia.

Size of the Penis

The size of the penis is normal in the majority of hypospadias patients. Patients with disorders of sex development constitute a different category. Avellán has found penile hypoplasia in 3% of his patients, half of which had associated chromosomal anomalies.[24]

The Proximal Urethra

The proximal urethra may be very thin for a variable distance down to the perineum. This is probably due to the absence of corpus spongiosum to a variable degree. Incomplete urethral valves may be present and render the introduction of an intraurethral catheter difficult.

In some patients with hypospadias, there may be accessory blind paraurethral tracts that open at the same urethral opening and end blindly after 1–2 cm. Classic posterior urethral valves may be present in about 10% of patients with hypospadias

The Scrotum

In the majority of hypospadias patients (90%), the scrotum is normal. A partially bifid or completely bifid scrotum is occasionally present in proximal forms of hypospadias.

Penoscrotal transposition, a condition in which the scrotal skin surrounds the root of the penis to a variable extent, is also not common. Avellán has reported different degrees of penoscrotal transposition in 20% of his group of patients.[24]

The Testes

The majority of hypospadias patients have normal testes in the scrotum. Retractile or undescended testes may be encountered in 10% of patients with hypospadias, usually in proximal forms.[24]

Patients with hypospadias associated with an undescended testis should have chromosomal and hormonal analysis, as well as ultrasound to exclude chromosomal anomalies and disorders of sex differentiation (DSD).

Müllerian Remnants and Enlarged Utricles

Cystoscopy in proximal hypospadias may reveal enlarged verumontanum and utricles. This may explain the occasional difficulty encountered in catheterisation of some patients with severe forms of hypospadias.

Other Urological Malformations

The majority of hypospadias patients have no other urological anomalies. Rarely, there may be vesicoureteric reflux, a double ureter, a double renal pelvis, a single kidney, or an ectopic kidney.

Classification

Consistent classification is necessary to standardise the terminology of hypospadias to enable improved treatment and comparison of results across centres and surgeons. Several classifications have been described for hypospadias. However, the simplest and the most practical classification has been described in 1886 by Kaufmann,[25] who classified hypospadias into first degree (glanular), second degree (penile), and third degree (proximal) (Figure 94.6). Duckett classified hypospadias into eight subgroups (glanular, coronal, subcoronal, distal penile, mid-penile, proximal penile, penoscrotal, and perineal).[26]

Note that the different degrees of hypospadias require different operations, have different complication rates, and have different prognoses. Glanular and penile hypospadias constitute about 85% of patients with hypospadias. There are no specific operations designed for mid-penile hypospadias. Depending on the exact site and presence or absence of chordee, one may use techniques designed for either distal or proximal hypospadias. Children with hypospadias, penile, and gonadal anomalies should be classified under DSD.

It is suggested that preoperative evaluation forms such as those shown in Figure 94.7 be completed at the first operation for proper assessment. However, a two-stage procedure may be necessary in some cases.

Clinical Features

Hypospadias is usually diagnosed early in life because of the peculiar appearance of the hooded prepuce that is deficient ventrally in 95% of patients. The parents may notice that urine comes out from the undersurface of the penis and that it usually splays out rather than exiting in a stream.

Hypospadias is usually asymptomatic. Occasionally, the urethral opening is narrow and the patient may pass a very narrow stream of urine, with difficulty.

Detailed clinical examination is needed with recording of

- meatus site and size;
- presence of chordee and severity;
- glans configuration;
- complete or incomplete prepuce;

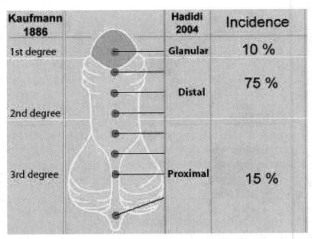

Source: Hadidi AT, Azmy AF, eds. Hypospadias Surgery: An Illustrated Guide, 1st ed. Springer Verlag, 2004. Reproduced with kind permission of Springer Verlag.

Figure 94.6: Classification of hypospadias.

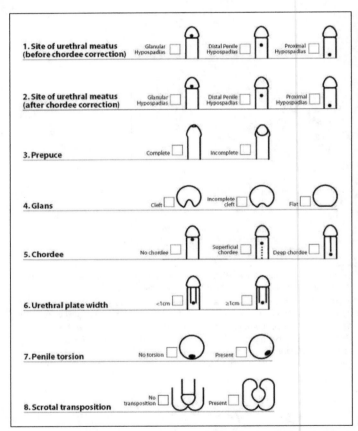

Source: Hadidi AT, Azmy AF, eds. Hypospadias Surgery: An Illustrated Guide, 1st ed. Springer Verlag, 2004. Reproduced with kind permission of Springer Verlag.

Figure 94.7: Hypospadias form.

- width of the urethral plate;
- presence of torsion;
- presence of bifid scrotum or penoscrotal transposition; and
- any associated anomalies (e.g., undescended testis).

Investigations

Healthy, asymptomatic patients with glanular and penile hypospadias may require no routine investigations.

Abdominal ultrasound and urinalysis are needed in patients with proximal hypospadias or urinary symptoms. Further investigations (e.g., micturating cystourethrogram) are indicated when the bladder, ureters, or kidneys are dilated. Chromosomal analysis is indicated when DSD is suspected.

Management

Parents Counselling

Once hypospadias is diagnosed, parent counselling is the first step that follows. The doctor should explain the condition in detail, emphasizing that it is not the fault of any of the parents and that familial incidence is about 7%.

It is also important to stress that circumcision is contraindicated in the presence of hypospadias because the preputial fascia and skin may be used to correct hypospadias. Circumcision may be required for medical, ethnic, or religious reasons (for more details on circumcision, see Chapter 95). Parents should be informed that complications can and may occur after surgery, but the majority are correctable.

Parents need assurance that patients with glanular and penile hypospadias have more than a 95% chance of normal functional and sexual life, provided that surgery is done by an experienced surgeon. The first operation has the best chance of success. Patients with penoscrotal hypospadias or intersex have a different prognosis, depending on the size of penis, chordee, and availability of healthy tissue.

Timing of Surgery

The penis grows less than 0.8 cm in the first 3 years of life: the phallus that is small at 3 months of age will still be small at 3 years of age.[27] Sexual identity is determined by 3 years of age. In older children, the psychological burden relating to this must not be underestimated (in some cases, this amounts to the sensation of being "different" from one's peers; in others, repeated operations on genitalia which may have a significant impact on the patient).

Studies[28] evaluating emotional, psychosexual, cognitive, and surgical risks have identified that there is an optimal window for surgery at 3–18 months of age (Figure 94.8).

However, anaesthesia in children younger than 6 months of age is technically demanding and requires experience. Hypospadias surgery in small children should be performed only in paediatric centres where experienced anaesthesia and intensive care services are available.

Referral Centres

Hypospadias surgery is a highly specialised surgery. Not every paediatric surgeon or urologist can perform it. Dedication, interest, experience, frequent surgery, and close follow-up of patients are key factors for success. There is no mild form of hypospadias that can be performed by an inexperienced surgeon. The best results of hypospadias surgery are obtained in centres that perform at least 50 hypospadias operations per year.

General Principles of Hypospadias Surgery

Preoperative Hormonal Treatment

Many surgeons advocate the routine preoperative use of local testosterone cream on the penis or intramuscular injection (1–2 mg/kg monthly for 3 months) up to one month before surgery to increase the size and vascularity of the penis.[17] However, the authors limit the use of preoperative hormones to severe cases of intersex with a very small phallus size. Hormonal therapy never acts locally, has several systemic side effects, makes the tissue oedematous, causes more bleeding, and does not improve the outcome.[29]

Instruments

A basic plastic surgery set of instruments is sufficient. Essential are 6–12 fine mosquito forceps, two finetooth dissecting forceps, fine sharp scissors, sharp scalpel, and fine needle holder.

Magnification

Urethroplasty is performed by using 6/0 or 7/0 sutures. The surgeon should be able to handle such fine sutures comfortably. Most surgeons

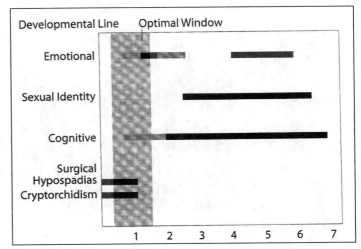

Source: Hadidi AT, Azmy AF, eds. Hypospadias Surgery: An Illustrated Guide, 1st ed. Springer Verlag, 2004. Reproduced with kind permission of Springer Verlag.

Figure 94.8: Timing of surgery.

prefer to use 2.5 or 3.5 magnifying loups.[30] Others, including the authors, prefer to use simple reading glasses. There is no evidence that supports the use of operating microscope in hypospadias repair.

Haemostasis

The penis is a very vascular organ. Haemostasis is an integral part of the operation. Some surgeons, including the authors, prefer to use a tourniquet whenever possible in order to reduce bleeding. The tourniquet should be released every 40 minutes. Swabs soaked in adrenaline (1:100,000) are also effective in hypospadias surgery. Bipolar diathermy, where available is useful and may reduce the need for a tourniquet. However, bipolar diathermy is not helpful when cutting through the glans, which is a sponge of blood. Monopolar diathermy is hazardous and is contraindicated because it may lead to thombosis and sloughing of the penis.

Degloving the Penis

Most surgeons perform degloving the penis as a primary step in hypospadias surgery to release any tethering causing superficial chordee.[31] The authors do not recommend routine degloving, but rather a 2-cm transverse incision proximal to the meatus to release superficial chordee.[32] Routine degloving is not only unnecessary, but may damage the blood supply of skin flaps, necessitate circumcision at the end of the operation, increase incidence of haematoma, and result in severe postoperative oedema of the penis.[32]

Suture Materials and Techniques

Fine 6/0 and 7/0 polyglactin absorbable suture (vicryl) are the standard sutures used in hypospadias repair. Several studies have shown that polydiaxanone (PDS) reacts with urine and causes a chemical reaction that increases the chances of fistula and complications.[33]

Different surgeons prefer different techniques, depending on which produces the best results for them. For urethroplasty, the authors prefer to use continuous extramucosal inverting sutures (Figure 94.9(A)). The idea is to reduce as much as possible the number of knots that act as a nidus for reaction and fistula. This technique helps to invert the epithelium into the lumen.[34] The surgeon should remember that healing occurs between the sutures. It is more important to have a well-vascularised urethroplasty than a water-tight suture line.

For glans closure, interrupted transverse mattress sutures using 7/0 vicryl help to avoid sutures cutting through the glans due to postoperative swelling and oedema (Figure 94.9(B)).

For skin closure, continuous mattress sutures using vicryl 6/0 or 7/0 usually give good results (Figure 94.9(C)).

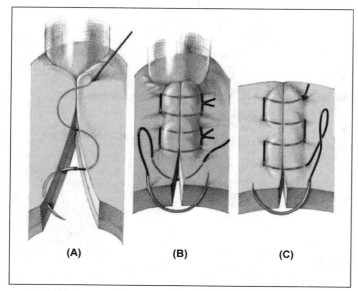

Figure 94.9: Different suturing techniques: (A) continuous subcuticular inverting suturing is suitable for urethroplasty; (B) interrupted transverse mattress is suitable for the glans closure; (C) continuous transverse mattress is suitable for skin closure.

Stents and Catheters

Stents and catheters are foreign bodies that irritate the urethral mucous membrane and may cause inflammation and fistula. The risk is less when silicon catheters or stents are used. In distal hypospadias, the first author does not leave catheters inside the urethra for more than 72 hours. In proximal hypospadias, the author prefers to use a suprapubic catheter for 12 days as a routine. Other surgeons use suprapubic catheters in complicated repair only. A suprapubic catheter leaves the patient symptom-free until the swelling disappears and allows the urethra to heal without having a foreign body (intraurethral stent or catheter) irritating the urethra. If the disposable suprapubic catheters are too expensive or are unavailable, one may use a simple size 10 Fr nelaton catheter introduced through a reusable trocar into the urinary bladder.

Dressings

There are more than 150 methods of dressing to cover the penis after hypospadias operations. Each has its advantages and disadvantages. A prospective randomised study perfomed in Cairo University showed that applying no dressing results in fewer complications than applying dressing for 5 days or more.[35] In places with hot, humid weather, and particularly in Africa, keeping the wound exposed and dry is much better than having a wet dressing on the wound. A dry wound is a clean wound.

The authors prefer to apply a simple dressing of dry gauze and local antibiotic ointment on the ventral aspect of the penis and to fix the penis, dressing, and catheter against the lower abdominal wall with good adhesive plaster for 1 or 2 days, according to the age of the patient. This allows adequate compression of the penis as well as mobilisation of the child who can sit and play a few hours after surgery. After a period ranging from 1 to 7 days, depending on the age of the child and the difficulty of the operation, the penis is left exposed, and local ointment is applied 4 times daily for 1 week.

Postoperative Analgesia

Caudal nerve block is ideal for postoperative pain relief. However, it requires an experienced anaesthetist and complete strict asepsis.

Alternatively, a local penile nerve block could be performed. The dorsal nerves of the penis arise from the pudendal nerves, pass directly under the symphysis pubis, and penetrate the suspensory ligament to

continue under the deep Buck's fascia. Three to four milliliters of 0.5% long-acting bupivacaine mixed with 1% quick-acting lidocaine is used. Palpate the symphysis pubis, insert a 22-gauge needle at 10 o'clock, feel the inferior border of the bone, withdraw slightly and move it so that it is just clear of the bone. Pop it through the Buck's fascia, aspirate, and inject. Repeat the same procedure at 2 o'clock.

Postoperative Antibiotics

A broad-spectrum antibiotic (e.g., cephalosporin) is recommended in hypospadias surgery.[36] The authors give the first intravenous (IV) dose after induction of anaesthesia. Oral cephalosporine antibiotics are continued for 1 week after distal hypospadias or until the suprapubic catheter is removed in proximal hypospadias. This protocol may decrease the risk of a complicating urinary tract infections after surgery, and probably reduces meatal stenosis and urethrocutaneous fistula rates.

Objectives of Surgery

The primary goal of hypospadias surgery is to have a good functioning penis. This means ensuring that the penis is straight and that the child can micturate from the tip of the penis in a straight adequately wide stream of urine. The second important goal is for the penis to have a normal or near-normal appearance with a slit-like meatus at the tip of the glans.

An alarming observation in recent literature is that the cosmetic appearance is taking priority over the function of the penis. Many patients with a good-looking penis are referred with recurrent fistula and difficulty to pass urine due to a narrow new urethra.

The steps of hypospadias correction are the following:

1. Assessment;
2. Chordee correction;
3. Urethroplasty;
4. Protective intermediate layer;
5. Meatoglanuloplasty;
6. Scrotoplasty; and
7. Skin cover.

Assessment under Anaesthesia

A thorough examination under anesthesia and after preparation and cover is a very important step. Based on this assessment, the surgeon should plan the operation and choose the appropriate technique suitable for this particular patient. The surgeon should evaluate the patient under good illumination with magnification, noting the following features:

1. glans configuration (cleft, incomplete cleft, or flat);
2. urethral opening (if narrow, it should be dilated or incised);
3. quality of the skin on the ventral aspect of the penis distal to the urethral meatus;
4. quality of the skin proximal to the urethral opening (sometimes it is very thin and requires incision); and
5. scrotum (ensure that both testes are in the scrotum and exclude bifid scrotum and penoscrotal transposition).

Chordee Assessment and Correction

The different forms of chordee have been discussed earlier in this chapter. There are two methods of assessing chordee. One method is to apply traction on a thread through the glans and check any tethering or limitation. This is considered by many surgeons to be inadequate because it does not detect chordee due to shortening of the tunica albuginea, but it has the advantage of being the least invasive method. The other method is application of the "artificial erection test" (Figure 94.10) described by Gittes and McLaughlin in 1974.[37] It is the most common method used. A red rubber catheter is used as a tourniquet at the base of the penis, and normal saline is injected into a corporal body or into the glans through a 23-G butterfly needle. Both corporeal bodies are filled and show the extent of curvature. This technique may be repeated after chordee correction to assess the completion of the correction of chordee before proceeding with urethral reconstruction. Many surgeons, including the authors, consider the artificial erection test invasive because it results in the overuse of tunica albuginea plication and unnecessary shortening of an already short penis.

About 80% of glanular and distal hypospadias have no chordee. Superficial chordee that is released by skin and fascia incision proximal to the urethral meatus can be seen in about 15% of patients with glanular or distal hypospadias.

However, about 50% of proximal hypospadias have deep chordee that requires incision and release distal to the urethral meatus. In such cases, the authors prefer to incise the urethral plate just proximal to the coronal sulcus. Note that the connective tissue tethering may extend proximally and laterally, and mobilisation should be complete.

If the child has proximal hypospadias and presents late, incision of the urethral plate may not be enough, and application of grafts ventrally or dorsal tunica albuginea plication (TAP) may be necessary.

There are different grafts used for correction of severe chordee, including dermal grafts, buccal mucosa, small intestinal submucosa (SIS), or tunica vaginalis (TV).[38] Dermal graft is usually harvested from the lower abdominal skin crease after removal of the epithelium. The tunica albuginea is incised at the point of maximum curvature, and the dermal graft is sutured to the edges of the tunica abluginea with continuous sutures.[39]

The dorsal TAP is advocated by many surgeons due to its simplicity (Figure 94.11). Baskin and Ebbers recommend the application of nonabsorbable sutures dorsally at 12 o'clock position. They suggest that would help to reduce the potential damage of nerves and vessels to the glans.[40] TAP has two major disadvantages, however: (1) a higher incidence of chordee recurrence, and (2) shortening of an already short penis. Most parents do not approve of shortening the penis.[41]

Surgery Options

More than 300 methods are described for hypospadias correction. This is partly because of the wide spectrum of hypospadias presentations and partly because no single method produces 100% satisfactory results.

Surgeons may use one of the following tissues to form the neourethra (Figure 94.12):[42]

1. mobilisation of the urethra;

2. skin distal to the meatus;

3. skin proximal to the meatus;

4. preputial skin;

5. combined prepuce and skin proximal to the meatus;

6. scrotal skin;

7. dorsal penile skin; and

8. different grafts.

In general, the surgeon should use the technique that is suitable for the patient and with which he is most conversant. The best operation for hypospadias correction is the operation that brings the best results. In addition, the surgeon should not shorten an already short penis. It cannot be overemphasized that the surgeon has to choose the technique that is suitable for each individual patients. In other words, the surgeon needs to master several techniques to use in different situations.

Figure 94.13 summarises the common techniques the authors prefer to use for hypospadias correction.

MAGPI Technique

The MAGPI technique[43] is suitable in selected patients with glanular hypospadias and a mobile urethral meatus that can be pushed to the tip of the glans. If the technique is used when the urethral meatus is not mobile, the urethra will retract back, in what is known as "retrusive meatus". If a fixed meatus is forcefully pushed forward, it will always go back to to its original position.

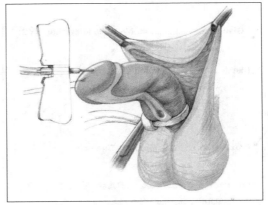

Source: Hadidi AT, Azmy AF, eds. Hypospadias Surgery: An Illustrated Guide, 1st ed. Springer Verlag, 2004. Reproduced with kind permission of Springer Verlag.

Figure 94.10: Artificial erection test.

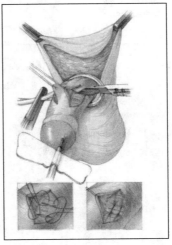

Source: Hadidi AT, Azmy AF, eds. Hypospadias Surgery: An Illustrated Guide, 1st ed. Springer Verlag, 2004. Reproduced with kind permission of Springer Verlag.

Figure 94.11: Tunica albuginea plication.

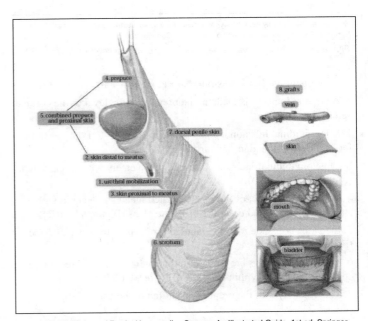
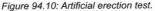

Source: Hadidi AT, Azmy AF, eds. Hypospadias Surgery: An Illustrated Guide, 1st ed. Springer Verlag, 2004. Reproduced with kind permission of Springer Verlag.

Figure 94.12: Tissues used for hypospadias repair.

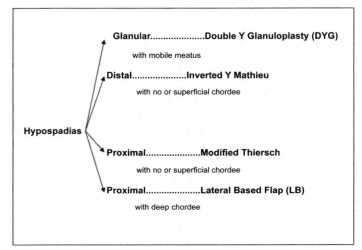

Source: Hadidi AT, Azmy AF, eds. Hypospadias Surgery: An Illustrated Guide, 1st ed. Springer Verlag, 2004. Reproduced with kind permission of Springer Verlag.

Figure 94.13: Authors' personal choice of operations.

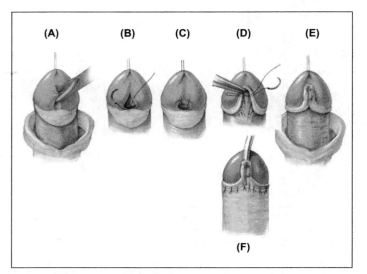

Source: Hadidi AT, Azmy AF, eds. Hypospadias Surgery: An Illustrated Guide, 1st ed. Springer Verlag, 2004. Reproduced with kind permission of Springer Verlag.

Figure 94.14: Meatal advancement and glanuloplasty incorporated (MAGPI).

The operative steps illustrated in Figure 94.14 are as follows:

1. A circular incision is made in the prepuce at the level of the coronal sulcus.

2. A longitudinal incision is made at the inner aspect of the meatus as far as the tip of the glans (Figure 94.14(A)).

3. This longitudinal incision is sutured transversely with single stitches (Figure 94.14(B),(C)).

4. The anterior aspect of the newly created meatus is secured with a stay suture and pulled up to the tip of the glans (Figure 94.14(D)).

5. Incisions are made in both glanular wings in an inverted V-shape (Figure 94.14(D)).

6. The glanular wings are sutured in the anteroposterior direction to enclose the urethra within the glans (Figure 94.14(E)).

7. The outer layer of the prepuce is sutured to the coronal sulcus (Figure 94.14(F)).

8. Preputial reconstruction, although possible, is not recommended at this stage.

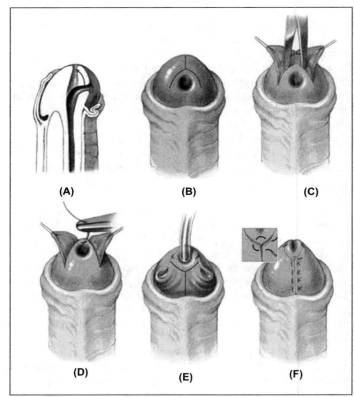

Source: Hadidi AT, Azmy AF, eds. Hypospadias Surgery, 2nd ed. Springer-Verlag, in press. Reproduced with kind permission of Springer Verlag.

Figure 94.15: Steps of double-Y glanuloplasty: (A) glanular hypospadias with mobile meatus; (B) inverted-Y incision; (C) three flaps elevated; (D) apex of meatus sutured to the tip of the glans; (E) Size Fr 10 catheter introduced inside the urethra and Y incision made that surrounds the meatus and extends down to the coronal sulcus; (F) glanular wings mobilised deep enough to wrap around the urethra and approximated in the midline. The 6 o'clock stitch (see inset) is a 3-point stitch that brings the urethra and the two medial edges of the glanular wings together. It is magnified in the inset.

Double-Y Glanuloplasty Technique

The double-Y glanuloplasty (DYG) technique (Figure 94.15) is suitable for selected patients with glanular hypospadias with mobile meatus in the absence of deep chordee. Those patients usually have a little ridge distal to meatus. This ridge can be pushed with a mosquito or toothed forceps to the tip of the glans.

If the distal edge of the urethral meatus is immobile and cannot be pushed to the tip of the glans, the child is not suitable for the DYG technique, and another technique suitable for distal hypospadias is performed (inverted-Y Mathieu technique in patients with flat glans or inverted-Y Thiersch in patients with cleft glans; see following two subsections, respectively).

1. A 5/0 nylon traction suture is placed on the glans, dorsal to the tip of the glans. A tourniquet is placed at the root of the penis and chordee is excluded by using the artificial erection test.

2. An inverted-Y incision is outlined on the glans. The centre of the inverted Y is just above the ridge distal to the meatus. The longitudinal limb extends to the tip of the glans where the tip of the neomeatus will be located. Each oblique limb of the inverted-Y is 0.5 cm long, and the angle between them is 60° (Figure 94.15(A,B)).

3. The incision is deepened and the flaps are mobilised to allow more mobility of the meatus (Figure 94.15(C)).

4. A 6/0 vicryl stitch is approximated and fixes the meatus at the tip of the glans (Figure 94.15(D)).

5. If the meatus is narrow or pinpoint, it is incised to make it wide

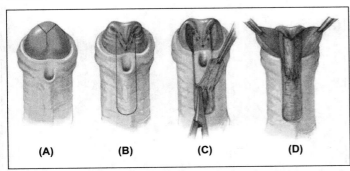

Source: Hadidi AT, Azmy AF, eds. Hypospadias Surgery: An Illustrated Guide, 1st ed. Springer Verlag, 2004. Reproduced with kind permission of Springer Verlag.

Figure 94.16: Y-V modified Mathieu technique.

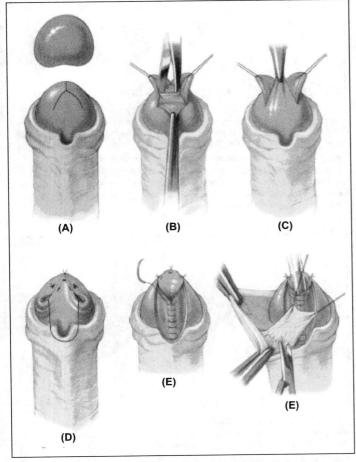

Source: Hadidi AT, Azmy AF, eds. Hypospadias Surgery, 2nd ed. Springer-Verlag, in press. Reproduced with kind permission of Spring Verlag.

Figure 94.17: Steps of inverted-Y Thiersch technique.

enough to accommodate a catheter size Fr 10 or larger according to the age of the patient and size of the penis. A transurethral Nelaton catheter size Fr 10 or larger is inserted into the bladder.

6. A Y-shaped incision is made proximal to the meatus (Figure 94.15(E)). The longitudinal limb of the Y incision extends from the meatus to the coronal sulcus. Extra care should be taken to avoid injury to the very thin urethra beneath the skin. The use of sharp scissors and traction helps to avoid injury of the distal urethra.

7. Traction is applied on the glanular wings, and the incision is deepened by using sharp scissors starting proximally at the coronal sulcus.

8. The glanular wings are mobilised off the urethra and are opened

like an open book. This is a very important step that helps to wrap the glanular wings around the urethra without any tension.

9. The incision is continued around the meatus to meet the lateral limbs of the inverted-Y incision (Figure 94.15(F)).

10. Local ointment is applied to the wound, a normal gauze is applied, and adhesive tape fixes the gauze, the catheter, and the penis against the lower abdominal wall. This allows free mobility of the patient and secures the catheter and penis against the lower abdominal wall.

The transurethral catheter is left for 1–2 days, depending on the degree of mobilisation and the degree of postoperative oedema of the penis. A caudal block is routinely used to reduce postoperative pain.

Inverted-Y Modified Mathieu Repair
The Mathieu technique is used for distal hypospadias. It is one of the oldest procedures, having withstood the test of time. It has a drawback, however—it results in a circular meatus that is not at the tip of the glans. The inverted-Y-V modification avoids the drawback of the original Mathieu repair and results in a slit-like meatus at the tip of the glans (Figure 94.16).

1. A Y-shaped incision is outlined on the glans (Figure 94.16(A)).

2. A catheter size 10 Fr or larger is inserted into the bladder.

3. The flap is outlined so that the distance between the meatus and the proximal end of the flap is slightly greater than the distance from the meatus to the tip of glans.

4. A U-shaped incision is made, extending from the tip of the V in the glans down to the lower end of the designed flap; this results in two glanular wings (Figure 94.16(B)).

5. The Mathieu flap is mobilised, preserving its fascial blood supply (Figure 94.16(C)).

6. Urethroplasty is performed by using continuous subcuticular polyglactin 6-0 sutures.

7. A protective intermediate layer is fashioned by using the flap fascia or dartos fascia (Figure 94.16(D)).

8. Both granular wings are sutured together around a neourethra by using interrupted mattress sutures.

Inverted-Y Modified Thiersch Technique
The inverted-Y tubularised plate technique[45] is a modification of the Thiersch technique. It is suitable in hypospadias patients without deep chordee. Thus, incision of the urethral plate is not needed to correct deep chordee. The original Thiersch technique is ideal in patients with cleft glans. However, it is necessary to modify the technique when the glans is flat or incompletely clefted in order to wrap the glanular wings around the new urethra (Figure 94.17).

1. A traction suture of 4/0 nylon is placed through the tip of the glans.

2. An inverted-Y-shaped incision is outlined on the glans. The tip of the longitudinal limb of the inverted-Y is at the tip of the glans, where the tip of the neomeatus will be located. The lower two limbs of the inverted Y are about 0.8 cm long, and the angle between them is 90°. The long vertical limb of the inverted-Y is 0.8 cm long (Figure 94.17(A)).

3. The inverted-Y-shaped incision is deepened to be able to wrap the glanular wings around the new urethra. This results in a median inverted-V flap and two lateral wings. The two lateral wings are elevated and the median flap is mobilised (Figure 94.17(B,C)).

4. A catheter, size 10 Fr or larger, is inserted into the bladder.

5. Using two fine surgical forceps, the adequate diameter of the new urethra is marked around the catheter.

6. A U-shaped skin incision is made by using sharp scissors or scalpel size 15. A transverse incision proximal to the meatus is cut by using sharp scissors (Figure 94.17(D)).

7. If the distal urethra is thin, it is incised until a healthy vascularised urethra is reached.

8. In the glans, the incision is deepened enough to create mobile lateral glanular wings to wrap around the new urethra.

9. Two or three sutures are tied along the length of the new urethra to reduce tension and help orientation.

10. The new urethra is constructed by using 6/0 vicryl on a cutting needle in a continuous subcuticular manner (Figure 94.17(E)).

11. A protective intermediate layer is fashioned from the preputial fascia under the foreskin (Figure 94.17(F)). (In proximal hypospadias without deep chordee, the authors prefer scrotal dartos/tunica vaginalis fascia.)

12. Closure of the glans follows, starting at the tip of the glans to ensure wide meatus.

Lateral-Based Flap Technique

The lateral-based flap technique[46] may be used in proximal hypospadias with deep chordee that necessitates incision of the urethral plate to straighten the penis. It has a double blood supply and allows extensive excision of ventral chordee. It may offer patients with proximal hypospadias a single-stage urethral reconstruction with a good success rate (91%) and relatively few complications. The operative steps for the lateral-based flap technique listed below are illustrated in Figure 94.18.

1. A deep Y-shaped incision is made on the glans that goes all the way down to the coronal sulcus (Figure 94.18(A)). This permits two deep glanular wings and a wide meatus.

2. The urethral plate is incised at the coronal sulcus and all the tissues that tether the corpora cavernosa and cause the penile curvature are removed (Figure 94.18(B)).

3. The edge of the lateral skin is then sutured at two points. Proximally, it is sutured to the hypospadias meatus (Figure 94.18(C)); distally, it approximates the lateral wall to the tip of the glans (Figure 94.18(D)), thus forming a "new urethral plate".

4. A 10 Fr catheter (or larger, depending on the size of the penis and the age of the patient) is introduced through the meatus.

5. A rectangular skin strip is outlined, extending proximally from the urethral meatus to the tip of the glans.

6. Several interrupted stitches assist in orientation, and the urethroplasty is carried out from proximal to distal in a subcuticular continuous manner.

7. The adjacent penile skin is elevated (rather than mobilising the flap) to preserve the vascular areolar tissue (Figure 94.18(E)).

8. The neourethra is covered with a protective intermediate layer (dartos or tunica) (Figure 94.18(F)).

9. The neomeatus is constructed by suturing the terminal end of the neourethra to the centre of the glans (Figure 94.18(G)).

10. The glanular wings are sutured around the neourethra by using interrupted mattress sutures (Figure 94.18(H)).

11. A percutaneous suprapubic cystocath is inserted into the bladder for 10–14 days.

12. A compression dressing is applied for 6–24 hours for haemostasis.

TIP Urethroplasty

The tubularised incised plate (TIP) is explained in detail by Snodgrass.[47] Incision of the urethral plate was first described by Reddy in 1975,[48] then by Orkiszewski[49] and Rich[50] in the 1980s, and popularised by Snodgrass in 1994.[51] The operative steps of TIP listed here are illustrated in Figure 94.19.

1. A circumscribing skin incision is made 1–2 mm proximal to the meatus.

2. The urethral plate is separated from the glans wings and distal penile skin by two parallel incisions running from the parameatal skin to the

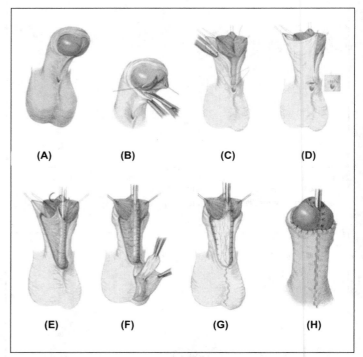

Source: Hadidi AT, Azmy AF, eds. Hypospadias Surgery: An Illustrated Guide, 1st ed. Springer Verlag, 2004. Reproduced with kind permission of Springer Verlag.

Figure 94.18: The lateral-based flap (LB flap) technique for proximal hypospadias: (A) Y-shaped deep incision of the glans; (B) three flaps are elevated and orthoplasty; (C) new urethral plate; (D) design of the LB flap; (E) urethroplasty; (F) mobilisation of dartos/tunica vaginalis fascia; (G) protective intermediate layer; (H) skin closure.

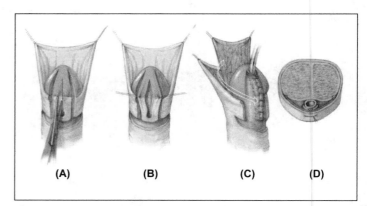

Source: Hadidi AT, Azmy AF, eds. Hypospadias Surgery: An Illustrated Guide, 1st ed. Springer Verlag, 2004. Reproduced with kind permission of Springer Verlag.

Figure 94.19: Tubularised incised plate (TIP).

tip of the glans (Figure 94.19(A)).

3. The penis skin is degloved to the penoscrotal junction.

4. The glans wings are mobilised, avoiding damage to the margins of the urethral plate.

5. A relaxing incision is made by using scissors in the midline from within the meatus to the end of the plate. The depth of this relaxing incision depends on the plate width and depth (Figure 94.19(B)).

6. Using a fine suture, preferably 7-0 polyglactin, the incised urethral plate is tubularised on the inserted catheter, placing the first stitch at approximately the midglans (Figure 94.19(C)).

7. The tubularisation is completed with a two-layer running subepithelial closure.

8. A dartos pedicle is developed from the dorsal shaft skin, button-holed, and transposed to the ventrum as skin cover for the new urethra (Figure 94.19(C)).

9. The skin edges of the tubularised glans are sutured together with the meatus (Figure 94.19(D)).

This method has become popular because of its simplicity. However, the long-term complication rate of the TIP procedure may be up to 35% in distal hypospadias and 66% in proximal hypospadias.[49,52]

Tubularised Preputial Island Flap

Figure 94.20 illustrates the operative steps of the tubularised preputial island flap procedure (Duckett operation), as outlined below.[53]

1. A neourethra is created by utilising the inner preputial layer. It is anastomosed proximally with the native urethra and distally with the glans.

2. A circular incision is made just proximal to the meatus and running through the inner preputial layer 0.3 cm behind the coronal sulcus (Figure 94.20(A)).

3. The urethral plate and chordee are excised completely, creating a ventral urethral defect (Figure 94.20(B)).

4. The length of the urethral defect is estimated while the penis is erect.

5. The prepuce is fixed with four holding sutures so that its inner layer is stretched out.

6. A flap is raised from the inner layer of the prepuce with dimensions that match those of the urethral defect. Particular care is taken not to injure its blood supply (Figure 94.20(C)).

7. The dissection of the vascular pedicle is conducted in such a way that rotation of the neourethra is possible in the anteroposterior direction without tension.

8. The neourethra is created by rolling up the inner preputial layer on a catheter as a tube and closing it with a running suture (Figure 94.20(D)).

9. The glans is then incised midline deeply to raise two large glanular wings to wrap around the new urethra (Figure 94.20(E)). A small V-flap is excised from the tip of the new urethra to help in fashioning a slit-like meatus (inset).

10. An oblique anastomosis is made between the neourethra and the native urethra in such a way that the suture line on the neourethra lies on the penile shaft.

11. The neourethra is pulled through the channel previously developed up to the glans tip and fixed to the glans.

12. The skin of the penis is closed on the shaft with a running suture (Figure 94.20(F)).

13. The defect created in the preputial skin is then closed with running sutures.

The recommendation is to avoid reconstruction and removal of the prepuce until a successful result is obtained.

Onlay Island Flap Procedure

Instead of creating a complete neourethra from the inner preputial layer, it is possible to complete the urethral plate with the layer itself. This is the onlay island flap procedure,[54] illustrated In Figure 94.21 and outlined here.

1. A semicircular skin incision is made along the urethral plate around the meatus.

2. A pedunculated flap is dissected from the inner preputial layer in the same way as for the Duckett's operation (see previous section).

3. The glans is split in line with the urethral plate.

4. The flap is transposed on the ventral aspect of the penile shaft, and both flap borders are sutured with the free borders of the urethral plate.

5. The skin and the glanular wings are then closed.

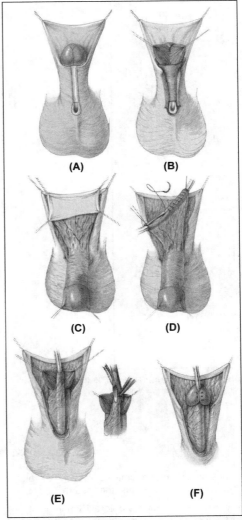

Source: Hadidi AT, Azmy AF, eds. Hypospadias Surgery: An Illustrated Guide, 1st ed. Springer Verlag, 2004. Reproduced with kind permission of Springer Verlag.

Figure 94.20: Duckett tubularised preputial island flap.

Urethral Reconstruction Using Buccal Mucosa

In redo operations, it is possible to resort to buccal mucosa to form a wide urethral plate as a first stage and to reconstruct a neourethra in the second stage. Bladder mucosa and one-stage repair using buccal mucosa are becoming less popular in complicated proximal hypospadias due to the high incidence of complications.

Complications

Hypospadias complications are not uncommon. The incidence depends on the experience of the surgeon and the technique employed. Common complications include meatal and urethral stenosis, fistula, diverticulum, and recurrent chordee.

Meatal and Urethral Stenosis

The incidence of meatal and urethral stenosis has increased in recent years due to employment of techniques that may result in narrow new urethra (e.g., the TIP technique).[51] Dilatation may work occasionally. However, if dilatation is needed frequently, a new wide urethra has to be reconstructed to avoid back pressure on the bladder and damage to the kidneys.

Fistula

Fistula used to be the most frequent complication after hypospadias surgery.[55] Several factors may be responsible for fistula, including distal stenosis, the technique applied, skin damage, tension on the sutures, infection, and overlapping of suture lines.

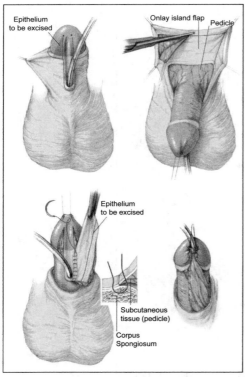

Source: Hadidi AT, Azmy AF, eds. Hypospadias Surgery: An Illustrated Guide, 1st ed. Springer Verlag, 2004. Reproduced with kind permission of Springer Verlag.

Figure 94.21: Onlay island flap procedure.

The four important steps for the correction of urethral fistula are:

1. exclusion and correction of distal stenosis;

2. wide excision of the fistula tract;

3. use of healthy, well-vascularised tissue; and

4. protection of fistula repair with a healthy vascular second protective layer.

Diverticulum

Diverticulum may occur after surgery for distal hypospadias and is probably due to a narrow new urethra. Diverticulum may also occur after proximal hypospadias, however, and is believed to be due to a lack of the supportive corpus spongiosum in patients with proximal hypospadias. This is supported by the finding that diverticulum is often encountered without distal obstruction in proximal hypospadias and may even recur after excision of the redundant urethra.[56]

Persistent or Recurrent Chordee

Persistent or recurrent chordee may occur due to inadequate orthoplasty during hypospadias correction or due to healing by scarring and fibrous tissue formation. In cases of scarring, the urethra is usually healthy, and excision of the fibrous tissue superficial to the urethra is sufficient to correct chordee. Correction of persistent chordee due to inadequate orthoplasty in the first operation is difficult and technically demanding. Some surgeons may opt for repeated tunica albuginea plication. Others, including the authors, would prefer to incise the urethra and correct the curvature from the ventral aspect to avoid shortening the penis.

Key Summary Points

1. Hypospadias is a wide spectrum of anomalies involving all the ventral structures of the penis and not just the urethra.

2. The ideal time to correct hypospadias is before 18 months of age. In fact, many surgeons correct hypospadias starting at age 3 months.

3. Surgeons need to master several techniques to suit the wide range of anomalies encountered.

4. The surgeon should use the technique that is suitable for the patient and not make the patient suitable for the technique he or she prefers.

5. Neourethra should be reconstructed around catheters of size 10 Fr or larger, depending on the age of the patient.

6. Tubularisation of the urethral plate without incision is suitable for more than 60% of hypospadias patients.

7. A second protective layer to cover and protect the new urethra is an essential part of hypospadias surgery.

8. With experience, the success rate in glanular and distal hypospadias has reached more than 95%. In proximal hypospadias, the complication rate is 10–20%.

References

1. Paulozzi L, Erickson D, et al. Hypospadias trends in two US surveillance systems. Pediatr 1997; 100:831–834.

2. Duckett JW, Baskin LA. In: Gillenwater J, et al., eds. Adult and Pediatric Urology, 3rd ed. Mosby Year Book, 1996.

3. Sadler T. Langman's Medical Embryology, 10th ed. Lippincott Williams & Wilkins, 2006, P 248.

4. van der Werff JFA, Nievelstein RAJ, Brands E, et al: Normal development of the male anterior urethra. Teratology 2000; 61:172–183.

5. Moore KL, Persaud TVN. The developing human, 5th ed. Saunders, 1993.

6. Wood-Jones F: The nature of the malformations of the rectum and urogenital passages. BMJ 1904; 2:1630–1634.

7. Glenister TW: The origin and fate of the urethral plate in man. J Anat 1954; 88:413–425.

8. Van Bagaert LJ. Surgical repair of hypospadias in women with symptoms of urethral syndrome. J Urol 1992; 147(5):1263–1264.

9. Gunn TR, Mora JD, Pease P. Antenatal diagnosis of urinary tract abnormalities by ultrasonography after 28 weeks gestation: incidence and outcome. Am J Obst Gynecol 1995; 172:479.

10. Hollowell JG Jr, et al. Embryonic considerations of diphallus and associated anomalies. J Urol 1977; 117:728.

11. Hinman FJ. Penis and male urethra. In: Hinman FJ, ed. Urosurgical Anatomy. WB Saunders, 1993.

12. Van der Putte SCJ, Neeteson FA. The normal development of the anorectum in the pig. Acta Morphol Neerl Scand 1983; 21:107–132.

13. Van der Putte SCJ. The development of the perineum in the human. Adv Anat Embryol Cell Biol 2005; 177:1e135.

14. van der Putte SCJ. Normal and abnormal development of the anorectum. J Pediatr Surg 1986; 21:434–440.

15. Kluth D, Lambrecht W, Reich P: Pathogenesis of hypospadias—more questions than answers. J Pediatr Surg 1988; 23:1095–1101.

16. Snodgrass WT, Shukla AR, Canning DA. Hypospadias. In: Docimo SG, ed. Clinical Pediatric Urology. Informa Health Care, 2007, P 1206.

17. Baskin LS. Hypospadias and urethral development. J Urol 2000; 163:951.

18. Hadidi AT. Morphology of hypospadis. In: Hadidi AT, Azmy AF. Hypospadias Surgery: An Illustrated Guide, 2nd ed. Springer Verlag, in press.

19. Hadidi AT. Classification of hypospadias. In: Hadidi AT, Azmy AF. Hypospadias Surgery: An Illustrated Guide, 1st ed. Springer Verlag, 2004, P 80.

20. Keating JM, Hamilton H. A New Pronouncing Dictionary of Medicine. Young J Pentland, 1892.

21. Smith CK. Surgical procedures for correction of hypospadias. J Urol 1938; 40:239.

22. Mosby´s Medical Dictionary, 8th ed. Elsevier, 2009.

23. Paul M, Kanagasuntheram R. The congenital anomalies of the lower urinary tract. Br J Urol 1956; 28:118–125.

24. Avellán L. Morphology of hypospadias. Scand J Plast Surg 1980; 14:239–247.

25. Kaufmann, C. Verletzungen und Krankenheiten der männlichen Harnröhre und des Penis. In: Bilrothe T, Luecke A. Deutsche Chirurgie. Lieferung 50a, 1886, Chap 5, Pp 18–39.

26. Duckett JW: Hypospadias. In: Gillenwater JY, Grayhack JT, Howards SS, Duckett JW, eds. Adult and Pediatric Urology, 3rd ed. Mosby Year Book, 1996, P 2550.

27. Schonfeld WA, Beebe CW. Normal growth and variation in the male genitalia from birth to maturity. J Urol 1942; 48:759.

28. Schulz JR, Klykylo WM, Wacksman J: Timing of elective hypospadias repair in children. Pediatr 1983; 71:342–351.

29. Hadidi AT. Editorial overview. In: Hadidi AT, Azmy AF Hypospadias Surgery: An Illustrated Guide, 2nd ed. Springer Verlag, in press.

30. Hadidi AT. Principles of hypospadias surgery. In: Hadidi AT, Azmy AF Hypospadias Surgery: An Illustrated Guide, 1st ed. Springer Verlag, 2004, P 100.

31. Wacksman J. Results of early hypospadias surgery using optical magnification. J Urol 1984; 131:516.

32. Hadidi AT. Principles of hypospadias surgery. In: Hadidi AT, Azmy AF. Hypospadias Surgery: An Illustrated Guide, 2nd ed. Springer Verlag, in press.

33. El-Mahrouky A, McElhaney J, Bartone FF, et al. In vitro comparison of the properties of polydioxanone, polyglycolic acid and catgut sutures in sterile and infected urine. J Urol 1987; 138:913–915.

34. Hadidi AT. Principles of hypospadias surgery. In: Hadidi AT, Azmy AF. Hypospadias Surgery: An Illustrated Guide, 1st ed. Springer Verlag, 2004, P 101.

35. Hadidi A, Abdaal N, Kaddah S. Hypospadias repair: is dressing important. Kasr El Aini J Surg 2003; 4(1):37–44.

36. Ben Meir D, Livne PM. Is prophylactic antimicrobial treatment necessary after hypospadias repair? J Urol 2004; 171:2621–2622.

37. Gittes R, McLaughlin Al. Injection technique to induce penile erection. Urol 1974; 4:473.

38. Leslie JA, Cain MP, Kaefer M, et al. Corporeal grafting for severe hypospadias: a single institution experience with 3 techniques. J Urol 2008; 160,1749–1752.

39. Caesar RE, Caldamone AA. The use of free grafts for correcting penile chordee. J Urol 2000; 164:1691.

40. Baskin LS, Ebbers MB. Hypospadias: anatomy, etiology, and technique. J Pediatr Surg 2006; 41:463.

41. Braga LHP, Lorenzo AJ, Bägli DJ. Ventral penile lengthening versus dorsal placation for severe ventral curvature in children with proximal hypospadias. J Urol 2008; 180:1743–1748.

42. Hadidi AT. Men behind principles and principles behind techniques. In: Hadidi AT, Azmy AF. Hypospadias Surgery: An Illustrated Guide, 1st ed. Springer Verlag, 2004, P 23.

43. Duckett JW: MAGPI (meatal advancement and glanuloplasty): a procedure for subcoronal hypospadias. Urol Clin North Am 1981; 8:513.

44. Hadidi AT. V modified Mathieu technique. In: Hadidi AT, Azmy AF. Hypospadias Surgery: An Illustrated Guide, 1st ed. Springer Verlag, 2004, P 149.

45. Hadidi AT. Inverted Y tubularised plate technique. In: Hadidi AT, Azmy AF. Hypospadias Surgery: An Illustrated Guide, 2nd ed. Springer Verlag, in press.

46. Hadidi AT. Lateral based flap with dual blood supply: a single stage repair for proximal hypospadias. In: Hadidi AT, Azmy AF. Hypospadias Surgery: An Illustrated Guide, 1st ed. Springer Verlag, 2004, P 209.

47. Snodgrass W. Tubularised incised plate urethroplasty. In: Hadidi AT, Azmy AF. Hypospadias Surgery: An Illustrated Guide, 1st ed. Springer Verlag, 2004, P 155.

48. Reddy LN. One-stage repair of hypospadias. Urol 1975; 5:475.

49. Orkiszewski M, leszniewski J. Morphology and urodynamics after longitudinal urethral plate incision in proximal hypospadias repairs. Long-term results. Eur J Pediatr Surg 2004; 14(1):35–38.

50. Rich MA, Keating MA, Snyder HM, Duckett JW. Hinging the urethral plate in hypospadias meatoplasty. J Urol 1989; 142:1551.

51. Snodgrass W. Tubularised incised plate urethroplasty for distal hypospadias. J Urol 1994; 151:464–465.

52. Chrzan R, Dik P, Klijn A, et al. Quality assessment of hypospadias repair with emphasis on techniques used and experience of pediatric urologic surgeons. Urol 2007; 70:148–152.

53. Duckett JW. The island-flap technique for hypospadias repair. Urol Clin North Am 1981; 8:503.

54. Elder JS, Duckett JW, Snyder HM. Onlay island flap in the repair of mid-and distal penile hypospadias without chordee. J Urol 1987; 138:376.

55. Hadidi AT. Fistula. In Hadidi AT, Azmy AF. Hypospadias Surgery: An Illustrated Guide, 1st ed. Springer Verlag, 2004, P 277.

56. Snodgrass WT. Hypospadias. In: Docimo SG, ed. Clinical Pediatric Urology. Informa Health Care, 2007, P 1234.

CHAPTER 95
CIRCUMCISION

Daniel Sidler
Christopher Bode
Ashish Desai

Introduction

Circumcision, the partial or complete removal of the male foreskin, is one of the most commonly performed surgical procedures.[1] It has been practiced since antiquity. The first record of male circumcision dates from the Sixth Dynasty of the Egyptian pharaohs, around 2420 BC.[1]

Circumcision for nonclinical reasons (nontherapeutic or prophylactic) has wide variations around the world. The United States has the highest rate of neonatal circumcision. In the past, about 90% of newborn boys were circumcised, but the rate has steadily declined, and currently is around 60–70%. More than 1 million neonatal male circumcisions are performed annually in the United States, and about 30% of all males are circumcised worldwide.[2,3] However, circumcision is very uncommon in northern European countries, Central and South America, and Asia. After Gairdner[4] published his landmark article in 1949, circumcision rates in the United Kingdom fell from about 30% to less than 10%.

Male circumcision is almost universally practiced in North Africa and most parts of West Africa. It is less common in East, Southern, and Central Africa, where its prevalence varies from country to country.

Circumcision Controversy

Less than 1% of all circumcisions are surgically indicated (see section "Indications for Circumcision"). Several medical bodies have long asserted the doubtful benefits of male circumcision in preventing known infection.[5–10]

The often referred benefit of circumcision in preventing penile cancer in men may be negligible, as this cancer is rare in most populations.[1,6] Male circumcision has been linked, however, to a low prevalence of cervical cancer in women living with circumcised spouses.[7] Circumcision excises the most erogenous part of the male anatomy, and its critics argue that this diminishes sexual performance and enjoyment for both partners.[1,11,12]

For surgeons in Africa and other countries where the practice of circumcision is entrenched, the question is not whether circumcision should be practiced. The challenge should be to ensure that circumcision is safely performed and to promote the teaching of its safe application in the community.

The Foreskin and Its Functions

Most boys have a nonretractile foreskin (phimosis) at birth.[1,4,13,14] The inner foreskin is attached to the glans. Foreskin adhesions break down and form smegma pearls, or "white cysts under the foreskin," which are then extruded. The process of retractability is spontaneous and does not require manipulation. The majority of boys will have a retractile foreskin by 10 years of age and 95% by 16–17 years of age.[4,13,14]

The prepuce has several possible functions:

• It prevents meatal ulceration.

• The foreskin is a complex and important sensory organ. It has a high concentration of encapsulated sensory receptors, mostly Meissner corpuscles containing nerve endings, similar to those found in the fingertips and lips. The unique sensory innervation of the prepuce establishes its function as an erogenous tissue.[15–17]

• The foreskin may have an immunological function, containing many Langerhans cells that produce langerin.

• As an easily available source of live human fibroblasts, the foreskin has become a favourite tissue source for cell-culture biologists doing basic scientific research.

• The prepuce has a useful function in reconstructive surgery due to its many advantages, including easy harvest, high viability, elasticity, and stem cells.

Indications for Circumcision

There are few surgical indications for circumcision, which altogether, according to one report,[16] constitute about 1% of all circumcisions performed.

Balanitis xerotica obliterans (BXO) is a lesion akin to lichen sclerosus et atrophicus; it is the cause of true scarring of the foreskin. It is rare before the age of 5 years, is associated with discomfort on voiding, and presents with a white firm scarring of the foreskin tip. The aetiology is unknown but may be of viral origin. This condition may also affect the glans and urethra. The techniques of intralesional steroid injection, long-term antibiotics, carbon dioxide laser therapy, and a radial preputioplasty alone or with intralesional injection of steroids have all been described in the literature. There are, however, no randomised trials to ascertain the efficacy and the long-term outcome of these techniques. There is a strong association between BXO in adults and penile carcinoma. Circumcision may be indicated.

Paraphimosis occurs when a tight retracted prepuce cannot be reduced, and thus forms a tight constricting band proximal to the glans. Although quite uncommon, this condition is an emergency because the ballooned glans penis is a painful condition and could be rendered ischaemic if left unreleased. Gentle compression with a saline-soaked swab followed by reduction of the prepuce over the glans is usually successful. Alternatives include multiple punctures in the oedematous foreskin or injection of hyaluronidase prior to compression reduction. A nitrous oxide and oxygen mixture is usually helpful and is available in some paediatric accident and emergency departments. Rarely, general anaesthesia may be required. A dorsal slit might be required for recurrent episodes or in acute conditions. Due to poor cosmesis after dorsal slit, or if there is scarring following reduction of paraphimosis, circumcision may be indicated. Circumcision is contraindicated in the acute situation.

Balanoposthitis is an inflammation of both the glans and foreskin. It may present with swelling and erythema of the distal penis and foreskin in association with discharge, bleeding from the prepuce, dysuria, and occasionally urinary retention. It occurs in about 4% of uncircumcised boys between 2 and 5 years of age.[18] The aetiology is unclear, although infection, contact allergy, and contact irritation have been described. Although balanoposthitis may be recurrent, the episodes decrease in frequency in older boys and reflect foreskin maturation. Simple bathing, appropriate antibiotics, and/or steroid treatment will suffice as treatment. Circumcision may be considered if recurrent severe episodes of inflammation occur.

Circumcision could be considered in boys with recurrent urinary tract infections (UTIs) and urogenital abnormality.[1] It has been shown that in children younger than 1 year of age, UTIs are more common in uncircumcised males.[19,20] As this may have a detrimental effect on a child with high-grade vesicoureteric reflux or obstructive uropathy, circumcision could be considered in this age group.

A hooded foreskin is an abnormal dorsal hemiforeskin that is deficient ventrally and may or may not be associated with hypospadias. A hooded foreskin without hypospadias is a cosmetic abnormality. A modified circumcision or a foreskin reconstruction is a possible consideration for treatment. Hooded foreskin with hypospadias needs treatment with correction of the hypospadia (see Chapter 94).

Contraindications to Circumcision

Circumcision is contraindicated in patients with hypospadia, in whom the foreskin is often used for repair of the proximally placed ventral urethral meatus (see Chapter 94).

Disorders of sex development should similarly be left uncircumcised until the proper gender assignment has been clarified.[21]

Other conditions for which a circumcision should be prevented are conditions such as a ventral or dorsal chordee with or without hypospadias; megameatus with an intact prepuce; megalourethra; and a webbed, small, or inconspicuous or buried penis.

Circumcision Procedure

Four principal factors are common to all forms of circumcision: asepsis, excision of adequate outer and inner preputial layers, proper haemostasis, and protection of glans penis. Circumcision may be complete or partial.

Complete circumcision may be performed in the newborn period by using the Gomco clamp, the PlastiBell, or the Mogen clamp. After the newborn period, surgical circumcision is recommended. General surgical guidelines include complete sterile dissection, complete separation of the glanular adhesions, and exclusion of hypospadias.

Bleeding is a common complication after circumcision unless meticulous haemostasis with bipolar diathermy is performed. Monopolar diathermy is contraindicated.

Facilities

The premises in which circumcisions are carried out must be suitable for the purpose. In particular, if general anaesthesia is used, full resuscitation facilities must be available.

Analgesia and Anaesthesia

Neonatal circumcision should always be performed with appropriate anaesthesia. The complicated innervation of the penis explains why a dorsal penile nerve block provides incomplete pain relief for neonatal circumcision. A eutectic mixture of local anaesthetics (EMLA), contraindicated on open wounds and mucous membranes, can cause methemoglobinaemia. Nonpharmacological methods (nonnutritive suckling, rocking, massaging, cuddling) or systemic analgesia with paracetamol are inadequate. Caudal analgesia is effective in anaesthetised boys but has not been studied in neonatal awake circumcisions.[1,18,22]

Methods

The most ideal method for circumcision has not yet been devised. However, circumcision should usually be done by using surgical techniques rather then the clamp method.

The open method developed from surgical standardisation of the ritual excision performed by traditional itinerant circumcision practitioners. Basically, it consists of protection of the penile glans and shaft from inadvertent injury, circumferential crushing of the foreskin at the corona to prevent bleeding, and safe excision of the foreskin distal to the crush. Three commonly used variations of the open method—the dorsal slit, the sleeve, and the guillotine methods—remain the predominant methods of circumcision.

The *dorsal slit method* involves the crushing and division of the two layers of the prepucial dorsum to enable the operator to free the prepuce circumferentially down to the corona. The slit is then extended to the corona and the prepuce is excised under direct vision, leaving a 2–3 mm skirt of prepucial rim.

The *sleeve method* is performed by excising each of the two layers of the prepuce under direct vision, starting with the outer layer to allow effective haemostasis as the bleeding vessels are ligated.

The *guillotine method* entails a circumferential release of the adherent prepuce, which is then pulled taut over the glans. The penis is retracted as far as possible, and a bone cutter or strong pair of artery forceps applied to crush the prepuce distal to the retracted glans penis for up to 10 minutes before the skin distal to the crush is trimmed off. It is a blind procedure.

Neonatal Circumcision

It is important to ensure safety and appropriate analgesia. The open dissection, Gomco, Plastibell, and the Mogen circumcision methods remain the most commonly used. For each baby to be circumcised, the surgeon should let the parents choose the procedure (except if it is medically indicated). Informed consent should be obtained. Whatever method of circumcision is employed, use of diathermy is contraindicated because it may lead to penile necrosis when employing a metallic circumcision device.[22,23]

The Gomco clamp (Figure 95.1), Mogen clamp, and the Plastibell (Figure 95.2) are the three commonly used kits for performing neonatal circumcision. They can be bulky. If the surgeon is not used to these clamps, they can present significant complications. The Gomco and Mogen clamps also need sterilisation.

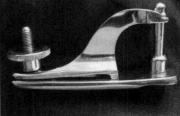
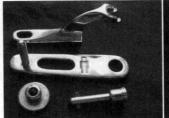

Figure 95.1: Gomco circumcision kit.

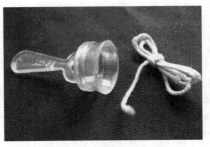

Figure 95.2: Plastibell circumcision kit.

The Plastibell, invented in 1956 by Kariher,[25] was fashioned after an earlier prototype. It is made entirely of plastic, comprising a protective bell with a ring grooved circumferentially. The bell is designed to fit over the glans while the ring is positioned under the foreskin around the corona. The conical end of the bell ends in an elongated detachable tab—a handle that is essential for stability during the circumcision, after which it is broken off.

1. The Plastibell ring is introduced under the prepuce following either a minimal dorsal slit or stretching of the prepucial opening.

2. The foreskin is pulled up to fit snugly over the ring up to a premarked position over the corona and then secured into place with the accompanying suture tied securely with a nonyielding ligature to crush the foreskin into the groove.

3. The prepucial skin distal to the ligature is trimmed off and the ring is left to fall off, often between 4 and 14 days, from ischaemic necrosis of the skin caught in the groove.

The Plastibell device, which comes in a sterile pack, is used for up to 60% of childhood circumcisions in the United States.[27] Youth, teen, and adult Plastibell devices are also available in Europe. It is the most popular circumcision kit in Nigeria, and is often specifically requested as "the ring method" by mothers wanting to circumcise their babies.

There is no formal way to measure what size is appropriate for each individual, so selection is based on the most likely fit. In its present format, the Plastibell ring protects the glans while the suture line helps ensure that the frenulum cannot be cut. There is also virtually no blood loss, and, in skilled hands, it can even be used on haemophiliac boys, a distinct advantage over all other methods.[27] The Plastibell is an ideal tool for use by medical personnel, such as midwives, junior doctors, and family practitioners relatively unskilled in surgery because the only real skill required is the ability to tie a surgical knot that will not come undone over a period of about 10 days. It creates an acceptable, smooth, bloodless margin. The device is easy to use. It does not have many parts and its disposable presentation allows for many cases to be quickly performed over a short period of time.

The long period of retention and/or usage of the wrong size of the Plastibell ring account for many of the complications associated with this device.[28] This device is more associated with infections than other devices[30] because the ischaemic foreskin becomes progressively more susceptible to bacterial invasion. Most of these infections are mild and are treated with dressings and antibiotics.[30] Some, however, are catastrophic with supervening cellulitis and sometimes necrotising fasciitis and Fournier's gangrene.[31,32] Glanular ischaemia, penile amputation, traumatic bladder rupture, and even death may occur.

Proximal migration and prolonged retention of the Plastibell ring have been associated with penile skin necrosis and urethrocutaneous fistula from the sustained pressure effect of the rigid plastic ring encasing the penile shaft eroding into the relatively subcutaneous penile urethra.[33] The Plastibell may occlude the urethra if wrongly applied and thus cause acute urinary retention. One report[23] found a 3% complication rate and a satisfaction rate of 96%. Due to these problems, it has been suggested that the Plastibell could be safely removed after 24 hours to obviate the many problems associated with prolonged retention.

Complete Circumcision after the Newborn Period

The steps in complete circumcision after the newborn period are outlined below (Figure 95.3).

1. The prepuce is widened with dissecting forceps and the coronal sulcus is exposed, removing any preputial adhesions.

2. The frenulum is clamped, separated from the prepuce, and reconstructed with two stitches.

3. The prepuce is repositioned and traction is applied by using two small artery forceps. The appropriate level of excision is marked on the skin just distal to coronal sulcus (gleams through the skin), drawing it obliquely, below from the back and above to the front.

4. A skin incision is made at the marked level, cutting only the outer cutaneous layer.

5. The prepuce is retracted and the inner layer is incised 2 mm proximal to the coronal sulcus.

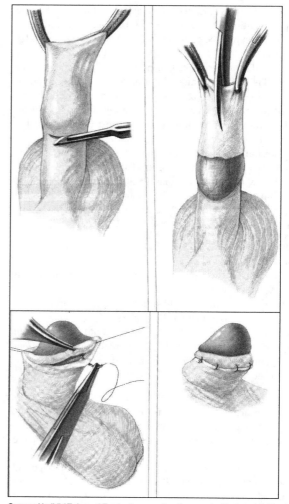

Source: Hadidi AT, Azmy AF, eds. Hypospadias Surgery: An Illustrated Guide, 1st ed. Springer Verlag, 2004. Reproduced with kind permission of Springer Verlag.

Figure 95.3: Complete circumcision.

6. Careful meticulous haemostasis is performed by using bipolar diathermy.

7. The inner and outer preputial layers are sutured together.

Partial Circumcision

Partial circumcision is performed in societies that want to preserve the foreskin. In such a case, some two-thirds of the prepuce must be left to cover the glans. The success of this operation essentially lies in the skin incision. The prepuce should be incised immediately below the stenotic ring to ensure that the scarred prepuce is completely removed.

Postcircumcision Care

The circumcision wound should be gently wrapped in petrolatum-soaked gauze for at least 24 hours; many mothers are reassured by the presence of a dressing over the wound. Thereafter, the dressing should be gently removed and the wound left open to dry. Antibiotics are not usually indicated for circumcision. Oral acetaminophen or paracetamol should be sufficient for analgesia. Oral promethazine may be required for a day or two if the baby is irritable. It is preferable to give a written set of instructions to mothers of circumcised babies detailing postoperative care. Follow-up is usually poor after the wound has healed, and thus, many delayed problems are discovered much later in childhood and at routine inspection.

After partial circumcision, gauze with local anaesthetic ointment is applied, and warm baths are encouraged from the 4th postoperative day, with cautious retraction of the remaining prepuce.

Complications

Complications of circumcision are few in skilled hands. Most circumcisions worldwide, however, are performed by junior trainees, general practitioners, and nurses. In Nigeria and most parts of Africa, medical personnel perform circumcision only in the big cities, whereas the majority of the population dwelling in the rural hinterland still rely on unskilled traditional circumcision by native doctors.[34] Many times, these doctors are itinerant, with little consideration for anaesthesia, haemostasis, or asepsis. The world literature on circumcision is rife with details of mutilation, sepsis, and sometimes death from this procedure.[28,35,36] Bailey et al. reported a 25% overall rate of adverse events following adult circumcisions in Kenya, with 6% of patients suffering permanent adverse sequelae.[37]

Early complications of circumcision include bleeding, infection, glanular laceration and partial amputation, urethrocutaneous fistula, and failure to remove enough skin. Other complications that may arise later include skin-bridge, implantation dermoid cyst, and meatal stenosis. With care, most of these complications are preventable. It is therefore a part of the duties of paediatric surgeons in Africa to advocate for a standardisation *of* and formal training *for* circumcision to reduce its associated morbidity and mortality.

Bleeding

Bleeding is the most common complication, occurring in up to 10% of all circumcisions. The bleeding is usually brisk and should stop with digital pressure applied for a few minutes; otherwise, a few well-placed sutures would suffice. Techniques of haemostasis, such as the use of adrenaline pack, are discouraged to prevent systemic effects of this drug, which can be absorbed through the operation site. Significant bleeding may occur, however, in babies with underlying bleeding disorder, and this may be severe enough to warrant hospitalisation and blood transfusion. Babies have been known to bleed to death from massive blood loss in this situation.

Laceration and Amputation

One series over four years in the United States reported 105 serious clamp-related complications, including laceration, penile amputation, and urethral injury. About 20 serious injuries are reported per year in the United States, with repeated warnings from the US Food and Drug Administration (FDA) between 1992 and 2002.[38,39] The Plastibell may lead to penile injuries from prolonged retention or proximal migration of its ring (Figure 95.4). Many more cases of significant penile trauma (Figures 95.5 and 95.6) have been recorded from circumcisions performed by native doctors and unskilled personnel in Africa.

Redundant Skin

Failure to remove enough skin is cosmetically unsightly and is the top reason for parental dissatisfaction.

Sepsis and Other Complications

• Infection remains an unacceptable complication of circumcision.

• Meatal stenosis may occur if the perimeatal glans is traumatised during circumcision.

• Chordee can be produced by a dense scar on the ventrum of the penis.

• Hesitancy and dysuria are seen in as many as 60% of older boys. Urinary retention may occur, leading to urosepsis, systemic infection, acute renal failure, or even bladder rupture.

Death may rarely occur after circumcision from haemorrhage, infection, or anaesthetic complications. Deaths have occurred in "initiation schools" for ritual circumcision, in South Africa.

Sexual and Psychological Consequences of Circumcision

A study testing subjects 4–7 years old shortly before and after circumcision reported that the procedure was "perceived by the child as an aggressive attack upon his body, which damaged, mutilated and, in

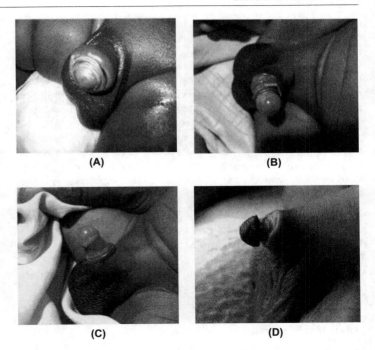

Source: J Pediatr Urol 2010; 6:23–27; reproduced with kind permission from Elsevier.

Figure 95.4: Complications from Plastibell circumcision: (A) prolonged retention of Plastibell (infant could not void urine); (B) penile skin loss resulting from proximal migration and prolonged retention of Plastibell ring; (C) after removal of the retaining ring in (B); (D) glanular nectosis from retained Plastibell.

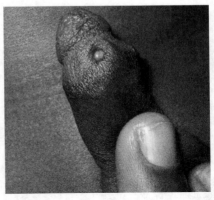

Source: J Pediatr Urol 2010; 6:23–27; reproduced with kind permission from Elsevier.

Figure 95.6: Urethrocutaneous fistula from open circumcision.

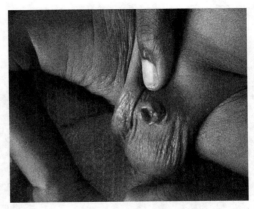

Figure 95.5: Partial penile amputation following circumcision by a traditional practitioner.

some cases, totally destroyed him." It resulted in increased aggressiveness and weakened the ego, causing withdrawal and reduced functioning and adaptation. In another study, children were observed to be "terribly frightened" during the procedure, leading to increased aggressive behaviour and nightmares afterwards. In a study of children in Turkey, most of whom underwent traditional circumcision at home, 66% did not remember anything, whereas 33% reported some bad sensations, such as fear, pain, and shame about the procedure.

An interesting psychological consequence of circumcision is *the perceived superiority* that may be felt by circumcised individuals or groups, which may create prejudice, discrimination regarding marriageability and property inheritance, and sometimes violence against noncircumcised individuals.[40,41] Many opinions on psychological complications can be found in the literature.[42]

Ethical Issues

This section is reproduced in part from the British Medical Association (BMA) document, The law and ethics of male circumcision.[43]

Male circumcision is generally assumed to be lawful provided that:

- it is believed to be in the child's best interests;
- it is performed competently; and
- there is valid *informed* consent.

Informed Consent/Assent and Refusal

Competent children may decide for themselves (assent). Different countries have different age restrictions. The wishes that children express must be taken into account. If parents disagree, nontherapeutic circumcision must not be carried out without the leave of a court. Consent should be confirmed in writing.

Best Interests

The views that children express are important in determining what is in their best interests. Parental preference must be weighed in terms of the child's interests. The child's lifestyle and likely upbringing are relevant factors to take into account. Parents must explain and justify requests for circumcision in terms of the child's interests. Parents do not have the right to demand a surgical procedure unless there is equivocal evidence of benefit and that the child would be harmed if the surgery is delayed and not performed. The need to belong to a particular religious or cultural group is relevant and needs to be considered. The question, however, arises, if the ritual could not be performed at a later time to give the child opportunity to decide for himself or herself.

Health Issues

In settings where circumcision is not universally practiced, parents seeking circumcision for their son for reasons of hygiene or health benefits should be fully informed of the lack of consensus within the profession over such benefits. The BMA considers there is insufficient evidence concerning health benefit from nontherapeutic circumcision. There is no urgent need to perform the circumcision before the consenting age.

Standards

The General Medical Council advises that circumcisers must "have the necessary skills and experience both to perform the operation and use appropriate measures, including anaesthesia, to minimise pain and discomfort." There is no legal requirement for nontherapeutic circumcisions to be undertaken by registered health professionals.

Conscientious Objection

Doctors are under no obligation to comply with a request to circumcise a child. Where the procedure is not therapeutic but a matter of patient or parental choice, there is no ethical obligation to refer on.

Key Summary Points

1. Circumcision is the most ancient surgical procedure known and has generated more controversy than any other operation.

2. The prevalence of circumcision in different populations varies, with approximately 80% of the world's population being uncircumcised.

3. Medical indications for circumcision develop in only 3–5% of boys.

4. Pathological phimosis occurs in less than 1.5% of boys at the age of 17, and is an indication for circumcision.

5. Recurrent paraphimosis and recurrent balanitis, especially in diabetic boys, are indications for circumcision.

6. Other valid medical indications are condylomata acuminata involving the foreskin and glans, and recurrent injury (or tears) of the prepuce.

7. The incidence of typical surgical complications after infant circumcision is high and reported from Africa as being greater than 20%.

8. The procedure should be performed only on infants who are stable and healthy, and adequate anaesthesia and analgesia should be provided.

9. Where circumcision is universally practiced, efforts should be made to teach safe methods to reduce the burden of complications.

References

1. Heyns CF, Krieger JN. Circumcision. In: Schill W-B, Comhaire FR, Hargreave TB, eds. Andrology for the Clinician. Springer-Verlag, 2006, Pp 203–212.

2. WHO information package on male circumcision and HIV prevention. Available at: http://www.who.int/hiv/mediacentre/infopack_en_2.pdf (accessed 12 November 2008).

3. Niku S, Stock J, Kaplan C. Neonatal circumcision. Urol Clin North Am 1995; 22:57–65.

4. Gairdner D. The fate of the foreskin. BMJ 1949; 2:1433–1437.

5. Leitch IOW. Circumcision: a continuing enigma. Aust Paediatr J 1970; 6:59.

6. Schoen E, Anderson G, Bohon C, et al. Report of the task force on circumcision. Paediatr 1989; 84:388–391.

7. Fetus and Newborn Committee, Canadian Paediatric Society. Neonatal circumcision revisited. CMAJ 1996; 154:769–780.

8. Beasley S, Darlow B, Craig J, et al. Position Statement on Circumcision. Sydney: Royal Australasian College of Physicians, 2002.

9. Task Force on Circumcision. Report of the Task Force of Circumcision. Pediatr 1989; 84:388–391.

10. Royal Dutch Medical Association (KNMG), Non-therapeutic Circumcision of Male Minors. KNMG, May 2010.

11. Sorrells M, et al. Fine-touch pressure thresholds in the adult penis. BJU Int 2007; 99:864–869.

12. Taylor JR, Lockwood AP, Taylor AJ. The prepuce: specialized mucosa of the penis and its loss to circumcision. Br J Urol 1996; 77:291–295.

13. Øster J. Further fate of the foreskin. Arch Dis Child 1968; 43:200.

14. Kayaba H, Tamura H, Kitajima S, Fujiwara Y, Kato T, Kato T. Analysis of shape and retractability of the prepuce in 603 Japanese boys. J Urol 1996; 156:1813–1815.

15. Winkelmann RK. The erogenous zones: their nerve supply and its significance. Proc Mayo Clinic 1959; 34:38–47.

16. Winkelmann RK. Nerve Endings in Normal and Pathological Skin. CC Thomas, 1960.

17. Halata Z, Munger B. The neuroanatomical basis for the protopathic sensibility of the human glans penis. Brain Res 1986; 371:205–230.

18. Fornasa CV, Calabro A, Miglietta A, et al. Mild balanoposthitis. Genitourin Med 1994; 70:345–346.

19. Wiswell TE, Hachey WE. Urinary tract infections and the uncircumcised state: an update. Clin Pediatr (Phila) 1993; 32:130–134.

20. Singh-Grewal D, Macdessi J, Craig J. Circumcision for the prevention of urinary tract infection in boys: a systematic review of randomised trials and observational studies. Arch Dis Child 2005; 90:853–858. Published online 12 May 2005. Review.

21. Mattson SR. Routine anesthesia for circumcision: two effective techniques. Postgrad Med 1999; 106:107–109.

22. Learman LA. Neonatal circumcision: a dispassionate analysis. Clin Obstet Gynecol 1999; 42:849–859.

23. Williams N, Kapila L. Complications of circumcision. Br J Surg 1993; 80:1231–1236.

24. Pearlman CK. Reconstruction following iatrogenic burn of the penis. J Pediatr Surg 1976; 11:121.

25. Kariher DH. Immediate circumcision of the newborn. J Obstet Gynaec 1956; 7(1):50–53.

26. Hobman J, Lewis E, Ringlar R. Neonatal circumcision techniques. Am Fam Physician 1995; 52:511–518.

27. Kaplan GW. Complications of circumcision. Urol Clin North Am 1983; 10:543–549.

28. Editorial: Astonishing indifference to deaths due to botched ritual circumcision. S Afr Med J 2003; 8:93.

29. Al-Samarrai AYI, Mofti AB, Crankson SJ, et al. A review of the Plastibell device in neonatal circumcision in 2000 instances. Surg Gynecol Obstet 1988; 167:342–343.

30. Adams JR Jr, Culkin DJ, Mata JA, Bocchim JA Jr, Venable DD. Fournier's gangrene in children. Urol 1990; 5:439–441.

31. Weinberger M, Haynes RE, Morse RS. Necrotizing fasciitis in a neonate. Arch Pediatr Adolesc Med 1972; 123:591–593.

32. Kirkpatric BV, Eitzman DV. Neonatal septicaemia after circumcision. Clin Pediatr (Phila) 1974; 13:767–768.

33. Bode CO, Ikhisemojie S, Ademuyiwa AO. Penile injuries from proximal migration of the Plastibell circumcision ring. J Pediatr Urol 2010; 6:23–27.

34. Bode CO, Kena-Ewulu. Complications of male circumcision in Lagos. Analysis of 90 cases. Nig Q J Hosp Med 1977; 7:129–133.

35. Limaye RD, Hancock RA. Penile urethral fistual as a complication of circumcision. J Pediatr 1968; 72:105–106.

36. Newell TEC. Judgement of inquiry into the death of McWillis, Ryleigh Roman Bryan. Burnaby, BC: British Columbia Coroner's Service, 19 January 2004.

37. Bailey RC, Egesah O, Rosenberg S. Bull World Health Organ 2008; 86:657–736.

38. Hazard: incompatibility of different brands of Gomco-type circumcision clamps. Health Devices 1997; 26:76–77.

39. Hazard: amputations with use of adult-size scissors-type circumcision clamps on infants. Health Devices 1995; 4:286–287.

40. Hammond T. A preliminary poll of men circumcised in infancy and childhood. BJU Int 1999; 83(Suppl 1):85–92.

41. Crowley JP, Kesner KM. Ritual circumcision (Umkwetha) among the Xhosa of the Ciskei. Br J Urol 1990; 66:318–321.

42. Johnson RC. Millions of "snips" will harm millions of men. Letter to the editor. SAMJ 2010; 100(3):133–134.

43. British Medical Association. The Law and Ethics of Male Circumcision: Guidance for Doctors. London: BMA, 2006.

CHAPTER 96
PHIMOSIS, MEATAL STENOSIS, AND PARAPHIMOSIS

Merrill McHoney

Kokila Lakhoo

Phimosis

Introduction

Phimosis is defined as a narrowing of the preputial ring that prevents retraction of the foreskin over the glans penis. It can be physiological (congenital) or pathological (acquired). Physiological phimosis is almost invariably present at birth. Most cases of phimosis presenting for surgical opinion are physiological and self-limiting.

Demographics

At birth, the foreskin is usually nonretractile (physiological phimosis), with no apparent racial differences in incidence. Physiological phimosis regresses with age, as the foreskin widens and gradually advances over the glans penis. Prepucial adhesions are sometimes present during regression of physiological phimosis, but these also resolve spontaneously in most cases as epithelial keratinisation occurs.

Aetiology/Pathophysiology

Physiological phimosis is a variant of normal prepucial development. Table 96.1 gives an indication of the natural history of physiological phimosis. Pysiological phimosis can persist up to, and resolve at puberty in some cases.

Table 96.1: Percentage of boys with retractile foreskin, by age.

Newborn Infants	4%
1-year old boys	50%
4-year old boys	90%

Pathological phimosis can be defined as a scarred and fribrotic foreskin that prevents its retraction and is unyielding. Pathological phimosis may very rarely be a primary or congenital anomaly, but is much more commonly secondary. One cause is repeated attacks of infection of the foreskin and/or glans (balanoposthitis) that cause scarring. The usual infecting organism is staphylococcus; flucloxacillin or co-amoxiclav is usually therapeutic. Poor foreskin hygiene may contribute to repeated infection. Recurrent or chronic inflammation may lead to a rigid, fibrous foreskin. Scarring from trauma, for example from zipper injuries, may also be causative.

Pathological phimosis is most often the result of balanitis xerotica obliterans (BXO).[1] In this condition, equivalent to lichen sclerosis atrophicus, the foreskin is thickened, inflamed, scarred, and unyielding. The exact aetiology of BXO is uncertain. Histologically, there is hyperkeratosis and basal layer degeneration with an infiltrate of lymphocytes, plasma cells, and histiocytes. The pathological process giving rise to BXO can also affect the urethra, giving rise to meatal and urethral stenosis. According to one study.[2] BXO is twice as common in blacks and Hispanics compared to whites. BXO is unusual before 2 years of age; usually peaking in presentation after 5 years.[3] The prevalence of pathological phimosis in boys up to 15 years of age is 0.6% in a Westernised population.[1]

Clinical Presentation

History

Phimosis usually presents with a history of inability to retract the foreskin, often with ballooning on urination. Other symptoms are uncommon. A misdirected urinary stream may be caused by the urine spraying off the foreskin, with complaints of wetting the toilet seat. A white or creamy discharge is consistent with a discharge of smegma associated with a physiological phimosis. There may be a history of recurrent discharge with or without an intermittent lump at the corona (smegmatous "cyst").

Mild inflammation of the tip of the foreskin is common and is due to ammoniacal irritation. This sometimes causes a history of redness confined to the tip. Overt infection of the foreskin causes swelling and redness of the entire foreskin and a yellow or greenish discharge. The child may complain of burning on urination. Urinary tract infection (UTI) should be ruled out.

BXO often presents with severe burning with urination. The patient or parent may also express the fact that the foreskin, which was once retractile, is no longer so. With severe disease, the pain can cause the child to inhibit urination and thus contribute to retention. There may be mild bleeding from the foreskin. With meatal or urethral involvement, the symptoms can progress to straining at urination and poor stream. Complete obstruction can ensue due to severe meatal stenosis.

Physical examination

In physiological phimosis, the foreskin is soft and supple. There is usually a sufficient prepucial meatus to be seen. Often, this can be accentuated by gentle stretching of the foreskin. In some cases the foreskin can be partially retracted to reveal part, if not most, of the glans, with supple glanular adhesion remaining. In physiological phimosis, the foreskin "pouts" or "mushrooms" on gentle retraction. Retraction should never be forceful.

In a rare variation of phimosis, the urine stream gets directed into the prepucial space, giving rise to the so-called "volcano penis" (Figure 96.1). In this condition, the prepuce stretches and covers most of the penis. The prepucial and suprapubic space expands with urine,

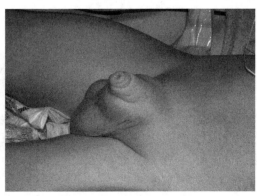

Figure 96.1: Volcano penis with a phimosis.

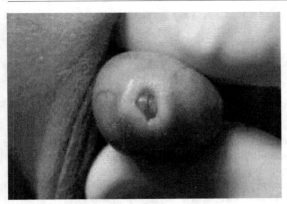

Figure 96.2: Pathological phimosis due to BXO.

stretching the tissue planes. Pressure on the large prepucial space can sometimes cause urine to be expressed from the foreskin meatus. This form of phimosis is best treated with a tri-radiate prepuitoplasty, as circumcision is difficult and can be disfiguring cosmetically.

With pathological phimosis, the foreskin is thickened and scarred and can be unyielding. In cases of BXO, the foreskin may be scaly, inflamed, and haemorrhagic, or it can be white and fibrotic (Figure 96.2). It can also be literally pinhole size.

Investigations

In cases of physiological phimosis, no investigation is usually required. If infection is suspected, a swab for culture should be taken. If UTI is suspected, a urine sample should be tested.

In cases of BXO and for those patients presenting with symptoms of meatal stenosis, a urine flow study is useful.

Management

Physiological phimosis

As already noted, most cases of physiological phimosis resolve spontaneously, sometimes as late as puberty. Conservative management is therefore the mainstay of treatment in these cases. Firm reassurance from the surgeon to the parents is required to avoid unnecessary circumcision. Routine foreskin care is all that is needed. When partial retraction of the foreskin becomes possible, the foreskin should be gently retracted in the bath, gently cleaned and then pulled back over the glans. This should never be forceful and should be done by the boy himself when possible, as he will normally stop retracting if there is any discomfort. Forceful retraction may create small tears and can create a pathological phimosis.

Topical steroids have been shown to be a viable, cost-effective outpatient means of treating physiological phimosis.[4] Occasionally a 4- to 6-week course of weak topical steroid administration (e.g., 0.05% betamethasone) is useful to demonstrate retractability. Parents should be warned, however, that recurrence is common after the course if routine foreskin care and retraction are not continued. The demonstration of what will soon ensue as a natural process in time is often sufficient treatment, and a second course should not be necessary.

Circumcision

Physiological phimosis alone is not an indication for circumcision. Indications for circumcision include:

- pathological phimosis;
- BXO;
- recurrent balanoposthitis;
- persistent painful erections associated with a phimosis; and
- physiological phimosis that persists into adolescence.

Circumcision is performed in the following steps (see also Chapter 95):

1. The foreskin is dilated to allow division of adhesions and full retraction.

2. The foreskin is marked at the coronal level where it will be incised, making sure that neither too much or too little is excised.

3. The foreskin and inner prepucial layer can be incised individually or together by using a knife.

4. The inner prepucial layer is then trimmed to leave a 5-mm cuff.

5. Haemostasis is achieved by using bipolar diathermy.

6. The shaft skin is then anastamosed to the inner layer by using fine interrupted absorbable sutures (e.g., 5/0 monocryl).

7. A haemostatic mattress suture can be placed on the frenulum to assist with haemostasis.

The most common complication of circumcision is bleeding. This is often minimal and self-limiting, requiring only a pressure dressing in most cases. Rarely, a return to the surgical theatre is needed to achieve haemostasis; either with suture or diathermy. The most common site for bleeding is the frenulum.

Infection is uncommon; usually a staphylococcus is causative. Topical (e.g., fucidin) or enteral (e.g., flucloxacillin or co-amoxiclav) antibiotics are usually needed for 5 days. Infection and sequelae of it are more common when untrained circumcisions are performed, a particular issue in African ritual circumcisions.[5;6] Severe infection can lead to penile gangrene and loss. Occasionally, overwhelming sepsis can lead to death.

Meatal stenosis can occur postcircumcision secondary to exposure of the meatus to trauma or ammoniacal dermatitis in the infant. If too much shaft skin is excised, painful erections can result. Removal of too much skin can also cause a partially buried appearance to the penis, and cosmetic dissatisfaction can occur.

Amputation of the glans is a rare complication of circumcision. This is more common in procedures being done by nontrained personnel.

Prognosis and Outcomes

There are no long-term aspects of physiological phimosis of note. If present after puberty at the age when sexual intercourse is started, however, it can cause interference with sexual activity.

Boys with BXO should be followed up to detect the development of urethral stenosis. Older patients and those with meatal involvement tend to have a more severe and complicated clinical course. Penile carcinoma in adulthood has been described as arising from BXO. Late-presenting or long-standing disease should include this differential diagnosis in the work-up.

Ethical Issues

The main ethical issue surrounds requests for circumcision in infants with physiological phimosis. Although there is sufficient evidence demonstrating the resolution with conservative management, there continues to be pressure from parents and doctors alike to circumcise these boys. There is also a group of patients who will be referred for consideration under religious and cultural reasons. The incidence of complications after circumcision is not negligible, but should be balanced against the higher incidence of complications if untrained personnel perform the surgery. There have been deaths and serious complications in both Western and African countries from untrained circumcisions. The paediatric surgeon may need to modify his practice based on local policies and outcomes as well as personal conviction.

Meatal Stenosis

Introduction

Meatal stenosis is a narrowing of the external urinary meatus, giving rise to difficulty passing urine. It is uncommon in the paediatric population, and most cases have an obvious cause that can be treated by simple intervention.

Demographics

The incidence of meatal stenosis varies alongside the aetiological causes. The international figure for meatal stenosis postcircumcision varies widely, from 1% to 20% of cases.

As mentioned earlier, BXO peaks in presentation after 5 years. Overall, between 15% and 30% of BXO cases have urethral involvement at presentation,[3] with an increasing prevalence of meatal stenosis with time. BXO seems to have a twice higher incidence in blacks compared to whites.

Aetiology/Pathophysiology

Meatal stenosis is almost always acquired. Congenital meatal stenosis is rare and usually associated with another congenital anomaly of the urinary tract, such as hypospadias or urethral duplication. These cases are not addressed in this chapter.

The most common natural cause of meatal stenosis in children is BXO. In these cases, foreskin disease (pathological, scarred, and fibrotic) is present as evidence of the aetiology. Meatal stenosis can also be secondary to iatrogenic trauma (e.g., catheterisations) or repeated trauma or inflammation from ammoniacal dermatitis (ammonia nappy rash) postcircumcision. Ischaemic damage during the circumcision itself is also possible due to excessive diathermy around the frenulum and meatus and posthypospadius repair.

Clinical Presentation

History

The history with meatal stenosis is that of severe difficulty urinating. The child forces and strains to pass urine, and produces a thin stream or sprays. Suprapubic pain may be present during micturation.

Lethargy, weight loss, vomiting, or symptoms of anaemia may be present in late-presenting cases of meatal stenosis when renal function may be affected.[7]

Physical examination

A meatus that is stenotic may be obvious on retracting the foreskin. If BXO is present, the foreskin and glans are thickened, inflamed, and scarred. If there is significant bladder outlet obstruction, the bladder may be palpable. The patient should be observed urinating. The urinary stream is thin and weak; often only a thin spray is produced. The child may seem to force and be in discomfort, and it takes an appreciably long time to empty the bladder.

In late-presenting cases, there may be detrusor failure, with a dribbling stream, distended bladder, and general ill health. There may be signs of renal failure (dry skin, weight loss, and pallor).

Investigations

A urine flow study is useful to assess the urine stream. It should also be repeated during follow-up after intervention. In meatal stenosis, the study can show a poor flow and there may be a significant residual volume after voiding.

Tests for renal function are required only if renal failure is suspected.

Cystoscopy is indicated only if urethral involvement is suspected from the severity of the symptoms.

Management

Meatal dilatation is an alternative in minor cases, but sometimes requires repeated dilatations, with a relatively high incidence of recurrence. Under general anaesthesia, serial urethral dilators are used to calibrate and then dilate the urethral meatus to an appropriate size for the child. A routine repeat dilatation can be scheduled, or the effect of a single dilatation can be assessed before proceeding to a repeat procedure. Severe or recurrent meatal stenosis is best treated by meatotomy.

At meatotomy, the following steps are taken:

1. Before incising the meatus, a fine mosquito clip can be used to gently crush the tissue for around 5 seconds to assist haemostasis.

2. An incision (approximately 3–5 mm) is made in the urethral meatus with a fine-tipped scissors or a knife to create an adequate meatal opening.

3. Careful bipolar diathermy can be used to achieve haemostasis if there are any vigorous bleeding points.

4. The edges of the incised urethra are then sutured to the glans by using a few fine absorbable sutures (e.g., 6/0 monocryl).

Postoperative Complications

Mild postoperative pain after meatotomy is common and can be treated by local pain-relieving gels along with oral pain relief. A soak in the bath is sometimes therapeutic.

Recurrence is the main postoperative complication. This can generally be treated successfully by repeat meatotomy. In cases of BXO, more extensive urethral disease should be considered, and referral made to a paediatric urologist or suitably experienced surgeon.

Prognosis and Outcomes

There are usually no long-term sequela in simple cases. However, boys with BXO should be followed up to identify any ongoing or progressive disease, with resulting urethral stenosis.

Rarely, meatal stenosis is discovered after a long clinical delay. There can be secondary effects on bladder function and secondary renal damage. These cases will need urological and/or nephrology follow-up as necessary.

Prevention

The main preventive measure to decrease the incidence of meatal stenosis will be the judicious practice of circumcision, especially in young boys, as well as attention to good surgical practice during circumcision. If circumcision is necessary, it should be performed by appropriately trained persons to give the lowest complication rate.

There is yet no known prevention of meatal stenosis in cases of BXO presenting without initial involvement. Prophylactic topical steroid use has not been shown to be efficacious enough in that vein.[8,9]

Paraphimosis

Introduction

Paraphimosis is defined as the inability to return a retracted foreskin back over the glans. This results in swelling of the glans and foreskin due to oedema from the resultant constriction.

Demographics

Paraphimosis can occur at any age after the foreskin becomes retractable over the glans. There is no specific age preference thereafter. Cases present from early childhood into adulthood. Overall, paraphimosis accounts for around 0.9% of boys presenting to hospital in a Western society.

Aetiology/Pathophysiology

There is sometimes, but not always, a partially tight foreskin in the history prior to the incident leading to the paraphimosis.

Clinical Presentation

History

The history is that of acute swelling of the glans penis after retraction of the foreskin, and the patient then not being able to return the foreskin to its normal position. Most cases in children occur after retracting the foreskin during micturation. In older children, it may be related to a sexual activity. There may or may not be a history of difficult retraction, due to a partial tightness, prior to the event.

Physical examination

The foreskin is retracted over the glans and is tight. The glans and foreskin are swollen and oedematous (Figure 96.3). With progression of time, the glans may become severely blue and swollen as evidence of venous engorgement. Gangrene is an extremely late sign.

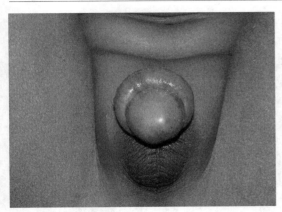

Figure 96.3: Paraphimosis.

Management

Paraphimosis is an emergency, requiring prompt reduction. In appropriate cases, this can be done with local and systemic pain relief and sedation in the emergency department. In some cases, general anaesthetic is needed.

Most cases of paraphimosis can be reduced with initial constant pressure applied to the glans and foreskin to "squeeze" out the oedema. Some pressure is maintained on the glans by forcefully pushing on the glans with the thumbs and pulling the foreskin over the glans with the fingers. In about 95% of cases, this is successful.

Severe cases may require a dorsal slit procedure, in which a dorsal incision is made along the length of the foreskin to release the tight band. The foreskin is then retracted over the glans. The incision can be left to heal by secondary intention after haemostasis is achieved.

Postoperative Complications

Postoperative dysuria is often mild. Pathological phimosis is rare. Recurrence is uncommon.

Prevention

Prevention of paraphimosis revolves around careful education of boys and their caregivers about routine foreskin care.

Evidence-Based Research

Table 96.2 presents an overview of foreskin development and its conditions, addressing indications for circumcision. Table 96.3 presents a randomised control study of the use of steroid cream for phimosis.

Table 96.2: Evidence-based research.

Title	The fate of the foreskin, a study of circumcision
Authors	Gairdner D
Institution	United Cambridge Hospitals, Cambridge, UK
Reference	British Medical Journal 1949; 2:1433–1447
Problem	The widespread and sometimes indiscriminate use of circumcision to treat phimosis is questioned and addressed in this paper.
Comparison/ control (quality of evidence)	Epidemiological and follow up study on foreskin development and conditions in childhood and the incidence of pathological conditions affecting the foreskin.
Outcome/ effect	Physiological phimosis is most often a self-limiting stage in prepucial development postnatally. Pathological phimosis is less common and is established as an indication for circumcision.
Historical significance/ comments	Establishes a basis of the incidence and natural history of physiological phimosis.

Table 96.3: Evidence-based research.

Title	Topical steroid application versus circumcision in pediatric patients with phimosis: a prospective randomized placebo controlled clinical trial
Authors	Esposito C, Centonze A, Alicchio F, Savanelli A, Settimi A
Institution	Department of Experimental and Clinical Medicine, Magna Graecia University, Campus SVenuta, Catanzaro, Italy
Reference	World J Urol 2008; 26(2):187–190
Problem	Phimosis.
Intervention	A prospective study was carried out over a 24-month period on an outpatient basis on patients with phimosis. One-hundred twenty patients applied a steroid cream twice a day for 4 weeks, and another group of 120 patients used a placebo cream twice a day for 4 weeks. Patients were assigned to either group by computer-generated random choice.
Comparison/ control (quality of evidence)	Randomised control study with placebo control
Outcome/ effect	This study showed that topical steroids represent a good alternative to surgery in case of phimosis. Steroid therapy gave better results than placebos, with an overall efficacy of 65.8%.

Key Summary Points

1. Physiological phimosis does not require circumcision.

2. Pathological phimosis and physiological phimosis presenting with complications or into puberty should be treated with circumcision.

3. Topical steroid therapy is an alternative therapy to circumcision for physiological phimosis in those requiring treatment.

4. BXO is a common cause of pathological phimosis and can also cause meatal stenosis.

5. Meatal stenosis is best treated by meatotomy as a daycase procedure, with good results.

6. Paraphimosis is an emergency often easily resolved with simple reduction of the glans through the foreskin, with little sequela.

References

1. Shankar KR, Rickwood AM. The incidence of phimosis in boys. BJU Int 1999; 84(1):101–102.

2. Kizer WS, Prarie T, Morey AF. Balanitis xerotica obliterans: epidemiologic distribution in an equal access health care system. South Med J 2003; 96(1):9–11.

3. Gargollo PC, Kozakewich HP, Bauer SB, et al. Balanitis xerotica obliterans in boys. J Urol 2005; 174(4 Pt 1):1409–1412.

4. Berdeu D, Sauze L, Ha-Vinh P, Blum-Boisgard C. Cost-effectiveness analysis of treatments for phimosis: a comparison of surgical and medicinal approaches and their economic effect. BJU Int 2001; 87(3):239–244.

5. Magoha GA. Circumcision in various Nigerian and Kenyan hospitals. East Afr Med J 1999; 76(10):583–586.

6. du Toit DF, Villet WT. Gangrene of the penis after circumcision: a report of 3 cases. S Afr Med J 1979; 55(13):521–522.

7. Sandler G, Patrick E, Cass D. Long standing balanitis xerotica obliterans resulting in renal impairment in a child. Pediatr Surg Int 2008; 24(8):961–964.

8. Webster TM, Leonard MP. Topical steroid therapy for phimosis. Can J Urol 2002; 9(2):1492–1495.

9. Das S, Tunuguntla HS. Balanitis xerotica obliterans—a review. World J Urol 2000; 18(6):382–387.

CHAPTER 97
UROLITHIASIS

Philip M. Mshelbwala

Hyacinth N. Mbibu

Introduction

Urinary stones are relatively uncommon in the paediatric age group; however, the prevalence seems to be on the increase and the tendency towards urinary lithiasis in males and females is the same in childhood.[1,2] The clinical features are often vague and nonspecific, so a high index of suspicion is usually required for diagnosis. Limited investigations tend to be performed in children presenting with urinary calculi,[3] and this may affect the prevalence of urinary stones in children. The prevalence is also affected by race, genetics, diet, and geographic location.[4]

Dermographics

The decreased prevalence in children may be due to the low rate of secretion of endogenous oxalate. Low levels of testosterone at childhood may protect children from forming the most common stones.[5] Stones have been found to be more common in Western countries and parts of Asia than in East and West Africa. The overall incidence in Africa is estimated at 2–3% of the general population, with lower figures reported in Nigeria.[6,7] The incidence may also vary within the same country.[8]

Aetiology/Pathogenesis

Urinary stones may be due to metabolic causes, congenital anomalies, or infections and can be found in any part of the urinary system, from the kidney to the urethra. They may also migrate from the upper urinary tract to lower sites.

In about 75% of cases of urinary stones in children, an identifiable predisposing cause can be found. It is not uncommon to find more than one factor in the same patient.[9] The causes are metabolic (40%), urinary tract abnormality (25%), urinary tract infection, or UTI (10%), with the remaining being idiopathic.[10] The hot climate in some parts of Africa has also been implicated.[11,12]

Metabolic Causes

The most common metabolic cause in children is hypercalciuria, occurring in 30–50% of cases in some series.[13] Certain diets and disorders of renal tubular transport may predispose to hypercalciuria, although high urinary calcium may be detected in 3–4% of normal children.[14] Cystinuria, hyperoxaluria, hyperuricosuria, hypocitric aciduria, and hyperxanthinuria are other metabolic causes.[15] change in diet and other social habits may have led to an increase of urinary stones in children. Improved health care has also led to the emergence of urinary stones in patients who previously would not have survived, such as premature infants with hypercalcinosis and children with cystic fibrosis presenting with urinary stones.[10]

Congenital Abnormalities

Genitourinary congenital abnormalities that cause obstruction to the free flow of urine also predispose to stone formation. These include posterior urethral valves, bladder exstrophy, vesicoureteric reflux, meatal stenosis, medullary sponge kidney, and pelviureteric junction obstruction. Neuropathic bladders from spinal bifida may lead to stone formation.

Urinary Tract Infection

UTI is an important predisposing factor in infants and younger children. The organisms commonly isolated are urease splitting species of *Proteus*, *Klebsellia*, *Pseudomonas*, *Staphylococcus*, and some anaerobes. These microbes split urea, leading to an increase in the urinary pH, which in turn raises the urinary concentration of magnesium ammonium phosphate ions, creating a favourable environment for stone formation. The presence of oxalate-splitting bacteria in urine has also been implicated.

Diet

Various foods and fluids that may result in the excessive excretion of substances that produce stones have a significant effect on the incidence of urinary stones. These include purines, oxalates, calcium, phosphates, and uric acid. Diets with excessive vegetables, high levels of animal protein (such as beef, chicken, and lamb), milk, and ice cream are associated with childhood lithiasis.[2]

Idiopathic

The cause of stone formation may be unidentifiable in a number of patients, especially in the adolescent age group; this situation is similar in adults. Due to the possibility of more than one predisposing factor, thorough clinical and exhaustive investigative parameters are desired in the proper assessment of these children.[8]

Pathophysiology

The pathophysiology of urinary stone formation is quite complex and involves the interaction of various factors,[16] including (Figure 97.1):

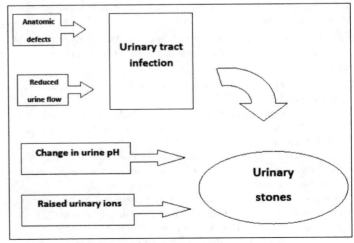

Figure 97.1: Pathophysiology of urinary stones.

• urinary concentration of stone-forming ions, such as calcium, phosphate, oxalates, and uric acid;

• urinary pH;

• rate of flow of urine;

• balance between promoter and inhibitory factors of crystallisation (e.g., citrate, magnesium, pyrophosphate, nephrocalcin, Tamm-Horsfall glycoproteins, and glycosaminglycans); and anatomic factors that predispose to urinary stais (e.g. congenital anomalies), foreign bodies, and some drugs such as acetazolamide.

All these factors should be treated if management is to be successful and recurrence minimised.

The chemical composition of urinary stones in children is similar to those found in adults. About 50% are calcium oxalate, 15–25% are calcium phosphate, and 10–15% are mixed (calcium oxalate and calcium phosphate). The others are struvite [magnesium ammonium, phosphate] (15–30%), cystine (6–10%), and uric acid (2–10%).[9,13]

Due to their relative high densities (based on their calcium content), most of these stones are visible on plain radiographs, some better than others.

Clinical Presentation

History

The average age at presentation is 8–10 years with a male-to-female ratio of 1.5:1.

The evaluation of a child with suspected urolithiasis requires a high index of suspicion because the symptoms may be vague and varied. These symptoms include:

1. Pain/colic: Pain is the most common symptom of urolithiasis in children. Frank renal colic is a feature in adolescents that waxes and wanes in severity; the pain may range from a mild ache to severe discomfort. The pain can last 20–60 minutes. Acute generalised abdominal pain is more common in younger children,[17] and diagnosis is made on work-up for UTI.

2. Recurrent UTI: A history of recurrent UTI, especially in younger children, should be a pointer and deserves further investigation.

3. Crying on micturition: Crying or pain on micturition (in older children) is also a common presenting feature; this may start early in life. The child may also tug at the penis during micturition.

4. Urinary retention: Urinary retention may be the initial symptom of urinary stones.

5. Gross haematuria: This alarming symptom, which is present in 30–50% of cases and may occur in combination with colic is the main presenting feature of urinary stones in older children. Haematuria may also be microscopic.

6. Nausea and vomiting: Unexplained nausea and vomiting may be due to stones. A deeper probing into the patient's history may reveal more symptoms.

7. Fever: Fever may occur in children with urinary stones, especially if associated with UTI.

Other symptoms include frequency of urination, tugging or pulling at the phallus, spontaneous passage of stones, failure to thrive, and rectal prolapse.[7]

A number of children with urinary stones, however, are asymptomatic, particularly those with staghorn stones; they are discovered only during investigation for other conditions, such as recurrent UTIs.

Review of medical and family history is pertinent because urinary stones may be recurrent or familial. The dietary history, especially high-protein foods, salts, and food and vitamin supplements, must be sought.

The daily fluid intake should be estimated because low fluid intake, especially in hot climates, has been shown to be a predisposing factor to urinary stones. A history of drugs that affect uric acid and calcium metabolism is also important.

Physical Examination

Findings on physical examination of a child with urinary stones vary widely.

• *Acute episode:* The patient most likely to present with acute colic is the older child in his teens; there is painful distress, listlessness, and there may be fever (if the cause is infective). Nonspecific generalised abdominal pain is encountered in younger children, and tenderness may be noted on examination.

• *Chronic stones:* The child may show signs of failure to thrive resulting from recurrent UTI and renal failure.

• *Normal child:* The child may appear grossly normal with no physical signs.

Investigations

Urine Tests

Both urinalysis and urine culture are indicated. Urine should be analysed for pH. A high pH points towards the presence of urea-splitting bacteria, whereas uric acid or cystine stones form in the presence of low pH. Levels of calcium, oxalate, citrate, uric acid, and cystine are also estimated. A 24-hour urine sample in older cooperative patients gives more information. Urine microscopy may reveal casts, crystals, haematuria, and pyuria. Urine culture would also be useful in isolating the offending organism when present, and the sensitivity pattern would guide antibiotic use. Clean midstream urine can be collected in older patients, but clean catheterisation or a suprapubic tap may be necessary to avoid contamination in some younger patients.[17,18]

Imaging

Imaging is useful in confirming the presence of a stone and also in detecting abnormalities of the urinary tract that may have predisposed to stone formation.

• *Plain radiographs* (Figure 97.2) can diagnose about 90% of urinary stones. In temperate countries, 60–70% of stones are renal at the time of diagnosis. When they are seen in the ureter, bladder, or urethra, the stones often have migrated from the kidney. In contrast, in hotter climates, more bladder stones are seen and have been referred to as endemic bladder stones.

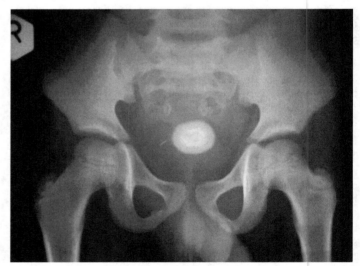

Figure 97.2: Plain radiograph showing stone.

• *Ultrasonography* (US) is useful in detecting kidney stones but less reliable for ureteric calculi. US can also evaluate the structural state of the urinary system, picking up congenital malformations that may predispose to stone formation. Obstructive features, such as hydro-ureters and hydronephrosis, are also diagnosed.

• *Intravenous urography* (IVU) would demonstrate less opaque or radio-lucent stones (not picked up by plain radiography) as filling defects in the urinary system. Renal functional status can also be assessed.

- *Helical computed tomography* (CT) scans have recently been shown to be useful in diagnosing urinary stones.[19] These give a three-dimensional image, are able to detect almost all types of stones, and can determine whether the stone is causing any obstruction.

- *Retrograde pyelgraphy* may rarely be needed if a radio-opaque stone is difficult to locate by other means.

Stone Analysis

Where the stone has been passed out spontaneously or obtained surgically, it should be analysed for its chemical composition. Apart from visualising the stone, other structural abnormalities that may predispose to calculi formation may be detected. Stones can also be extracted during the procedure.

Endoscopy

Urethrocystoscopy is used with increasing frequency in children; this assesses the urethra, bladder, and ureteric orifices.

Blood Analysis

The serum levels of calcium, phosphate, creatinine, uric acid, sodium, potassium, alkaline phosphate, albumin, and bicarbonate should be estimated. Elevated levels may suggest the cause of the stones in metabolic cases and provide useful information regarding treatment.

Treatment

The definitive treatment of urinary stones in children should be directed at the specific cause; however, general and medical measures are important in all patients.[1]

Medical

A high fluid intake is encouraged to ensure good urinary output, especially in patients living in hotter climates. This increased intake is continued after definitive treatment to reduce the chance of recurrence.

The older child is more likely to present with typical acute ureteric colicky abdominal pain. The pain in the younger child is more usually a generalised abdominal ache. Acute pain may be managed with narcotic analgesics and antispasmodics. The agitated child necessarily needs to be calmed; otherwise, further evaluation may be difficult.

Appropriate antibiotic therapy where UTI has been established is mandatory. Bacteria commonly may be trapped in the core of calculi and therefore be inaccessible to antibiotics. Treatment may continue over prolonged periods to achieve permanent cure and to reduce the risk of renal scarring and recurrent UTIs.

Patients with hypercalciuria are advised to reduce dietary sources of calcium such as milk and cheese; low sodium and potassium-enhanced diets are also beneficial. Those with hyperoxalouria are to avoid nuts, spinach, tea, and cocoa-based drinks and foods. In patients with citric acid deficiency, dietary supplementation of sodium and potassium citrate increases urinary citrate level, thus decreasing the chance of stone formation.[20]

Potassium citrate is commonly used as an effective calcium stone inhibitor. It is readily absorbed from the gastrointestinal tract, and after excretion in the urine, inhibits the crystallisation of stone-forming calcium salts by binding the calcium ion, thus decreasing its urinary saturation and inhibiting the nucleation and crystal growth of calcium oxalate.

Extracorporeal Shock-Wave Lithotripsy

Extracorporeal shock-wave lithotripsy (ESWL), a noninvasive mode of treatment, was initially reserved for adult patients but is used with increasing frequency and success in children.[9,21,22] The stone is localised by US scan or x-ray, and ultrasonic shock waves are beamed at the site to disintegrate the stone, which is subsequently passed out or extracted.

Indications for the use of ESWL are growing; they commonly include a large single stone and no evidence of urinary tract obstruction that may impede expulsion of fragments. Obesity and other concomitant medical illnesses may be relative contraindications.

Surgery

A wide range of surgical options are available for the treatment of urinary stones in children; these may be open or minimally invasive. Indications for surgery include failed medical treatment and failed or contraindicated ESWL. Surgery can also be used in conjunction with other forms of therapy. Surgery directed at correcting structural abnormalities is also indicated because this can serve to reduce the risk of recurrence.

Minimally invasive surgery

Endoscopic procedures such as ureteroscopic, cystoscopic, and nephroscopic lithotomy are commonly used to treat stones in children, especially in the developed countries. These techniques may be used alone or together with ESWL. Percutaneous nephrolithotomy is also a popular treatment option. More recently, laser has also been used to treat urinary stones.[19]

Open Surgery

In developing countries due to the limited availability of endoscopic equipment, treatment of urinary stones is most commonly by open procedures. Pyelolithotomy, nephrolithotomy, ureterolithotomy, or cystolithotomy are used to extract the stones, depending on the site.[7]

The most common nonanatomic cause of paediatric lithiasis is hypercalciuria. This must be diligently searched for and treated. If not, it remains an important cause of recurrent lithiasis in children. Treatment must also be directed towards the management of the underlying cause of the stone where this is identified.[1] Anatomic anomalies such as posterior urethra valves, vesicoureteric reflux, and pelviureteric junction obstruction should be corrected.

Prevention

Long-term follow-up of children with urinary stones is necessary to detect recurrence. Adequate fluid intake and dietary adjustment, along with infection control if used in concert, help to reduce the rate of recurrence.

Regular imaging, such as ultrasonography, urinalysis, and other means of monitoring may be indicated in these patients.

Key Summary Points

1. Urinary stones are relatively uncommon in children.

2. Changes in diet and other social habits may have led to an increase of urinary stones.

3. In a majority of patients, an identifiable predisposing cause can be found, and more than one factor may be responsible in the same patient.

4. Presentation may be acute or nonspecific and varied; thus, diagnosis is often difficult or delayed.

5. A wide range of imaging techniques as well as urine and serum biochemical analysis are needed for evaluation.

6. Helical noncontrast CT is useful in confirming the presence of a stone and also in detecting abnormalities of the urinary tract.

7. Treatment should be directed towards removing the underlying cause(s) of the stone, where this is identified, as well as dealing with the pathological effects of the stone.

8. Long-term follow-up of children with urinary stones is necessary to detect recurrence.

References

1. Mshelbwala PM, Ameh EA, and Mbibu HN. Urinary stones in children: Review article. Niger J Surg Res 2005; 79(3–4):238–243.

2. Holmes RP, Goodman HD, Assimos DG. The distribution of urinary calcium excretion in individuals on control diets. J Uol 1995; 153:350. Abstract, 468.

3. Hulton SA. Evaluation of urinary tract calculi in children. Arch Dis Child 2001; 84:320–323.

4. Schwarz RD, Dwyer NT. Pediatric kidney stones: long-term outcomes. Urology 2006; 67:812–816.

5. Brockis JG, Bowyer RC, McCulloch RK. Pathophysiology of endemic bladder stones. In: Brocks JG, Finlayson B, eds. Urinary Calculus. PGS Publishing, 1981.

6. Hassan I, Mabogunje OA. Urinary stones in children in Zaria. Ann Trop Paediatr 1993; 13:269–271.

7. Abubakar AM, Mungadi IA, Chinda JY, Ntia IO, Jalo I, Obianno SK. Paediatric urolithiasis in Northern Nigeria. Afr J of Paed Surg 2004;1:2–5.

8. Rodgers, A. The riddle of kidney stone disease: lessons from Africa. Urol Res 2006; 34:92–95.

9. Milliner DS. Calculi. In: Kaplan BS, Meyers KE, eds. Pediatric Nephrology and Urology: The Requisites in Pediatrics, 1st ed. Mosby, 2004, Pp 361–374.

10. Milliner DS, Murphy ME. Urolithiasis in pediatric patients. Mayo Clin Proc 1993; 68:241–248.

11. Duvie SOA, Endeley EML, Dahinya MA. Urolithiasis in Maiduguri. The Nigerian Savannah Belt Experience. West Afr J Med 1988; 7:148–156.

12. Jones TW, Henderson TR. Urinary calculi in children in Western Australia: 1972–86. Austral Paediatr J 1989; 25:93–95.

13. Polinsky MS, Kaiser BA, Balnarte HJ. Urolithiasis in childhood. Pediatr Clin North Am 1987; 34:683–710.

14. Moore ES. Hypercalciuria in children. Contrib Nephrol 1981; 27:20–32.

15. Ratan SK, et al. Urinary citrate excretion in idiopathic nephrolithiasis. Indian Pediatr 2002; 39:819–825.

16. Angwafo FF III, Daudon Dado M, Wonkam A, Kuwong PM, Kropp KA. Pediatric urolithiasis in sub-Saharan Africa: a comparative study in two regions of Cameroon. Eur Urol 2000; 37:106–111.

17. Davenport M. ABC of general surgery in hildren: acute abdominal pain n children. BMJ 1996; 312:498–501.

18. Zelikovic I, Adelman RD, Nancarrow PA. Urinary tract infections in children. An update. West Afr J Med 1992; 157:554–561.

19. Williams JC. Progress in the use of helical CT for imaging urinary calculi. J Endourology 2004; 18(10):937–941.

20. Pak CYC, Fuller C, Sakhaee K, Preminger GM, Britton F. Long term treatment of calcium nephrolithiasis with potassium citrate. J Urol 1985; 134:11–19.

21. Frick J, Kohle R, Kunit G. Experience with extracorporeal shock wave lithotripsy in children. Eur Urol 1988; 14:181–183.

22. Kroovand RL, Harrison LH, McCullough DL. Extracorporeal shock wave lithotripsy in childhood. J Urol 1987; 138:1106–1108.

CHAPTER 98
UNDESCENDED TESTIS

John Lazarus
John R. Gosche

Introduction

Undescended testis (UDT; also known as cryptorchism) can be defined as a failure of the testis to descend normally from the abdominal cavity into the scrotum. UDT is the most common genital problem seen in children. Despite this fact, many conclusions about UDT, its aetiology, and ideal management, remain controversial.

Consequences of UDT

UDT is associated with a variety of potential consequences: neoplasia, testicular carcinoma, infertility, torsion of testis, and inguinal hernia. Treatment of UDT is aimed at minimising these risks.

Neoplasia

UDT is associated with an increased risk of germ cell tumour of the testis. It has been suggested that males with UDT have a 40 times increase in the rate of neoplasia above the general population.[1] Although this number is debatable, these data need to be interpreted with caution because testicular malignancy is very rare in Africa.[2] The role of orchiopexy in reducing malignancy is controversial, but it makes self-examination easier.

Infertility

Unsurprisingly, reduced fertility and attendant poor-quality semen analysis is seen in men with UDT.[1] Subfertility is observed in 40% of patients with unilateral and 70% of patients with bilateral cryptorchism. There appears to be an advantage to early orchiopexy to improve the fertility potential.[3] This guides the timing of surgery, with an ideal window being between 6 and 24 months of age.

Inguinal Hernia and Testicular Torsion

A patent processus vaginalis is found in 90% of UDT.[1] The hernia is routinely repaired at the time of orchiopexy. Torsion of the testis is rarely associated; if it occurs, a tumour is often present.

Demographics

UDT occurs in approximately 30% of premature and 3–5% of full-term males.[1] In 80% of cases, the UDT migrates into the correct position without intervention during the first year, most in the first 3 months. This leaves the incidence from 1 year of age to adulthood at 1%. The condition occurs bilaterally in about 10% of cases. The right side is twice as commonly affected.

The causes of UDT are multifactorial, but risk factors include low birth weight (the most important factor), twins, prematurity, small for gestational age, and maternal exposure to estrogen during the first trimester.[1] Hereditary factors appear to play a role, with fathers and brothers being more commonly affected than the general population. No definite racial differences in incidence are reported.

UDT can be associated with other congenital anomalies, including epididymal cyst (90%), hypospadias, and genital ambiguity. The presence of hypospadias and an undescended testis warrant work-up for intersex.[4]

Aetiology/Pathophysiology

Testicular differentiation occurs during the 7th week of gestation. The testis-determining factor is the *SRY* gene (sex-determining region on the Y chromosome). Hormones that control male sexual differentiation include testicular androgen from Leydig cells and Müllerian-inhibiting substance (MIS) from the Sertoli cells.

Androgens (testosterone and dihydroxytestosterone) mediate the differentiation of paired wolffian ducts into seminal vesicles, epididymis, vas deferens, and ejaculatory ducts. MIS causes degeneration of the Müllerian structures. The testis lies dormant in the abdomen until the 28th week of gestation; thereafter, it descends into the scrotum.

The multifactorial mechanism of testicular descent involves:

• hormonal factors: the hypothalamus-pituitary-gonadal axis;

• the gubernaculum and genitofemoral nerve;

• increased abdominal pressure; and

• development/maturation of the epididymis.

Heyns et al. of South Africa have helped elucidate the role of the gubernaculum in testicular descent.[5]

There is presently no unified theory of testicular maldescent. Anomalies of the above-mentioned normal mechanism have all been implicated in the development of cryptorchism.

Clinical Presentation

UDTs can be classified into testes that are truly undescended, retractile, ectopic, absent, or ascended.[1] Eighty percent of UDTs are palpable (undescended, retractile, ectopic), and 20% are impalpable (intraabdominal or absent). Those impalpable UDTs that are truly absent at surgical exploration represent an in utero vascular event.

It is critical to identify the retractile testis, which result from an overactive cremasteric reflex and can be manipulated without tension into the scrotum. Retractile testes are regarded as a variant of normal; however, recent suggestions are that ascent may occur, and annual follow-up is now recommended.[1] The acquired ascending testis and the congenital UDT have been shown to share the same histopathology as germ cells.[6]

An ectopic testis follows an abnormal path of descent below the external ring and in this way differs from a typical UDT.

UDT is usually diagnosed during the newborn examination. It is critically important to differentiate between retractile and truly UDT. Warm hands covered in soapy water help reduce skin friction and ease pick-up.

Investigations

Imaging studies looking for an impalpable UDT are of no value.

In the setting of a unilateral UDT with an associated hypospadias, intersex should be considered and a karyotype would be indicated.

Where bilateral impalpable UDTs are present, endocrine work-up is required. Elevated gonadotrophins, especially follicle-stimulating hormones (FSHs), likely represent bilateral anorchia. A human chorionic gonadotropin (HCG)-stimulation test has clinical use where gonadothrophins are normal. However, no matter what the results of the test, surgical exploration remains indicated.[1] Typically, this involves injection of HCG (100 IU/kg or 2940 IU/body surface area) with a post-testosterone level taken 72 hours after injection.

Management

The ideal timing of intervention is at 6 months of age (Figure 98.1). Few UDTs will descend thereafter, with early management enhancing fertility potential.

Hormonal therapy is used in the management of UDT, yet it achieves success in only 20% of the cases. Surgery remains the gold standard. Typically, HCG (250 IU/dose in young infants, 500 IU/dose for children 6 years or younger, and 1000 IU/dose for individuals older than 6 years) is given intramuscularly twice a week for 5 weeks. The total dose should not exceed 15,000 IU.[7]

Orchiopexy for the palpable UDT is a well-established operation. The following pointers aid in surgical success:

1. After anesthesia is established, it is useful to re-examine the child to establish the site of the UDT. A previously nonpalpable testis may become palpable, thus avoiding abdominal exploration.

2. An incision is made in the groin crease. Careful dissection exposes the external oblique aponeurosis, the inguinal ligament, and the external ring.

3. The latter is opened in line with the fascia. Rolling the cord structures under a finger may help confirm the exact site of the canal. Care inside the canal is taken to identify and preserve the ilioinguinal nerve.

4. The cord is isolated by sweeping the cremasteric fibres off it. The gubernaculum is divided, and the patent processus is dissected off the vas and vessels.

5. A high ligation of the hernia sac is performed, and the remaining structures are skeletonised.

6. Manoeuvres to gain sufficient length include dissection of retroperitoneal attachments of the cord, known as the Prentiss manoeuvre. Divide (or pass the testis under) the inferior epigastric vessels after opening the floor of the canal (transversalis fascia), allowing a more medial and thus direct route to the scrotum.

7. The testis is placed in a superficial dartos pouch. Fixation sutures should be avoided, as they have been demonstrated to cause testicular damage.[1]

Impalpable UDTs are explored either via extending the above-mentioned inguinal incision, or an abdominal incision (vertical midline or Pfannenstiel incision), or—preferable if facilities allow—via diagnostic and potentially therapeutic laparoscopy. This exploration will reveal three possible findings:

1. An intraabdominal UDT is seen in roughly 40%.

2. Blind-ending vas and vessels occur in 40%. This implies a vanishing testis syndrome—a foetal vascular event. However, dissection of the retroperitoneum up to the kidney is suggested to confirm absence of a testis where no vessels are seen.

3. Vas and vessels entering the canal occur in 20%. Here inguinal exploration may be warranted to remove the testicular nubbin or remnant and fix the contralateral testis to prevent testicular torsion. This

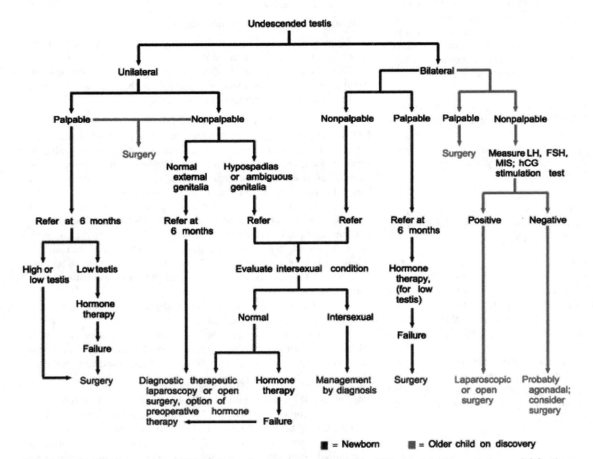

■ = Newborn   ▨ = Older child on discovery

Note: LH = luteinizing hormone; FSH = follicle-stimulating hormone; MIS = Müllerian inhibiting substance; hCG = human chorionic gonadotropin.

Source: Reprinted from Docimo SG, Silver RI, Cromie W. The undescended testicle: diagnosis and management. Am Fam Physician 2000; 62(9): 2037–2044.

Figure 98.1:. Management of the infant with cryptorchism, including suggested times for referral to a paediatric urologist. Older children should be referred on discovery of an undescended testicle.

action is debated because the risk for malignant transformation is low.[1]

Options for dealing with the intraabdominal UDT include:

1. A two-stage Fowler-Stephens orchiopexy via either open surgery or laparoscopy. Here the tethering testicular artery is divided at some distance from the testis. The rationale of using Fowler-Stephens orchiopexy is that the testicular arterial supply comes from three sources (testicular, artery to the vas, and cremasteric). At a 2nd stage (after 6 months of age, when collaterals have formed), the testis is brought down on a wide pedicle of peritoneum containing the remaining vessels.

2. The above surgery can also be performed as a one-stage operation where the artery is divided at the same sitting. Temporary occlusion of the testicular artery can give the surgeon confidence to proceed with division and mobilization. A recent multicentre review suggests a significantly higher atrophy rate than with the two-stage repair.[8]

3. Occasionally, the testis can be brought down in a single stage without division of the vessels.

4. Orchiectomy is usually reserved for postpubertal men with a contralateral normally positioned testis.

Postoperative Complications

Standard orchiopexy is associated with the following complications: haematoma, infection, unsatisfactory position (requiring revision), ilioinguinal nerve injury, damage to the vas, testicular atrophy, and torsion testis.

Prognosis and Outcomes

A meta-analysis found an 8% failure rate of orchiopexy, even in the distal UDT. A failure of more than 25% of orchiopexies for intraabdominal testes was seen.[9]

The rate of malignancy has been suggested to be as high as 22 times the incidence of the normal population, yet this represents only 1% of men with UDT. Ten percent of testicular tumours occur in men with a history of UDT.[1]

Prevention

Early diagnosis and management of the UDT is needed to preserve fertility and improve detection of potential testicular cancer. In the African context, primary health care standards need to improve to meet these goals and prevent the all too common presentation of an UDT in adulthood.

Evidence-Based Research

Table 98.1 presents a study that compared laparoscopic orchiopexy to other approaches to correct UDT.

Table 98.1: Evidence-based research.

Title	A multi-institutional analysis of laparoscopic orchidopexy
Authors	Baker LA, et al.
Institution	Multicentre
Reference	BJU Int 2001; 87(6):484–489
Problem	Multi-institutional review of the outcomes of laparoscopic orchiopexy.
Intervention	Laparoscopy.
Comparison/ control (quality of evidence)	A questionnaire was distributed to participating paediatric urologists.
Outcome/ effect	Single-stage Fowler-Stephens laparoscopic orchiopexy resulted in a significantly higher atrophy rate than the two-stage repair.
Historical significance/ comments	First muticentre review of its kind. The laparoscopic approach gave greater success than previously reported for the same open approaches.

Key Summary Points

1. The retractile testis is important to differentiate on examination from the UDT because no surgery is required for a retractile testis. However, annual follow-up is advised.

2. Eighty percent of UDTs are palpable and 20% are impalpable.

3. Therapy for UDT is motivated by a chance to improve fertility, to ease examination for potential malignancy, and for cosmesis.

4. The ideal time for ochiopexy is at 6 months of age, with an aim to complete staged repairs by 2 years of age.

5. The most significant complication of orchiopexy is testicular atrophy.

References

1. Walsh PC, et al. Campbell-Walsh Urology, 9th ed. Elsevier Health Sciences, 2007.

2. Gajendran V, Nguyen M, Ellison L. Testicular cancer patterns in African-American men. Urology 2005; 66(3): 602–605.

3. McAleer IM, Packer MG, Kaplan GW, Scherz HC, Krous HF, Billman GF. Fertility index analysis in cryptorchidism. J Urol 1995; 153:1255–1258.

4. Rajfer J, Walsh PC. The incidence of intersexuality in patients with hypospadias and cryptorchidism. J Urol 1976; 116:769–770.

5. Heyns CF, Human HJ, Werely CJ, De Klerk DP. The glycosaminoglycans of the gubernaculum during testicular descent in the foetus. J Urol 1990; 143(3):612–617.

6. Rusnack SL, Wu HY, Huff DS, Snyder HM 3rd, Zderic SA, Carr MC, Canning DA. The ascending testis and the testis undescended since birth share the same histopathology. J Urol 2002; 168(6):2590–2591.

7. Docimo SG, Silver RI, Cromie W. The undescended testicle: diagnosis and management. Am Fam Physician 2000; 62(9):2037–2044.

8. Baker LA, Docimo SG, Surer I, Peters C, Cisek L, Diamond DA, Caldamone A, Koyle M, Strand W, Moore R, Mevorach R, Brady J, Jordan G, Erhard M, Franco I. A multi-institutional analysis of laparoscopic orchidopexy. BJU Int 2001; 87(6):484–489.

9. Docimo SG. The results of surgical therapy for cryptorchidism: a literature review and analysis. J Urol 1995; 154:1148–1152.

CHAPTER 99
DISORDERS OF SEX DEVELOPMENT

Mohammed A. Latif Ayad
Alaa F. Hamza

Introduction

Sexual differentiation is the process of development of the differences between male and female from an undifferentiated zygote (fertilised egg). Sex and gender are both important determinants of health. The term "gender" describes those characteristics of females and males that are largely socially created, whereas "sex" encompasses those characteristics that are biologically determined.

Disorders of sex development (DSDs) have been endorsed by the Chicago Consensus to replace the term "intersex". The proposed changes in terminology are summarised in Table 99.1. DSD is defined as a congenital condition in which development of chromosomal, gonadal, or anatomical sex is atypical. Approximately 1 in 2,000 children globally is born with a DSD condition. This term uses chromosomes, rather than gonads, as the most important classifier of an individual's sex. In some DSDs, there is an associated obvious genital ambiguity at birth, whereas in others, the external genitalia are typically male or typically female, but the internal anatomy is discordant. Associated endocrinal and other congenital anomalies are always present.

Table 99.1: Proposed revised nomenclature.

Previous	Proposed
Intersex	DSD
Male pseudohermaphrodite, undervirilisation of an XY male, and undermasculinisation of an XY male	46,XYDSD
Female pseudohermaphrodite, overvirilisation of an XX female, and masculinisation of an XX female	46,XXDSD
True hermaphrodite	Ovotesticular DSD
XX male or XX sex reversal	46,XX testicular DSD
XY sex reversal	46,XY complete gonadal dysgenesis

DSDs are always challenging to manage. Choosing the optimal gender is difficult when the genitalia are ambiguous. There is the risk that childhood and adolescence for affected individuals will be compromised by gender dysphoria "dissatisfaction" (unhappiness with assigned sex, which occurs more frequently in individuals with DSD than in the general population, but is difficult to predict from karyotype, prenatal androgen exposure, degree of genital virilisation, or assigned gender). In addition, psychosexual difficulties, defined and noted to be influenced by factors including androgen exposure, sex chromosome genes, brain structure, social context, and family dynamics, may carry over into adult life.

Demographics

DSDs occur more commonly in developing countries. Certain areas of the world have a high incidence for certain genetic forms of DSD (see section on "Aetiology and Classification" for a discussion of gene deficiencies). 5α-reductase deficiency was first reported on one island in the Dominican Republic. It is also prevalent in southern Lebanon and the Eastern Highlands Province of Papua New Guinea, but is relatively rare in caucasians. 17β-Hydroxysteroid dehydrogenase deficiency is very common in the Gaza Strip. Both of these conditions can lead to a gradual transition in gender identity from female to male. In southern African blacks, 46,XX ovotesticular DSD has an unusually high prevalence.

Important Considerations in Africa and Developing Countries

Traditional Values and Beliefs

Traditional values and beliefs are often strong in certain cultures. They can play a very crucial role, especially in situations such as those presented by DSD, which is difficult to explain scientifically and poorly understood by the common man. This is often compounded by the fact that sexual issues are taboo subjects in certain societies, and parents do not want to discuss them even with medical professionals. Resorting to faith healers, shrines, and purveyors of magic is more natural for some cultures.

Family Issues

The lack of social security provisions in developing countries means that when they are no longer able to do productive work, parents are totally dependent on their children for survival. In many cultures, the eldest son has special responsibilities for both the physical and spiritual welfare of his parents; this is one powerful reason why sons may be valued more highly than daughters.

Consanguinity

Conditions such as congenital adrenal hyperplasia (CAH), which are perpetuated by autosomal recessive inheritance, are likely to affect multiple family members and to occur with greater frequency in countries where consanguinity is common.

Discrimination

It is extremely common for parents of children with DSDs to experience guilt, anxiety, and depression after the diagnosis has been made. Their natural reaction is to keep the child's condition a closely guarded secret, even from close relatives. This serves to further isolate these children and aggravate their distress. The parents' fear is that if the child's condition becomes widely known, both they and the child will suffer from being the subjects of rumour and discrimination.

Table 99.2: Classification of DSD.

Sex chromosome DSD	46,XY DSD	46,XX DSD
45,XO (Turner syndrome and variants)	*Disorders of gonadal (testicular) development* 1. complete gonadal dysgenesis (Swyer syndrome) 2. partial gonadal dysgenesis; 3. gonadal regression 4. ovotesticular DSD	*Disorders of gonadal (ovarian) development* 1. ovotesticular DSD 2. testicular DSD (e.g., SRY_, duplicate SOX9) 3. gonadal dysgenesis
47,XXY (Klinefelter syndrome and variants)	*Disorders in androgen synthesis or action* 1. androgen biosynthesis defect (e.g., 17-hydroxyster-oid dehydrogenase deficiency, 5αRD2 deficiency, StAR mutations) 2. defect in androgen action (e.g., CAIS, PAIS) 3. luteinising hormone receptor defects (e.g., Leydig cell hypoplasia, aplasia) 4. disorders of anti-Müllerian hormone and anti-Müllerian hormone receptor (persistent Müllerian duct syndrome)	*Androgen excess* 1. foetal (e.g., 21-hydroxylase deficiency, 11-hydroxylase deficiency) 2. foetoplacental (aromatase deficiency, POR _P450 oxido-reductase_) 3. maternal (luteoma, exogenous, etc.)
45,XO/46,XY (MGD, ovotesticular DSD)		*Other* (e.g., cloacal exstrophy, vaginal atresia)
46,XX/46,XY (chimeric, ovotesticular DSD)		

Notes: CAIS = complete androgen insensitivity syndrome; DSD = disorder of sex development; MGD = mixed gonadal dysgenesis; PAIS = partial androgen insensitivity syndrome; StAR = steroidogenic acute respiratory (protein function).

Aetiology and Classification

Abnormalities of sex determination and differentiation result from mutations of any of the genes involved in male or female sex development. Some of these mutations are well-established, but additional mechanisms remain to be described. In addition to the adequate expression of these genes, proper timing of their expression is also important. For example, normal but delayed androgenic effects result in incomplete masculinisation of genitalia, whereas the persistent presence of Müllerian remnants results from normal but delayed Müllerian-inhibiting substance (MIS) action. For clinical purposes, DSDs are classified according to karyotype and based on the various steps of sex differentiation and development (Table 99.2).

Sex Chromosome DSD

The peripheral karyotypes of sex chromosome DSD show marked variation. Approximately 60% are 46,XX; 15% are 46,XY; and 25% show various forms of mosaicism. Less than 1% show 46,XX/46,XY chimerism or the existence of two or more cell lines, each of which has a different genetic origin.

DSDs and sex chromosome aneuploidy

In Klinefelter (47,XXY) and 47,XYY syndromes, normal male external genitalia are typically present at birth. However, rare cases of the syndromes have presented with ambiguous genitalia. In newborns affected by the Turner (45,XO) syndrome, the external genitalia appear female, regardless of whether the remaining X chromosome is maternal or paternal in origin. Rare cases of genital ambiguity observed with the Turner syndrome are probably related to a hidden 46,XY cell line.

Ovotesticular DSD

Ovotesticular DSD refers to the presence of a gonad that contains both ovarian follicles and testicular tubular elements in the same individual. Ovotestes are the most frequent gonad present in sex chromosome DSD (60%), followed by the ovary and then the testis (Figures 99.1 and 99.2). Most newborns with ovotesticular DSD possess a 46,XX chromosome complement and present with ambiguous genitalia; however, some possess a 46,XY chromosome complement or 46,XX/46,XY mosaicism. In newborns with ovotesticular DSD, the risk of germ cell tumours is believed to be low (3%) and no recommendation of testicular tissue removal is offered at this time.

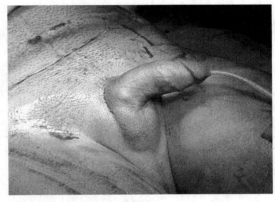

Figure 99.1: Ovotesticular DSD.

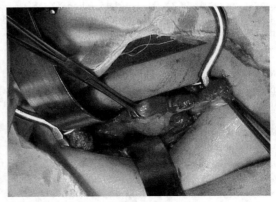

Figure 99.2: Müllerian remnant and ovotestis.

Mixed gonadal dysgenesis

Also known as asymmetrical gonadal differentiation, mixed gonadal dysgenesis is characterised by unique anatomical abnormalities. On one side of the body, a poorly developed testicular gonad exists, usually accompanied by wolffian duct structures. On the other side of the body is a gonadal streak. Most patients with mixed gonadal dysgenesis have deficient testosterone production related to their poorly developed testicular gonad, resulting in ambiguous external genitalia. These cases can be considered a subgroup of the larger group of partial gonadal dysgenesis. Newborns affected by mixed gonadal dysgenesis can present with a 46,XY karyotype, but they can also present with a 45,XO/46,XY karyotype. Gonadectomy is recommended for these patients, regardless of whether they possess a 46,XY or 45XO/46,XY chromosomal complement.

46,XY DSD

Ambiguous genitalia in a 46,XY newborn are due to either abnormal formation of the early foetal testes, low production of testosterone, deficient 5α-reductase activity, or the inability to respond to androgens (androgen insensitivity syndrome). Depending on the degree of abnormality, clinical presentation of the external genitalia can be categorised according to the following phenotypes: female-appearing, ambiguous genitalia with a small phallus and hypospadias, or a micropenis without hypospadias.

46,XY DSD due to disorders in gonadal development

Gonadal dysgenesis is defined as an impairment of the formation of the primordia of the gonads involving the two major elements of the foetal testes, the Sertoli cells that secrete MIS, and the Leydig cells that secrete testosterone. Gonadal dysgenesis can result from a mutated or deleted SRY gene.

Complete gonadal dysgenesis in 46,XY DSD (Swyer syndrome)

Complete gonadal dysgenesis is characterised by a total absence of functional testicular tissue in a 46,XY newborn resulting in the inability to produce both testosterone and MIS. Newborns affected by complete gonadal dysgenesis present with fully formed Müllerian structures, bilateral streak gonads, and female external genitalia. Affected newborns are reared as females as a result of their female genital phenotype. Gonadectomy is recommended.

Partial gonadal dysgenesis in 46,XY DSD

In partial gonadal dysgenesis, it is presumed that a gene mutation results in a partial abnormality of testicular formation from the early urogenital ridge or bipotential gonad. Partial gonadal dysgenesis could also involve a mutation of a gene such as SRY needed to differentiate the bipotential gonads into testes. The phenotypic result of this particular category of DSD is partial masculinisation of the external genitalia along with variable degrees of Müllerian and wolffian duct maintenance and development.

Mixed gonadal dysgenesis in 46,XY DSD and 45,XO/46,XY DSD

This condition has been discussed previously under the heading "Mixed gonadal dysgenesis".

Embryonic testicular regression syndrome

In embryonic testicular regression syndrome (ETRS), most of the patients present with ambiguous genitalia or severe micropenis associated with complete regression of testicular tissue in one or both sides. The variable degree of masculinisation of the internal and external genitalia is a consequence of the duration of testicular function prior to its loss. Familial cases have been reported, but the nature of the underlying defect is still unknown.

Disorders in androgen synthesis or action

46,XY DSD due to deficiency of testosterone biosynthesis

Complete testosterone biosynthetic defect in 46,XY DSD refers to a complete inactivity of any of the enzymes required for the biosynthesis of testosterone from cholesterol. Similar to complete gonadal dysgenesis, newborns affected by a complete testosterone biosynthetic defect are typically reared female as a result of their female external genital phenotype. Partial testosterone biosynthetic defect in 46,XY DSD refers to conditions in which there is reduced activity of any of the enzymes required for the biosynthesis of testosterone from cholesterol. Similar to partial gonadal dysgenesis, a partial testosterone biosynthetic defect results in ambiguous external genitalia and variable degrees of

wolffian duct development. However, unlike partial gonadal dysgenesis, Müllerian ducts are not maintained in newborns with a partial testosterone biosynthetic defect.

46,XY DSD due to 5α-reductase-2 deficiency

Deficiency of the 5α-reductase enzyme results from mutations in the steroid 5α-reductase type 2 (SRD5A2) gene. Affected newborns possess fully functioning Leydig and Sertoli cells, but due to the inability to convert testosterone to dihydrotestosterone (DHT), they present with undermasculinised external genitalia. The phenotype can range from a clitoral-like phallus with labio-scrotal folds to a penile urethra with testes located in the inguinal canal. At puberty, the testes of affected individuals are capable of spermatogenesis because, unlike testosterone, DHT is not required for germ cell maturation. Therefore, fertility is possible with the use of intrauterine insemination, and as a result, male sex rearing is recommended.

46,XY DSD due to a defect in androgen action

A defect in androgen action is either complete or partial, which is due to androgen receptor (AR) gene mutations. Newborns with complete androgen insensitivity syndrome (CAIS) present with female external genitalia and are therefore raised as girls. These newborns possess normally functioning testes, but they are unresponsive to the androgenic effects of their testosterone. Due to the risk, albeit low (<5%), of germ cell malignancy, removal of both testes following the completion of pubertal breast development is advised. After the testes are removed, estrogen replacement is required to maintain secondary sexual characteristics and to protect against osteoporosis. Individuals with partial androgen insensitivity syndrome (PAIS) experience variable degrees of end-organ unresponsiveness to androgens, resulting in variable degrees of wolffian duct and external genital ambiguity. Newborns affected by PAIS are considered to be at high risk (50%) for developing gonadal tumours, and bilateral gonadectomy is recommended at the time of diagnosis.

Luteinising hormone receptor defects in 46,XY DSD

Leydig cell aplasia or hypoplasia can be considered as a variant of gonadal dysgenesis. It is a condition of decreased numbers of Leydig cells, which leads to a decrease in androgen production. The phenotype resulting from Leydig cell hypoplasia is incomplete masculinisation of the external genitalia accompanied by incomplete development of the wolffian ducts.

Congenital micropenis without hypospadias in 46,XY DSD

Congenital micropenis refers to a penis that forms normally during the first trimester of foetal development, followed by a failure to lengthen in an appropriate manner during the second and third trimesters. In male newborns, a stretched penile length of 1.9 cm or less without hypospadias is considered a micropenis.

46,XX DSD

A foetus with a 46,XX chromosomal complement and normal ovarian organogenesis can be exposed to excessive amounts of androgens originating either from the foetus itself or from the mother. Timing of exposure is important. If androgen exposure occurs after the 8th week of gestation but before the 12th week, the vaginal opening may fuse posteriorly and appear slitlike. Exposure to androgen after the 12th week of gestation (e.g., exogenous administration to the mother) will result in clitoromegaly without fusion of the labioscrotal folds. On occasion, multiple congenital malformations may be present in a 46,XX newborn with ambiguous genitalia.

Abnormal foetal androgen production: congenital adrenal hyperplasia

Congenital adrenal hyperplasia (CAH) is a family of inherited disorders of adrenal steroidogenesis due to a mutation of one of the enzymes necessary for the biosynthesis of cortisol from cholesterol (Table 99.3). These abnormalities result in increased adrenocorticotropic hormone (ACTH) secretion by the pituitary gland that can, in turn, result in the

Table 99.3: Congenital adrenal hyperplasia.

Deficiency	Newborn Phenotype	Postnatal Virilisation	Other
StAR (steroidogenic acute regulatory protein function, also called lipoid congenital adrenal hyperplasia)	Infantile female	–	Salt loss
3ß-Hydroxylase	Ambiguous in XY and XX	+	Salt loss
17α-Hydroxylase (P450c17)	Infantile female	–	Delayed puberty
11ß-Hydroxylase (P450c11 ß)	Male in XY, ambiguous in XX	+	Hypertension
21 Hydroxylase (P450c21) (most common form)	Male in XY, ambiguous in XX	+	Salt loss
18 Hydroxylase (P450c11B2)	Normal	–	Salt loss

increased secretion of cortisol precursors and adrenal androgens. CAH is considered to exist in classic (salt wasting and simple virilising) and nonclassic forms.

Classic CAH
Males with classic CAH may not be diagnosed clinically at birth because they do not have genital ambiguity except for scrotal hyperpigmentation and phallic enlargement. Virilisation in boys due to CAH is distinguished from true precocious puberty by the testicular size, which is <4mls in prepubertal boys affected with CAH.

Females with classic CAH due to salt wasting or simple virilising forms will have virilised genitalia at birth, ranging from clitoral enlargement, rugated labioscrotal folds (with or without posterior fusion; Figure 99.3), to complete fusion of labioscrotal folds, urogenital sinus, and a single opening typical of a male (Figure 99.4).

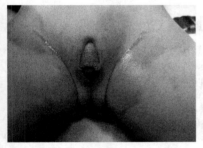

Figure 99.3: Classic CAH.

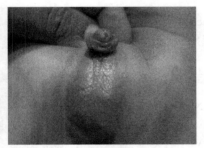

Figure 99.4: Severe virilisation.

Inadequate secretion of the mineralocorticoid aldosterone causes salt wasting in approximately three-quarters of all classic CAH patients. It is characterised by hyponatremia, hyperkalemia, inappropriate natriuresis, and low serum and urinary aldosterone with concomitantly high plasma renin activity. Affected male newborns with the salt-wasting phenotype usually are undiagnosed at birth, and they present 2–3 weeks later or earlier, if stressed, in salt-wasting adrenal crisis.

Simple virilising is prenatal virilisation and progressive postnatal masculinisation with accelerated growth and advanced bone ages but no evidence of mineralocorticoid deficiency. Affected males with the simple virilising form, if not diagnosed at birth, will present at 2 years of age or older with early development of pubic, auxillary, and facial hair, penile enlargement, body odor, and growth acceleration with bone age advancement.

Nonclassic CAH
Nonclassic 21-hydroxylase deficiency is one of the most common autosomal recessive diseases in the world. This form of CAH results from a mild deficiency of the 21-hydroxylase enzyme and is diagnosed by serum elevations of 17-hydroxypregnenolone (within the range of levels for unaffected individuals and levels observed for classic CAH patients). Patients with nonclassic CAH do not have symptoms at birth. Clinical presentation during childhood may include early pubic hair development, growth acceleration, and bone age advancement. Hirsutism is the most common symptom (60%), followed by irregular menses (54%), and acne (33%) in adolescent or adult women with nonclassic CAH.

Excess maternal androgen production
Because excessive androgen production adversely affects fertility due to anovulation, cases of maternal androgen production during pregnancy are extremely rare. The origin of these maternal androgens is usually the ovaries or adrenal glands.

Placental aromatase deficiency
During foetal development, the adrenals produce large amounts of 17-hydroxypregnenolone and 16-hydroxy-DHA. These steroids are transferred to the placenta, which then converts these steroids into androgens and then estrogens. If an aromatase enzyme deficiency exists, then androgen precursors accumulate and return to foetal circulation, resulting in masculinisation of female foetuses.

Clinical Presentations of DSD
DSDs may cause changes that are immediately visible in the newborn infant, or they may cause changes that are detected and presented to the doctor only when the child is older or has even reached adolescence. The range of presentations in relation to the most common causes is summarised in Table 99.4.

Work-up of Infants Born with Ambiguous Genitalia

General Concepts of Care
The consensus conference, comprising members of the Lawson Wilkins Pediatric Endocrine Society (LWPES) and the European Society for Paediatric Endocrinology (ESPE), highlighted several standards of care recommendations:

Table 99.4: Correlation between mode of clinical presentation and underlying cause.

Mode of presentation	Most common causes
Child with ambiguous genitalia.	• 46,XX DSD due to CAH (21 hydroxylase deficiency) • Sex chromosome DSD (e.g., 45,XO/46,XY partial gonadal dysgenesis and ovotesticular DSD) • 46,XY PAIS • 46,XY 5α-Reductase-2 deficiency • 17β-hydroxysteroid dehydrogenase deficiency
Y(+) girl found to have either testes or dysgenetic gonads.	• 46,XY DSD due to CAIS • 46,XY DSD due to complete gonadal dysgenesis
Adolescent girl with primary amenorrhoea who is found to have no uterus and/or vagina. She may be 46,XX and have ovaries or be 46,XY and have testes.	• 46,XX Müllerian agenesis • 46,XY CAIS
46,XY boy with impalpable or inguinal testes who is found at surgery to have a uterus and fallopian tubes.	• 46,XY persistent Müllerian duct syndrome
Boy with impalpable gonads who is found to have ovaries and a uterus. Or older boy with impalpable gonads who presents with isosexual precocious puberty.	• 46,XX DSD due to CAH (21-hydroxylase deficiency)
Girl who, although born with typical female genitalia, undergoes progressive clitoral enlargement and other signs of virilisation during childhood or adolescence.	• 46,XY DSD due to 17β-hydroxysteroid dehydrogenase deficiency

1. gender assignment for all;

2. avoidance of assignment before expert evaluation;

3. open communication;

4. a multidisciplinary team approach; and

5. confidentiality and attention to patient and family concerns (adolescent patients should be given opportunities to ask questions and discuss their condition confidentially, without their parents being present).

A key point to emphasize is that the child with DSD has the potential to become a well-adjusted, functional member of society. Although privacy needs to be respected, a DSD is not shameful. It should be explained to the parents that the best course of action may not be clear initially, but the health care team will work with the family to reach the best possible set of decisions in the circumstances. The health care team should discuss with the parents what information to share in the early stages with family members and friends. Parents need to be informed about sexual development in a balanced simple way.

The multidisciplinary team

Optimal care for children with DSDs requires an experienced multidisciplinary team generally found in tertiary care centres and ideally including paediatric subspecialists in endocrinology, surgery or urology, psychology or psychiatry, gynecology, genetics, and neonatology. The multidisciplinary team can play a critical role in creating a climate of commitment to the health and welfare of children born with DSDs, as well as to their families.

Clinical evaluation

The evaluation and initial management of the newborn with ambiguous genitalia must be regarded as a medical and psychosocial emergency and be handled with great sensitivity toward the family. In obtaining the history, certain pieces of information may be particularly valuable. A history of infant death within the family might suggest the possibility of CAH, and infertility, amenorrhea, or hirsutism might also suggest possible familial patterns of disorders. Maternal use of medications during the pregnancy, in particular steroids or contraceptives, is of great importance.

The initial physical examination should begin with an assessment of the general health of the patient and an evaluation for malformations or dysmorphic features because ambiguous genitalia can occur in conjunction with several other congenital malformations. It is necessary to look for signs of dehydration with vomiting and diarrhoea because these are symptoms of a salt-losing crisis. A careful examination of the external genitalia must also be performed. A genital exam must include a measure of stretched phallic length, evaluation of the quality of the corpora, and inspection of the labia, labio-scrotal folds, or scrotum. The position of the urethral opening (and vaginal opening, if applicable) should be documented, as well as the presence and location of palpable gonads.

Investigations

Within the immediate newborn period, a karyotype should be obtained. Typically this requires 2–3 days to perform. Serum studies should be immediately sent to rule out a salt-wasting form of CAH. In addition to serum electrolytes, testosterone and DHT should be measured early because their levels may drop quickly. In addition, serum 17-hydroxyprogesterone should not be measured until day 3 or 4 to rule out 21-hydroxylase deficiency because the stress of delivery may result in a physiologic elevation of this steroid precursor in the first 1 or 2 days of life. The suggested schedule for hormone studies in an infant with ambiguous genetalia is as follows:

• At day 2 of life, measure plasma androstenedione, testosterone, and dihydrotestosterone. These androgens must be measured from a single blood sample so that the ratios of androstenedione/testosterone and testosterone/DHT can be calculated.

• At day 3 or 4 of life, measure plasma 17-hydroxyprogesterone, 17-hydroxypregnenolone, and progesterone.

• At day 6 or 7 of life, measure plasma MIS and obtain white cells for deoxyribonucleic acid (DNA) studies, such as androgen receptor gene mutations.

• At day 8 of life, repeat androstenedione, testosterone, DHT, and 17-hydroxyprogesterone measures.

A sonogram or magnetic resonance imaging (MRI) can be helpful in identifying both the type and extent of internal sex organ development. Imaging can also detect associated abnormalities of the urinary tract. Laparotomy or laparoscopy and gonadal biopsy are usually the next definitive clinical step required when a firm diagnosis based on the aforementioned data is impossible. Laparotomy or laparoscopy in this setting remains a diagnostic manoeuvre; removal of gonads or reproductive organs should be deferred until the final pathology report is available and a gender has been assigned. Detection of AR gene mutations may help, although current molecular diagnosis is limited by cost, accessibility, and quality control.

Finally, anatomic definition of the urogenital sinus and ductal structures contributes to the correct diagnosis and is necessary before any surgical intervention. The urogenital sinus and ductal structures are well imaged by genitogram, which defines the entry of urethra and vagina into the sinus and outlines the cervical impression within the vagina. Endoscopy can define these relationships further, but is usually not necessary until surgical reconstruction becomes imminent.

Gender Assignment

The basis of gender assignment should include:

• The most likely adult gender identity based on impression of foetal androgen exposure, parents' expectations, and expected impact of sexual differentiation;

• diagnosis;

• genital appearance;

• genital surgical options (potential for functional, sensitive genitalia);

• potential for fertility (considering assisted fertility techniques);

• social and cultural pressures; and

• family dynamics (parents' desires, expectations, malleability, and reactions to genital ambiguity).

The relative weight of the gender assignment interrelated factors differ in each situation. The magnitude of the impact of each factor upon the others is also variable over time. Depending on the degree of unpredictability of outcome, deference is given to psychosocial factors.

This approach recognizes the powerful influence of parental input on outcomes. Medical decisions in the DSD patient are usually made in what has been referred to as the category III level of evidence (opinions of respected authorities based on clinical experience, descriptive studies and case reports, or reports of expert committees). Thus, major limitations exist in making recommendations for DSD patients for most issues. Guidelines for gender assignment are addressed only for those DSD patients with substantial outcome data (Table 99.5).

Table 99.5: Current diagnosis-based recommendations for sex of rearing.

Diagnosis	Sex of rearing
46,XY CAIS	Female
46,XY PAIS	Dependent upon judgment of degree of masculinisation and parental input
46,XX CAH	Female, realizing that there are anecdotal reports, but not verified documentation, of those with essentially male external genitalia raised satisfactorily as male
5α-reductase deficiency	Strongly consider male assignment
17β-hydroxysteroid dehydrogenase deficiency	Strongly consider male assignment
Cloacal exstrophy	Conflicting outcome data; reports from the United States show high rates of self-reassignment to male
Ovotesticular DSD	Consider external genital development and fertility potential; given outcome uncertainties, potential for fertility (assuming consistent genitalia) is a major factor

Management of Patients with DSD

The consensus conference recognised the role of various entities in decision making for the DSD child, including the parent, the child, and the medical system. A practical application of these roles and ways to resolve potential conflicts between decision makers were not addressed, however. Decision making should be based on ethical, human rights,

and legal grounds. Some important universally applicable ethical principles can be followed, such as minimising physical risk (e.g., malignancy) to the child; minimising psychosocial risk (e.g., social isolation) to the child; preserving potential for fertility; preserving or promoting capacity to have satisfying sexual relations; and leaving options open for the future.

Surgical Management

The surgeon has a responsibility to outline the surgical sequence and subsequent consequences from infancy to adulthood. Only surgeons with expertise in the care of children and specific training in the surgery of DSD should perform these procedures. The consensus, based upon the recommendations of the surgical subgroup, agreed that the primary goal of genital surgery was to improve functional rather than cosmetic outcome to enhance sexual function and romantic partnering.

Rationale for early reconstruction includes the beneficial effects of estrogen on infant tissues, avoiding complications from anatomic anomalies, satisfactory outcomes, minimising family concern and distress, and mitigating the risks of stigmatisation and gender-identity confusion of atypical genital appearance. Adverse outcomes have led to recommendations to delay unnecessary genital surgery to an age of patient-informed consent, although relative risks and benefits are unknown.

Feminising genital surgery involves external genitalia reconstruction and vaginal exteriorisation, with early separation of the vagina and urethra. Clitoral reduction is considered with severe virilisation and performed in conjunction with common urogenital sinus repair. Total urogenital mobilisation and clitoplasty is the procedure of choice in the authors' unit and is done in infancy starting from 6 months of age (Figure 99.5). Long-term follow-up of more than 50 cases reveals a very good cosmetic outcome, no urinary sequel, and very few complications (Figure 99.6).

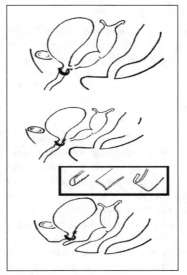

Figure 99.5: Total urogenital sinus mobilisation.

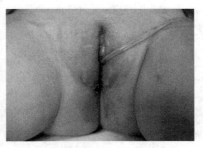

Figure 99.6: Postoperative view.

Vaginal dilatation should not be performed during childhood. Refinement is sometimes necessary at puberty for other procedures. Surgery should emphasize functional cosmetic appearance and be designed to preserve erectile function and innervation. Substitution vaginoplasty should be performed in the teenage years; each of the techniques (self-dilatation, skin or bowel substitution) has specific advantages and disadvantages, and all carry potential for scarring that would require modification before sexual function.

Masculinising genital surgery involves more surgical procedures and urologic difficulties than feminising genitoplasty. Standard surgical repair involving hypospadias includes chordee correction, urethral reconstruction, and judicious testosterone supplementation. If needed, adult-sized testicular prostheses should be inserted after sufficient pubertal scrotal development. The enormity of the undertaking and complexity of phalloplasty must be considered during the initial counselling period. Care should be taken to avoid unrealistic expectations about penile reconstruction.

Gonadectomy is indicated in patients at high risk of developing germ cell malignancy. The highest tumour risk is found in testis-specific protein Y (TSPY)-encoded positive gonadal dysgenesis and PAIS with intraabdominal gonads, whereas the lowest risk (<5%) is found in ovotestis and CAIS. Specifically:

- For patients with CAIS or PAIS raised female, the testes should be removed to prevent malignancy in adulthood. The availability of estrogen-replacement therapy allows for the option of early removal at the time of diagnosis.

- The streak gonad in patients with MGD raised male should be removed laparoscopically (or by laparotomy) in early childhood. Bilateral gonadectomy is performed in early childhood in females (bilateral streak gonads) with gonadal dysgenesis and Y-chromosome material.

- For patients with androgen biosynthetic defects raised female, gonadectomy should be performed before puberty.

- A scrotal testis in patients with gonadal dysgenesis is at risk for malignancy. Current recommendations are testicular biopsy at puberty, seeking signs of the premalignant lesion termed carcinoma in situ or undifferentiated intratubular germ cell neoplasia. If positive, the option is sperm banking before treatment with local low-dose radiotherapy that is curative.

Sex-Steroid Replacement

Hormonal induction of puberty stimulates replication of normal pubertal maturation to induce secondary sexual characteristics, a pubertal growth spurt, and optimal bone mineral accumulation, together with psychosocial support for psychosexual maturation. Intramuscular depot injections of testosterone esters are commonly used in males; another option is oral testosterone. Transdermal preparations are also available. Patients with PAIS may require supraphysiologic doses of testosterone for optimal effect. Females with hypogonadism require estrogen supplementation to induce pubertal changes and menses. A progestin is usually added after breakthrough bleeding develops or within 1–2 years of continuous estrogen. There is no evidence that the addition of cyclic progesterone is beneficial in women without a uterus.

Lifelong glucocorticoid replacement therapy is the mainstay of treatment for classic and symptomatic nonclassic CAH patients. Glucocorticoids not only replace cortisol but also reduce the overstimulation of the adrenal cortex by reducing the release of ACTH, thereby suppressing the overproduction of adrenal androgens. Hydrocortisone is usually chosen for infants and children, as it is shorter acting than prednisone or dexamethasone, and thus less likely to compromise growth. Excessive glucocorticoid administration should be avoided because it can cause Cushingoid facies, growth retardation, and inhibition of epiphyseal maturation. Patients with salt-wasting CAH may also require mineralocorticoid replacement.

Psychosocial Management

Psychosocial care provided by mental health staff with expertise in DSD should be an integral part of management to promote positive adaptation. This expertise can facilitate team decisions about gender assignment/reassignment, timing of surgery, and sex-hormone replacement. Gender identity (a personal concept of oneself as male or female, or, rarely, both or neither) development begins before the age of 3 years, but the earliest age at which it can be reliably assessed remains unclear. The generalisation that the age of 18 months is the upper limit of imposed gender reassignment should be treated with caution and viewed conservatively. Atypical gender-role behavior (the outward manifestations of personality that reflect the gender identity) is more common in children with DSD than in the general population, but should not be taken as an indicator for gender reassignment. In affected children and adolescents who report significant gender dysphoria, a comprehensive psychological evaluation and an opportunity to explore feelings about gender with a qualified clinician are required over a period of time. If the desire to change gender persists, the patient's wishes should be supported.

The process of disclosure of all aspects of the DSD and its clinical care should be collaborative, ongoing, and planned with the parents from the time of diagnosis. Medical education and counselling are recurrent gradual processes of increasing sophistication that take into account the patient's changing cognitive and psychological development. Quality of life encompasses dating, falling in love, ability to develop intimate relationships, sexual functioning, and the opportunity to marry and to raise children, regardless of biological indicators of sex. Because of fears of rejection in intimate relationships, a focus of psychological care should be interpersonal relationships. Frequent problems encountered in patients with DSD are sexual aversion and lack of arousability, often misinterpreted as low libido. Repeated examination of the genitalia, including medical photography, may be experienced as shaming and should be undertaken when the patient is under anaesthesia whenever possible.

Outcomes

As a general statement, information across a range of assessments is insufficient in DSD. With regard to surgical outcome, some studies suggest satisfactory outcomes from early surgery; however, other studies on clitoroplasty identify problems related to decreased sexual sensitivity, loss of clitoral tissue, and cosmetic issues. Interpretation of published reports on the risk of gonadal tumours is hampered by unclear terminology and by the effects of normal cell maturation delay.

Concerning cultural and social factors, DSD may carry a stigma. Gender role change occurs at different rates in different societies, suggesting that social factors may also be important modifiers of gender role change. In the West, when selection of the optimal gender is being considered, a great deal of attention will be paid to whether the child will grow up able to enjoy sexual pleasure and fulfillment. Eastern thinking, in contrast, is more concerned with ensuring that the individual (especially if brought up as a girl) will be capable of having sexual intercourse to satisfy a partner.

In some societies, female infertility precludes marriage, which also affects employment prospects and creates economic dependence. Religious and philosophical views may influence the parents' response to the birth of an infant with a medical condition. Poverty and illiteracy negatively affect access to health care.

Evidence-Based Research

The impact of reduction of the enlarged clitoris on adult sexuality has not been sufficiently evaluated in CAH or other DSDs. Follow-up studies in childhood have not been able to assess sexual function. A few previous reports considered surgical outcomes but they were small case series, and methodical assessment of genital sensitivity and sexual function were not performed. Table 99.6 presents a study of genital sensitivity following feminising genitoplasty for CAH.

Table 99.6: Evidence-based research.

Title	Sexual function and genital sensitivity following feminizing genitoplasty for congenital adrenal hyperplasia
Authors	Crouch NS, Liao LM, Woodhouse CRJ, Conway GS Creighton SM
Institution	The Middlesex Centre, University College London, Institute of Women's Health, Elizabeth Garrett Anderson and Obstetric Hospital, and Institute of Urology, University College London Hospital (CRJW), London, UK
Reference	J Urol 2008; 179:634–638
Problem	Evaluation of the effect of feminising genital surgery on genital sensation and sexual function in women with CAH.
Intervention	Sensitivity thresholds for temperature and vibration for the clitoris and upper vagina were measured by using a GenitoSensory Analyzer. Sexual function was assessed by using a mailed questionnaire incorporating the Golombok Rust Inventory of Sexual Satisfaction.
Comparison/control (quality of evidence)	This was a cross-sectional study of genital sensitivity in 28 women with CAH, 17 to 39 years old (mean age, 25.4); and 10 normal controls, 23 to 38 years old (mean age, 25.3). Four women with CAH had not undergone prior genital surgery. None of the normal controls was known to have any endocrine abnormality or history of genital surgery. The study consisted of two parts: (1) sensitivity testing of the clitoris and upper vagina, and (2) completion of a mailed sexual function questionnaire.
Outcome/effect	Sensitivity is decreased in genital areas where feminising genitoplasty has been done. Surgery is also associated with sexual difficulties. A moderate but significant linear relationship between impaired clitoral sensitivity and the severity of sexual difficulties has been identified.
Historical significance/comments	1. All patients in this study underwent their surgical correction in the early 1980s. The results of this study cannot be generally applied to current patients. Today, the neuroanatomy of the clitoris is better understood than it was 25 or more years ago, and current techniques give more concern to preserve the neurovascular bundle of the clitoris, so the clitoral sensation is much less affected. 2. If possible, no clitoral surgery should be performed, as no evidence suggests that a large clitoris is detrimental to sexual function. However, in most cases, the clitoris is quite large, appearing like a penis. In such cases clitoral reduction should be discussed with the parents after detailed consent. 3. The sexual function assessment in this study was dependent on a subjective method (a mailed questionnaire). The answers, and hence the final assessment, will be greatly affected by cultural and behavioural factors. Eastern thinking is more concerned with ensuring that the female will be capable of having sexual intercourse to satisfy her partner. In contrast, in the West, great concern is paid to whether the child will grow up able to enjoy sexual pleasure and fulfillment. 4. A large cohort of studies, in addition to accurate objective measures, are needed to justify the final outcome of feminising surgery, and hence outline the guidelines more precisely.

Key Summary Points

1. Disorders of sex development (DSD) is new terminology that replaces the well-known terminology "intersex".

2. DSD is a congenital condition characterised by atypical development of chromosomal, gonadal, or anatomical sex.

3. DSD is classified as sex chromosome DSD, 46,XY DSD, and 46,XX DSD.

4. Management of infants suffering from DSD is challenging, especially in Africa and developing countries due to educational, financial, and behavioural factors.

5. Cases should be managed through a multidisciplinary team.

6. No assignment should be offered before full work-up, and reassignment should be considered in some cases.

7. Surgical correction should be based on anatomical and functional bases rather than a cosmetic one, although the importance of cosmesis should not be ignored.

8. Early correction is advised in congenital adrenal hyperplasia; otherwise, delay of surgery is advisable in most cases.

9. Gonadectomy should be performed in cases at high risk to develop gonadal carcinoma as well as in cases suffering gonadal dysgenesis or PAIS with intraabdominal gonads.

Suggested Reading

American Academy of Pediatrics, Committee on Genetics. Evaluation of the newborn with developmental anomalies of the external genitalia. Pediatrics 2000; 106:138–142.

American Academy of Pediatrics, Section on Urology. Timing of elective surgery on the genitalia of male children with particular reference to the risks, benefits, and psychological effects of surgery and anesthesia. Pediatrics 1996; 97:590–594.

Cohen-Kettenis P. Psychological long-term outcome in intersex conditions, Horm Res 2005; 64:27–30.

Crouch NS, Minto CL, Laio LM, Woodhouse CR, Creighton SM. Genital sensation after feminizing genitoplasty for congenital adrenal hyperplasia: a pilot study. BJU Int 2004; 93:135–138.

Diamond DA. Sexual differentiation: normal and abnormal. In: Wein AJ (ed). Campbell-Walsh Urology, Saunders, Elsevier, 2007, Pp 3799–3829.

Dreger AD, Chase C, Sousa A, Grupposo PA, Frader J. Changing the nomenclature/taxonomy for intersex: a scientific and clinical rationale. J Pediatr Endocrinol Metab 2005; 18:729–733.

Eroğlu E, Tekant G, Gündoğdu G, et al. Feminizing surgical management of intersex patients. Pediatr Surg Int 2004; 20:543–547.

Hamza AF, Soliman HA, Abdel Hay SA, Kabesh AA, Elbehery MM. Total urogenital sinus mobilization in the repair of complex female genital anomalies. J Pediatr Surg 2001; 36:1656–1668.

Houk CP, Lee PA. Disorders of sex development: making ambiguity less ambiguous. Growth, GeneticHormones J 2007; 23:33–39.

Houk CP, Hughes IA, Ahmed SF, Lee PA, Writing Committee for the International Intersex Consensus Conference. Summary of consensus statement on intersex disorders and their management. Pediatrics 2006; 118:753–757.

Intersex Society of North America. Clinical guidelines for the management of disorders of sex development in childhood, Consortium on the Management of Disorders of Sex Development. Available at www.dsdguidelines.org/htdocs/clinical/index.html (accessed 2006).

Kuhnle U, Krahl W. The impact of culture on sex assignment and gender development in intersex patients. Perspect Biol Med 2002; 45:85–103.

Lee PA, Houk CP, Ahmed SF, Hughes IA, in collaboration with the participants in the International Intersex Consensus Conference. Consensus statement on management of intersex disorders, 2006, 118:e488–e500.

Maharaj N, Dhai A, Wiersma R, Moodley J. Intersex conditions in children and adolescents: surgical, ethical, and legal considerations. J Pediatr Adolesc Gynecol 2005; 18:399–402.

Martin CL, Ruble DN, Szkrybalo J. Cognitive theories of early gender development. Psychol Bull 2002; 128:903–933.

Merke D, Cutler G. New ideas for medical treatment of congenital adrenal hyperplasia. Endocrinol Metab Clin North Am 2001; 30:121–135.

Migeon CJ, Krishnan S, Wisniewski AB. Ambiguous genitalia in the newborn. Available at http:www.endotext.org/pediatrics/pediatrics10/pediatricsframe10.htm (accessed 2007).

Mouriquand PD, Mure PY. Current concepts in hypospadiology. BJU Int 2004; 93:26–34.

New MI, 21-hydroxylase deficiency: classical and nonclassical congenital adrenal hyperplasia. Available at: http://www.endotext.org/pediatrics/pediatrics8a/pediatricsframe8a.htm (accessed 2006).

Warne GL, Raza J. Disorders of sex development (DSDs), their presentation and management in different cultures. Rev Endocr Metab Disord 2008; 9:227–236.

Warne GL, Grover S, Zajac JD. Hormonal therapies for individuals with intersex conditions: protocol for use. Treat Endocrinol 2005; 4:19–29.

Wisniewski AB, Migeon CJ, Meyer-Bahlburg HF, et al. Complete androgen insensitivity syndrome: long-term medical, surgical and psychosexual outcome, J Clin Endocrinol Metab 2000; 85:2664–2669.

CHAPTER 100
BLADDER OUTLET OBSTRUCTION

Lukman O. Abdur–Rahman
Rowena Hitchcock

Introduction

Bladder outlet obstruction (BOO) is the impedance or blockage of urine outflow from the bladder into the urethra. This may be due to anatomical or functional causes. The anatomical causes can be intraluminal, intramural, or extrinsic. The functional causes may be neurogenic or nonneurogenic. The causes are frequently overlooked in children because they present typically with lower urinary tract symptoms that are associated with other more common forms of voiding disorders, which are often wrongly treated and delay presentation until adulthood.[1,2] Many of the underlying conditions lend themselves to medical or minimally invasive therapy, but in recent years, sophisticated techniques have become available to accurately diagnose the site and extent of obstructive uropathy.[2] These techniques are out of reach at many centres in African countries, and the diagnosis still may be missed. Subsequent treatment with a variety of empiric modalities may ultimately fail, leading to permanent damage of the urinary system, renal failure, or detrusor failure.

Demographics

The causes of BOO are numerous and vary in incidence from one region to another. In Africa, reports on the incidence are scanty, probably due to lack of documentation. Voiding dysfunction is a general term to describe abnormalities in either the filling and/or emptying of the bladder. It is a common problem in children and constitutes up to 40% of paediatric urology clinic visits.[3] The International Children's Continence Society (ICCS) has issued standardised definitions for voiding dysfunction symptoms to facilitate classification and treatment.[4] The peculiar demography of each cause is discussed next.

Embryology of Lower Urinary Tract

The development of the lower urinary tract is closely interrelated with that of the genital tract and the hindgut.[5] By the 3rd week of gestation, the cloaca, an endodermal structure, meets the ectoderm of the body wall at the cloacal membrane, and by the 5th week, the cloaca is divided by the urorectal septum to form the primitive rectum posteriorly and urogenital sinus anteriorly (Figure 100.1). The allantois, bladder, pelvic, and phallic portions of the urogenital system are recognisable in the 6th week. By the 7th week, the mesonephric ducts (vas deferens) are shifted further caudal in the sinus and come to lie close to each other at Müller's tubercle. The metanephric buds (ureters) arise from the mesonephric ducts, and are incorporated and shift cephalad and laterally into the bladder, forming the trigone.[6]

By the 9th week of gestation, the bladder cavity expands and the urachus elongates and continues with the allantoic stalk at the umbilicus. The extra embryonic allantois degenerates, and the urachus closes by the 12th week, forming the median umbilical ligament. Closure of the urachus permits any bladder outlet obstruction to become manifest in some foetuses, but delayed closure may protect others.

The early bladder epithelium initially consists of a single cell layer, but by this point has become transitional. Meanwhile, the bladder muscle arises from mesenchyme as a longitudinal layer on the dorsal

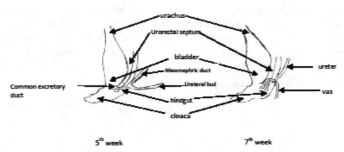

Source: Drawing by Abdur-Rahman, LO.

Figure 100.1: Embryonic development of lower urinary tract

surface of the bladder and spreads cephalad from the bladder to the intrarenal collecting system.[7] The bladder epithelium over the ureteral orifice—Chwalla's membrane—temporarily covers and occludes the ureteral orifice, but later perforates, and the ureter becomes continuous with the bladder.[8] By the 16th week of gestation, the bladder is completely muscularized and the urachus is closed.

Agenesis of the bladder is a rare anomaly that may arise because the allantoic stalk fails to develop. Most urachal anomalies (e.g., patent urachus, urachal cyst, urachal sinus, and urachal diverticula) seem to result from delayed closure of the urachus, which may also arise from lower urinary tract obstruction at less than 12 weeks gestation. Some anomalies result from a general mesodermal failure (the urachal diverticulum of the Prune belly syndrome).[6] Intravesical (simple) ureterocoeles are thought to be due to the persistence of Chwalla's membrane beyond the time when urine flow begins.[8]

Bladder outlet obstruction caused by the urethral obstruction of posterior urethral valves or urethral hypoplasia may be detected from 4 weeks gestation concurrent with the absorption of the mesonephric duct and the resorption of the urogenital membrane. Abnormal dilatation of Cowper's glands may give rise to an obstructive urethral syringocele.

Physiology of Voiding

The control of voiding is at three levels: the central nervous system (CNS), the spinal cord, and the peripheral nervous systems from the sacral cord.

Normal voiding essentially is a spinal reflex modulated by the CNS (brain, pontine micturition centre, and spinal cord), which coordinates the functions of the bladder and urinary sphincter. The bladder and sphincter are innervated by three sets of peripheral nerves arising from the autonomic nervous system (parasympathetic (S2–S4) and sympathetic (T11–L2)) and somatic nervous system (pudendal nerve (S1–S4)).

In infants, the higher CNS network that controls voiding is not sufficiently mature to command the bladder, and control of urination in infants and young children comes from signals sent from the sacral cord. When urine fills the infant bladder, an excitatory signal is sent to the sacral cord (a spinal reflex center), which automatically triggers the detrusor to contract involuntary, and voiding results. As the child's brain matures and develops, it gradually dominates the control of the bladder and the urinary sphincters to inhibit involuntary voiding until complete control is attained. Voluntary continence is affected by the environment, but it is usually attained by age 3–4 years.

Bladder filling is primarily a passive event determined by its intrinsic viscoelastic properties and inhibition of the parasympathetic nerves reducing detrusor tone. The sympathetic nerves facilitate urine storage by inhibiting the parasympathetic nerves, thereby causing relaxation and expansion of the detrusor muscle and closing the bladder neck by constricting the internal urethral sphincter.

As the bladder fills, the pudendal nerve becomes excited, resulting in contraction of the external urethral sphincter. The continence mechanism is achieved by contraction of the external sphincter and the internal sphincter, which maintains urethral pressure (resistance) above normal bladder pressure. The storage phase of the urinary bladder can be switched to the voiding phase either involuntarily (reflexively) or voluntarily.

Aetiology

The primary causes of BOO in children are anatomical or functional and may be congenital or acquired in both males and females (Table 100.1). The causes may be grouped further into primary urogenital tract abnormalities and secondary causes from adjacent structures, and may be neurogenic or nonneurogenic.[9]

Congenital Causes of BOO

Congenital urethral developmental anomalies may present early with features of congenital obstructive uropathy, or later with voiding dysfunction. These include urethral hypoplasia, urethral agenesis, urethral valves, syringocele, and urethral duplications. The severity of presentation depends on the gestational age at onset and the degree of obstruction. In surviving patients with severe obstruction, an accompanying vesicorectal fistula or patent urachus may be present,[10–12] as this would have been protective of the foetus.

Table 100.1: Causes of bladder outlet obstruction.

Congenital urinary anomalies	
Male	**Female**
Posterior urethral valve	Vaginal obstruction (e.g., vaginal atresia with hydrometrocolpos, haematometrocolpos)
Anterior urethral valve	
Urethral diverticulum	Urogenital sinus
Urethral duplication	Cloacal abnormalities
Urethral atresia	Urethral atresia
Posterior urethral polyp	Urethral diverticulum
Urethral stricture	Urethral duplication
Ureterocoele	Ureterocoele
Cowper's gland duct cysts	Prune belly syndrome
Prune belly syndrome	
Congenital urethral hypoplasia	
Congenital giant diverticulum of the bladder	
Hypertrophic utriculus masculinus	

Acquired urogenital tract anomalies	
Anomaly	**Example**
Bladder neck fibrosis	Schistosomiasis and other infections
Stones	
Tumours	Soft tissue sarcomas (rhabdomyoblastoma), squamous cell cancer of bilharziasis
Urethral stricture	Trauma and infection
	Postinstrumentation (endoscopy, catheterisation)
Marian's disease	A neural disorder of the urethral sphincters due to excessive fibrosis
Neurogenic bladder dysfunction	Associated with hypertrophy of the bladder neck
Postoperative obstruction	Ablation of posterior urethral valve (PUV) or ureterocoele, internal urethrotomy, bladder neck sling
Trauma	Haematoma, urethral transaction
Gastrointestinal tract (GIT)	Severe constipation including Hirschsprung's disease with faeculoma
	Rectal duplication
Pelvic tumours	Neuroblastomas
	Sacrococcygeal teratomas (types III, IV)
	Anterior (pelvic) meningocele/myelolipoma
	Currarino's triad (anal stenosis, sacral defect, anterior meningocele)
Some dysfunctional voiding disorders	
Neuropathic bladder with fixed sphincter resistance or detrusor sphincter dyssynergia	
Dysfunctional voiding: sphincter dyssynergia with no apparent neurological lesion (Hinman's syndrome)	

Posterior urethral valves

Posterior urethral valves occur in 0.25–0.5 per 10,000 births. In Europe, this condition may represent 10% of all urological anomalies detected by prenatal ultrasound, and the overall mortality is 25–50%. Many foetuses are lost antenatally, and renal failure is present in 45% of survivors. Foetuses with obstructive uropathy can also have other associated anomalies, such as chromosomal abnormalities (especially trisomies 13, 18, and 21), and some deformations related to the oligohydramnios. In Africa, the severity of this diagnosis and the complexity of treatment may preclude effective management in many infants.

Congenital urethral polyps

Congenital urethral polyps are a rare anomaly of the male urethra that may present with features of voiding dysfunction or obstruction. The exact incidence is unknown because many cases are asymptomatic; their diagnosis requires a high index of suspicion due to the variability of presentation.[13] Many reports favour a congenital aetiology of the polyps, though; infective, irritative, traumatic, and obstructive causes have also been proposed.[13–15]

Congenital giant diverticulum of the bladder

Congenital giant diverticulum of the bladder is a consequence of deficiency in the detrusor musculature and has been reported in infants as a rare cause of bladder outlet obstruction.[16] A giant congenital bladder diverticulum, when noted on voiding cystourethrogram (VCUG) to descend below the bladder neck, may lead to bladder outlet obstruction. Children with connective tissue disorders may be predisposed to this disorder.

Ureterocoeles

A ureterocoele is an abnormal dilatation of the terminal intravesical or extravesical portion of the ureter, most commonly associated with distally ectopic and upperpole duplex ureters. The aetiology may include:

• incomplete dissolution of Chwalla's membrane;[8]

• inadequate muscularisation;

• infection (especially schistosoma haematobium);

• trauma leading to fibrosis and subsequent stenotic ureterocoele; and

• incomplete distal ureteral obstruction by tumour or calculus, causing a pseudoureterocoele due to fibrosis.

Ureterocoeles are common in females (the male-to-female ratio is 1: 4–7), with incidence of 1 in 4,000 live births, but could be as high as 1 in 500 in autopsies.[17] Ureterocoeles are more common in caucasian than black infants. A ureterocoele is the most common cause of bladder outlet obstruction in the female, and 80% are associated with the upper pole ureter of a duplex kidney. A ureterocoele may be confused with a bladder base mass or bladder diverticulum, as it may evert on filling where the associated bladder wall is thin; early filling phase images on MCUG are therefore recommended.

Urethral duplication

Urethral duplication is a rare congenital anomaly with varied presentation, including urinary tract infection (UTI), infertility, penile deviation during erection, urinary incontinence, and abnormal urethra. The embryologic development is poorly understood, but proposed theories suggest cloaca membrane–genital tubercle and urogenital sinus anomalies.[18,19] Effmann types IIA2 and IIB are known to cause outflow obstruction due to a mucous plug in the orthotopic urethra or by proximal dilatation of the dorsal urethra that compresses the ventral urethral during micturition.[19]

Acquired and Extrinsic Causes of BOO

Bladder stones

Bladder stones forming in the absence of underlying uropathy are termed primary or endemic bladder stones. Children account for only 2–3% of all calculous disease patients, endemic in the developing nations of Asia (Turkey, India, and Thailand) and northern Africa.[20]

Until recently, bladder stones were relatively rare in the Western Hemisphere. Boys and girls are equally affected. The mean age at presentation is 6.9 years for girls and 5.2 years for boys.[21,22] Insufficient diuresis, stasis, and infection associated with malnutrition seem to be the most common causes. Bladder schistosomiasis and foreign bodies may form niduses for stone formation.[23] The foreign bodies can be either iatrogenic or noniatrogenic (e.g., suture material, shattered Foley catheter balloons, staples, ureteral stents, and regimen of clean intermittent catheterisation (CIC) of Mitrofanoff conduit).[23] Endemic paediatric bladder stones are not usually associated with renal stones and are relatively less likely to reoccur after treatment.[24] In the paediatric population, the rate of recurrence of stones ranges from 3.6% to 68%, with the highest rates in children with underlying metabolic risk factors.[25] Endemic stones are composed mainly of ammonium acid urate, calcium oxalate, or an impure mixture of ammonium acid urate and calcium oxalate with calcium phosphate. The schema proposed by Smith and Segura[26] is one of the most comprehensive and useful systems for classification.

Extrinsic bladder outlet compression

Extrinsic compression of the bladder outlet is not common but may occur in association with sacrococcygeal teratoma, anterior sacral myelolipoma/meningocele, hydrometrocolpos, faeculoma of constipation or Hirschsprung's disease, pelvic neurofibromatosis or neuroblastoma, and genitourinary rhabdomyosarcoma. These conditions present a great challenge to the surgeon[27–29] (Figures 100.2 and 100.3).

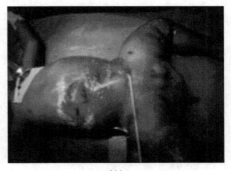

(A)

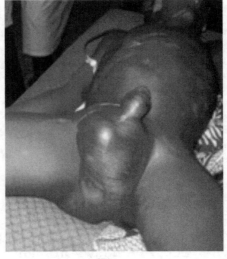

(B)

Figure 100.2: (A) Seven-month-old girl with growing type III sacrococcygeal teratoma causing BOO and constipation, which necessitated suprapubic cystostomy and transverse loop colostomy. Note the gross vulva and bilateral thigh oedema. (B) Thirteen-year-old boy with genitourinary rhabdomyosarcoma. Note suprapubic fullness and overflow urinary and faecal incontinence.

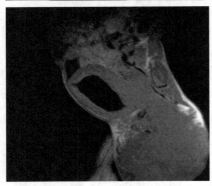

Figure 100.3: Eleven-year-old girl with sacrococygeal mass (histology: neurofibromatosis) since birth. MRI (below) shows that the bladder and the rectum are surrounded and compressed by the mass, causing BOO and constipation.

Secondary Pathologies from UTI

Urethral stricture

Urethral strictures are not common in children. When they do occur, they are usually posttraumatic or iatrogenic from urethral catheterisation and instrumentation.[30,31] The use of equipment should be carefully monitored for the size and suitability for the patient and suitable lubrication and care taken to avoid this complication. The congenital form results from abnormal junction between the proximal and distal urethra and may have a neonatal and postpubertal presentation. Recurrent infection may lead to bladder neck fibrosis, contracture, and resultant BOO. This may also occur from urinary schistosomiasis.[32]

Dysfunctional voiding

Dysfunction of the lower urinary tract in children can be secondary to derangement of nervous control, disorder of detrusor and sphincteric muscle function, structural abnormalities, and unclassified conditions.[9] Where there is loss of coordinated relaxation of the sphincter when there is detrusor contraction, a functional BOO occurs. This may be associated with congenital pathologies of the spinal cord, spinal trauma, or presacral nerve injury associated with surgery or tumour, or may be physiological in origin with no identifiable neurological deficit (nonneurogenic bladder dysfunction).[9,33,34] Nonneurogenic functional bladder disorders in children are observed in 5–15% of the paediatric population. Depending on the balance between the detrusor activity and the sphincter leak pressure, the patient may present with retention, overflow incontinence, or, in rare cases, a small, high-pressure bladder with vesicoureteric reflux and obstructive uropathy, Hinman's syndrome, or nonneurogenic neurogenic bladder dysfunction).[9,35,36] Video urodynamics is useful in the diagnosis and management of these conditions but is not available in many parts of Africa.[33,34]

Pathophysiology of BOO: Obstructive Uropathy

An obstruction of the bladder outlet (mechanical or functional) results in an elevation of intravesical pressure, which is followed by excessive force generation by the detrusor muscles against outlet resistance. This results in massive hypertrophy of the detrusor muscles with resultant sacculation, trabeculation, and ultimately diverticula formation. The trigone may be preserved, but in many instances the antireflux mechanism

of the ureterovesical junction becomes incompetent, ureteral peristalsis is overcome, and increased hydrostatic pressures are transmitted directly to the nephron, causing resultant impairment of renal development and function. The ureters respond to the outlet obstruction by changes similar to the detrusor macroscopically by showing dilatation, elongation, and tortuousity.[33]

As pressures in the proximal tubule and Bowman space increase, glomerular filtration rate (GFR) falls. After 12–24 hours of complete obstruction, intratubular pressure decreases to preobstruction levels. If complete obstruction is not relieved, a depressed GFR is maintained by decreases in renal blood flow mediated by thromboxane A2 and angiotensin II. With continued obstruction, there is a progressive fall in renal blood flow, ischaemia, and nephron damage. GFR falls, but tubular function is particularly severely affected, with a high water and sodium loss resulting in the high output renal failure of obstructive nephropathy.

In the foetus, the placenta functions as the primary excretory organ in place of the kidney throughout gestation. Hence, in the newborn with BOO, the renal function is usually similar to the normal maternal levels initially because of the placental function. The kidneys commence gradual glomerular filtration by the 11th to 12th weeks of gestation. About 90% of amniotic fluid is produced in the kidneys, and only 10% comes from the GIT, lungs, and skin. In the absence of adequate foetal urine production, oligohydramnios results, restricting lung movement and decreasing fluid in the bronchial tree, and thereby causing poor acinar growth and decreased surfactant production. The newborn may have compressed limbs, Potter's facies, and pulmonary hypoplasia presenting with respiratory distress and pneumothorax.

The renal compromise affects the homeostatic, hormonal, and enzymatic functions of the kidney and may manifest as disturbances of water, electrolytes and acid-base balance, anaemia, UTI, septicaemia, circulatory collapse or hypertension, growth retardation, azotaemia, chronic acidosis, and renal osteodystrophy.

Clinical Presentation

History

Many of the cases of BOO may be asymptomatic for a long time or present with constitutional features that often are misleading to an unsuspecting practitioner. The presentation may be acute or chronic urinary retention, overflow incontinence, UTI, or renal failure. In the neonate, the presentation is characterised by abdominal distention; palpable suprapubic or flank masses (bladder and the kidneys); and urachal cyst, fistula, or abscess. Neonatal sepsis and respiratory distress

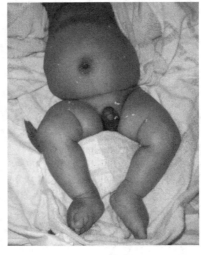

Figure 100.4: Six-week-old infant who presented with progressively reducing urine output, feed intolerance, failure to thrive, abdominal distenion, and gross lower limbs pitting oedema. Bilateral flank masses on abdominal palpation and ultrasound confirmed bilateral urinoma with hydroureteronephrosis.

may also be present. Parents may give a history of urine dribble, poor stream, and failure to thrive in the young infant.

In infants and other children, there may be enuresis, weight loss, vomiting, and diarrhoea. Constipation may be present in cases of dysfunctional voiding, faecal impaction, Hirschsprung's disease, or compression from pelvic masses. Other features include urine dribbling, incontinence, straining, frequency, and intermittency or "staccato" stream. The history should elicit prenatal health, birth and development, perinatal complication, and bowel and bladder habits.

Physical Examination

In the African setting, due to late presentation and lack of prenatal diagnosis, many children present with complications such as small stature for age, anaemia, gross pitting pedal oedema, ascites, and abdominal masses (Figure 100.4). Other features depend on primary or secondary causes. The spine should be examined for defects, and the lower extremities for reflexes, muscle mass and strength, sensation, and gait. The perineum should be checked for gluteal fold symmetry, natal cleft depth, absent coccyx, perineal sensation, tone and reflexes. The CNS should be checked for handedness as well as fine and gross motor coordination. A digital rectal examination should be done for anal sphincteric tone, faecal impaction, distended rectum, and presacral and pelvic masses.

Investigations

Before putting forward diagnostic pathways, consideration must be given to which investigative methods are available and what they can achieve. Hence, the algorithm shown in Figure 100.5 can be followed in the choice of investigative tools for diagnosis of the cause of BOO.

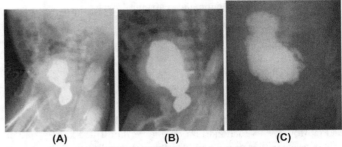

Figure 100.6: MCUG showing (A) dilated posterior urethral and bladder diverticulum around the neck; (B) multiple saculation and diverticula of the bladder wall; and (C) distorted bladder wall and giant fundal diverticulum (a multiple streak of contrast suggests extravasations).

A good bladder function diary and urinary flow rate form the basis of BOO diagnosis, but a variety of tests may be required to confirm the diagnosis and determine the extent of damage. Imaging studies such as ultrasonography (US), plain radiography, and contrast radiography such as MCUG, retrograde urethrocystogram, and intravenous urography (IVU) are relatively inexpensive and easily accessible modalities in many parts of Africa. Where available, magnetic resonance imaging (MRI), computed tomography (CT), scintigraphy, and angiography are modalities of choice. Such imaging may be sufficient to define:

• site and extent of an obstructing pathology;

• extent of urinary tract reaction to the BOO (renal pop-off mechanisms);

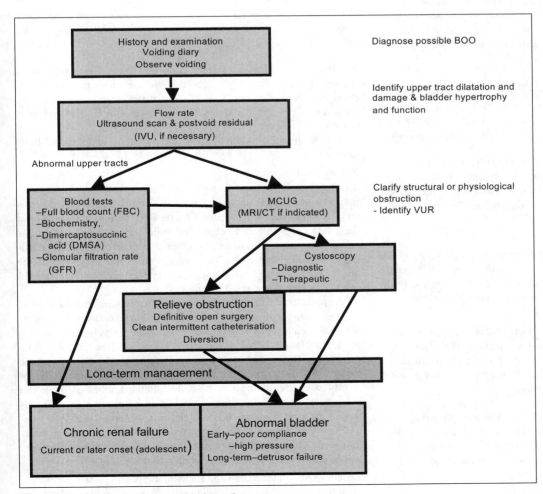

Figure 100.5: Algorithm for bladder outlet obstruction.

• split and total renal function and scarring;

• presence and degree of reflux; and

• associated anomalies, where present.

Useful Imaging Modalities

Plain radiography

Plain radiography can identify radio-opaque stones. It may suggest an enlarged or poorly emptying bladder, displacement of the bowel shadow from the hypochondrium by a large fluid-filled kidney, and/or outline associated vertebral and other bony anomalies.

Ultrasonography

Ultrasonography can demonstrate filling, dilated, or narrow posterior urethra or the presence of intraluminal lesions. US can demonstrate the size and shape of the kidneys and bladder as well as dilated pelvicaliceal system and ureter. US should be performed with a moderately filled urinary bladder, and if an anomaly is found, US should be repeated with the bladder empty. It can be used to estimate the post voidresidual volume of urine, and a spinal ultrasound in children younger than 3 months of age is useful for spinal lesions (tethering, defects, or masses)

Micturating cystourethrography

MCUG is essential for demonstration of bladder shape and capacity, including diverticulum (Figure 100.6) and vesicoureteric reflux and grading, posterior urethral dilatation, and possible filling defects and urinary incontinence. A filling phase is important to identify ureterocoele.

Intravenous urogram

An IVU study gives all the information needed about the morphology of the urinary tract, provided the kidney is working well enough. IVUs in young infants are often disappointing and sometimes dangerous. In the neonate, due to the low GFR, the urinary tract does not opacify well. The x-ray exposure for IVU is relatively high, and US scans are performed where possible.

Scintigraphy

Dimercaptosuccinic acid (DMSA) scintigraphy is a radionuclide technique that provides a functional cortical map of the kidney, quantifying renal tubular cell mass. It is particularly useful for identifying scars of reflux nephropathy and for estimating differential function, provided there is no obstruction.

In a diethylenetriamine penta-acetic acid (DTPA) scintigram, the DTPA is filtered by the glomerulus and gives a dynamic study similar to an IVU. It identifies dilatation and obstruction, and in the latter stages of the study it can give information concerning reflux. Differential renal function can also be quantified.

CT scan/MRI

CT scan and MRI with or without contrast enhancement are very precise in providing anatomical details of the lesion and the extent of damage, but they are quite expensive and not readily available in most African centres. Good-quality ultrasound with Doppler is a good substitute.

Urodynamic studies

Urodynamic studies of the physiologic function of the bladder mechanics during filling and voiding have been used to ascertain the aetiology and epidemiology of nonneurogenic bladder sphincter dysfunction (NNBSD) with the aid of x-ray screening.[35] Examples of such studies include uroflowmetry and cystometrogram.

Uroflowmetry

Uroflowmetry should precede urodynamics to determine the urine flow rate in the child. Structural BOO is associated with a low-amplitude plateau flow rate, detrusor sphincter dyssynergia may be associated with staccato voiding or nonsustained flow with detrusor failure. The careful observer can identify this just by watching.

Cystometrogram

Cystometrogram investigates the pressures during the filling and emptying phases of bladder function and may be used to measure external urethral sphincter activity. Bladder volumes and pressures allow detrusor stability and compliance, and voiding pressures may be assessed.

Cystourethroscopy

Cystourethroscopy is the approach of choice for the identification and treatment of structural abnormalities. Posterior urethral valves, syringoceles, and ureterocoeles may be definitively treated, and polyps may be biopsied or resected. In the African setting, however, appropriate scopes may not be readily available or accessible for either adults or paediatric surgical services.[37]

Ancillary Investigations

Ancillary investigations include the following:

• Haemogram to quantify anaemia, white cell counts, and differentials in UTI. The platelet count may also drop.

• Serum biochemistry to assess the electrolytes, urea, creatinine, and acid-base balance to reveal the level of renal function and allow prompt correction. Attention should be paid to the age-related, lower-than-adult creatinine levels in a child, lest significant renal impairment be missed.

• Urinalysis for blood or infection and urine specific gravity for renal concentration ability and albuminurea.

• Urine culture and antibiotic sensitivity.

• Biopsy and histology for potential bladder tumours and schistosoma granules.

• Urinary stone analysis to determine composite content and hence predict aetiology.

Management

The degree and duration of obstruction are the chief determinants of bladder dysfunction. Early recognition and treatment are the keys to preventing renal function loss. Bladder outlet obstruction should be viewed as a potentially curable form of lower urinary tract and renal disease.

Efforts should be made to probe the symptoms and signs of BOO in children.

Initial Treatment

Treatment of BOO depends on the underlying cause of the obstruction. For most cases, there is a need to control superimposed sepsis and urgently relieve the obstruction pending definitive diagnosis of the cause. The empirical choice of antibiotic includes intravenous amoxyl-clavulanic acid or an ampicillin-sulbactam combination, pending arrival of culture results. The cephalosporins and quinolones can be used as well. Aminoglycosides (e.g., gentamicin) are contraindicated in cases of compromised renal function.

A nonballoon catheter inserted through the urethra into the bladder will relieve the obstruction temporarily. The bladder may be drained by suprapubic catheter or vesicostomy or the upper tracts by ureterostomy or nephrostomy. Loop ureterostomy protects the kidneys from persistent reflux of infected urine and permits early recovery of the tone of dilated ureters while allowing the bladder to cycle normally. A postobstructive diuresis is possible following relief or bypass of obstruction, particularly chronic bladder outlet obstruction, and may lead to massive fluid depletion and electrolytes derangement.

In nonneurogenic dysfunctional voiding disorder, surgery is rarely indicated. Adoption of a conservative regimen, such as that presented below, may prevent further deterioration of this disorder.[9,36]

1. Behavioural modification and standard urotherapy, which includes good fluid intake and timed voiding schedules and double voiding,

and a nonpharmacologic and nonsurgical combination of cognitive, behavioural, and physical therapy with the aim to normalise the micturition pattern.

2. Biofeedback and pelvic floor rehabilitation to build self-perception on the detrusor contraction and pelvic floor relaxation in the patient.

3. Bowel management by use of diets, laxatives, enema, and regular elimination.

4. Clean intermittent catheterisation, which is indicated in upper tract dilatation, thickened bladder wall, and significant residue. This can be combined with medications.

5. Medications, such as anticholinergics and α-adrenergic blockers. Anticholinergics (e.g., oxybutynin, 0.2 mg/kg b.d.; propantheline, 0.5 mg/kg b.d.; and hyoscyamine) are used to reduce or abolish uninhibited bladder contracture and increase functional bladder capacity but do not overcome BOO and may make bladder empting worse. Thus, they may need to be used with CIC. α-adrenargic blockers (e.g., doxazin mesylate, prazosin, terazocin) are used to cause detrusor smooth muscle relaxation and decrease outlet resistance.

6. Botulinum A toxin injection into the urethral urinary sphincter has been used in children with NNBSD,

Surgical Treatment

The definitive treatment of mechanical causes of BOO is mostly surgical. Noninvasive and minimally invasive approaches have less morbidity compared with open surgery. Many centres in Africa still have to contend with an open approach to treat and relieve obstruction, which can be done with endoscopy, laparoscopy, or extracorporeal lithotripsy where available.

Surgical diverticulectomy, often with ureteral reimplantation, is the preferred treatment for bladder diverticulum, and this gives excellent long-term results if the underlying cause of BOO has been treated.[16]

Endoscopic incision of ureterocoeles (intravesical and ectopic) as a primary form of treatment diminishes the need for upperpole heminephroureterectomy. Open deroofing of a ureterocoele may require bladder wall reconstruction or in the presence of poor detrusor support of the ureterocoele, puncture is preferred.[17,38] Endoscopic subureteric injection of polytetrafluoroethylene (PTFE) gives good results for associated reflux after relief of BOO.

The majority of vesical calculi in children are treated by open surgery because the removal per-urethrally with the use of ultrasonic or pneumatic lithotripsy devices is restricted in paediatric patients by the narrow calibre of the urethra.[20–24] A percutaneous suprapubic cystolithotripsy as an alternative to open surgery circumvents the problem of urethral calibre in children.[39] It is safe; in addition, it reduces morbidity and hospital stay, and thus reduces the cost of treatment.

In urinary schistosomiasis, medical treatment with praziquantel is used in the acute phase, whereas in the late forms, transurethral incision can be successful in treating bladder neck contracture.

Excision of a duplicated poorly functioning urethra and or urethroplasty is successful in urethral duplication. However, individual cases should be selected by adequate investigation to avoid postoperative incontinence or urinary retention.[18,19] The more hypospadiac urethra is usually the better functioning channel.

Extrinsic compression by masses should be treated accordingly by surgical excision and/or the use of cytotoxic drugs as either adjuvant or neoadjuvant where indicated. Some rhabdomyosarcomas respond to radiation therapy, but care must be taken to avoid postradiation damage with bladder neck contracture.

Subsequent reconstruction, including bladder augmentation and urinary diversion, may be necessary and demand expert care to reduce morbidity.

Concomitant medical treatment for correction of accompanying pathophysiologic derangements, such as control of cardiovascular risk factors, diabetic nephropathy, drug dosage adjustment, and renal replacement therapy, is very important for early recovery of function and patient recovery.[40]

Postoperative Complications

- Reparative operations will fail if the underlying cause of BOO has not been treated. Urinary fistula (vesicocutaneous, perineal) requires catheterisation and/or prompt repair. Treat UTI as much as possible before surgery.

- Wound infection requires adequate dressing, maintenance of sterile procedure rules, and appropriate use of antibiotics.

- Urinary incontinence from damage to pelvic innervation during pelvic dissection, weakness of the bladder neck, or bladder neck fibrosis and contracture require careful plane dissection during surgery.

- Urethral stricture may be treated by dilatation, optical urethrotomy, or urethroplasty.

- Vesicoureteric reflux may suggest a need for reimplantation.

- Psychological disturbance and disruption in the family and social cycle demands social and religious support.

Prognosis and Outcome

Early diagnosis and prompt appropriate treatment of most causes of BOO give good results. Any untreated obstruction to the developing renal tract can lead to irreversible damage to the developing kidneys and accounts for 25% of chronic renal failure seen in childhood.[40]

Even complete early relief of a severe structural obstruction such as posterior urethral valves may not prevent the later onset of long-term detrusor failure, increasing postvoid residual volumes, UTI, and upper tract dilatation with obstructive nephropathy.

Improved nutrition, better prenatal and postnatal diagnosis and care, and improved awareness of the problem improve the prognosis.

Prevention

Parents should be educated on proper toilet training of their children and to look out for any abnormal patterns. In all cases, early referral and a team approach improve the outcome. The routine antenatal US scan should be upgraded and is the key to early diagnosis. Follow-up should be life-long because urological status may change rapidly.

Ethical Issues

In view of the poor outcome of late diagnosed BOO, a general debate on ethical grounds concerns whether prenatal diagnosis, early and repeated postnatal screening, and even treatment can be used in children to prevent the occurrence of complications. The cost of the screening, unwarranted exposure to radiation, and sometimes invasive techniques in search of the pathology in a relatively small population of children calls for caution. More specifically, the question is whether every child with UTI needs a MCUG and where does the DMSA scan fit into our evaluation? In the UK, MCUGs are now more rarely performed, and national guidelines no longer routinely call for DMSA unless there is a US scan abnormality or the child is younger than 3 months of age. The questions of how long prophylactic antibiotics should be used or whether they are useful at all are as controversial in Europe as they are in Africa.

Key Summary Points

1. A high index of suspicion is needed for early detection and prevention of inappropriate treatment.

2. Dysfunctional elimination syndrome describes the association between voiding and bowel dysfunction.

3. Progressive bladder outlet obstruction (BOO) leads to obstructive nephropathy and renal failure.

4. Urethral instrumentation in children should be under a sterile technique, choosing appropriate-size material and using gentle manoeuvres to avoid strictures.

5. Patients should have sepsis controlled and obstruction relieved while investigating the cause of the obstruction to prevent further damage.

6. Treatment may consist of behavioural modification, standard urotherapy, biofeedback, pelvic floor rehabilitation, neuromodulation, bowel management, drug therapy, and/or surgery.

7. An open surgical approach may suffice to correct anatomical BOO in many instances.

8. There should be medical treatment of concomitant obstructive nephropathy.

9. Many patients would benefit from prolonged follow-up and a team approach.

References

1. Honkinen O, Jahnukainen T, Mertsola J, Ruuskanen O. Bacteraemic urinary tract infection in children. Pediatr Infect Dis J 2000; 19:630–634.

2. Grafstein NH, Combs AJ, Glassberg KI. Primary bladder neck dysfunction: an overlooked entity in children. Curr Urol Rep 2005; 6(2):133–139.

3. Farhat W, Bagli DJ, Capolicchio G, O'Reilly S, Merguerian PA, Khoury A, et al. The dysfunctional voiding scoring system: quantitative standardisation of dysfunctional voiding symptoms in children. J Urol 2000; 164:1011–1015.

4. Nevéus T, von Gontard A, Hoebeke P, Hjälmås K, Bauer S, Bower W, et al. The standardisation of terminology of lower urinary tract function in children and adolescents: report from the Standardisation Committee of the International Children's Continence Society. J Urol 2006; 176:314–324.

5. Sadler TW. Urogenital system. In: Longman's Medical Embryology, 10th ed., Lippincott, Williams & Wilkins, 2006, Pp 236–238.

6. Mackie GC, Stephens FD. Duplex kidneys: a correlation of renal dysplasia with position of the ureteral orifice. J Urol 1975; 114:274–280.

7. Baker LA, Gomez RA. Embryonic development of the ureter and bladder: acquisition of smooth muscle. J Urol 1998; 140:545–550.

8. Chwalle R, The process of formation of cystic dilatations of the vesical end of the ureter and of diverticular at the ureteral ostium. Urol Cutan 1972; 31:499.

9. Yeung CK, Sihoe JDY, Bauer SB. Voiding dysfunction in children: non-neurogenic and neurogenic. In: Wein AJ, Kavoussi LR, Novisk AC, Partin AW, Peters CA, eds. Campbell-Walsh Urology, 9th ed. Saunders-Elsevier, 2007, Pp 3604–3655.

10. Kumar B, Sharma SB, Agrawal LD. Congenital urethral hypoplasia with urethral fistula without imperforate anus: report of two cases. Afr J Pediatr Surg 2008; 5:37–39.

11. Passerini-Glazer G, Araguna F, Chiozza L, Artibani W, Robinwitz R, Firlit CF. The PADUA (progressive augmentation by dilating the urethra anterior) procedure for treatment of severe urethral hypoplasia. J Urol 1998; 140:124–129.

12. Rich RH, Hardy BE, Filler RM. Surgery for anomalies of the urachus. J Pediatr Surg 1983; 18:370–372.

13. Tsuzuki T, Epstein JI. Fibroepithelial polyp of the lower urinary tract in adults. Am J Surg Pathol 2005; 29:460–466.

14. Eziyi AK, Helmy TE, Sarhan OM, Eissa WM, Ghaly MA. Management of male urethral polyps in children: experience with four cases. Afr J Pediatr Surg 2009; 6:49–51.

15. Tsuang W, Rapp DE, Feinstein KA, Orvieto MA, Close CE. Urethral polyp in asymptomatic male infant with prenatal hydronephrosis. Urology 2006; 67(5):1085.e9–e11.

16. Shukla AR, Bellah RA, Canning DA, Carr MC, Snyder HM, Zderic SA. Giant bladder diverticula causing bladder outlet obstruction in children. J Urol 2004; 172(5, pt 1):1977–1979.

17. Cooper CS, Synder HM. Ureteral duplication, ectopy and ureterocele. In: Gearhart JP, Rink RC, Mouriquard PDE, eds. Pediatric Urology, WB Saunders, 2001, Pp 430–449.

18. Abdur-Rahman LO, Nasir AA, Agboola JO, Adeniran JO. Penile shaft sinus: a sequelae of circumcision in urethral duplication. Indian J Urol 2009; 25:134–136.

19. Bogaert GA. Urethral duplication and other urethral anomalies. In: Gearhart JP, Rink RC, Mouriquard PDE, eds. Pediatric Urology, WB Saunders Company, 2001, Pp 607–619.

20. Kroovand RL. Pediatric urolithiasis. Urol Clin North Am 1997; 24:173–184.

21. Abubakar AM, Mungadi IA, Chinda JY, Ntia IO, Jalo I, Obianno SK. Paediatric urolithiasis in Northern Nigeria. Afr J Pediatr Surg 2004; 1:2–5.

22. Angwafo FF, Daudon M, Wonkam A, Kuwong PM, Kropp KA. Pediatric urolithiasis in sub-Saharan Africa: a comparative study in two regions of Cameroon. Eur Urol 2000; 37:106–111.

23. Barroso U, Jednak R, Fleming P, Barthold JS, González R. Bladder calculi in children who perform clean intermittent catheterisation. BJU Int 2000; 85:879–884.

24. Rizvi SAH, Naqvi SAA, Hussain Z, Hashmi A, Hussain M, Zafar MN, et al. Pediatric urolithiasis: developing nation perspectives. J Urol 2002; 168:1522–1525.

25. Van Reen R. Idiopathic urinary bladder stones of childhood. Aust NZ J Surg 1980; 50:18–22.

26. Smith L, Segura J. Urolithiasis. WB Saunders, 1990, Pp 1327–1352.

27. Adetiloye VA, Adejuyigbe O, Adelusola KA. Presacral myelolipoma: sonographic appearance. Pediatr Radiol 1996; 26:271–272.

28. Leung AK, Rubin SZ, Seagram GF, Hwang WS. Sacrococcygeal teratoma. Aust Pediatr J 1985; 21:123–125.

29. Ekenze SO, Ezegwui HU. Hydrometrocolpos from a low vaginal atresia: an uncommon cause of intestinal and urinary obstruction. Afr J Pediatr Surg 2008; 5:43–45.

30. Shittu OB. Urethroplasty for stricture in Nigerian children. Nigerian J of Surg Res 2002; 4:80–83.

31. Baskin LS, McAninch JW. Childhood urethral injuries: perspective on outcome and treatment. Br J Urol 1993; 72:241–246.

32. Salah MA, Böszörmenyi-Nagy G, Alsaaidi AA, Nagi MA. Bladder neck obstruction in young males with history of Bilhazial infection. Int Urol Nephrol 1999; 31:781–786.

33. Yeung CK. Pathophysiology of bladder dysfunction. In: Gearhart JP, Rink RC, Mouriquard PDE, eds. Pediatric Urology, WB Saunders, 2001, Pp 453–469.

34. Bauer SB. Pediatric urodynamics: lower tract. In O'Donnel B, Koff SA, eds. Pediatric Urology, Butterworth Heinemann, 1997, Pp 125–151.

35. Hoebeke P, Van Laecke E, Van Camp C, Raes A, Van De Walle J. One thousand video-urodynamic studies in children with non-neurogenic bladder sphincter dysfunction. BJU Int 2001; 87:575–580.

36. Hinman F Jr. Nonneurogenic neurogenic bladder (the Hinman syndrome)—15 years later. J Urol 1986; 136:769–777.

37. Salako AA, Badmus TA, Sowande OA, Adeyemi BA, Nasir AA, Adejuyigbe O. Endourology in a Nigerian tertiary hospital—current level of practice and challenges (short report). Nigerian J Surg Res 2005; 3–4:268–270.

38. Blyth B, Passerini-Glazel G, Camuffo C, Snyder HM, Duckett JW. Endoscopic incision of ureteroceles: intravesical versus ectopic. J Urol 1993; 149:556–559.

39. Agrawal MS, Aron M, Goyal J, Elhence IP, Asopa HSI. Percutaneous suprapubic cystolithotripsy for vesical calculi in children. J Endourol 1999; 13:173–175.

40. Clothier J, Hulton S-A. Urological disorders in children that progress to chronic renal failure. Medicine 2007; 35:447–449.

CHAPTER 101
ACUTE SCROTUM

William Appeadu-Mensah
Ashish P. Desai

Introduction

Acute scrotum is defined as an acutely painful and/or swollen scrotum. One of the possible causes, torsion of the testis or epididymis requires urgent surgical intervention to salvage the testis. There are, however, no pathognomonic signs that clearly differentiate torsion of the epididymis from other possible diagnoses.[1] The acute scrotum should therefore be assumed to be due to torsion of the epididymis until proven otherwise.

Demographics

The incidence of the various causes of acute scrotum varies across studies.[1-4] Torsion of the testis, torsion of a testicular appendage, and epididymitis are the most common causes of acute scrotum, contributing more than 85% of the causes. The aetiology and pathophysiology of these and other, less frequent causes are discussed in the next section.

The incidence of torsion of the epididymis accounts for 10–40% of the causes of acute scrotum in children, and is more common in the neonatal and adolescent years. It occurs with an incidence of about 1 in 4,000 boys aged less than 25 years. It is often unilateral, more often on the left side, but it also may be bilateral.

Torsion of a testicular appendage occurs at a frequency of 30–45% of causes of acute scrotum and is common in the prepubertal period.

Epididymitis occurs in 30–50% of causes of acute scrotum and usually affects postpubertal boys worldwide. It may also occur in infancy. There are no studies that show the incidence in Africa, but there also is no evidence that the frequency is different.

Aetiology/Pathophysiology

Causes of acute scrotum include torsion of the testis, torsion of a testicular appendage, epididymitis, trauma, Henoch-Schönlein purpura, varicocoeles, hernias, hydrocoeles, idiopathic scrotal oedema, and testicular tumours.

Torsion of the Testis

Torsion of the testis refers to a twist of the spermatic cord. This could be extravaginal or intravaginal. The precipitating factor that causes the twist is not known for sure but there may be a history of trauma.

Extravaginal torsion occurs when the spermatic cord twists at a site proximal to the tunica vaginalis. This is due to lack of attachment of the tunica vaginalis to the scrotal wall. It usually occurs in utero before the tunica vaginalis has fixed to the scrotal wall. The child is therefore born with an infarcted testis; this may be bilateral. It may, however, also occur soon after birth in the neonatal period. Metachronous bilateral torsion of testis has also been recognised.

Intravaginal torsion occurs when the cord twists at a site within the tunica vaginalis. It is often associated with a high attachment of the tunica to the cord rather than close to the testis (the "bell clapper" anomaly). This anomaly is usually bilateral. The testis often has a transverse lie, and this allows the cord to twist.

Torsion of the testis may also be associated with undescended testis due to poor fixation to the scrotum. Torsion is usually away from the midline and leads initially to venous obstruction and then to arterial obstruction, ischaemia, and infarction. About 720 degrees of torsion is required for ischaemic damage to occur.

Torsion of a Testicular Appendage

Torsion of a testicular appendage occurs when there is a twist in either the appendix testis, which is a remnant of the Müllerian duct, or the appendix epididymis, which is a remnant of the wolffian duct. The appendix testis is attached to the superior pole of the testis, whereas the appendix epididymis is attached to the superior pole of the epididymis.

Epididymitis

Epididymitis is inflammation of the epididymis and may be due to reflux of urine, urinary tract infection (UTI), or a sexually transmitted disease (STD). In children, reflux of urine or a UTI is more likely to be the cause and is usually associated with an anomaly of the urinary system. The organisms involved in the younger child may be those that usually cause UTIs, such as *Escherichia coli*. In the postpubertal child, the causative organisms are usually those that cause STDs such as gonorrhoea and chlamydia. Schistosomiasis may, however, be a rare cause of epididymitis in endemic regions.[5] Epididymitis may eventually lead to orchitis.

Trauma

Trauma to the scrotum due to blunt or penetrating injury may result in an acute scrotum. Blunt injury may be as a result of a blow to the scrotum or a straddle injury. The trauma may lead to a hematocele, a ruptured testis, or a haematoma in the testis. A penetrating injury is usually accompanied by an entry and exit wound.

Henoch-Schönlein Purpura

Henoch-Schönlein purpura is a generalised vasculitis that affects the skin, joints, gastrointestinal tract (GIT), and kidneys. It causes inflammation of the scrotal wall and a vasculitis, which may involve the epididymis or testis. The cause is not known, but may be due to an abnormal reaction of the immune system to normal antigens.[6]

Varicocoeles

Varicocoeles are dilated tortuous veins in the scrotum due to a failure of the valves draining the testicular veins. Varicocoeles may lead to pain, swelling, subfertility, oligospermia, or reduced sperm motility. The warm environment created in the scrotum is believed to contribute to subfertility.

Hernias and Hydroceles

Hernias and hydroceles occur as a result of a patent processus vaginalis that allows abdominal viscera or fluid to move in and out of the processus. When viscera such as bowel are involved, it may become irreducible, obstructed, or strangulated, leading to a painful scrotal swelling.

Idiopathic Scrotal Oedema

Idiopathic scrotal oedema is sudden onset of oedema and redness of the scrotum in children, usually not associated with pain. The aetiology is not known for certain, but it is suspected to be an allergic reaction.

Testicular Tumours

Testicular tumours may present as painful scrotal swellings in children, probably due to bleeding into them. Teratomas are a common cause of tumours in children.

Clinical Presentation

Although no pathognomonic signs differentiate torsion of the epididymis from other diagnoses, a complete history, physical examination, and necessary investigations help to narrow down the possibilities and thus reduce the number of unnecessary explorations.[7] Table 101.1 summarises the clinical presentations for torsion of the epididymisis, torsion of a testicular appendage, and epididymitis.

History

The age at presentation is important in the differential diagnosis of acute scrotum. In the neonatal period, torsion of the testis is likely, whereas Henoch-Schönlein purpura or torsion of a testicular appendage may occur in the prepubertal period. In the postpubertal period, torsion of the testis and epididymitis are more common. No childhood age is exempt, however, from any of these pathologies, and all children should be treated promptly.

Symptoms in patients with acute scrotum may include pain, swelling, nausea and vomiting, urinary symptoms, or fever.

Pain is an important symptom in the history of acute scrotum. Sudden onset of severe scrotal pain in a patient who has been well suggests torsion of the testis. Gradual onset of pain becoming severe over a number of days suggests epididymitis or torsion of a testicular appendage. The site of pain may be the abdomen or scrotum in torsion of the testis or epididymitis. Hence, the testes should be examined in all cases of pain in the abdomen, especially in smaller children. Pain localised to the top of the scrotum may be due to torsion of a testicular appendage. Joint pains associated with abdominal pain, bloody stool, and sometimes haematuria suggests Henoch-Schönlein purpura.

A history of a scrotal swelling that appears on straining and then disappears on relaxation suggests a hernia, whereas a recurrent swelling that appears while awake and disappears when sleeping may suggest a varicocoele or a hydrocoele. Swelling that occurs after severe pain suggests torsion of the testis.

Nausea and vomiting may occur at the onset of torsion of the epididymis.

Urinary symptoms, such as frequency and dysuria, may suggest a UTI and epididymitis, whereas a urethral discharge suggests epididymitis due to a sexually transmitted infection. A previous history of urinary instrumentation or urinary anomaly suggests epididymitis.

A history of fever suggests epididymitis.

A history of trauma may suggest injury but may also suggest torsion of the testis, especially if the severity of symptoms is not explained by the nature of the trauma. A previous history of recurrent pain in the scrotum that subsides without much intervention suggests torsion of the testis.

Physical Examination

A thorough physical examination is mandatory. As previously mentioned, fever suggests epididymitis.

Abdominal distention may be present in a patient with an obstructed hernia and may be associated with visible peristalsis. Tenderness and rebound tenderness suggest peritonitis, which may be due to a strangulated hernia.

The scrotum may be enlarged in torsion of the testis, torsion of a testicular appendage, epididymitis, trauma, hydrocoele, hernias, idiopathic scrotal oedema, varicocoele, and testicular tumours. The enlargement is inguinoscrotal in hernias but purely scrotal in the others. In torsion of the testis, the testis may be visibly high and lying transversely, although this is not invariably the case.

In lighter-skinned individuals, the scrotum may look red and oedematous in torsion of the testis, torsion of a testicular appendage, epididymitis, trauma, strangulated hernias, Henoch-Schönlein purpura, and idiopathic scrotal oedema. A blue dot may be noted at the superior end of the testis in light-skinned individuals in torsion of a testicular appendage, and this finding in addition to localised tenderness at this spot is pathognomonic of this condition.

Tenderness in the scrotum is elicited in torsion of the epididymis, torsion of a testicular appendage, epididymitis, strangulated inguinal hernias, trauma, and Henoch-Schönlein purpura. Tenderness may be localised to the top of the scrotum in torsion of a testicular appendage, where a nodule may also be palpated. It may be localised to the epididymis posterior to the testis in early epididymitis, but the whole testis becomes tender and enlarged in late epididymitis. In torsion of the epididymis, tenderness affects both testis and epididymis early in the history. There is no tenderness in idiopathic scrotal oedema.

Lack of relief of pain on lifting the scrotum upwards suggests torsion of the testis (Prehn's sign). Relief of pain on rotating the testis toward the midline in an attempt to detort the epididymis suggests torsion of the testis. The cremasteric reflex, which is elicited by stroking the medial aspect of the thigh, suggests torsion of the epididymis when absent, but suggests torsion of the appendix testis or epididymitis when present.

An enlarged, firm, well-circumscribed swelling that may or may not be tender may be palpated in testicular tumours.

A palpable "bag of worms" suggests varicocoele.

Table 101.1: Clinical presentations.

Clinical feature	Torsion of the epididymis	Torsion of a testicular appendage	Epididymitis
Pain in the scrotum	Sudden severe onset	Gradually getting severe over days	Gradually getting severe over days
Nausea and/or vomiting	May be present at onset	Not usually present at onset	Not usually present at onset
Urinary symptoms	Usually absent	Usually absent	May be present
Urethral discharge	Usually absent	Usually absent	May be present
History of trauma	May be present	Usually absent	Usually absent
Previous history of recurrent pain	May be present	Usually absent	Usually absent
Previous history of instrumentation or urinary anomaly	Usually absent	Usually absent	May be present
Fever	Usually absent	Usually absent	May be present
Swollen tender testis and epididymis	Occurs early	Occurs late	Occurs late
Localised tenderness	Usually not localised	Localised to nodule at top of testis at the onset	Localised to epididymis posterior to testis at the onset
Prehn's sign	Negative	Positive	Positive
Cremasteric reflex	Absent	Present	Present

Investigations

Investigations may be helpful if there is a great likelihood that the acute scrotum is not due to torsion of the testis or if presentation is late. The time spent on this, however, may lead to the demise of a viable testis. Early exploration is therefore mandatory if torsion of the testis cannot be ruled out clinically.[3]

Routine urine examination may show pyuria and bacteriuria or pyuria alone and support the diagnosis of epididymitis in a patient with other suggestive clinical signs. However, the presence of microscopic pyuria alone does not rule out other conditions.

Colour Doppler ultrasonography (US) may show absence of blood flow or reduced flow to the testis in torsion of the testis while showing normal or increased flow in patients with torsion of the appendix testis or epididymitis. This investigation may not, however, be easily available in Africa, and the need to explore should be based on clinical findings rather than any investigation. In centres where it is available, colour Doppler US is used to rule out torsion of the testis in cases where this is not likely. Colour Doppler US may confirm the diagnosis of varicocoele.[3] Doppler is operator-dependent, however, and needs a well-trained operator to diagnose these patients.

Radioisotope scan may show blood flow to the testis in epididymitis or torsion of a testicular appendage, and absent or reduced blood flow in torsion of the epididymis. This scan, however, is not 100% sensitive or specific, and may lead to delay in exploration of the scrotum. Its absence in most parts of Africa makes it unavailable to most clinicians. Where available, it may be used in patients who present late or have symptoms that do not suggest torsion of the epididymis.

Ultrasonography may help confirm the diagnosis of a hernia, hydrocoele, varicocoele, or testicular tumour.

Management

The aim of management is to save all viable testes in cases due to torsion while minimising unnecessary explorations. It is important to explore the scrotum early in those patients in whom the diagnosis of torsion is likely or cannot be ruled out clinically. As much as possible, exploration should be done within 6 hours of the onset of symptoms. An attempt may be made to detort the testis, which causes immediate relief if successful. The testis may then be fixed later. In neonates, however, presentation is almost always late, and an elective exploration may be planned to remove the nonviable testis and to fix the viable testis.

Epididymitis, Henoch-Schönlein purpura, and idiopathic scrotal oedema are managed conservatively. Bed rest and scrotal elevation allow the inflammation to subside. Analgesics may be necessary for pain, and antibiotics for infection. US and micturating cystourethrogram (MCUG) are necessary to rule out any urinary anomaly in prepubertal children with epididymitis.

Hernias and hydroceles are treated surgically electively unless a hernia cannot be reduced or there is a high likelihood of gangrenous viscera.

Testicular tumours are excised through an inguinal approach. Where frozen section is available, this may help to confirm the diagnosis before excision.

In children with varicocoeles, Palomo's operation of high ligation of testicular vessels could be performed either open or laparoscopically.

Torsion of a testicular appendage, if confirmed preoperatively, may be treated conservatively. However, it is difficult to diagnose torsion of appendix testis, and hence this should be treated by early exploration of scrotum. Scrotal exploration should also be performed if the child has severe pain.

If in doubt about the diagnosis, urgent scrotal exploration and bilateral fixation of the testes should be the treatment of choice.

Technique of Surgery for Torsion of Epididymis

1. A midline scrotal incision or two longitudinal incisions in each hemiscrotum are made. The involved testis is brought out and inspected. Any twist is reduced and the testis is observed for improvement in colour. While waiting for colour change, the other testis could be fixed.

2. If the colour does not improve, if the blood from the testis on incising the tunica albuginea remains black, and if the onset of symptoms is more than 24 hours, the testis may be excised. Otherwise, it is fixed.

3. The tunica vaginalis is incised and the testis sutured to the scrotal wall by using 3-point fixation with nonabsorbable stitches. Alternatively, the edges of the opening in the tunica vaginalis could be sutured to the tunica albuginea to expose a wide surface of the albuginea directly to the subcutaneous tissue of the scrotum, thus allowing fixation to a wider area.

Management of Neonatal Torsions

Most neonatal torsions are present when the child is born and are antenatal events. They are usually unilateral and hence are traditionally treated by a wait-and-watch approach if there is no sign of acute onset of torsion.

Recently, however, multiple reports of bilateral neonatal torsions have been noted. In 33% of the cases, the torsion can be metachronous. If diagnosis is delayed, the salvage rate is very low. Hence, urgent exploration and fixation of the testis should be the treatment of choice in neonatal torsions.[8]

Postoperative Complications

Infection, abscess formation, reactive hydrocoele, haematoma, infarction, and atrophy of the testis are possible complications. These resolve with rest and relevant antibiotics. An infarcted testis may have to be excised later.

Prognosis

The ability to salvage the testis following torsion of the epididymis depends on the time interval between the onset of symptoms and exploration of the scrotum. Exploration done within 6 hours of the onset gives the best results. A few testes may still be viable after 12 hours; however, beyond 24 hours the probability of having viable testes drops to almost nil. It is important, therefore, that exploration be done as soon as possible.

In Africa, this is a particular problem due to the time it takes for a patient to see a relevant specialist who could explore the scrotum. Distance from hospitals, cultural practices, delay in referrals, and economic considerations contribute to this late presentation and thus reduce the number of viable testes obtained. More often than not, exploration is done to remove the infarcted testis and fix the normal one.

Prevention

Prevention of the loss of viable testes depends on early diagnosis and exploration of the scrotum. Acute scrotum is a surgical emergency and everything must be done to make it possible for patients to reach relevant experts in time. Education of the general public is therefore very important to make them recognise the possible dangers of presenting to the hospital late with an acute scrotum. The media, various political leaders, religious groups, and nongovernmental organisations may play key roles in increasing awareness of this condition. Inclusion of this topic in school health education programs may also help increase awareness of this condition.

Lack of enough medical personnel as well as financial and other resources make this difficult in the African setting. Training of medical officers and other primary health care providers to recognise the condition and refer as quickly as possible to a surgeon who could manage the condition is important.

The provision of an efficient emergency ambulance service may make it possible for patients to reach a relevant specialist on time. In the absence of an ambulance service, it may be necessary to transport patients in any available vehicle to the nearest surgeon. All surgeons should be trained to recognise and fix the testis, because enough subspecialists may not be available close enough to all patients.

Evidence-Based Research

Table 101.2 presents a large retrospective study that reviewed clinical diagnosis of acute scrotum.

Table 101.2: Evidence-based research.

Title	The diagnosis and treatment of acute scrotum in children and adolescents
Authors	Knight PJ, Vassy LE
Institution	Departments of Surgery of St. Francis Regional Medical Centre, Wesley Medical Centre, and St. Joseph Medical Centre, Wichita, Kansas, USA; Children's Hospital and Mount Carmel Hospital, Columbus, Ohio, USA
Reference	Ann Surg 1984; 200:664
Problem	The difficulty in the diagnosis of acute scrotum.
Intervention	The use of specific symptoms, physical signs, and investigations to guide decision making.
Comparison/ control (quality of evidence)	The clinical signs suggesting a particular diagnosis were compared with the findings at surgery and on follow-up.
Outcome/ effect	Patients with a previous history of recurrent scrotal pain benefited from scrotal exploration, even when physical findings were normal, because most were due to recurrent torsion. Patients with at least three suggestive symptoms and signs of epididymitis almost always had epididymitis. Watchful observation in doubtful cases was not beneficial when the diagnosis was unclear. Investigation was not usually helpful when the diagnosis of torsion of the testis could not be ruled out.
Historical significance/ comments	This study showed that, with careful history and examination, it is possible to make a reasonable diagnosis of epididymitis in some children with acute scrotum. It also showed that exploration of testes in those with recurrent pain could help salvage a number of testes before they become irreversibly torsed. No investigation is foolproof, although it may be helpful when clinical signs point to epididymitis. It may however delay the appropriate treatment of a torsed testis. In Africa, where this may be difficult to obtain, the use of clinical signs to rule out cases of epididymitis where possible and the early exploration of doubtful cases are more appropriate.

Key Summary Points

1. There is no pathognomonic sign that helps in making a definite diagnosis of acute scrotum.

2. In a number of patients, the history and physical findings together may make it possible to make a definite diagnosis of either torsion of the testis (sudden onset of pain, transverse lie of the testis, etc.), torsion of the appendix testis (palpable blue tender nodule at superior end of testis), or epididymitis (frequency of micturition, fever, urethral discharge, etc.). These may be treated accordingly.

3. In most patients, no definite diagnosis can be made based on history and physical examination, and early exploration without further investigation is the diagnostic and usually therapeutic procedure of choice.

References

1. Cavusoglu YH, Karaman A, Karaman I, et al. Acute scrotum—aetiology and management. Indian J Pediatr 2005; 72:201–203.

2. Sidler D, Brown RA, Millar AJW, Rode H, Cywes S. A 25 year review of acute scrotum in children. South Afr Med J 1997; 87:1606–1698.

3. Lee JW, Kim YT, Lee HM. Evaluation of the acute scrotum by colour Doppler ultrasonography and radioisotope imaging in children. Korean J Uro 1996; 37:671–676.

4. Varga J, Zivkovic D, Grebeldinger F, Somer D. Acute scrotal pain in children—10 years' experience. Urol Int 2007; 78:73–77.

5. Yakubu AA, Mohammed AZ, Sheshe AA, Edino ST, Alhassan SU. Testicular schisotsomiais. An unusual cause of acute scrotal pain. Afr J Urol 2005; 11:258–260.

6. Najmaldin A, Burge DM. Acute idiopathic scrotal oedema: incidence, manifestations, aetiology. Br J Surg 1987; 74:634–635.

7. Philip JK, Vassy LE. The diagnosis and treatment of acute scrotum in children and adolescents. Ann Surg 1984; 200:664–673.

8. Baglaj M, Carachi R. Neonatal bilateral testicular torsion: a plea for emergency exploration. J Urol 2007;177(6):2296–2299.

Suggested Reading

Chokoto T. Case report: unusual cause of acute painful scrotal swelling. Malawi Med J 2005; 17:28.

Dakum K, Ramyil VM, Sani AA, Kidmas AT. The acute scrotum: aetiology, management and early outcome—preliminary report. Nigerian J Med 2005; 14:267–271.

Davenport M. ABC of general surgery in children: acute problems of the scrotum. BMJ 1996; 312:435–437.

Hegarty PK, Walsh E, Corcoran MO. Exploration of the acute scrotum: a retrospective analysis of 100 consecutive cases. Ir J Med Sc 2001; 170:181–182.

Kass EJ, Lunbak B. The acute scrotum. Pediatr Clin North Am 1997; 44:1251–1266.

Koester MC. Initial evaluation and management of acute scrotal pain. J Athletic Training 2000; 35:76–79.

Kuranga SA, Rahman GA. Testicular torsion: experience in the Middle Belt of Nigeria. Afr J Urol 2002; 8:78–82.

Makela E, Lahdes-Vasama T, Rajakorpi H, Wikstrom S. A 19-year review of paediatric patients with acute scrotum. Scand J Surg 2007; 96:62–66.

McAndrew H, Pemberton R, Kikiros C, Gollow I. The incidence and investigation of acute scrotal problems in children. Paediatr Surg Int 2002; 18:435–437.

Ugwu BT, Dakum NK, Yiltol SJ, et al. Testicular torsion on the Jos Plateau. West Afr Med J 2003; 2:120–123.

Watkin NA, Reiger NA, Moisey CU. Is the conservative management of acute scrotum justified on clinical grounds? Br J Urol 2003; 78:623–627.

TUMOURS

CHAPTER 102
KIDNEY TUMOURS

Sebastian O. Ekenze
Hugo A. Heij
George G. Youngson

Introduction

A variety of benign and malignant tumours can arise in the kidney in children. With minor variations, the spectrum of tumours has world-wide distribution. Wilms' tumour (WT; also known as nephroblastoma) is the most common kidney tumour in childhood, and may represent the most common abdominal tumour presenting in infants and children in sub-Saharan Africa. In the past decade, considerable advances have been made in the management and elucidation of the molecular biology of Wilms' tumour. Multidisciplinary collaboration has led to the forma-tion of cooperative study groups in Europe and North America, and has resulted in standardisation of treatment and a remarkable improvement in the outcome of this tumour.[1,2] The treatment of children with WT is considered the paradigm for management of most childhood tumours.

In Africa as well as some other developing countries, WT remains a challenge to the oncologist, with a significantly poorer outcome of treatment than in developed countries.[3-5]

This chapter highlights the demographics, aetiology, and pathology of this typical kidney tumour, followed by a presentation of the diagnosis, treatment, outcome, and challenges in Africa. A brief overview of other tumours of the kidney is also highlighted.

Demographics

The overall incidence of Wilms' tumour is 7.6 cases per million chil-dren younger than 15 years of age, or 1 case per 10,000 infants. In Africa, it accounts for about 4–26% of all malignant solid tumours in childhood.[6,7] The hospital-based reports suggest that 4 to 10 new cases of Wilms' tumour are seen every year in most tertiary referral cen-tres.[5,7–9] The incidence in Africa is probably underestimated, however, because some of the affected children are not brought to the attention of trained medical practitioners.[3]

There is no gender predilection; the peak age at presentation is 2–5 years.[3,5] Other malignant renal tumours (e.g., rhabdoid tumour of the kidney; clear cell carcinoma; renal cell carcinoma) occur in older children.

Aetiology/Pathology

In about 10% of the cases, WT is associated with congenital syndromes, for example:

- isolated hemihypertrophy;

- Beckwith-Wiedemann syndrome (visceromegaly, hypoglycaemia, macroglossia, midline defects);

- WAGR (an acronym for WT, Aniridia, Genito-urinary malforma-tions, mental Retardation); and

- Denys-Drash syndrome (protein-losing nephropathy, disorders of sexual development, WT).

These associations have led to the discovery of genetic mutations in WT. In WAGR patients, a deletion has been found on band p13 of chromosome 11, and it has been hypothesised that a Wilms' tumour suppressor gene, WT1, is located there. In Beckwith-Wiedemann patients, another deletion has been found on band p15 of chromosome 11, which has been designated as the WT2 gene. To date, there is no evidence that WT1 and WT2 are correlated with the prognosis, and research is ongoing in this field. Loss of heterozygosity of chromosome 16q has been observed in 15–20% of patients with WT and found to be associated with a 3.3 times higher relapse risk and a 12 times higher risk of death.[10]

The presence of embryonal nephrogenic rests (NR) increases the risk of developing WT. NR can be solitary or multiple (nephroblastomatosis). NR may regress, remain dormant, or become hyperplastic and progress to WT.

WT consists of three types of tissue: embryonal blastema, epithelial tissue, and mesenchymal tissue. Glassberg gives a thorough review on developmental aspects in relation to renal oncogenesis.[11]

According to the SIOP (Société Internationale d'Oncologie Pédiatrique) classification,[12] there are three risk categories for kidney tumours.

1. Low-risk tumours are mesoblastic nephroma and nephroblastoma that has become completely necrotic after chemotherapy (see the later section "When to Operate: NWTSG versus SIOP").

2. Intermediate-risk tumours are triphasic nephroblastoma, including those with focal anaplasia.

3. High-risk tumours are nephroblastoma with blastemal predominance or with diffuse anaplasia and other tumours such as clear cell sarcoma and rhabdoid tumour of the kidney.

Staging of WT in the SIOP and National Wilms' Tumour Study Group (NWTSG) protocol is established after surgery. SIOP staging is as follows:

Stage I:	tumours with an intact capsule that have been removed completely.
Stage II:	tumours with penetration of the capsule that have been removed completely without lymph node metastases.
Stage III:	tumours with microscopic residue, either because of rupture (before or during operation), intravas-cular extension, ingrowth into other organs that cannot be excised, or lymph node metastases.
Stage IV:	tumours with distant metastases, most common in the lungs but also in the liver or brain.
Stage V:	bilateral tumours, each of which should also be staged according to local characteristics.

The histological classification as well as clinico-pathological staging is correlated to the outcome. Hadley emphasized the relevance of this risk assessment in the Third World.[4] In the Western world, the prognosis for stage I and II with low- or intermediate-risk histology is excellent, with 95% survival.

Clinical Presentation

The main presentation is painless abdominal mass in an otherwise healthy child. The mass in the sub-Saharan African setting is in most cases of a considerable size (Figure 102.1). Other, less common presentations include weight loss, fever, haematuria, or hypertension. The presence of weight loss is common among African patients compared to caucasian children and may indicate an advanced stage of the disease at presentation.[3,5]

A significant number of children in Africa have delayed presentation. The average duration of symptoms before attendance to a mainstream hospital is reported to be 4.7 months.[3] This delay in presentation is related mainly to lack of knowledge or familiarity of the condition and resource deficiency. Some children may be taken initially by their parents to a herbalist and present to hospital only when there is no improvement with herbal treatment (Figure 102.2). The late presentation may thus be responsible for the unique distribution of the stages of the disease in Africa (Table 102.1).[3,7–9]

Table 102.1: Average distribution in Africa of the stages of Wilms' tumour at operation.

Stage of disease at operation	Average percentage
Stage I:	6.9
Stage II:	25.2
Stage III:	42.4
Stage IV:	22.9
Stage V:	2.6

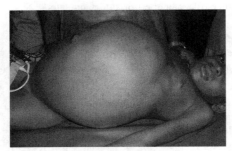

Figure 102.1: A 4-year-old girl presenting with a 6-month history of abdominal mass. At operation, a 6.5-kg left Wilms' tumour was excised.

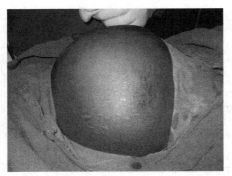

Figure 102.2: A 3-year-old boy with left Wilms' tumour. He presented with a 7-month history. The scarification was inflicted during herbal treatment.

In clinical evaluation of affected children, it may be necessary to exclude associated syndromes such as aniridia, hypospadias, macroglossia, intersex, and the recently described sex-linked Simpson-Golabi-Behmel syndrome (macroglossia, coarse facial features, viceromegaly, diaphragmatic and heart defects, and polydactyly).

Evaluation

Definition of the abdominal mass, status of the contralateral kidney, and involvement of surrounding or distant structures can be achieved with ultrasonography (US), intravenous urography (IVU), chest radiograph, computed tomography (CT), and magnetic resonance imaging (MRI). CT and MRI exceptionally characterise the tumour and the extent of spread, especially with respect to patients with intracaval involvement (Figure 102.3), and bilateral Wilms' tumour. Unfortunately, CT and MRI are not readily available in many centres in Africa. Surgeons working in those centres need a high index of suspicion and appreciation of the diagnostic findings on the readily available US, chest radiograph, and IVU. It is important to determine function on the contralateral kidney and to exclude other retroperitoneal tumours, and in the African setting this can be reasonably achieved by using IVU. A chest radiograph is required to exclude pulmonary metastasis.

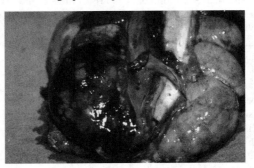

Figure 102.3: Autopsy specimen demonstrating extension of tumour along the right renal vein and into the inferior vena cava.

If any diagnostic uncertainty exists, needle biopsy (Trucut®) will help to confirm tissue diagnosis. This is particularly relevant in the evaluation of retroperitoneal masses to distinguish WT from Burkitt lymphoma.[13]

Treatment

Definitive treatment of Wilms' tumour involves surgery, chemotherapy, and radiotherapy. The treatment modalities used can be modified by stage of the disease, age of the patient, size of the tumour, and the clinical state of the patient. Prior to the commencement of therapy, it is imperative to correct anaemia and malnutrition, which are relatively common in the African setting.

Role of Surgery

Despite the advances in chemotherapy, surgery is still critical in the therapy of Wilms' tumour. Complete resection of the tumour and accurate staging of the disease, both of which are crucial in effecting cure, can be achieved only through surgery. Optimal outcome with surgery will require a generous transperitoneal incision, thorough exploration of the abdomen, biopsy of the lymph nodes in the renal hilum and along the vena cava or aorta, and nephroureterctomy. Migration of the tumour along the renal vein and into the vena cava requires proximal and distal venous control to permit temporary occlusion sufficient to allow removal of the intravascular tumour. Postoperative complications may include intestinal obstruction, haemorrhage, wound infection, and vascular injury.

Role of Chemotherapy

Based on a series of studies by NWTSG in North America and SIOP in Europe, standard chemotherapy regimens have been established. Effective agents currently in use include actinomycin-D, vincristine, cyclophosphamide, doxorubicin, iphosphamide, and etoposide. Unfortunately, these drugs are not readily available in some centres in Africa. Additionally, in a number of centres where the drugs are available, some patients may not be able to afford them.[3,5] These factors are considered responsible for poor compliance with therapy.

Chemotherapy can be administered preoperatively in all patients (SIOP) or in selected patients with solitary kidney, bilateral tumours, intravascular tumour extension, inoperable tumours, or tumour in a horseshoe kidney (NWTSG). Pretreatment biopsy may be necessary in these cases. Agents used include vincristine and actinomycin-D given weekly over a 4-week period.[14]

Adjuvant chemotherapy is advocated by all the protocols. Here the agents used and the duration of therapy depend on the stage of the disease and the histology of the tumour. Advanced stages and cases with unfavourable histology require more intense therapy (Table 102.2).

Role of Radiotherapy

Preoperative radiotherapy may be used to achieve the same effects as preoperative chemotherapy: minimise intraoperative tumour rupture; shrink huge tumours to respectable size; and preserve maximum renal parenchyma in bilateral, solitary, or horseshoe kidneys.

Postoperative radiotherapy has been shown to significantly reduce local recurrence in stages III and IV disease. Radiotherapy facilities and trained personnel are not available, however, in many centres in Africa. Some of the patients requiring this modality of treatment are therefore referred to centres where they are available. Because some of these centres are hundreds of miles away from the referral hospitals,

Table 102.2: Postoperative treatment commonly used for various stages of Wilms' tumour.

Stage of disease at operation	Optimal treatment
Stage I:	Vincistine, actinomycin-D
Stage II:	Vincristine, actinomycin-D
Stage III:	Vincristine, actinomycin-D, doxorubicin, x-ray therapy (XRT)
Stage IV:	Vincristine, actinomycin-D, doxorubicin, cyclophosphamide, XRT

compliance may be difficult to achieve.

When to Operate: NWTSG versus SIOP

Whereas SIOP promotes the use of preoperative chemotherapy or radiotherapy for all cases of Wilms' tumour, NWTSG advocates preoperative therapy for only a select category of patients. Issues such as lack of staging information, modification of tumour histology, and potential for inappropriate use of chemotherapy in nonmalignant disease have been raised against the routine preoperative treatment.[15] A critical appraisal[9,16] of the clinical state of cases in Africa suggests that this SIOP protocol may indeed be suited for the African setting. Some centres have reported better outcome with SIOP protocol when compared with immediate nephrectomy.[8,9,16] Israels and Molyneaux have published several papers on this subject based on Malawi data.[17]

Prognosis and Outcome

In the West, the prognosis depends on the stage and histology (see the section "Aetiology/Pathology" for risk classification), but in Africa additional factors are equally important: nutritional and general condition of the child, comorbidity, availability of chemotherapy and radiotherapy, and compliance with completion of postoperative treatment. Some paediatric surgeons therefore advocate keeping these children in hospital from the start of preoperative chemotherapy until they have finished the postoperative courses.

Challenges in Africa

The results of treatment of WT in most centres in Africa are poor, with an overall survival of less than 50%. Although a few centres have reported overall survival approaching 70%, numerous challenges confront the management of this tumour in Africa. Prominent among these is late presentation, inadequate facilities and trained personnel, and

poor compliance to therapy. Lack of multidisciplinary collaboration, inadequate drug supply, and comorbidity (human immunodeficiency virus/ acquired immune deficiency syndrome (HIV/AIDS), tuberculosis (TB)) may also play an important role.[4]

Prevention

There is no primary prevention for WT, but early detection is an important tool to improve outcome. Routine screening of patients with relevant syndromes (such as Beckwith-Wiedemann or WAGR) and immediate investigation of patients with abdominal masses have to be advocated by surgeons to paediatricians, general practitioners, underfive clinics staff, and other health care workers.

Ethical Issues

The balance between cost and benefit in WT in Africa is delicate. Expensive diagnostic procedures and drugs, sophisticated surgery, and extended postoperative treatment will place a heavy burden on the resources of the family and the country. However, in view of the good prognosis in children with stage I or II WT and favourable histology, an active surgical approach is commended. More debatable are patients with advanced disease, relapses, or with severe comorbidity (TB, HIV) because these patients will not only need more treatment but also have less of a chance of survival.

Other Kidney Tumours

With the exception of Burkitt lymphoma, the other tumours found in the kidney are extremely rare in Africa. They include mesoblastic nephroma, cystic nephroma, clear cell sarcoma, malignant rhabdoid tumour, renal cell carcinoma, and renal teratoma. These can be distinguished by histology of biopsy specimen. Sometimes differentiating between WT and retroperitoneal Burkitt may be challenging, especially in parts of Africa where Burkitt is endemic.[13] Definitive treatment is in accordance with the histology of the tumour. Burkitt lymphoma can be managed exclusively with chemotherapy with good outcome. The outcome of treatment for the other tumours is variable. For mesoblastic and cystic nephroma, the prognosis is quite good if completely excised. In contrast, the outlook for clear cell sarcoma and rhabdoid tumours is rather dismal; even with multimodal treatment.[18]

Evidence-Based Research

Table 102.3 presents the results of the 9th SIOP Wilms' tumour trial and study on the optimal duration of preoperative chemotherapy in Wilms' tumour.

Table 102.3: Evidence-based research.

Title	Optimal duration of pre-operative therapy in unilateral and nonmetastatic Wilms' tumour in children older than 6 months: Results of the Ninth International Society of Pediatric Oncology Wilms' tumour trial and study
Authors	Tournade MF, Com-Nougue C, de Kraker J, et al
Institution	SIOP
Reference	J Clin Oncol 2001; 19:488–500
Problem	Optimal duration of preoperative chemotherapy in WT.
Intervention	4 weeks vincristine and actinomycin-D.
Comparison/ control (quality of evidence)	8 weeks vincristine and actinomycin-D.
Outcome/ effect	No difference in event-free or overall survival.
Historical significance/ comments	Demonstrates that in Western settings, 4 weeks of chemotherapy is sufficient. Longer treatment may be associated with more complications.

Key Summary Points

1. Cytological or histological (needle biopsy) diagnosis of abdominal tumours in Africa may be an imperative addition to ultrasonography.

2. Preoperative chemotherapy will enable reduction of the bulk of most Wilms' tumours (WT), thereby reducing the risk of surgical complications, in particular tumour rupture.

3. The optimal duration of preoperative chemotherapy in Africa has yet to be established.

4. Surgery remains the only certain way to cure WT, and surgical technique is of utmost importance.

5. Every effort has to be made to complete the postoperative treatment.

6. Multidisciplinary, and multiinstitutional collaborations may help to standardise treatment in Africa.

References

1. Spreafico F, Bellani FF. Wilms' tumour: past. present, and (possibly) future. Expert Rev Anticancer Ther 2006; 6:249–258.

2. Gommersall LM, Arya M, Mushtaq I, Duffy P. Current challenges in Wilms' tumour management. Nat Clin Pract Oncol 2005; 2:298–304.

3. Ekenze SO, Agugua-Obianyo NE, Odetunde O. The challenge of nephroblastoma in a developing country. Ann Oncol 2006; 17:1598–1600.

4. Hadley GP, Govender D, Landers G. Wilms' tumour with unfavourable histology: implications for clinicians in the Third World. Med Pediatr Oncol 2001; 36:652–653.

5. Abuidris DO, Elimam ME, Nugud FM. Wilms tumour in Sudan. Pediatr Blood Cancer 2008; 50:1135–1137.

6. Nkanza NK. Paediatric solid malignant tumours in Zimbabwe. Cent Afr J Med 1989; 35:496–501.

7. Aguehounde C, da Silva-Anoma S, Roux C. Nephroblastoma at the hospital unit in Abidjan. Apropos of 60 cases. J Urol (Paris) 1994; 100:196–199.

8. Rogers T, Bowley DM, Poole J, et al. Experience and outcomes of nephroblastoma in Johannesburg, 1998–2003. Eur J Pediatr Surg 2007; 17:41–44.

9. Amel L, Leila BF, Lamia K, et al. Histologic and prognostic study of nephroblastoma in central Tunisia. Ann Urol (Paris) 2003; 37:164–169.

10. Grundy PE, Breslow NE, Li S, et al. Loss of heterozygosity for chromosomes 16q and 1p is an adverse prognostic factor in favorable-histology Wilms' tumour. J Clin Oncol 2005; 23:7312–7321.

11. Glassberg KI. Normal and abnormal development of the kidney: a clinician's interpretation of current knowledge. J Urol 2002; 167:2339–2351.

12. Vujanic GM, Sandstedt B, Harms D, et al. Revised International Society of Paediatric Oncology (SIOP) working classification of renal tumours of childhood. Med Pediatr Oncol 2002; 38:79–82.

13. Wilde JC, Lameris W, van Hasselt EH, et al. Challenges and outcome of Wilms' tumour management in a resource-constrained setting. Afr J Paediatr Surg 2010; 7:159–162.

14. Tournade MF, Com-Nougue C, de Kraker J, et al. Optimal duration of pre-operative therapy in unilateral and nonmetastatic Wilms' tumour in children older than 6 months: results of the ninth International Society of Pediatric Oncology Wilms' tumour trial and study. J Clin Oncol 2001; 19:488–500.

15. Zoeller G, Pekrun A, Lakomek M, Ringert RH. Wilms' tumour: the problem of diagnostic accuracy in children undergoing preoperative chemotherapy without histological tumour verification. J Urol 1994; 151:169–171.

16. Madani A, Zafad S, Harif M, et al. Treatment of Wilms tumour according to SIOP 9 protocol in Casablanca, Morocco. Pediatr Blood Cancer 2006; 46:472–475.

17. Israëls T, Molyneux EM, Caron HN, et al. Preoperative chemotherapy for patients with Wilms tumor in Malawi is feasible and efficacious. Pediatr Blood and Cancer 2009; 53(4):584–589.

18. Shamberger RC. Renal tumours. In: Carachi R, Grosfeld JL. Azmy AF. The Surgery of Childhood Tumours. Springer, 2008, Ch 10, Pp 171–199.

CHAPTER 103
TERATOMAS

Shilpa Sharma
Devendra K Gupta
Jean-Martin Laberge
Kokila Lakhoo

Introduction

The term teratoma, derived from the Greek *teraton* meaning "a monster", was coined by Virchow in 1869 for a tumour originating in the sacrococcygeal region. Teratomas are composed of multiple tissues foreign to the organ or site in which they arise. Although teratomas are sometimes defined as having the three embryonic layers (endoderm, mesoderm, and ectoderm), recent classifications also include monodermal types.

The term germ cell tumour (GCT) is also frequently used to describe these tumours, although this term encomprises a larger group including the mature and the immature teratomas, germinomas, embryonal carcinomas, yolk sac tumours, and choriocarcinomas. The germ cell tumours may arise in the gonads or in extragonadal sites, including the brain, face, neck, mediastinum, retroperitoneum, and sacrococcygeal region.

Aetiology

Three theories are postulated for the aetiology of teratomas. The first theory supports the origin from the totipotent primordial germ cells. These cells develop among the endodermal cells of the yolk sac near the origin of the allantois and migrate to the gonadal ridges during weeks 4 and 5 of gestation. Some cells may miss their target destination and give rise to a teratoma anywhere from the brain to the coccygeal area, usually in the midline. The second theory has teratomas arising from remnants of the primitive node. During week 3 of gestational development, midline cells at the caudal end of the embryo divide rapidly, giving rise to all three germ layers of the embryo. By the end of week 3, the primitive streak shortens and disappears. This theory would explain the more common occurrence of teratomas in the sacrococcygeal region. The third theory has teratomas as an incomplete twinning.

Classification

Teratomas are anatomically classified as gonadal (testis or ovary) or extragonadal (brain, face, neck, mediastinum, retroperitoneum, and sacrococcygeal region). Histologically, teratomas are classified as mature or immature on the basis of the presence of the immature neuroectodermal elements within the tumour. Mature teratomas comprise only mature elements, such as the skin, hair, fat tissue, cartilage, bone, and glands. Immature teratomas contain immature elements, such as neuroepithelial tissue and immature mesenchyme. The presence of microscopic foci of the yolk sac tumour, rather than the histological grade of immaturity, is a valid predictor of recurrence. The grading of immature teratomas is unnecessary in children because the management is not altered by the grade.

Teratomas may also contain or develop foci of malignancy; and a malignant germ cell tumour may be found in sites typical for teratomas, such as the mediastinum or sacrococcygeal area. Whether the lesion was malignant from the onset or the malignant cells destroyed and replaced the benign teratoma component is often difficult to differentiate. The most common malignant component within a teratoma is a yolk sac tumour. Malignancy at birth is uncommon, but increases with age and with incomplete resection. An apparently mature teratoma may recur several months or years after resection as a malignant yolk sac tumour, illustrating the difficulties in histologic sampling of large tumours and the need for close follow-up.

Tumour Markers

Alpha-fetoprotein (AFP) is a tumour marker secreted by most yolk sac tumours and some embryonal carcinomas. It can be measured in the serum and noted in cells by immunohistochemistry. This marker is particularly useful for assessing the presence of residual or recurrent disease. AFP levels are normally very high in neonates and decrease with time. The postoperative half-life is about 6 days. Persistently high levels may be an indication of the need for further surgical procedures or chemotherapy. Other markers that may be elevated are β-human chorionic gonadotropin (β-hCG), produced by choriocarcinomas, and, rarely, carcinoembryonic antigen. The lactate dehydrogenase (LDH) isomer of LDH-1 is present in many tumours with the histologic features of an endodermal sinus tumour, yolk sac tumour, dysgerminoma, and choriocarcinoma.

Genetics

The genetic basis for teratomas is not well understood, and the clinical usefulness of chromosome mapping for teratomas is unclear. Deletions on chromosomes 1 and 6 were reported in children but noted on chromosome 12 in adults. N-myc gene expression was noted in immature teratomas, but not in the mature group.

Associated Anomalies

Teratomas are mainly isolated lesions but may form part of the Currarino triad (anorectal malformation, sacral anomaly, and a presacral mass) as the presacral mass. Other associated anomalies reported are urogenital (hypospadias, vesicoureteral reflux, and vaginal or uterine duplications); congenital dislocation of the hip; central nervous system lesions (anencephaly, trigonocephaly, Dandy-Walker malformations, spina bifida, and myelomeningocele); Klinefelter syndrome (strongly associated with mediastinal teratoma); and the very rare associations with trisomy 13, trisomy 21, Morgagni hernia, congenital heart defects, Beckwith-Wiedemann syndrome, pterygium, cleft lip and palate; as well as such rare syndromes as the Proteus and Schinzel-Giedion syndromes.

Tumour Sites

Testicular Teratoma

Teratomas of the testes are the most common type of benign neoplasms, usually occurring in boys under 3 years of age. These tumours can be managed successfully with radical orchiectomy and do not require any adjunctive treatment. Small encapsulated cystic teratomas may also be enucleated much like their ovarian counterpart (see the next subsection); the cord should be occluded atraumatically until a frozen section confirms the benign nature of the lesion. However, for the purpose of treatment, all testicular tumours should be assumed malignant unless proven otherwise on histopathology.

The operation is performed through a groin incision.

1. The external inguinal ring is identified and the inguinal canal incised to identify the internal ring.

2. The cremasteric bundle is opened, the spermatic cord is carefully mobilised at the internal inguinal ring, and it is controlled by an occlusive vascular clamp. This prevents lymphatic and haematogenous spread of the tumour during manipulation.

3. The testis is delivered into the wound, and if the mass is solid, a radical orchiectomy is completed with ligation of the spermatic cord at the level of the internal ring.

4. If the malignant tumour was biopsied through the scrotum before referral, a hemiscrotectomy is generally performed, although recent evidence suggests that chemotherapy could adequately treat tumour seeding.

Ovarian Teratoma

Mature teratoma, a benign neoplasm, is the single most common ovarian tumour, representing approximately 40% of all ovarian tumours. It may be cystic, solid, or mixed with calcification (noted in 50% of cases on plain abdominal radiograph). Ten percent are bilateral.

Abdominal pain, the presence of a mass, and occasionally an acute abdomen as a result of torsion or rupture of the tumour are known clinical presentations. Some are discovered incidentally with imaging. Tumours that are predominantly cystic (dermoid cysts) may be safely excised, preserving a rim of normal ovarian tissue. Controversy exists about the safety of laparoscopic excision because rupture of the cyst often occurs, leading to potential peritoneal implantation of cells. Solid teratomas are more often immature, and the treatment of choice is salpingo-oophorectomy. Chemotherapy is reserved for tumours with a higher grade of immaturity. Serum AFP levels may be elevated preoperatively and should be monitored after operation. In such cases, careful sectioning of the specimen may reveal microscopic foci of a yolk sac tumour; this does not alter management as long as AFP levels return to normal.

Sacrococcygeal Teratoma

Sacrococcygeal teratoma is the most common congenital tumour, accounting for 35–60% of all teratomas. The estimated incidence is 1 per 35,000 to 40,000 live births, with a female-to-male ratio of 4:1. Altman et al. have classified these tumours into four types:

• Type I tumours are predominantly external with a minimal presacral component—this is the most common type.

• Type II tumours are external but have a significant intrapelvic component.

• Type III tumours are external but pelvic and extend significantly into the abdomen.

• Type IV tumours are entirely presacral.

Recently, an increasing number of sacrococcygeal teratomas have been detected by antenatal ultrasonography (US) examination of the fetus. Prenatal US is useful in making a differential diagnosis between sacrococcygeal teratoma, myelomeningocele, and other tumours. Antenatal US helps to establish tumour extension into the pelvis and the presence or absence of polyhydramnios, foetal hydrops, and intratumoural haemorrhage. Massive haemorrhage into the tumour may occur spontaneously in utero, resulting in anaemia and hypoproteinaemia followed by foetal hydrops.

In countries where prenatal US is not readily available, a sacrococcygeal teratoma is seen as a visible mass at birth, making the diagnosis obvious (Figure 103.1). Although many neonates with sacrococcygeal teratomas do not have symptoms, some require intensive care because of prematurity, high-output cardiac failure, disseminated intravascular coagulation, and tumour rupture or bleeding within the

tumour. Lesions with a large intrapelvic component may cause urinary obstruction. Besides looking for signs of a myelomeningocele, the physical examination should always include a rectal examination to evaluate any intrapelvic component. The most useful imaging is a US scan looking for intrapelvic extension and meningomyelocoele. The diagnosis of purely intrapelvic teratomas is often delayed. Children have constipation, urinary retention, an abdominal mass, or symptoms of malignancy such as failure to thrive.

Age is a predictor of malignancy in sacrococcygeal teratomas. The risk of malignancy is <10% at birth but >75% after the age of 1 year for sacrococcygeal tumours (Figure 103.2), with the exception of familial presacral teratomas. The risk of malignancy also is high for incompletely excised lesions. Complete excision of the tumour with the coccyx should be carried out as soon as the neonate is stable enough to undergo the procedure. An abdominoperineal approach may be necessary for tumours with pelvic extension. Serum markers (AFP and β-hCG) should be determined before the operation for later comparison.

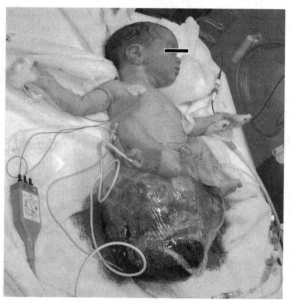

Figure 103.1: Giant ruptured sacrococcygeal teratoma.

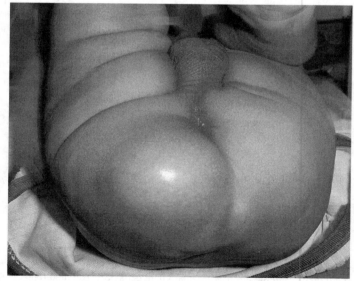

Figure 103.2: Malignant sacrococcygeal teratoma presenting at 3 months of age.

Postoperatively, it is important to monitor all patients with physical examination, including rectal examination and serum markers, every 2 or 3 months for at least 3 years, because most recurrences occur within 3 years of operation.

In older patients, treatment of malignant tumours involves excision, chemotherapy, and monitoring with imaging studies and serum markers. For unresectable tumours, biopsy and chemotherapy are followed by excision of the primary tumour after adequate reduction has been obtained. Radiation therapy is usually reserved for local recurrence of malignant tumours. Patients with malignant tumours should be enrolled in a paediatric cooperative study or treated according to their guidelines.

Poor prognosis is noted in prenatal hydrops, dystocia, tumour rupture, prematurity, highly vascular lesions, and lesions >10 cm. In the absence of severe prematurity and intrapartum complications, the prognosis is dependent on the presence of malignancy and is therefore related to age at operation, completeness of resection, tumour type, and tumour stage.

Functional results in survivors are excellent in most patients, with the exception of reports of faecal and urinary continence problems as well as lower limb weakness in some series.

Mediastinal Teratoma

The mediastinum is the second most frequent site of extragonadal teratomas. Mediastinal teratomas occur in newborns to adolescents, and arise predominantly in the anterior mediastinum, occasionally in the posterior mediastinum, and rarely in the pericardial and intracardiac region. Mediastinal teratomas typically manifest on computed tomography (CT) scans as a heterogeneous mass containing soft tissue, fluid, fat, or calcification. Some patients are asymptomatic, and diagnosis is made incidentally on chest x-ray. However, affected children usually manifest symptoms such as dyspnea, cough, or chest pain. When the tumour causes severe respiratory distress in neonates, mimicking congenital diaphragmatic hernia, emergency surgery to relieve lung compression and postoperative care supporting respiration are required. Surgical approaches to mediastinal teratomas are either lateral thoracotomy or median sternotomy; the latter is necessary in some patients with large, bilaterally invasive lesions. Small lesions have been resected by using video-assisted thoracic surgery (VATS). Large lesions may cause airway compromise and require intubation and care in the intensive care unit. Many of these large tumours are best managed with initial biopsy, neoadjuvant chemotherapy, and delayed complete resection.

Other sites for thoracic teratomas are intrapericardial, cardiac, and pulmonary.

Gastric Teratomas

Gastric teratomas (Figure 103.3) are rare tumours, accounting for less than 2% of abdominal teratomas and 1% of all teratomas. They occur mainly in neonatal boys and are almost always benign in nature with an excellent prognosis. The tumour is predominantly exogastric (67%). The endogastric type (33%) grows into the lumen of the stomach and erodes mucosa, causing gastric outlet obstruction, haematemesis, and melaena. The exogastric type is an exophytic mass in the lesser curvature or posterior wall of the stomach; the entire stomach may be involved. The exogastric variant may present with respiratory distress and abdominal distention. Diagnostic modalities include plain radiograph, US, CT scan, and serum markers. Plain radiograph may show a soft tissue mass with calcification in the upper abdomen. Surgical excision is curative. Recurrence and malignancy are rare, despite local infiltration or nodal metastasis. Periodic follow-up, including AFP measurements, is important.

Other rare sites of abdominal teratomas include liver, gallbladder, pancreas, kidney, intestine, bladder, prostate, uterus, mesentery, omentum, abdominal wall, and diaphragm.

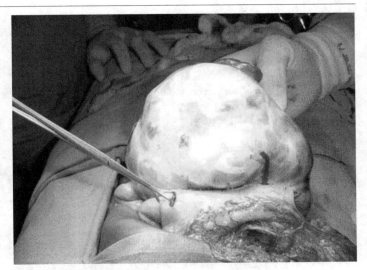

Figure 103.3: Gastric teratoma.

Retroperitoneal Teratomas

Retroperitoneal teratomas represent 5% of all childhood teratomas and occur outside the pelvis in the suprarenal location.The tumour presents as an abdominal mass with symptoms of vomiting and constipation. Diagnosis is made by imaging with calcification on plain radiograph, US, CT scan, and serum markers. Surgical excision is often easily performed, and malignancy is uncommon. The retroperitoneum site is the most common for the foetus in foetu malformations.

Intracranial Teratomas

Intracranial teratomas generally present with symptoms of space-occupying lesions. These lesions account for only 2–4% of all teratomas, but they represent nearly 50% of brain tumours in the first 2 months of life. Most are benign in neonates but malignant in older children and young adults. These teratomas can appear in utero and cause massive hydrocephalus. The pineal gland is the most common site of origin, but intracranial teratomas may be seen in different areas, such as the hypothalamus, ventricles, cavernous sinus, cerebellum, and suprasellar region.

Cervical Teratomas

Cervical teratomas represent up to 8% of all teratomas. Large tumours can be seen in utero with US. These tumours are initially seen as a partly or completely cystic neck mass, which may compromise the airway and require immediate intubation or tracheostomy. Extension of the tumour to the mediastinum or displacement of the trachea may cause pulmonary hypoplasia and increase respiratory morbidity and mortality. The tumour is usually well defined and may contain calcifications. The differential diagnosis includes cystic hygroma, congenital goiter, foregut duplication cyst, and branchial cleft cyst. Investigation should include plain radiographs, US, and measurement of AFP and β-hCG, as well as urinary catecholamine metabolites. CT and magnetic resonance imaging (MRI) may be useful to establish the diagnosis and to define the anatomic relations.

Craniofacial Teratomas

Craniofacial teratomas include a spectrum of lesions that may be life threatening. The spectrum includes epignathus (teratoma from palate), orbital, pharyngeal, oropharyngeal, and middle ear teratomas.

Miscellaneous Sites

Teratomas have been reported in other sites, such as the skin, parotid, vulva, perianal region well away from the coccyx, spinal canal, umbilical cord (possibly associated with omphalocele), and placenta.

Key Summary Points

1. Teratomas comprise multiple tissues foreign to the organ or site in which they arise.

2. Most teratomas are benign and have excellent surgical outcomes.

3. Sacrococcygeal teratoma is the most common neonatal tumour with a worst prognosis in delayed presentation and recurrence.

4. Serum tumour markers assist in the diagnosis of recurrent tumours.

References

Altman RP, Randolph JG, Lilly JR. Sacrococcygeal teratoma: American Academy of Pediatrics Surgical Section survey. J Pediatr Surg 1974; 9:389–398.

Azizkhan RG, Haase GM, Applebaum H, Dillon PW, Coran AG, King PA, King DR, Hodge DS. Diagnosis, management, and outcome of cervicofacial teratomas in neonates: a Children's Cancer Group study. J Pediatr Surg 1995; 30:312–316.

Basu S, Rubello D. PET imaging in the management of tumours of testis and ovary: current thinking and future directions. Minerva Endocrinol 2008; 33:229–256.

Bernbeck B, Schneider DT, Bernbeck B, Koch S, Teske C, Lentrodt J, Harms D, Göbel U, Calaminus G, on behalf of the MAKE Study Group. Germ cell tumours of the head and neck: report from the MAKEI Study Group. Pediatr Blood Cancer 2008; 52:223–226.

Certo M, Franca M, Gomes M, Machado R. Liver teratoma. Acta Gastroenterol Belg 2008; 71:275–279.

Chaganti RSK, Rodriguez E, Mathew S. Origin of adult male mediastinal germ-cell tumours. Lancet 1994; 343:1130–1132.

Chen Y, Xu H, Li Y, Li J, Wang D, Yuan J, Liang Z. Laparoscopic resection of presacral teratomas. J Minim Invasive Gynecol 2008; 15:649–651.

Gupta DK, Carachi R, eds. Pediatric Oncology—Surgical and Medical Aspects. Jaypee Brothers, 2007.

Gupta DK, Kataria R, Sharma MC. Prepubertal testicular teratomas. Eur J Pediatr Surg 1999; 9:173–176.

Gupta DK, Sharma S. Granulosa cell tumour of the ovary. In: Gupta DK, Carachi R, eds. Pediatric Oncology—Surgical and Medical Aspects. Jaypee Brothers, 2007, Chap 30, Pp 308–316.

Gupta DK, Sharma S, Carachi R. Neonatal tumours. In: Gupta DK, Carachi R, eds. Pediatric Oncology—Surgical and Medical Aspects. Jaypee Brothers, 2007. Chap 11, Pp 48–57.

Herman TE, Siegel MJ. Congenital gastric teratoma. J Perinatol 2008; 28:786–787.

Ikeda H, Tsuchida Y. Germ cell tumours. In: Gupta DK, Carachi R, eds. Pediatric Oncology—Surgical and Medical Aspects. Jaypee Brothers, 2007, Chap 27, Pp 271–286.

Ishiguro T, Tsuchida Y. Clinical significance of serum alpha-fetoprotein subfractionation in pediatric diseases. Acta Paediatr 1994; 83:709–713.

Kaplan GW, Cromie WC, Kelalis PP, Silber I, Tank ES. Prepubertal yolk sac testicular tumours: report of the Testicular Tumour Registry. J Urol 1988; 140:1109–1112.

Noudel R, Vinchon M, Dhellemmes P, Litré CF, Rousseaux P. Intracranial teratomas in children: the role and timing of surgical removal. J Neurosurg Pediatr 2008; 2:331–338.

Rintala R, Lahdenne P, Lindahl H, Siimes M, Heikinheimo M. Anorectal function in adults operated for a benign sacrococcygeal teratoma. J Pediatr Surg 1993; 28:1165–1167.

Shimizu K, Nakata M, Hirami Y, Akiyama T, Tanemoto K. Teratoma with malignant transformation in the anterior mediastinum. J Thorac Cardiovasc Surg 2008; 136:225–227.

Swamy R, Embleton N, Hale J. Sacrococcygeal teratoma over two decades: birth prevalence, prenatal diagnosis and clinical outcomes. Prenat Diagn 2008; 28:1048–1051.

Treiyer A, Blanc G, Stark E, Haben B, Treiyer E, Steffens J. Prepubertal testicular tumours: frequently overlooked. J Pediatr Urol 2007; 3:480–483.

CHAPTER 104
LYMPHOMAS

Larry Hadley
Kokila Lakhoo

Introduction

Lymphoma is a generic term used to describe malignant expansion of any of the lymphoid cell series. The nosology of lymphoma is an evolving science with clinical, morphological, and phenotypic studies contributing to the final diagnosis. The historical classification of lymphomas based purely upon morphological appearances under the light microscope has led to confusion and had little prognostic significance, so the Revised Euro-American Lymphoma (REAL) classification is in current use,[1] albeit modified by the World Health Organisation (WHO) to include cytogenetic factors.[2]

Currently, about 15% of lymphomas are regarded as Hodgkin's disease, defined by the presence of Reed-Sternberg cells on light microscopy, and the remaining 85% as non-Hodgkin's lymphoma (NHL). NHL may stem from cells that have B-cell or T-cell, including natural killer (NK) cell, lineage. Amongst NHL, B-cell phenotypes account for about 85% of the diagnosed cases, and within Africa, Burkitt lymphoma is the most common B-cell tumour. REAL divides lymphomas into high-, intermediate-, and low-grade tumours, giving prognostic information that is of value. Burkitt lymphoma is regarded as a high-grade tumour and is one of the fastest-growing neoplasms known, with a tumour doubling time of between 24 and 48 hours.[3]

Aetiology/Pathophysiology

The transformation of cellular behaviour from "normal" to a pattern that we recognise as "malignant" occurs when the genes controlling cellular behaviour are altered in some way. In lymphoid cells, this commonly occurs as a result of chromosomal translocations (e.g., t(8;14) in Burkitt lymphoma, in which a proto-oncogene *cmyc* is moved from its normal site on chromosome 8 to a site on chromosome 14), chromosomal deletions, or oncogenic viruses.

There is a strong association between the Epstein-Barr virus (EBV) and endemic Burkitt lymphoma; although a causal relationship is not certain, EBV antigen can be detected in up to 90% of children affected by Burkitt lymphoma. Many viruses may, through chronic antigenic stimulation, result in chronic B-cell proliferation, thereby increasing the probability of spontaneous chromosomal aberration. It is possible that the origin of the genomic injuries in endemic Burkitt lymphoma is more complex, involving malaria, EBV, arborviruses,[4] and possibly also plant products.[5]

In only 15% of patients with sporadic Burkitt lymphoma seen outside Central Africa is there an associated EBV infection. Sporadic Burkitt lymphoma also has a different pattern of presentation but is histologically identical to the endemic form. It is likely that sporadic Burkitt lymphoma is a disease different from the African form that shares a similar cellular morphology.

Within each subgroup of NHL, cell size and pattern of growth (nodular or diffuse) reflect the gene products of the altered genome, and these in turn determine the innate aggression of the tumour. Anatomical staging also contributes to treatment decisions.

In Africa, the human immunodeficiency virus (HIV) pandemic has greatly altered the epidemiology of lymphoma, resulting in a considerable increase in primary cerebral lymphoma and a substantial increase in the numbers of patients with B-cell NHL.[6,7] Burkitt lymphoma is regarded as an acquired immune deficiency syndrome (AIDS)-defining disease in HIV-infected individuals.[8] HIV-related Burkitt lymphoma seems to be biologically closer to sporadic Burkitt than to the endemic form and is less responsive to chemotherapy, even for those patients in whom the HIV status allows full chemotherapy doses.[3]

Clinical Presentation

Patients with lymphoma may present with the following symptoms:
- Lymphadenopathy similar to tuberculosis
- Mediastinal mass
- Pleural effusion
- Splenomegaly
- Maxillary mass (Burkitt lymphoma)
- Right iliac fossa mass
- Intussusception
- Bowel obstruction
- Bowel perforation
- Fever, weight loss, night sweats
- Pel-Ebstein fever

Hodgkin's lymphoma is primarily a disease of lymph nodes, and the clinical presentation largely depends upon which group of nodes is predominantly affected. The classical presentation is of painless lymph node swelling that proceeds to displace structures and may reach massive proportions, causing secondary pressure effects (Figures 104.1–104.3).

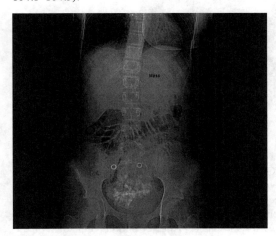

Figure 104.1: Abdominal radiograph with a mass.

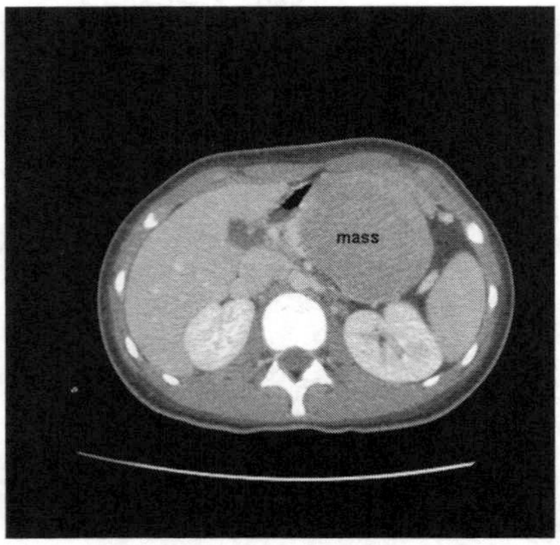

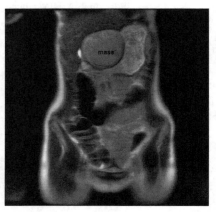

Figure 104.2: Abdominal computed tomography (CT) scan with a mass.

Figure 104.3: Abdominal magnetic resonance imaging (MRI) with a mass.

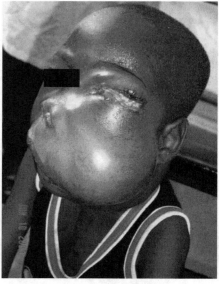

Figure 104.4: Burkitt lymphoma.

In NHL, extra-nodal disease is common and is often related to the gastrointestinal (GI) tract or other lymphoid organs, such as the spleen. Lymphoblastic lymphoma, which is difficult to differentiate from a lymphoblastic leukaemia, typically presents with a mediastinal mass or pleural effusion.

In Equatorial Africa, the classic picture of Burkitt lymphoma (Figure 104.4) is of a rapidly growing jaw or maxillary tumour in a small child under the age of 5 years. Additional abdominal disease is seen in about half of the patients. Endemic Burkitt lymphoma rarely presents as a right iliac fossa mass that can be confused with an inflammatory lesion, but intestinal involvement can provoke intussusception, intestinal obstruction, and occasionally intestinal perforation, although these symptoms are more common in sporadic cases. However, the pattern of disease presentation varies widely across relatively small geographic areas, suggesting that environmental factors may play a role.[9]

Constitutional symptoms of fever, weight loss, and night sweats, known as B symptoms, are associated with extensive extranodal disease and a poorer prognosis, irrespective of the lymphoma subtype.[10] B symptoms are more commonly present in patients with HIV-related lymphoma. The well-known Pel-Ebstein fever seen occasionally in patients with Hodgkin's lymphoma is simply a B symptom with a name.

Investigation and Staging

Appropriate treatment can only follow tissue diagnosis and accurate staging. Because the intranodal pattern of growth still has an important bearing on classification, an entire node should be submitted for examination. Fine needle aspirates and needle biopsies give limited information, but they may suffice in areas where more detailed studies are not available or are irrelevant to management decisions. In children with jaw tumours clinically thought to be Burkitt lymphoma, the diagnosis can often be confirmed by removing one of the free-floating teeth that are characteristic of the lesion. Usually this can be achieved without an operation, as the tooth can be extracted digitally, and the tissue attached to the tooth is adequate for diagnosis.

Cytogenetic studies allow lymphoma to be categorised more precisely, but therapeutic decisions can be made on morphological assessment alone combined with clinical staging. The St. Jude modification of the Ann Arbor Hodgkin's staging system based on clinical assessment, plain radiology, and ultrasound (Table 104.1) can be applied to NHL.

Burkitt lymphoma should be staged according to the Uganda Cancer Institute staging system. This reflects the high incidence of abdominal disease, even in patients presenting primarily with jaw disease, and recognises the effect of complete surgical resection when this is possible (Table 104.2).

All lymphomas should further be categorised as to the presence or absence of B symptoms. The presence of B symptoms should be signified by an addition of the suffix "B" after the stage shown in Table 104.1. If present, B symptoms would justify an increase in treatment intensity.

Table 104.1: St. Jude modification of the Ann Arbor staging system for non-Hodgkin's lymphoma.

Stage	Description
Stage 1	• Single nodal or extranodal tumour, excluding the mediastinum and abdomen
Stage 2	• Single extranodal tumour with regional lymph nodes affected
	• Primary gastrointestinal tract disease; regional nodes may or may not be affected
	• Lymphoma in two or more areas of lymph nodes on the same side of the diaphragm
Stage 2R	• Primary abdominal tumour that has been completely removed by surgery
Stage 3	• Two single extranodal tumours on opposite sides of the diaphragm
	• Origin in the lungs, chest, or thymus gland
	• Two or more nodal areas affected on opposite sides of the diaphragm
Stage 3A	• Abdominal tumour only that cannot be removed by surgery
Stage 3B	• Tumour affecting more than one organ within the abdomen
Stage 4	• Any of the above, plus—at the time of diagnosis—the central nervous system (CNS; brain and spinal cord) and/or the bone marrow also affected

Table 104.2: Uganda Cancer Institute staging system for Burkitt lymphoma.

Stage	Description
Stage A	• Single extraabdominal tumour
Stage AR	• Completely resected abdominal tumour without extraabdominal disease
Stage B	• Multiple extraabdominal tumours
Stage C	• Intraabdominal tumour with or without a single jaw tumour
Stage D	• Intraabdominal tumour with extraabdominal sites other than a single jaw tumour

Serum lactate dehydrogenase (LDH) is a useful marker of tumour activity and can be measured serially to assess response to treatment. Most high-risk lymphomas have initially high levels of LDH; a rapid fall reflects tumour responsiveness and is associated with a more favourable prognosis.[11]

Treatment

The actual treatment of lymphoma does not usually involve the surgeon, as it is based primarily on chemotherapy with selective use of radiotherapy. The surgeon may be involved in the diagnosis of lymphoma, particularly in differentiating between tuberculosis nodal enlargement and lymphoma in the HIV-positive child, the definition and resection of localised intraabdominal disease, as well as in the management of complications of either the disease itself or its treatment.

High-grade lymphomas, by virtue of their rapid cell proliferation, generally respond well—often dramatically—to chemotherapy. Indeed, the rapidity of cell death after initiating treatment may present the kidney with unmanageable quantities of purines, pyrimidines, phosphate, and other cellular detritus, leading to tumour lysis syndrome. Oncology treatment protocols should include measures, such as prophylactic urate oxidase, hyperhydration, and urine alkalinisation[12] to minimise this occurrence.

The outcome for children with Burkitt lymphoma is clearly related to access to effective chemotherapy. This is such a rapidly growing tumour that those in whom there is a delay—either pending histopathology confirmation or pending recovery from laparotomy at which extensive disease precluded total resection—fare worse.[13] In addition to systemic chemotherapy, intrathecal methotrexate should be given to reduce the risk of CNS relapse.[14]

A considerable amount of energy has been expended in attempting to develop a low toxicity, high efficacy regimen for the treatment of Burkitt lymphoma that would be practicable in a resource-limited environment.[14] This effort is being cofunded by the International Society for Pediatric Oncology (SIOP). Resource limitations not only impact the actual affordability of treatment drugs but also the availability of supportive care, such as antibiotics, and the ability to manage treatment-related toxicity, particularly bone marrow suppression with, among others, blood component therapy. An ideal regimen should therefore be nontoxic as well as effective, inexpensive, and easy to administer.[15] The results of the SIOP studies have been encouraging, and relapse, should it occur, can also be effectively treated within a resource-constrained service.[16]

Patients with HIV-related lymphomas, excluding cerebral lymphomas, can tolerate effective chemotherapy protocols when treatment is given in conjunction with highly active antiretroviral therapy (HAART).

Surgery

The surgeon may be required to biopsy either a nodal mass, gonad, or mediastinal tumour, although frequently in Africa the diagnosis can be reached with sufficient precision to allow rational treatment following needle biopsy or bone marrow biopsy.

The role of the surgeon in the primary management of children with B-cell lymphoma remains controversial. In endemic areas, localised intraabdominal disease is, unfortunately, not as frequent as it is in sporadic cases occurring outside Equatorial Africa. There is, however, no doubt that on rare occasions abdominal disease is localised, complete resection is beneficial but biopsy only or debulking does not improve survival.[17,18] As chemotherapy regimens become more successful and more widely available, pressure on the surgeon is easing.[19]

In patients who present with an abdominal emergency, such as perforation, obstruction, or intussusception, the decision to operate is easy. The procedure that can be performed is defined by the findings at the time of surgery. Complete resection is ideal if circumstances allow, but the extent of disease may limit this ambition to a bypass procedure or biopsy alone. In patients with residual intraabdominal disease after laparotomy, delay in the administration of chemotherapy should be avoided.[17]

In patients in whom there is no crisis but an abdominal mass is palpable, the likelihood of complete resection must be judged from clinical assessment and preoperative imaging.

If abdominal disease is associated with extraabdominal lymphoma, then the initial strategy should be chemotherapy.[20] If the tumour is judged by the surgeon to be unresectable, the initial treatment should also be chemotherapy.

Staging laparotomy is not required. Even in the absence of sophisticated radiological techniques, it is usually possible to define the extent of disease within the abdomen with ultrasound, and, if necessary, to obtain tissue by using a needle biopsy. In some patients, a diagnostic laparotomy will have been indicated for symptoms at presentation. It is not necessary to remove the spleen or any other organ in order to stage or effectively treat the tumour.

In patients with primary bowel lymphoma, chemotherapy can be so effective that the tumour regresses, leaving a hole in the bowel.[21] This constitutes a surgical emergency. Surgical management will depend upon the clinical status of the patient as well as the findings at laparotomy. Exsanguinating haemorrhage from the bowel has also been reported in patients while on treatment for intestinal lymphoma. If the bleeding does not respond to conventional resuscitation, operative treatment may be necessary.[21]

Outcomes

Patients with T-cell and large-cell lymphomas fare worse than those with lymphomas of B-cell lineage.[22] Generally, patients with lymphoma and coexistent HIV disease do less well than patients who are not HIV-infected. The advent of HAART may change this perception, as improvement in immune status will allow HIV-infected individuals to tolerate more aggressive chemotherapy with shorter rest periods.[10,23]

Patients in the developed world have a higher incidence of resectable abdominal disease, and treatment with aggressive chemotherapy, including stem cell rescue, is available. With such aggressive treatment, 5-year survival rates reach 90% for localised disease and 70% for disseminated disease.[3]

In Africa, outcomes vary according to local geographic and economic factors. The most convincing data come from the Malawi Burkitt Lymphoma Project, which used initial cyclophosphamide monotherapy and later introduced intrathecal methotrexate for CNS prophylaxis. Initially, 63% of those with lesions in the head and neck secured complete remission with monotherapy, but only 33% of those with abdominal or other sites did so.[14] More recent studies have shown a 53% event-free survival for stage 3 patients[13] and a 71% complete clinical remission in those who relapsed or had primarily resistant tumours.[15]

These results are encouraging and show that much can be achieved even in the most resource-constrained countries.

Key Summary Points

1. The most common type of lymphoma is non-Hodgkin's lymphoma, which includes Burkitt type in association with the Epstein-Barr virus.

2. Presentation is variable.

3. Tissue diagnosis is essential.

4. Staging is best done by following the Uganda Cancer Institute staging system (see Table 104.2).

5. Chemotherapy is the mainstay of treatment.

6. Surgical input is mainly for tissue sampling and for acute abdominal presentation.

7. The prognosis is good where a chemotherapy programme is available.

References

1. Armitage JO, Weisenburger DD. New approach to classifying non-Hodgkin's lymphomas: clinical features of the main histologic subtypes: Non-Hodgkin's Lymphoma Classification Project. J Clin Oncol 1998; 16:2780–2795.

2. Harris NL, Jaffe E, Diebold J, Flaudrin G, Muller-Hermelink HK, Vardiman J. Lymphoma classification: from controversy to consensus: the REAL and WHO classification of lymphoid neoplasms. Ann Oncol 2000; 11(Suppl 1):S3–S10.

3. Ferry JA. Burkitt's lymphoma: clinicopathological features and differential diagnosis. The Oncologist 2006; 11(4):375–383.

4. van den Bosch C, Lloyd G. Chikungunya fever as a risk factor for endemic Burkitt lymphoma in Malawi. Trans Royal Soc Tropical Med Hyg 2000; 94(6):704–705.

5. van den Bosch C. Is endemic Burkitt's lymphoma an alliance between three infections and a tumour promoter? Lancet Oncol 2004; 5(12):738–746.

6. Stein L, Urban MI, O'Connell D, Yu XQ, Beral V, Newton R, et al. The spectrum of human immunodeficiency virus-associated cancers in a South African black population: results from a case-control study, 1995–2004. Int J Cancer 2008; 122(10):2260–2265.

7. Sinfield RL, Molyneux EM, Banda K, Borgstein E, Broadhead R, Hesseling P, et al. Spectrum and presentation of pediatric malignancies in the HIV era: experience from Blantyre, Malawi, 1998–2003. Pediatr Blood & Cancer 2006; 4(5):515–520.

8. Sissolak G, Abayomi EA, Jacobs P. AIDS defining lymphomas in the era of highly active antiretroviral therapy (HAART): an African perspective. Transfus Apher Sci 2007; 37(1):63–70.

9. Mwanda WO, Orem J, Remick SC, Rochford R, Whalen C, Wilson ML. Clinical characteristics of Burkitt's lymphoma from three regions of Kenya. East Afr Med J 2005; 82(9 Suppl):S135–S143.

10. Ratner L, Lee J, Tang S, Redden D, Hamzeh F, Herndier B, et al. Chemotherapy for HIV-associated non-Hodgkins lymphoma in combination with highly active antiretroviral therapy. J Clin Oncol 2001; 19(8):2171–2178.

11. Schneider RJ, Seibert K, Passe S, Little C, Gee T, Lee B, et al. Prognostic significance of serum lactate dehydrogenase in malignant lymphoma. Cancer 2006; 46(1):139–143.

12. Wössmann W, Schrappe M, Meyer U, Zimmermann M, Reiter A. Incidence of tumor lysis syndrome in children with advanced stage Burkitt's lymphoma/leukaemia before and after introduction of prophylactic use of urate oxidase. Ann Hematol 2003; 82(3):160–165.

13. Stein JE, Schwenn MR, Jacir NN, Harris BH. Surgical restraint in Burkitt's lymphoma in children. J Pediatr Surg 1991; 26(11):1273–1275.

14. Hesseling PB, Broadhead R, Molyneux E, Borgstein E, Schneider JW, Louw M, et al. Malawi pilot study of Burkitt lymphoma treatment. Med Pediatr Oncol 2003; 41(6):532–540.

15. Kazembe P, Hesseling PB, Griffin BE, Lampert I, Wessels G. Long term survival of children with Burkitt's lymphoma in Malawi after cyclophosphamide monotherapy. Med Pediatr Oncol 2003; 40(1):23–26.

16. Hesseling P, Molyneux E, Kamiza S, Broadhead R. Rescue chemotherapy for patients with resistant or relapsed endemic Burkitt's lymphoma. Trans Royal Soc Tropical Med Hyg 2008; 102(6):602–607.

17. Abbasğlu L, Gün F, Salman FT, Celik A, Unüvar A, Görgün O. The role of surgery in intra-abdominal Burkitt's lymphoma in children. Euro J Pediatr Surg 2003; 13(4):236–239.

18. Gahukamble DB, Khamage AS. Limitations of surgery in intraabdominal Burkitt's lymphoma in children. J Pediatr Surg 1995; 30(4):519–522.

19. Davidson A, Desai F, Hendricks M, Hartley P, Millar A, Numanoglu A, et al. The evolving management of Burkitt's lymphoma at Red Cross Children's Hospital. South Afr Med J 2006; 96(9):951–954.

20. Shamberger RC, Weinstein HJ. The role of surgery in abdominal Burkitt's lymphoma. J Pediatr Surg 1992; 27(2):236–240.

21. The role of surgery in the management of American Burkitt's lymphoma and its treatment. Ann Surg 1982; 196(1):82–86.

22. Kimm BS, Kim T-Y, Kim CW, Kim JY, Heo DS, Bang Y-J. Therapeutic outcome of extranodal NK/T-cell lymphoma initially treated with chemotherapy. Acta Oncologica 2003; 42(7):779–783.

23. Blinder VS, Chadburn A, Furman RR, Mathew S, Leonard JP. Improving outcomes for patients with Burkitt's lymphoma and HIV. AIDS Patient Care and STDs 2008; 22(3):175–187.

CHAPTER 105
NEUROBLASTOMAS

Larry Hadley
Kokila Lakhoo

Introduction

Neuroblastomas, along with most other paediatric solid tumours, should no longer be considered a single disease. Within the histological appearance of small round blue cells with rosette formation and background neuropil are an infinite number of behaviour patterns, each reflecting the genomic characteristics of the tumour cells. Thus, in some patients with neuroblastomas, the tumour spontaneously disappears or matures into a benign ganglioneuroma. In other patients with histologically identical neuroblastomas, the tumour rapidly disseminates and is resistant to even the most aggressive treatment. Refinements in nosology will ultimately recognise that these are different diseases that share morphological characteristics and a common cell of origin.

As morphological characteristics alone are insufficient to allow a prediction of behaviour, the concept of "risk stratification"—a process that encompasses assessment of the innate aggression of the tumour—has become important. Prediction of behaviour is an inexact science, but it is becoming more precise as genomic markers of aggression are identified. Thus, loss of part of chromosome 1p, amplification of N-Myc oncogene, and abnormalities of chromosomes 6p22, 2p, 11q, and 17q deletions in the malignant cell are all thought to code for aggressive behaviour.[1] Not only do tumour genomics affect behaviour, but certain features of the host, most notably age, are also critical in determining outcome.

Demographics

Neuroblastoma is, fortunately, infrequent in Africa.[2] Whether this reflects a low prevalence or a low rate of diagnosis is uncertain. It may be that neuroblastoma is another noncommunicable disease that is in some way influenced by industrialisation and the environmental insults associated with the process.[3]

In Europe and North America, neuroblastomas are the most common solid tumours of childhood; in Africa, however, the incidence of neuroblastomas lags far behind that of lymphomas, retinoblastomas, Wilms' tumours, and sarcomas.[4] The tumour may be recognised antenatally, but the median age at diagnosis is 2 years.

Pathophysiology

Sites of Origin

Neuroblastomas arise from neural crest cells. These are the cells that populate the adrenal medulla, the sympathetic ganglia, and the olfactory apparatus. They demonstrate a wide range of neuronal differentiation, but their distribution defines the sites at which primary neuroblastomas may occur. The most common site is the adrenal gland. Tumours arising from the sympathetic ganglia may occur in the abdomen, commonly around the origin of the celiac axis, or in the pelvis around the organ of Zukerkandl. In the chest, they present as posterior mediastinal tumours. Occasional tumours arise in the neck from the cervical sympathetics. Tumours arising from olfactory elements are termed esthesio-neuroblastomas.

Paraneoplastic Effects

Neuroblastomas may secrete catecholamines or their precursors. Thus, hypertension and diarrhoea are common. Opsomyoclonus occurs in 2–3% of affected children.[5]

Maturation

Neuroblastomas are unique in their potential to "mature" towards benign ganglioneuromas. It is also likely that a histological picture indistinguishable from neuroblastoma forms part of the normal maturation of the adrenal medulla, as "neuroblastoma-in-situ" has been found in autopsies in premature babies dying of unrelated causes.[6] Maturation is more likely to be seen in neonates and infants with stage 4S disease.

Histology

Neuroblastomas clearly demonstrate the limitations of the light microscope as a means of predicting cellular behaviour. Nonetheless, histological findings of ganglioneuroma presage a benign clinical course. Shimada defined histological features that predict poor behaviour, which have been incorporated into risk stratification protocols.[7] Frequently, in the absence of immunohistochemical stains, the pathologist can offer little beyond "small round blue cell tumour", and the clinical features must be considered when making a diagnosis.

Staging

The concept of staging as a predictor of outcome is being replaced by the concept of risk stratification, which incorporates cytogenetic markers and histological appearance as well as patient characteristics. Such studies allow the risk of treatment-related morbidity to be matched to the risk of progressive disease, and to avoid aggressive treatment in children who have biologically favourable tumours.[8] "Surgical risk factors", which predict the ease of resectability, are defined by preoperative imaging,[9] and should carefully be reviewed before any surgery is attempted.

Staging, however, is still important to allow comparisons between studies and experiences, as well as contributing to risk stratification.

The current international neuroblastoma staging system (INSS) is shown in Table 105.1.

Table 105.1: International neuroblastoma staging system.

Stage	Description
Stage 1	Localised tumour with complete gross resection; ipsilateral nonadherent lymph nodes negative
Stage 2A	Incomplete gross resection; nodes negative
Stage 2B	Either stage 1 or stage 2A with ipsilateral nodes positive
Stage 3	Tumour crossing midline or unilateral tumour with contralateral nodes positive
Stage 4	Metastatic disease
Stage 4S	Patient younger than 18 months of age with specific disease pattern

This system depends upon the surgeon understanding that the "lymphatic" midline lies along the aorta and that nodes between the aorta and the cava are ipsilateral to right-sided tumours and contralateral to left-sided tumours.[10]

The system also draws attention to stage 4S, which describes children younger than 18 months of age with a primary adrenal tumour that would otherwise be stage 1, but with metastases limited to the liver, skin ("blue berry" nodules) (Figure 105.1), and bone marrow. Less than 10% of the marrow cells should be blast cells. Such patients do much better than expected. In these patients, the liver may be massive and interfere with the mechanics of breathing. Under such circumstances, chemotherapy may be indicated, or, rarely, surgery may be needed to temporarily house the liver in a silo.[11]

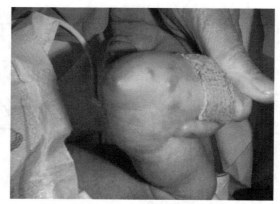

Figure 105.1: "Blue berry" nodules.

Clinical Presentation

Presentation depends upon the site of the primary tumour as well as the stage of disease. Many children will have obvious metastatic disease when they are first seen. In addition to liver secondaries, neuroblastomas have a propensity to metastasize to the orbits, causing exophthalmos and "raccoon eyes" (Figure 105.2); to the skull and long bones, causing painful swellings and increasing the risk of pathological fractures; and into the epidural space through intervertebral foramina, leading eventually to paraplegia. The bone marrow is very frequently invaded. Additionally, some patients present with paraneoplastic syndromes such as hypertension and opsomyoclonus.

Cervical neuroblastoma may present as Horner's syndrome.

Abdominal neuroblastoma has a characteristic nodularity, akin to palpating a bag of potatoes, which may help the clinician differentiate it from a nephroblastoma. Neuroblastoma also is frequently a central abdominal tumour (Figure 105.3).

The challenge is the patient who presents with an abdominal or posterior mediastinal mass with no other clues to its origin. In such a child, urgent investigation is required.

Presenting complaints may include any from Table 105.2; a nonspecific range of symptoms makes diagnosis difficult.

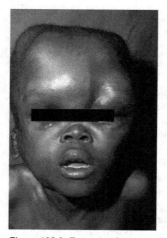

Figure 105.2: Example of raccoon eyes.

Investigations

In many instances, little more is needed than a needle biopsy of the primary or metastatic site. Few African centres currently have facilities for cytogenetic studies, or for metiodobenzylgaunidine (MIBG) radio-isotope imaging, magnetic resonance imaging (MRI; Figure 105.4), or axial tomography. Plain abdominal x-rays often show a mass with speckled calcification displacing bowel. Intravenous pyelography may show displacement of the kidney and help to differentiate neuroblastoma from an upper pole nephroblastoma, although clinical features are also important.[12] In cases of difficulty, urine can be assessed for catecholamines or their precursors. Ultrasound may help in the localisation of the tumour as well as in the assessment of retroperitoneal lymph nodes and liver.

In patients who present with spinal compression, it is useful to have some idea of the extent of disease within the spinal canal so that a surgical approach can be planned if possible. This may involve myelography if no other imaging is available (Figure 105.5).

Skeletal x-rays will reveal bony cortical metastases, and a bone marrow biopsy will define marrow involvement. A chest x-ray with a lateral view is important in the assessment of thoracic lesions (Figure 105.6).

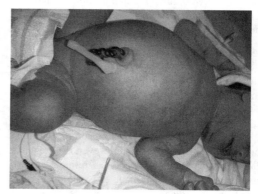

Figure 105.3: Abdominal mass.

Surgical Management

The mainstay of treatment for neuroblastoma is chemotherapy. In most patients presenting in Africa, neuroblastoma is manifestly a systemic disease that requires a systemic treatment; at best, surgery can provide local control. Surgery has, however, an important role in palliation and, infrequently, in cure.

The surgeon may be called upon to obtain biopsy material to establish the diagnosis of neuroblastoma, although this can usually be

Table 105.2: Presenting complaints with neuroblastoma.

• Mass	• Myoclonus/opsoclonus
• Limp/ bone pain/refusing to walk	• Neurological
• Generally unwell	• Constipation
• Decreased appetite	• Diarrhoea
• Vomiting	• Skin lesions
• Hypertension	• Proptosis
• Anaemia	• Antenatally diagnosed mass
• Fever	• Incidental (e.g., single incidence of urinary tract infection)
• Abdominal pain	• Horner's syndrome
• FTT/ weight loss	• Urinary retention

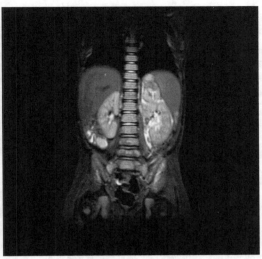

Figure 105.4: MRI showing left adrenal neuroblastoma marked "T".

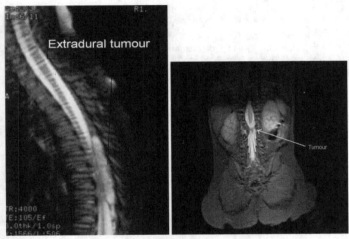

Figure 105.5: Imaging showing spinal extension.

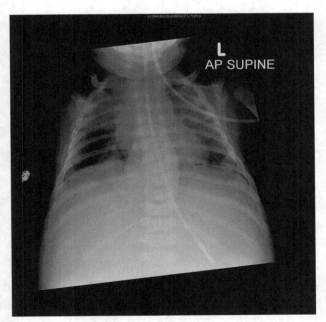

Figure 105.6: Chest radiograph showing posterior mediastinal mass.

achieved by bone marrow aspiration or other noninvasive means. In Europe and North America, biopsy is used for assessment of MYCN gene status. In Africa, however, it is usually impossible to assess risk in greater detail than considerations of stage of disease and histological appearance. In the absence of immunohistochemistry, it is important to correlate the pathologist's finding of a small round blue cell tumour with the clinical pattern of disease in order to reach a diagnosis.

Surgery may also be required to decompress the spinal canal in children who present with a short history of cord compression. Paraplegia of more than a few days duration is unlikely to be reversible.

Pathological fractures of long bones may require internal fixation to improve quality of life and to facilitate nursing care. Single-dose radiotherapy, as little as 5 Gy, resolves the pain of bony metastases.

Uncommonly, there is a need to resect localised primary tumours in patients who have responded well to either chemotherapy or *per primam* (with little scarring). As neuroblastomas tend to surround the major abdominal vessels, especially the coeliac trunk and the superior mesenteric artery, such resections can be mammoth undertakings,[13] and careful review of imaging studies should precede any such operations. Even in the most experienced hands, aortic and other major vessel injuries occur.[13] Intractable diarrhoea following retroperitoneal nerve injury occurs postoperatively in 30% of resections.[14] In infants younger than 18 months of age, surgical resection is more frequently possible.

Resection of the primary tumour in children with metastatic disease that has responded to chemotherapy remains controversial and is not thought to improve survival.[15]

Outcomes

In the authors' experience, without the resources for bone marrow transplantation and high-risk chemotherapy, metastatic neuroblastoma is a lethal disease, with the exception of babies with stage 4S disease. Even in centres with the proper resources, the outlook is dismal.[16] The role of the surgeon is palliative.

In patients with localised disease (stages 1 and 2), surgery may be curative, but sadly, such patients are few. It is believed that such tumours have favourable biological characteristics, and this limits their growth potential and confers a favourable prognosis. Patients with stage 3 intraabdominal disease may be made surgically curable by preoperative chemotherapy when this is available.

Key Summary Points

1. Neuroblastoma is rare in Africa.

2. Neuroblastoma is of neural crest origin and usually secretes catacholamines.

3. Neuroblastoma may mature into benign ganglioneuroma.

4. The clinical presentation is nonspecific as well as site and stage dependent.

5. In the absence of sophisticated imaging, plain radiographs may reveal a soft tissue mass with or without calcification.

6. Molecular biology and cytogenetics are key to the diagnosis; however, if these are not available, histopathology may be the only diagnostic tool.

7. Surgery for neuroblastoma in Africa is mainly palliative.

8. Neuroblastoma in Africa, with the continent's limited resources, is a lethal disease.

References

1. Kushner BH, Cheung NV. Neuroblastoma—linking a common allele to a rare disease. NEJM 2008; 358(24):2635–2637.

2. Stiller CA, Parkin DM. Human cancer: international variations in the incidence of neuroblastoma. Int J Cancer 2006; 52(4):538–543.

3. Bickler S, De Maio A. Western diseases: current concepts and implications for pediatric surgery research and practice. Pediatr Surg Int 2008; 24(3):251–255.

4. Gyasi R, Tettey Y. Childhood deaths from malignant neoplasms in Accra. Ghana Med J 2007; 41(2):78–81.

5. Hildebrandt T, Traunecker H. Neuroblastoma: a tumour with many faces. Current Paediatr 2005; 15(5):412–420.

6. Grosfeld J. Risk-based management of solid tumors in children. Amer J Surg 2000; 18(5):322–327.

7. Altungoz O, Aygun N, Tumer S, Ozer E, Olgun N, Sakizli M. Correlation of modified Shimada classification with MYCN and 1p36 status detected by fluorescence in situ hybridization in neuroblastoma. Cancer Genet Cytogenet 2007; 172(2):113–119.

8. Nuchtern JG. Perinatal neuroblastoma. Sem Pediatr Surg 2006; 15(1):10–16.

9. Cecchetto G, Mosseri V, De Bernardi B, Helardot P, Monclair T, Costa E, et al. Surgical risk factors in primary surgery for localized neuroblastoma; the LENSG1 study of the European International Society of Pediatric Oncology, Neuroblastoma Group. J Clin Oncol 2005; 23(3):8483–8489.

10. Rouviere H. Anatomie des Lymphatiques de l'Homme. Masson, Paris, 1932

11. Harper L, Perel Y, Lavrand F, Brissaud O. Surgical management of neuroblastoma-related hepatomegaly: do material and method really count? Pediatr Hematol Oncol 2008; 25(4):313–317.

12. Dickson PV, Sims TL, Streck CJ, McCarville MB, Santana VM, McGregor LM. Avoiding misdiagnosing neuroblastoma as Wilms tumour. J Pediatr Surg 2008; 43(6):1159–1163.

13. Kiely E. A technique for excision of abdominal and pelvic neuroblastoma. Ann Royal College Surg Engl 2007; 98(4):342–348.

14. Rees H, Markley MA, Kiely EM, Pierro A, Pritchard J. Diarrhea after resection of advanced abdominal neuroblastoma: a common management problem. Surgery 1998; 123(5):568–572.

15. Kiely EM. The surgical challenge of neuroblastoma. J Pediatr Surg 1994; 29(2):128–133.

16. Escobar MA, Grosfeld JL, Powell RL, West KW, Scherer LR, Fallon RJ. Long-term outcomes in children with stage IV neuroblastoma. J Pediatr Surg 2006; 41(2):377–381.

CHAPTER 106
MALIGNANT SOFT TISSUE TUMOURS

Sam Moore
Hugo Heij

Introduction

Tumours of soft tissue are mostly benign lesions of connective tissue in children. A number of aggressive malignant tumours that require multimodal therapy do occur, however, usually including surgical management. These malignant soft tissue sarcomas (STSs) are relatively rare in childhood, contributing approximately 5–8% of childhood malignancies (approximately 850–900 children and adolescents are diagnosed in the United States each year).[1] STSs arise predominantly from the embryonic mesoderm and mostly present as an asymptomatic mass in an extremity in older children or adults.

Demographics

The prevalence of STS appears to vary among population groups worldwide. In ethnic groups representing mainly caucasian populations, an age-standardised STS annual incidence rate of 5–9 per million can be expected, but this rate has recently been observed to be increasing in Europe. In Asia, the age-standardised STS annual incidence rate is less than 6 per million. Due to the paucity of data, the age-standardised STS annual incidence rates for Africa remain uncertain, but there is a widely held view that they are as common—if not more frequent—in black African children and adolescents than in Western population groups. A Nigerian study has reported STS as making up as much as 11.3% of all childhood cancers.

Rhabdomyosarcomas (RMSs) and fibrosarcomas predominate; fibrosarcomas were found to be more prevalent in black African Americans than in caucasians (both males and females) in the United States.[2] A similar spectrum is thought to exist in Africa. This interethnic variation in rhabdomyosarcoma and fibrosarcoma occurrence, together with their genetic and inheritable associations, suggest that genetic dysfunction is important in the pathophysiology. Viral exposure may also play a role, and Kaposi sarcoma (KS) rates are peaking in African children, mostly those from eastern and southern Africa in association with the acquired immune deficiency syndrome (AIDS) epidemic.

Aetiology and Pathophysiology

Sarcomas are malignant tumours of mesenchymal origin and derive from a variety of cell types. Their pathology usually relates to their site and cell of origin. Although they represent only 1% of tumours seen in an adult oncology clinic, their prevalence in childhood appears higher.

Although the aetiology of sarcomas remains obscure, a possible genetic origin is proposed, as there is an association with the alternative lengthening of telomeres (ALT) mechanism in about half of the osteosarcomas, STSs, and glioblastomas. Familial transmissability is a possibility, an example of which is the complex cancer predisposition Li-Fraumeni association (the molecular basis of which is a germline TP53 (tumour protein 53) mutation).[3] Impaired differentiation of myoblasts in RMS is associated with a tumour suppressor-like action due to reconstitution of miR-29, which promotes cellular differentiation and inhibits tumour growth in animals.[4]

Clinical Presentation

STSs occur in numerous sites, including the trunk, retroperitoneum, or the head and neck, in addition to the extremities. No aetiologic factors have been identified in the majority, even though a variety of predisposing or associated factors have been identified.

From a clinical point of view, at least three separate clinical groups of malignant STSs are encountered in childhood:

- congenital fibrosarcoma (CFS);
- rhabdomyosarcoma (RMS); and
- nonrhabdomyosarcoma soft tissue sarcoma (NRSTS).

Fibrosarcoma may warrant a separate group in the classification, but fibrosarcomas that occur in childhood have a very different biological behavior, despite their malignant histological appearance. In contrast to the situation in adults, where fibrosarcoma was the most frequent STS, rhabdomyosarcoma predominates in children in Africa as well as worldwide.

Findings on physical examination depend on the type and site of the tumour.

Investigations

For the most part, investigations are presented in this chapter under the specific type of STS.

Histological grading of STS is often difficult, with more than 70 histologic types currently being identified, including RMS, KS, and vascular tumours predominantly in the paediatric and adolescent age groups. RMSs and undifferentiated sarcomas are the most frequent types, making up more than 50% of STSs in most series of childhood tumours, with the remainder falling into the heterogeneous NRSTS group.

Management

The role of the surgeon is to

- establish a diagnosis;
- perform timely and adequate removal (often following chemotherapy);
- assess spread with a view towards staging; and
- provide supportive care (e.g., long-term venous access, feeding, etc.).

Prognosis

The outcome of STS has shown a marked improvement over the past 30 years, with a decrease in radical surgical procedures, improved 5-year survival, and a decrease in morbidity. This improvement can largely be attributed to teamwork within national and international study groups and the establishment of clear treatment protocols.

The age at diagnosis of STS appears to be a fairly major predictor of survival. Up to 77% of tumours occurring before the age of 1 year are surgically resectable, having the lowest occurrence of invasive or high-grade tumours. As a result, a 5-year survival of 93% has been reported in this age group.[5] The good prognosis of this group drops significantly with increasing age, and is probably below 50% event-free survival for children aged 5 years, and less than one-third for older children (>11 years of age).

Fibrosarcoma

The age-standardised STS annual incidence rate for malignant fibromatous tumours is 1–2 per million in the United States. Fibrosarcoma is the most common NRSTS in the <1 year age group.

Congenital fibrosarcoma usually occurs in the extremities (Figure 106.1) or trunk, and although histologically it appears malignant, it behaves benignly and rarely metastasizes.

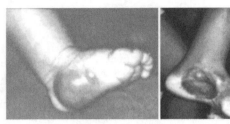

Figure 106.1: Congenital fibrosarcoma of the foot in an infant (left) and the result of wide excision at 7 years of age (right).

In children older than 4 years of age, the natural history of fibrosarcomas approximates that of the adult tumour, and the treatment is more radical than for younger children.

In US population groups, a higher incidence of fibrosarcoma has been reported among black people compared to white people for both sexes, suggesting that fibrosarcoma may be more prevalent in African populations.

Malignant fibrous histiocytoma (MFH) also occurs in children.

Inactivation of the RB1 gene has been shown to be involved in tumours such as fibrosarcoma, osteogenic sarcomas, and melanomas in early adult life. Of interest is the association of this gene with infantile fibrosarcoma via the ETV6-NTRK fusion protein.[6]

Since the 1980s, the identification of balanced translocations in STSs has changed the face of histopathological identification to a combination of histopathological and molecular genetic identification. Sarcomas that are known to have identifiable gene fusions include synovial sarcomas (SYT-SSX), Ewing's sarcomas (EWS-Fli1), clear cell sarcomas (EWS-ATF1), and myxoid liposarcomas (FUS-CHOP), among others.[7] The ETV6-NTRK fusion associated with infantile fibrosarcoma may link it to mesoblastic nephroma. Considered to be disease-specific, the identification of sarcoma translocations and their fusion is possible, but limited by availability of specific resources. Fibrosarcomas of bone may also occur.

The prognosis for infantile fibrosarcomas is excellent following surgical excision. The survival rate drops to 60% in the older child, however.

Rhabdomyosarcoma

Rhabdomyosarcoma is a malignant tumour of striated muscle, which usually displays early local invasiveness and may later metastasize via lymphatic and haematogenous pathways. It is derived from mesenchymal cells that differentiate along rhabdomyoblastic lines, often displaying cross striations on histopathological examination. It is the most common STS encountered in childhood, occurring even in the perinatal period[8] (10% of neonatal malignancies[9]). RMS may arise from any site during childhood but the most common sites include the head/neck (25.6%), leg/foot (26.7%), and thigh (19%) in an African series.[10]

Although the aetiology of RMS is still unclear, familial STSs do occur, and RMS may be associated with a number of syndromes (e.g., Beckwith-Wiedeman, Li-Fraumeni, and WAGR (Wilms' tumour, Aniridia, Genito-urinary malformations, mental Retardation)) as well as neurofibromatosis (type 1) and the basal cell naevus syndrome. Whereas the majority of the alveolar RMS subtypes show

reciprocal chromosomal translocations ['t(2;13)(q35;q14) or t(1;13)(p36;q14).t(2;13)], embryonal subtypes show a loss of heterozygosity (LOH) on the short arm of chromosome 11 [11p15.5]. The latter shows the suppression of the tumour-suppressor gene H19 on 11p15.5, which results in insulin growth factor II (IGFII) gene overexpression. In keeping with this observation, rhabdomyosarcoma (as well as retinoblastoma), has been shown to be positively associated with increased intrauterine growth, suggesting a possible role of foetal growth factors in its pathogenesis.[11] Rhabdomyosarcomas are also associated with a number of other genetic variations (e.g., mutations in the p53 tumour suppressor gene and adverse outcome, as well as the loss of 1p36, which corresponds to the locus for PAX 7, a paired home box characteristically altered in alveolar RMS tumours).

The PAX/FKHR fusion gene is found in as many as 60% of alveolar RMS cases, but a further 10% of patients with particularly poor prognosis histological types may carry the Ewing's sarcoma EWS/ETS fusion genes (occasionally along with the PAX/FKHR gene).

RMS Prevalence and Demographics

In Western countries, STSs have an annual prevalence of 8.4 per million in caucasian populations, and the American Cancer Society estimates about 8,680 new cases per year.[12] This would give RMSs an occurrence between 10% and 15% of paediatric solid malignancies. A male predilection (male-to-female ratio of 3:2) has been reported, and the peak age group is 2–5 years with a second peak occurring in adolescence.

Ethnic differences have been reported, with RMS in the United States being more frequent in caucasian than in black patients. Although it is possible that RMS is underreported worldwide in black communities, a suggestion that there is an increased preponderance in black African children is not supported by US data; one study showed that out of 5,623 cases of STS reported in whites and blacks living in the United States, only 574 cases (10.2%) were reported in blacks. This appears to be mainly in females, as RMS prevalence has been found to be only half of the caucasian rate in black girls in the United States, as opposed to a similar rate in both black and white boys. Furthermore, certain studies have shown no striking differences between blacks and whites concerning anatomic sites, histologic types, histologic grades, or clinical stages. This has led to the conclusion that there are no really significant differences in occurrence or survival between white and black STS patients. The prevalence in mixed races in Africa is unknown.

Clinical Presentation

RMS tumours occur in numerous sites, including the trunk, retroperitoneum, or the head and neck in addition to the extremities (Figure 106.2).

The most common clinical presentation is that of an asymptomatic mass (often noted by the parents). The precise signs and symptoms usually vary, depending on the anatomical site of the primary tumour.

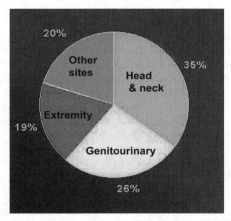

Figure 106.2: Approximately 35% of primary RMS occurs in the head and neck region, 19% in the genitourinary region, and the same in the extremities. Other sites are approximately 20% of the total.

Head and Neck Tumours

Head and neck RMS tumours are classified as those occurring in the orbit and in the parameningeal and nonparameningeal sites.[13.]

Orbit

Primary RMS of the orbit presents with proptosis, loss of vision, chemosis, and swelling. Ophthalmoplegia may occur in advanced disease. A mass may be present on the eyelid or subconjunctivally. This site usually demonstrates embryonal histological features, and has the best prognosis, given appropriate management.

Parameningeal sites

Parameningeal sites include the external auditory meatus, the middle ear, the nasopharynx, and other sites around the pharynx and larynx, where erosion of bone is a feature. RMS may present with a bleeding mass and/or meningeal symptoms with possible cranial nerve involvement. Complete surgical extirpation may be difficult, so these tumours not infrequently require radiotherapy. Parameningeal tumours mostly have a poor outcome because their deep situation leads to delay in presentation and hence extensive local infiltration as well as early distant metastases (15%) due to the rich lymphatic and blood networks in these areas.

Nonparameningeal sites

Nonparameningeal sites include the cheeks, oral cavity, and oropharynx, scalp, and thyroid, among others. _

Genitourinary Tumours

Genitourinary tumours include primary sites from the vulva, vagina, uterus, or bladder/prostate. Patients may present with a mass or may present with haematuria and/or bladder outlet obstruction (Figure 106.3).

Patients also may have an abdominal or pelvic mass. These masses may be large, making identification of the primary site difficult.

Paratesticular RMS

Paratesticular RMS tumours present with nontender scrotal masses but may present with a large abdominal mass of retroperitoneal lymph nodes. These tumours may be spindle-shaped, being embryonal in 93%,[14] and having a good prognosis on the whole. Whereas, in the past, an extensive dissection of the retropertitoneal nodes was required, these patients may present with lung metastases (see Figure 106.4).

Sarcoma botryoides

Sarcoma botryoides is a particular form of genitourinary RMS that presents with grape-like structures (Figure 106.5) protruding from the vulva or causing bladder neck obstruction in a child younger than 4 years of age. The histopathology is usually embryonal and the prognosis usually good due to chemosensitivity of the tumour.

Tumours of the Body Wall

Tumours of the body wall occur either in the chest wall or paraspinally. Tumours of the chest wall are of considerable interest due to the possibility of an extra-osseous Ewing's tumour of soft tissue or a primitive neuroectodermal tumour (PNET; the so-called Askin tumour) in the differential diagnosis (Figure 106.6).

Tumours of the abdominal wall are rare. They have a high rate of local (as opposed to lymph node) recurrence and are often chemoresistant.

Other sites where RMS can occur include the retroperitoneum (10%), and other, rarer sites such as the perineum, biliary tract, and GIT.

Imaging

In Western countries, computed tomography (CT) and magnetic resonance imaging (MRI) are considered essential for the staging of RMS as it often affects deep organs, and clinical assessment of the local and regional involvement as well as the relationship to other neighbouring structures may prove difficult. Imaging of RMS remains a problem in poorly resourced parts of the world, including Africa, where many of the imaging modalities taken for granted in the West are often not

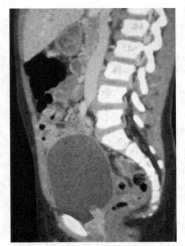

Figure 106.3: RMS of bladder neck presenting with bladder outlet obstruction.

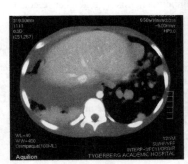 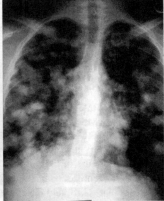

Figure 106.4: Chest x-ray and CT scan of pulmonary metastases from a 12 year-old-boy with a para-testicular RMS tumour.

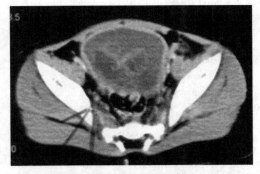

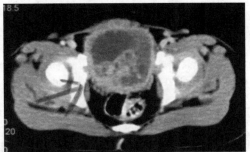

Figure 106.5: Sarcoma botryoides of the bladder. Note the grape-like structures in the lumen.

available. Where they are available, however, they should be used to evaluate these tumours.

Clinical procedures such as cystoscopy, examination under anaesthesia, and lumbar puncture for tumours affecting the spinal canal gain importance as alternatives in many African centres. When used in association with Doppler ultrasound (US) investigation, reasonable results can be obtained to guide the clinician in management decisions.

MRI is the preferred modality in many centres due to its good definition of regional anatomy and the absence of artifacts on CT scanning. For example, MRI holds the added benefit of special signal characteristics in certain tumours that may assist in the diagnostic work-up of the patient. Examples of this are lipoma versus liposarcoma, vascular lesions, and fibromas. Nevertheless, it is highly debatable whether imaging per se can identify malignant as opposed to benign tumours.

Histopathology

Arising from immature striated muscle, RMS is one of the small blue round cell tumours of childhood, along with neuroblastoma, Ewing's family of tumours, and lymphoma. Histopathology may be difficult, and many subtypes exist. Cross-striations may be visualised even on light microscopy to indicate the myogenic origin of the tumour. Subtypes may, however, be difficult to distinguish without highly sophisticated tools such as immunocytochemistry and even electron microscopy and genetic studies.

There are three main histological types of RMS: embryonal, alveolar, and pleomorphic.

Embryonal RMS

Embryonal RMS is the most common RMS, making up about 66% of all childhood RMS, virtually all in the <8 year age group. Embryonal RMS makes up at least 80% of genitourinary RMS and 60% of head and neck tumours in the younger child. Two very favourable subtypes have been identified: (1) the spindle cell embryonal variant seen in paratesticular RMS, and (2) some head and neck tumours and sarcoma botryoides of the genitourinary tract.

Sarcoma botryoides, discussed previously (see Figure 106.5), is a specific embryonal subtype occurring in children younger than 4 years of age in muscular cavities such as the nasopharynx, vagina (appearing as grape-like lesions protruding from the vulva), and biliary tree. The histopathological picture includes small, round, or possibly spindle-shaped cells surrounded by myxoid material. It has a very good prognosis, generally responding well to chemotherapy.

Alveolar RMS

The alveolar RMS type (20%) occurs mostly on the trunk or extremities and mostly has a poorer outcome.[15] The less well defined histological subtypes include undifferentiated sarcomas and the pleomorphic (adult) type. There may be occasional difficulties in subtyping RMS tumours, which explains the origin of the term *sarcoma, type indeterminate* in the histopathological classification. Currently, the use of immunocyto-chemistry, electron microscopy, and cytogenetics for further subtyping of difficult tumours is currently in practice in the Western world due to the importance of correctly identifying subtypes on management stratification and prognosis.

Pleomorphic RMS

Pleomorphic RMS is virtually unknown in childhood, mostly present-ing in adults.

Pretreatment Investigation

Pretreatment investigation includes, but is not limited to

- *blood tests:* full blood count, platelet count, urea and electrolytes, liver function tests, and urinanalysis;

- *bone marrow biopsy and aspirate:* usually bilateral;

- *radiology:* chest x-ray, skeletal survey, CT chest (if available), MRI

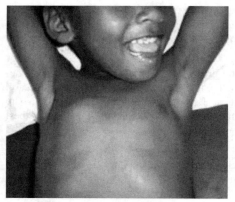
Figure 106.6: Anterior chest wall tumour.

Table 106.1: IRSG staging of RMS, based on residual after surgical resection.

Group	Description
Group I	Localized disease, completely resected
	Absence of regional lymphadenopathy
	a. confined to muscle of origin
	b. infiltration outside muscle or organ of origin
Group II	Total macroscopic resection, but evidence of regional spread
	c. grossly resected tumour with microscopic residual
	d. regional disease with involved nodes—completely resected with no microscopic residual
	e. regional disease with involved nodes—grossly resected but with microscopic residual and/or histologic involvement of the most distal node in the dissection
Group III	Incomplete resection or biopsy with presence of macroscopic disease
Group IV	Distant metastases

of primary site (with contrast);

- *scintigraphy:* bone scan (if available); and

- *lumbar puncture:* cerebrospinal fluid (CSF) cytology if parameningeal.

Staging

Staging depends on such factors as the primary site and the extent of dis-ease as determined by one of a number of staging systems. These include the International Society of Pediatric Oncology (SIOP), the tumour, nodes, metastases (TNM), or the Intergroup Rhabdomyosarcoma Study Group (IRSG) staging systems (see Table 106.1).

In some respects, RMS staging must be site-specific due to individual aspects of local invasion, regional lymph node spread, and biologic tumour response.

IRSG classification

The current staging system used in the United States is the IRSG system. Table 106.1 refers to the IRSG postsurgical classification (in contrast to the presurgical classification, which depends on special investigations).

SIOP classification

More recently, patients have been classified into low-, intermedi-ate-, and high-risk categories by SIOP/IRS (IRS is the Intergroup Rhabdomyosarcoma Study Group), based on studies of clinical out-comes in order to direct treatment protocols.[16]

- *Low-risk tumours* include stage 1, groups I and II (N0) (and orbit eyelid up to group III) as well as stage 2 of group I tumours.

• *Intermediate-risk tumours* include the rest of stage 1 (group II (N1) and group III (nonorbit)), and stages 2 and 3.

• *High-risk tumours* consist mainly of group IV.

Treatment

The overall aim of treatment in patients with RMS is to optimize survival, minimize toxicity, and maximize the quality of life. The possibility of cure is a realistic goal in patients with localized early tumours. On the African continent, this mostly applies to the few patients who are not in advanced stages on presentation.

The correct pathologic diagnosis as well as the correct histologic subtype will determine much of the treatment, so they are important in RMS management. Site-specific issues, such as the specific patterns of local invasion, regional lymph node spread, and therapeutic response, as well as histopathological subtyping, require physicians to be familiar with site-specific staging and treatment details. They require clear protocols as well as attention to the significant acute toxicities and long-term effects that may occur in young children.

Chemotherapy

All patients with RMS require chemotherapy. Generally speaking, embryonal RMS is more responsive to treatment than the alveolar subtype. A regimen of vincristin, actinomycin D, and cyclophosphamide (VAC) is generally administered.

A 5-year survival rate of about 72% can be achieved on this regime. Large variations in the 5-year survival, however, depend on patient age and tumour characteristics. Children who survived the first 5 years after diagnosis have an excellent long-term prognosis.[15] When patients with metastatic disease are removed from the analysis (i.e., localized disease) and more advanced chemotherapeutic regimens are used, the 5-year survival rate exceeds 80%.

Surgical aspects of RMS management

The surgeon is an integral part of the oncology team for three reasons:

• to establish a diagnosis and to obtain a pathological sample;

• many, if not most, tumours rely on surgery to achieve local control; and

• support in terms of vascular access, etc.

The surgical management of RMS has altered fairly dramatically over the past few decades from radical surgical treatment to preoperative chemotherapy followed by wide surgical excision. This is justified by the considerable improvement in 5-year survival and a marked decrease in morbidity.

RMS is treated with adjuvant chemotherapy, whereas chemotherapy is mostly reserved for NRSTS that is high grade or unresectable. Surgery appears to be a major therapeutic modality, although radiation may also play a role in certain circumstances. The possibility of NRSTS should be considered when resecting a soft tissue mass in children, and diagnostic incisional biopsy followed by wide local excision with negative microscopic margins should be the surgical goal for localized tumours.

Surgery is best suited to areas where both a good cosmetic result and wide excision can be achieved. It must be borne in mind that primary surgery is probably best reserved for easily resectable small lesions (e.g., extremity, trunk, anterior wall), where an excision biopsy can be achieved. In the IRSG trials, 64% of group III, who demonstrated more than a 50% response to the chemotherapy, were found to have no residual tumour at surgery.

In general, surgical treatment now rests on the principles of diagnosis (biopsy), neoadjuvant chemotherapy, and a primary re-excision of any remaining tumour. Second-look surgery may not be required, depending on posttherapy reassessment. It is generally true that younger patients have a significantly better response to chemotherapy and a longer survival than do their older counterparts.

Diagnostic

Tumours of the extremity lend themselves to initial biopsy. This procedure should be performed through a longitudinal incision so as not to compromise later surgical excision.

There is no place for debulking procedures, which usually result in an incomplete excision.

Primary re-excision

In tumours with a good biological response to chemotherapy, the residual tumour may be quite small, favoring conservative surgery with preservation of vital functions. Excision of the entire organ of origin is no longer the standard. Complete macroscopic and microscopic clearance gives rise to the best long-term results.

Second-look surgery

Some debate still exists about the value of second-look surgery in the presence of radiological clearance of disease. In patients with an incomplete chemotherapeutic response or doubt, second-look surgery still appears to have a role, as survival is bound to a disease-free outcome. It is of limited value in stage IV disease.

Management of recurrence

The recurrence/relapse rate for RMS is as high as 30%,[13] with a mortality of 50–90% in these patients. These recurrences may be localized or widespread.

Grade alone does not determine the rate of local recurrence. In both low- and high-grade tumours, a pathological margin of resection greater than 1 cm reduced local recurrence. The effect of margin of tumour resection and postoperative radiation therapy (RT) on local tumour recurrence is not yet clear in children .

Histology and tumour biology plays a major role in determining the outcome of these recurrences. Sarcoma botryoides recurrences have a 5-year survival of 64%, pleomorphic tumours 26%, and alveolar tumours only 5% (depending on IRSG).

Radiotherapy

Although radiation therapy is of considerable use in controlling local recurrence, its use varies considerably worldwide. Attempts to minimize side effects by avoiding radiation therapy have been very successful in the SIOP trials, where its use is limited to salvage therapy or local relapse. In the MMT89 (Malignant Mesenchymal Tumour 1989) protocol study,[17] this applied to only 23% who required local therapy to achieve complete control.

Radiotherapy is particularly used where either microscopic disease remains after surgical resection or in areas where wide excision would result in a very poor cosmetic result (e.g., parameningeal, orbit, etc.).

Benefits of radiotherapy in preserving organs must be weighed against the long-term side effects, which include secondary malignancies (e.g., thyroid) and features such as xerostomia, abnormal dental development, poor facial bone development, and neuroendocrine abnormalities, as well as hearing and visual loss in head and neck lesions. In the pelvic region, impaired gonadal function, poor pelvic bone development, and intestinal obstruction may ensue. Growth disturbance, bone and nerve damage, as well as limitation of function may result in the extremities.

Prognosis

The prognosis of STS is largely determined by the degree of spread at the time of diagnosis, the biology of the tumour, the histological features, the site of origin, and the treatment given. Because much of the management of paediatric soft tissue sarcomas (NRSTS) is extrapolated from adult studies, the treatment is debated, due to their varying chemosensitivity.

Nevertheless, a 5-year survival rate greater than 70% has been reported in recent trials of localised rhabdomyosarcoma. Survival for group I is 93%; group II, 81%; group III, 73%; and group IV, 30%. Patients presenting with metastatic disease (20% of patients with newly diagnosed RMS) still have a poor outcome (Figure 106.7).

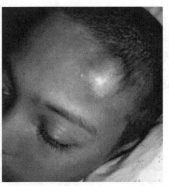

Figure 106.7: Metastatic RMS lesion on forehead from an extremity primary.

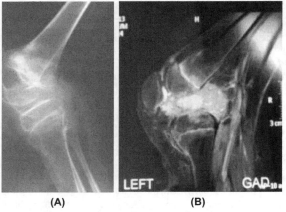

(A)   (B)

Figure 106.8: (A) X-ray of left knee in a 13-year-old female with a synovial sarcoma. (B) MRI image demonstrates the extent of the tumour.

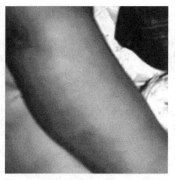

Figure 106.9: Malignant fibrous histiocytoma of the upper limb in a 6-year-old child.

In the future, risk-adapted classification of rhabdomyosarcoma will likely be based on biologic features, such as the presence of chromosomal translocations or specific gene expression profiles.

Nonrhabdomyosarcoma Soft Tissue Tumours

Whereas RMS predominates in children younger than 14 years of age, NRSTS occurs less commonly, making up less than 3% of childhood malignancies.[5] They are somewhat more common in boys than girls (ratio is 2.3:1) and occur mostly in adolescents (median age, 12 years) and young adults. They may also present in infancy, usually occurring in the trunk or lower limbs. Pathologically, they make up a heterogeneous group, with the most common types being synovial sarcomas (42%), fibrosarcoma (13%), malignant fibrous histiocytoma (12%), and neurogenic tumours (10%). Age appears to be important, as synovial sarcomas, peripheral nerve sheath tumours, and malignant fibrous histiocytoma most frequently occur in patients aged 10–15 years as opposed to those younger than 1 year of age, who mostly had a congenital fibrosarcoma.

The lower limb is the most common primary site of NRSTS in childhood, but the site does not appear to correlate with age. Prognosis is related to size, spread (stage), and biologic and histological features.

Complete surgical excision remains the mainstay of therapy in more than 70% of NRSTS, making it of considerable interest to surgeons. A multidisciplinary team approach with avoidance of mutilating procedures has become the standard for the treatment of STS in children and results in cure for many.

Postoperative adjuvant chemotherapy significantly improves the overall and disease-free survival for patients with large-size and high-grade sarcomas.

NRSTSs are less responsive to radiotherapy than the more common paediatric STS, RMS, and Ewing's sarcoma of soft tissue. However, radiation therapy does play an important role in the treatment of NRSTS, including synovial sarcoma. Limb preservation with adjuvant radiation thereby is standard, and there is a greater incentive to reduce long-term complications of radiation in younger patients. Techniques such as using smaller margins, lower doses, and conformal techniques have changed the practice in many centres. Where paediatric NRSTS patients have had an initial unplanned or incomplete resection, a wide re-excision should precede any further adjuvant treatment.

Synovial Sarcoma

Synovial sarcoma is an uncommon malignant soft tissue neoplasm that accounts for 7–8% of all malignant soft tissue tumours.[18] Approximately 30% of synovial sarcoma patients are younger than 20 years of age. Synovial sarcoma is the most common NRSTS in paediatric patients. It is a high-grade malignancy and tends to spread to the lungs.

Clinically, synovial sarcoma classically arises from the knee or upper leg, closely related to joints, tendons, or bursae (Figure 106.8). The upper extremity, trunk, abdomen, and head and neck regions may also be involved. It is also associated with a nonrandom chromosomal translocation t(X, 18)(p11; q11).

Initial biopsy should be incisional unless a very localized tumour is present, and should be longitudinal to allow for later wide excision. A wide surgical excision with clear margins remains the treatment of choice for synovial sarcoma in children, as microscopic residual has a major influence on local recurrence and survival. Amputation may be required in a limb to ensure adequate margins.

Regional lymphadenopathy may occur, and lymph nodes should be evaluated for local regional disease.

Adjuvant radiation therapy may assist in containing residual disease and should possibly be considered in patients with clear margins (IRSG group I) and in patients with microscopic residual tumour (IRSG group II). Overall, chemotherapy does not seem to improve the outcome, although chemotherapeutic drugs such as ifosfamide appear fairly effective in advanced disease. Survival of metastatic disease is rare.

Leiomyosarcoma

Leiomyosarcoma arises from smooth muscle and is the most common retroperitoneal tumour STS in the paediatric age group. It may arise from the GIT, and is occasionally being seen in association with HIV infection and immunosuppression (e.g., renal transplantation). Leiomyosarcoma is associated with a t(12;14)(q14;q23) translocation.

Neurofibrosarcoma

Neurofibrosarcoma is a tumour of the nerve sheath with a strong association with neurofibromatosis, occurring in 16% of patients with an NF1 gene variation (up to 50% of cases with NF1). Other reported genetic variations include 22q11-q13, 17q11, and p53 mutations. It mostly occurs in the trunk or major plexuses (e.g., brachial plexus) in the periphery. It is locally invasive.

Surgical excision remains the mainstay of treatment, as it is largely chemo- and radio-resistant.

Malignant Fibrous Histiocytoma

Like fibrosarcoma, malignant fibrous histiocytoma arises from fibroblasts, mostly occurring in the trunk and extremities (Figure 106.9). Pathologically, it occurs deep in the subcutaneous layer, displaying a number of histopathological variants (giant cell, myxosis, storiform, and angiomatoid). The angiomatoid variant occurs in younger patients.

Malignant fibrous histiocytoma is surgically curable by excision. A wide surgical excision is the treatment of choice. Chemotherapy may be required for advanced cases in the older child.

Liposarcoma

Liposarcoma is very rare in childhood, but has been described in the peripheries and retroperitoneally. It is sometimes difficult to distinguish from lipoblastoma, a benign condition; any fatty tumour with unusual features, such as poorly localized, invading fascia, should be evaluated.

It may be difficult to distinguish between lipoblastoma and liposarcoma on histopathology alone and may require karyotyping in order to make the distinction. Histological features are suggestive of malignancy with the formation of poorly defined larger lobules and/or nuclear pleomorphism, hyperchromasia, and atypical mitoses. Liposarcoma typically may be associated with a nonrandom gene translocation, t(12;16)(13;p11); it may be of myxoid lipoblastoma; or other genetic abnormalities may occur.

Liposarcoma tends to be locally invasive and rarely spreads to distant sites. Wide surgical excision is the treatment of choice.

Vascular Tumours and Kaposi Sarcoma

Kaposi sarcoma

Kaposi sarcoma in a child is usually regarded as a rare and unexplained condition. Essentially, KS is a multicentric neoplasia of microvascular origin arising in association with HIV-affected individuals. It presents as brown, reddish, or purple cutaneous spots in HIV-positive patients.

The risk is known to be elevated in association with HIV-positive patients, immunosuppression, and human herpes virus 8 (HHV-8) infections.[19] Children are also at risk for KS following renal transplantation.

Kaposi sarcoma rates are rapidly increasing in African children, mostly in association with the AIDS epidemic. In endemic regions, KS represents as much as 25–50% of STS in adult men and 2–10% of all childhood cancers.[20] A further difference in children is a similar male-to-female ratio, as opposed to the male predominance in adults.

Clinically, KS presents on the feet or ankles, thighs (Figure 106.10), arms, hands, or face as a brown, reddish, or purple cutaneous spot but may involve any other part of the body. It can involve skin, mucous membranes, and lymph nodes, as well as viscera (e.g., liver). Apart from the skin lesions, KS often presents with lymphadenopathy in childhood as well as wasting and anaemia.

Although rare in most parts of the world, KS has become an increasing problem in areas of high HIV prevalence in Africa. This is particularly true of the highland areas of Zaire, Kenya, Tanzania, and Southern Africa. The incidence is increasing; for instance, in Zambia the incidence has risen from 2.63 per million in 1982 to 19% 10 years later. Equally, in South Africa, a threefold increase in the incidence of KS has been reported from 1988 to 1996 and continues to increase as the HIV epidemic in this area continues.[20] African KS is fairly common in young adult males living near the equator. One form is also common in young African children.

Kaposi sarcoma is also associated with immunosuppression, and an increased KS-associated herpes virus (KSHV) seroprevalence, the risk being highest in children of KSHV-seropositive mothers.

The status of KS as a true soft tissue malignancy is still unclear, and many still regard it as an opportunistic neoplasm rather than a genuine malignancy. Management decisions are governed by the extent and location of the lesions, as well as the symptoms and degree of immunosuppression. Diagnosis can be confirmed on skin biopsy.

The outlook depends on the immune status and patient's HIV viral load. Antiretroviral therapy can shrink the lesions, but the treatment of

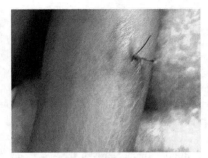

Figure 106.10: Kaposi sarcoma of leg with evidence of biopsy.

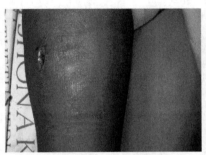

Figure 106.11: Poor healing in a biopsy wound of a haemangiopericytoma of the thigh.

KS does not improve the outcome from HIV itself.

Radiotherapy or cryotherapy have both been used for the local lesion. Chemotherapy also has to be used in certain circumstances.

Lesions may return after treatment, however.

Haemangiopericytoma

Haemangiopericytoma is an uncommon soft tissue tumour that arises from small pericapillary spindle-shaped cells (capillary pericytes). It may be benign or malignant, depending on the tumour biology, and it has a variable and unpredictable malignancy risk. Haemangiopericytoma is exceedingly rare in childhood. It mostly occurs in the lower limbs (Figure 106.11) or retroperitoneally, but may also occur in the head and neck, particularly in older patients (but also is reported in childhood). It has been associated with certain chromosomal translocations (e.g., t(12;19)(q13;q13) or t(13;22)(q22;q11)).

Haemangiopericytoma may be difficult to diagnose clinically due to its rarity. It usually presents as a soft tissue mass but may have unusual clinical presentations as hypoglycaemia or hypophosphataemic rickets.

Total surgical excision is the treatment of choice, and curative surgery is the most important predictor of survival. The role of chemotherapy in treatment is not well established.

Haemangioendothelioma

Haemangioendothelioma (congenital haemangioma) may occur in viscera (e.g., liver, lung) or in soft tissue elsewhere.

Hepatic epitheloid haemangioendothelioma is an uncommon, low-grade vascular tumour with uncertainties about the best treatment. It usually has a favorable prognosis but may develop complications such as thrombocytopaenia and cardiac failure, due to its size. This may lead to a poorer prognosis and may require liver transplantation.

Epithelioid haemangioendothelioma, in contrast, is a distinctive vascular soft tissue tumour that has been previously considered a tumour of borderline malignancy and low-grade angiosarcoma. It occurs in the extremities as well as the head and neck, mediastinum, trunk, genitals, and retroperitoneum. Most tumours occur in adults, affecting females predominantly, but some have been reported at 9 years of age. Although many run a benign clinical course and respond to wide local excision, tumours with more than 3 mitoses/50 high-power fields (HPF) and a size greater than 3.0 cm have a significantly worse prognosis.

Angiosarcoma

Angiosarcoma is an extremely rare tumour in childhood. At least one-third arise within the skin, and about 25% in soft tissue. Other sites (e.g., liver, breast, or bone) make up about 25% of occurrences. There is an association with the NF1 gene and neurofibromatosis, particularly with thoracic sites. Survival is generally poor, although long-term survival has been reported.

Miscellaneous Tumours

Alveolar Soft Part Sarcoma

Alveolar soft part sarcoma is a tumour that occurs in the head and neck or extremities and grows very slowly, tending to metastasize (to the lung and brain) some years after diagnosis. It possibly arises from muscle. Complete surgical resection is the treatment of choice

Ewing's Sarcoma Family of Tumours

Long regarded as a tumour of the bone (Figure 106.12), the Ewing's sarcoma family of tumours (ESFT) remains a not uncommon malignancy of children, adolescents, and adults younger than 25 years of age. Ethnic disparities in incidence (more common in caucasians) as well as sex-related differences in outcome (caucasian females do better) have been reported.[21]

Although better known as Ewing's sarcoma of the bone, there is a distinct extra-osseous group of Ewing's sarcomas that originate from soft tissues (including PNET and the Askin tumour of the chest wall).

Prognostic factors used to stratify patients include

- tumour-related stage (metastases), site, size, serum lactic dehydrogenase (LDH), chromosomal translocation (type and position), and fusion transcripts (blood and bone marrow);

- treatment (e.g., local surgical control, chemotherapy protocol, chemotherapeutic response), both histological and radiological; and

- patient factors (e.g., gender, age).

Ewing's sarcoma is treated successfully in many cases by a combination of chemotherapy, surgery, and radiotherapy.[22] Patients with small peripheral tumours without distant spread have been reported to have a high rate of cure (>70%) . Large, centrally located tumours and those with advanced stage disease have a very much less successful outcome (<33% 5-year survival).

Newer chemotherapeutic agents are currently being investigated, and there is now increasing interest in the identification of molecular targets in ESFT, which include the mammalian target of rapamycin (mTOR) and insulin growth factor-1 (IGF-1) receptor pathways, that could be exploited therapeutically.

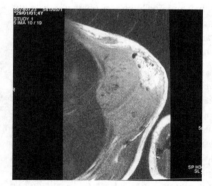

Figure 106.12: Ewing's sarcoma of the rib.

Evidence-Based Research

A number of aggressive malignant tumours occur that require multi-modal therapy, usually including surgical management. Table 106.2 presents a review of management strategies for rhabdomyosarcoma in children.

Table 106.2: Evidence-based research.

Title	Optimal management strategies for rhabdomyosarcoma in children
Authors	Walterhouse D, Watson A
Institution	Division of Hematology/Oncology, Children's Memorial Hospital, Northwestern University Feinberg School of Medicine, Chicago, Illinois, USA
Reference	Paediatr Drug 2007; 9(6):391–400
Problem	Rhabdomyosarcoma is the most common sarcoma of childhood. Fortunately, the goal of cure is realistic for the majority of patients with localized tumours. However, management of these patients remains challenging. The fact that the tumour arises in a wide variety of primary sites, some of which are associated with specific patterns of local invasion, regional lymph node spread, and therapeutic response, requires physicians to be familiar with site-specific staging and treatment details. In addition, rhabdomyosarcoma requires multimodality therapy that can be associated with significant acute toxicities and long-term effects, particularly when administered to young children. These factors sometimes present a dilemma as to the best approach to optimize the chance of cure, minimize toxicity, and respect quality of life.
Intervention	The purpose of this review is to discuss "optimal" management of this complicated tumour. Since the tumour is relatively rare and requires highly specialized care, and important management questions remain to be answered, optimal management of rhabdomyosarcoma includes enrollment in clinical trials whenever possible.
Comparison/ control (quality of evidence)	Appropriate management begins with establishing the correct pathologic diagnosis, histologic subtype, primary site, extent of disease (International Society of Pediatric Oncology (SIOP)-TNM-Union Internationale Contre le Cancer stage or Intergroup Rhabdomyosarcoma Study Group (IRSG) stage), and extent of resection (IRSG). Cooperative groups throughout North America and Europe have defined risk-adapted treatment based on these factors; this treatment requires a coordinated management plan that includes surgery, chemotherapy, and usually radiotherapy. The surgical approach for rhabdomyosarcoma is to excise the primary tumour, whenever possible, without causing major functional or cosmetic deficits. Wide excision is difficult in some primary sites and can be complicated by the fact that the tumour grows in a locally infiltrative manner so that complete resection is often neither possible nor medically indicated. Incompletely resected tumours are generally treated with radiotherapy. The cooperative groups reduce the dose of radiation based on the response of the tumour to chemotherapy and delay primary resection to differing degrees. Response-adjusted radiation administration may reduce the long-term effects of radiotherapy, such as bone growth arrest, muscle atrophy, bladder dysfunction, and induction of second malignant neoplasms; however, it may also be associated with an increased risk of tumour recurrence. All patients with rhabdomyosarcoma require chemotherapy. A backbone of vincristine and actinomycin D with either cyclophosphamide (VAC) or ifosfamide (IVA) has been established. Risk-adapted treatment involves reducing or eliminating the alklyating agent for patients with the most favourable disease characteristics.
Outcome/ effect	Clinical trials are ongoing to improve outcomes for higher risk patients; newer agents, such as topotecan or irinotecan, in combination with VAC or the use of agents in novel ways, are being investigated. Acute and long-term toxicities associated with these chemotherapy regimens include myelosuppression, febrile neutropaenia, hepatopathy, infertility, and second malignant neoplasms. A 5-year survival rate >70% has been achieved in recent trials for patients with localized rhabdomyosarcoma. However, the outcome for patients who present with metastatic disease remains poor.
Historical significance/ comments	In the future, risk-adapted classification of rhabdomyosarcoma will likely be based on biologic features, such as the presence of chromosomal translocations or specific gene expression profiles. It is hoped that newer therapies directed at specific molecular genetic defects will benefit all patients with rhabdomyosarcoma.

Key Summary Points

1. Tumours of soft tissue are mostly benign lesions of connective tissue in childhood.

2. Malignant soft tissue sarcomas (STSs) arise predominantly from the embryonic mesoderm deriving from a variety of cell types.

3. STSs are relatively rare—approximately 5–8% of childhood malignancies per year.

4. STSs mostly present as an asymptomatic mass in an extremity in older children.

5. There are at least three clinically relevant groups in childhood: congenital fibrosarcoma, rhabdomyosarcoma, and nonrhadomyosarcoma STS.

6. Nonrhabdomyosarcoma STS includes synovial sarcoma, liposarcoma, vascular tumours (e.g., Kaposi sarcoma, haemangiopericytoma, angiosarcoma), and alveolar soft part sarcoma.

7. Treatment is multimodal, usually involving neoadjuvant chemotherapy and conservative surgery. Radiotherapy is required only under certain circumstances.

8. The role of the surgeon is to establish a diagnosis; perform timely, adequate removal; assess metastatic spread; and provide supportive care (e.g., long-term venous access).

9. Although STSs are often highly malignant tumours, the prognosis has improved significantly over the last three decades. Up to 77% of tumours in children younger than 1 year of age are surgically resectable following neoadjuvant chemotherapy.

References

1. Loeb DM, Thornton K, Shokek O. Pediatric soft tissue sarcomas. Surg Clin North Am 2008; 88(3):615–627.

2. Gurney JG, Severson RK, Davis S, Robisin L. The incidence of cancer in children in the United States: sex, race and 1 year age-specific rates by histological type. Cancer 1995; 75:2186–2195.

3. Upton B, Chu Q, Li BD. Li-Fraumeni syndrome: the genetics and treatment considerations for the sarcoma and associated neoplasms. Surg Oncol Clin N Am 2009; 18(1):145–156.

4. Wang H, Garzon R, Sun H, Ladner KJ, Singh R, Dahlman J, et al. NF-kappaB-YY1-miR-29 regulatory circuitry in skeletal myogenesis and rhabdomyosarcoma. Cancer Cell 2008; 14(5):369–381.

5. Hayes-Jordan AA, Spunt SL, Poquette CA, Cain AM, Rao BN, Pappo AS, et al. Nonrhabdomyosarcoma soft tissue sarcomas in children: is age at diagnosis an important variable? J Pediatr Surg 2000; 35(6):948–953.

6. Minard-Colin V, Orbach D, Martelli H, Bodemer C, Oberlin O. Soft tissue tumors in neonates. Arch Pediatr 2009; 16(7):1039–1048.

7. Miettinen M. From morphological to molecular diagnosis of soft tissue tumors. Adv Exp Med Biol 2006; 587:99–113.

8. Plaschkes J. Epidemiology of neonatal tumours. In: Puri P, ed. Neonatal Tumours. Springer-Verlag, 1996, Pp 11–22.

9. Azizkhan RC. Neonatal tumours. In: Carachi R, Azmy A, Grosfeld JL, eds. The Surgery of Childhood Tumours, 1st ed. Arnold, 1999, Pp 107–123.

10. Mandong BM, Kidmas AT, Manasseh AN, Echejoh GO, Tanko MN, Madaki AJ. Epidemiology of soft tissue sarcomas in Jos, North Central Nigeria. Niger J Med 2007; 16(3):246–249.

11. Laurvick CL, Milne E, Blair E, de KN, Charles AK, Bower C. Fetal growth and the risk of childhood non-CNS solid tumours in Western Australia. Br J Cancer 2008; 99(1):179–181.

12. Gurney JG, Young JL, Roffers SD, et al. Soft tissue sarcomas. In: Gloeker Ries IA, Smith MA, Gurney JG, et al., eds. SEER Paediatric Monograph: Cancer Incidence and Survival among Children and Adolescents, United States SEER Program, 1975–1995. National Cancer Institute, 1999, Pp 111–124.

13. Paulino AC, Okcu MF. Rhabdomyosarcoma. Curr Probl Cancer 2008; 32(1):7–34.

14. Leuschner I, Newton WA, Jr, Schmidt D, Sachs N, Asmar L, Hamoudi A, et al. Spindle cell variants of embryonal rhabdomyosarcoma in the paratesticular region. A report of the Intergroup Rhabdomyosarcoma Study. Am J Surg Pathol 1993; 17(3):221–230.

15. Punyko JA, Mertens AC, Baker KS, Ness KK, Robison LL, Gurney JG. Long-term survival probabilities for childhood rhabdomyosarcoma. A population-based evaluation. Cancer 2005; 103(7):1475–1483.

16. Raney RB, Maurer HM, Anderson JR, Andrassy RJ, Donaldson SS, Qualman SJ, et al. The Intergroup Rhabdomyosarcoma Study Group (IRSG): Major lessons from the IRS-I through IRS-IV studies as background for the current IRS-V treatment protocols. Sarcoma 2001; 5(1):9–15.

17. Stevens MC, Rey A, Bouvet N, Ellershaw C, Flamant F, Habrand JL, et al. Treatment of nonmetastatic rhabdomyosarcoma in childhood and adolescence: third study of the International Society of Paediatric Oncology—SIOP Malignant Mesenchymal Tumor 89. J Clin Oncol 2005; 23(12):2618–2628.

18. Andrassy RJ, Okcu MF, Despa S, Raney RB. Synovial sarcoma in children: surgical lessons from a single institution and review of the literature. J Am Coll Surg 2001; 192(3):305–313.

19. Viejo-Borbolla A, Schulz TF. Kaposi's sarcoma-associated herpesvirus (KSHV/HHV8): key aspects of epidemiology and pathogenesis. AIDS Rev 2003; 5(4):222–229.

20. Sitas F, Newton R. Kaposi's sarcoma in South Africa. J Natl Cancer Inst Monogr 2001; 28:1–4.

21. Jawad MU, Cheung MC, Min ES, Schneiderbauer MM, Koniaris LG, Scully SP. Ewing sarcoma demonstrates racial disparities in incidence-related and sex-related differences in outcome: an analysis of 1631 cases from the SEER database, 1973–2005. Cancer 2009; 115(15):3526–3536.

22. Subbiah V, Anderson P, Lazar AJ, Burdett E, Raymond K, Ludwig JA. Ewing's sarcoma: standard and experimental treatment options. Curr Treat Options Oncol 2009; 10(1–2):126–140.

Further Reading

Carachi R, Grosfeld JL, Azmy AF, eds. The Surgery of Childhood Tumours. Springer, 2008.

Soliman H, Ferrari A, Thomas D. Sarcoma in young adult population: an international overview. Semin Oncol 2009; 36(3):227–236.

Walterhouse D, Watson A. Optimal management strategies for rhabdomyosarcoma in children. Paediatr Drugs 2007; 9(6):391–400.

CHAPTER 107
LIVER TUMOURS

Graeme Pitcher
V. T. Joseph

Introduction

The burden of tumours on African communities is often overshadowed by the immediacy of problems such as social and political instability and civil wars. Health problems such as communicable diseases and diseases borne from deprivation are in most places the priority of clinical care and the primary thrust for preventive strategies. Liver tumours, both benign and malignant, are uncommon in children and constitute only 3% of all solid organ lesions. Furthermore, overall figures show that malignant liver tumours account for less than 2% of all childhood malignancies. The incidence of the different histological types varies geographically and is related to hepatitis B and human immunodeficiency virus (HIV) prevalence.

In communities in Africa where access to medical care and sophisticated imaging technologies is limited, deep-seated visceral tumours often grow to an enormous size before they are detected and treated. In most areas, the facilities for the provision of good-quality, modern, multimodal and multidisciplinary care, which is so critical for a good outcome in these patients, simply do not exist. Little is known about the epidemiology and the outcomes of the management of liver tumours in children on the African continent as a whole because good-quality reports and registry data are generally lacking. The unique milieu of predisposing infectious diseases and other environmental influences and carcinogens results in a different pattern of malignant tumours on the continent, making research into their causes and treatment all the more pressing.

Demographics

Data reviewed recently from a tumour registry of paediatric oncology services in South Africa[1] provides a scarce and much-needed insight into the problem. An 18-year review provided 274 malignant liver tumours in children under the age of 14 years—amounting to 1 case per million at-risk children per year, in keeping with data from the United States.[2] The incidence of benign primary liver tumours is not known, but is probably similarly rare.

Of the malignant tumours, hepatoblastoma (HB) is the most common, occurring in 48% of tumour patients.[1] This tumour shows a distinct male preponderance (male-to-female ratio of 2:1), occurring at a mean age of 2.1 years of age and without any ethnic predeliction. Interestingly, in this series, no patient older than 4 years of age presented, and all patients had markedly elevated levels of alpha-foetoprotein (AFP).

Hepatocellular carcinoma is the second most common tumour, occurring in 27% of patients and showing a definite ethnic and gender bias.[1] The distribution of the other malignant tumours seen in the registry is depicted in Table 107.1. The incidence of HB is lower than reported from Western series (where the incidence appears to be increasing), which may be due to lower rates of such recognized risk factors as low birth weight and low maternal age,[3] genetic differences, or failure of diagnosis.

The study showed an interesting trend.[1] Over the course of the period of study, vascular tumours and Kaposi sarcoma seemed to increase in incidence, whereas hepatocellular carcinoma seemed to be occurring less commonly. The authors attributed this to the beneficial effect of the introduction of mandatory immunisation against hepatitis B in South Africa during the course of the period of study and possibly to the growing impact of the HIV epidemic in the country.

Aetiology

A thorough description of all the known causes and risk factors for liver tumours is beyond the scope of this book. This chapter therefore concentrates on the factors that are known or suspected of impacting the unique pattern of tumours seen on the African continent. The role of hepatitis B coinfection is well recognized as the most important risk factor for liver tumours in Africa.[4] Factors such as aflatoxin exposure, membranous vena caval obstruction, and excessive iron ingestion may play minor roles in placing African children at risk for liver tumours.

Table 107.1: Demographic of malignant liver tumours in childhood.

Tumour	Incidence of HB (%)	Gender bias (male-to-female ratio)	Age (years)	Racial distribution	Alpha-foetoprotein	Comments
Hepatocellular carcinoma	48	1.95:1	2.16	Equal	All ↑	Less than 4 years of age
Hepatocellular carcinoma	27	2.09:1	10.5	Black	85%↑	fibrolamellar variant, 12%; hepatitis B positive, 69%
Liver sarcoma	6	0.4:1	7.6			
Vascular tumours						
Kaposi sarcoma	5					All HIV positive
Haemangio-endothelioma	5					

Source: Moore SW, Davidson A, Hadley GP, Kruger M, Poole J, Stones D, Wainwright L, Wessels G. Malignant liver tumors in South African children: a national audit. World J Surg 2008; 32(7). Modified with permission.

The reasons for the lower-than-expected incidence of HB in Africa are not well understood, as mentioned above. The relationship between the Beckwith-Weidemann syndrome (BWS) and hemihypertrophy and the risk of HB (and more commonly Wilms' tumour and adrenocortical carcinoma) are well known. Regular screening of affected infants by three-monthly US and AFP monitoring is recommended. AFP is a serum protein produced by foetal liver cells, yolk sac, and the gastrointestinal tract.

The aetiology of most benign liver tumours is obscure. Adenomas associated with high-dose estrogen administration in oral contraceptives have become much less common after these drugs were reformulated. Patients with glycogen storage disease due to glucose-6-phosphatase deficiency or Fanconi anaemia are at risk for adenomas and should be monitored.

Clinical Presentation

Mass Presentation
In the majority of cases, the presentation of liver tumours in childhood is one of a progressively enlarging mass. The poor access of many children on the African continent to quality tertiary health care as well as the relatively hidden subcostal position of the liver result in many patients presenting with extraordinarily large tumours. Sometimes patients are erroneously referred for pulmonology assessments due to diaphragmatic elevation or to orthopaedics for apparent scoliosis. Patients with hepatoblastoma will occasionally show evidence of thrombocytosis and fever. Jaundice is usually not present except in the case of obstructing hilar tumours. As seen more frequently with Wilms' tumour, some unfortunate children will present in a very poor nutritional state with advanced cancer cachexia.[5]

Cirrhosis Presentation
In the Western world, most patients with de novo hepatocellular carcinoma (HCC) do not have underlying cirrhosis.[6] In sub-Saharan Africa, where the prevalence of hepatitis B is so much greater, the presentation with cirrhosis is much more common. Cirrhotic patients may present with symptoms of the underlying disease. In these cases, the presenting symptoms may be those of upper gastrointestinal haemorrhage due to varices, nosebleeds from thrombocytopaenia, lethargy, fatigue, failure to thrive, weight loss, or jaundice. In many patients with cirrhosis, the tumour will be detected on US or computed tomography (CT) scan screening at the time of the patient's first presentation with symptoms, but occasionally these will be detected during routine screening in larger centres.

Haemorrhage or Rupture Presentation
Intraperitoneal bleeding can rarely be the presenting symptom, either as a result of spontaneous rupture or more commonly after misguided attempts at needle biopsy. Rupture of large undifferentiated embryonal sarcomas has been described in older children. Newborns with ante-natally undiagnosed hepatoblastoma or haemangioma are at particular risk of death during delivery.[7]

Prenatal Presentation
Routine antenatal US screening is not available to the vast majority of mothers on the African continent. In larger centres, both HB and haemangiomas may be diagnosed by antenatal US. This obviously aids in the overall care of the patient by directing the place and mode of delivery to diminish the risk of rupture and to expedite postnatal management. Large tumours (typically mesenchymal hamartomas and haemangiomas) can compromise foetal well-being and cause hydrops foetalis or even foetal death.[7,8]

Haematological Presentation
Rarely, infants with cutaneous or visceral haemangiomas may develop a consumptive coagulopathy. This has been named the Kasabach-Merritt syndrome. It can occur with any histological type of vascular lesion, but usually occurs in the kaposiform haemangioendothelioma or in the tufted angioma variants.[9] Its hallmarks are thrombocytopaenia and consumptive coagulopathy, which can be life threatening.

Investigations

Haematological Studies
All children with a suspected liver mass should be investigated by haematological and imaging studies. A full blood count, coagulation profile, and liver function tests, as well as a screen for tumour markers (AFP and β-HCG, or β-human chorionic gonadotropin) should be performed. Infants with haemangiomas should have thyroid function screening. AFP is the most useful single test. The results need to be interpreted in the light of normal high levels in the neonatal period. The 95% confidence intervals for AFP levels is 15.7–146.5 μg/ml.[10] Levels usually return to the normal adult range of <10 ng/ml by the age of 2 years. An encountered pitfall is that neonates with HB may have AFP levels scarcely higher than normal for their age. This limits its value as a screening tool but can also mislead the clinician. An elevated level can also occur in other tumours, such as mesenchymal hamartoma or in the face of hepatocellular regeneration.

If cirrhosis is suspected, viral studies seeking hepatitis A, B, C; cytomegalovirus; and Epstein-Barr virus should be included. In all patients, the HIV serology should be determined, either to aid in the diagnosis (e.g., for patients with vascular tumours) or to be able to optimize their condition for a potential major resection. In cases where parasitic disease is possible, hydatid serology should be considered.

Imaging
In the Western experience, imaging includes US, contrast-enhanced CT scan, and MRI. US is the most commonly used imaging modality for all masses in the liver. Haemangiomas are echogenic but cannot be differentiated from other vascular lesions such as tumours. The scan may be improved if colour Doppler is employed but US is probably most useful in follow-up of lesions that are being treated conservatively. US performed by an experienced operator is an excellent tool for the diagnosis of liver tumours and may be the only modality available in many African centres.

Contrast-enhanced CT provides good imaging of hepatic haemangiomas. The lesion shows peripheral enhancement during the arterial phase, which progresses towards the central area during the portal venous phase. For the planning of surgery, CT scanning is essential. It shows the operating surgeon the relationship of the tumour to major vessels and its exact location in the liver with greater accuracy, allowing a better assessment of resectability. In addition, the appearance may suggest the tumour type. Large, low-density lesions in the right lobe suggest mesenchymal hamartomas or undifferentiated embryonal sarcoma (Figure 107.1). Hepatoblastoma typically appears as a heterogenous solid tumour with ill-defined borders and may contain areas of calcification (Figure 107.2).

MRI provides the most accurate diagnosis of haemangiomas. Gadolinium can be given intravenously to produce enhancement of the lesion. In planning surgical resections, MRI can be extremely useful in defining the margins of the lesion in relation to adjacent vascular structures. Unfortunately, MRI is not routinely available in the African setting.

Radionuclide studies and hepatic angiograms are not used routinely in the imaging of haemangiomas in the liver.

Positron emission tomography (PET) scanning is not available in most African centres. Hepatic scintigraphy is no longer indicated except in the unusual incidence of differentiating uptake in an area of focal nodular hyperplasia (FNH) to distinguish it from an adenoma.

All patients with malignant tumours should receive chest x-rays as screening for metastases, and chest CT scans should be performed if any abnormality is detected. In patients with HCC, the screen should include a bone scan as well as CT of the brain.[11]

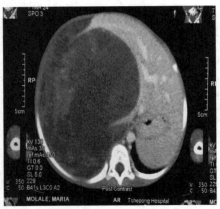

Figure 107.1: CT appearance of a large mesenchymal hamartoma in the right lobe of the liver

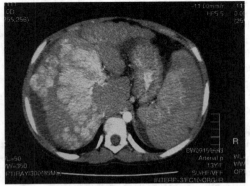

Figure 107.2: A large hepatoblastoma in the right lobe of the liver prior to neoadjuvant therapy.

Table 107.2: Main categories of liver tumours.

Malignant	Benign
Hepatoblastoma	Vascular neoplasm
Hepatocellular carcinoma	Haemangioma
Sarcoma	Haemanioendothelioma
Undifferentiated	Mesenchymal hamartoma
Angiosarcoma	Adenoma
Rhabdomyosarcoma	Focal nodular hyperplasia
	Adenoma
	Simple cyst

Types of Liver Tumours

The main categories of liver tumours are presented in Table 107.2.

Malignant

The two most important childhood liver malignancies are hepatoblastoma and hepatocellular carcinoma. The relative frequencies of these diseases shows a wide geographical variation and is influenced by the presence of environmental and genetic factors.

Hepatoblastoma

HB is a rare malignant neoplasm of the liver that occurs in children between the ages of 1 to 3 years. It is the most common primary malignant liver tumour, accounting for two-thirds of all cases. There is a male preponderance, with boys being twice as commonly affected as girls.

The prognosis for HB has improved in recent years, but the maxim still holds true that at some time in the course of the patient's treatment, a resection with complete peritumoural clearance is necessary for a good outcome.

The characteristic laboratory finding is the presence of an elevated AFP. At birth, it is normal to have high levels of AFP, which then decline over a period of time. In HB, the AFP is markedly elevated in at least 90% of the cases, and it can be also used as a marker to follow the response to therapy as well as to detect recurrence. The half-life of AFP is 4 to 9 days, and it returns to normal values approximately 6 weeks after tumour resection. Very high or very low levels of AFP in HB usually are associated with a poor prognosis.

A number of imaging studies are used in the diagnosis of children presenting with an abdominal mass that may be HB:

Plain abdominal x-ray shows a soft tissue mass in the right hypochondrium and occasionally may also show calcification within the mass.

Ultrasound shows HB as a hyperechoic mass in the liver; US is particularly good for showing the vascular anatomy using colour Doppler.

CT with contrast shows lesion contrast enhancement during the portal venous phase (Figure 107.3).

• *MRI* is the investigation of choice, but unfortunately for most children in this age group it will require general anaesthesia and it is not generally available in Africa. The images are sequenced after administration of gadolinium-based contrast agents, and three-dimensional (3D) reconstruction can be performed to provide an accurate anatomical picture (Figure 107.4).

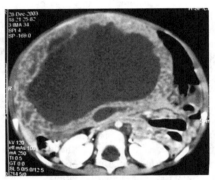

Figure 107.3: CT scan of hepatoblastoma.

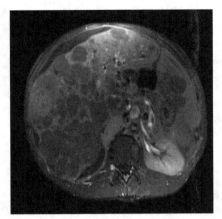

Figure 107.4: MRI of hepatoblastoma.

• *CT chest* is always performed to detect the presence of lung metastases.

• *Bone scans* are usually done to exclude any metastatic involvement.

The HB tumour is derived from immature liver precursor cells and it is usually a single lesion situated in the right lobe. On microscopic examination, microvascular invasion is often present, which must be taken into account when surgical resections are planned. The tumour has a pseudocapsule, and the surrounding liver tissue does not show evidence of cirrhosis. Metastatic spread usually occurs to the lungs only, with bone secondaries being very rare.

Histologically, several subtypes have been described.

- Epithelial (56%)
  - Foetal (31%)—this has a good prognosis if completely resected
  - Embryonal + foetal (19%)
  - Macrotrabecular (3%)
  - Small cell undifferentiated (3%)
- Mixed epithelial/mesenchymal (44%)
  - Teratoid features present
  - Teratoid features absent

A large amount of data has now confirmed that HB is associated with a number of other conditions that are known to have a genetic basis. This is consistent with evidence that HB is derived from a pluripotent stem cell and arises as a result of developmental error during the formation of the liver.

- Beckwith-Wiedemann syndrome and hemihypertrophy: In these syndromes, there is loss of heterozygosity (LOH) of chromosome 11p.

- Familial adenomatosis polyposis (FAP): Mutations in the adenomatous polyposis coli (APC) supressor gene lead to alterations in the Wnt/Bcatenin signalling pathway contributing to the development of tumour.

- Talipes equinovarus

- Patent ductus arteriosus

- Tetralogy of Fallot

- Extrahepatic biliary atresia

Also, studies in Germany have shown the association with very low birth weight infants, and this has been confirmed elsewhere.

Two major staging systems have been used in the treatment of HB: The North American system, which uses postsurgical staging; and the European SIOPEL/PRETEXT,[12] which is a presurgical staging system. PRETEXT stands for PRETreatment EXTent of disease.

According to the PRETEXT system, which is assessed by CT scan, patients are divided into risk groups on the basis of the PRETEXT type and the behaviour of the tumour. The PRETEXT staging system involves dividing the liver into four sections (Figure 107.5):

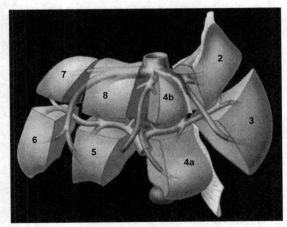

Figure 107.5: Anatomical liver segmentation.

- Segments 2 + 3 (left lateral section)
- Segments 4a + 4b (left medial section)
- Segments 5 + 8 (right anterior section)
- Segments 6 + 7 (right posterior section)

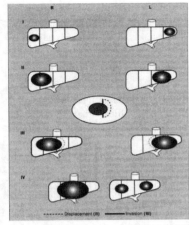

Figure 107.6: Four liver sections for PRETEXT staging.

The PRETEXT number (Figure 107.6) is derived by subtracting the number of adjacent sections not involved with a tumour from the number 4. Thus,

- PRETEXT I: One section involved, three sections free
- PRETEXT II: One or two sections involved, two adjoining sections free
- PRETEXT III: Two or three sections involved, one adjacent section free
- PRETEXT IV: All four sections involved

Additional criteria include:

- caudate lobe involvement;
- inferior vena cava involvement;
- hepatic veins;
- portal veins;
- extraabdominal disease;
- tumour rupture/intraperitoneal haemorrhage;
- lymph node metastases; and
- distant metastases.

Based on these criteria, patients can be classified into high-risk and standard-risk groups. Standard-risk patients are those classified as PRETEXT I, II, and III with no spread outside of the liver. High-risk patients are those classified as PRETEXT IV or with extrahepatic spread, distant metastases, or vascular invasion.

Most patients are asymptomatic, and the first indication of the tumour may be an enlarging abdomen. This accounts for the finding that 40% of cases are in an advanced stage at the time of presentation and 20% already have pulmonary metastases. Among other symptoms are:

- anorexia, loss of weight, and failure to thrive;
- osteopaenia;
- rupture with haemorrhage; and
- precocious puberty associated with β-hCG secreting tumours.

The HB tumour is usually fairly responsive to chemotherapy with cisplatin and doxorubicin (known as PLADO), and in most cases, resection is facilitated by using these drugs as neoadjuvant chemotherapy. In high-risk cases, carbopalatin is often added to the regimen. These approaches have yielded high resection rates and 3-year tumour-free survival rates of 89% for standard-risk patients and 48% for high-risk patients.[13] Liver transplantation, in countries where that modality is available, has greatly improved the outcome of patients with extensive high-risk disease. Recent data clearly show that posttransplant outcomes are much more favourable in borderline patients who were subjected to primary transplantation compared to those in whom transplantation was attempted after unsuccessful resection (i.e., as rescue therapy).[14,15] Recently, liver transplantation has been shown to play a significant role in the treatment of unresectable HB with 5-year disease-free survivals of 80%.

Hepatocellular carcinoma

HCC accounts for only 23% of paediatric malignant liver tumours, but the actual incidence varies in different geographical areas. In countries where hepatitis B and HIV are prevalent, the incidence can rise to almost 50%. Two peak age groups can be identified: the first from 0 to 4 years and the second from 10 to 14 years. Unlike HB, this tumour is associated with cirrhosis of the liver. Predisposing factors therefore include metabolic liver disease, hepatitis B, biliary atresia, and total parenteral nutrition.

Clinically, patients present with an abdominal mass, pain, weight loss, anaemia, and fever. The AFP is elevated in 50% of cases. Imaging studies are similar to HB, and tissue diagnosis by liver biopsy is required for confirmation of the disease and to assess the extent of cirrhotic involvement of the liver.

The outlook for the African child with HCC remains dismal. The majority present with multicentric disease, and most tumours (85%) are not amenable to resection from the outset.[5,16] Most patients with unresectable disease are best treated by palliation. Response rates to chemotherapy with or without radiation treatment tend to be poor, although newer agents that have been tried in adults with HCC in the developed world may improve the outlook. Transplantation has been offered to a small, select group of patients with exclusively intrahepatic disease in whom resection is not possible, but results have been mixed.

Hepatic sarcoma

Undifferentiated embryonal sarcoma is the third most common malignant tumour in the liver. These tumours occur in children between 5 and 10 years of age. They are mesenchymal in origin and are closely related to the vascular tumours. Angiosarcoma of the liver is a highly malignant tumour and has a poor outlook. Embryonal rhabdomyosarcoma arises from intrahepatic biliary ducts and often presents clinically as obstructive jaundice. The treatment and outcomes follow those of the rhabdomyosarcoma protocols.

As these are rare tumours, it is essential to have tissue diagnosis before appropriate therapy can be instituted. Although US-guided percutaneous biopsy has been advocated, it is safer to do an open biopsy or laparoscopic-assisted biopsy due to the risk of bleeding. This approach will also provide better tissue samples for histology and specialised examination.

The undifferentiated embryonal sarcoma classically presents with a large, usually right-lobed, low-density or sometimes frankly cystic lesion on imaging, which may easily be mistaken for a simple liver cyst,[17] or hydatid disease[18] in high prevalence areas for that disease. AFP levels are usually normal in this tumour. Careful planning to enhance the possibility of complete resection is mandatory, with misdiagnosis significantly diminishing the chance of cure.

The only hope of cure in patients presenting with one of the variants of sarcoma is complete resection. Neoadjuvant treatment may be helpful in rendering tumours resectable, particularly in embryonal rhabdomyosarcoma and in some cases of undifferentiated embryonal sarcomas.[19] Results in patients in whom resection can be achieved are good, with cure achieved in 20–30% of cases and useful palliation achieved in many[5] (Figure 107.7).

Kaposi sarcoma and malignant vascular tumours in AIDS patients

Malignant vascular lesions in the HIV-positive patient tend to be more aggressive, being more commonly anaplastic and frequently metastatic at presentation. This is commonly a terminal manifestation of severe immunodeficiency and carries a very poor prognosis.

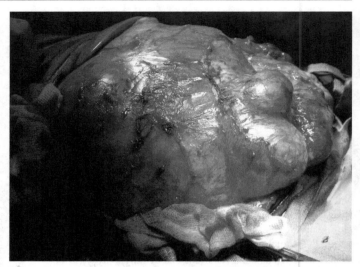

Figure 107.7: Massive undifferentiated embryonal sarcoma, successfully resected with adjuvant chemotherapy and disease-free at 2 years.

Benign Tumours

Benign lesions of the liver presenting as tumours account for one-third of all hepatic masses. Most of these lesions are not neoplastic in origin and may be better regarded as malformations. Benign tumours can be divided into two groups:

- Mesenchymal
  - Haemangioma
  - Hamartoma
- Epithelial
  - Cysts
  - Focal nodular hyperplasia
  - Hepatic adenoma

Haemangiomas

Haemangiomas are the most common benign lesions seen in the liver and are frequently seen in the first 6 months of life. They vary from small lesions that are incidentally detected on scans done for other reasons to massive lesions that may precipitate high-output cardiac failure. Large lesions that are symptomatic present with abdominal pain, abdominal mass, or with complications of which bleeding is the most frequent.

The natural history is one of spontaneous regression, and in asymptomatic cases a conservative approach with regular monitoring may be all that is needed. In the presence of symptoms that may be life-threatening, treatment is initiated with high-dose steroids. Alpha interferon has also been used, but it is toxic and the response is slow, occuring over a period of months. Focal lesions may be resected or controlled with hepatic artery embolisation. Hepatic irradiation and radio frequency ablation have been successfully used to treat large lesions in some cases, but the experience is limited. Extensive lesions that cannot be managed in this way may require liver transplantation.

Infantile haemangioendothelioma

Infantile haemangioendothelioma is the third most common liver tumour in childhood (12% of all paediatric liver tumours in the Western world), and is the most common liver tumour in infancy. It is usually seen in infants younger than the age of 6 months; 85% of cases present within this age group. There is a female preponderance with a female-to-male ratio of 2:1. Fifty percent have cutaneous haemangiomas and the lesions themselves may show calcifications. They are usually benign, but malignant sarcoma can occur.

The natural history of these tumours is that they grow in the first year of life and then start regressing probably due to thrombosis in the vascular channels. Histologically, they are mesenchymal tumours with vascular channels lined by endothelial cells. Two subtypes are recognised:

• *Type 1* consists of multiple small vascular channels with calcification and a fibrous stroma containing bile ductules.

• *Type 2* consists of vascular channels with disorganised endothelial lining and there is no stroma containing bile ductules.

Haemangioendothelioma is generally managed conservatively, as spontaneous regression will usually occur. Intervention is required if the lesion becomes symptomatic or due to its size. Steroids have been used to induce regression, but they are not usually effective. Surgical resection provides cure and is the treatment of choice when feasible.

Mesenchymal hamartoma

Mesenchymal hamartoma is a rare benign tumour of the liver that is more properly classified as a malformation. In the Western world, it accounts for only 6% of liver tumours in childhood and generally occurs between the ages of 1 to 2 years. The right lobe of the liver is almost always the site of involvement (Figure 107.8).

Histologically, the lesion consists of an overgrowth of mesenchymal tissue with a marked tendency to cyst formation. This is reflected in the CT findings of a heterogenous, complex mass with multiple cystic spaces. The treatment is either marsupialisation of the cysts or surgical resection, which can be successfully done because the tumour is always confined to one lobe only.

All mesenchymal hamartomas are best treated by complete resection. Incomplete resection has been associated with the development of sarcoma.[20] Infantile haemangiomas can be managed expectantly without biopsy if their imaging appearance is typical. Careful medical management, consisting of treatment of cardiac failure and occasionally hypothyroidism (due to expression of type 3 iodothyronine deiodinase in the tumour, resulting in consumption of thyroxine) is critical to a good outcome.

Liver cysts

Nonparasitic cysts of the liver may be simple cysts or part of the spectrum of polycystic disease (Figure 107.9). Simple cysts are usually incidental findings and are generally single. They vary in size from small lesions to very large ones that occupy the whole lobe of the liver. The wall is thin and composed of mature connective tissue. The treatment of large, symptomatic simple liver cysts is surgical, as percutaneous aspiration is always associated with recurrence. Most cysts can be unroofed, leaving the interior open to the peritoneal cavity. This may be done laparoscopically with good results. It may sometimes be necessary to carry out hepatic resection if the cyst is very large and occupies the whole lobe of the liver.

The cysts of Caroli's disease arise from the intrahepatic biliary ducts and are filled with bile. They may involve a single lobe, in which case hepatic resection is the treatment of choice. However, both lobes of the liver may also be involved, and transplantation is then the only possible mode of treatment.

Polycystic liver disease is associated with polycystic kidney disease in 50% of cases. The cysts may be diffuse throughout the liver or may occupy one lobe. The hepatic parenchyma between the cysts is normal and liver function is well preserved.

Liver abscesses may present as cystic lesions, or an infected cyst may subsequently appear as an abscess. The aetiology may be pyogenic or amoebic. Pyogenic abscess is usually secondary to infection from the biliary tract. It may sometimes be associated with immune deficiency states, especially chronic granulomatous disease. Rarely, tuberculous abscess of the liver may occur without any evidence of lung disease.

Amoebic abscess is endemic in certain parts of Africa and Asia. The parasite enters the portal venous channels through the intestine and lodges in the liver, causing abscess formation.

Simple liver cysts can be treated expectantly unless they are large or symptomatic, in which case they should be treated by resection if possible

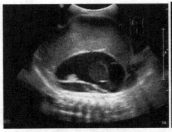
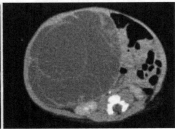

Figure 107.8: Mesenchymal harmatoma.

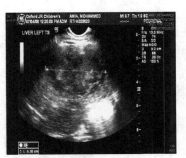

Figure 107.9: Liver cyst.

or by aspiration, sclerotherapy or fenestration as circumstances permit.[21]

Focal nodular hyperplasia

FNH represents a localised proliferation of hepatocytes in response to a vascular malformation. It is the second most common benign tumour of the liver, accounting for 8% of the lesions seen; it has a predilection for females. The lesions usually present as solitary, well-defined nodules, and the characteristic feature is the presence of a central scar with radiating fibrous septa. Bile duct proliferation is seen on histology.

Two types of FNH have been described:

• Classic (80%) contains all three components: abnormal nodular architecture, malformed vessels, and cholangiolar proliferation.

• Nonclassic (20%) contains two of the three components of the classic type but always includes bile duct proliferation and is further subdivided into three subtypes: telangiectatic FNH, FNH with cytologic atypia, and mixed hyperplastic and adenomatous FNH.

Clinically, most FNHs are asymptomatic and are discovered during routine scanning. They can, however, present with abdominal pain and with a palpable mass. Although oral contraceptives do not cause these lesions, they may aggravate them and precipitate complications such as infarction and bleeding.

The diagnosis can be made on imaging studies when the characteristic central scar with a stellate appearance is seen. Unfortunately, a positive diagnosis can be achieved in only two-thirds of the patients, and other lesions (particularly hepatocellular carcinoma) can mimic the appearance on scans. It is therefore advisable that in all cases where the diagnosis is not clear and in patients who are symptomatic, surgical exploration and biopsy or resection of the affected area should be carried out.

Hepatic adenoma

Hepatic adenoma is a rare, benign tumour arising from liver cells. It most often occurs in young women and is associated with the use of oral contraceptives. The lesions are generally solitary (80%) but may be multiple (20%). Histologically, the tumour is composed of sheets of hepatocytes containing fat and glycogen with an absence of bile ducts and portal tracts. These lesions have a propensity to rupture and bleed and may rarely also undergo malignant transformation to hepatocellular carcinoma.

The diagnosis in the Western experience is made on the history and imaging findings on CT and gadolinium-enhanced MRI. Typically, adenomas show arterial phase enhancement and the presence of fat and haemorrhage. Nuclear medicine studies are also helpful.

Surgical exploration is advised in all cases due to the risk of haemorrhage. Withdrawal of oral contraceptive use does not lead to regression of the lesions. Solitary lesions are managed by localised resections. Multiple lesions may require biopsy and follow-up evaluation.

Other benign tumours

Some tumours, most recently described as the diffuse type,[22] are large, occupying almost the entire liver (Figure 107.10); these will require systemic steroid or alpha-2A-interferon therapy. In life-threatening circumstances, hepatic artery embolisation (or ligation at open operation) can show dramatic results. Adenomas of the liver are considered premalignant and should be resected where possible. Patients with FNH should be treated expectantly because this condition has no premalignant potential.

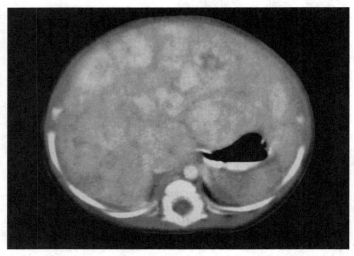

Figure 107.10: Typical CT scan appearance of large, diffuse infantile hepatic haemangioma, typical of the type associated with cardiac failure, coagulopathy, and life threat.

Management

Work-up should be expeditious, and children should be aggressively nutritionally supported, particularly in neglected cases. Treatment depends on the suspected histological type of the tumour (see Table 107.2), its resectability, the presence of metastatic or extrahepatic spread, and the general condition of the patient, including the presence or absence of cirrhosis. Social factors, such as parental compliance, concordance of beliefs with respect to the cause of illness, and access to medical services, need to be assessed. In some cases, these factors will sadly mitigate against any attempt at curative treatment.

Biopsy

The role of biopsy is somewhat controversial. For patients with a typical clinical picture of HB (between 6 months to 3 years of age, elevated AFP more than three times the normal for age, and perhaps fever and thrombocytosis), chemotherapy can usually be started without biopsy confirmation,[23] although not all units follow this approach. All other patients must be submitted to histological biopsy, either by submission of the completed resection specimen if the tumour is deemed safely resectable, or by a percutaneous, laparoscopically guided, or open biopsy at laparotomy. A core-cutting (Trucut®) needle usually gives adequate tissue for the pathologist to make an accurate assessment. It is very important for the clinician to liase closely with the pathologist if there is any doubt as to the diagnosis. A serious pitfall of management

is to falsely assume one kind of pathology and to treat incorrectly. A typical example is the management of HB in a young infant or neonate as a presumed haemangioma.

Surgery

Liver surgery is a major undertaking and requires a specialist team for both the intraoperative and postoperative care of the patient. Thorough preoperative evaluation using appropriate imaging studies is carried out to plan the surgery. The abdomen is opened through an upper transverse or bilateral subcostal incision. Special retractors are available that are clamped to the sides of the operating table and hold the blades to retract the costal margins. The liver is mobilised by dividing the falciform and both triangular ligaments (Figure 107.11). The line of resection is then marked on the surface, and division of the hepatic paenchyma is started. This can be done in several ways: finger fracture, crushing with clamps, bipolar diathermy, LigaSure™, harmonic scalpel, or Cavitron® ultrasonic surgical aspirator (CUSA®). As the division proceeds, the vessels need to be controlled with coagulation or ligatures. The procedure can be made easier by vascular control. Usually, only portal triad occlusion with a clamp that controls hepatic artery and portal venous inflow into the liver is all that is required. The clamp must be released after 30 minutes, and then it may be reapplied after a short interval. The operation should be completed by that time to avoid ischaemic damage to the liver. With very large or vascular tumours, particularly in the right lobe, it may be necessary to obtain total vascular control by clamping the suprahepatic and infrahepatic vena cava as well. Bleeding from the cut surface can also be reduced by keeping the central venous pressure low. At the end of the procedure, the cut surface is sealed with fibrin glue, and the right subhepatic space is drained (Figure 107.12).

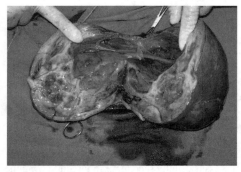

Figure 107.11: Operative view of right lobe hepatoblastoma.

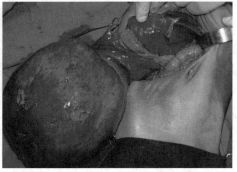

Figure 107.12: Cross section of the tumour from Figure 107.11.

Resection Techniques

Liver resection surgery should always be performed by a surgeon with operative experience with the liver and a thorough knowledge of its segmental anatomy. Before embarking on any liver resection, it is vitally important to assemble the required personnel and facilities as these are not universally available in developing countries (see the checklist in Table 107.3). The most important facilitator of surgical safety and comfort is good exposure. Optical magnification in the form of 2.5 to 3.5 loupes is essential. A headlight illuminates the darker corners and enhances safety. The bilateral subcostal incision affords excellent exposure, and when combined with a strong mechanical retractor such as a Thompson retractor, usually suffices without the necessity for a midline extension except in older children with narrow subcostal angles. On entering the abdomen, a routine inspection of the abdominal cavity and assessment of extrahepatic spread is performed. The liver should be completely mobilised, allowing access and slinging of the inferior vena cava both above (subdiaphragmatically) and below the liver and to the hepatoduodenal ligament. Although the "Pringle manoeuvre" should be avoided, if possible, to ensure normal liver function and production of coagulation factors during the procedure, it is best to have it exposed preemptively in the event that it is required.

Table 107.3: Checklist of essential equipment, personnel, and drugs for liver resection

Surgical equipment	Personnel and facilities	Drugs, blood, pumps
Vascular instruments	Experienced anaesthetist	Good venous access
Mechanical retractor	Able first assistant	Packed cells and fresh frozen plasma (FFP)
Optical magnification	Able scrub nursing team	Blood pumps
Electrocautery	Postoperative intensive care unit (ICU)	Infusion pumps for inotropes
Sutures	Warming device	
Parenchymal dividers	Intraoperative ultrasound	
Argon beam	Pathologist	
Topical haemostatic agents		

Most resections are best carried out anatomically. This has the advantage of minimising blood loss, injury to biliary structures, and inadequate resections leaving a residual tumour.[11] Hilar dissection prior to parenchymal transection facilitates the performance of major resections by determining the anatomical location of vital structures providing inflow and bile drainage from the liver remnant. It is not necessary to perform cholangiography routinely.

A slightly head-down position lowers the inferior vena caval venous pressure, minimising bleeding, and facilitates venous return, optimising the patient's haemodynamic stability. The line of transection is marked on the liver capsule with electrocautery. An almost bloodless field can be achieved by the placement of pledgeted sutures through the hepatic parenchyma prior to starting division.[24] If this is not possible in larger tumours, then the first assistant can usually achieve very useful bimanual liver compression, which provides haemostasis as well as stabilising and exposing the plane of transection.

Parenchymal division can be safely achieved by a number of techniques, according to the availability of specialised equipment or the surgeon's individual preference. Instruments such as the ultrasonic dissector, LigaSure, harmonic scalpel, and TissueLink™ are useful adjuncts to a good operation, but safe transection of the parenchyma can be achieved by the use of electrocautery alone in most cases. Large veins (both portal and hepatic) will be encountered periodically and are best suture ligated, or clipped with a clip applicator. For this purpose, the LigaSure certainly facilitates an easier and safer division of such vessels. Transecting the parenchyma in the direction of the

inferior liver margin up towards the hepatic veins is preferred because it allows for maximal exposure (towards the end of tissue transection) of the most dangerous area of the procedure at the hepatic veins. These veins are most commonly suture ligated with a polypropylene suture. Raw surface bleeding can be managed by a combination of suture, electrocautery, argon beam laser (if available), or various topical haemostatic agents. The liver bed is always drained by an active suction drain, as it is an area of negative pressure.

Postoperative Complications

A vast number of complications can potentially occur following major liver resection. Among the most important and specific to the operation are postoperative haemorrhage and postoperative liver dysfunction due to an insult to an insufficient-sized liver remnant—the "small for size syndrome". A safe remnant liver is usually considered to be >25% of the functional liver volume, or 0.8–1.0% of body mass. As long as that guideline is respected and there has not been a significant insult to the remnant, then this complication should occur very rarely.[25] Postoperative bleeding can usually be avoided by maintaining liver function by limiting periods of cross-clamping, judicious blood and product use, and maintenance of normal haematological parameters and meticulous haemostasis of all areas, including the liver raw surface.

Other less dangerous but more common problems include bile leaks, prolonged ascitic drainage, pleural effusions, atelectasis, and pulmonary infections. These can be managed on their merits. Limiting the use of postoperative ventilation can dramatically reduce pulmonary complications and is safe if used with discretion.

Prognosis and Outcomes

The prognosis for benign tumours is excellent overall. The two exceptions to this rule are large mesenchymal hamartomas and infantile haemangiomas. Children with large central mesenchymal hamartomas (Figure 107.13) present a specific challenge; these can be resected with innovative nonanatomic resections and by a technique of dissection in the immediate peritumoural plane in order to avoid injury to major portal or venous structures.[5] Concerns about malignant transformation of the residual tumour should not override safety concerns. Multimodal therapy combined with medical treatment and embolotherapy or hepatic artery ligation of the infant with diffuse haemangioma have improved the outcomes for these infants as well. Whereas transplantation has been used in that scenario in the developed world,[26] it will rarely be feasible on the African continent, even in transplant centres.

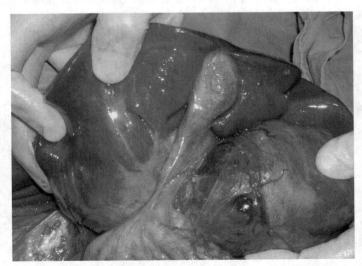

Figure 107.13: Intraoperative appearance of central mesenchymal hamartoma in a 2-year-old child.

Prevention

Immunisation against hepatitis B provides a wonderful opportunity for the prevention of hepatocellular carcinoma in childhood. For example, compulsory hepatitis B immunisation commenced in the United States in 1992,[27] and it has been predicted that deaths in children due to hepatitis B could be decreased by 80% as a result of effective vaccine programs.[28] Within the last few years, many African countries have commenced hepatitis B immunisation programs.[29,30] Although some encouraging reports of declining hepatocellular carcinoma incidence are emerging, the full benefit will probably not be seen until the next decade.

Hepatocellular carcinomas are well known to be associated with diseases such as biliary atresia, hereditary tyrosinaemia type I, progressive familial intrahepatic cholestasis (PFIC), Alagille syndrome, and other causes of cirrhosis in children.[31] Although these patients probably represent only a small percentage of tumours in African children, it is important that they are provided surveillance in appropriately staffed and funded units.

With the mainly unchecked progression of the HIV epidemic in many countries on the African continent, the upsurge of Kaposi sarcoma contributing to the malignant tumour burden of African children is to be expected.[1] The management of this epidemic should be accorded top priority to prevent the millions of deaths occurring annually in children and to contribute to improving the quality of life of these children.

Ethical Considerations

In most instances, the treatment of children with liver tumours follows the lines of maximum effort (with available resources) to help the patient with the presumption of beneficence (i.e., that the patient will benefit from the treatment). The treatment of patients with advanced and unresectable hepatocellular carcinoma certainly falls within the ambit of *futile treatment*. This term is used advisedly, as no care (such as the provision of analgesia, tapping ascitic collections) is futile, but no heroic measures should be adopted in the oncologic treatment of these children. Similar considerations exist in the patient with AIDS who presents with an aggressive malignant vascular tumour.

A controversial and difficult circumstance arises when treatment by transplant would be advisable but the child and the family are deemed unsuitable due to either geographic, educational, or financial reasons, or are expected not to adhere to the rigorous posttransplant treatment and surveillance strategies. This scenario occurs not uncommonly, and the usual outcome is exclusion of the child from access to such treatment. The harsh realities of transplantation in the developing world often offer no other solution.

Evidence-Based Research

Table 107.4 presents an observational study of different patterns of disease in malignant liver tumours based on African children's cancer registry data. Table 107.5 presents a review of the current state of the art in management of liver tumours in children in Germany.

Table 107.4: Evidence-based research.

Title	Malignant liver tumors in South African children: a national audit
Authors	Moore SW, Davidson A, Hadley GP, Kruger M, Poole J, Stones D, Wainwright L, Wessels G
Institution	Multiinstitutional in South Africa—children's cancer registry data
Reference	World J Surg 2008; 32(7):1389–1395
Problem	Epidemiology and outcomes of treatment in South Africa for malignant tumours.
Intervention	Collation of registry data.
Comparison/ control (quality of evidence)	Observational study.
Outcome/ effect	Showed different patterns of disease.
Historical significance/ comments	This is the largest registry-based study of malignant liver tumours in Africa and provides unique insights into the problem of malignant disease in an area with high seroprevalence of HIV and hepatitis B.

Table 107.5: Evidence-based research.

Title	Management of liver tumors in childhood
Authors	Von Schweinitz D
Institution	Paediatric surgery clinic, University of Munich, Germany
Reference	Semin Pediatr Surg 2006; 15(1):17–24
Problem	Review of management of liver tumours in children.
Intervention	Review.
Outcome/ effect	Education.
Historical significance/ comments	An excellent review of the current state of the art from a developed country.

Key Summary Points

1. The prevalence of liver tumours related to infection with HIV and hepatitis B, the Kaposi sarcoma, and hepatocellular carcinoma is higher in African children than in the Western world, with poor prognosis.

2. The most common presentation is an enlarging abdominal mass, but practitioners should be wary of the other modes of presentation.

3. Carefully performed work-up with haematological investigation as well as good-quality imaging are the critical first steps in evaluation.

4. Many patients with advanced multicentric hepatocellular carcinoma as well as patients who have terminal AIDS and aggressive malignant vascular tumours are best treated by palliation.

5. Good results can be achieved by combining good-quality surgery with multimodal treatment for hepatoblastoma, and for sarcomas even in partially resource-deprived communities.

6. Prevention by promoting hepatitis vaccination programs and encouraging specific treatment and support for patients with HIV infection are critical.

References

1. Moore SW, Davidson A, Hadley GP, et al. Malignant liver tumors in South African children: a national audit. World J.Surg 2008; 32(7):1389–1395.

2. Darbari A, Sabin KM, Shapiro CN, Schwarz KB. Epidemiology of primary hepatic malignancies in US children. Hepatology 2003; 38(3):560–566.

3. McLaughlin CC, Baptiste MS, Schymura MJ, Nasca PC, Zdeb MS. Maternal and infant birth characteristics and hepatoblastoma. Am J Epidemiol 2006; 163(9):818–828.

4. Kew MC. Prevention of hepatocellular carcinoma. HPB (Oxford); 2005; 7(1):16–25.

5. Hadley GP, Govender D, Landers G. Primary tumours of the liver in children: an African perspective. Pediatr Surg Int 2004; 20(5):314–318.

6. Czauderna P. Adult type vs childhood hepatocellular carcinoma—are they the same or different lesions? Biology, natural history, prognosis, and treatment. Med Pediatr Oncol 2002; 39(5):519–523.

7. Isaacs H Jr. Fetal and neonatal hepatic tumors. J Pediatr Surg 2007; 42(11):1797–1803.

8. Catanzarite V, Hilfiker M, Daneshmand S, Willert J. Prenatal diagnosis of fetal hepatoblastoma: case report and review of the literature. J Ultrasound Med 2008; 27(7):1095–1098.

9. Hall G W. Kasabach-Merritt syndrome: pathogenesis and management. Br J Haematol 2001; 112(4):851–862.

10. Bader D, Riskin A, Vafsi O, et al. Alpha-fetoprotein in the early neonatal period—a large study and review of the literature. Clin Chim Acta 2004; 349(1–2):15–23.

11. Von Schweinitz D. Management of liver tumors in childhood. Semin Pediatr Surg 2006; 15(1):17–24.

12. Roebuck DJ, Aronson D, Clapuyt P, et al. 2005 PRETEXT: a revised staging system for primary malignant liver tumours of childhood developed by the SIOPEL group. Pediatr Radiol 2007; 37(2):123–132.

13. Perilongo G, Shafford E, Maibach R, et al. Risk-adapted treatment for childhood hepatoblastoma. Final report of the second study of the International Society of Paediatric Oncology—SIOPEL 2. Eur J Cancer 2004; 40(3):411–421.

14. Otte JB, Pritchard J, Aronson DC, et al. Liver transplantation for hepatoblastoma: results from the International Society of Pediatric Oncology (SIOP) study SIOPEL-1 and review of the world experience. Pediatr Blood Cancer 2004; 42(1):74–83.

15. Czauderna P, Otte JB, Aronson DC, et al. Guidelines for surgical treatment of hepatoblastoma in the modern era—recommendations from the Childhood Liver Tumour Strategy Group of the International Society of Paediatric Oncology (SIOPEL). Eur J Cancer 2005; 41(7):1031–1036.

16. Moore SW, Millar AJ, Hadley GP, et al. Hepatocellular carcinoma and liver tumors in South African children: a case for increased prevalence. Cancer 2004; 101(3):642–649.

17. Chowdhary SK, Trehan A, Das A, Marwaha RK, Rao KL. Undifferentiated embryonal sarcoma in children: beware of the solitary liver cyst. J Pediatr Surg 2004; 39(1):E9–E12.

18. Charfi S, Ayadi L, Toumi N, et al. Cystic undifferentiated sarcoma of liver in children: a pitfall diagnosis in endemic hydatidosis areas. J Pediatr Surg 2008; 43(6):E1–E4.

19. Bisogno G, Pilz T, Perilongo G, et al. Undifferentiated sarcoma of the liver in childhood: a curable disease. Cancer 2002; 94(1):252–257.

20. Stringer MD, Alizai NK. Mesenchymal hamartoma of the liver: a systematic review. J Pediatr Surg 2005; 40(11):1681–1690.

21. Rogers TN, Woodley H, Ramsden W, Wyatt JI, Stringer MD. Solitary liver cysts in children: not always so simple. J Pediatr Surg 2007; 42(2):333–339.

22. Christison-Lagay ER, Burrows PE, Alomari A, et al. Hepatic hemangiomas: subtype classification and development of a clinical practice algorithm and registry. J Pediatr Surg 2007; 42(1):62–67.

23. Von Schweinitz D, Burger D, Mildenberger H. Is laparatomy the first step in treatment of childhood liver tumors?—the experience from the German Cooperative Pediatric Liver Tumor Study HB-89. Eur J Pediatr Surg 1994; 4(2):82–86.

24. Sandler A, Kimura K, Soper R. Nonanatomic hepatic resection with a pledgetted suturing technique. J Pediatr Surg 2001; 36(1):209–212.

25. Yigitler C, Farges O, Kianmanesh R, Regimbeau JM, Abdalla EK, Belghiti J. The small remnant liver after major liver resection: how common and how relevant? Liver Transpl 2003; 9(9):S18–S25.

26. Nudo CG, Yoshida EM, Bain VG, et al. Liver transplantation for hepatic epithelioid hemangioendothelioma: the Canadian multicentre experience. Can J Gastroenterol 2008; 22(10):821–824.

27. Goldstein ST, Alter MJ, Williams IT, et al. Incidence and risk factors for acute hepatitis B in the United States, 1982–1998: implications for vaccination programs. J Infect Dis 2002; 185(6):713–719.

28. Goldstein ST, Zhou F, Hadler SC, Bell BP, Mast EE, Margolis HS. A mathematical model to estimate global hepatitis B disease burden and vaccination impact, Int J Epidemiol 2005; 34(6):1329–1339.

29. Shatat H, Kotkat A, Farghaly A, Omar S, Zayton S. A study of hepatitis B vaccine efficacy 10 years after compulsory vaccination in Egypt. J Egypt Public Health Assoc 2005; 80(5–6):495–508.

30. Viviani S, Carrieri P, Bah E, et al. 20 years into the Gambia Hepatitis Intervention Study: assessment of initial hypotheses and prospects for evaluation of protective effectiveness against liver cancer. Cancer Epidemiol Biomarkers Prev 2008; 17(11):3216–3223.

31. Finegold MJ, Egler RA, Goss JA, Guillerman RP, Karpen SJ, Krishnamurthy R, O'Mahony CA. Liver tumors: pediatric population. Liver Transpl 2008; 14(11):1545–1556.

Suggested Reading

Awan S, Davenport M, Portmann B, et al. Angiosarcoma of the liver in children. J Pediatr Surg 1996; 31:1729–1732.

Burrows PE, Dubois J, Kassarjian A. Pediatric hepatic vascular anomalies. Pediatr Radiol 2001; 31:533–545.

Chen JC, Chang ML, Lin JN, et al. Comparison of childhood hepatic malignancies in a hepatitis B hyper-endemic area. World J Gastroenterol 2005; 11:5289–5294.

Czauderna P, Otte JB, Aronson DC, et al. Guidelines for surgical treatment of hepatoblastoma in the modern era—recommendations from the Childhood Liver Tumour Strategy Group of the International Society of Paediatric Oncology (SIOPEL). Eur J Cancer 2005; 41:1031–1036.

Czauderna P, Otte JB, Roebuck DJ, et al. Surgical treatment of hepatoblastoma in children. Pediatr Radiol 2006; 36:187–191.

Otte JB, de Ville de Goyet J, Reding R. Liver transplantation for hepatoblastoma: indications and contraindications in the modern era. Pediatr Transplant 2005; 9:557–565.

Pritchard J, Brown J, Shafford E, et al. Cisplatin, doxorubicin, and delayed surgery for childhood hepatoblastoma: A successful approach—results of the first prospective study of the International Society of Pediatric Oncology. J Clin Oncol 2000; 18:3819–3828.

Prokurat A, Kluge P, Chrupek M, et al. Hemangioma of the liver in children: proliferating vascular tumor or congenital vascular malformation. Med Pediatr Oncol 2002; 39:524–529.

Roebuck DJ, Aronson D, Clapuyt P, et al. 2005 PRETEXT: A revised staging system for primary malignant liver tumours of childhood developed by the SIOPEL group. Pediatr Radiol 2007; 37:123–132.

Selby DM, Stocker JT, Waclawiw MA, et al. Infantile hemangioendothelioma of the liver. Hepatology 1994; 20:39–45.

Siddiqui MA, McKenna BJ. Hepatic mesenchymal hamartoma: a short review. Arch Pathol Lab Med 2006; 130:1567–1569.

Tiao GM, Bobey N, Allen S, et al. The current management of hepatoblastoma: a combination of chemotherapy, conventional resection, and liver transplantation. J Pediatr 2005; 146:204–211.

Tomlinson GE, Douglas EC, Pollock BH, et al. Cytogenetic evaluation of a large series of hepatoblastomas: numerical abnormalities with recurring aberrations involving 1q12-q21. Genes Chromosomes Cancer 2005; 44:177–184.

Van Tornout JM, Buckley JD, Quinn JJ, et al. Timing and magnitude of decline in alpha-fetoprotein levels in treated children with unresectable or matastastic hepatoblastoma are predictors of outcome: a report from the Children's Cancer Group. J Clin Oncol 1997; 15:1190–1197.

CHAPTER 108
PRIMARY BONE TUMOURS

Kant Shah
Kokila Lakhoo

Introduction

Bone tumours in childhood cause considerable anxiety to both the affected child and the parents. They may present with vague symptoms or a fracture and can easily be confused with osteomyelitis or some tumour-like lesions that may be developmental in origin. Benign lesions account for 50% of all bone lesions; some may be large enough to cause significant disability. Primary malignant tumours of the bone make up for 6% of all childhood malignancies[1] and are indeed the most common malignancy of adolescence after leukaemias and lymphomas. Overall diagnosis depends on factors such as age of patient, site of lesion, imaging (plain x-rays, computed tomography (CT), nuclear studies, magnetic resonance imaging (MRI)), and, if possible, the histopathology and immunohistochemistry. Thus, a multidisciplinary team approach is vital to the diagnosis and management of bone tumours.

The mainstay of treatment of benign lesions is surgery to limit disability, with reconstruction as needed. As chemotherapy has become more advanced with fewer side effects, the focus of treatment of bone malignancies has changed from surgery to neoadjuvant chemotherapy followed by wide excision and then chemotherapy or radiotherapy as appropriate.

The aim of this chapter is to acquaint the reader with the common lesions of the bone,[2] and the differential diagnosis, investigations, and management of the common malignancies. For simplicity in this chapter, the demographics, pathophysiology, clinical presentation, investigations, prognosis, and outcomes are listed together, and management of individual lesions is described separately.

Classification of Bone Tumours

Bone tumours are primarily classified according to the type of tissue they produce. Hence, they may be osteogenic, chondrogenic, etc. The World Health Organization (WHO) classification (Table 108.1) is extensive. The tumours that affect children and adolescents are marked with an asterisk (*) in the table.

Demographics

The common benign tumours of childhood are osteochondroma, enchondroma, osteoid osteoma, osteoblastoma, chondroblastoma, and haemangioma. In addition, tumour-like lesions such as nonossifying fibroma, simple bone cyst, and fibrous dysplasia are also common in the developing child. Primary bone malignancies are rare, however, with osteosarcoma (54%) and Ewing's sarcoma (34%) being the most common.[1] The overall age-adjusted incidence of bone malignancy increases with age and peaks at 20 cases per million at 15–19 years of age.

In North America, the overall incidence rate among caucasian American children was 8.8 per million compared with 6.8 per million for African American children. This racial difference is further highlighted as the two tumour types are compared[1] (Figure 108.1). The reason for this difference is not known. Males have a slightly higher and delayed peak of incidence of osteosarcoma compared to females, which correlates to their relative rates of growth.

Table 108.1: WHO classification of bone tumours.

Cartilage-forming tumours	
Benign:	Enchondroma;* osteochondroma;* periosteal chondroma; chondroblastoma;* chondromyxoid fibroma*
Malignant:	Chondrosarcoma: conventional; juxtacortical; mesenchymal;* dedifferentiated; clear cell
Bone-forming tumours	
Benign:	Osteoma, osteoid osteoma,* osteoblastoma*
Malignant:	Osteosarcoma: intramedullary* (conventional; telangiectatic; small cell; well differentiated); surface (parosteal; periosteal; high grade surface)
Fibrous/fibrohistiocytic tumours	
Benign:	Nonossifying fibroma;* desmoplastic fibroma;* myofibromatosis;* benign fibrous histiocytoma
Malignant:	Fibrosarcoma/malignant fibrous histiocytoma
Ewing's sarcoma/primitive neuroectodermal tumour of bone*	
Giant cell tumours of bone	
	Giant cell tumour of bone; giant cell reparative granuloma (GCRG) of jaw*; GCRG small bones*
Vascular tumours	
Benign:	Haemangioma*; lymphangioma; glomus tumour; angiomatosis;* Gorham-Stout disease*
Malignant:	Haemangiopericytoma; haemangioendothelioma; angiosarcoma
Other primary tumours	
	Smooth muscle tumours Lipogenic tumours Neural tumours Chordoma Adamantinoma of long bone
Miscellaneous tumour-like lesions	
	Simple bone cyst* Aneurysmal bone cyst* Fibrous dysplasia* Fibrocartilaginous dysplasia* Osteofibrous dysplasia* Langerhans cell histiocytosis* Mesenchymal hamartoma of chest wall*
Joint lesions	
	Synovial chondromatosis

* Childhood tumours

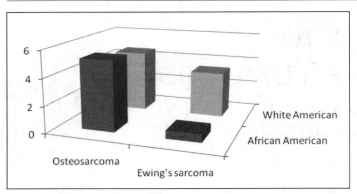

Source: United States Surveillance, Epidemiology and End Results (SEER) Program, 1975–1995. National Cancer Institute, 1999.

Figure 108.1: Age-adjusted incidence rates of bone tumours showing a remarkable dip in Ewing's sarcoma in the African American population

Pathophysiology

To date, no causative factors for bone tumours are known in general. However, associations have been found between osteosarcoma and retinoblastoma, osteosarcoma and Li-Fraumeni syndrome, and enchondroma and soft tissue and skin haemangiomas (Maffucci syndrome). These associations are uncommon, and the majority of tumours are isolated. A distinct feature of bone tumours is that many may be multiple in nature at the time of presentation (i.e., synchronous), such as osteosarcoma, Ewing's sarcoma, fibrous dysplasia (not a neoplasia), and enchondromatosis.[3] Another feature typical of bone tumours is that they have a predilection for certain bones and certain locations within the bones[4] (Table 108.2).

Table 108.2: Distribution of common bone tumours according to site.

Small tubular bones	Enchondroma Periosteal chondroma Osteoid osteoma Osteoblastoma Giant cell reparative granuloma
Long tubular bones	Most primary benign and malignant bone tumours and tumour-like lesions Metastasis (e.g., neuroblastoma)
Ribs/sternum	Benign/malignant cartilage tumours Fibrous dysplasia Mesenchymal hamartoma of the chest wall Eosinophilic granuloma Metastasis
Spine	Aneurysmal bone cyst Osteoblastoma Osteoid osteoma Haemangioma Metastasis
Skull/facial bones	Fibrous dysplasia "Fibro-osseous lesions" of the jaw Osteoma Giant cell reparative granuloma Haemangioma Eosinophilic granuloma Osteosarcoma Mesenchymal chondrosarcoma Metastasis
Pelvis	Osteochondroma Chondrosarcoma Ewing's sarcoma Metastasis

Presentation

History

Usually a child presents with nonspecific symptoms, such as limping, weakness, oedema of an extremity, or swelling of an associated joint, all of which make the diagnosis confusing. Pain is the most common symptom, and 50% of all malignancies are associated with minor trauma. Bone pain is typically dull, constant, severe at rest, and worse in the night. Fever may be present in Ewing's sarcoma, which is often confused with osteomyelitis.

Physical Examination

A swelling or mass is frequently present; however, lesions in the pelvis may be obscure. There may be venous engorgement or peripheral oedema, which points towards a malignancy. Benign lesions may cause a deformity or fracture.

Investigations

Blood investigations may show anaemia, a high erythrocyte sedimentation rate, and a high white cell count. Serum alkaline phosphatase and lactate dehydrogenase may be higher and associated with a poorer prognosis in malignancy.[5]

Primary radiological investigations may be inconclusive or confusing, and special or oblique view x-rays or CT may be needed. A high index of suspicion and careful review of radiology is adequate to pick up most malignancies. Multiple lesions may be present in multifocal osteosarcoma, and multiple primary lesions in Ewing's sarcoma or osteomyelitis apart from secondary malignancies. Hence, biopsy or further imaging may be necessary in the form of MRI or bone scintigraphy.

X-rays

Some features on a plain radiograph assist in differentiating benign from malignant lesions[4] (Table 108.3).

Table 108.3: Radiological features of benign and malignant bone tumours.

Feature	Benign	Malignant
Periosteal reaction	Variable	Common
Margin of lesion/zone of transition	Well-defined and sclerotic	Poorly defined
Cortical destruction	Rare	May be present
Pattern of osteolysis	Geographic	Expansile, moth-eaten, permeative
Soft tissue involvement	Variable	Common
Size	Variable	Usually extensive
Multiple lesions	Unlikely	May be present especially around the primary
Involvement of joint	Unlikely	Effusion may be present

Computed Tomography

CT scans help in the diagnosis of bone tumours as well as planning of biopsy, surgery, and chemotherapy. Information is obtained at various levels. Local disease extent is defined, the nature of the tumour is classified, and the amount of soft tissue involvement can be judged. In addition, neurovascular structures can be studied around the tumour; this information aids in the plan for reconstruction of the limb. Also CT of the chest can detect pulmonary metastases <3 mm, which have a significant prognostic value.

Magnetic Resonance Imaging

MRI is now the gold standard investigation for bone tumours in the Western world, mainly for its ability to pick up marrow extension and delineate the level of surgery. Also multiplanar and three-dimensional (3D) imaging allows the surgeon to accurately choose between wide excision and amputation because it gives details on neurovascular bundles, availability of soft tissue for cover, and it visualises skip metastases.

Bone Scintigraphy

Nuclear medicine has a vast beneficial diagnostic advantage both in primary and secondary bone lesions. Tecnitium-99m (Tc-99m) labelled scans are widely used in the Western world for identifying synchronous tumours as well as metastases of primary bone malignancies. Combined with CT, bone scintigraphy is a good tool to manage most primary bone malignancies.

Management

Great strides have been made in the past two to three decades in the management and survival of children with malignant bone tumours. This is attributable to worldwide unity in conducting research due to low numbers of malignant bone tumours in individual centres. 3D radiological investigations, advances in pathological understanding of tumours and their origins, newer chemotherapeutic agents, better reconstructive surgery, and a multidisciplinary approach have all contributed.

Staging

The Musculoskeletal Tumour Society staging system[6] (Table 108.4), originally developed by Enneking, depends on the tumour's histological grade, local extent, and metastasis.

Table 108.4: Musculoskeletal Tumour Society staging system.

Stage	Grade	Local extent	Metastasis
IA	Low	Intraompartmental	None
IB	Low	Extraxcompartmental	None
IIA	High	Intraompartmental	None
IIB	High	Extraxcompartmental	None
III	Any	Any	Present

The significance of staging for malignant tumours is as follows:

- *Stage IA tumours* are treated with wide excision and are usually amenable to limb salvage procedures.

- *Stage IB tumours* may be treated with wide excision, but the choice between amputation and limb salvage depends on the estimated amount of residual tumour left behind after a limb salvage procedure.

- *Stage II tumours* are high grade, are usually extracompartmental, and have significant risks for skip metastases. They usually are not amenable to limb salvage operations and require radical amputation or disarticulation in most patients. However, bone tumours responsive to chemotherapy may be treated successfully by using wide excision and adjuvant therapy.

- *Stage III tumours* are responsive to chemotherapy and may be treated with aggressive resection. Those that are not responsive to adjuvant therapy should be treated with palliative resection.

Individual Tumours

Benign

Osteochondroma

Osteochondroma is a cartilage-capped bony outgrowth arising from the external surface of a bone. It is the most common benign bone tumour, accounting for almost 60% of all bone tumours. A lesion may be asymptomatic, and hence may not need any treatment except for careful observation.

Enchondroma

Enchondroma is a benign bone tumour. Radiologically, enchondroma is metaphyseal in location and does not have a soft tissue mass, periosteal reaction, or bone destruction, which differentiates it from chondrosarcoma.

Osteoid osteoma

Osteoid osteoma is a benign tumour that occurs mostly in the second decade of life, affecting males at a rate twice that of females. It arises commonly in the femur and tibia, presenting with typical bone pain that is worse at night. X-rays show a radiolucent core with sclerotic margins, but this tumour is best seen on CT scan. Complete removal of the lesion is recommended with grafting and cementing.

Osteoblastoma

Osteoblastoma is an uncommon benign tumour in children slightly younger than those with osteoid osteoma. It may not have a sclerotic rim and may involve short bones as well. It may also have systemic symptoms such as fever and weight loss. A particular variety is aggressive and can resemble low-grade osteosarcoma radiologically and pathologically. Careful follow-up is needed.

Nonossifying fibroma

Nonossifying fibroma is a common fibrohistiocytic lesion that may be large and involve the medulla of metaphyses. Radiologically, it is a lytic lesion with a well-defined sclerotic border. If symptomatic or vulnerable to fracture, excision may be necessary.

Simple bone cyst

Although benign, a simple bone cyst has a tendency to recur as it affects the growth plate. It often presents as a metaphyseal fracture of tubular bones and hence needs excision. Radiologically, it is an osteolytic lesion with trabeculations.

Fibrous Dysplasia

Fibrous dysplasia is a relatively common benign fibro-osseous lesion that is not a true neoplasm. It is thought to be developmental and is composed of fibrous tissue with irregular woven bone trabeculae. Radiologically, this lesion is well defined, with a ground-glass appearance and a sclerotic rim. Surgical excision or curettage with careful follow-ups is necessary because this lesion tends to recur often. Polyostotic fibrous dysplasia affects multiple bones and can be crippling, even needing radiotherapy. A sarcomatous change to a fibrous, osteoid, or cartilage component may occur in this setting.

Malignant

Chondrosarcoma

Chondrosarcoma is the third most common primary bone malignancy. It can occur in the setting of a benign lesion, such as exostosis or enchondroma; also, it occurs in patients older than 30 years of age, compared to benign lesions that can occur in childhood. There may be cortical destruction or a soft tissue mass, which may be the only differentiating factor between a benign active lesion and a low-grade malignant chondrosarcoma. Histology shows chondrosarcoma can be clear cell, dedifferentiated, or mesenchymal in origin. The treatment of these lesions is primary surgical excision followed by chemotherapy for the mesenchymal variety and radiation for pain control.

Osteosarcoma

Classic high-grade osteosarcoma is a highly malignant osteoid-forming spindle cell sarcoma of the bone. It is the most common primary malignant bone tumour in children and is the third most common malignant disease after leukaemia and lymphoma in adolescence. The incidence in Africa may be lower, however, due to underreporting, as shown in a large study in Nigeria.[5] It is still a rare tumour, and there appears to be no race- or sex-related predominance in incidence. Prevalence is higher in patients affected with retinoblastoma (40% in bilateral disease)[7] and those who have undergone radiation therapy or Paget's disease (secondary osteosarcoma).

Osteosarcoma can occur in any bone, but is most common in the metaphyses of long bones (80–90% of tumours), with particular predilection for distal femoral metaphyses (35%), proximal tibial metaphyses (20%), and proximal humeral metaphyses (10%).[5] Pain and swelling or mass are the most common presenting features, along with fever, weakness, and limping. Pelvic masses may be obscured.

Investigations

Radiologically, osteosarcoma appears as a destructive lesion of a metaphysic of a long bone, exhibiting mixed lytic and blastic areas (Figure 108.2). There is cortical destruction and a wide transitional zone. There is often soft tissue involvement with irregular densities. At the margins there may be reactive periosteal bone formation forming Codman's triangles, which are the mark of an aggressive destructive process.

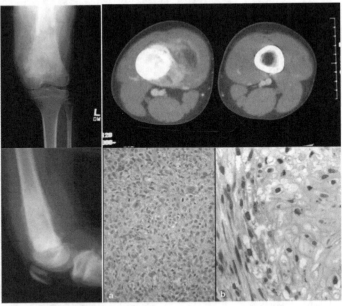

Figure 108.2: Osteosarcoma. X-rays (left panes) showing Codman's triangles, soft tissue invasion, and cortical destruction. The CT scan (upper right pane) shows a similar picture and is superior in defining the extent of the tumour. Histopathology (lower right panes, a and b) shows osteoid-forming highly mitotic cells.

The tumour is staged preoperatively by using oblique-view x-rays and CT. In the West, MRI is the gold standard because it shows accurate marrow extension, which helps in determining the surgical intervention. The multiplanar views of these instruments help in finding the appropriate surgical route for the biopsy as well as in identifying viable areas. A CT scan of the chest can identify small pulmonary metastatic lesions, which are of significant prognostic value. Bone scintigraphy, where available, helps in finding areas of skip metastases and sites of synchronous metastases.

Gross pathology of the tumour shows a heavily mineralised soft tissue mass extending from the marrow through the cortex to the soft tissues. Intraarticular extension typically occurs along ligaments. Microscopy shows frankly malignant pleomorphic cells producing osteoid. The background contains fibrous or chondroid stroma and many areas of necrosis (see Figure 108.2). The radiological and clinical correlation of histology is extremely important in differentiating malignant bone tumours from reactive, infective, and benign processes, as pure histology may be confusing.

Variants

High-grade central osteosarcoma is the classic type, described above. Surface or juxtacortical (parosteal, periosteal) osteosarcoma can be low to intermediate grade with variable response to chemotherapy, and wide surgical excision gives higher survival rates than for the classic type.

Treatment

In the past, surgery alone gave high metastatic rates with abysmal survival of less than 20%. Accurate clinical staging, vast strides in chemotherapy, and appropriate surgery have increased survival dramatically in the past few decades and also limited morbidity significantly. The current protocol for a suspected malignant bone tumour is radiology

(x-rays, and, where available, CT, MRI, and bone scintigraphy); biopsy of the tumour; preoperative (neoadjuvant) chemotherapy; wide resection or amputation; and postoperative (adjuvant) chemotherapy.[7]

The benefits of neoadjuvant chemotherapy are manifold. It prevents the development of resistant clones, especially in the setting of the rapid doubling time in osteosarcoma, and it kills microscopic metastases and shrinks the primary tumour-inducing necrosis. The degree of necrosis thus induced is an important prognostic marker for long-term survival. The drugs commonly used are doxorubicin, cisplatin, and high-dose methotrexate. Recently, ifosfamide has been used.

Wide excision may be limb sparing and prevent morbidity; however, survival is not affected. Amputation may be particularly necessary in cases where tumour extent or grade are inadequately known, preoperative chemotherapy response is poor, or the surgical stump may not be adequate for prosthesis. Occasionally, reconstruction may be embarked upon by using allografts, metal prosthesis, or composites.

Prognosis

Concurrent to the improvement in strategy and introduction of neoadjuvant chemotherapy, the 5-year survival rates for osteosarcoma have gone up to 60–80% in different series.[8,9] In patients with apparent metastatic disease prior to surgery the survival is much poorer, at 10–20%. If the pulmonary metastases can be resected, this figure can go up to 40%.[7,10] The factors that affect or predict prognosis are tumour necrosis after neoadjuvant chemotherapy and presence or absence of metastases at time of presentation. A larger tumour size, raised lactate dehydrogenase and alkaline phosphatase levels, and tumours located in the pelvis and proximal femur or humerus are poor prognostic signs.[7]

In the future, antivascular growth factor antibodies and a vascular endothelial growth factor inhibitor may be beneficial as well as directed therapies against overexpressed tumour-related genes, such as Rb (retinoblastoma) gene and Her2/erb-2.

Ewing's sarcoma

Ewing's sarcoma is a malignant round-cell bone tumour of neuroectodermal origin. It accounts for 10% of all primary malignant bone tumours. Eighty percent of patients are younger than 20 years of age. This tumour is rare in Africa;[11–13] however, it is discussed in detail here because it is still the second most common tumour, and is probably the most common for children younger than 5 years of age.

The Ewing's sarcoma tumour presents usually in the lower limbs and pelvis, although it can occur in any bone. It belongs to a family of tumours of common neuroectodermal origin, along with primitive neuroectodermal tumour (PNET), atypical Ewing's tumour, and Askin tumour. This confers susceptibility of these tumours to chemotherapy, with increased survival noted in the past few decades .

Ewing's tumour frequently presents with a painful soft tissue mass and with fever, resembling osteomyelitis.

Investigations

Radiologically, Ewing's sarcoma appears as a soft tissue mass eroding through bone, and hence it may be confused with an acute reactive process or osteomyelitis. Indeed, a biopsy may show "pus", and it is important to send the biopsy material for histology or frozen section along with microbiology. Pathological fractures may occur. Rib involvement may cause malignant pleural effusion, and vertebral involvement may cause scoliosis due to the soft tissue mass. The primary tumour in the limbs may show a mottled, or "onion skin" appearance (Figure 108.3).

Special-view radiographs and a CT scan will help define the extent of the tumour as well as pulmonary metastases, if any. Bone scintigraphy may be particularly useful, as 10% patients may have multiple lesions. The scans are repeated after several cycles of chemotherapy; hence, MRI is more useful, especially in children.

Gross morphology shows a grey-white mass with extensive areas of necrosis and haemorrhage mimicking "pus formation". Microscopically the neuroectodermal origin is confirmed with numerous malignant

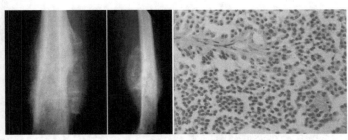

Figure 108.3: Ewing's sarcoma: x-rays (left) show onion-skin appearance (right).

small blue cells with sparse stroma. All such tumours also exhibit the MIC2 gene, which differentiates them from lymphomas and rhabdomyosarcoma. A commercial kit available for this investigation has a 95% sensitivity for detecting Ewing's sarcoma.

Treatment

Over the past two decades, the Intergroup Ewing Sarcoma Study has demonstrated a dramatic improvement in survival by modifying chemotherapeutic agents and the intensity of their dosage regimen. The society has recommended high-dose vincristine, actinomycin, cyclophosphamide, and adriamycin (VACA).[7,10] Recently, the Children's Cancer Group and the Paediatric Oncology Group have shown that the addition of ifosfamide and etoposide improved the morbidity of the survivors.

Surgical excision of the primary tumour, where possible, markedly improves the outcome, possibly due to the removal of chemotherapy-resistant clones. Radiotherapy may be added where surgical margins may not be adequate, but in sites where this is the only postoperative treatment possible, the outcome is poorer (34%). Indeed, the risk of radiation-induced malignancies and crippling disabilities are coming to light in this era. Patients who have received doses of more than 60 Gy have the maximum lifetime risk. Aggressive excision with reconstruction is now being favoured in difficult sites such as the proximal femur, pelvis, and spine.[3]

Prognosis

As with osteosarcoma, the presence of distal metastases at time of diagnosis of Ewing's sarcoma, initial tumour size >8 cm, and central lesions such as in the pelvis fare worse. The overall survival has increased from 5% in the 1980s to >70% currently.

Postoperative Complications

Surgical complications may be related to the amputation stump or the distal end of the limb. Additionally, functional inability to fit a prosthesis or adapt to a restricted lifestyle causes severe mental and emotional as well as physical disability. Implants have their own risk of wear and tear and can fracture, but this is certainly more acceptable than the risks of radiotherapy, which may be multiple. Radiotherapy has limited use in delimiting preoperative disease and treating tumours difficult to resect. It has a serious life time malignancy risk, and complications such as limb-length discrepancy or joint contracture are more pronounced in the skeletally immature. Chemotherapy risks are minimised by the addition of multiple agents and by worldwide consortiums offering research into newer molecules.

Ethical Issues

In Africa, the management of bone tumours is more complex, as specialist oncology, pathology, or radiology centres may not be available; surgical experience also may be limited in rural areas.[12] Of special note are patients who have a rather unusual story of osteomyelitis or those who have a sudden onset or presence of other systemic features and require a high index of suspicion and multiple radiological investigations to determine the nature of the tumour. Telemedicine and digital radiology are able to offer expert radiological opinions to many centres.

In addition, the balance between wide-excision surgery and limited resection to preserve function has greater meaning in Africa, where reconstructive surgery and rehabilitation are not always possible. Greater planning prior to surgery and the use of expert help can prevent many a disability, which, in turn, would save many disability-adjusted life years.[4]

Evidence-Based Research

Table 108.5 presents a detailed description of various bone lesions. Table 108.6 is a monograph on the incidence and prevalence of bone tumours, with an emphasis on racial differences.

Table 108.5: Evidence-based research.

Title	Radiological and pathological diagnosis of paediatric bone tumours and tumour-like lesions
Authors	Vlychou M, Athanasou NA
Institution	Nuffield Department of Pathology and Nuffield Department of Orthopaedic Surgery, University of Oxford, Nuffield Orthopaedic Centre, Oxford, United Kingdom
Reference	Pathology 2008; 40(2):196–216
Problem	Radiological and pathological diagnosis.
Comparison/ control (quality of evidence)	Benign with malignant tumours.
Historical significance/ comments	A detailed description of various bone lesions. The focus is on radiology and includes various modalities and their advantages. Its feature on pathology illustrates immune-histochemical differences and the basis for adjuvant therapy in malignancies.

Table 108.6: Evidence-based research.

Title	SEER paediatric monograph
Authors	Gurney JG, Swensen AR, Bulterys M
Institution	National Cancer Institute, Bethesda, Maryland, USA
Reference	Gurney J, Swensen A, Bulterys M. Malignant bone tumors. In: Ries L, Smith M, Gurney J, et al., eds. *Cancer Incidence and Survival among Children and Adolescents: United States SEER Program 1975– 1995.* National Cancer Institute, SEER Program, 1999, Pp 99–110.
Problem	Incidence and prevalence of bone tumours.
Outcome/ effect	Racial differences in bone tumour incidence is highlighted.

Key Summary Points

1. Malignant bone tumours are the third most common malignancy in adolescence.

2. Presentation and radiological findings of benign and malignant bone lesions may be similar and be confused with reactive or infective processes.

3. The site of the tumour and age of the patient are the most important factors in differential diagnosis.

4. Accurate preoperative staging, aggressive neoadjuvant chemotherapy, and surgical resection are the cornerstones of management of primary malignant bone tumours.

5. Even though survival has increased in the Western world from 20% to >70% due to modern chemotherapy, the key factors to survival in Africa are the availability of chemotherapy, selection of patients, surgical complications, and rehabilitation.

6. Newer drugs, telemedicine, and the availability of mobile radiological services have tremendous roles to play in providing cancer services in Africa.

References

1. Gurney J, Swensen A, Bulterys M: Malignant bone tumors. In: Ries L, Smith M, Gurney J, et al., eds. *Cancer Incidence and Survival among Children and Adolescents: United States SEER Program 1975–1995*. National Cancer Institute, SEER Program, 1999, Pp 99–110.

2. Dorfman HD, Vanel D, Czerniak B, Park YK, Kotz R, Unni KK, WHO classification of tumours of bone: introduction. In: Christopher DM, Fletcher K, Unni K, Mertens F. Pathology and Genetics. Tumours of Soft Tissue and Bone. World Health Organization, 2006, Pp 226–232.

3. Heare T, Hensley MA, Dell'Orfano S. Bone tumors: osteosarcoma and Ewing's sarcoma. Curr Opin Pediatr 2009; 21(3):365–372.

4. Vlychou M, Athanasou NA. Pathology, radiological and pathological diagnosis of paediatric bone tumours and tumour-like lesions, J Bone Joint Surg Am 2008; 40(2):196–216.

5. Omololu AB, Ogunbiyi JO, Ogunlade SO, Alonge TO, Adebisi A, Akang EE. Primary malignant bone tumour in a tropical African University teaching hospital. West Afr J Med 2002; 21(4):291–293.

6. Musculoskeletal Tumor Society. Staging of musculoskeletal neoplasms. Skeletal Radiol 1985; 13(3):183–194.

7. Gibbs CP Jr, Weber K, Scarborough MT. Malignant bone tumors. Instr Course Lect 2002; 51:413–428.

8. Foster L, Dall GF, Reid R, Wallace WH, Porter DE. Twentieth-century survival from osteosarcoma in childhood. Trends from 1933 to 2004. J Bone Joint Surg Br 2007; 89(9):1234–1238.

9. Mariotto AB, Rowland JH, Yabroff KR, et al. Long-term survivors of childhood cancers in the United States. Cancer Epidemiol Biomarkers Prev 2009; 18(4):1033–1040.

10. Ilić I, Manojlović S, Cepulić M, Orlić D, Seiwerth S. Osteosarcoma and Ewing's sarcoma in children and adolescents: retrospective clinicopathological study. Croat Med J 2004; 45(6):740–745.

11. Stiller CA, Parkin DM. Geographic and ethnic variations in the incidence of childhood cancer. Br Med Bull 1996; 52(4):682–703.

12. Polednak AP. Primary bone cancer incidence in black and white residents of New York State. Cancer 1985; 55(12):2883–2888.

13. Bahebeck J, Atangana R, Eyenga V, Pisoh A, Sando Z, Hoffmeyer P. Bone tumours in Cameroon: incidence, demography and histopathology. Int Orthop 2003; 27(5):315–317.

CHAPTER 109
BRAIN AND SPINAL CORD TUMOURS

Bello Bala Shehu
Muhammad Raji Mahmud
Saurabh Sinha
Jayaratnam Jayamohan

Introduction

Brain and spinal cord tumours are increasingly being diagnosed in Africa and other developing countries as more centres acquire more sophisticated and less invasive diagnostic facilities. Improvement in the number and expertise of medical personnel also plays a significant role. In addition, advances in anaesthesia and surgical techniques have allowed for increased survival of children with these otherwise dismal clinical conditions. However, the situation in Africa is still far from the ideal, that obtains in the developed nations because only very few centres have the facilities and manpower to manage these conditions. Even in developed centres, however, the poor prognoses of some tumour types have not changed despite all the advances.[1]

Brain tumours are much more common than spinal tumours; this is more so in the paediatric age group. Available data show brain tumours as the second most common tumour after leukaemia (20%), and the most common solid paediatric tumours.[2,3,4] Brain tumours comprise 40–50% of all tumours.[5] One-quarter of all childhood cancer deaths is caused by brain tumours.[1] Although paediatric brain tumours are predominantly infratentorial (60%), the location of tumours depends highly on age. Children under 6 months of age are more likely to have a supratentorial tumour (75%).

The nature of the tumour also depends on location as well as age. In the infratentorial region, there is a relatively equal incidence of primitive neuroectodermal tumour (PNET); most commonly, medulloblastoma); brain-stem gliomas; and pilocytic astrocytomas. In the supratentorial region, astrocytomas are significantly more common. Concerning age, congenital tumours presenting in neonates are more likely to be neuroectodermal in origin, with teratomas being most common, whereas in older children, astrocytomas, PNET, and ependymomas predominate. Some glial tumours, such as mixed gliomas, are unique to children. They are located more frequently in the cerebellum (67%) and are usually benign.

Demographics

The exact incidence or prevalence of central nervous system (CNS) tumours in most African countries is largely unknown. More new cases are seen now than previously, perhaps due to a true increase in incidence, or to increased awareness by the communities and medical workers, with more people presenting now than before. In addition, improvements in diagnostic techniques may be partly responsible for this increase.

From unpublished statistics obtained from Regional Centre for Neurosurgery in Sokoto, Nigeria, paediatric (age <15 years), brain tumours accounted for 22% of all the brain tumours with a male-to-female ratio of 4:1. Another centre in Nigeria found that the most common types of tumours encountered are the astrocytomas, medulloblastomas, craniopharyngiomas, and ependymomas.[6]

Aetiopathogenesis

Like most neoplasms elsewhere in the body, the exact cause of craniospinal tumours in humans is unknown. In animal models, however many environmental agents have been used to induce tumours. Whether this can be extrapolated to the humans remains to be verified. Associated factors include the following:

- *Genetics:* Brain tumours in general are not believed to be inherited genetic disorders, except in von Recklinghausen's disease and some gliomas. Some chromosomal abnormalities may be associated in part with specific tumour types. Astrocytomas may be associated with abnormalities of chromosomes 7, 9, 10, 17, 19 and deletion of p53 gene and amplification of the epidermal growth factor (EGF) gene.

- *Chemical agents:* Many chemicals show carcinogenic properties in animals and produce CNS tumours, especially ethyl and methyl nitrosourea and anthracine derivatives, but this is yet to be proven in humans.

- *Viruses:* There have been reports of patients with JC virus (JCV)-induced demyelination who have developed multifocal astrocytomas, but again the evidence is not firm.

- *Radiation:* There is increasing evidence that exposure to excessive radiation plays a role in causing brain tumours. There is increased incidence of brain tumours in those who have had irradiation to the head and neck for different conditions.

- *Immunosuppression:* Immunosuppression is known to increase the risk of primary lymphoma of the brain, particularly in transplant patients, but it is unlikely that it plays a significant role in the development of cerebral tumours in general.

- *Trauma:* The concept that head trauma leads to the development of meningioma has been controversial. Although epidemiological studies do not support trauma as an aetiological factor, there have been case reports of meningiomas developing at the site of substantial meningeal trauma.

Pathophysiology

As brain tumours increase in size, they acquire new blood vessels from surrounding blood vessels. Sometimes they grow so rapidly that they overwhelm the blood supply and undergo ischaemic necrosis. Many of the tumours cause surrounding oedema, which may be responsible for the mass effect produced by the tumour. Brain tumours rarely metastasize except for some such as medulloblastoma and ependymomas, which become carried along the cerebrospinal fluid pathways to the spinal cord—a phenomenon sometimes referred to as drop metastasis.

Classification of Craniospinal Tumours

Classification of craniospinal tumours has evolved over the years. Currently, the most widely used classification system is the World Health Organisation (WHO) system, based on the cell of origin.[7] Detailed classification is beyond the scope of this chapter, but an abridged version (Table 109.1) is given to highlight the major groups.

Clinical Presentation

The clinical presentations of brain tumours are those of features of raised intracranial pressure from the mass effect of the tumour or obstructive hydrocephalus, focal neurological deficit referrable to the

Table 109.1: WHO classification system (abridged).

	Craniospinal tumours	Examples
Tumours of neuroepithelial tissue	Astrocytomas	Grades i-iv with the anaplastic type and glioblastoma multiformes carrying the worst prognosis
	Oligodendroglial tumours	Oligodendroglioma
	Ependymal tumours	Ependymoma and subependymoma
	Mixed gliomas	
	Choroid plexus tumours	
	Neuronal and mixed neuronal-glial tumours	Ganglioglioma
	Pineal tumours	Pineoblastomas
	Embryonal tumours	Neuroblastoma and retinoblastoma
Tumours of cranial and spinal nerves	Schwannoma	
	Neurofibroma	
	Malignant peripheral nerve sheath tumour	Malignant schwannoma
Tumours of the meninges	Tumours of meningothelial cells	Meningiomas
	Mesenchymal, nonmeningothelial tumours	Fibrous histiocytoma, mesenchymal chondrosarcoma
	Primary melanocytic lesions	Malignant melanoma
	Tumours of uncertain origin	Haemangioblastoma
Haemopoietic neoplasms		Malignant lymphomas
Germ cell tumours		Germinomas, choriocarcinoma, yolk sac tumours, teratomas
Cysts and tumour-like lesions		Rathke's cleft cyst, dermoid and epidermoid cysts, colloid cyst of 3rd ventricle
Tumours of the pituitary		
Local extension from regional tumours		Craniopharyngioma, chondroma, chordoma
Metastatic tumours		

site of the brain affected, and/or seizure. Children with brain tumours often experience a long delay between the onset of symptoms and diagnosis because the symptoms are nonspecific and the patients are treated for conditions other than the brain tumour.

Historical findings include intermittent headache and nausea that is worse in the early mornings. As the disease progresses, the headache becomes persistent and there is associated vomiting. Depending on age, the child may present with worsening irritability and progressive head enlargement due to ensuing hydrocephalus. The child may also present with drowsiness, gait disturbance, visual impairment, limb weakness, stunting of growth or precocious puberty, and seizures.

Examination findings are age specific. The infant may present with features of hydrocephalus with tense fontanelles. There may be failure to thrive, cranial nerve deficits, and limb weakness. There may be hypertonia with exaggerated deep tendon reflexes. Visual assessment may show loss of some visual fields and the presence of papilloedema.

The diagnosis of craniospinal tumours requires a high index of suspicion and meticulous examination to elicit subtle changes that may give away the diagnosis; herein lies the need for commitment and patience.

Diagnostic Investigations

Before the advent of computed tomography (CT) and magnetic resonance imaging (MRI) in the mid 1970s and 1980s, respectively, the diagnoses of brain tumours were based largely on x-rays and angiographic findings. The findings were often nonspecific. X-ray features include erosion of the clinoid processes, widening of the sella turcica, thinning of the skull bone with a copper beaten appearance, osteolytic or osteosclerotic lesions, and calcifications, among others.

CT scans have revolutionised neurosurgery and have now made it possible to diagnose most intracranial pathologies. CT also gives very good bony definition. It is able to give the site and size of the tumour and presence of surrounding oedema.

MRI gives a far better soft tissue definition than the CT scan and clearly defines the extent of the tumour and oedema. It also allows for the image to be taken in different planes. Modifications of this technique have increased the sensitivity and specificity of this diagnostic tool, including MR angiography (MRA), MR spectroscopy, and functional MRI (fMRI).

A lumbar puncture (to be avoided in the presence of raised intracranial pressure (ICP)) could be done to sample for tumour cells in cerebrospinal fluid (CSF) in suspected tumours such as medulloblastomas.

Conventional angiography is important to assess the vascularity of a tumour, look for the feeding vessels, and plan for possible tumour embolisation prior to surgery, thus minimising blood loss at surgery and easing surgical tumour resection.

Management

The management of brain tumours begins with an adequate history and detailed clinical examination, followed by relevant investigations, as outlined earlier. These findings not only help to establish the diagnosis but also determine the extent to which the disease has affected the anatomy and function of the individual. Further, these findings identify those patients requiring emergency intervention.

Patients present as emergencies in the following settings:

- acute raised intracranial pressure due to tumour expansion, surrounding oedema causing mass effect, or acute hydrocephalus from tumour obstruction of the CSF pathway;

- haemorrhage into a tumour cyst, leading to sudden neurological deterioration (e.g., pituitary apoplexy); and

- any of the above leading to herniation, especially of the brain stem, which could be rapidly fatal.

Raised intracranial pressure can be managed nonsurgically, surgically, or a combination of both. Nonsurgical methods include the following:

- *head elevation* to 15°–30° with the head in a neutral position, which ensures adequate venous return and reduces congestion in the brain;

- *oxygen administration and controlled hyperventilation*, which causes cerebral vasoconstriction and reduces congestion within the brain;

- *use of diuretics* (e.g., mannitol and frusemide); and

- *steroids (dexamethasone)*, which are very useful for intracranial mass lesions with surrounding oedema. The effect is often dramatic with quick resolution of symptoms, which gives the surgeon a period of time to prepare for the definitive treatment.

The surgical methods for reducing raised intracranial pressure include the insertion of a shunt for hydrocephalus, excision of the tumour, or debulking where total excision is not feasible.

When patients do not present in an emergency setting, they are optimised for the definitive treatment, which includes correction of nutritional deficiencies, blood levels, dyselectrolytaemia, and cardiovascular and respiratory problems. The definitive treatment modalities include surgery, radiotherapy, chemotherapy, and immunotherapy. These modalities are either used singly or in various relevant combinations.

Surgery

Surgery for childhood tumours is usually done for histological confirmation, total excision or maximum cytoreduction, neural decompression, and CSF pathway restoration. Surgical resection is usually the primary treatment modality; in fact, most benign brain tumours can be cured by surgical resection only. Patients with malignant tumours also benefit from maximal tumour debulking because it allows for better response to chemotherapy and radiotherapy.

Surgical resection has been improved by advances in surgical techniques and instrumentation, such as microsurgery, surgical lasers, and ultrasonic aspirators. Stereotaxy and intraoperative ultrasonography enable the surgeon to precisely localise the tumour based on a previously taken CT scan or MRI. Despite these advances, some tumours still pose great challenges. These include brain-stem tumours, optic chiasmal tumours, and diencephalic tumours, which are operable but often not completely resectable.

Complications of surgery include postoperative haemorrhage, major or minor neurological deficits, brain swelling, and infection. Fortunately, children tend to do better with rehabilitation, even from major postoperative neurological deficit. The success of surgery depends not only on the surgeon, but also on a coordinated and dedicated team that includes the neurosurgeon, anaesthetist, paediatrician, nurses, and physiotherapist, among others.

Radiotherapy

Radiotherapy is required for children with malignant brain tumours or unresectable benign tumours because of a microscopic residual tumour, even when there is macroscopic total tumour excision. Some tumours, such as ependymomas, medulloblastomas and other PNETs are carried along the CSF pathway to the spine necessitating irradiation of the whole neuroaxis.

External beam radiotherapy entails giving high-energy radiation that passes through the scalp and skull to the brain. Anything along its path is irradiated. Complications include the effect on rapidly dividing cells, leading to transient hair loss, bone marrow suppression with anaemia, thrombocytopaenia, and leucopaenia. Endocrine dysfunction and progressive cerebral vascular thrombosis, which may present as a stroke 10–20 years after irradiation, have all been reported. Another complication is the induction of secondary tumours in the brain, which may occur 5–15 years after the irradiation.

A very serious complication of radiotherapy is its deleterious effect on the intellectual development of the child. About 80% of the development of the child's brain occurs in the first 2 years of life. Therefore, radiotherapy is generally not recommended in children younger than 3 years of age. An alternative is the use of chemotherapy in these young children.

Stereotaxic irradiation, such as that provided by a gamma knife or a linear accelerator, delivers focally intensified radiation with minimum damage to the surrounding tissues. A single large dose is usually given.

Another method is the use of brachytherapy or interstitial radiotherapy. In this modality, radioactive seeds are implanted in the tumour intraoperatively by using a catheter or by stereotactic means. The seeds are then removed after they have delivered the calculated required dose.

Chemotherapy

Chemotherapeutic antineoplastic agents also affect rapidly dividing cells and give rise to complications similar to those produced by radiotherapy. They are often given in combination, and act by inhibiting cellular metabolism. They could be given intraarterially through the vertebral or carotid arteries (the use in children is still being evaluated), or intrathecal, to deliver high doses of the drug at the target site. Intrathecal chemotherapy can be given by use of spinal needles. A subcutaneous Ommaya reservoir can be used for intralesional, intracystic, or intraventricular administration of cytotoxic medications.

Intraarterial injection may be complicated by blindness and stroke.

Individual Tumours of the Brain

The general features of tumours have been given earlier. The peculiarities of some specific tumours are noteworthy and are presented here.

Infratentorial Tumours

Infratentorial, or posterior fossa, tumours are more common in the paediatric age group than in adults. The common posterior fossa tumours include medulloblastoma, cerebellar astrocytomas, ependymomas, and brain-stem gliomas.

Primary neuroectodermal tumours

PNETs include medulloblastomas, medulloepitheliomas, pigmented medulloblastomas, ependymoblastomas, pineoblastomas, and cerebral neuroblastomas. These tumours originate from undifferentiated cells in the subependymal region in the foetal brain. The frequency of PNETs is similar to that of pilocytic astrocytoma.

Medulloblastomas

Medulloblastomas initially arise in the inferior medullary velum (possibly from remnants of the external granular layer) and grow to fill the 4th ventricle, infiltrating the surrounding structures (Figure 109.1). They are the most common malignant posterior fossa tumour in the paediatric population. They are characterised by their tendency to seed along the neuro-axis, following CSF pathways, and rarely can metastasise to extraneural tissues.[8,9] Ten to thirty percent of affected patients will have evidence of "drop-mets" at the time of diagnosis. Extracranial metastases account for 5% of cases, involving bone, liver, and lymph nodes.

Medulloblastomas are highly cellular, vascular tumours with a deeply basophilic nucleus and multiple mitoses ("small blue cell tumour"). These histological features are commonly seen in the other variants of PNET.

The male-to-female ratio is approximately 3:1. Medulloblastomas demonstrate a bimodal age distribution: a larger peak occurs at 5–9 years of age, and a smaller peak occurs at 20–30 years of age.

Gross surgical excision followed by craniospinal irradiation remains the ultimate goal in these patients. Any attempt to remove the tumour from the floor of the 4th ventricle, however, can lead to significant morbidity. Up to 30% of tumours will have invaded the floor, and care must be taken not to damage this very eloquent region.

Children with nondisseminated medulloblastoma and old enough to have radiation therapy have a 5-year survival rate of about 70%. In the presence of dissemination, adjuvant chemotherapy (CCNU (lomustine), vincristine, and prednisolone) can be given, but the survival rates are significantly lower. Neurological, endocrine, and cognitive deficits are not uncommon in this latter group.

Piloctyic astrocytoma

Low-grade astrocytomas occur more often in children and young adults than in adults. They are the most common astrocytic tumours in children, accounting for 80–85% of cerebellar astrocytomas and 60% of optic gliomas. They comprise about 33% of all posterior fossa tumours in children and represent about 25% of all paediatric tumours.

Pilocytic astrocytomas usually arise in the cerebellum, brain stem, hypothalamic region, or optic pathways, but they may occur in any area where astrocytes are present, including the cerebral hemispheres and the spinal cord.

There is an association of pilocytic astrocytomas with neurofibromatosis; optic nerve gliomas are common tumours in patients with this condition and may present bilaterally. Patients with optic pilocytic astrocytomas associated with NF1 usually have better outcomes than patients with juvenile pilocytic astrocytomas.

These tumours are usually discrete, indolent lesions associated with cyst formation. The cysts may be unilocular or multilocular, with an associated tumour nodule. CT scan reveals a hypodense or isodense nodular mass that homogeneously enhances with contrast with a cystic component in 60–80% of cases. Calcification is present in 10% of juvenile pilocytic astrocytomas. MRI shows a contrast enhancing hypointense lesion on T1WI and hyperintense on T2WI (Figures 109.2 and 109.3).

Histologically, the tumour contains fibrillary astrocytes with associated Rosenthal fibres (intracellular eosinophilic rod-shaped bodies). The tumour is named after the "hair-like" bipolar (piloid) astrocytes. Features more typically seen in higher grade gliomas can be seen (e.g., nuclear atypia, mitoses, endothelial proliferation, and necrosis) but they have no proven prognostic significance.

The peak incidence of pilocytic astrocytoma is in patients 5–14 years of age; it has no gender predilection.

Posterior fossa pilocytic astrocytomas are typically treated with surgery and completely resected whenever possible. Optic nerve tumours can often be managed conservatively, and surgery is usually indicated in an attempt to preserve vision in the unaffected eye. There has been some success treating these tumours with chemotherapy (particularly platinum-based regimes), but this is used only for unresectable progressive tumours, or progression of remnants.

Patients with juvenile pilocytic astrocytoma have a better prognosis than patients with most other types of astrocytomas. If gross total resection is possible, the 10-year survival rate is as high as 90%.[10] After subtotal resection or biopsy, the 10-year survival rate is as high as 45%. Morbidity is related to the location of the tumour and to the associated complications of tumour resection.

Ependymoma

Ependymomas account for 1–8% of paediatric brain tumours. There is a female preponderance with a female-to-male ratio of approximately 2:1. The median age of presentation is in the second decade, but there is a bimodal peak with the younger peak at about age 5 years. Ependymomas are derived from ependymal cells and occur most commonly in the ependymal lining of the ventricles. These tumours can also arise in the conus (myxopapillary) and spinal canal. The majority of ependymomas are located in the posterior fossa with a predilection for the 4th ventricle; 20% arise from the floor. Extension through the foramina of Magendie and Luschka is not uncommon. Approximately 10% will have spinal metastases at the time of diagnosis, although

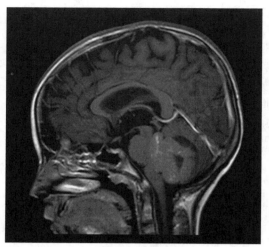

Figure 109.1: Medulloblastoma. Note the tumour filling the 4th ventricle and extending up the cerebral aqueduct.

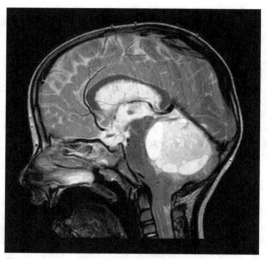

Figure 109.2: Large posterior fossa pilocytic astrocytoma. Hydrocephalus has been treated by external ventricular drainage (EVD), but tonsillar herniation remains.

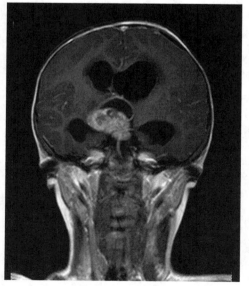

Figure 109.3: Large suprasellar pilocytic astrocytoma encircling the basilar artery. This could not be completely removed at surgery.

this is more common with the anaplastic variants. Tumours presenting supratentorially are more common in adults and are usually located in the trigone of the lateral ventricles. Symptoms of ependymomas are similar to those of medulloblastoma, but there may also be cranial nerve deficits.

Ependymomas of the posterior fossa present as solid mass lesions. Histologically, they are uniform ependymal cells forming true rosettes and perivascular pseudorosettes. It is not uncommon to have associated calcification, cysts, and haemorrhage. Anaplastic ependymomas tend to have histological features of a higher grade tumour with vascular proliferation and necrosis. Ependymomas of the spinal cord and conus are more likely to be low grade, and total excision may be curative.

A CT scan of the tumour shows an isodense mass that may enhance slightly but irregularly with contrast.

Gross total surgical excision, where possible, with adjuvant radiotherapy is the treatment of choice.

Combined treatment leads to a 35–60% 5-year survival rate. Although adults have an increased tendency to anaplastic variants, their survival rate is better than that of children. This is most likely due to the fact that craniospinal radiation therapy is limited to children older than the age of 5 due to the adverse effects on the developing nervous system.

Brain-Stem Gliomas

Brain-stem gliomas require special mention because they present a peculiar challenge to the neurosurgeon. Their total resection is difficult and often impossible, except in expert hands.

In children, brain-stem gliomas represent 10–20% of all brain tumours. Most brain-stem gliomas are low-grade astrocytomas and can be conservatively managed. Surgical debulking is reserved for exophytic portions of tumour.

Ninety percent of diffuse pontine gliomas are, however, more aggressive (anaplastic astrocytoma or glioblastoma) with a very short survival. They present with rapidly deteriorating symptoms such as dysarthria, hemiparesis, ataxia, and facial and abducens nerve palsies.

MRI shows enlargement of the pons, with a lesion hypointense on T1WI and hyperintense on T2WI that is contrast enhancing. CT also shows an enhancing lesion (Figure 109.4).

Because of the danger and difficulty of obtaining a biopsy in this condition, the patient could be commenced on radiotherapy even without a biopsy. However, some authorities have completely resected such tumours.

Supratentorial Tumours

Craniopharyngioma

Craniopharyngiomas arise from remnants of the Rathke's pouch. They account for 2–4% of all brain tumours, occurring mostly in the age group 5–15 years. Craniopharyngiomas are slow growing and may attain a large size before manifesting. They present with visual impairment due to compression of the optic nerves; endocrinopathy, especially diabetes insipidus and obesity; and features of hydrocephalus due to extension to the floor of the 3rd ventricle.

CT scan shows a sellar or parasellar mass with cystic and solid components and sometimes calcification. A preoperative hormonal work-up is very important. Teamwork with an endocrinologist and ophthalmologist is invaluable.

Surgery is the primary treatment modality and may employ the use of endoscopic trans-sphenoidal resection or craniotomy and excision.

Radiotherapy, especially intracystic injection, has been found useful in incompletely resectable or nonresectable lesions; also effective is the intracystic injection of bleomycin. Systemic chemotherapy has not been found useful.

Pilocytic astrocytoma

Pilocytic astrocytoma differ markedly from infiltrating fibrillary or diffuse astrocytomas in terms of their ability to invade tissue and for malignant degeneration. They occur throughout the neuraxis and are

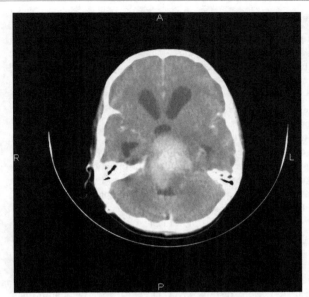

Figure 109.4: Post contrast CT of a 12 year-old-girl with brain-stem glioma. Note the enhancing lesion with dilated lateral and 3rd ventricles.

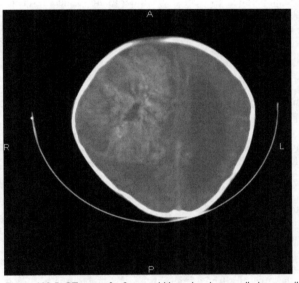

Figure 109.5: CT scan of a 6-year-old boy showing a well-circumscribed huge right fronto-parietal contast-enhancing astrocytoma. Note the effacement of the right ventricle, mild oedema, midline shift, and left lateral ventriculomegaly.

more common in children and young adults than in adults. Malignant transformation has been reported after many years, even without radiotherapy. Cerebral gliomas, optic gliomas, and thalamic and hypothalamic gliomas tend to occur in young adults.

Hemispheric lesions give rise to headaches, seizures, and focal weakness. Chiasmal tumours present with visual deficits, endocrine dysfunction, or symptoms of hydrocephalus.

CT or MRI show these tumours as well-circumscribed, contrast-enhancing lesions (Figure 109.5) with cystic components and a mural nodule, having little or no surrounding oedema.

Surgery is the most recommended treatment modality, with an aim to total excision, including especially the mural nodule. Radiotherapy is controversial, but can be used after a subtotal resection in a patient older than 3 years of age. Chemotherapy is given to younger patients.

Complete resection yields 100% recurrence-free survival without adjuvant therapy.[11] After subtotal resection and radiotherapy, 10- and 20-year freedom from progression rates are 74% and 41%, respectively, and 10- and 20-year survival rates are 81% and 54%, respectively.

Choroid plexus papilloma and carcinoma
Choroid plexus papilloma and carcinoma represent 0.4–0.6% of all intracranial tumours. They represent approximately 3% of childhood brain tumours and are more likely to occur in the lateral ventricle. Although these tumours can occur in the 4th ventricle, this feature is more commonly seen in adults. Approximately 85% of tumours present in children under 5 years.

Symptoms can be due to hydrocephalus, which is likely to be due to the presence of increased protein and xanthochromia within the CSF, causing diminished absorption. Overproduction of CSF is not uncommon, but does not explain the persistence of hydrocephalus after tumour removal. These tumours may also present with mass effect, particularly in the case of papilloma.

Although macroscopically, choroid plexus papilloma appears as a reddish solid tumour, histologically, it can be difficult to differentiate from a normal choroid. As with the malignant variants of a tumour, the presence of nuclear atypia, mitoses, and necrosis is suggestive of carcinomatous change.

Surgical resection results in a cure for benign papillomas. These tumours are very vascular, and in the presence of carcinoma, preoperative chemotherapy or embolisation may have roles in shrinking tumour size and reducing vascularity in order to aid surgical resection.

Five-year survival rates of about 80% have been described. The main late morbidity arises from persistent subdural collections due to a ventriculo-subdural fistula.

Spinal Cord Tumours
Spinal cord tumours are relatively rare in the paediatric age group when compared to brain tumours.[12] They could be extradural or intradural. The intradural tumours can be intramedullary or extramedullary, with intramedullary tumours more common than extramedullary. Intramedullary tumours in children include astrocytomas, ependymomas, gangliogliomas, diffuse leptomeningeal tumours, and haemangiomas. The more common childhood extramedullary tumours consist of meningiomas, schwanomas, and neurofibromas; extradural tumours comprise lipomas and dermoid and epidermoid cysts.

Astrocytomas
Astrocytomas are by far the most common childhood spinal tumours. They are mostly benign, but can be malignant in 10–15% of cases. They may remain asymptomatic for a long time, reaching large sizes before presentation. The onset of symptoms is usually insidious and may appear at the time of a trivial injury. An early symptom is back pain, which is usually diffuse.

Extramedullary tumours
Radicular pain may be suggestive of an extramedullary lesion.

Children present with frequent falls, lower limb weakness or motor regression, or gait abnormalities. About a third present with kyphoscoliosis. Sphincteric involvement occurs late in the disease. A few may present with features of hydrocephalus, which is thought to be due to increased protein secretion by the tumour cells into the CSF, leading to obstruction. Examination reveals varying degrees of motor weakness and upper motor neurone features.

MRI is the diagnostic tool of choice because it clearly defines the lesion. CT myelography may be done where MRI is contraindicated or not available. Plain radiographs are mandatory for those with scoliosis. Again, extramedullary tumours may show as thinning or sclerosis of the pedicles. There may also be enlargement of the neural foramina in dumbbell tumours.

Adjuncts for spinal cord surgery include ultrasonic aspirator and lasers.

Astrocytomas are excised after performing a laminectomy or laminotomy. The outcome depends on the neurological state of the patient prior to surgery. Those with incomplete injury are likely to

benefit more than those who have a complete injury. The majority of extramedullary tumours are benign, and gross total excision is possible in most cases.

Management

General Principles
Mass lesions in children and adults present in one (or more) of the following ways:

- raised ICP, which can be due to the mass lesion or hydrocephalus;

- seizures, which can be focal or generalised;

- focal neurological deficits, which are specific to the location of the tumour; and

- pituitary tumours and craniopharyngiomas, which may present with either a neurological deficit (in particular visual loss) or endocrine dysfunction.

Classic neurological features of raised ICP in older children and adults include headache, vomiting, and blurred vision. Papilloedema/ataxia is another feature. Nonspecific features in infants and children, as previously mentioned, include poor feeding/failure to thrive, irritability, behavioural disturbance, and deterioration in schoolwork.

Remember ABC when assessing any acutely unwell patient: airway, breathing, circulation. This is particularly relevant in children who may have a decreased conscious level, or may be dehydrated due to anorexia and vomiting.

Work-ups
The general work-up is the same as for hydrocephalus.

Specific work-ups include the following:

- MRI of the brain and spine is preferable prior to any surgical intervention; is useful to assess suitability for endoscopic management (e.g., endoscopic third ventriculostomy (ETV) or biopsy); allows better evaluation of the tumour and its relation to eloquent structures; and allows assessment of any spinal disease (e.g., drop metastases). A CT scan can, of course, be used as an alternative—it is not quite as good, but with reconstructions in the sagittal plane, is a realistically achieved alternative.

- Tumour markers are obtainable from CSF and serum, and are essential for optimising management of pineal region tumours.

- Endocrine assessment should be used for pituitary and craniopharyngioma patients, who may need preoperative hormone replacement.

- Opthalmology and visual field assessment is most commonly required for pituitary patients, and is recommended for any child with a tumour along the visual pathway.

Treatment Options
Previous series have described carrying out treatment for symptomatic hydrocephalus first. This has the advantage of rapidly improving such symptoms as headache and vomiting, and also allows investigation of CSF markers. In the presence of an aqueductal stenosis due to an offending tumour, an initial endoscopic approach may be used to create a third ventriculostomy and biopsy the tumour at the same sitting.

In recent years, however, in the case of a posterior fossa tumour, the pendulum has swung back towards single-sitting surgery. This option is aimed at opening up the CSF pathways and avoids the added risks of a third ventriculostomy or shunt. An EVD may be placed during the early part of the procedure if there is grossly raised ICP. A drawback is that this regime relies on an operating theatre being available at the time of presentation or deterioration, whereas the two-stage procedure allows more leeway from the organisational point of view.

Surgical excision is carried out wherever tumour location makes it possible. Unlike for adult cases, the free use of chemo- and radiotherapy is not possible for young children. Children under the age of 5 years have a significant long-term morbidity with whole brain (with or without spine) radiotherapy. Outcomes are improved in children older than 5 years of age at diagnosis with no evidence of disseminated disease and maximal surgical resection.

Brain-stem and optic tract gliomas are usually low-grade astrocytomas and are predominantly managed conservatively.

Follow-up Imaging

MRI within the first 24 hours after surgery provides a baseline for further follow-up and optimises any adjuvant therapy. The artefact produced from surgical intervention makes radiological assessment of any residual tumour after 48 hours exceptionally difficult; therefore, if imaging cannot be performed within this time period, it should be deferred for at least 6 weeks.

Key Summary Points

1. Central nervous system tumours are the most common childhood tumours worldwide.

2. More cases are reporting to health facilities, but the challenges in Africa are inadequate facilities and manpower to manage these conditions appropriately.

3. Presentation commonly involves features of raised intracranial pressure, seizure, or focal neurological deficit.

4. Africans typically present at the late stage of brain and spinal cord disease.

5. CT scan and MRI are the investigations of choice, but tissue diagnosis is required for treatment (except in the few instances in which this is not feasible due to the site of the tumour).

6. Full resection is not always the aim—the histology and location of the tumour should dictate the surgical aim.

7. Pre- and postsurgical adjuvant treatment will become increasingly important as their efficacy increases.

8. Patients with incomplete neurological deficit are more likely to benefit from spinal surgery than those with complete deficits.

References

1. Tindall GT, Cooper PR, Barrow DL. Management of brain tumours of glial and neuronal origin in infants and children. In Tindall GT, Cooper PR, Barrow DL, eds. The Practice of Neurosurgery. Williams & Wilkins, 1996, Section 54.

2. Stiller CA, Nectoux J. International incidence of childhood brain and spinal tumours. Inter J Epidemiol 1994; 23(3):458–464.

3. Tomita T, Bowman RM. Craniopharyngiomas in children: surgical experience at Children's Memorial Hospital, Chicago. Child's Nerv Syst 2005; 21(8–9):729–746. Epub 26 July 2005.

4. Allen JC: Childhood brain tumours: current status of clinical trials in newly diagnosed and recurrent disease. Ped Clin N Am 1985; 32:633–651.

5. Laurent JP, Cheek WR. Brain tumours in children. J Pediatr Neurosci 1985; 1:15–32.

6. Aghadiuno PU, Adeloye A, Olumide AA, Nottidge VA. Intracranial neoplasms in children in Ibadan,Nigeria. Child's Nerv Syst 1985; 1(1):39–44.

7. Crockard A, Hayward R, Hole, J, eds. Classification of tumours of the CNS; In: Crockard A, Hayward R, Hole, J, eds. Neurosurgery: The Scientific Basis of Clinical Practice, 2nd ed. Blackwell Scientific Publication, 1992, Pp 519–520.

8. Buckner JC, Brown PD, O'Neill BP, Meyer FB, Wetmore CJ, Uhm JH. Brain tumours—children. In: Medline Plus Medical Encyclopaedia, 2007, Vol 10, Pp 1271–1286.

9. Adeloye A. Intracranial neoplasms. In: Adeloye A. Neurosurgery in Africa. Ibadan University Press, 1989, Pp 218–232.

10. Kuratsu JI, Ushio Y. Epidemiological study of primary intracranial tumours in childhood. Paediatr Neurosurg 1996; 25:240–247.

11. Wallner KE, Gonzales MF, Edwards MSB, et al. Treatment results of juvenile pilocytic astrocytoma. J Neurosurg 1988; 69:171–176.

12. Winn RH. Intraspinal tumours in infants and children. In: Winn, RH. Youman's Neurological Surgery, 5th ed. Saunders, 1995, Chap 240.

Suggested Reading

Paediatric neurosurgery is a constantly evolving science. The most up-to-date reviews are to be found in journals, many of which are available online. In the authors' opinion, the best are Child's Nervous System (published by Springer), Paediatric Neurosurgery (published by Karger), and Journal of Neurosurgery (Pediatrics).

Many textbooks are available; two that cover many aspects of both diagnostic and operative management of paediatric neurosurgical patients are:

Albright AL, Pollack IF, Adelson PD. Principles and Practice of Pediatric Neurosurgery. Thieme Medical Publishers, Inc., 2008.

McLone DG, ed. Pediatric Neurosurgery: Surgery of the Developing Nervous System, 4th ed. Saunders, 2001.

Vascular System

CHAPTER 110
LYMPHANGIOMAS

Emmanuel A. Ameh
Louise Caouette-Laberge
Jean-Martin Laberge

Introduction

Lymphangiomas are developmental defects of the lymphatic channels that belong to a large spectrum of vascular malformations. They are most commonly located in the head and neck region, and to a lesser extent on the axilla and trunk, but can occur anywhere there are lymphatic vessels. Even though they are congenital defects, they may not become apparent until several years after birth. Although benign, lymphangiomas frequently present surgical difficulties and challenges due to their propensity to infiltrate and extend around neighbouring structures.

Lymphatic malformations encompass entities other than lymphangiomas. The goal of this chapter is to address the lesions known as lymphangiomas or hygromas. This chapter does not discuss pulmonary and intestinal lymphangiectasia and peripheral lymphoedema, which may be congenital or acquired, or lymphangiomatosis, an ill-defined disease usually implying the coexistence of lymphangiectasia and multiple lymphangiomas in several sites.

Demographics

The incidence of lymphangiomas is difficult to ascertain. Some authors have quoted an incidence of 1.5 to 2.8 per 1,000,[1] but this applies to foetal nuchal translucency, which is a different pathology (see subsection on "Prenatal Presentation"). Others have reported an occurrence of 1 in 12,000 births for cystic lymphangiomas.[2] There are no reported racial or ethnic predispositions; the male-to-female ratio is equal in most large reviews,[3–6] but some authors have described a male predominance.[7,8] In most of Africa, incidence data are not available, but hospital-based reports suggest that at least 1–3 children with lymphangiomas are seen every year in most teaching centres.[4,5,7,9–11]

These lesions are apparent in 50–70% children at birth or prenatally, and 80–90% present within 5 years. However, presentation may occur as late as adolescence or adulthood.[2,3,12,13]

Embryology

The lymphatic system starts to develop by the end of the 5th week of gestation, 2 weeks after the primordia of the cardiovascular system are recognisable and 1 week after coordinated contractions of the primitive heart initiate unidirectional blood flow.[14,15] The lymphatic vessels are thought to be derived from the venous system as endothelial outgrowths.[14–16] By the 8th week of gestation, six lymphatic sacs are formed: two jugular, two iliac, the retroperitoneal sac at the root of the mesentery, and the cysterna chyli, which is dorsal to the latter. From these form new sprouts that grow to the periphery of the embryo, passing along veins. Bilateral thoracic ducts connect the cysterna chyli to the jugular sacs in the 9th week; a large anastomosis forms between the two thoracic ducts, and the final thoracic duct comes from the right duct in the lower chest and the left duct in the upper chest and neck, where it connects with the venous system at the junction between the left internal jugular and subclavian veins.

The majority of lymphangiomas arise from parts of lymph sacs that are pinched off during development or that fail to establish connections with the main lymphatic or venous channels. A small proportion appears to arise from localised lymphatic malformations or obstruction.

Pathology

Lymphangiomas are cysts or pockets of lymphatic fluid collection, which may consist of multiple cysts connected to each other by small lymphatic channels. They usually contain clear, straw-coloured fluid unless infection or bleeding has occurred.

Microcystic lymphangiomas have the propensity to infiltrate and extend into and around neighbouring structures, making complete excision difficult.

Microscopically, the cysts are lined by endothelium, supported by stroma of varying thickness and containing smooth muscle elements and lymphoid tissue. The endothelial lining is quite vulnerable to infection and chemical irritants. This observation forms the basis for sclerotherapy.

Nomenclature

Many misconceptions exist about lymphatic anomalies, and classifications are confusing. The suffix –oma is generally associated with tumours and a notion of cellular division and invasion, which does not apply to lymphangiomas. Used in the broad sense of a "space-occupying lesion", such as a haematoma or seroma, the term lymphangioma continues to be used, but it should not be considered a tumour in the neoplastic sense.

Cystic hygroma is a term coined in 1843 by Wernher, which was perpetuated since the classification proposed by Landing and Farber in 1956.[17] Because hygroma means a fluid-filled mass, the term "cystic hygroma" is redundant and should be abandoned. Hygromas are often used to describe cystic lymphangiomas occurring in the cervical area. In the abdomen, mesenteric cysts are generally synonymous with lymphangioma of the mesentery in the paediatric literature, even though some authors distinguish the two entities. The former is thought to occur mainly in adults, whereas mesenteric lymphangiomas usually present at birth or in infancy.

Furthermore, the classification of lymphangiomas into capillary, cavernous, and cystic has no clinical usefulness, as the various types may coexist in the same lesion. This nomenclature has been largely replaced by the unifying classification of Mulliken,[18] which

Table 110.1: Classification of lymphatic malformations.

Lymphatic malformation classification	Types
Primary lymphoedema	
Lymphangioma	Macrocystic (formerly cystic hygroma) Microcystic (formerly cavernous lymphangioma) Mixed
Diffuse lymphatic anomalies	Pulmonary or pleural or intestinal lymphangiomatosis Gorham-Stout disease (the so-called "vanishing bone disease")
Combined/complex malformations	Klippel-Trenaunay syndrome (capillary-lymphatico-venous malformation) Proteus syndrome Maffucci syndrome

was adopted by the International Society for the Study of Vascular Anomalies in 1996.[19] However the term "lymphatic malformation" used by Mulliken in this classification is very broad (Table 110.1).

The term "lymphangioma" continues to be used by most clinicians and will be used in this chapter. Lymphangiomas can be divided into macrocystic, microcystic, and mixed forms on the basis of imaging studies (see Table 110.1). This classification has important therapeutic and prognostic implications, as will be seen in this chapter.

Natural History

Lymphangiomas tend to grow slowly with the child, but sudden enlargement may be seen during a viral infection or when bacterial infection or spontaneous bleeding occurs in some cysts. Spontaneous resolution is uncommon but has been reported in up to 15% of cases.[8,12,16,20] Resolution may occasionally follow infection.

Clinical Presentation

History

Generally, lymphangiomas are asymptomatic at diagnosis; however, presentation may be delayed in Africa, particularly if the lymphangioma is outside the head and neck region.

The most common site of involvement is the neck, with other common sites being the head (especially the tongue), the axilla and chest wall, the abdominal wall and flank, and the extremities (Figure 110.1, Table 110.2). Internal organs are involved in 10% of patients, the most common being the bowel mesentery.

Presentation depends on the site. Reasons for presentation include disfigurement; mass lesion; pain (and fever); pressure effect (e.g., respiratory obstruction or dysphagia); and acute abdomen or intestinal obstruction.

Physical Examination

Patients presenting with uncomplicated lymphangiomas usually look healthy otherwise. Local warmth and tenderness with pyrexia generally signify infection of the lesion. In such circumstances, the skin may be erythematous (in light-skinned patients), or simply appear shiny. Tachypnea and cyanosis may be present in those with airway obstruction.

In the neck, 85% of lymphangiomas are unilateral. There may be extension into the ipsilateral face or floor of the mouth in some patients. Fifteen percent are midline or extend to both sides of the neck.[6] The lesion may be quite large; some may attain massive proportions.

Diagnosis is based on the finding of a soft, multiloculated mass, which transilluminates brilliantly. However, lymphangiomas with infection or intracystic haemorrhage may not transilluminate. Microcystic lymphangiomas, due to the significant amount of stroma, may have solid areas that could create diagnostic difficulty.

Prenatal Presentation

Lymphangiomas are increasingly being diagnosed by prenatal ultrasonography (US), particularly when located in the neck. Posterior nuchal translucency, confusingly called nuchal cystic hygroma, is not the same as lymphangioma.[21] Foetal nuchal translucency is an important marker for aneuploidy in the first trimester and early part of the second; it may be associated with pleural effusion and hydrops. It is usually bilateral and posterior, whereas lymphangiomas are lateral or anterior and are diagnosed in the second and third trimesters. In the absence of chromosomal anomalies, 80% of foetuses with first-trimester nuchal translucency have a normal outcome unless there is spontaneous abortion; in favorable cases, the translucency usually resolves spontaneously by the end of the second trimester. Turner and Noonan syndromes are often accompanied by nuchal translucency; the prenatal diagnosis of the latter is difficult to make because the karyotype would be normal.[22]

The differential diagnosis of cervical cystic lesions includes cystic teratomas, thymic and branchial cysts, and congenital fibrosarcomas. In the abdomen, ovarian cysts are most common, followed by enteric duplications; cystic renal masses are also common but are usually readily distinguishable. Rare abdominal cystic lesions in the foetus

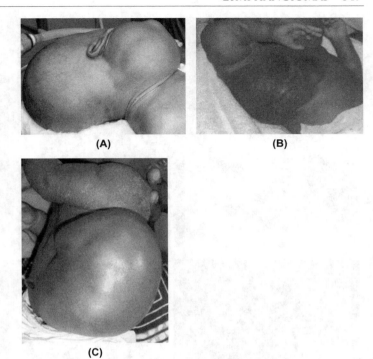

(A)   (B)

(C)

Figure 110.1: Lymphangiomas at various sites: (A) cervical, (B) axillary, (C) left flank.

Table 110.2: Anatomic distribution of lymphangiomas in two large paediatric series.

Site	Number	Percentage
Cervical	116	31
Craniofacial	72	19
Trunk (including axilla and genitalia)	89	23
Extremities	59	16
Intraabdominal and mediastinal	43	11
Totals	379	100

Sources: Hancock BJ, St-Vil D, Luks FI, Di Lorenzo M, Blanchard H. Complications of lymphangiomas in children. J Pediatr Surg 1992; 27: 220–224. Alqahtani A, Nguyen LT, Flageole H, Shaw K, Laberge JM. 25 years' experience with lymphangiomas in children. J Pediatr Surg 1999; 34:1164–1168.

include cystic teratomas, mesenchymal hamartomas of the liver, choledochal cysts, urachal cysts, and congenital fibrosarcoma.[21]

Prenatal diagnosis is especially important for large lymphatic malformations because they may cause dystocia. Prenatal aspiration of selected macrocystic lesions may allow for vaginal delivery or facilitate caesarean section in some cases. Prenatal diagnosis is even more important for large cervical lesions, which may cause respiratory distress at birth. When tracheal obstruction is predicted on prenatal imaging, an EXIT procedure is the safest way to deliver the baby.[23] EXIT, which stands for EX-utero Intrapartum Treatment, is essentially a large caesarean section done under deep maternal general anesthesia; the foetal head is delivered and an airway is secured while placental circulation maintains foetal oxygenation. Sometimes a tracheostomy will be required, but often the baby can be intubated successfully with the help and confirmation of flexible bronchoscopy. Prenatal imaging is usually accurate in predicting airway compression and the need for caesarian section (Figure 110.2).

Prenatal treatment of foetal lymphatic malformations with sclerosants, such as OK-432 (see subsection "Types of Lesions"), has been advocated by some authors, but its role remains to be determined.[24,25] The problem is that the rate of incorrect prenatal diagnosis of lymphatic malformations may be as high as 38–50%.[21,26]

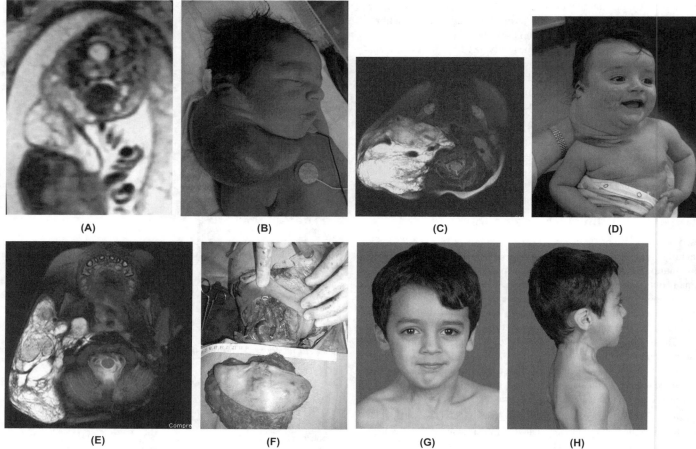

Figure 110.2: Giant cervical lymphangioma (unilateral supra and infra hyoid, mixed macro and microcystic): (A) Prenatal MRI, showing right cervical cysts (white on this T-2-weighted image, right eye seen in top part of picture). (B) Child after delivery by caesarian section, with paediatric surgeon in attendance. (C) MRI at 4.5 months of age. (D) Child at 4.5 months of age; note scarring from Ethibloc extrusion on lower neck. (E) MRI at 18 months of age, prior to surgical resection (after two sclerotherapies with Ethibloc and one streptococcal infection). (F) Cervical dissection with cranial nerves VII, X, XI, XII, and phrenic nerve, hugely dilated dysplastic jugular vein, and resected specimen. (G) Frontal view, 3.5 years postoperatively. (H) Lateral view, 3.5 years postoperatively.

Investigations

Although the diagnosis of most lymphangiomas is clinical, various modalities are required for confirmation of the diagnosis, planning of treatment, and follow-up.

Ultrasonography

US helps in classifying the lesion (macrocystic, microcystic, or mixed), as well as ascertaining the extent of the disease. This should be the minimum imaging modality for evaluation. Neighbouring and susceptible regions of the body should also be assessed adequately by US.

Plain Radiography

Plain radiography is useful when the lymphangioma may extend into or is located in a body cavity, particularly in the absence of computed tomography (CT) scan and magnetic resonance imaging (MRI). For example, normal chest radiographs exclude any significant mediastinal extension of large cervical lymphangioma. Plain radiographs may also be useful in evaluating the trachea in such patients, as this will be helpful during anaesthesia and tracheal intubation.

CT Scan and MRI

CT scan and MRI are being used increasingly for evaluation. MRI is now considered to be the most accurate imaging modality for evaluation. However, these imaging modalities have limited application in resource-limited settings due to cost and availability. The CT scan is superior to US in detecting small areas of calcifications or fat, which would change the diagnosis to teratoma.

Needle Aspiration and Culture

Needle aspiration and cytological examination of the fluid should be done in any patient who will be treated by sclerosants or who will be observed for a period of time. This will avoid delaying resection of a teratoma, with its inherent risk of malignant transformation (Figure 110.3).

Needle aspiration may also be used in situations where intracystic haemorrhage is suspected (rapid increase in size), or infection has occurred and abscess formation is suspected. In the latter instance, culture of the pus will help to direct antibiotic treatment; in the former, aspiration may decompress the lesion until definitive treatment is undertaken.

In patients presenting with airway obstruction, needle aspiration may be performed as a temporising measure. Any aspirated fluid in all situations should be sent for microbiological culture, cell count (the differential will show at least 80–90% lymphocytes in lymphangiomas), and cytology.

Complications

In Africa, many children with lymphangiomas present with complications, which can be life threatening, particularly in the cervical area.[4,7]

Respiratory Obstruction

Respiratory obstruction is a feared complication of head and neck lymphangiomas and can be due to the infiltration of the malformation in the tongue, pharynx, or larynx, or compression of a normal airway by large cysts. Emergency management includes cyst aspiration, positional nursing, endotracheal intubation, and tracheostomy. Aspiration of a macrocystic lesion is a temporary measure and carries a risk of

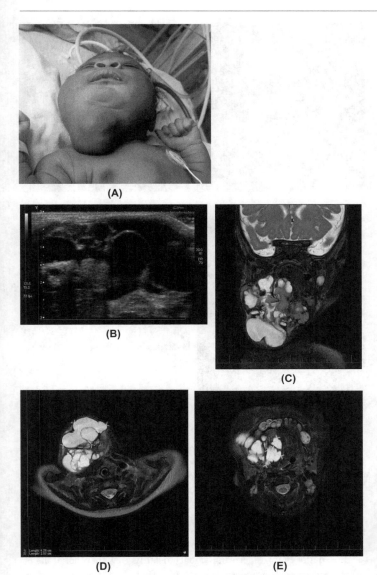

Rapid Size Increase

A rapid increase in the size of the lymphatic malformation can occur in reaction to a viral or bacterial infection anywhere in the body, but it is more frequent with upper airway infection. This is due to increased lymphatic flow. This usually resolves as the primary infection is controlled. The increase in size may cause airway obstruction, discomfort, transient nerve compression, or pressure necrosis, which in turn increases the risk of infection. A sudden increase in size may also be due to intracystic haemorrhage. In large cysts, bleeding due to the rupture of a blood vessel normally present in intracystic septae can be severe and necessitate transfusions.

Infection

Infection of the lymphatic malformation should be treated promptly. The incidence of infection in cervical lymphatic malformations varies in different series from 17% to 71%.[6,7,28] Since infection often follows an episode of upper respiratory tract infection, initial antibiotic therapy should be directed at the prevalent bacteria in the nasopharynx, particularly group B streptococcus. Parenteral administration of ampicillin (or amoxicillin) and gentamicin is usually effective. A cephalosporin may be used as a single agent. In patients who develop infection following cyst aspiration, coverage for staphylococcus is essential, and metronidazole can be added to cover for anaerobes. When an abscess is suspected, aspiration is indicated to confirm diagnosis and obtain cultures; often a drainage procedure (percutaneous or incisional) will be required. Ultrasonographic guidance may be helpful, particularly in the cervical area, to decrease the risk of damage to adjacent structures.

Ulceration

Ulceration is due to pressure necrosis. The ulcerated area often rapidly becomes infected, and the infection may extend into the cyst (Figure 110.4). This should be managed by dressings and the use of antibiotics if infected. To decrease the risk of postoperative wound infection, it is usually safer to wait until the ulceration has healed before embarking on surgical excision.

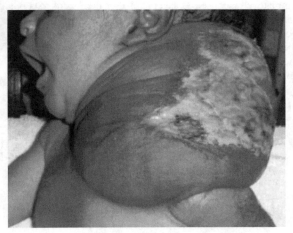

Figure 110.4: Ulcerated left cervical cystic lymphangioma.

Figure 110.3: Difficulties in diagnosis: (A) A large lobulated neck mass in a newborn. (B) US showing multicystic lesion; patient was initially observed, but was readmitted with feeding difficulty. (C) MRI (coronal view, T-2 weighted) showing extent in the floor of the mouth. (D) Axial view demonstrating an intact trachea. (E) Proximally, the mass displacing the larynx and base of the tongue. The patient failed two attempts at sclerosis with doxycycline and required nasogastric tube feedings and a tracheostomy following an episode of bronchiolitis. Excision carried out at 5 months of age revealed a mature teratoma.

Feeding and Speech Difficulties

Feeding and speech difficulties can be present in lesions of the suprahyoid area with tongue involvement or can occur sporadically during episodes of rapid increase of the size of the lesion. Tube feeding or a gastrostomy may be required to maintain adequate nutrition.

Mortality

Reported mortality as a result of one or a combination of these complications, particularly in neonates, ranges from 0% to 2%[7,12] and may be much higher in the African setting.[4] The incidence in other reports may be underestimated, as many of the severely obstructed neonates may never reach the tertiary centres where case series are reviewed.

infection. It can be repeated once or twice while preparing for definitive treatment. A sterile technique is mandatory, and US guidance helps to achieve efficient aspiration.

Positional nursing on the ipsilateral side (if unilateral) or on the more affected side (if the cyst extends to both sides of the neck) helps to take the pressure and weight off the trachea and to temporarily relieve airway obstruction. Endotracheal intubation or tracheostomy may be necessary, especially when the larynx is directly involved by the lymphangioma. Endotracheal intubation can be maintained for a few weeks to relieve the obstruction by cyst aspiration, antibiotherapy, sclerotherapy, or early surgical resection. Tracheostomy carries a significant risk for early and late complications in neonates and should be avoided as much as possible, but it is unavoidable in certain circumstances.[27] If a tracheostomy is done, it should be left in place until definitive treatment is achieved. Oxygen supplementation should always be given in patients with airway obstruction.

Other Complications

Skeletal overgrowth and maxillary malocclusion are also well documented.[28,29]

Treatment

Lymphangiomas are benign vascular malformations; therefore, growth is not a concern, although the size of the lesions varies over time, depending on inflammation, infection, bleeding, or fluid accumulation in the cysts. Once the diagnosis has been established, observation during the first years of life is adequate unless the lesion causes severe deformity or a complication occurs. Reports of spontaneous resolution, sometimes following an episode of infection, have been published,[8,12,16,20] but it remains uncommon. The mainstays of treatment are sclerotherapy and surgical excision. Radiation therapy, although occasionally used in the past, carries a risk of growth retardation and malignancy and is not recommended. Before considering surgery, the feasibility of complete excision and the risks of postoperative complications and damage to adjacent structures, as well as the scarring involved, should be carefully weighed against the advantages and risks of sclerotherapy. In recent years, many centres have switched to using sclerotherapy as a primary treatment, followed by surgery if needed, rather than using sclerotherapy as rescue treatment. The prognosis varies with the type of malformation (macrocystic, microcystic, or mixed lesion) and its location.

Types of Lesions

Macrocystic lesions

Macrocystic lesions have the best prognosis for successful treatment with sclerotherapy or surgery.[13,30–32] The large cysts are more easily removed completely, and there is less infiltration of the adjacent structures, which can usually be completely preserved. If sclerotherapy is done, the large cysts provide an easy access for successful treatment. The two treatment modalities can be combined if necessary.

Mixed lesions

In mixed lesions, the large cysts provide an access for sclerotherapy and the inflammatory response reduces the size of the macrocysts but may also have a positive effect on the microcystic components adjacent to the macrocysts. It is therefore essential not to surgically remove the large cysts before addressing the microcystic component infiltrating adjacent structures. Mixed lesions of the suprahyoid region are not completely resectable due to the infiltration of the tongue, floor of the mouth, pharynx, and larynx. Sclerotherapy has significantly improved the prognosis for such patients (Figures 110.2 and 110.5).

Microcystic lesions

Microcystic lesions are infiltrating lesions that are more difficult to treat both surgically and with sclerotherapy. There is little space available for the sclerosing material, and surgical resection is limited by the infiltration of important structures. Residual malformation is the rule in the majority of cases unless the lesion is well delineated and completely excised. When the skin overlying the lesion is involved (angiokeratosis or lymphangiomata circumscriptum), it should be removed whenever feasible.

Treatment Modalities

Percutaneous sclerotherapy

Percutaneous sclerotherapy is performed with a sterile technique, usually under sedation or general anaesthesia, depending on the age of the child, with US guidance. Fluid is aspirated and sent for cell count and cytological examination to confirm the diagnosis. A contrast medium may be injected to identify and quantify the number of cysts and intercystic communications under fluoroscopy. The sclerosing material is then introduced into the cysts. Many sclerosing agents have been used, including absolute ethanol (98%); doxycycline;[33–36] OK-432 (Picibanil, Chugai Pharmaceutical, Tokyo, Japan);[31,32,37–40] bleomycin;[41–46] and Ethibloc (Ethicon, Norderstedt, Germany).[13,47] Doxycycline has been used by radiologists as well as surgeons for cervical lesions as well as

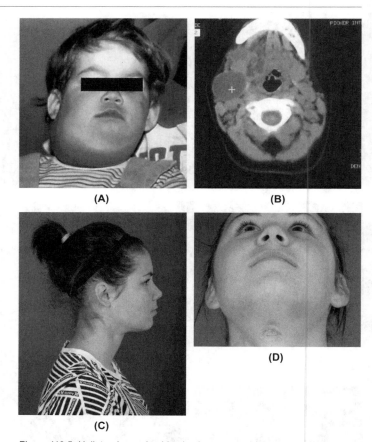

(A) **(B)**

(C) **(D)**

Figure 110.5: Unilateral suprahyoid, mixed macro- and microcystic: (A) At age 2 years, inflammatory response postsclerotherapy with Ethibloc. (B) CT scan at age 2 years; note microcystic infiltrating lesions anterior to large cyst. (C) 13 years follow-up after two sclerotherapies with Ethibloc and one infection at age 2 years. (D) Residual submental scar from Ethibloc extrusion.

for those on the extremities and trunk, including intraabdominal/retroperitoneal lymphangiomas.

The majority of sclerosing agents destroy the endothelial layer of the cysts and produce a marked inflammatory reaction. The use of prophylactic antibiotics, nonsteroidal anti-inflammatory drugs (NSAIDS), or systemic steroids to minimise swelling and the risk of infection are recommended by some authors. OK-432, an inactivated (by incubation with benzathine penicillin) strain of human *Streptococcus pyogenes* has a theoretical advantage over other sclerosants because it produces little or no perilesional fibrosis. However, surgery after other types of sclerosants has been reported without complications.[13] Significant swelling of the lesion is expected following sclerosis; therefore, in lesions of the cervical and oral area, the children should be monitored closely and endotracheal intubation should be performed if the airway is compromised.

Even though OK-432 appears to be a "magic bullet" in many series that advocate its use as a first-line treatment, others have not found it as effective.[39] Furthermore, it has been difficult to obtain at times; contacting a paediatric surgical colleague in Japan may be helpful. As with any sclerosing agent, repeat sclerotherapy is required in most cases, at intervals varying from a few weeks to a few months. In some patients, sclerotherapy has no effect and has to be abandoned.

Surgical resection

Surgical resection should follow the precise documentation of the lesion with MRI or CT scan and should remove the entire lesion whenever feasible.[48] One complete excision is technically easier than repeat surgical excisions of the same area. In cases where the lesion is too extensive for complete resection in one procedure, anatomic areas are resected in staged procedures.[49] The skin presenting intradermal involvement with visible angiokeratosis and clear vesicles should be resected when feasible because it increases the risk of infection and recurrence and may lead to persistent lymphatic cutaneous fistulas.

Important structures, such as nerves, major vessels, and muscles, are dissected free from the cysts under loupe magnification and kept intact. The use of a nerve simulator in an unparalysed patient makes nerve identification easier, particularly in the head and neck area. A bipolar cautery is helpful to coagulate afferent lymphatic and blood vessels and limit injury to adjacent structures. A suction drain is left in place, and antibiotics are kept until the drain is removed. In cases of prolonged drainage, sclerotherapy can be used as an adjunct to surgery. Conversely, in cases where regression of the lymphatic malformation following sclerotherapy is incomplete, surgical resection of the residual lesion can be done. The surgery is done once the inflammation has completely subsided after the last sclerotherapy. Contrary to a widely accepted belief, the authors find that the procedure is often easier than for an untreated lesion because the cysts are smaller and their walls are thicker and easier to identify. The child is also generally older (see Figure 110.2).

Specific Locations

Lymphangiomas of the tongue usually require partial glossectomy. Those involving the pharyngeal and laryngeal mucosa cannot be resected or sclerosed, but may improve with laser ablation. Mediastinal lesions have been traditionally resected, but the positive results obtained with sclerosants for extensive retroperitoneal lymphangiomas may shift the treatment strategy.

Complete resection of mesenteric lymphangiomas generally requires resection of the adjacent bowel (Figure 110.6), but sometimes this is not possible. In such circumstances, as well as for multiple intestinal lesions, as much as possible of the cyst walls is resected, and the remnant can be cauterised, ideally with an argon beam coagulator. Fibrin glue has also been used.

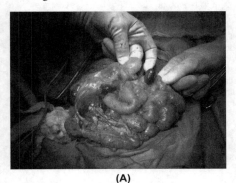

(A)

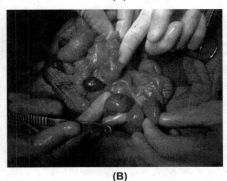

(B)

Figure 110.6: This patient had an incomplete excision of a mesenteric lymphangioma of the sigmoid in the neonatal period. She presented at 3 years of age with an acute abdomen and fever. At operation, a large infected lymphangioma (A, top left) required resection of the descending colon and sigmoid, as well as multiple other lesions, both mesenteric and antimesenteric, most containing serous fluid, others haemorrhagic; two were chylous (B).

Complications Following Treatment

As a rule, the same complications already discussed (airway obstruction, bleeding, infection) can occur after sclerotherapy or surgical excision, and the treatment is the same. Complications more specific to either treatment are discussed next.

Postsclerotherapy

Pain, oedema, and localised inflammation as well as mild fever, are expected for 24 to 48 hours postsclerotherapy. In large neck lesions, this may cause airway obstruction, and careful monitoring is essential. Depending on the agent used, skin necrosis, nerve damage and cardiac arrhythmia (ethanol), skin erosion, material extrusion (see Figures 110.2 and 110.5) and infection (Ethibloc), staining of unerupted teeth (doxycyclin), alopecia, skin discolouration, and pulmonary fibrosis (bleomycin) have been reported, although this latter serious complication did not occur in a series of 200 patients with long-term follow-up.[46]

Postoperative

Postoperative complication rates vary significantly among published series,[3,4,6,7,9,12] but the location of the lesion, mucosal involvement,[8,27] and the type of malformation (macrocystic, microcystic, or mixed) significantly affect the prognosis. For cervical lymphangiomas that are suprahyoid, bilateral, mixed, or microcystic, the complication and recurrence rate is close to 100%.[6] Conversely, with unilateral macrocystic infrahyoid lesions or with lymphangiomas located outside the head and neck area, complete excision is often possible, and the complication rate is low (Table 110.3).

Table 110.3: Complications of surgical excision of cystic lymphangiomas in African series.

All sites (n = 47)*	Number (%)	Cervical location (n = 60)**	Number (%)
Wound infection	14 (29.8)	Respiratory obstruction	11 (18.3)
Seroma	11 (23.4)	Wound infection	7 (11.7)
Respiratory obstruction	9 (19.1)	Facial nerve palsy	6 (10.0)
Pneumonia	7 (14.9)	Skin disfigurement	4 (6.7)
		Hypoglossal nerve palsy	2 (3.3)
Nerve palsies	6 (12.8)	Injury to pharynx	2 (3.3)
Skin disfigurement	4 (8.5)	Recurrent laryngeal nerve palsy	1 (1.7)
Injury to pharyn	1 (2.1)	Parotid duct injury	1 (1.7)
		Injury to internal jugular vein	1 (1.7)

*Sources: Uba AF, Chirdan LB. Management of cystic lymphangioma in children: experience in Jos, Nigeria. Pediatr Surg Int 2006; 22:353–356. Sowande OA, Adejuyigbe O, Abubakar AM. Management of cystic lymphangiomas in Ile-Ife, Nigeria. Niger J Surg Res 2003; 5:32–37.

**Sources: Ameh EA, Nmadu PT. Cervical cystic hygroma: pre-, intra-, and postoperative morbidity and mortality in Zaria, Nigeria. Pediatr Surg Int 2001; 17:342–343. Sowande OA, Adejuyigbe O, Abubakar AM. Management of cystic lymphangiomas in Ile-Ife, Nigeria. Niger J Surg Res 2003; 5:32–37.

The presence of a complication at the time of initial presentation and the age at surgery (neonates versus older children) also affect the prognosis. Newborns have a high risk of laryngeal oedema and airway obstruction following extensive neck dissection. The endotracheal tube should be left in place in susceptible infants and ventilation maintained for 48–72 hours to allow oedema to subside. Airway obstruction is the leading cause of postoperative mortality in Africa, particularly in children younger than 1 year of age.[4,5,7]

Prolonged drainage and seroma (9.8%) are more frequent after incomplete excision, although they can occur after a macroscopically complete excision. They can be treated with repeat aspiration or sclerotherapy.

Infections occur even with the use of perioperative antibiotics (6.6% to 27%). Children presenting with an ulcerated lesion have a higher risk of infection.

Damage to nerves (VII, X, XI, XII, recurrent laryngeal, phrenic, sympathetic chain) during excision of large cervical lymphangiomas is reported to occur in 1% to 25% of cases and represents a significant morbidity. This includes facial asymmetry, speech impairment, and Horner's syndrome.

Recurrence or enlargement of residual lesions occurs frequently. A series of 144 patients reported a 17% recurrence rate in completely excised lesions compared to 40% after incomplete excisions.[12] Some of these "recurrences" are actually due to the enlargement of preexisting microscopic lesions neighbouring the surgical resection margins.[5,8,28,50]

Prognosis and Outcome

In large series, considering all sites and types of lymphangiomas, complete excision of the malformation can be obtained with one surgical procedure in >70% of the children.[3,12] For cervicofacial lymphangiomas, recurrence and complications depend on the initial extent of the lesion.[6,27] Depending on the size, location, and symptomatology of residual or recurrent lesions, more than one surgery may be necessary. It is important to understand that some lesions (e.g., suprahyoid microcystic infiltrating lesions) will never be completely resectable, however, and research for other means of treatment is essential.

The use of sclerotherapy has markedly increased in the recent years. However, not all sclerosing materials are available in every country, and studies comparing the different sclerosing agents are missing. Many centres have published very good results with 50% or more regression of the lesions in >75% of the cases.[8,13,30-32,41] Unfortunately, not all lesions are amenable to sclerotherapy; as for the surgical treatment, the macrocystic lesions have the best prognosis (see Figure 110.5). There is some indication, however, that sclerotherapy of the macrocysts included in the mixed lesions has improved the microcystic component. A multidisciplinary team approach and the combination of sclerotherapy and surgery offer many advantages.

Evidence-Based Research

At the present time, there are no prospective, randomised studies comparing surgical excision and sclerotherapy. Available guidelines have to be based on reports of large retrospective experiences. Table 110.4 presents a study comparing the usage of bleomycin and OK-432 with surgery in two time periods.

Table 110.4: Evidence-based research.

Title	Treatment of lymphangiomas in children: our experience of 128 cases
Authors	Okazaki T, Iwatani A, Yanai T, et al.
Institution	Department of Pediatric General and Urological Surgery, Juntendo University School of Medicine, Tokyo 113-8421, Japan
Reference	J Pediatr Surg 2007; 42:386–389
Problem	Role of surgical excision and sclerotherapy in the management of lymphangiomas.
Intervention	Surgical excision, sclerotherapy.
Comparison/ control (quality of evidence)	Two periods of treatment divided arbitrarily into period I (1979–1988, n = 53) and period II (1989–2005, n = 75). Bleomycin was used as sclerosant in period I, and OK-432 was introduced in period II. Sclerotherapy was used as the primary treatment in 64% of patients in period II.
Outcome/ effect	Effectiveness of sclerotherapy in single cysts, macrocystic, microcystic, and cavernous (mixed) types was 90.9%, 100%, 68%, and 10%, respectively. Seventeen patients who had primary sclerotherapy required surgical excision with good outcome. Primary surgical excision was significantly more successful than sclerotherapy (88.5% versus 64.0%, p < 0.01). Complications after sclerotherapy included transient fever and swelling (32%), infection (6%), airway obstruction (4%), and nerve palsy (2%). In comparison, complications after surgical excision were more serious: lymphorrhea (27%), nerve palsy (9%), infection (6%), airway obstruction (1%), and persistent pain (1%).
Historical significance/ comments	This report of a large series of children with various types of lymphangiomas at various sites (head and neck, 53.9%), provides a useful practice guide. Although both surgical excision and sclerotherapy were used for more than two decades, sclerotherapy became increasingly used in later years. Irrespective of site, primary surgical excision was more effective than sclerotherapy, and the latter was more effective for single cysts and macrocystic lesions. It is noted that surgical excision may still be required after primary sclerotherapy, with good outcome. The complication rate following surgical excision and sclerotherapy was similar (44%), but it fell to 12% after sclerotherapy if transient fever and swelling were excluded. The authors of the study recommend sclerotherapy alone (using OK-432) for single cysts and macrocystic lesions and surgical excision after initial sclerotherapy for microcystic and cavernous lesions. The findings of this report have important implications for the African setting: primary surgery is effective, but initial sclerotherapy should be considered in patients at risk of postoperative complications (e.g., neonates and infants with large cervical lymphangiomas). In the African setting, bleomycin and doxycycline may be more readily available for sclerotherapy, and the latter is relatively inexpensive.

Key Summary Points

1. Cystic lymphangiomas are not common.

2. Cervical location is the most common and important site.

3. Airway obstruction and infection are common complications in cervical lymphangioma, both before and after surgery.

4. Ultrasonography is the minimum evaluation modality and is necessary to categorise and ascertain the extent of the lesion.

5. Surgical excision is effective, particularly in macrocystic malformations, and can be combined with sclerotherapy.

6. Sclerotherapy is more effective in single cysts and macrocystic lesions.

7. Cystic teratoma should be excluded by imaging and cytology if nonoperative management is initially chosen.

8. Morbidity can be high after surgery: complete excision should not be performed if injury to important structures is likely. Sclerotherapy should be the first-line treatment if complete surgical excision does not appear likely from imaging studies.

9. Morbidity and mortality are most common in cervical lymphangiomas and in infants younger than 1 year of age.

10. In infants younger than 1 year of age presenting without complications, surgery should be delayed to minimise operative morbidity and mortality.

References

1. Filston HC. Hemangiomas, cystic hygromas, and teratomas of the head and neck. Semin Pediatr Surg 1994; 3:147–159.

2. Fonkalsrud EW. Congenital malformations of the lymphatic system. Semin Pediatr Surg 1994; 3:62–69.

3. Hancock BJ, St-Vil D, Luks FI, Di Lorenzo M, Blanchard H. Complications of lymphangiomas in children. J Pediatr Surg 1992; 27:220–224.

4. Uba AF, Chirdan LB. Management of cystic lymphangioma in children: experience in Jos, Nigeria. Pediatr Surg Int 2006; 22:353–356.

5. Adeyemi SD. Management of cystic hygroma of the head and neck in Lagos, Nigeria; a 10-year experience. Int J Pediatr Otorhinolaryngol 1992; 23:245–251.

6. de Serres LM, Sie KC, Richardson MA. Lymphatic malformations of the head and neck. Arch Otolaryngol Head Neck Surg 1995; 121:577–582.

7. Ameh EA, Nmadu PT. Cervical cystic hygroma: pre-, intra-, and post-operative morbidity and mortality in Zaria, Nigeria. Pediatr Surg Int 2001; 17:342–343.

8. Kennedy TL, Whitaker M, Pellitteri P, Wood WE. Cystic hygroma/lymphangioma: a rational approach to management. Laryngoscope 2001; 111:1929–1937.

9. Miloundja J, Manfoumbi Ngoma AB, Mba ER, Nguema EB, N'Zouba L. Cystic cervicofacial lymphangioma in children in Gabon. Ann Otolaryngol Chir Cervicofac 2007; 124:277–284.

10. Ofodile FA, Oluwasanmi JO. Lymphangiomas in Nigeria. East Afr Med J 1980; 57:279–284.

11. Sowande OA, Adejuyigbe O, Abubakar AM. Management of cystic lymphangiomas in Ile-Ife, Nigeria. Niger Jour Surg Res 2003; 5:32–37.

12. Alqahtani A, Nguyen LT, Flageole H, Shaw K, Laberge JM. 25 years' experience with lymphangiomas in children. J Pediatr Surg 1999; 34:1164–1168.

13. Emran MA, Dubois J, Laberge L, Al-Jazaeri A, Butter A, Yazbeck S. Alcoholic solution of zein (Ethibloc) sclerotherapy for treatment of lymphangiomas in children. J Pediatr Surg 2006; 41:975–979.

14. Moore KL, Persaud TVN. Development of the lymphatic system. In: Moore KL, Persaud TVN, eds. The Developing Human: Clinically Oriented Embryology. Saunders, 1998, Pp 398–401.

15. Breugem CC, van der Horst CM, Hennekam RC. Progress toward understanding vascular malformations. Plast Reconstr Surg 2001; 107:1509–1523.

16. Chappuis JP. Current aspects of cystic lymphangioma in the neck. Arch Pediatr 1994; 1:186–192.

17. Landing BH, Farber S. Tumors of the cardiovascular system. In: Atlas of Tumor Pathology. Armed Forces Institute of Pathology, 1956.

18. Mulliken JB, Glowacki J. Hemangiomas and vascular malformations in infants and children: a classification based on endothelial characteristics. Plast Reconstr Surg 1982; 69:412–422.

19. Enjolras O, Mulliken JB. Vascular tumors and vascular malformations (new issues). Adv Dermatol 1997; 13:375–423.

20. Williams HB. Hemangiomas and lymphangiomas. Adv Surg 1981; 15:317–349.

21. Marler JJ, Fishman SJ, Upton J, et al. Prenatal diagnosis of vascular anomalies. J Pediatr Surg 2002; 37:318–326.

22. Longaker MT, Laberge JM, Dansereau J, et al. Primary foetal hydrothorax: natural history and management. J Pediatr Surg 1989; 24:573–576.

23. Bouchard S, Johnson MP, Flake AW, et al. The EXIT procedure: experience and outcome in 31 cases. J Pediatr Surg 2002; 37:418–426.

24. Chen M, Chen CP, Shih JC, et al. Antenatal treatment of chylothorax and cystic hygroma with OK-432 in nonimmune hydrops fetalis. Fetal Diagn Ther 2005; 20:309–315.

25. Sasaki Y, Chiba Y. Successful intrauterine treatment of cystic hygroma colli using OK-432. A case report. Fetal Diagn Ther 2003; 18:391–396.

26. Fisher R, Partington A, Dykes E. Cystic hygroma: comparison between prenatal and postnatal diagnosis. J Pediatr Surg 1996; 31:473–476.

27. Hartl DM, Roger G, Denoyelle F, Nicollas R, Triglia JM, Garabedian EN. Extensive lymphangioma presenting with upper airway obstruction. Arch Otolaryngol Head Neck Surg 2000; 126:1378–1382.

28. Padwa BL, Hayward PG, Ferraro NF, Mulliken JB. Cervicofacial lymphatic malformation: clinical course, surgical intervention, and pathogenesis of skeletal hypertrophy. Plast Reconstr Surg 1995; 95:951–960.

29. Mulliken JB, Fishman SJ, Burrows PE. Vascular anomalies. Curr Probl Surg 2000; 37:517–584.

30. Dubois J, Garel L, Abela A, Laberge L, Yazbeck S. Lymphangiomas in children: percutaneous sclerotherapy with an alcoholic solution of zein. Radiology 1997; 204:651–654.

31. Luzzatto C, Lo PR, Fascetti LF, Zanon GF, Toffolutti T, Tregnaghi A. Further experience with OK-432 for lymphangiomas. Pediatr Surg Int 2005; 21:969–972.

32. Sichel JY, Udassin R, Gozal D, Koplewitz BZ, Dano I, Eliashar R. OK-432 therapy for cervical lymphangioma. Laryngoscope 2004; 114:1805–1809.

33. Burrows PE, Mitri RK, Alomari A, et al. Percutaneous sclerotherapy of lymphatic malformations with doxycycline. Lymphat Res Biol 2008; 6:209–216.

34. Mabrut JY, Grandjean JP, Henry L, et al. Mesenteric and mesocolic cystic lymphangiomas. Diagnostic and therapeutic management. Ann Chir 2002; 127:343–349.

35. Nehra D, Jacobson L, Barnes P, Mallory B, Albanese CT, Sylvester KG. Doxycycline sclerotherapy as primary treatment of head and neck lymphatic malformations in children. J Pediatr Surg 2008; 43:451–460.

36. Shiels WE, Kenney BD, Caniano DA, Besner GE. Definitive percutaneous treatment of lymphatic malformations of the trunk and extremities. J Pediatr Surg 2008; 43:136–139.

37. Banieghbal B, Davies MR. Guidelines for the successful treatment of lymphangioma with OK-432. Eur J Pediatr Surg 2003; 13:103–107.

38. Claesson G, Kuylenstierna R. OK-432 therapy for lymphatic malformation in 32 patients (28 children). Int J Pediatr Otorhinolaryngol 2002; 65:1–6.

39. Hall N, Ade-Ajayi N, Brewis C, et al. Is intralesional injection of OK-432 effective in the treatment of lymphangioma in children? Surgery 2003; 133:238–242.

40. Giguere CM, Bauman NM, Sato Y, et al. Treatment of lymphangiomas with OK-432 (Picibanil) sclerotherapy: a prospective multi-institutional trial. Arch Otolaryngol Head Neck Surg 2002; 128:1137–1144.

41. Baskin D, Tander B, Bankaoglu M. Local bleomycin injection in the treatment of lymphangioma. Eur J Pediatr Surg 2005; 15:383–386.

42. Mathur NN, Rana I, Bothra R, Dhawan R, Kathuria G, Pradhan T. Bleomycin sclerotherapy in congenital lymphatic and vascular malformations of head and neck. Int J Pediatr Otorhinolaryngol 2005; 69:75–80.

43. Okazaki T, Iwatani S, Yanai T, et al. Treatment of lymphangioma in children: our experience of 128 cases. J Pediatr Surg 2007; 42:386–389.

44. Muir T, Kirsten M, Fourie P, Dippenaar N, Ionescu GO. Intralesional bleomycin injection (IBI) treatment for haemangiomas and congenital vascular malformations. Pediatr Surg Int 2004; 19:766–773.

45. Sanlialp I, Karnak I, Tanyel FC, Senocak ME, Buyukpamukcu N. Sclerotherapy for lymphangioma in children. Int J Pediatr Otorhinolaryngol 2003; 67:795–800.

46. Zhong PQ, Zhi FX, Li R, Xue JL, Shu GY. Long-term results of intratumorous bleomycin-A5 injection for head and neck lymphangioma. Oral Surg Oral Med Oral Pathol Oral Radiol Endod 1998; 86:139–144.

47. Baud AV, Breton P, Guibaud L, Freidel M. Treatment of low-pressure vascular malformations by injection of Ethibloc. Study of 19 cases and analysis of complications. Rev Stomatol Chir Maxillofac 2000; 101:181–188.

48. Fung K, Poenaru D, Soboleski DA, Kamal IM. Impact of magnetic resonance imaging on the surgical management of cystic hygromas. J Pediatr Surg 1998; 33:839–841.

49. Marler JJ, Mulliken JB. Current management of hemangiomas and vascular malformations. Clin Plast Surg 2005; 32:99–116, ix.

50. Ricciardelli EJ, Richardson MA. Cervicofacial cystic hygroma. Patterns of recurrence and management of the difficult case. Arch Otolaryngol Head Neck Surg 1991; 117:546–553.

CHAPTER 111
HAEMANGIOMAS

N. Marathovouniotis

Introduction

Haemangiomas are benign tumours of vascular endothelium. Larger haemangiomas, especially those appearing on the face, could cause anxiety and psychological distress for both parents and child, a factor that has to be considered in treatment. Complications such as ulceration and infection, and sometimes bleeding, can occur. Haemangiomas are vascular tumours, different than vascular malformations (see Table 111.1).

Table 111.1.: Classification of vascular tumours and vascular malformations.

Vascular Tumours	Haemangioma
	Haemangioendothelioma
	Tufted angioma
	Glomangioma
	Pyogenic granuloma
Vascular Malformations	Capillary vascular malformation
	Venous malformations
	Arteriovenous
	Lymphatic malformations
	Combined vascular malformations

Demographics

Haemangiomas are the most common tumours at infancy. They are present in 1.1–2.6% of newborns. They appear even more frequently among premature babies. The female-to-male ratio is 3:1.

Aetiology/Classification

The cause of haemangiomas has not been determined. The parents should not feel guilty for the occurrence or appearance of one of these vascular birthmarks. They show a dynamic growth and a dynamic regression. Angiogenic factors appear to play an important role in the growth and involution of haemangiomas.

According to a new classification, the most common haemangiomas are the focal haemangiomas, which progress from a central focus to a round vascular tumour. Less common are segmental haemangiomas, which spread within a body growing segment. These lesions are difficult to treat and show a number of complications. The type of haemangioma needs to be considered when deciding the timing and modality of therapy. Those haemangiomas that cannot be classified in one or the other group are called nondetermined haemangiomas.

Haemangiomas can appear within 1 to 4 weeks of age (30% of all haemangiomas), or they are visible immediately after birth as a small red macula (70% of all haemangiomas). These vascular tumours develop a rapid proliferation in the first 6 months of life and undergo a slow involution after the first year of life. The rapid proliferative phase can last even longer, and the involution is variable and may be incomplete years later. How large these lesions will grow in the proliferative phase is not known. Certain sites show a regression less frequently than other sites. The involution is complete in only 50–60% of all the haemangiomas, which means that about 50% of these tumours would need treatment due to partial involution and a remaining disturbing part such as a remaining scar or teleangiectasy.

Clinical Presentation

The common sites of haemangiomas are:

• 60% at the head and neck;

• 25% at the trunk; and

• 15% at the extremities.

Critical sites are the face, especially the eyelids, the lips, and the anogenital area.

Problems and Complications

Large haemangiomas, especially those appearing on the face, could cause anxiety and psychological distress.

Complications such as ulceration and infection are quite common. The risk of bleeding is usually overestimated. However, a special form of haemangioma, pyogenic granuloma, is the only type that could be termed an emergency due to acute bleeding. Periorbital haemangiomas can cause astigmatism, ptosis, strabismus, amblyopia, or even blindness.

Lip haemangiomas could destroy a part of the soft tissue, so that suckling or drinking is impaired. Ear or nose haemangiomas could destroy a part of the cartilage or cause a deviation. Haemangiomas at the airways could cause airway obstruction.

Ulceration occurs more frequently at the anogenital area than at other parts of the body.

Huge haemangiomas can cause cardiac problems. Platelet trapping can cause coagulopathy (the Kasabach-Merritt syndrome) or disseminated intravascular coagulations.

The appearance of more than five cutaneous haemangiomas is called haemangiomatosis. Ultrasound (US) examination of the abdominal organs to exclude other vascular tumours in the liver, spleen, or pancreas should be performed.

Focal haemangiomas at the body trunk, at the hairy part of the head, or at the extremeties cause few complications.

Investigations

Physical examination and US with colour Doppler for the assessment of the haemangioma dimensions, especially for subcutaneous haemangiomas, are standard for diagnosis. MRI should be considered for haemangiomas in the deeper soft tissue layers, or when vascular tumours are suspected in the chest or in the skull. Biopsy is indicated only in rare cases when the clinical signs indicate a possible malignancy.

Treatment

The aim of treatment is to stop the progression of the haemangioma with minimal side effects and to induce involution. A complete involution in the first 2 years of life is not the main goal of the treatment. If the haemangioma shows regression after initial therapy, further natural involution after the 12th month of life could be expected.

Intervention may be required for lesions that interfere with a vital structure or function. These include:

• lesions in the airway, liver, or gastrointestinal tract;

• lesions in the periorbital region;

- lesions of the nose, lip, or ear;

- large segmental haemangiomas on the face; and

- lesions complicated by ulceration.

The cosmetic result for progressive haemangiomas are generally better the sooner initial therapy begins. Haemangiomas at critical sites, such as the lips, eyelids, nose, ears, or anogenital area, should be treated as soon as possible (4–8 weeks of age).

Focal haemangiomas at the body trunk, upper or lower limbs, or even the hairy part of the head hardly cause any cosmetic or functional problems. Active nonintervention should be suggested for these uncomplicated haemangiomas; this means observation with serial photography and measurement of the lesion to monitor the clinical course. In these cases, waiting for spontaneous involution is suggested. The cosmetic result after spontaneous involution is sometimes better than after surgical interventions.

The choice of treatment depends on factors such as:

- type (flat, voluminous, subcutaneous, focal, or segmental);

- size;

- rate of growth and involution;

- location (e.g., face or body trunk); and

- age of the child.

Treatment modalities include:

- cryotherapy;

- laser treatment;

- surgery;

- intralesional steroids;

- systemic steroid treatment;

- systemic B-blocker treatment;

- intralesional bleomycin; and

- intralesional fibrin glue.

Cryotherapy

The freezing process of cryotherapy damages the endothelial cells of the haemangioma and stops the proliferation of the haemangioma. This is the most suitable treatment for small focal superficial haemangiomas (Figure 111.1). Treatment is possible with liquid nitrogen; the metal probe is frozen at −180°C, and is held on the surface of the haemangioma for 10 seconds. New electrical devices enable cryotherapy at a constant temperature of −32°C with a contact time of 20 seconds. The electrical devices cause fewer complications such as ulcerations and discolouration of the skin. This makes cryotherapy advisable even for flat, small haemangiomas on the face.

The great advantage of cryotherapy is using local anaesthetics (eutectic mixture of local anaesthetics, or EMLA) instead of general anaesthetics, which is usually necessary for laser treatment. EMLA

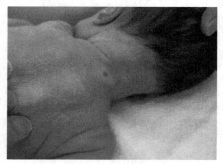

Figure 111.1:Focal haemangioma at the back of the neck.

cream should be applied in small quantities and on small surfaces. EMLA contains prilocaine hydrochloride, which has been associated with infantile methemoglobinemia.

In cases of incomplete regression of the haemangioma after cryotherapy, repeating the treatment in 6 weeks time should be recommended.

If the haemangioma has a height of more than 2 mm, cryotherapy would manage a reduction of the redness or even an ulceration, but not a regression.

Laser Treatment

The neodymium:yttrium aluminium garnet (Nd:YAG) laser (1060 nm) is the most common laser device for the treatment of haemangioma because it penetrates deeper in the tissue and is not readily absorbed by haemoglobin or water. Through selective thermolysis, the laser beam destroys the haemangioma vessels.

Laser treatment is suitable for haemangiomas that have a large surface and large volume and are superficial (flat and reddish) or deep (beneath the skin surface and bluish).

The Nd:YAG laser beam could be applied over an ice cube, with the special handpiece through the skin (transcutaneous). The ice cube cools the skin surface and avoids blistering. The heat reaches a depth of about 8 mm under the skin surface.

Another option is an intralesional application with the bare laser fibres. In this modality, the light reaches the vascular tumour without any absorption, reflexion, or refraction. Thermolysis is much more effective than the transcutaneous application, but the side effects are more obvious.

Treatment with the Nd:YAG laser is painful, so general anaesthesia is necessary. During this treatment, the eyes of the child have to be closed and protected.

The laser treatment has to be repeated in intervals of 6 to 8 weeks; haemangioma on the face, lip, or eyelid needs 3–5 laser sessions (Figure 111.2).

The pulsed dye laser (PDL; 585 nm) penetrates no deeper than 1–2 mm and is mainly used for reducing the redness of a haemangioma. It could be used in certain devices as a combination with a Nd:YAG laser for the treatment of large haemangiomas.

PDL alone is mainly used for the treatment of a "port-wine stain", or nevus flameus, a vascular malformation of the capillaries.

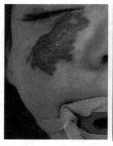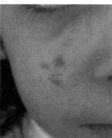

Figure 111.2: Haemangioma of the face before (left) and after (right) five Nd:YAG laser treatments.

Surgical Treatment

Surgical treatment is mainly performed after laser treatment or after an incomplete spontaneous regression when a haemangioma rest causes a cosmetic problem. Large haemangiomas at the neck or trunk, especially those under the skin, usually undergo surgical treatment. The incision lies in the skin tension lines, the skin closure causes no problem, and the result is very satisfactory. Some authors advocate circular excision and insertion of a purse-string suture, which can be performed serially.

Bulky haemangiomas at the hairy part of the head can be removed surgically if they cause cosmetic problems. The wound closure will leave a thin scar, which would be covered by the hair. The surgical removal of haemangiomas at the extremities is limited due to the difficult skin-defect cover. Operation of a haemangioma in childhood requires a general anaesthetic. The advantage of the surgical procedure is the definite complete removal of this vascular tumour in most cases in one session of general anaesthetics. The results are very satisfactory if the size and location of the haemangioma are considered. The remaining scar should be discussed with the parents before surgery.

Injury of other structures, such as nerves and important vessels, can be avoided through meticulous operative technique and loupe magnification.

Systemic or Intralesional Steroid Treatment

The positive effect of systemic steroids in the treatment of haemangiomas is well known, especially in rapid progressive haemangiomas on the face or other critical locations. The side effects of systemic steroids (e.g., weight gain, growth arrest, cataracts, and cardiomyopathy) are also well known. These side effects are usually reversible. The recommended systemic steroid treatment is 3–5 mg/kg per day. This dosage should be taken for no less than 6 weeks and for as long as 12 weeks.

The use of intralesional steroids with success is mainly reported in ophthalmic cases of periorbital haemangiomas. The use of a mixture of triamcinolone acetonide (cristalloid) and betamethesone acetate is related to severe complications, such as vascular occlusion of the retina and eyelid necrosis. Therefore, this method is mainly used only by experienced ophthalmologists.

Systemic Beta-Blocker Treatment

In 2008, successful treatment of complicated haemangiomas with the systemic beta-blocker propranolol was reported. Propranolol should be given, after cardiological examination with US and electrocardiogram (ECG), under blood-pressure monitoring in the hospital at a dose of 2 mg/kg per day in 3 daily divided doses. Severe side effects are not reported. The results are very encouraging, so propranolol could substitute for systemic steroid application in the treatment of complicated haemangiomas (Figure 111.3).

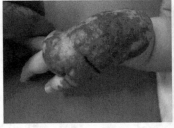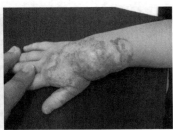

Figure 111.3:Before (left) and after (right) beta-blocker systemic therapy

Intralesional Bleomycin

Intralesional bleomycin has been reported for the treatment of large complicated haemangiomas. Bleomycin is a sclerosant and an antineoplastic agent that has an apoptotic effect on rapidly growing immature cells. This method requires multiple general anaesthetics in children. Scarring with overlapping hyperpigmentation is a common side effect.

Intralesional Fibrin Glue Treatment

The use of fibrin glue injections in vascular tumours and vascular malformations is occasionally reported with encouraging results.

Systemic Interferon Alpha Treatment

Interferon alpha therapy is reserved for life-threatening haemangiomas due to its severe side effects (e.g., fever, leucopaenia, nephritis, nephrotic syndrome, and autoimmune diseases such as thyroiditis and spastic paresis).

Evidence-Based Research

To date, no studies compare the different treatment modalities, considering the wide range of vascular tumours and vascular malformations.

Key Summary Points

1. Haemangiomas are the most common benign tumours in infancy.

2. Sixty percent of haemangiomas appear at the head and neck.

3. The standard for diagnosis of haemangiomas is a physical examination, using ultrasound with colour Doppler for the assessment of tumour dimensions.

4. The choice of treatment depends on factors such as type, size, rate of growth, location of haemangioma, and age of the child.

5. The usual treatment modalities are cryotherapy, laser treatment, surgery, systemic treatment with steroids, and beta blockers.

Suggested Reading

Cremer H, Hämangiome (vaskuläre Tumoren)- neue Klassifizierung [Hemangiomas (vascular tumours) new classification]. Kinder und Jugendartz 2008; 39(9).

Höger P. Vaskuläre Tumoren und Malformationen. In: Höger P. Kinderdermatologie. Schattauer, 2005, Pp. 247–280.

Pienaar C, Graham R, Geldenhuys S, Hudson DA. Intralesional bleomycin for the treatment of hemangiomas. Plast Reconstr Surg 2006;117(1):221–226.

Stringel G. Hemangiomas and lymphangiomas, In: Ashcroft KW, Pediatric Surgery, 3rd ed. Saunders, 2000, Chap 71, Pp 965–986.

Wiese K, Kirchhoff L, Merten H-A, Orofaziale Hämangiome und Lymphangiome [Orofacial hemangiomas and lymphangiomas]. CHAZ 2006; 7(10):428–438.

CHAPTER 112
ARTERIOVENOUS MALFORMATIONS

Phuong D. Nguyen
Oriana D. Cohen
Evan P. Nadler

Introduction

An arteriovenous malformation (AVM) is defined as an abnormal communication between an artery and vein that bypasses a capillary bed. These lesions may present as isolated, innocuous cutaneous naevi, or they rarely may take the form of life-threatening systemic shunts involving large portions of the body. They may occur at any site, involve any organ, and violate normal tissue planes. AVMs are present at birth, and are neither neoplastic nor proliferative. As such, they grow commensurate with the child.

AVMs are best characterised by the type of abnormal vascular channel, the degree of blood flow, and the structures involved. The most common sites of these lesions are the pelvis, extremities, and intracranial circulation.[1] Cutaneous AVMs are usually noted at birth but are given little attention due to their innocent appearance. A standard approach to management of AVMs does not exist due to the rare need for treatment. Furthermore, AVMs are frequently associated with additional findings and fall under the auspices of multiple syndromes[2] (Table 112.1).

Table 112.1: Syndromes with associated arteriovenous malformations

Syndrome	Arteriovenous malformation
von Hippel-Lindau disease	Cerebelloretinal haemangioblastomatosis
Klippel-Trenaunay syndrome	Naevus, varicose veins, limb hypertrophy
Kasabach-Merritt syndrome	Platelet consumption, kaposiform haemangioendothelioma, or tufted angiomas
Parkes-Weber syndrome	Microfistulous arteriovenous communication
Maffucci syndrome	Cavernous haemangioma, dyschndroplasia, osteochondromas
Sturge-Weber syndrome	Encephalotrigeminal haemangiomatosis
Servelle-Martorell syndrome	Cavernous haemangioma, limb hypotrophy
Rendu-Osler-Weber syndrome	Hereditary haemorrhagic telangiectasia
Louis-Bar syndrome	Ataxia telangiectasia
Sturge-Weber syndrome	Facial capillary malformations
Riley-Smith syndrome	Macrocephaly, pseudopapilloedema, lymphaticovenous malformation

Demographics

The prevalence of congenital AVMs is unknown. Differences in nomenclature and the lack of an accepted classification contribute to the inability to collectively analyse reported cases. In the Western world, congenital AVMs account for only 1 in 10,000 hospital admissions.[2] This rate likely represents an underestimate of the true prevalence because most lesions are initially asymptomatic. Although congenital AVMs are present at birth, they are often not diagnosed and treated until later in life as they become more clinically apparent. One-half of all congenital AVMs occur in the extremities, with two thirds of these occurring in the lower limb.[3] There is a paucity of epidemiologic data from Africa and it is unclear whether the data provided from the West are appropriate for the African region. Diarra et al. described 20 cases of vascular malformations at a single African institution over a 4-year period with a female-to-male ratio of 1.5:1 and an average patient age of 15.5 years at presentation.[4] However, little other data regarding the incidence or prevalence of AVMs on the African continent are available.

Embryology and Pathology

Embryology

During the third week of foetal life, mesenchymal cells differentiate into primitive capillary clusters. By the 48th day of gestation the capillary clusters connect with feeding arteries and draining veins. AVMs are a result of structural abnormalities formed during foetal development and are therefore not neoplasms. Vascular malformations occur as a result of hypoplasia, hyperplasia, aplasia, or any combination of any of these vascular structures. In the foetus, an AVM can be detected only on prenatal ultrasound if the AVM is very large or results in foetal hydrops.

Pathology

AVMs contain enlarged vascular spaces lined by nonproliferating endothelium, and not the mitotically active endothelial cells of a haemangioma. Thus, AVMs do not undergo the different stages of growth and involution seen in haemangiomas. They have an increased ratio of endothelial cells to smooth muscle cells of 214:1, as compared to a ratio of 10:1 to 62:1 found in normal vessels.[5] Histologic features include:

- ectatic capillaries, veins, or lymphatics;
- thin basement membranes; and
- absence of rapid endothelial turnover.

Natural History

In contrast to haemangiomas, AVMs do not improve nor resolve with time. Generally, an AVM will grow in parallel with the child's growth.

Clinical Presentation

History

Vascular malformations are present at birth but are not necessarily obvious. The presentation of the lesion differs, depending on the aetiology of the lesion and its location. In 1982, a biologic classification of vascular anomalies was proposed that separated true haemangiomas (neoplasms) from vascular malformations and was based on cellular characteristics correlated with both physical examination and natural growth history.[6]

Unlike haemangiomas, vascular malformations do not undergo rapid growth and involution; rather, they grow in proportion to the body. AVMs are often high-flow lesions. Fast flow typically becomes evident in childhood; hormonal changes during puberty or minor trauma may trigger expansion. A cutaneous AVM presents as a mass under the skin with noted warmth, a dermal stain, palpable thrill, audible bruit, or visible pulsation (Figure 112.1). Capillary vascular malformations appear to follow sensory nerve distribution and have a purplish hue. Venous malformations are easily compressible and swell with dependent positioning. Unlike malignant tumours, AVMs are lined by mature endothelial cells, which do not proliferate to a greater extent than normal cells. Enlargement occurs as a result of blood flowing through "paths of least resistance," and the voluminous blood flow accounts for the progressive dilatation of the preexisting channels. If flow through the fistula is large enough, the distal organ may suffer permanent ischaemic changes, such as wasting or gangrene due to "stealing" of blood through the fistula. A clinical staging system introduced by Schobinger is useful for documentation of AVM in any anatomic site[7] (Table 112.2).

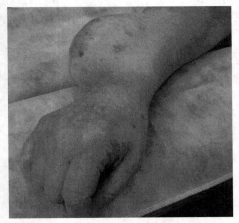

Figure 112.1: Upper extremity AVM presenting as a large mass under the skin in an adult.

Table 112.2: Schobinger staging for arteriovenous malformations.

Stage	Description
I (quiescence)	Pink bluish stain, warmth, and arteriovascular shunting
II (expansion)	Same as stage I, plus enlargement, pulsations, thrill, bruit, and tortuous/tense veins
III (destruction)	Same as stage II, plus dystrophic skin changes, ulceration, bleeding, persistent pain, or tissue necrosis
IV (decompensation)	Same as stage III, plus cardiac failure

Physical Examination

A palpable thrill and bruit are often present in large fistulas. The distal arterial blood flow may be limited, depending on the size of the fistula shunt, which may present as a diminished distal pulse with or without symptoms of ischaemia. Frank gangrene of the end-organ occasionally can be seen. The resultant venous hypertension also may result in brawny oedema, stasis skin changes, and, ultimately, chronic venous ulcers. When large or multiple arteriovenous communications affect an entire extremity during early life, before epiphyseal closure, increased bone growth and limb hypertrophy or hypotrophy may occur, such as in the Klippel-Trenaunay syndrome.

Complications

Overlying ischaemic ulcers, adjacent bone destruction, or local hypertrophy may occur. In rare instances, the increased venous return to the heart combined with an increase in plasma volume may produce cardiac enlargement and congestive heart failure. Placental AVMs may result in a significant shunt from the maternal to the foetal circula-tion, producing hydrops foetalis.[8] Further complications include pain, haemorrhage, ulceration, cardiac effects, and destruction of surrounding structures. Therefore, treatment requires elimination of this lesion.

Investigations

Most congenital AVMs are recognised easily on physical examination and do not warrant further investigation. However, in patients requiring therapy, diagnostic studies are often useful to determine the type and extent of the lesion. However, the clinician must balance the utility of imaging with the cost in areas where resources are limited. Several imaging options are effective, as discussed here.

Ultrasonography

Ultrasonography (US) is a useful screening examination, but is highly operator dependent. When combined with colour-flow imaging (duplex scan), it can be helpful in differentiating slow-flow anomalies (mainly venous and lymphatic types) from fast-flow arterial anomalies. Comparison with the normal contralateral limb will demonstrate a sharp contrast with the arterial signal at a corresponding level. Due to its relatively low cost, US may be the modality best suited to the African setting for cases that require imaging. However, the major drawback to this technique is limited delineation of the size of the lesion and its relation to adjacent structures.

Computed Tomography

Contrast-enhanced computed tomography (CT) may give the practitioner additional information not available on US. The appearance of vascular malformations on CT vary, depending on their origin and location, but the full extent of the lesion is often delineated. Venous malformations typically have heterogeneous enhancement and sometimes calcifications. The cost of CT scanning may be prohibitive in developing regions; thus, its use should be reserved for cases for which a surgical resection is to be undertaken and the extent of the lesion is in question.

Magnetic Resonance Imaging and Angiography

Magnetic resonance imaging and angiography (MRI/MRA) is perhaps the most accurate radiologic study to evaluate vascular lesions. Magnetic resonance is able to differentiate vascular malformations from haemangiomas and is able to easily distinguish high-flow lesions from low-flow lesions. An additional advantage is that MRI avoids the use of contrast agents and exposure to radiation. Again, however, the cost of this study may render it of limited value in the African setting.

Angiographic Evaluation

Angiographic evaluation, consisting of arteriography, venography, or fistulography, may be the most useful diagnostic tool for AVMs. It is also useful as a therapeutic adjunct in certain instances. Arteriographic findings suggestive of AVMs include:

• arterial dilatation and tortuosity;

• blushing or puddling of dye in the vascular channels;

• visualisation of the arteriovenous fistula itself;

• early venous filling; and

• dilatation of the draining venous channel.

Treatment

Therapy for AVM should be adapted to the extent, location, and degree of disability produced by the lesion. Treatment is rarely indicated during infancy or early childhood for a stage I AVM, unless postnatal high output heart failure caused by shunting is evident. In this circumstance, prompt embolisation or surgical excision may be necessary. In general, treatment is usually reserved for symptomatic lesions (e.g., recalcitrant ulceration, ischaemic pain, bleeding, increased cardiac output), cosmetically unacceptable lesions, and lesions in critical locations (e.g., encroaching on orifices or key organ structures, including the mouth or eye) that may otherwise be asymptomatic.

The disability from the lesion must be weighed against the extent of disfigurement caused by excisional therapy and the cost and availability of the various nonsurgical techniques. Port wine stains are best ablated by using laser photocoagulation. Venous malformations of the extremities with symptoms of venous hypertension may benefit from the use of external compression stockings. Additionally, they may sometimes be treated by using laser therapy, sclerotherapy, or surgical removal.

Therapy for arteriovenous malformations consists of angiography with selective embolisation or complete surgical excision. Embolisation is particularly useful for lesions not accessible to surgery, such as in deep tissue planes, or in patients for whom resection would cause a significant deformity. Transcatheter embolisation alone, although often necessary multiple times, is sufficient to eliminate or improve symptoms in a high percentage of patients.[1] The most effective agents for embolisation seem to be cyanoacrylate adhesives administered through the technique of superselective catheterisation of arterial branches allowing access to the nidus of the AVM. Absolute alcohol seems to be an effective agent for sclerotherapy of lower flow venous malformations. Simple ligation is ineffective, with high rates of recurrence.

Embolisation has generally failed for large lesions but is useful when performed within 24 hours preceding operation to reduce blood loss at the time of excision. Occasionally, hypothermia and cardiac bypass are required to minimise blood loss during surgical excision of large lesions. If it is feasible to remove the entire mass and preserve limb function, complete excision should be attempted and should include ligation of all feeding vessels. Proximal ligation of feeding vessels in AVMs without resection of the nidus often results in continued enlargement of the AVM and increased recruitment of smaller feeding and draining vessels.[1] Furthermore, proximal ligation may make subsequent transcatheter therapy impossible by obstructing access. The nidus and usually the involved skin must be excised widely (Figure 112.2). However, if the overlying skin is normal, it can be saved. The most accurate way to determine the completeness of the resection is observing the pattern of bleeding from the wound edges.[9] The defect should be primarily closed with either local tissue or distant tissue free-transfer using a microsurgical technique. If there is any question about the adequacy of resection, depending on the location of the defect, temporary coverage with a split thickness skin graft is often the best strategy.

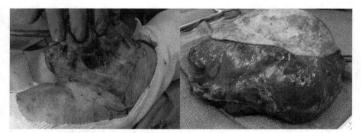

Figure 112.2: Dissection of AVM from upper extremity (left); AVM specimen including resected overlying skin, en bloc (right).

Postoperative Complications

Surgical site infection and local wound complications, as seen in any skin or soft tissue procedure, may be seen with resection of cutaneous AVMs. Unless the lesion is completely resected, there is a reasonable chance for recurrence. For sclerotherapy, direct puncture of the nidus is required in conjunction with local arterial and venous occlusion from embolisation of feeding arteries. There is a high risk of severe neurologic and soft tissue damage with this combined method. For AVMs found in solid organs, the complications associated with resection mirror those seen after resection for other pathology.

Prognosis and Outcome

The surgeon must be aware that surgical resection may still result in residual arteriovenous connections, as congenital AVMs are almost never confined to a single anatomic segment of the arterial tree or to circumscribed anatomic regions. Patients may be followed for years by clinical examination, US, or MRI for signs of occult recurrence. However, clinical examination is likely the most cost-effective method in developing regions such as Africa.

Ethical Considerations

In consideration of limited resources and patient follow-up, procedures that may require multiple visits, such as transcatheter embolisation, may not be accessible or practical. Surgical resection thus remains the primary modality of treatment in these circumstances, ideally as a single-stage definitive treatment. In addition, diagnostic technologies such as MRI may not be readily available, and less expensive strategies such as clinical examination and US may determine the extent of surgical resection.

Evidence-Based Research

At this time, no prospective randomised studies exist that compare surgical excision to angiographic embolisation in peripheral and organ-based AVMs. Often, these modalities are used in an adjunctive fashion. Furthermore, the majority of evidence-based literature pertains to intracranial AVMs. Tables 112.3 and 112.4 report experiences in AVM management.

Table 112.3: Evidence-based research.

Title	Vascular malformations of the upper limb: a review of 270 patients
Authors	Upton J, Coombs CJ, Mulliken JB, et al.
Institution	Division of Plastic Surgery, Department of Surgery, and the Division of Vascular and Interventional Radiology, Children's Hospital, Harvard Medical School, Boston, Massachusetts, USA
Reference	J Hand Surg Am 1999; 24(5):1019–1035
Problem	Evaluation and categorisation of 270 vascular malformations in the upper extremity over a 28-year period.
Intervention	During the study period, 260 surgical resections in 141 patients were completed. Magnetic resonance imaging with and without contrast best demonstrated the site, size, flow characteristics, and involvement of contiguous structures for all types of malformations. Resections were restricted to well-defined regions and often completed in stages.
Comparison/ control (quality of evidence)	The surgical strategy in all groups was to thoroughly extirpate the malformation with preservation of nerves, tendons, joints, and uninvolved muscle, and to perform microvascular revascularisation and skin replacement as required. Preoperative angiographic assessment with magnified views were an important preoperative adjunct before well-planned resection of fast-flow AVMs.
Outcome/ effect	Symptomatic slow-flow malformations and types A and B fast-flow anomalies were resected without major sequelae. Type C arterial anomalies, which included diffuse, pulsating lesions with distal vascular steal, progressed clinically and resulted in amputation in 10 of 14 patients. The complication rate was 22% for slow-flow lesions and 28% for fast-flow lesions.
Historical significance/ comments	The role of selective angiography and embolisation is still evolving, and this retrospective study suggests a preoperative algorithm that includes these techniques before planned excisions of most fast-flow lesions. Although this study did not directly compare head-to-head imaging modalities or even therapy that did or did not include surgery, it is valuable in that it reviews one of the largest reported experiences in a highly specialised and renowned vascular malformation treatment center.

Table 112.4: Evidence-based research.

Title	Transcatheter embolization of extremity vascular malformations: the long-term success of multiple interventions	**Outcome/ effect**	Predominantly venous lesions were treated by sclerotherapy with injection of ethanol. Arteriovenous and arterial lesions were treated by embolisation via the arterial branch feeding vessels with cyanoacrylate. The most common vessels involved and treated were branches of the profunda femoris and tibial arteries (83% of lower-extremity lesions), and branches of the brachial and radial arteries (82% of upper-extremity lesions). Patients required a mean of 1.6 embolisation procedures (range 1–5) over a mean period of 57 months. Sixteen patients (32%) underwent more than one embolisation procedure. Of these, 1 was a planned staged procedure and 15 were performed secondary to residual or recurrent symptoms. Adjunctive surgical procedures were performed subsequent to embolisation in three cases (6%). Ninety-two percent of patients remained asymptomatic or improved at a mean follow-up of 56 months. There was one case of limb loss (2%). Diffuse extremity vascular malformations are difficult to eradicate completely, and recurrences are common.
Authors	Rockman CB, Rosen RJ, Jacobowitz GR, et al.		
Institution	Department of Vascular Surgery, New York University Medical Center, New York, New York, USA		
Reference	Ann Vasc Surg 2003; 17(4):417–423		
Problem	Alternative therapy for management of congenital vascular malformation in the extremity.		
Intervention	Superselective catheterisation of feeding vessels and transcatheter administration of embolic agents were performed in 50 patients. Indications for therapy included severe pain, haemorrhage, congestive heart failure, distal extremity ischaemia or ulceration, and mass effect causing significant oedema or other functional disturbance of the extremity. Embolic agents used for arteriovenous malformations included rapidly polymerising acrylic adhesives (n-butyl cyanoacrylate (NBCA) or isobutyl cyanoacrylate (IBCA)) and polyvinyl alcohol foam particles (Ivalon).	**Historical significance/ comments**	As a retrospective review, this study lacks predictive power of the proposed treatment strategy of transcatheter embolisation. However, this study still retains value, as it is one of the largest studies reporting the outcome of transcatheter embolisation. The authors acknowledge that for patients in whom significant symptoms do develop, the optimal treatment is probably complete surgical resection of the superficial, limited lesion when this is possible. However, they further suggest that even though transcatheter embolisation is not a cure, it is highly successful for symptom relief in complex lesions, albeit this may require multiple procedures. Subsequently, with the knowledge that surgical extirpations are difficult and perhaps even impossible for some larger lesions, they assert that transcatheter embolisation is the treatment of choice in these situations.
Comparison/ control (quality of evidence)	Retrospective review of 50 patients over 15 years of upper- and lower-extremity arteriovenous malformations utilising transcatheter embolisation therapy.		

Key Summary Points

1. Lesions are present at birth and are nonproliferative, unlike haemangiomas.

2. Arteriovenous malformations may be observed unless they become symptomatic.

3. Investigative measures help identify the extent of the lesion and include ultrasound, computed tomography with contrast, and magnetic resonance imaging.

4. Treatment, if necessary, consists of complete surgical excision when possible.

5. If the lesion is not easily accessible or resection would cause undue morbidity, selective embolisation may improve symptoms.

6. Recurrence is not uncommon if the lesion is not completely resected.

References

1. Riles TS, Jacobowitz GR. Surgical management of vascular malformations. In: Rutherford RB, ed. Vascular Surgery, vol. 2, 6th ed. Elsevier Saunders, 2005, Pp 1646–1650.

2. Kasirajan K, Ouriel K. Vascular malformation and arteriovenous fistula. In: Greenfield LJ, ed. Surgery: Scientific Principles and Practice, Vol. 3, 3rd ed. Lippincott Williams & Wilkins, 2001, Pp 1859–1871.

3. Tice DA, Clauss RH, Keirle AM. Congenital arteriovenous fistulae of the extremities. Archiv Surg 1963; 86:460.

4. Diarra O, Ba M, Ndiaye A, et al. Vascular dysplasia in vascular surgery in an African area: 28 cases at the Dakar teaching hospital. J Maladies Vasculaires 2003; 28:24–29.

5. Sheehan M, Bambini DA. Hemangiomas and vascular malformations. In: Arensman RM, Bambini DA, Almond PS, eds. Vademecum Pediatric Surgery. Landes Bioscience, 2000, Pp 65–68.

6. Mulliken JB, Glowacki J. Hemangiomas and vascular malformations in infants and children: a classification based on endothelial characteristics. Plastic Reconstruct Surg 1982; 69:412–422.

7. Kohout MP, Hansen M, Pribaz JJ, et al. Arteriovenous malformations of the head and neck: natural history and management. Plastic Reconstruct Surg 1988; 102:643–654.

8. Liechty KW, Flake AW. Pulmonary vascular malformations. Sem Pediatr Surg 2008; 17:9–16.

9. Connors JP III, Mulliken JB. Vascular tumors and malformations in childhood. In: Rutherford RB, ed. Vascular Surgery, vol. 2, 6th ed. Elsevier Saunders, 2005, Pp 1626–1645.

CHAPTER 113
UNILATERAL LIMB ENLARGEMENT

Charles F.M. Evans
Jacob N. Legbo

Introduction

Unilateral limb enlargement (ULE) is a challenging diagnostic and management problem. Treatment options are often complex and are dependent upon accurately determining the correct aetiology for each individual case. Although the enlargement may be mild and may pass unrecognised, it can attain a tragically distorting and grotesque dimension, leading to significant functional, cosmetic, and psychological complications. The complex nature of this problem, combined with the rarity in presentation, has led to inconsistencies in management that need to be addressed.

Demographics

The exact incidence of ULE within Africa is not fully known. This is due to both the difficulties in obtaining accurate epidemiological studies for any rare condition within Africa and a lack of consistency in the actual diagnosis of the problem, with frequently misused terminology and nomenclature especially relating to the causes of this condition.[1]

Limb Embryology

Limb development takes place over a 5-week period from the 4th to 8th weeks of embryological life.[2] Development of the upper and lower limbs is similar, although morphogenesis of the upper limb is usually about 1–2 days ahead of the lower limb, and at 7 weeks the limbs rotate in opposite directions (the upper ones rotating laterally 90°, so that the extensor muscles lie on the lateral and posterior surface and the thumbs lie laterally, whereas the lower ones rotate 90° medially, placing the extensor muscles on the anterior surface and the big toe lies medially).[3]

Upper limb buds form on the ventrolateral wall at about the level of C5 to T1, and lower limb buds form at about L1 to L5. Each bud consists of a mesenchymal core (derived from lateral plate mesoderm) covered by a layer of cuboidal ectoderm. This ectoderm thickens to form an apical ectodermal ridge along the distal margin of the limb bud to maintain outgrowth of the limb bud along the proximal-distal axis.[3]

The terminal portions of the limb buds become flattened to form the handplates and footplates, which are separated from the proximal segment by a circular constriction. Digital rays appear on the hand and foot plates, with fingers and toes formed by a process of programmed cell death between these rays.[2] A second constriction divides the proximal portion into two segments, enabling the main parts of the extremities to be recognised.[3] The bones, tendons, and other connective tissues of the limb arise from the lateral plate mesoderm, but the limb muscles and endothelial cells arise in the somatic mesoderm and migrate into the limb buds.[2]

Congenital limb anomalies are rare, occurring in approximately 6 per 100,000 births.[3] Anomalies fall into four categories:[2]

- *reduction defects*—either the entire limb (amelia) or part of the limb (meromelia) is missing;

- *duplication defects*—supernumary of limb elements, such as polydactyly (presence of extra digits);

- *dysplasias*—limb fusions, such as syndactyly (digit fusion); or

- *disproportionate growth*—limb is abnormally larger, smaller, longer, or shorter.

Primary limb enlargement may be associated with conditions such as Beckwith-Wiedemann syndrome, McCune-Albright syndrome, Proteus syndrome, macrodactyly, and isolated hemihypertrophy.[4,5] To date, no definite documented report of a teratogen-induced limb enlargement has appeared.

Aetiology

A wide range of differentials can cause ULE, both congenital and acquired. It may occur as an isolated abnormality or as part of a syndrome (hemihyperplasia syndromes are a heterogenous group of disorders with asymmetric limb growth being the primary finding).[6] The most common cause for ULE in the developing world is secondary lymphoedema as a result of lymphatic filariasis. Worldwide, more than 120 million people have been affected by the disease, of which more than 40 million are seriously incapacitated and disfigured. One-third of all cases occur within Africa.

Although ULE is primarily thought to be a disease of adulthood, occurring only sporadically in children, the increasing sensitivity of tests to detect the responsible parasites has demonstrated that infection often occurs in childhood but remains subclinical for many years.[7] Given the wide range of differentials causing ULE in children, it is helpful to consider the anatomical structures within the limb when attempting to determine the cause (see Table 113.1).

Lymphoedema

Lymphoedema is a progressive pathological condition in which there is interstitial accumulation of protein-rich fluid and subsequent inflammation, adipose tissue hypertrophy, and fibrosis. It is caused by lymphatic transport dysfunction and most commonly affects the limbs, with the resulting swelling potentially leading to disfigurement as well as decreased mobility and function.[8] Lymphoedema can be either congenitally determined (primary) or as a consequence of acquired lymphatic failure due to obstruction or damaged lymphatics (secondary).[9] The lymphatics could be aplastic, hypoplastic, or hyperplastic.

Primary lymphoedema is rare, affecting 1.5 per 100,000 population younger than 20 years of age.[10] It is subdivided into categories according to the onset of symptoms:[8]

- congenital hereditary lymphoedema (Milroy disease) presents at birth or within the first two years of life;

- familial lymphoedma praecox (Meige disease) typically presents during puberty; and

- lymphoedema tarda presents spontaneously after 35 years of age.

Worldwide, secondary lymphoedema accounts for about 90% of both paediatric and adult cases of lymphoedema. The most prevalent cause of secondary lymphoedema is filariasis secondary to infection with the filarial worms *Wuchereria banrofti* and *Brugia malayi*. Secondary lymphoedema is a mosquito-borne disease in which adult filarial worms lodge in the lymphatic systems, thus obstructing lymphatic vessels and

Table 113.1: Causes of unilateral limb enlargement in children.

System	Cause of limb enlargement

Lymphatics	**Primary lymphoedema**
	  Congential lymphoedema (Milroy disease)
	  Lymphoedema praecox (Meige disease)
	Secondary lymphoedema
	  Infection—filariasis, mycobacterium
	  Inflammation—dermatitis, sarcoidosis,
	    psoriasis, rheumatoid arthritis
	  Trauma—lymphadenectomy, burns,
	    radiotherapy, scarring
	  Obstructing tumour

Vascular	**Vascular tumours**
	  Haemangioma, tufted angioma (TA),
	  Kaposiform haemangioendothelioma (KHE)
	Slow-flow vascular malformations
	  Capillary malformations (CM), venous malforma-
	tions (VM), lymphatic malformations (LM).
	Fast-flow vascular malformations
	  Arteriovenous fistula (AVF)
	  Arteriovenous malformation (AVM)
	Combined/complex vascular malformations
	  Klippel-Trenaunay syndrome (CLVM)
	  Parkes-Weber syndrome (CAVM)
	  Proteus syndrome.
	  CLOVE syndrome

Soft tissue/ neuromuscular	Lipoblastoma—lipoblastomatosis Neurofibromatosis type 1 Macrodystropyhia lipomatosa Hemihyperplasia multiple lipomatosis syndrome Syringomyelia
Skeletal	Osteomyeltis Bone tumours

disrupting lymphatic transport.[8] In Africa, scarring of inguinal/axillary lymph nodes from repeated nonspecific infections is also a common occurrence. Occasionally, chronic, specific infection from organisms such as *Mycobacterium tuberculosis* may result in lymphoedema of the limb. In the Western world, nearly all cases of secondary lymphoedema are related to malignancy or its therapy (surgery and/or radiotherapy), and paediatirc cases are nearly always classified as primary.[9]

Vascular

In an attempt to prevent confusion and inappropriate treatment, vascular anomalies are now classified by using a system based upon their physical characteristics, natural history, and cellular features (see Table 113.1).[11,12] Haemangiomas are benign neoplasms characterised by vascular endothelium that proliferates. In contrast, vascular malformations (capillary, venous, lymphatic, arterial) are characterised by mature endothelial cells that do not grow rapidly, proliferate, or involute.[12,13] Although rare with haemangiomas, vascular malformations involving the limbs have been found to be associated with hypertrophy of the underlying soft and skeletal tissues.

Several clinical syndromes involve complex vascular malformations with an associated ULE. Klippel-Trenaunay syndrome is a slow-flow malformation involving abnormal capillaries, lymphatics, and veins characterised by a triad of portwine stain, varicose veins, and skeletal and soft tissue hypertrophy.[14] Parkes-Weber syndrome is similar, except for a combined fast-flow vascular arteriovenous malformation (AVM) in association with a cutaneous capillary malformation and skeletal or soft tissue hypertrophy.[1] Proteus syndrome is a progressive sporadic overgrowth disorder that is extremely rare and of unknowm aetiology.[15] Overgrowth can affect any tissue, but most commonly involves bone, connective tissue, and fat. Vascular malformations are frequently seen and are usually capillary or venous. The overgrowth in Proteus is distinct in that it causes distortion of the skeletal system.[15,16] Proteus overlaps with several other asymmetric overgrowth syndromes, including hemihyperplasia-multiple lipomatosis (HHML) syndrome and congenital lipomatous overgrowth, vascular malformations,

and epidermal naevi (the so-called CLOVE syndrome, standing for Congenital Lipomatous Overgrowth, Vascular alformations, and Epidermal naevi).[16]

Soft Tissue/Neuromuscular

Excessive deposition of fatty/fibrous tissue can result in limb enlargement, especially if deep and diffuse.[17] There is also growing evidence that the peripheral nervous system has an important role in limb size regulation, with peripheral nerve abnormalities resulting in limb overgrowth.[4] Soft tissue overgrowth can affect skin, fat, lymphatic, or nerve structures, although flexor tendons and blood vessels may be spared. This means that although the tissues may be abundant in a limb, they have a relatively poor blood supply.

Lipoblastoma and lipoblastomatosis are rare benign soft tissue tumours that occur almost exclusively in infants and children, resulting from proliferation of primitive adipocytes. Lipoblastoma is encapsulated and more likely to be superficial, whereas lipoblastomatosis is infiltrative and likely to be deeply situated.[18,19] Neurofibromatosis type 1 is an autosominal dominant condition with several clinical forms including elephantiasis nervorum, which includes neurofibromas of the extremities that cause greatly thickened skin stimulating limb hypertrophy.[20] Macrodystrophia lipomatosa is a rare form of localised gigantism characterised by progressive overgrowth of all the mesenchymal elements with a disaproportionate increase in the fibroadipose tissues. This congenital abnormality occurs most frequently in the distribution of the median nerve in the upper extremity and in the distribution of the planter nerves in the lower extremity.[21] HHML syndrome is a rare hemihyperplasia syndrome that is similar in presentation to the Proteus syndrome except that patients show only moderate abnormalities of asymmetry and overgrowth combined with subcutaneous lipomata.[22]

Syringomyelia is another rare cause of limb enlargement that can result in hypertrophy of the soft tissue and skeletal components of the limb. Neurogenic hypertrophy has been postulated to be the result of stimulation of the sympathetic nervous system, causing defective circulation and oedema; others believe muscle hypertrophy occurring in syringomyelia is secondary to neural abnormalities.[23–25]

Skeletal

In infants, acute haematogenous osteomyelitis may be complicated by the arrest of growth and shortening of the bone or limb due to physeal damage. In older children, however, the bone (along with the soft tissues) occasionally grows too long because of metaphyseal hyperaemia, which subsequently stimulates the growth plate. This, however, leads more to limb length discrepancy, as transverse enlargement is usually minimal.

Primary bone tumours are rare but account for a significant proportion of cancers occurring in children. The most common primary malignant tumours are osteosarcoma and Ewing's sarcoma. The most common benign bone tumours are osteochondroma, enchondroma, osteoid osteoma, osteoblastoma, chondroblastoma, chondromyxoid fibroma, and haemangioma.[26] Tumours can result in soft tissue swelling and localised enlargement of the extremity (osteosarcoma).[27] In advanced stages, tumour swelling may also cause skin changes, including prominent veins, striation, hyperthermia, and eventually ulceration.[27]

Clinical Features

The clinical presentation of children with ULE is varied and depends on the cause and extent of the enlargement (Figures 113.1–113.3). Commonly, there is an overgrowth (limb length discrepancy), which may impede function or be of cosmetic concern to the child and/or the parents. Overgrowth may be localised or diffuse, regular or irregular, rapidly or slowly progressive; it may or may not cause deformity.

Determining the underlying pathology causing ULE is vital for offering the correct management. Important factors for assessing aetiology include identifying the time of presentation (e.g., from birth or later in childhood) and whether the ULE is an isolated problem or part of broader

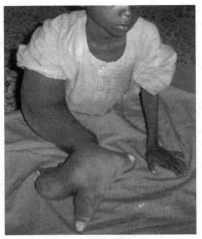

Figure 113.1: Vascular malformation of the right upper limb in a young boy.

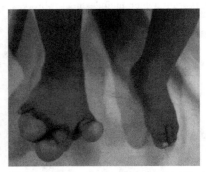

Figure 113.2: Lipofibromatosis of the right lower limb in a young girl. Note the slight discrepancy in the diameter of the legs, and pedal macrodactyly of the medial 3 toes.

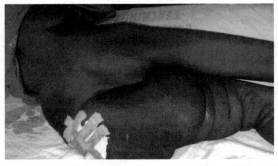

Figure 113.3: Plexiform neurofibroma of the left lower limb in a teenage girl. Note the hyperpigmentation. The dressing is covering a pressure ulcer.

syndrome. Specific clinical features are seen with the different causes.

In the early stages of lymphoedema, there is swelling that subsides with elevation, and pitting oedema is seen with peau d'orange skin changes. In later stages, tissue fibrosis develops, preventing pitting, and ultimately lymphostatic elephantiasis develops, combined with trophic skin changes such as acanthosis, fat deposits, and warty overgrowths.[8]

Childhood cases of lymphatic filariasis may be unrecognised because they may be clinically asymptomatic, with symptoms developing only after puberty. However, affected children may suffer with adenitis or lymphadenopathy, and (although uncommon under the age of 10 years) children have been reported to have the same chronic clinical manifestations as adults, including hydrocele, lymphoedema, and elephantiasis.[7]

Haemangiomas, neurofibromas, and other vascular anomalies could be associated with pigmentary changes of the overlying skin[1,17] (see

Figure 113.3). Complications of pain, ulceration, and bleeding may herald late presentation.[13] Most vascular malformations will empty on gentle pressure, as opposed to the case for haemangiomas and lipofibromatosis. Some children with complex vascular malformations could also present with features of high output cardiac failure.[1]

Osteomyelitis and bone tumours can present with clinical features relatively similar to ULE, the most common being bone pain followed by localised tissue swelling.[28] Children with osteomyelitis often show systemic signs of infection, including fever, malaise, and weight loss, with the infected area of bone likely to be sore, warm, and swollen. Most children with bone tumours are well systemically, although symptoms such as fever, weight loss, anorexia, and malaise can be present in advanced disease.[29] As with osteomyelitis, there may be the presence of a localised soft tissue mass with raised temperature that grows in size.[26]

Investigations

The choice of investigations carried out should be determined by the clinical history and features. Imaging techniques often have an important role in identifying the cause of ULE.[1,30] Although advanced, expensive radiological investigations may be required to obtain an accurate diagnosis, more basic tests also can be of significant use. As an example, the diagnosis of lymphatic filariasis had been extremely difficult because parasites had to be detected microscopically in the blood, and in most parts of the world, the parasites have a "nocturnal periodicity" that restricts their appearance in the blood to only the hours around midnight. However, there is now a very sensitive, very specific simple "card test" to detect circulating parasite antigens without the need for laboratory facilities and using only finger-prick blood droplets taken any time of the day.[31]

Radiography

Plain radiographs are used to assess any bone pathology and to document limb length discrepancies, which can be performed serially. Plain radiographs remain the mainstay for the initial evaluation of a primary bone tumour, providing information on the anatomical site of the lesion, the nature of the host bone in which the tumour has arisen, the presence of any mineralised matrix that may represent areas of calcification or ossification within the tumour, the nature of the interface between the tumour and the surrounding host bone, and the reaction of the host bone to the presence of the tumour.[26] Plain x-ray bone changes lag osteomyelitis by 10–20 days but include osteolysis, sequestra (islands of necrotic bone), and bone abscess (Brodie's abscess, pineda vargos), but earlier findings include soft tissue swelling and periosteal reaction.[32]

Ultrasonography

Ultrasonography (US) is an imaging modality with a wide application spectrum in the paediatric population due to its lack of ionising radiation.[26] US combined with Doppler imaging is an excellent tool to visualise the soft tissue and vascular structures of the limbs. It is able to determine the flow rate of the vascular lesions and differentiate one from another. Although haemangiomas can be characterised by fast flow as well, the history and age at onset should distinguish them from AVMs and other vascular malformations.[1] US may also be used to identify bone lesions and it has been demonstrated to be of use in diagnosing the early signs of osteomyelitis in children, identifying soft tissue abscesses or fluid collections, and identifying periosteal elevation.[32] US is also a useful tool in diagnosing lymphatic filariasis.[7]

Magnetic Resonance Imaging

Magnetic resonance imaging (MRI) is a particularly useful imaging modality in the assessment of ULE because it accurately visualises bone, soft tissue, and vascular structures without radiation exposure.[26] Indeed, MRI and MR angiography (MRA) are the most useful tools to demonstrate the full extent of vascular malformations.[33] MRI provides the foundation for describing the type and extent of each of the vascular malformation components. MRI can demonstrate fatty, muscular, and bony overgrowth, with generalised enlargement of the normal named arteries and veins within the affected limb. MRI is also routinely used in the assessment of bone tumours to define the lesion and soft tissue reactions and is effective in the detection and surgical localisation of osteomyelitis.[34]

Diagnositic imaging is not usually helpful in the diagnosis of lymphoedema. MRI, however, might be useful to distinguish between lymphoedema, tissue overgrowth, or vascular malformation when there is a mixed clinical picture. Qualitative lymphoscintigraphy can also be helpful to understand whether swelling is (or is not) lymphatic in origin and, if so, what the mechanism might be. For example, Milroy disease shows no peripheral uptake of tracer as there due to an absence of initial lymphatics.[9]

Treatment

The treatment of unilateral limb enlargement requires a systematic approach. Generally, the goal is to treat the problem as conservatively as possible. Surgical intervention is usually reserved for advanced disease because it is often technically challenging, requiring meticulous dissections to preserve vital structures, and it frequently has a risk of severe complications. Surgery is required primarily for cosmetic purposes and to restore function. However, it may also be required to address the complications of ulceration, bleeding, and limb-length discrepancy.

Conservative Treatment

The cornerstones to the treatment of lymphoedema are compression therapy, manual lymph drainage, and exercise in order to reduce pitting oedema, encourage lymph flow transport, and maintain mobility, respectively. This includes elevation and compression stockings/bandaging, massage techniques to stimulate collateral lymph drainage, and encouragement of children to perform as many normal recreational activites as possible.[9] Most studies have not found significant improvement with the use of diuretics.[35]

Antiparasite treatment is necessary for patients with lymphatic filariasis. Both albendazole and diethylcarbamazine (DEC) have been shown to be effective in killing the adult-stage filarial parasites. This treatment in itself can result in improvements of lymphoedema symptoms. Conservative measures to improve lymphatic flow combined with rigorous hygiene to prevent bacterial and fungal "superinfection" of the affected tissues also play vital roles in prevention of disease progression and even clinical improvement.[36]

Most cases of haemangiomas are best handled by reassuring the parents because significant numbers will involute before the first decade of life. Antiangiogenic treatment for haemangiomas include oral, systemic, or intralesional steroids as first-line drugs and recombinant interferon alfa, 2a or 2b, as a second-line drug. The overall response rate following steroid or interferon treatment is 80–90%, but no synergism has been demonstrated when steroids and interferon are used simultaneously.[1] Live vaccines, such as polio, measles, rubella, mumps, and varicella, should be withheld while children are taking the steroids. Low-flow vascular malformations, especially venous and macrocystic lymphatic malformations, are effectively treated by percutaneous intralesional injection of sclerosant drugs such as ethanol and detergent sclerosant drugs. The commonly used agents include 95% ethanol, 1–3% sotradechol, doxycycline, and sodium tetradecyl sulphate, all of which produce scarring and collapse of the cysts.[37] Shoe lifts are recommended for children with lower limb length discrepancy if the discrepancy is greater than 1.5 cm at the age of 2 years.[1]

Osteomyelitis is primarily treated by using antibiotics, preferably or at least initially intravenously, generally given over a prolonged period of time ranging from 4 to 6 weeks.

Minimally Invasive Treatment

The use of lasers has not found much place in the management of limb enlargement, unlike the treatment of head and neck haemangiomas. Preoperative embolisation is used as part of a strategy for the management of AVMs. Angiographic embolisation facilitates the operation by decreasing bleeding, although this does not reduce the extent of tissues to be resected.[38] It is also useful in large and extensive vascular lesions that are not amenable to surgical treatment.

Surgical Treatment

Surgical treatment is indicated when conservative/minimally invasive methods are contraindicated or have failed, when there are complications, or for correction of significant lower limb length discrepancy. Surgical excisions of soft tissues aim to resect as much abnormal and excessive tissues as possible while making an effort to preserve vital structures. Staged contour resection/debulking can be used to treat areas of limb overgrowth and lymphoedema. Following some excisional surgeries, primary closure may not be possible without tissue-transfer techniques. Vacuum-assisted closure devices can also be useful in wounds with large soft tissue loss precluding linear closure.[1]

Surgical intervention for paediatric bone tumours depends upon the type of tumour, particularly whether it is benign or malignant. Depending upon the type of benign tumour, it may be simply observed or it may require curettage out of the bone, with bone grafting used to fill the debrided space. Malignant tumours require excision, which may be combined with preoperative chemotherapy. There is a growing use of limb-sparing surgery; however, there may be the need for amputation. Surgical intervention may also be required to treat osteomyelitis, including debridement and washout.

Occasionally, epiphysiodesis of the distal femoral growth plate could be performed at about the age of 12 years to correct overgrowth, but such a procedure for arm-length discrepancies is usually unnecessary. Amputation may be a last option in late presentation (see Figure 113.1) where the limb enlargement is massive (not amenable to resection/debulking) and limited to the distal extremity.

Intraoperative tips to avoid morbidity and mortality include the following:

1. Staged surgical approach is usually required.

2. Remove as much abnormal/excessive tissue as possible.

3. Avoid injury to vital structures by avoiding overzealous excision.

4. Limit blood loss to less than the patient's total blood volume.

5. Employ special tissue transfer techniques, when necessary, to close the wound.

Western Management

The underlying pathophysiology of ULE within the developed world is different from that of the developing world. The Western world has an increased incidence of congenital versus acquired causes, particularly with the absence of lymphatic filariasis and other secondary causes of lymphoedema. Generally, a multidisciplinary team approach is necessary to carefully assess the patient, sequentially evaluate limb inequalities, and formulate the appropriate management plan. Despite greater access to interventional radiology and advanced surgical techniques, treatment is still focused upon conservative measures unless severe symptoms or complications arise.

Prognosis

The outcome of unilateral limb enlargement depends on the cause of enlargement, the extent of the lesion, and the treatment that is available to the patient. The condition is essentially from benign causes, and malignant transformation is very rare. However, sarcomatous change can occur in a small percentage of patients. Those with chronic ulcerations may transform to Marjolin's ulcers. The recurrent rate after surgical intervention ranges from 15% to 40%. Death is usually from bleeding, infections, and high output cardiac failure.

Evidence-Based Research

Table 113.2 presents an extensive review of information available on lymphatic filariasis as well as problems still to be addressed.

Table 113.2: Evidence-based research.

Title	Lymphatic filariasis: an infection of childhood
Authors	Witt C, Ottesen EA
Institution	Lymphatic Filariasis Elimination, World Health Organisation, Geneva, Switzerland
Reference	Trop Med Inter Health 2001; 6(8):582–606
Problem	New, highly sensitive diagnostic tests have now revealed that lymphatic filariasis (LF) is first acquired in childhood, often with as many as one-third of children infected before age 5. Recognising that the disease starts its development in childhood has immediate practical implications both for its management and prevention in individual patients and for the broader public health efforts.
Intervention	This review aims to bring together in a comprehensive fashion much of the information already available on LF in children and to focus attention on those critical uncertainties that still need to be resolved.
Comparison/ control (quality of evidence)	A medline-based literature search covering the years 1966–2000 was carried out by exploring the identifier "filariasis" with the terms "child", "children", "paediatric", and '"adolescent". Retrieved articles were supplemented by bibliographic references from these articles and reports and documents published by the World Health Organization (WHO). Of all the publications assessed, 83 were selected for inclusion in this review because they met the following criteria: they were published either in peer-reviewed journals or in official government documents; they described age-delineated populations endemic for either *Wuchereria bancrofti* or *Brugia malayi* infection that had not been subjected to antimalarial measures during at least the previous 5 years; and they included a complete description of the relevant diagnostic methods used.
Outcome/ effect	Across all endemicity levels, the prevalence of LF infection in children is proportional to that of the adults in each population; those younger than 10 years of age have prevalence rates averaging 30% of the adult rate, and 10–19-year-olds have about 69% of the adult rate. The enhanced effectiveness of antigen detection, vis-à-vis microfilaria detection, to diagnose LF infection is greatest in very young children, many of whose infections had been previously undiagnosed. The new, recently codified approaches to managing filarial lymphoedema and hydrocoele in adults have also been used successfully with children.
Historical significance/ comments	LF is a frequent and common infection of children in all LF-endemic areas. It causes both subclinical lymphatic damage and eventual overt clinical disease. It is critically important to learn how to reverse these early lesions and thereby prevent future development of lymphoedema and hydrocoele in older children and adults.

Key Summary Points

1. Unilateral limb enlargement is uncommon in day-to-day practice.

2. Unilateral limb enlargement has numerous aetiological factors.

3. A common presentation is for enlargement, limb length discrepancy, cosmesis, and complications.

4. Imaging techniques are the mainstay of investigations.

5. Staged contour resection is the mainstay of treatment.

6. The recurrence rate is between 15% and 40%.

References

1. Smithers CJ, Fishman. SJ. Vascular anomalies. In: Ashcroft KW, Holcomb GW, Murphy JP, eds. Pediatric Surgery, 4th ed. Elsevier Saunders, 2005. Pp 1038–1053.

2. Schoenwolf GC, Bleyl SB, Brauer PR, Francis-West PH. Development of the limbs. In: Schoenwolf GC, Bleyl SB, Brauer PR, Francis-West PH, eds. Larsen's Human Embryology, 4th ed. Churchill Livingstone Elsevier, 2001, Pp 617–644.

3. Sadler TW. Skeletal system. In: Sadler TW, ed. Langman's Medical Embryology. 10th ed. Lippincott, Williams & Wilkins, 2006, Pp 125–142.

4. Romero-Ortega MI, Ezaki M. Nerve pathology in unregulated limb growth. J Bone Joint Surg Am 2009; 91(Suppl 4):53–57.

5. Firth HV, Hurst JA, Hall JG. Clinical approach. In: Firth HV, Hurst JA, Hall JG, eds. Oxford Desk Reference: Clinical Genetics. Oxford University Press, 2009, Chap 3, Pp 278–282.

6. Litani C, Engel G, Piette WW. Tumescent liposuction in the treatment of hemihyperplasia multiple lipomatosis syndrome. Dermatol Surg 2009; 35(7):1147–1151.

7. Witt C, Ottesen EA. Lymphatic filariasis: an infection of childhood. Trop Med Int Health 2001; 6(8):582–606.

8. Warren AG, Brorson H, Borud LJ, Slavin SA. Lymphedema: a comprehensive review. Ann Plast Surg 2007; 59(4):464–472.

9. Damstra RJ, Mortimer PS. Diagnosis and therapy in children with lymphoedema. Phlebology 2008; 23(6):276–286.

10. Dale RF. The inheritance of primary lymphoedema. J Med Genet 1985; 22(4):274–278.

11. Mulliken JB, Glowacki J. Classification of pediatric vascular lesions. Plast Reconstr Surg 1982; 70(1):120–121.

12. Mulliken JB, Glowacki J. Hemangiomas and vascular malformations in infants and children: a classification based on endothelial characteristics. Plast Reconstr Surg 1982; 69(3):412–422.

13. Marler JJ, Mulliken JB. Vascular anomalies: classification, diagnosis, and natural history. Facial Plast Surg Clin North Am 2001; 9(4):495–504.

14. Jacob AG, Driscoll DJ, Shaughnessy WJ, Stanson AW, Clay RP, Gloviczki P. Klippel-Trenaunay syndrome: spectrum and management. Mayo Clin Proc 1998; 73(1):28–36.

15. Biesecker L. The challenges of Proteus syndrome: diagnosis and management. Eur J Hum Genet 2006; 14(11):1151–1157.

16. Sapp JC, Turner JT, van de Kamp JM, van Dijk FS, Lowry RB, Biesecker LG. Newly delineated syndrome of congenital lipomatous overgrowth, vascular malformations, and epidermal nevi (CLOVE syndrome) in seven patients. Am J Med Genet A 2007; 143A(24):2944–2958.

17. Papendieck CM, Barbosa L, Pozo P, Vanelli C, Braun D, Iotti A. Lipoblastoma-lipoblastomatosis associated with unilateral limb hypertrophy: a case report in a newborn. Lymphology 2003; 36(2):69–73.

18. Bourelle S, Viehweger E, Launay F, Quilichini B, Bouvier C, Hagemeijer A, et al. Lipoblastoma and lipoblastomatosis. J Pediatr Orthop B 2006; 15(5):356–361.

19. Dilley AV, Patel DL, Hicks MJ, Brandt ML. Lipoblastoma: pathophysiology and surgical management. J Pediatr Surg 2001; 36(1):229–231.

20. Laberge J, Shaw KS, Nguyen LT. Teratomas, dermoids, and other soft tissue tumours. In: Ashcroft KW, Holcomb GW, Murphy JP, eds. Pediatric Surgery, 4th ed. Elsevier Saunders, 2005, Pp 972–996.

21. Goldman AB, Kaye JJ. Macrodystrophia lipomatosa: radiographic diagnosis. AJR Am J Roentgenol 1977; 128(1):101–105.

22. Biesecker LG, Peters KF, Darling TN, Choyke P, Hill S, Schimke N, et al. Clinical differentiation between Proteus syndrome and hemihyperplasia: description of a distinct form of hemihyperplasia. Am J Med Genet 1998; 79(4):311–318.

23. Mehta J, Khanna S. Syringomyelia as a cause of limb hypertrophy. Neurol India 2002; 50(1):94–96.

24. Negri S, Pacini L. Association of muscular hypertrophy and syringomyelia. Riv Neurol 1960; 30:325–335.

25. Sudarshana Murthy KA, Ravishankar SB. Localized hypertrophy of hand in syringomyelia. J Assoc Physicians India 2001; 49:1203–1204.

26. Vlychou M, Athanasou NA. Radiological and pathological diagnosis of paediatric bone tumours and tumour-like lesions. Pathology 2008; 40(2):196–216.

27. **Wittig** JC, **Bickels** J, Priebat D. **Osteosarcoma**: a multidisciplinary approach to diagnosis and treatment. Am Fam Physician. 2002; 65(6):1123–1132.

28. World Health Organization. Classification of Bone Tumours. In: Fletcher CDM, Unni K, Mertens F, eds. Pathology and Genetics of Tumours of Soft Tissue and Bone. World Health Organization, 2002, Pp 225–234.

29. Bernstein M, Kovar H, Paulussen M, Randall RL, Schuck A, Teot LA, et al. Ewing's sarcoma family of tumors: current management. Oncologist 2006; 11(5):503–519.

30. Pearn J, Viljoen D, Beighton P. Limb overgrowth—clinical observations and nosological considerations. S Afr Med J 1983; 64(23):905–908.

31. Weil GJ, Lammie PJ, Weiss N. The ICT Filariasis Test: A rapid-format antigen test for diagnosis of bancroftian filariasis. Parasitol Today 1997; 13(10):401–404.

32. Termaat MF, Raijmakers PG, Scholten HJ, Bakker FC, Patka P, Haarman HJ. The accuracy of diagnostic imaging for the assessment of chronic osteomyelitis: a systematic review and meta-analysis. J Bone Joint Surg Am 2005; 87(11):2464–2471.

33. Breugem CC, Maas M, Reekers JA, van der Horst CM. Use of magnetic resonance imaging for the evaluation of vascular malformations of the lower extremity. Plast Reconstr Surg 2001; 108(4):870–877.

34. McAndrew PT, Clark C. MRI is best technique for imaging acute osteomyelitis. BMJ 1998; 316(7125):147.

35. Keeley V. Pharmacological treatment for chronic oedema. Br J Community Nurs 2008; 13(4):S4, S6, S8–S10.

36. Addiss D, Critchley J, Ejere H, Garner P, Gelband H, Gamble C. Albendazole for lymphatic filariasis. Cochrane Database Syst Rev 2004; (1):CD003753.

37. Burrows PE, Mason KP. Percutaneous treatment of low flow vascular malformations. J Vasc Interv Radiol 2004; 15(5):431–445.

38. Lee BB, Do YS, Yakes W, Kim DI, Mattassi R, Hyon WS. Management of arteriovenous malformations: a multidisciplinary approach. J Vasc Surg 2004; 39(3):590–600.

PAEDIATRIC GYNAECOLOGY

CHAPTER 114
HYDROMETROCOLPOS

Bankole S. Rouma
Jennifer H. Aldrink
Julia B. Finkelstein
Howard B. Ginsburg

Introduction

Hydrocolpos is an uncommon congenital disorder consisting of cystic dilatation of the vagina caused by obstruction of the distal genital tract, resulting in retained fluid. If there is also associated uterine enlargement, the term hydrometrocolpos is applied. Vaginal obstruction may result from a high vaginal septum, varying degrees of vaginal atresia, cloacal malformations, or an imperforate hymen. Hydrocolpos may manifest at birth as a palpable mass or it may present at puberty as progressive accumulation of menstrual blood, causing haematometrocolpos. Hydrocolpos and hydrometrocolpos are the third most common causes of all abdominal masses in the newborn, accounting for 15% of all abdominal masses in female newborns, with an estimated occurrence rate of 1 in 16,000 female deliveries.

The clinical features of hydrometrocolpos in the newborn are dominated by the abdominal mass with regional compression (Figure 114.1). An overly distended vagina can compress the adjacent organs and cause abdominal pain, intestinal obstruction, ureteral obstruction, hydronephrosis, bladder perforation, respiratory distress, and lower extremity venous stasis. Accordingly, presentation of hydrometrocolpos depends on the degree of compression of the surrounding structures by the uterovaginal swelling. Although the rarity and variable presentation of hydrometrocolpos can lead to delayed diagnosis and erroneous management, it should be considered in the differential diagnosis if a female neonate is found to have a large abdominal mass.

Early diagnosis and treatment of hydrocolpos or hydrometrocolpos is important to minimise various complications of mechanical pressure exerted on surrounding structures. The most important step is a comprehensive perineal examination. Cross-sectional imaging and dye studies help in early diagnosis and demarcating the exact anatomy as well as revealing associated renal anomalies.[1] Comprehensive management is necessary, usually involving surgical treatment, to provide normal phenotypic appearance and to preserve reproductive potential.

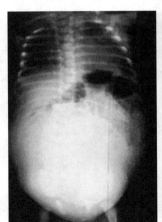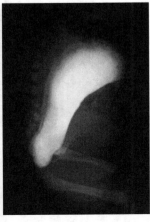

Figure 114.1: Abdominal radiograph showing a mass density in a 3-day-old infant (left); abdominal radiograph on lateral view showing a hydrometrocolpos in a 3-day-old infant (right).

Demographics

Prevalence data for Africa were not available. In general, the prevalence of hydrocolpos is estimated to be approximately 1 in 16,000 births.[2] Imperforate hymen is the most frequent congenital malformation of the female genital tract.[3] The incidence is estimated to be 0.1%.[4] However, manifestations of imperforate hymen presenting as an abdominal mass in the perinatal or neonatal age are extremely rare, with an estimated incidence of 0.006%.[4] Vaginal atresia is estimated to occur in 1 in 5,000 to 1 in 10,000 live female births; approximately 1 in 70,000 to 1 in 80,000 females are born with a transverse vaginal septum, with septa more frequently occurring in the middle and upper third of the vagina.[5] Persistent cloaca has an incidence of 1 in 250,000 live born infants. Twenty-five percent of patients with persistent cloaca present with associated hydrocolpos.[6]

Embryology

Both the urinary system and the genital system develop from a common mesodermal ridge along the posterior wall of the abdominal cavity. The excretory ducts of both systems initially enter a common cavity, the cloaca. The cloaca divides into the urogenital sinus anteriorly and the anal canal posteriorly during the 4th to 7th weeks of gestational development. By the 7th week, there is a layer of mesoderm—the urorectal septum—between the primitive anal canal and the urogenital sinus. Three portions of the urogenital sinus can be distinguished:

1. The superior and largest vesicle part becomes the urinary bladder. As the bladder grows, it absorbs the proximal segment of the mesonephric ducts into its posterior wall, forming the trigone of the bladder. Absorption of the mesonephric ducts continues until the ureters open directly into the bladder.

2. The middle segment of the urogenital sinus is a narrow canal, the pelvic portion of the urogenital sinus.

3. The remaining part is the phallic area of the urogenital sinus, which is flattened from side to side.[7]

During the 2nd month of prenatal development, paramesonephric ducts arise as longitudinal invaginations of epithelium on the anterolateral surface of the urogenital ridge, and as tubular invaginations of the coelemic mesothelium parallel to the mesonephric ducts. In the absence of male gene products, the mesonephric ducts disappear. Meanwhile, under the influence of oestrogens, the paramesonephric ducts remain. At first, three different parts can be distinguished in each paramesonephric duct. The first two parts develop into the uterine tube with the descent of the ovary. The caudal part of each contralateral paramesonephric duct is initially separated by a septum, but they later fuse to form the uterine canal. The caudal tip of the combined ducts projects into the posterior wall of the urogenital sinus, where it causes a small swelling, the paramesonephric tubercle. The paramesonephric ducts then fuse in the midline to form a tube with a single lumen, which will form the uterus, cervix, and superior end of the vagina.

Shortly after the tip of the paramesonephric ducts reaches the urogenital sinus, two solid evaginations—the sinovaginal bulbs—grow out from the pelvic part of the sinus. These evaginations proliferate and form a solid vaginal plate. Proliferation continues at the cranial end of the vaginal plate, increasing the distance between the uterus and the urogenital sinus. The vaginal plate canalises to form the lower two-thirds of the vagina. This is completed by the 20th gestational week. Accordingly, the vagina has a dual origin, from the paramesonephric ducts (mesoderm) and from the urogenital sinus (endoderm). The hymen, a thin tissue plate, separates the lumen of the vagina from the urogenital sinus. The hymen consists of an epithelial lining of the urogenital sinus and a thin layer of vaginal cells. At 5 gestational months, it usually begins to degenerate to establish a connection between the vaginal lumen and perineum. A remnant usually persists postnatally. The tissue superior to the vagina begins to enlarge and extend inferiorly to separate the bladder from the vagina, forming the urovaginal septum.[7,8]

Pathology

Vaginal outflow obstruction and subsequent hydrocolpos may be secondary to a transverse vaginal septum, atresia of the vagina, imperforate hymen, or a persistent urogenital sinus. Associated anomalies are relatively rare with an imperforate hymen but are common with vaginal atresia, urogenital sinus, or cloacal malformations.

Vaginal Atresia

If the sinovaginal bulbs fail to develop, vaginal atresia results. Females with vaginal atresia lack the lower portion of the vagina but otherwise have normal external genitalia. Fibrous tissue develops in place of the vagina. In some females, nearly the entire length, beginning at the perineum and extending to the cervix, may be fibrotic. However, as the primary defect is in the sinusal contribution to the vagina, the contiguous superior structures, especially the uterus, are well differentiated.[8] Accordingly, a small vaginal pouch originating from the paramesonephric ducts usually surrounds the opening of the cervix. Before hydrocolpos will develop, there must be sufficient oestrogenic stimulation to provoke secretion from the glands in the reproductive tract. For this reason, both oestrogenic stimulation and vaginal obstruction must coexist.

Transverse Vaginal Septum

A transverse vaginal septum results when there is failure of either fusion of the urogential sinus and paramesonephric ducts or canalisation of the vaginal plate. There is a well-developed vagina in which a thick intervening septum separates the lower from the upper vagina. The septum may be obstructive, with accumulation of mucus or menstrual blood.[9] In neonates and infants, an obstructive transverse vaginal septum has been associated with fluid and mucus collection in the upper vagina, resulting in a mass that that may be large enough to compress abdominal or pelvic organs. The external genitalia appear normal, but internally the vagina is a shortened, blind pouch. A transverse vaginal septum can develop at any level within the vagina but is more common in the upper portion, at the junction between the sinovaginal plate and the caudal end of the fused paramesonephric ducts.[9] The thickness of the septum may be variable. However, thicker septa tend to be located nearer the cervix.

Imperforate Hymen

Hymenal anomalies are derived from incomplete degeneration of the central portion of the hymen. Imperforate hymen is one of the most common obstructive lesions of the female genital tract. It is almost always an isolated finding. In the presence of vaginal outflow obstruction, there is potential for significant accumulation of cervico-vaginal secretion during foetal life, occurring secondary to circulating maternal oestrogens. In infants, the obstructed vagina may distend from mucus accumulation, with the mucocolpos causing a bulging hydrocele membrane. More commonly, symptoms of cyclic pelvic pain present during adolescence after menarche. Trapped menstrual blood behind the imperforate hymen may create a bluish bulge at the introitus.[9]

Persistent Urogenital Sinus

Persistent urogenital sinus is an important, but often missed, cause of hydrocolpos. A persistent urogenital sinus represents failure of urethro-vaginal septation at 6 weeks of gestation. This developmental arrest leads to a common channel for the urinary and genital tracts, with drainage of the bladder and the vagina through one orifice. Therefore, there is distal vaginal atresia and a proximal urethrovaginal fistula. The urethrovaginal communication allows urine to empty into the vagina, which subsequently dilates. When the defect occurs at an early stage, the result is a long urogenital sinus with a short vagina and a high urethral opening. A short urogenital sinus with almost normal length of vaginal vestibule and low urethral opening results when the defect occurs later in development. The perineum exhibits two distinctive orifices, a ventral urogenital sinus and a dorsal anus.

Persistent Cloaca

Persistent cloaca results from partial or total failure of the urorectal septum to descend and divide the cloaca during month 2 of gestation. The anatomic findings in each case may be related to septal differentiation. In the patient for whom the fold develops but fails to make contact with the cloacal membrane, the cloaca will be small and the urinary, genital, and alimentary tracts, which are well separated, will open into the cloaca adjacent to the external orifice. In the case where septal development was incomplete, the cloaca will be larger; separation of urinary, genital, and alimentary tracts will be variable and may be incomplete; and the fistulous communications tend to be remote from the external orifice. Either way, there is junction of the urinary tract, genitalia, and rectum into a single channel, opening onto the perineum in a single orifice.[6]

Clinical Presentation

Associated Malformations

The McKusick-Kaufman syndrome is a rare autosomal recessive disorder mapped to 20p12 characterised by hydrometrocolpos, polydactyly, and congenital heart defects.[10,11] The Bardet-Biedl syndrome is a genetic name for a heterogeneous group of autosomal recessive disorders with at least four loci in 16q13q22, 11q13, 3p11-p13, and 15q22.[10] It is characterised by retinal dystrophy or retinitis pigmentosa, postaxial polydactyly, obesity, nephropathy, and mental disturbances or mental retardation. It is also associated with hydrometrocolpos, usually as a consequence of vaginal atresia or transverse vaginal septum. Its diagnosis is typically delayed to the teenage years. Rarely, hydrometrocolpos can be associated with Pallister-Hall syndrome, an autosomal dominant trait with variable expressivity, characterised by postaxial polydactyly, hypothalamic hamartoma, imperforate anus, intrauterine growth retardation, and several visceral anomalies.[12]

Persistent cloaca is the most severe malformation of anorectal anomalies in girls and is associated with complex pelvic malformation and frequent hydrocolpos.[13,14] Hydrometrocolpos due to a urogenital sinus malformation may be associated with ureteral duplication, ectopic ureter, urethral membrane, imperforate anus, hypoplastic or multicystic dysplastic kidney, and bifid clitoris.

Symptoms

Hydrocolpos or hydrometrocolpos can be asymptomatic if only a small amount of fluid is accumulated, which is the case with most obstructions. Asymptomatic imperforate hymen that does not show a cystic mass can easily be overlooked and undiagnosed until adolescence, when menarche does not appear and the young girl complains of lower abdominal pain.[9]

The condition will be symptomatic if a large cyst is formed, causing urine retention, hydronephrosis and renal impairment, constipation, abdominal mass, ascites, oedema, and even cyanosis of low extremities. The upward pull of the enlarging vagina elongates and makes the urethra angulated, producing dysuria and acute urinary retention. This may result in infection of the urinary tract or of the fluid retained in the vagina. Moreover, hydronephrosis and hydroureter may result from pressure of the vagina on the ureters crossing the pelvic brim.[15] Foetal urine may drain through the uterine tubes into the peritoneal cavity, giving rise to ascites. In addition, the patient may experience vomiting as a result of intestinal obstruction.

History

Maternal hormones profoundly affect the reproductive tract of the female infant both in utero and during the early neonatal period. In response to maternal oestrogens, vaginal and cervical epithelium secretes mucus, which pools in the obstructed vagina. Thus, hydrocolpos is usually detected in infancy when there is a high level of maternal hormones. However, uncomplicated hydrocolpos may be initially asymptomatic. The early symptoms associated with hydrocolpos are nonspecific indications of discomfort followed by urinary, venous, or intestinal obstruction, respiratory distress, or superimposed infection of the urinary tract or of the fluid retained in the vagina.[16] Conversely, if there is a low level of maternal hormones, hydrocolpos may not be detected until early puberty, when the female begins to produce oestrogenic hormones. In many of these cases, hydrocolpos is not symptomatic until haematocolpos is superimposed at the time of menarche. Specifically, in the case of vaginal atresia, adolescents often present with primary amenorrhea accompanied by cyclic pelvic pain.[15]

Physical

Close inspection of the perineum is required in all cases of suspected hydrocolpos or hydrometrocolpos. This may require a general anaesthetic to obtain a thorough evaluation in infants and children. In vaginal atresia, the vaginal orifice may be retraced upward into the pelvis. Hydrocolpos associated with an imperforate hymen presents with a thin translucent membrane bulging between the labia. It may have a bluish color when seen in adolescent females, associated with haematometrocolpos (Figure 114.2). A transverse septum higher in the vagina may protrude through a normally perforated hymen. With this situation, the external genitalia appear normal, but internally the vagina is shortened as a blind pouch.[15] A vaginal dimple may be noted on external examination of a patient with vaginal atresia.

A single perineal orifice may be noted on external examination of a patient with a persistent urogenital sinus or cloaca. In the case of a persistent cloaca, the single perineal orifice will usually be located at the site of the normal urethra and there will also be an imperforate anus as well as partially fused labia.[6] A urine sample will be green and contain meconium due to the admixture of urinary and alimentary products in the cloaca.

Regardless of the pathology, the upper vagina becomes distended in hydrocolpos and, as a result, a tense, round abdominal mass arising from the pelvis may be palpated on abdominal examination.

Investigations

Current management emphasizes prenatal diagnosis with ultrasonography (US) or magnetic resonance imaging (MRI). US remains the most widely used diagnostic imaging technique for routine evaluation of the foetus.[17] As US becomes increasingly reliable, prenatal diagnosis of hydrocolpos is possible as early as the second trimester.

The most common sonographic finding is a median intraabdominal or pelvic cystic structure. US may demonstrate significant echogenic fluid accumulation in the vagina (Figure 114.3). In addition, targeted foetal US may show the site of obstruction and continuation of the pelvic mass with both the cervical canal and uterine cavity, confirming hydrocolpos.

Diagnosis of transverse vaginal septum is confirmed by either US or MRI. Both investigations help to define the location and thickness of a transverse vaginal septum. However, MRI is most helpful prior to surgery to determine the thickness and depth of the transverse septum. Both US and MRI also facilitate the differentiation between a high septum and

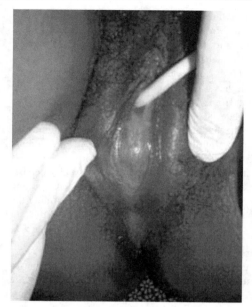

Figure 114.2: Imperforate hymen in a 15-year-old girl.

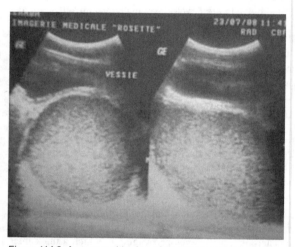

Figure 114.3: A sonographic view of the pelvis showing a hydrometrocolpos in a 15-day-old infant.

congenital absence of the cervix. In particular, for vaginal atresia, MRI is a more accurate diagnostic tool, as the length of the atresia, the amount of upper vaginal dilatation, and the presence or absence of a cervix can be identified. US cannot clearly differentiate between imperforate hymen and transverse vaginal septum. Consequently, foetal MRI is used to assist in the ultimate diagnosis of imperforate hymen. For these reasons, MRI has the capability to provide more accurate anatomical information in hydrocolpos than other diagnostic methods.[17]

A single orifice corresponding to a persistent urogenital sinus can be investigated by cystovaginoscopy. A voiding cystourethrogram (VCUG) is used by many as an initial tool in the evaluation of a single perineal orifice. This radiologic study can demonstrate the entrance of the vagina into the urogenital sinus. It can also evaluate the size and configuration of the vaginal remnant.

In the case of a persistent cloaca, a high-pressure distal colostogram should be performed. A Foley catheter is passed through the mucous fistula (distal stoma), the balloon is inflated with water, and hydrosoluble contrast material is injected under fluoroscopy while applying traction to the balloon to avoid leakage of the contrast material. By doing this, the anatomy of the malformation can be delineated.

Management

Temporising Measures

Percutaneous uterostomy or vaginostomy for temporary drainage may be an important temporising measure in neonates. Failure to drain a hydrocolpos exposes the patient to persistent hydronephrosis and/or infection of the hydrocolpos (pyocolpos). Antibiotic prophylaxis may be given to prevent urinary tract infections (UTIs). Pyocolpos and possible subsequent perforation of a hydrocolpos is a serious event that requires emergency laparotomy and may severely and permanently damage the vagina.[6] Percutaneous US-guided drainage of fluid from the hydrocolpos has also been suggested to decompress the distended organs. This may be performed prenatally if needed. Percutaneous nephrostomy may be necessary to salvage renal function. For persistent cloaca, a descending colostomy is indicated.

Definitive Measures

1. Surgical intervention for isolated hydrocolpos with lower tract obstruction is associated with excellent results. Surgery for persistent urogenital sinus, however, is more complex and uncertain.[18] Commonly utilised treatment options include the following. The treatment goal for most females with vaginal atresia is the creation of a functional vagina. This may be accomplished conservatively or surgically. Each of the several conservative approaches attempts to progressively invaginate the vaginal dimple to create a canal of adequate size. The McIndoe vaginoplasty creates a canal within the connective tissue between the bladder and rectum. A split-thickness skin graft obtained from the patient's buttocks or thigh is then used to line the neovagina. This technique is believed to have a functional success rate >80%.[5] Alternatively, cutaneous or musculocutaneous flaps have been used to line the neovagina. The Williams vaginoplasty creates a vaginal pouch by using labial skin flaps. All surgical methods require a commitment to scheduled postoperative dilatation to avoid significant vaginal stricture.[8] In the case of a very short or small vagina located high in the pelvis, vaginal replacement is necessary. Most often, a length of diverted colon is used to replace the vagina. If the colon cannot be used, the small bowel or a portion of dilated rectum is used.[6]

2. Surgical repair of an imperforate hymen involves an elliptical or cruciate incision in the membrane close to the hymenal ring followed by evacuation of the obstructed material.[9] The vaginal mucosa is then sutured to the hymenal ring to prevent adhesion and recurrence of obstruction. Uncommonly, the hymeneal edges may re-epithelialise, and a repeat procedure may be required. Bleeding, scarring, and stenosis of the vaginal orifice are major complications of this procedure.

3. A thin transverse vaginal septum can be resected, followed by end-to-end anastamosis of the upper to lower vaginal mucosa. As an alternative to end-to-end anastomosis, a Z-plasty technique can be employed that may minimise scar formation. In contrast, a thick septum is more difficult to excise and repair. Preoperative use of vaginal dilators may thin the septum and thereby facilitate reanastomosis. With higher-level septums, diagnostic needle aspiration of the suspected haemato- or hydrocolpos can help to locate the upper vagina to determine the direction of dissection. Once this is complete, the vaginal vault is incised transversely to avoid laceration of the urethra, bladder, or rectum.[9] The septum is transected, and the cervix is then identified. The vaginal mucosa is undermined, and the cephalic mucosal edge is sutured to the opposite caudal edge. A circumferential ring of interrupted sutures is constructed by using absorbable suture. The septum is excised widely to its base to minimise postoperative stricture.

4. If the urogenital sinus is low, with a short common channel, a U-flap vaginoplasty is an effective surgical procedure. If the vagina enters the urogenital sinus higher up, a division of vaginal orifice from the urogenital sinus is required, together with pull-through vaginoplasty. Some of these cases with a long common channel may require additional manoeuvres, such as creation of a neourethra from the anterior vaginal wall, to complete the reconstruction.

5. In correction of a persistent cloaca, the operation consists of separating the rectum from the genitourinary tract and bringing it down to be placed within the limits of the sphincter. This procedure is beyond the scope of this chapter.

Postoperative Complications

Successful reconstruction of the vagina is a difficult task. The optimal surgical strategy provides the patient with an adequate vaginal introitus positioned correctly, a vestibule with appropriately innervated skin, and an acceptable external cosmetic appearance.[19] Complications include graft failure, wound infection, haematoma, and fistula formation. In the Williams vaginoplasty, the labia majora are created from hair-bearing skin, which will usually result in an undesirable cosmetic result. Excision of hymenal tissue may occur too close to the vaginal mucosa, causing stenosis of the introitus and dyspareunia. Nevertheless, according to Rock et al., no complaints of dyspareunia were elicited from sexually active women after surgery.[20] In cases of imperforate hymen where retrograde blood flow through the uterus and fallopian tubes occurs, pelvic endometriosis may develop with a subsequent negative impact on fertility.

With correction of a transverse vaginal septum, a common complication of resection of thick septa is scar contracture and vaginal stenosis.[5] Dyspareunia seems to be the most common complaint after surgery for a transverse vaginal septum.[21]

With very high vaginal entrance into the urogenital sinus and/or cloaca, there is a significant incidence of urinary incontinence. When the patient reaches the age of urinary control, she may require a complex urinary reconstruction and diversion.

Prognosis and Outcomes

Endometriosis and infertility are the most prominent late consequences reported in vaginal obstruction. Early diagnosis and treatment of the vaginal obstruction might enhance pregnancy success by reducing the risk of haematometra and haematosalpinx with the subsequent development of pelvic endometriosis.[21] The general prognosis for hydrocolpos is good, especially in early diagnosed and treated cases. However, late onset of sexual development, ability of the vagina to expand, a normal-appearing vaginal orifice in a mid- and high-transverse vaginal septum, and limited access to expert medical facilities in the developing world can delay the presentation.

The prognosis of isolated imperforate hymen is normally excellent. Although some patients in one particular follow-up suffered from dysmenorrhea and irregular menstruation, most patients progressed well in terms of fertility and sexual function.[22,23] Rock et al. have shown that women with an imperforate hymen had a high success rate in pregnancies, with no infertility.[20] Moreover, obstetric outcome in treated imperforate hymen is no different from that of the general population.[20] When the imperforate hymen occurs with a constellation of other findings, prognosis largely depends on the presence of the associated findings. Associated congenital anomalies involving the urogenital (incidence of 30–50%), gastrointestinal, skeletal, and cardiovascular systems are common in patients with complex anomalies.[24]

Females with imperforate hymen had better pregnancy success than those with complete transverse septum following the surgical correction of obstructive defects.[20] Patients with middle or upper complete transverse septum were less likely to conceive than those with a septum in the lower vagina.[20]

Long-term follow-up after reconstruction is essential because many patients may experience sexual difficulties, menstrual irregularities, infertility, spontaneous abortion, or premature delivery. Infertility is probably due to endometriosis and pelvic adhesion in patients with outflow obstructions. Rock et al. have reported a pregnancy rate of 47% in cases of lower obstruction, 43% in middle-third obstructions, and only 25% in upper-third obstructions.[20] The rate of spontaneous abortions has been reported to be as high as 50% in cases of transverse vaginal septum and 6% due to imperforate hymen.[21]

Ethical Issues

Many surgeons in developing countries are constrained by late presentation and lack of facilities. The diagnosis of hydrometrocolpos is often delayed because of its rarity. Moreover, in these countries, neonates often have prolonged investigations to exclude more common causes of intestinal and urinary obstruction. In the African population, this is complicated by the absence of ultrasound facilities.[10] This may prevent preoperative diagnosis because emergency US is not available at the time of presentation. Consequently, the provision of basic diagnostic services such as US is essential. It is also important to educate health care workers about the need for early referral.

Key Summary Points

1. Vaginal anomalies range from relatively common to relatively rare.

2. The rarity and variable presentation of congenital obstruction of the vagina can lead to delayed diagnosis and erroneous management.

3. It is important to be aware of the differential diagnoses and associated anomalies, including the consideration of hydrocolpos or hydrometrocolpos, in a female newborn with an abdominal mass and urinary obstruction.

4. A thorough physical genital examination and appropriate imaging can aid in achieving the correct diagnosis.

5. Ultrasonography and magnetic resonance imaging are diagnostic modalities of choice and can reveal associated renal anomalies and the anatomy of complex lesions, although further evaluation may require voiding cystourethrogram.

6. Delayed diagnosis may impair normal functions of urogenital systems and cause compression of surrounding structures.

7. Early surgical intervention will reduce long-term morbidity.

References

1. Khan RA, Ghani I, Wahab J. Hydrometrocolpos due to persistent urogenital sinus mimicking neonatal ascites. Iran J Pediatr 2008; 18(1):67–70.

2. Romero R, et al. Prenatal Diagnosis of Congenital Anomalies. Appleton and Lange, 1988, Pp 307–309.

3. Messina M, Severi FM, Bocchi C, et al. Voluminous perinatal mass: a case of congenital hydrometrocolpos. J Matern Fetal Neonatal Med 2004; 15:135.

4. Tseng JJ, et al. Prenatal diagnosis of isolated fetal hydrocolpos secondary to congenital imperforate hymen. J Chin Med Assoc 2008; 71(6):325–328.

5. Miller RJ, Breech LL. Surgical correction of vaginal anomalies. Clinical Obstet and Gynecol 2008; 51(2):223–236.

6. Pena A, et al. Surgical management of cloacal malformations: a review of 339 patients. J Pediatr Surg 2004; 39(3): 470–479.

7. Sadler TW. Langman's Medical Embryology, 10th ed. Lippincott Williams & Wilkins, 2006, Chap 15, Pp 229–256.

8. DeUgarte CM, et al. Embryology of the urogenital system and congenital anomalies of the female genital tract. In: DeCherney AH, et al. Current Diagnosis and Treatment: Obstetrics and Gynecology, 10th ed. McGraw-Hill, 2007, Chap 4. Available at http://www.accessmedicine.com/content.aspx?aID=2382989.

9. Schorge JO, et al. William's Gynecology. McGraw-Hill, 2008, Chap 18, Anatomic Disorders. Available at http://www.accessmedicine.com/content.aspx?aID=3157418. Chap 41, Surgeries for Benign Gynecologic Conditions. Available at http://www.accessmedicine.com/content.aspx?aID=3166442.

10. David A, Bitoun P, Lacombe D, Lambert J, Nivelon A, Vigneron J, et al. Hydrometrocolpos and polydactyly: a common neonatal presentation of Bardet-Biedl and McKusick-Kaufman syndromes. J Med Gent 1999; 36:599–603.

11. Tekin I, Ok G, Genc A, Tok D. Anaesthetic management in McKusick-Kaufman syndrome. Pediatr Anes 2003; 13:167–170.

12. Kos S, Roth K, Korinth D, Zeilinger, G, Eich G. Hydrometrocolpos post axial polydactyly, and hypothalamic hamartoma in a patient with confirmed Pallister-Hall syndrome: a clinical overlap with McKusick-Kaufman syndrome, Pediatr Radiol 2008; 38:902–906.

13. Shimada K, Hosokawa S, Matsumoto F, Johnun K, Naitoh Y, Harado Y. Urology management of cloacal anomalies. Intl J Urol 2001; 81:282–289.

14. Shono T, Teguchi T, Suita S, Nakanami N, Nekane H. Prenatal ultrasonographic and magnetic resonance imaging findings of congenital cloacal anomalies associated with meconium peritonitis. J Pediatr Surg 2007; 42:681–684.

15. Laufer MR. Diagnosis and management of congenital anomalies of the vagina. Available at http://www.uptodate.com (accessed 2008).

16. Spencer R, Levy DM. Hydrometrocolpos: report of three cases and review of the literature. Ann Surg 1962; 155(4):558–571.

17. Hayashi S, et al. Prenatal diagnosis of fetal hydrometrocolpos secondary to cloacal anomaly by magnetic resonance imaging. Ultrasound Obstet Gynecol 2005; 26:577–579.

18. Dhombres F, et al. Contribution of prenatal imaging to the anatomical assessment of fetal hydrocolpos. Ultrasound Obstet Gynecol 2007; 30:101–104.

19. Powell DM, Newman KD, Randolph J. A proposed classification of vaginal anomalies and their surgical correction. J Pediatr Surg 1995; 30(2):271–275.

20. Rock JA, et al. Pregnancy success following surgical correction of imperforate hymen and complete transverse vaginal septum. Obstet Gynecol 1982; 59:448–452.

21. Joki-Erkkila MM, Heinonen PK. Presenting and long-term clinical implications and fecundity in females with obstructing vaginal malformations. J Pediatr Adolesc Gynecol 2003; 16:307–312.

22. El-Messidi A, Fleming NA. Congenital imperforate hymen and its life-threatening consequences in the neonatal period. J Pediatr Adoles Gyn 2006; 19(2):99–103.

23. Cunningham FG, Leveno KJ, Bloom SL, et al. Williams Obstetrics, 22nd ed. McGraw-Hill, 2005, P 685.

24. Nazir Z, et al. Congenital vaginal obstructions: varied presentation and outcome. Pediatr Surg Int 2006; 22:749–753.

Suggested Reading

Ahment G, et al. Prenatal ultrasonographic features of persistent urogenital sinus with hydrometrocolpos and ascites. Gynecol Obstet 2008; 278:493–496.

Arena F, et al. The neonatal management and surgical correction of urinary hydrometrocolpos caused by a persistent urogenital sinus, BJU Intl 1999; 84:1063–1068.

Ekenze SO, Ezegwui HU. Hydrometrocolpos from a low vaginal atresia: an uncommon cause of neonatal intestinal and urinary obstruction. Afr J Paediatr Surg 2008: 5(1):43–45.

Pena A, Levitt M. Surgical management of cloacal malformations. Sem Neonatology 2003; 8:249–257.

CHAPTER 115
VAGINAL AND UTERINE DUPLICATIONS

Nkeiruka Ameh

Alaa Fayez Hamza

Hesham Mohamed AbdElkader

Introduction

Congenital anomalies of the vagina, cervix, and uterus arise from errors in embryogenesis and are characterised by diversity in anatomic features, clinical presentation, and reproductive performance.[1] Uterine anomalies are associated with both normal and adverse reproductive outcomes.

Demographics

The true prevalence of vaginal and uterine duplications is unknown because the anomaly may not manifest until the reproductive years of the individual.[2] Although a prevalence of 3.2% in the healthy fertile population has been quoted in one study, another study quoted an incidence of 0.1–0.5%.[3,4] Rackow and associates reported an incidence of 3–4% in fertile and infertile women, 5–10% in women with early recurrent pregnancy loss (RPL), and up to 25% in women with late first and second trimester pregnancy loss or preterm delivery.[3,4] Uterine and vaginal duplications can present at birth, in childhood, in adolescence, or in adulthood.[5,6,7]

Aetiology/Pathophysiology

The aetiology of uterine anomalies is embryological in nature. Both male and female embryos initially have two pairs of genital ducts, the mesonephric and paramesonephric ducts. The paramesonephric duct arises as a longitudinal invagination of the coelomic epithelium of the anterolateral surface of the urogenital ridge in a 5- to 7-week embryo. Cranially, the duct opens in the coelomic cavity with a funnel-like structure; caudally, it runs first lateral to the mesonephric duct, but then crosses it ventrally to grow in a caudomedial direction. In the midline,

it comes in close contact with the paramesonephric duct from the opposite side.[3,4] The two ducts are initially separated by a septum but later fuse to form the uterine canal. The caudal tips of the combined ducts project into the posterior wall of the urogenital sinus.

With the descent of the ovary, the upper two-thirds of the fused paramesonephric ducts develops into the uterine tube, and the lower third develops into the uterine canal. The fused walls of the paramesonephric ducts break down to form the cavity of the uterus. Defects in the fusion

Figure 115.1: Diagrammatic representation of the AFS classification of Müllerian duct anomalies.

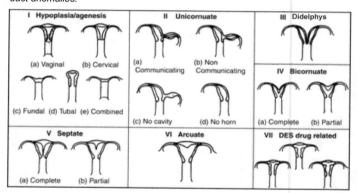

Source: The American Fertility Society Classification of adnexal adhesions, distal tubal occlusion, tubal occlusion secondary to tubal ligation, tubal pregnancies, Müllerian anomalies and intrauterine adhesions. Fertility and Sterility, 1988; 49(6):944–955. Reproduced with kind permission of Elsevier®.

Table 115.1: The AFS classification.

Classification	Clinical Finding	Description
I	Segmental or complete agenesis or hypoplasia	Agenesis and hypoplasia may involve the vagina, cervix, fundus, tubes, or any combination of these structures. Mayer-Rokitansky-Kuster-Hauser (MRKH) syndrome is the most common example in this category.
II	Unicornuate uterus with or without a rudimentary horn	When an associated horn is present, this class is subdivided into communicating (continuity with the main uterine cavity is evident) and noncommunicating (no continuity with the main uterine cavity). The noncommunicating type is further subdivided on the basis of whether an endometrial cavity is present in the rudimentary horn. These malformations have previously been classified under asymmetric lateral fusion defects. The clinical significance of this classification is that they are invariably accompanied by ipsilateral renal and ureter agenesis.
III	Didelphys uterus	Complete or partial duplication of the vagina, cervix, and uterus characterises this anomaly.
IV	Complete or partial bicornuate uterus	Complete bicornuate uterus is characterised by a uterine septum that extends from the fundus to the cervical os. The partial bicornuate uterus demonstrates a septum, which is located at the fundus. In both variants, the vagina and cervix each have a single chamber.
V	Complete or partial septate uterus	A complete or partial midline septum is present within a single uterus.
VI	Arcuate uterus	A small septate indentation is present at the fundus.
VII	Diethylstilbesterol (DES)-related abnormalities	A T-shaped uterine cavity with or without dilated horns is evident.

Source: The American Fertility Society Classification of adnexal adhesions, distal tubal occlusion, tubal occlusion secondary to tubal ligation, tubal pregnancies, Müllerian anomalies and intrauterine adhesions. Fertility and Sterility, 1988; 49(6):944–955. Reproduced with kind permission of Elsevier®.

of the two paramesonephric ducts and failure of the breakdown of the fused middle walls gives rise to congenital anomalies of the uterus.[3,4,8] The upper third of the vagina is derived from the uterine canal, and the lower two-thirds is of urogenital sinus origin. Shortly after the solid tips of the paramesonephric ducts reach the urogenital sinus, two solid evaginations grow out from the pelvic part of the sinus. These evaginations, the sinovaginal bulbs, proliferate strongly and form a solid plate. The proliferation continues at the cranial end of the plate, thus increasing the distance between the uterus and the urogenital sinus. By the 5th gestational month, the vaginal outgrowth is entirely canalised. The wing-like expansions of the vagina are of paramesonephric origin.[8] Duplication and atresia of the uterine canal, or lack of fusion of the paramesonephric ducts in a localised area or throughout the length of the ducts, may explain all the different types of duplication of the uterus. In its extreme form, the uterus is entirely double (uterus didelphys).[8]

Classification

In 1979, Buttram and Gibbons[9] proposed a classification arranged into six subgroups. This classification was revised in 1988 by the American Fertility Society (AFS) (Figure 115.1, Table 115.1).

Clinical Presentation

Complete duplication of the urogenital system in girls is a very rare congenital anomaly. It is characterised by widely variable modes of presentation, depending on the anomaly. Some children present early in the newborn period with abnormalities of the external genitalia, anorectal malformation, or urinary tract obstruction.[3]

Other groups remain asymptomatic for many years, and the anomalies are found during evaluation for infertility or as incidental findings in otherwise healthy young women.[7] They are also most likely to have a higher rate of spontaneous abortion (about 32.2%), preterm birth rate (28.3%), RPL, foetal abnormalties, presentations, and obstructed labours.[4]

Patients with uterine duplication may also present with menorrhagia because of the increased surface area of the two endometrial cavities, dysmenorrhoea, and pelvic pain. Associated anomalies of the urinary system may be coexistent. Other findings include obstructed labour and antepartum and postpartum hemorrhage.

Physical examination may reveal the presence of two vaginal orifices.[7]

Investigation

Several radiologic techniques are useful for evaluating anomalies of the female reproductive tract. Modalities employed include hysterosalpingography, ultrasonography (US), sonohysterography, computed tomography (CT) scan, and magnetic resonance imaging (MRI).[10]

Hysterosalpingography

Hysterosalpingography, commonly used to assess the patency of the fallopian tubes, can provide further information about the contour of the endometrial cavity and the presence of any complex communication in the setting of a Müllerian anomaly[3,4] (Figure 115.2).

Pelvic Ultrasound Scan

Definitive diagnosis of a uterine abnormality requires assessment of the external uterine contour. Transabdominal, transvaginal, or transperineal US effectively evaluates the internal and external uterine contour; detects a pelvic mass, haematometra, or haematocolpos; confirms the presence of ovaries; and assesses the kidneys. Transrectal US has been reported to help in defining the pelvic anatomy, which can be especially useful in young patients.[11] Timing the study to the secretory phase of the menstrual cycle provides better visualisation of the endometrium and thus the internal uterine contour[4] (Figure 115.3).

Sonohysterography

Sonohysterography can further delineate the intracavitary space and internal and external uterine contours. Three-dimensional (3D) US (Figure 115.4) is a highly accurate imaging modality that provides

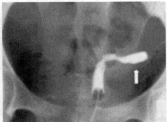
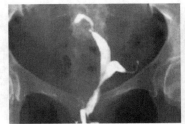

Figure 115.2: Hysterosalpingography of bipartite (left) and unicornuate (right) uteri.

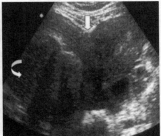
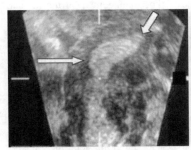

Figure 115.3: Sonographic appearance of Müllerian duct anomaly.

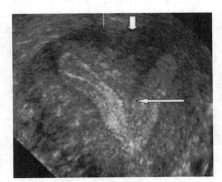

Figure 115.4: 3D sonographic view of a bicornuate uterus.

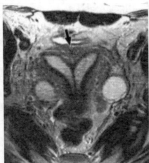
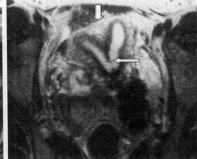

Figure 115.5: Magnetic resonance imaging appearance of bicornuate uterus.

thorough views of the pelvic anatomy and detailed visualisation of the uterus. This is a reliable method of evaluating Müllerian anomalies.[10]

A combination of sonohysterography and laparoscopy will sufficiently diagnose a uterine anomaly. The urinary system also needs to be evaluated by using US scan and an intravenous urography because of the coexistence of uterine anomalies and urinary abnormalities.[10]

Magnetic Resonance Imaging

MRI is considered the gold standard technique for diagnosing Müllerian anomalies; it is both sensitive and specific. This modality provides excellent delineation of internal and external uterine contours. MRI (Figure 115.5) can distinguish a myometrial versus a fibrous uterine division and thus distinguish among bicornuate, didelphic, and septate uterus as well as determine the extent of a uterine or vaginal septum. MRI can also identify a rudimentary uterine horn and determine whether functional endometrium is present. However, in low-resource settings such as those found in the African continent, MRI may not be available, or if available may be unaffordable to some patients.[4,5,11]

Management

The initial management of a patient with uterine and urinary duplication is to investigate and determine the degree of the anomaly and associated anomalies of the urinary system. A serum electrolytes and urea and blood cross match are needed.[7,11] The management of uterine and urinary duplication in the younger group when associated with anorectal anomalies is done at the time of the repair of the anorectal anomaly.[7]

Management of these conditions typically relates to three primary issues: menstrual problems, fertility problems, and sexual function problems. The presence and severity of these areas, along with the type of anomaly present, will help to dictate the appropriate management. It should be stated that the mere presence of an abnormality does not necessitate treatment unless the patient is symptomatic as a result of it.[4]

Menstrual disturbances typically relate to outflow anomalies most commonly represented by a transverse or blocking septum, but also are seen with an absence of the vagina or cervical anomalies. In these circumstances, menstrual blood builds up behind the blockage and can result in pain. Additionally, it has been found that patients with blocked outflow are at increased risk of developing endometriosis—likely secondary to increased retrograde menses. The major concern in treating these patients is to create a passageway through which the menses can flow.

As mentioned previously, infertility is probably the most common presenting complaint in affected patients. This may be the result of problems relating to fertilisation (due to blockage of the sperm's path), implantation, or pregnancy maintenance. The type of abnormality will guide the approach to treatment. Many assisted reproductive techniques are now available.

Sexual function can be affected in a couple of ways. The most obvious is in the situation of a complete absence of the vagina. In this circumstance, normal intercourse would be impossible and creation of a neovagina may be appropriate. In the case of both a transverse and longitudinal septum, a physical barrier may make intercourse difficult, painful, or even impossible, as the calibre and length of the vagina may be altered.[4]

After consideration of the above, a decision can be made by both the patient and physician as to how to proceed. In cases of minor abnormalities, such as a uterine partial septum or even a complete septum, hysteroscopic resection can be an appropriate choice, particularly if fertility is an issue. The advantages of hysteroscopy include the shorter duration of surgery, smaller blood loss, lower costs, reduced morbidity, and shorter hospital stay compared with abdominal surgery.[1,3] In select women with RPL or preterm delivery, uterine reconstruction with Strassman metroplasty achieves unification of two endometrial cavities in a divided uterus and is associated with a live birth rate >80%.[4]

Attempts to unify a double cervix or a septate cervix are not recommended because of the possibility of causing cervical incompetence. However, a double or septate cervix can adversely affect the outcome of delivery if vaginal delivery is attempted, and delivery should be by caesarean section if it appears that the cervix will cause dystocia.[12]

Vaginal septum, if the patient is symptomatic, can usually be treated with a simple resection if small.[4]

In cases of absence of the vagina, surgical and nonsurgical methods can be used to create a neovagina.[13] An appropriate choice in this circumstance depends on the presence or absence of a uterus. If the uterus is present, then creation of a neovagina, along with a communication to the cervix, would be important if menstrual abnormalities exist. If these do not exist, or if there is no uterus, then nonsurgical methods should be employed initially.[13] The nonsurgical approach entails the use of subsequently larger vaginal dilators to stretch the area where the vagina is to be created.

Multiple surgical procedures have been described. The McIndoe surgical procedure for vaginal agenesis is the most well known. A space is dissected between the rectum and the bladder, and a split-thickness skin graft from the buttocks is used to form the vagina; a specially crafted dilator at the time of the procedure creates continuous dilatation of the vagina while the graft heals. Other procedures include Williams vulvovaginoplasty, musculocutaneous flaps, and free intestinal grafts, which are easier and with better results due to the absence of stenosis and need for lubrication.[12] The disadvantage of the intestinal conduits can be excess mucus production and the magnitude of surgery. The decision of which approach to take is dictated by the patient's characteristics and needs.

Given the major advances in infertility treatments, it is possible to perform an in vitro fertilisation (IVF) cycle through the myometrial wall. Therefore, a direct connection of the uterine cavity to the vagina through the cervix may not be an issue when considering fertility problems. When fertility is not an issue and the patient is suffering from menstrual problems, hysterectomy can be a consideration.[14]

Laparoscopy should be used to excise obstructed, rudimentary uterine horns and adjacent tubes in patients with a unicornuate uterus. It should also be used for hysterectomy in cases of cervical agenesis and in neovaginoplasty procedures in cases of vaginal agenesis. In many women, the malformation results in obstructed and retrograde menstruation, thereby facilitating the development of endometriosis. During laparoscopy, this diagnosis may be confirmed and the endometrial foci may be resected.[1]

Postoperative Complication

The complication of pelvic infection can be prevented by administering broad spectrum antibiotics intra- and postoperatively. Haemorrhage may occur if the sutures are not properly applied; therefore, meticulous application of sutures intraoperatively is very important.[12]

Prognosis and Outcome

A good prognosis with improvement in reproductive performance subsequently has been documented.[15,16] The pregnancy outcome has improved following unification procedures. Other causes of infertility have to be excluded by investigation, however, before embarking on this procedure.[16]

Ethical Issues

In Africa, genital surgery is a taboo for some patients and their families. Delayed presentation is very common, and refusal of treatment is common in some communities. One of the major challenges is convincing the patients and their families to perform vaginal dilatations; that is why the choice of surgery depends mainly on social conditions.

Evidence-Based Research

Table 115.2 presents a randomised study of two different techniques in surgical excision of a uterine septum.

Table 115.2: Evidence-based research.

Title	Small-diameter hysteroscopy with Versapoint versus resectoscopy with a unipolar knife for the treatment of septate uterus: a prospective randomized study
Authors	Colacurci N, De Franciscis P, Mollo A, Litta P, Perino A, Cobellis A
Institution	Department of Gynecology, Obstetrics and Reproductive Sciences, Second University of Naples, Naples, Italy
Reference	J Minim Invasive Gynecology 2007; 14(5):622–627
Problem	Role of two different techniques of metroplasties were analysed in surgical excision of a uterine septum.
Intervention	Small diameter hysteroscope with Versapoint™, resectoscope with unipolar knife.
Comparison/ control (quality of evidence)	Two groups of patients. In group A (n = 80), a 26F hysteroscope with unipolar knife was used for excision of the uterine septum. In group B (n = 80), a 5-mm hysteroscope with Versapoint device was used. The study was conducted in 2001–2005.
Outcome/ effect	Operative time and fluid absorption were significantly lower in group A (23.4±5.7 vs 16.9±4.7). The complication rate was significantly lower in group B than in group A. No difference in any of the reproductive parameters was observed between the two groups: pregnancy and delivery rates were 70% and 81.6%, respectively, in group A versus 76.9% and 84%, respectively, in group B. Nine women (18.4%) from group A and 8 women (16%) from group B experienced spontaneous abortions.
Historical significance/ comments	This report randomly compared two hysteroscopic techniques in performing metroplasties for a large group of women having uterine septa. The study used a variety of parameters to compare the two groups: operative parameters were operative time, fluid absorption, complications, and need for second intervention; reproductive outcome parameters were pregnancy, abortion, term and preterm delivery, modality of delivery, and cervical cerclage. Most patients (54/82) delivered by caesarean section without differences according to the hysteroscopic technique used for metroplasty (65% in group A vs 67.7% in group B) or to the gestational age (65.1% of term and 68.7% of preterm deliveries). Small-diameter hysteroscopy with bipolar electrode for the incision of the uterine septum is as effective as resectoscopy with a unipolar electrode regarding reproductive outcome and is associated with a shorter operating time and a lower complication rate.

Key Summary Points

1. Müllerian anomalies are congenital defects of the female reproductive tract resulting from failure in the development of the Müllerian ducts and their associated structures. Their cause has yet to be fully clarified; it is currently believed to be multifactorial.

2. The embryological development of the female reproductive system is closely related to the development of the urinary system, and anomalies in both systems may occur in up to 25% of these patients. Other associated malformations may affect the gastrointestinal tract (12%) or musculoskeletal system (10–12%).

3. Müllerian anomalies are frequently asymptomatic and are often missed in routine gynecological examinations. Nevertheless, a history of pelvic pain following menarche, dysmenorrhea, and an increase in abdominal volume are complaints suggestive of uterine anomalies. In addition, primary amenorrhea and changes to menstrual flows may be present.

4. Due to the complexity of presentations, diagnosing Müllerian malformations requires the use of more than one imaging method in 62% of the cases.

5. The treatment for Müllerian anomalies varies according to the specific type of malformation found in each patient.

6. Müllerian anomalies consist of a wide range of defects that may vary from patient to patient. Therefore, their management must also be individual, taking anatomical and clinical characteristics into consideration, as well as the patient's preference.

References

1. Patton PE, Novy MJ, Lee DM, Hickok LR. The diagnosis and reproductive outcome after surgical treatment of the complete septate uterus, duplicated cervix and vaginal septum. Am J Obstet Gynecol 2004;190:1669–1678.

2. Adeyinka AO, Ibinaiye PO. Bicornuate unicollis uterus with left renal agenesis. Trop J Obstetr Gynaecol 2006; 23:72–74.

3. Troiano RN, McCarthy MS. Mullarian duct anomalies: imaging and clinical issues. Radiology 2004; 233:19–34.

4. Rackow BW, Aydin A. Reproductive performance of women with Mullerian anomalies. Curr Opin Obstet Gynecol 2007;19:229–237.

5. Tolete-velcek F, Hansbrough F, Kugaczewski J, Coren CV, Klotz DH, Price AF, Laungani G, Kottmeier PK. Utero vaginal malformations: a trap for the unsuspecting surgeon. J Pediatr Surg 1989; 24:736–740.

6. Goh DW, Davey BR, Dewan PA. Bladder, urethral and vaginal duplication. J Pediatr Surg 1995; 30:125–126.

7. Gastol PM, Baka-Jakubiak M, Skobejko-Wlodarska L, Szymkiewicz C. Complete duplication of the bladder, urethra, vagina and uterus in girls. Urology 2000; 55:578–581.

8. Moore KL, Persaud TVN. The developing human: clinically oriented embryology. Saunders, 1998, Pp 305–345.

9. Buttram VC Jr, Gibbons WE. Müllerian anomalies: a proposed classification. (An analysis of 144 cases). Fertil Steril 1979; 32:40–46.

10. Alborzi S, Dehbashi S, Parsanezhad ME. Differential diagnosis of septate and bicornuate uterus by sonohysterography eliminates the need for laparascopy. Fertil Steril 2002; 78:176–178.

11. Mazouni C, Girard G, Deter R, Haumonte JB, Blanc B, Bretelle F. Diagnosis of Mullerian anomalies in adults: evaluation of practice. Fertil Steril 2008; 89:219–222.

12. Rock JA, Breech LL. Surgery for anomalies of the Mullerian ducts. In: Rock JA, Jones WH, eds. Te Linde's Operative Gynecology, 9th ed. Lippincott Williams & Wilkins, 2003, Pp 705–752.

13. Edmonds DK. Normal and abnormal development of the genital tract. In: Edmonds DK, ed. Dewhurst's Textbook of Obstetrics and Gynaecology for Postgraduates. Blackwell Science, 1999, Pp 1–11.

14. Heinonen PK. Complete septate uterus with longitudinal vaginal septum. Fertil Steril 2006; 85:700–705.

15. Zlopasa G, Skrablin S, Kalafatic D, Banovic V, Lesin J. Uterine anomalies and pregnancy outcome following resectocope metroplasty. Int J Gynecol Obstet 2007; 98:129–133.

16. Heinonem PK. Clinical implications of the didelphic uterus: long-term follow-up of 49 cases. Eur J Obstet Gynencol Reprod Biol 2000; 91:183–190.

CHAPTER 116
LABIAL ADHESIONS/AGGLUTINATION

Adesoji O. Ademuyiwa
Safwat S. Andrawes
Modupe Odelola
Kokila Lakhoo

Introduction

Labial agglutination, also known as labial adhesions, vulvar fusion, or vulvar synachia, describes the apposition of the labia minora, which may be complete or partial.[1] It constitutes one of the minor gynaecological conditions in prepubertal girls that may present to the paediatric surgeon.

Demographics

There are few reports from Africa on epidemiology of labial agglutination. A hospital-based study from Nigeria has put the prevalence at 3%.[2] In the United States, the incidence is between 1% and 5%;[3,4] however, the incidence is likely to be higher because most patients are asymptomatic and will not present to the hospital. Although labial agglutination is a disease that affects prepubertal girls, there are reports that it may occur in postpubertal girls, but these cases usually follow trigger factors such as trauma and sexual abuse.[5] The peak age of incidence is the second year of life.[3]

Aetiology and Pathophysiology

The aetiology of labial agglutination is unknown; however, low oestrogen levels are a possible cause in this age group.[6] Other causes include vulvitis, trauma, and—in Africa—the practice of female genital cutting (mutilation) (FGC(M)), which predisposes to labial fusion as a complication.[7,8]

Labial agglutination is an acquired disorder. Studies on newborns did not show any infants with this condition.[3] Inflammation of the labial epithelium from either trauma or infection in a background of low levels of oestrogen results in denuded epithelium. Healing of the epithelium thereafter results in the adhesion.

Clinical Presentation

Labial agglutination is often asymptomatic. Most who present to hospital do so after their parents observe that the "vaginal opening" is not visible (Figure 116.1). Others will present because of urinary leakage from a small hole during micturition or difficulty in micturition. Some adolescent girls present with haematocolpos following menarche.

Presentation in hospital may be for another condition, and the physician (paediatrician or general practitioner) may pick up the labial agglutination. There is usually extreme parental anxiety, but this is disproportionate to the simple nature of the lesion.

Careful physical examination should be made in all cases. The labia majora are usually present and easily separated The labia minora are fused together in the midline; fusion is complete if it is from the clitoris to the posterior vestibule and partial if there is some separation between the labia minora. The diagnosis of labial agglutination is clinical, and investigation of the upper genital tract is not necessary.

Differential diagnoses include imperforate hymen or scarring of the labia minora in girls who have had FGC(M), in which the labia majora may have been excised partially or completely. Others include absent vagina and scarring of the labia minora following sexual abuse and certain forms of intersexuality and cloacal malformation.

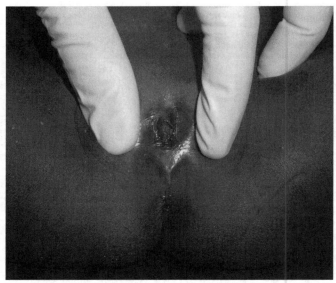

Figure 116.1: Preseparation appearance of labial agglutination.

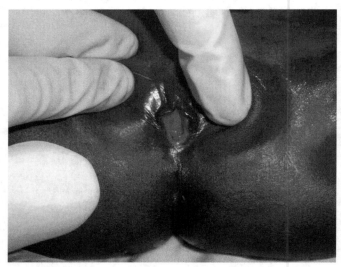

Figure 116.2: Postseparation appearance of labial agglutination.

Management

The care of the female child with labial minora should include the relief of parental anxiety as well as health education on perineal hygiene, especially in the African setting. Wiping the perineum from the front to the back after defecation, frequent change of diapers, and avoidance of irritant ones are important to the overall success of the treatment given to the child.[9]

Specific treatment measures can be medical or surgical. Gentle application of oestrogen cream topically to the fused labia twice daily for a variable period of between 2 to 6 weeks has been found to lead to separation of the labia.

Surgical separation (Figure 116.2) using a topical anaesthetic agent such as a eutectic mixture of local anaesthetics (EMLA) cream (in this case, lidocaine and prilocaine) or xylocaine cream with the separation effected using "mosquito" artery forceps can be carried out in the clinic. In older children who may not cooperate, separation under general anaesthesia can be done in the theatre. There may be slight bleeding, but this resolves spontaneously. Postoperatively, petroleum jelly, such as Vaseline®, may be applied to prevent recurrence or it can be combined with medical treatment using oestrogen cream.

Postoperative Complications

Minor haemorrhage may occur postoperatively, but it is unusual for it to be troublesome. Recurrence is the most common complication (with rates of up to 39% in some series), especially if the other supportive measures are not meticulously followed. Treatment of recurrent labial agglutination can be managed either medically by oestrogen cream or surgically. Hyperpigmentation of the skin may result from the application of topical oestrogen cream, but it usually resolves with discontinuation after treatment.

Prognosis and Outcome

The prognosis is good. Most asymptomatic cases usually resolve at puberty with the increase in circulating oestrogen levels. For symptomatic cases following separation, the outcomes are equally good.

Prevention

Health education for the parents is important to promote good hygienic practice to prevent irritation of the perineum in their child, with clear instructions on what to do in order to prevent recurrence as well as the same condition in their other children.

Evidence-Based Research

Table 116.1 presents a prospective study that compares the outcomes of treatment using conservative treatment methods with topical application of oestrogen cream alone with surgical manual separation of the labia and a combination of surgery with adjuvant application of oestrogen cream.

Table 116.1: Evidence-based research.

Title	Topical estrogen therapy in labial adhesions in children: therapeutic or prophylactic?
Authors	Soyer T
Institution	Ankara Güven Hospital, Department of Pediatric Surgery, Ankara, Turkey
Reference	J Pediatr Adoles Gynecol 2007; 20:241–244
Problem	Role of topical oestrogen application and surgery in treatment of labial agglutination
Intervention	Topical application of oestrogen, surgical separation, combination of surgery and oestrogen application.
Comparison/ control (quality of evidence)	Forty-nine patients were grouped into three groups: 18 were treated with oestrogen cream alone, 14 were treated by surgical separation of the fused labia minora, and 17 had surgical separation followed by topical application of oestrogen cream.
Outcome/ effect	The success rate in those treated with oestrogen cream alone was 66.6% at the third month and 55.5% in the ninth month. Recurrence was experienced in 2 (11%) patients. There was a success rate of 85.7% in those who had surgical separation only, both in the 3rd and 9th months, and recurrence was 14.2%. All of the patients (100%) treated by manual separation with prophylaxis (MSP) recovered when followed up at 3 and 9 months. The topical oestrogen group had significantly lower success rates when compared to the other two groups (P = 0.002). There was no statistical difference between those who had surgery alone and those who had surgery and adjuvant oestrogen cream application and the MSP groups (P = 0.196).
Historical significance/ comments	Labial agglutination can be successfully managed with oestrogen cream alone; however, the success rates are significantly lower when compared with surgical separation. Recurrence can be treated successfully with either topical oestrogen or surgery. A combination of surgical separation and adjuvant topical oestrogen may have a superior outcome. Larger series, however, may be necessary to validate this finding.

Key Summary Points

1. Labial agglutination is one of the gynaecological conditions in prepubertal girls that may present to the paediatric surgeon.

2. Although the aetiology is unknown, low levels of oestrogen have been implicated.

3. In Africa, female genital mutilation practices and sexual abuse of children are important causal factors.

4. Labial agglutination is often asymptomatic; however, urinary leakage following micturition and urinary tract infection can be the presenting complaints.

5. Diagnosis of labial agglutination is clinical, and invasive investigation of the genital tract should be avoided.

6. Differential diagnosis includes atresia of the vagina, imperforate hymen, and ambiguous genitalia and cloacal malformation.

7. Treatment includes use of topical oestrogen or surgical separation or a combination of both, which has lower recurrence rates.

8. Health education on perineal hygiene is vital to prevention of the condition and avoids recurrence after treatment.

9. An important aspect of the treatment of this simple condition is to relieve parental anxiety.

References

1. Leung AK, Robson WLM, Wong B. Labial fusion. Pediatr Child Health 1996; 1:216–218.

2. Bobzom DN, Mai MA, Akpede GO, Chama CM. Paediatric and teenage gynaecological disorders in northern Nigeria. Ann Trop Paediatr 1997; 17(3):229–232.

3. Leung AK, Robson WL, Tay-Uyboco J. The incidence of labial fusion in children. J Paediatr Child Health 1993; 29:235–236.

4. Alagiri M. Labial adhesions. Available at www.emedicine.com (accessed September 2008).

5. Kumar RK, Sonika A, Charu C, Sunesh K, Neena M. Labial adhesion in post-pubertal girls: case report. Obstet Gynaecol Forum 2005; 15(4):22–23.

6. Omar HA. Management of labial adhesions in prepubertal girls. J Pediatr Adolesc Gynecol 2000;13:183–186.

7. Ekenze SO, Ezegwui HU, Adiri CO. Genital lesions complicating female genital cutting in infancy: a hospital-based study in south-east Nigeria. Ann Trop Paediatr: Intl Child Health 2007; 27(4); 285–290.

8. Odelola MA, Bode CO. Labial agglutination in prepubertal girls in Lagos. J Clinic Sci 2003; 3(1):35–37.

9. Kumetz LM, Fisseha S, Quint EH, Haefner HK, Smith YR. Common pediatric vulvar disorders: vulvovaginitis, lichen sclerosus, and labial agglutination. Available at http://www.medscape.com/viewprogram/4406 (accessed September 2008).

CHAPTER 117
OVARIAN LESIONS

Emily Stamell
Adekunle O. Oguntayo
Evan P. Nadler

Introduction

Ovarian lesions in paediatric patients require special considerations that may not be applicable in adult patients with comparable diseases. Importantly, these lesions do not follow the same histologic distribution as those seen in adults. They range from benign cysts that can regress spontaneously to bilateral malignancies that require aggressive treatment. Gynecological malignancies account for about 1–2% of all paediatric cancers, and roughly 60–70% of gynecological malignancies are ovarian in origin.[1,2] The diagnosis of ovarian malignancies can often be challenging. Early detection is vital not only for fertility preservation, but also for cure or disease-free remission. Early detection may be even more difficult in developing countries, where access to health care may be limited.

Demographics

Worldwide and African incidence of ovarian lesions has not been reported; however, the incidence of all ovarian masses in childhood in the United States is approximately 2.6 cases per 100,000 girls per year, and malignancy is reported in 16–55% of cases.[2] In North America, the frequency of ovarian cancer has actually decreased due to the identification of tumour markers, newer diagnostic imaging modalities, and reclassifying the pathology, which allows better identification of all gonadal masses.[3] Laboratory tests for tumour markers and the newer imaging modalities are not readily available or are too expensive to be commonly used in many African regions, however. The frequency of ovarian lesions is greatly influenced by age in North America. Table 117.1 provides the age of peak incidence for ovarian neoplasms in the paediatric population.[4]

Table 117.1: Age of peak incidence for common ovarian neoplasms.

Tumour	Age of peak incidence
Mature cystic teratomas	>5 years
Granulosa cell tumour	< 9 years
Yolk sac tumours	10–14 years
Surface epithelial tumours	>10 years

Aetiology/Pathophysiology

Ovarian lesions can arise from different cell types, so the aetiology can vary; however, there is a consistent trend of normal tissue underlying the abnormal lesions. Ovarian cysts arise from mature follicles, and neonatal and prepubertal children have been shown to have active follicular growth in the appropriate hormonal millieu. Neoplastic ovarian tumours can arise from germinal epithelium surrounding the urogenital ridge, stromal tissue comprising the urogenital ridge, or germ cells from the yolk sac. The cells dedifferentiate, proliferate, and then undergo malignant transformation. Surface epithelial tumours are more common in women who ovulate more frequently over their lifetime, whereas germ cell tumours are most common in younger children.

It is proposed that the more times a follicle ruptures, the more times the ovary epithelium repairs itself, which can increase cellular errors, in turn allowing for increased malignant transformation. This principle

may explain why it is believed that pregnancy confers some protection against ovarian cancer, especially in women with high parity. The relevance of this theory in young children is unclear because they either have not begun to ovulate or have ovulated very few times. Sex cord-stromal tumours arise from mesenchymal stem cells below the surface epithelium of the urogenital ridge. These cells have not committed to a cell lineage; therefore, they can differentiate into different cell lines.[5]

A number of syndromes are associated with ovarian tumours. Examples include, but are certainly not limited to, Peutz-Jeghers syndrome and granulosa cell tumours, Ollier's disease and juvenile granulosa cell tumours, Sertoli-Leydig cell tumours, and Maffucci syndrome and fibrosarcoma.[6–8] In nonfamilial cases of ovarian malignancy, infertility and nulliparity have been shown to increase the risk.[8,9] Conversely, multiparity and the use of oral contraceptive pills have been shown to decrease the risk.[10] Other, more controversial, factors that increase the risk of ovarian cancer include the use of ovulation-induction medications and diets that include animal fats, dairy products, and lactose.[5] Genetics have been shown to predispose women to breast and ovarian cancer in roughly 5–10% of patients. The tumour suppressor genes BRCA1 and BRCA2 have been unequivocally linked to ovarian cancer.[11,12] Although other genes are likely responsible for hereditary ovarian cancer, they remain unknown.

Pathology

The term "ovarian lesion" encompasses a number of nonneoplastic and neoplastic lesions that can be distinguished based on histological features. Tables 117.2 and 117.3 list the nonneoplastic and neoplastic lesions, respectively. The neoplastic lesions comprise both benign and malignant tumours. Nonneoplastic ovarian cysts are included in the spectrum of ovarian lesions because they can produce symptoms mostly related to mass effect and endocrinopathies.[13]

Table 117.2: World Health Organization histologic classification of nonneoplastic ovarian lesions.

Solitary follicle cyst	Stromal hyperplasia
Multiple follicle cyst	Stromal hyperthecosis
Large solitary luteinised follicle cyst of pregnancy and puerperium	Massive oedema
	Fibromatosis
Hyperreactio luteinalis	Endometriosis
Corpus luteum cyst	Cyst, unclassified
Pregnancy luteoma	Inflammatory lesions
Ectopic pregnancy	

Source: Templeman C, Fallat M. Ovarian tumours. In: Grosfeld JL, O'Neill JA Jr, Coran AG, Fonkalsrud EW, Caldamone AA, eds. Pediatric Surgery, Sixth Edition. Mosby Elsevier, 2006, Pp 593–621.

Table 117.3: World Health Organization classification of tumours of the ovary.

Surface epithelial-stromal tumours	Germ cell tumours
Serous tumours	Primitive germ cell tumours
Mucinous tumours	Dysgerminoma
Endometriod tumours	Yolk sac tumour
Clear cell tumours	Embryonal carcinoma
Transitional cell tumours	Polyembryoma
Squamous cell tumours	Nongestational choriocarcinoma
Mixed epithelial tumours	Mixed germ cell tumours
Undifferentiated and unclassified tumours	Biphasic or triphasic teratomas
Sex cord–stromal tumours	Immature
Granulosa–stromal cell tumours	Mature
Granulosa cell tumour group	Monodermal teratomas
Tumours in thecoma-fibroma group	**Germ cell sex cord-stromal tumours**
Sertoli-stromal cell tumours	Gonadoblastoma
Sex cord–stromal tumours of mixed or unclassified cell types	Mixed germ cell–sex cord–stromal tumour of nongonadoblastoma type
Sex cord tumour with annular tubules	**Tumours of rete ovarii**
Gynandroblastoma	**Miscellaneous tumours**
Steroid cell tumours	Small-cell carcinomas, hypercalemic type
	Gestational choriocarcinoma
	Soft-tissue tumours not specific to ovary
	Tumourlike conditions
	Lymphoid and haematopoietic tumours
	Secondary tumours

Source: Templeman C, Fallat M. Ovarian tumours. In: Grosfeld JL, O'Neill JA Jr, Coran AG, Fonkalsrud EW, Caldamone AA, eds. Pediatric Surgery, Sixth Edition. Mosby Elsevier, 2006, Pp 593–621.

Clinical Presentation

The presentation of an ovarian lesion can vary depending on the pathological classification; however, benign and malignant lesions often will have similar clinical presentations.[14] Abdominal pain and/or distention are the most common symptoms in patients with an ovarian lesion regardless of the tumour pathology. Pain can be a result of torsion, rupture, or perforation (Figure 117.1). The most common initial diagnosis based on these symptoms is appendicitis, which must be carefully excluded. Some signs and symptoms can be more indicative of a benign or malignant lesion. Benign lesions will rarely cause vaginal bleeding, whereas malignant ones will often have early bleeding in their development due to hormonal imbalance. Other nonovarian lesions can cause bleeding, most commonly vulvo-vaginitis, but in children the presence of bleeding should prompt a work-up for an ovarian tumour.[15] Other symptoms relating to ovarian neoplasms include anorexia, nausea, vomiting, and urinary frequency.[5]

Endocrine disorders can be detected in roughly 10% of both neoplastic and nonneoplastic ovarian lesions and may be the first sign of disease. Isosexual precocious puberty occurs with ovarian cysts and sex cord–stromal tumours, most commonly granulosa cell tumours, but can also occur in Sertoli-Leydig cell tumours, due to the production of oestrogen. Patients with central precocious puberty or premature thelarche can also develop similar signs and symptoms.[16] Granulosa-theca cell tumours can be differentiated from true sexual precocious puberty, gonadotropin-secreting lesions, or feminising adrenal tumours by increased serum and urinary oestrogen levels, which are low in the other three conditions.[5] Precocious pseudopuberty can occur in patients with germ cell tumours that produce human chorionic gonadotropin. Heterosexual precocious puberty can be seen in Sertoli-Leydig cell tumours, dysgerminomas with syncytial trophoblastic giant cells, yolk sac tumours, steroid cell tumours, and polycystic ovaries.[5] Patients with heterosexual precocious puberty present with the following signs, depending on the stage of development: defeminisation then masculinisation, breast atrophy, oligomenorrhea then amenorrhea, voice-deepening, hirsuitism, male pattern hair growth, and clitoromegaly.[16]

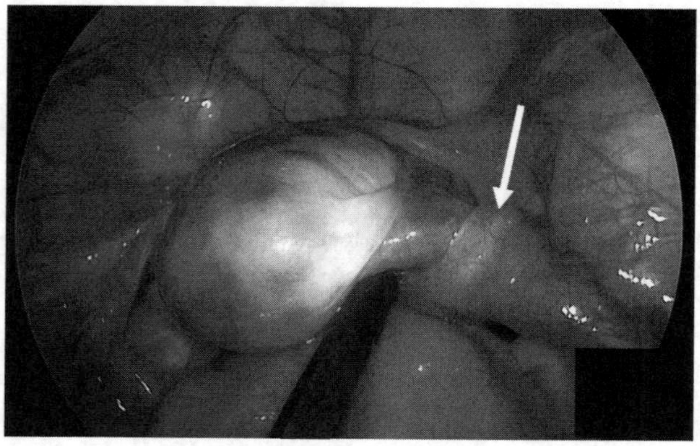

A thorough physical exam should be the first step in evaluating any patient suspected of having a potential ovarian lesion. More than 60% of patients with ovarian tumours have a palpable abdominal mass below the pelvic brim, with or without tenderness.[14] A bimanual examination between the lower abdomen and rectum can assist in palpating smaller lesions. In general, vaginal examination is reserved for sexually active women.

Investigations

Laboratory tests consisting of specific tumour markers or hormones can be useful in the diagnosis and follow-up of an ovarian lesion; however, these tests may not be available in all regions. Although neither tumour markers nor hormones are specific to an ovarian lesion, they are inexpensive methods of evaluating a possible diagnosis. Tables 117.4 and 117.5 list the ovarian tumours with their associated tumour markers and serum hormone levels, respectively.

Imaging plays a central role in the diagnosis of ovarian lesions. Ultrasound (US) is the gold standard imaging technique. It is quick and cost-effective with no radiation exposure. Transabdominal US should be used with a distended bladder. Alternatively, transvaginal US, which entails placement of a high-frequency transducer in the mid to upper portion of the vagina, is utilised in nonvirginal teenagers, but should not be used in children. Transperineal imaging—placement of a transducer directly on the introitus—may be used for children. The normal ovarian size fluctuates throughout a woman's life-span.[17] The structural appearance of the ovaries also varies. Both are important factors in evaluating the ovaries in different age groups. Children younger than 8 years of age usually have solid and ovoid ovaries with a homogeneous echogenic texture. During and after puberty the ovaries develop cystic structure, reflecting the ovulatory cyle. These normal follicular cysts appear anechoic and thin-walled and have strong acoustic enhancement.[18]

Figure 117.1: Laparoscopic view of torsion of the right ovary in a peripubertal female. Note the twisting of the fallopian tube (arrow).

Table 117.4: Ovarian tumours and tumour markers.

Histological subtype	Tumour marker
Endometrioma	CA-125
Epithelial	
Borderline	CA-125
Carcinoma	CA-125
Germ cell (pure tumours)	
Dysgerminoma	b-hCG, LDH
Yolk sac	AFP, b-HCG
Immature teratoma	
Choriocarcinoma	b-hCG
Embryonal	AFP, b-hCG
Endodermal sinus	AFP
Sertoli-Leydig	AFP

Table 117.5: Ovarian tumours and hormones.

Histological subtype	Hormone
Ovarian cyst	
Simple	Increased estradiol
Follicular	Increased estradiol
Luteal	Increased estradiol
Sex cord–stromal	
Juvenile granulosa	Increased estradiol, increased testosterone
Sertoli-Leydig	Increased estradiol, increased testosterone
Luteinised thecoma	Increased estradiol, increased testosterone
Sex cord tumour with annular tubules	Increased estradiol
Steroid cell tumour	Increased testosterone, increased urinary 17-ketosteroid
Gonadoblastoma	Increased estradiol, increased testosterone, increased urinary 17-ketosteroid, decreased gonadotropins
Choriocarcinoma	Increased estradiol, increased gonadotropins

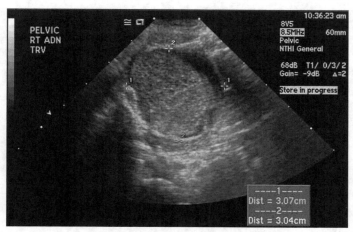

Figure 117.2: Ultrasound view of an in utero torsion of the right ovary diagnosed in a one-month-old infant. The mass is echogenic without any evidence of blood flow.

Ovarian masses have a variety of appearances on US. In general, benign tumours are complex hypoechoic masses with peripheral echogenic mural nodules that may produce acoustic shadowing. Specifically, classic benign cysts will have sharp posterior walls, have strong acoustic enhancement, and be echoless. Benign cysts can be distinguished from haemorrhagic cysts, which have diffuse, homogeneous, or complex internal echoes and decreased acoustic enhancement. Mature teratomas have a large cystic component in addition to at least one mural nodule. Additionally, they can be homogeneously echogenic due to the presence of calcifications, fat, sebaceous material, or matted hair. Teratomas are bilateral 25% of the time, so the contralateral ovary should be evaluated. Malignant ovarian tumours are usually complex masses with an average size of 15 cm, but are at least larger than 10 cm. The solid component is not hyperechoic and is usually nodular or papillary, and there are often thick septations. Color or power Doppler can be useful in identifying blood flow to the ovary to rule out torsion as well as in the solid component of the tumour (Figure 117.2). Other signs of malignancy include ascites, omental or peritoneal implants, lymphadenopathy, and hepatic metastases. Ovarian tumours can contain calcifications, which appear stippled in dysgerminomas and coarse in malignant teratomas.[17]

Other imaging modalities may play a role in the diagnosis of ovarian lesions. Computed tomography (CT) scans and magnetic resonance imaging (MRI) are superior to US for tumour staging, when the origin of the pelvic masses is unclear on US, or when the extent of a noncystic lesion cannot be fully assessed by US[17] (Figure 117.3). However, these modalities add cost to the evaluation and may not be necessary. Although CT does have utility (it easily identifies direct extension of tumours into other pelvic, abdominal, or chest structures), the benefits should be weighed against the risk of radiation exposure and the cost of the exam.

MRI is useful, especially in patients with ample subcutaneous fat, but again, it is expensive and often unnecessary. MRI is extremely accurate in determining the origin of a lesion and can demonstrate specific characteristics. Even though MRI has no radiation exposure, it requires more imaging time, which can often be difficult in paediatric patients who necessitate the use of sedation.[5] Both CT and MRI are far more costly than US and may have limited use in African hospitals, where US is able to narrow down the differential diagnosis and guide care in a majority of cases.

Management

The management of ovarian lesions depends on the histological classification of the lesion. In paediatric patients, treatment of ovarian lesions should attempt to preserve the most reproductive function while also providing complete treatment of the lesion. These considerations are often irrelevant in adult patients with comparable disease because

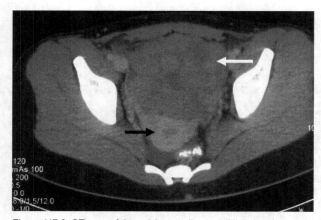

Figure 117.3: CT scan of the pelvis revealing a multilobulated mass (white arrow) in a 17-year-old girl. The mass is separate from the uterus (black arrow). Contrast is seen in the rectum. Final pathology revealed a dysgerminoma.

childbearing has often been completed. Treatment can be modified to the individual patient to preserve reproductive and menstrual functions.[13] A general algorithm can be applied, with the caveat that the treatment depends on the aggressiveness of the specific histological subtype and, of course, on the individual patient.

Nonneoplastic Ovarian Lesions

The management of ovarian cysts is controversial. Nonneoplastic ovarian cysts should rarely be treated surgically in patients other then neonates; however, if surgical intervention is warranted, it should always be conservative.

Follicular cysts

Neonatally diagnosed follicular cysts will generally regress on their own, necessitating only observation with serial ultrasounds. The management of follicular cysts in prepubertal children with acute symptoms and endocrine activity may require more invasive treatment. Operative intervention has been indicated for acute, severe abdominal pain, symptoms persisting for more than 24 hours, imaging studies indicating a neoplasm, a cyst increasing in size, or failure to regress on follow-up ultrasound. The use of US has increased the detection of cysts in children. One study found that large cysts in children, defined as greater than 5 cm, can be followed with serial US due to the high rate of spontaneous regression. Surgical intervention should be based on US characteristics, symptomatology, evidence of a neoplasm, and failure of cyst to regress.[19]

Corpus luteum cysts

Corpus luteum cysts develop only in ovulating women and usually will regress spontaneously. Persistent corpus luteum cysts can rupture, undergo torsion, or cause menstrual irregularities or dysfunctional uterine bleeding. Surgical intervention is indicated if there are acute symptoms or if the cyst persists for 4–6 weeks after the initial diagnosis. Ovarian cystectomy is the procedure of choice; however, if the manipulation necessary to remove the lesion threatens either gonad, then the cyst should be unroofed, debulked, and excised to the extent possible. Unilateral oophorectomy is indicated only if there is no possibility of preserving normal tissue, but the ipsilateral fallopian tube should not be resected since it can still transport ova from the contralateral ovary.

Parovarian cysts

Parovarian cysts do not arise from gonadal tissue; however, their location generates the same concerns regarding treatment. Parovarian cysts are often small and asymptomatic. Cysts less than 3 cm can be treated with bipolar coagulation of the cyst wall, but those greater than 3 cm should be enucleated via the mesosalpinx.[20]

Neoplastic Ovarian Lesions

Neoplastic ovarian tumours have a range of treatment modalities based on the pathogenesis of the histological tumour type. In general, lesions limited to one ovary can be treated with a unilateral salpingo-oophorectomy. Lesions limited to both ovaries can be managed with a bilateral salpingo-oophorectomy (BSO), preserving the uterus for future fertility options. Unfortunately, assisted reproductive endocrinology is an expensive option and therefore may be limited in Africa. Extensive disease requires BSO with a total abdominal hysterectomy, omentectomy, lymph node sampling, and peritoneal washings. Adjuvant therapies are variable, providing the best outcomes in certain ovarian cancers.

Surface epithelial-stromal tumours

The stage of the tumour, as determined by the International Federation of Gynecology and Obstetrics for surface epithelial-stromal tumours,[5] dictates treatment (Table 117.6). Stage IA tumours (one ovary) are treated with unilateral salpingo-oophorectomy, whereas stage IB tumours require BSO. Hysterectomy is not necessary. Studies have shown that epithelial borderline tumours can be treated with fertility-sparing surgery in fertile woman without an increased risk of recurrence.[21] Unfortunately, more advanced stages of surface epithelial tumours require total abdominal hysterectomy with BSO along with omentectomy, intraperitoneal debulking, if necessary, and peritoneal washings. In addition, advanced stages require adjuvant chemotherapy.[22] The current recommended systemic chemotherapy regimen includes a platinum agent (cisplatin or carboplatin) and a taxane (paclitaxel or docetaxel).[23]

Tumours of low malignant potential

Epithelial tumours of low malignant potential generally occur in younger patients and have a better prognosis than epithelial tumours. Usually, these tumours behave in a benign manner; however, they do have the potential to recur as many as 10 to 15 years after the primary tumour and cause metastatic disease. Conservative therapy is recommended for stage I tumours, and more recently for advanced-stage disease. Surgical management should include unilateral salpingo-oophorectomy or cystectomy. The risk of recurrence following conservative therapy is greater than with a total abdominal hysterectomy with BSO; however,

Table 117.6: International Federation of Gynecology and Obstetrics surgical staging of ovarian carcinoma.

Stage	Extent of disease
I	Tumour limited to the ovaries
IA	Tumour limited to one ovary; no tumour on the external surface, capsule intact
IB	Tumour limited to both ovaries; no tumour on external surface, capsule intact
IC	Stage IA or IB but with tumour on surface of one or both ovaries, with ruptured capsule, or ascites or peritoneal washings containing malignant cells
II	Tumour involving one or both ovaries with pelvic extension or metastases
IIA	Extension and/or metastases to the uterus, fallopian tubes, or both
IIB	Extension to other pelvic tissues
IIC	Stage IIA or IIB but with tumour on the surface of one or both ovaries, with ruptured capsule, or ascites or peritoneal washings containing malignant cells
III	Histologically confirmed metastases outside the pelvis, superficial liver metastases, positive retroperitoneal or inguinal lymph nodes, or tumour limited to the true pelvis but with histologically verified malignant extension to small intestines or omentum
IIIA	Gross tumour limited to the true pelvis with negative lymph nodes but with histologically confirmed microscopic tumour outside pelvis
IIIB	Histologically confirmed abdominal peritoneal metastases that extend beyond the pelvis and are <2 cm in diameter with negative lymph nodes
IIIC	Abdominal peritoneal metastases that extend beyond the pelvis and are >2 cm in diameter and/or with positive retroperitoneal or inguinal lymph nodes
IV	Distant metastases, including parenchymal liver metastases; if pleural effusion is present, cytologic test results must be positive to signify stage IV

Source: Templeman C, Fallat M. Ovarian tumours. In: Grosfeld JL, O'Neill JA Jr, Coran AG, Fonkalsrud EW, Caldamone AA, eds. Pediatric Surgery, Sixth Edition. Mosby Elsevier, 2006, Pp 593–621.

Table 117.7: Children's Oncology Group staging of ovarian germ cell tumours

Stage	Extent of disease
I	Limited to the ovary
II	Microscopic residual disease, but peritoneal evaluation is negative
III	Lymph node involvement; gross residual or biopsy only; contiguous visceral involvement; peritoneal evaluation positive for malignancy
IV	Distant metastases

Source: Templeman C, Fallat M. Ovarian tumours. In: Grosfeld JL, O'Neill JA Jr, Coran AG, Fonkalsrud EW, Caldamone AA, eds. Pediatric Surgery, Sixth Edition. Mosby Elsevier, 2006, Pp 593–621.

salvage therapy has been shown to have good outcomes. Although controversial, the laparoscopic surgical approach has been shown to be effective in conservative management as long as there is no suggestion that the mass may be malignant. Initial surgery should include limiting staging, which involves peritoneal exploration, washings, and biopsies in addition to contralateral ovarian biopsy. Roughly 50% of tumours occur bilaterally; bilateral oophorocystectomy or salpingo-oophorectomy therefore would be appropriate in these situations.[21]

Sex cord–stromal tumours

Each subtype of sex cord–stromal tumour has specific management requirements. The juvenile form of granulosa-theca cell tumours must be treated differently from adult lesions, which are far more indolent. The juvenile type is very aggressive; the aggressiveness of each tumour can be determined by tumour size, stage of disease, whether the tumour has ruptured, and the amount of nuclear atypia and mitotic figures.

These tumours are staged following the same guidelines outlined in Table 117.6. If a patient is diagnosed with an early-stage lesion, unilateral oophorectomy or salpingo-oophorectomy is adequate due to the low rate of bilateral disease. Advanced-stage lesions are best treated with a multidisciplinary treatment plan, including hysterectomy with BSO, 3000 cGy whole-abdominal radiation with a boost to areas of residual disease, and multidrug chemotherapy including methotrexate, actinomycin D, cyclophosphamide, bleomycin, and vinca alkaloids. These agents may not be available in African regions, however. Generally, even patients who undergo this aggressive treatment plan will relapse.[5]

Patients with Sertoli-Leydig cell tumours are treated according to their stage. Stage IA tumours should be managed with unilateral salpingo-oophorectomy unless childbearing is complete, at which point the contralateral ovary should be removed. If more advanced disease is present, then a more aggressive approach similar to that used in granulosa cell tumours should be utilised.[16] Fibromas and steroid cell tumours are benign tumours that can be treated conservatively. Unilateral lesions can be managed with a unilateral oophorectomy; however, if there is bilateral ovarian involvement, the entire tumour should be removed while preserving normal-appearing tissue.[24]

Germ cell tumours

Germ cell tumours encompass a number of tumour subtypes; however, their treatment can be generalised. As with all other ovarian lesions in children, the primary goal of germ cell tumour management is to preserve reproductive function. Surgery is performed to evaluate disease extent, remove the tumour, and preserve uninvolved reproductive organs. Benign lesions can be treated with ovarian cystectomy or unilateral oophorectomy. Staging is recommended for any tumour that is either known to be or may be malignant. This includes cytologic evaluation of ascitic fluid or peritoneal washings with lactated Ringer's solution, careful inspection of the contralateral ovary and other pelvic and abdominal organs, and biopsy of suspicious omental or liver lesions and retroperitoneal lymph nodes. The affected ovary should be removed, and

if a lesion is found in the contraleral ovary, a BSO should be performed. Omentectomy is indicated if tumours are found on the omentum, and debulking of retroperitoneal adenopathy should be performed, if necessary. Peritoneal disease should also be removed if possible. If the extent of disease is so overwhelming that debulking will cause more harm, then neoadjuvant chemotherapy (if it is available) should be offered prior to surgical intervention. Postsurgical treatment depends on the stage of the tumour (Table 117.7).[5] Patients with stage I tumours may be managed with observation alone. Although a significant number may relapse, salvage treatment is effective. The chemotherapy regimen of choice for all stages is cisplatin, etoposide, and bleomycin (PEB), which has been shown to be extremely effective, especially in stage I and II tumours.[25]

Postoperative Complications

Any surgery to the abdomen or pelvis has associated postoperative complications. Wound infection and fluid imbalances can occur and should be monitored in all surgical patients. Intraabdominal surgery can also produce adhesions that can cause pain, impair fertility, cause bowel obstruction, and make reoperative procedures more difficult.

Rupture of a malignant ovarian tumour during initial surgery can change the prognosis. A stage IA tumour becomes a stage IC if the tumour is ruptured at the time of surgery. One study found that the survival of patients with stage IC due to a ruptured tumour is 20%, versus 3% in patients with stage IA for epithelial ovarian tumours.[26] While stage IA tumours may not require chemotherapy, stage IC tumours usually do, so special care should be taken to avoid tumour rupture.

Patients who receive a BSO initial surgery, which can eventually produce pelvic pain or a pelvic mass. The incidence of ovarian remnant syndrome (ORS) has not been determined, although it has been shown to be rising over the past four decades. The residual ovarian tissue generally requires surgical removal; however, premenopausal patients can be treated with medications suppressing ovarian function. Blunt dissection of ovarian adhesions should be avoided during the initial BSO because it has been shown to increase the development of ORS. Additionally, failure to open the retroperitoneum during adnexectomy increases the risk; therefore, making an incision in the peritoneum lateral to the ovarian vessels to ensure access to the retroperitoneum is recommended.[27] Obviously, in any patient where all of the ovarian tissue is removed, postoperative hormone replacement may be required, depending on the age of the patient.

Prognosis and Outcome

Patients with nonneoplastic ovarian lesions have extremely favorable outcomes, with little, if any, long-term sequelae. The prognosis for neoplastic lesions depends on the specific type of tumour and the stage at which the tumour was diagnosed. In the African setting, many patients present late in the course of their disease, which negatively impacts outcome. The prognosis of surface epithelial tumours can vary. Although low-stage tumours have promising long-term survivals, for advanced stages requiring chemotherapy, the prognosis is very poor. Only about one-third of the patients with stage IA have long-term survival. Tumours of low malignant potential have extremely good outcomes, producing >90% 10-year disease-free survivals, which is considerably better than their carcinoma counterparts.[21] Patients with early stages of juvenile granulosa cell tumours have a favorable outcome, whereas the prognosis of patients with stage II or greater lesions is very poor. These patients will usually die regardless of the treatment plan. The prognosis for fibromas is very good, with little chance of tumour recurrence. The prognosis of Sertoli-Leydig cell tumours highly depends on patient age, degree of tumour differentiation, and stage of tumour. Most of these tumours are diagnosed at stage IA and have an excellent prognosis.[5] The prognosis for stage I and II germ cell tumours treated with surgery and adjuvant chemotherapy is very high, with a 6-year event-free survival much greater than 90% for both stages I and II.[25]

Prevention

Little can be done to prevent ovarian lesions in paediatric patients or even in adults. However, one of the most important factors for long-term survival is early diagnosis. Early-stage diseases can often be treated with surgery alone; in many instances, some fertility can be preserved. This may be difficult to achieve in any community, but may be even more difficult in Africa, where access to imaging may be limited. Therefore, it is important to have a high index of suspicion for ovarian lesions. An ovarian lesion should be on the differential for a young girl who presents with abdominal pain and a clinical picture that is consistent with appendicitis. Endocrine disorders, anorexia, weight loss, and other vague symptoms may guide the practitioner to consider ovarian pathology. If US is available and there is the suspicion of a pelvic or abdominal mass, early use is recommended because most lesions can be well characterised with this relatively inexpensive modality.

Ethical Issues

Fertility can be affected by both the extent of the initial disease as well as the treatment course. Studies have shown that conservative treatment is an option for many paediatric lesions, but there is still a risk of recurrence, which can increase the cost of treatment overall. In Africa, therefore, it may be more cost effective to treat the disease with aggressive surgery. In such cases, patients may thus sacrifice their future fertility, unless the ova can be stored for assisted conception. Additionally, sparing the uterus in hopes of future in vitro fertilisation may not be reasonable. Each practitioner must take into account local regional factors when deciding which surgical option is best.

Evidence-Based Research

Although no prospective, randomised studies exist on the role of conservative management versus aggressive therapy, large retrospective studies have produced valuable information. Tables 117.8 and 117.9 present two such studies on the role of conservative management in ovarian germ cell tumours and in large ovarian cysts, respectively.

Table 117.8: Evidence-based research.

Title	The influence of conservative surgical practices for malignant ovarian germ cell tumours
Authors	Chan JK, Krishnansu ST, Sarah W, et al.
Institutions	Department of Obstetrics, Gynecology, and Reproductive Sciences, University of California, San Francisco School of Medicine, San Francisco, California, USA; Department of Obstetrics and Gynecology and Department of Medicine, University of California, Orange, California, USA; Department of Obstetrics and Gynecology and Department of Radiation Oncology, Stanford University School of Medicine, Stanford, California, USA
Reference	J Surg Oncol 2008; 98:111–116
Problem	Role of conservative management in ovarian germ cell tumours.
Intervention	Fertility-sparing surgery, standard surgery.
Comparison/ control (quality of evidence)	Patients with germ cell tumours from 1988 to 2001 (n=760) on the Incidence-SEER 9 Regs Public-Use Database from February 2006 were compared based on standard surgical treatment (n=222) versus fertility-sparing surgery (n=313).
Outcome/ effect	The difference in survival rates for patients who received fertility-sparing surgery was not statistically significant when compared to the rates for patients who received standard therapy (97.6% versus 95.6%, p=0.26).
Historical significance/ comments	Although this manuscript is specific for germ cell tumours, it serves as an example of how fertility-preserving surgery can be utilised without decreasing survival. In addition, germ cell tumours are the most common ovarian malignancies in the paediatric age group. Fertility-sparing surgery in this study included ovarian cystectomy, unilateral salpingo-oophorectomy with or without hysterectomy, and bilateral salpingo-oophorectomy. Even though a number of cases did preserve at least one ovary and the uterus, some patients were left with only a uterus or an ovary. This implies that there is access to assisted reproduction techniques. As common as in vitro fertilisation is in Western countries, there is very limited access to it in African countries. Thus, the definition of fertility-sparing surgery may need to be redefined for Africa due to the lack of access to expensive fertility methods. In this study, 76% of the patients presented with stages I–II whereas 24% presented with stages III–IV. The 5-year disease-free survival for patients with stages I–II was 97.6%, and the survival in the same time period for patients with stages III–IV was 85.5%. Finally, this study found that the improved survival over time with fertility-sparing surgery is partially a result of in-depth surgical staging. Thus, staging should be utilised in all surgeries regardless of the presumed stage.

Table 117.9: Evidence-based research.

Title	Conservative management of large ovarian cysts in children: the value of serial pelvic ultrasonography
Authors	Warner BW, Kuhn JC, Barr LL
Institution	Department of Surgery and Radiology, University of Cincinnati, Cincinnati, Ohio, USA
Reference	Surgery 1992; 112:749–755
Problem	Role of conservative management in large ovarian cysts.
Intervention	Conservative management, surgical intervention.
Comparison/ control (quality of evidence)	Three groups of patients were compared based on indications for ultrasonography (US), menarchal status, age, average cyst volume, and type of cysts. Group 1 (n=10) comprised patients who received surgery with neoplastic findings, group 2 (n=13) comprised patients who had surgery with nonneoplastic findings, and group 3 (n=46) comprised patients who had no surgical intervention and on follow-up had cysts that decreased in size or completely resolved.
Outcome/ effect	No statistical significance was found among the three groups in the indications for US, menarchal status, or age. The cyst volume in the neoplastic cyst group (group 1) was significantly greater than for the cysts in group 3. There was no statistical difference between cyst volume in the two groups that underwent surgery or between groups 2 and 3. There were no differences in the type of cyst in all groups.
Historical significance/ comments	This study found that large cysts (greater than 4–5 cm), could not be distinguished based on the character of the cyst, patient age, or mencharchal status. Even though cyst volume in neoplastic lesions tended to be larger, this finding was not universal. As a result, there is no clear way to distinguish neoplastic from benign lesions that will regress. Of 51 patients who did not receive surgical management and received follow-up within 1 to 2 weeks of diagnosis, 46 were noted to have either a decrease in cyst size or complete regression. Of the remaining five patients, two were found to have an increase in size and three had unchanged. Furthermore, this study concluded that large ovarian cysts in paediatric patients can be safely followed with serial pelvic ultrasounds to monitor for decrease in size and eventual resolution. Surgical intervention should be based not only on size but on a number of clinical observations, which includes symptoms that do not resolve after 12–24 hours of observation, signs and symptoms of a large mass associated with complications, evidence of neoplasm, ovarian cause uncertain, and increase or failure to decrease in size on follow-up US. The study recommends US follow-up after 1 to 2 weeks. It is important to consider observation in large ovarian cysts because spontaneous regression eliminates surgery and its complications as well as the possibility of future fertility problems, although this may not be applicable to regions where resources are limited.

Key Summary Points

1. Ovarian lesions are uncommon in children.

2. Children with ovarian neoplasms are often first diagnosed with appendicitis; thus, ovarian lesion should be included on the differential for any child who presents with a history consistent with appendicitis.

3. The presence of a lesion can represent either benign or malignant pathology—both of which need to be considered.

4. Management of ovarian lesions is multimodal and depends on the extent of the disease—early identification is vital to decreasing mortality and preserving future fertility.

5. Ovarian cysts that are incidentally identified without notable symptomatology, even if they are larger than 5 cm, can be managed with serial ultrasounds. Symptoms consistent with torsion, lack of regression, and possibility of a neoplasm are all indications for surgery.

6. Low-grade malignant ovarian tumours can often be managed with fertility-sparing surgery, whereas high-grade lesions require aggressive surgery followed by radiation and chemotherapy.

7. The prognosis depends on the specific tumour type and grade.

References

1. Piver MS, Patton T. Ovarian Cancer in Children. Semin Surg Oncol 1986; 2:163–169.

2. von Allmen D. Malignant lesions of the ovary in childhood. Semin Pediatr Surg 2005; 14:100–105.

3. Gribbon M, Ein SH, Mancer K. Pediatric malignant ovarian tumours: a 43-year review. J Pediatr Surg 1992; 27:480–484.

4. Lack EE, Young RH, Scully RE. Pathology of ovarian neoplasms in childhood and adolescence Pathol Annu 1992; 27:281–356.

5. Templeman C, Fallat M. Ovarian tumours. In: Grosfeld JL, O'Neill JA Jr., Coran AG, Fonkalsrud EW, Caldamone AA, eds. Pediatric Surgery, Sixth Edition. Mosby Elsevier, 2006, Pp 593–621.

6. Dozois RR, Kempers RD, Dahlin DC, Bartholomeew LG. Ovarian tumours associated with the Peutz-Jeghers syndrome. Ann Surg 1970; 172:233–238.

7. Ablin AR, Krailo MD, Ramsay NKC, et al. Results of treatment of malignant germ cell tumours in 93 children: a report from the Children's Cancer Study Group. J Clin Oncol 1991; 9:1782–1792.

8. Christman JE, Ballon SC. Ovarian fibrosarcoma associated with Maffucci's syndrome. Gynecol Oncol 1990; 37:290–291.

9. Weiss NS. Measuring the separate effects of low parity and its antecedents on the incidence of ovarian cancer. J Epidemiol 1988; 128:451–455.

10. Hartge P, Devesa S. Ovarian cancer, ovulation and side of origin. Br J Cancer 1995; 71:642–643.

11. Modan B, Hartge P, Hirsh-Yechezhel G, et al. Parity, oral contraceptives, and the risk of ovarian cancer among carriers and noncarriers of a BRCA1 or BRCA2 mutation. N Engl J Med 2001; 345:235–240.

12. Easton DF, Ford D, Bishop DT. Breast and ovarian cancer incidence in BRCA1-mutation carriers. Breast cancer linkage consortium. Am J Hum Genet 1995; 56:265–271.

13. Breen JL, Maxson WS. Ovarian tumours in children and adolescents. Clin Obstet Gynecol 1977; 20:607–623.

14. Brown MF, Hebra A, McGeehin K, Ross AJ III. Ovarian masses in children: a review of 91 cases of malignant and benign masses. J Pediatr Surg 1993; 28:930–933.

15. Imai A, Furui T, Tamaya T. Gynecologic tumours and symptoms in childhood and adolescence: 10-years' experience. Int J Gynaecol Obstet 1994; 45:227–234.

16. Sachdeva P, Arora R, Dubey C, Sukhija A, Daga M, Singh DK. Sertoli-Leydig cell tumour: a rare ovarian neoplasm. Case report and review of literature. Gynecol Endocrinol 2008; 24:230–234.

17. Ratani RS, Cohen HL, Fiore E. Pediatric gynecologic ultrasound. Ultrasound Q 2004; 20:127–139.

18. Siegel MJ, Surratt JT. Pediatric gynecologic imaging. Obstet Gynecol Clin North Am 1992; 19:103–127.

19. Warner BW, Kuhn JC, Barr LL. Conservative management of large ovarian cysts in children: the value of serial pelvic ultrasonography. Surgery 1992; 112:749–755.

20. Darwish AM, Amin AF, Mohammad SA. Laparoscopic management of paratubal and paraovarian cysts. JSLS 2003; 7:101–106.

21. Crispens MA. Borderline ovarian tumours: a review of the recent literature. Curr Opin Obstet Gynecol 2003; 15:39–43.

22. Ayhan A, Celik H, Taskiran C, Bozdag G, Aksu T. Oncologic and reproductive outcome after fertility-saving surgery in ovarian cancer. Eur J Gynaecol Oncol 2003; 24:223–232.

23. Markman M. Antineoplastic agents in the management of ovarian cancer: current status and emerging therapeutic strategies. Trends Pharmacol Sci 2008; 29(10):515–519.

24. Howell CG Jr, Rogers DA, Gable DS, Falls GD. Bilateral ovarian fibromas in children. J Pediatr Surg 1990; 25:690–691.

25. Rogers PC, Olson TA, Cullen JW, et al. Treatment of children and adolescents with stage II testicular and stages I and II ovarian malignant germ cell tumours: a pediatric Intergroup Study—Pediatric Oncology Group 9048 and Children's Cancer Group 8891. J Clin Oncol 2004; 22:3563–3569.

26. Sainz de la Cuesta R, Goff BA, Fuller AF Jr, Nikrui N, Eichhorn JH, Rice LW, Prognostic importance of intraoperative rupture of malignant ovarian epithelial neoplasms. Obstet Gynecol 1994; 84:1–7.

27. Magtibay PM, Magrina JF. Ovarian remnant syndrome. Clin Obstet Gynecol 2006; 49:526–534.

Surgical Rehabilitation

CHAPTER 118
GENERAL DISABILITY: THE CONCEPTS

Richard Bransford

Introduction

Webster's New World Dictionary of American English[1] makes the following distinctions of terms related to general disability:

Disable: (1) to make unable, unfit, or ineffective; cripple; incapacitate; (2) to make legally incapable; disqualify legally

Disability: (1) a disabled condition; (2) that which disabled, as an illness, injury, or physical handicap; (3) a legal disqualification or incapacity; (4) something that restricts; limitation; disadvantage

Cripple: (1) a person or animal that is lame or otherwise disabled in a way that prevents normal motion of the limbs or body: somewhat offensive when used to refer to a person

Handicap: (2a) something that hampers a person; disadvantage; hindrance; (2b) physical disability

In the present age of "enlightenment", many terms have been suggested to describe a person with a disability. However, the terminology used can be politically sensitive and abruptly change from decade to decade. For example, should we say "disabled child" or "child with a disability"? While remaining sensitive to others, we must also utilise terms that can be understood by the audience to whom we address these terms. When trying to describe the work being done in Africa, compromise may be necessary. When directing letters to friends in North America and referring to working with the handicapped, I often receive inquiries about whether these were people with alcohol- or drug-related problems. One hospital in Africa providing care for children with disabilities was named Bethany Crippled Children's Centre. Many were aghast that the word "crippled" had been used with such indiscretion. The explanation usually given was that the name was an attempt to communicate the type of work being done to the "least educated in the most rural village". Disabled, handicapped, and various other terms did not communicate to these nearly as effectively as "crippled", which seemingly was a term that many understood.

Demographics

Some studies estimate that 1% of the people in the world are disabled.[2] Africa is likely a different scene, however. Due to wars, civil strife, various religious beliefs, economic constraints, a relative lack of medical care, and a greater incidence of infectious diseases, the incidence of disabilities in Africa is likely greater than 1%. Some estimate an incidence of as low as 3%, whereas others, such as Dr. Rodney L. Belcher, the former chief of orthopaedics at Mengo Hospital in Kampala, Uganda, have suggested that the figure is actually as high as 10%. Regardless of the exact number, it is likely that the incidence of disabilities in Africa is greater than for the world in general. In the early 1990s, Dr. Belcher estimated that 10% of the population of Uganda had some disability; he also commented: "Each week in Kampala we have approximately three new cases of culture-proven polio." The level of disability in that country was undoubtedly related to nearly two decades of civil strife and the breakdown of the economic and health systems.

The Kenya scene in 2008 is far different in certain respects from that of many other countries. Even though the number of medical practitioners is large by sub-Saharan African standards, it falls far short of that of nearly all Western countries. Polio is rarely seen in its acute phase, even though it probably is not eradicated. The incidence of talipes, spina bifida, cleft lips and palates, and various other congenital abnormalities in Kenya is not known, but it would appear that their presence is as plentiful as it is in other African countries. There are more than 40 tribal groups in Kenya, and patients with clubfeet, spina bifida, and cleft lips come from nearly all of those tribal groups.

Children with disabilities seem to abound in nearly all sub-Saharan African countries. Few have been adequately treated, and most have had no treatment.

Aetiology

Disabilities in general can be identified as either congenital or acquired. One could further break down the congenital disabilities into those of genetic aetiologies (e.g., Down syndrome); those related to a nutritional deficit (e.g., neural tube defects); those associated with some inciting event (e.g., rubella); and random expression. Moreover, some defects that may appear identical could be, in reality, either "familial" or ran-

Table 118.1: Recurrence risks for some defects.

Defect	Normal parent of one affected child*	Recurrence risk for: Future males	Future females
Cleft lip with or without cleft palate	4–5%		
Cleft palate alone	2–6%		
Cardiac defect (common type)	3–4%		
Pyloric stenosis	3%	4%	2.4%
Hirschsprung's anomaly	3–5%		
Clubfoot	2–8%		
Dislocation of hip	3–4%	0.5%	6.3%
Neural tube defects—anencephaly, meningomyelocele	3–5%		
Scoliosis	10–15%		

Source: Jones KL. Smith's Recognizable Patterns of Human Malformation. Saunders, 1997, Table 4-1.
*Range of recurrence risks observed.

Table 118.2: Ratio of males versus females for various disorders.

Disorder	Male-to-female ratio
Pyloric stenosis	5:1
Clubfoot	2:1
Cleft lip with and without palate	2:1
Cleft palate alone	1:1.3
Meningomyelocele	1:1.5
Anencephaly	1:3
Congenital dislocated hip	1:5.5

Source: Jones KL. Smith's Recognizable Patterns of Human Malformation. Saunders, 1997, Figure 4-14.

dom. Among family members it is not uncommon for more than one member to be affected with clubfeet, cleft lips, cardiac defects, pyloric stenosis, Hirschsprung's disease, hip dislocation, neural tube defects, scoliosis, or other problems (Table 118.1).[3] The gender distribution may also vary in various malformations (Table 118.2).[3]

One of the most commonly identified defects related to a nutritional deficit are neural tube defects. A deficit of folate creates an environment in which this defect is manifested more commonly. In countries where nutritional fortification with folate has occurred, the incidence of this problem has diminished by 66–75%. In North America, the incidence of children born with spina bifida has diminished due to folate fortification. The incidence of children conceived who have spina bifida may be considerably underreported, however, due to the frequent abortion of fetuses identified by ultrasonography (US) as having neural tube defects.

Other disabilities, such as burn contractures and polio, are generally preventable either by improved living standards or immunisation. Improved community education should promote the reduction of many disabilities as people learn basic steps they can take to prevent disabilities from occuring. Genetic counselling can also assist in diminishing the number of children born with disabilities.

Clinical Presentation

History
A good history and physical examination usually will lead to an accurate diagnosis and can often save time and money. A disproportionate number of those described as disabled come from families who are poor and/or less educated. Many, if not most, of these children are born at home with, at best, a traditional birth attendant (TBA) in attendance. Most newborns will not have had that early evaluation, even briefly, that usually occurs in a hospital birth; this initial physical can lead to early diagnosis and a better informed attempt at seeking appropriate care. Often, these families have little access to appropriate medical care, even if they were to recognise that "something can be done".

Parents of children from poor and less educated families will also frequently not understand the importance of immunisations and early care.

Physical Examination
The variation in physical findings parallels the diseases encountered and the timing at which the child arrives for care. Burns, spina bifida, hydrocephalus, clubfeet, polio, and the various other disabilities often arrive late in the course of their disease.

A routine physical examination will easily identify most of the overt disabilities, but the less obvious associated conditions (e.g., cardiac, renal, and liver problems) often go undiscovered longer, frequently complicating their management.

Investigations
In the case of late arrival, the diagnosis often declares itself. Yet, for certain infants, a differentiation of aetiology must be determined. An example of this is the clinical presentation of a child with clubfeet. In differentiating among the congenital clubfoot, a nearly identical foot with polio, and the "clubfoot" associated with spina bifida, a few

questions can clarify the aetiology: "Was the child born with this deformity?" "At what age did the child demonstrate this deformity?" "Does the child seem to have sensation and motor activity in the leg?"

In other situations—for example, in the hydrocephalic patient—one might seek to identify the aetiology of the condition (i.e., infectious, congenital, or other). The aetiology may dictate the extent of brain damage and what can, or should, be done. If the fontanelle is open, ultrasound (US) can clarify the size of the ventricles as well as identify the amount of cortex; this may suggest the potential long-term outcome. US is relatively inexpensive, whereas computed tomography (CT) and magnetic resonance imaging (MRI) can be costly. Often, however, none of these exams are available. If they are unavailable, in the case of hydrocephalus, the head circumference should be measured and compared to the normal range for that age (Figure 118.1). The size of the fontanelle, together with the history, and general impression are important. In most cases, this is sufficient to determine the presence of hydrocephalus.

In the case of an occipital encephalocele, US may help clarify the contents and the potential viability of the infant if this is to be repaired; the size of the ventricles is also important to determine whether there is an accompanying hydrocephalus needing shunting.

A good examination of patients with congenital talipes equinovarus (CTEV) can suggest the best pathway for treatment without expensive tests. Similarly, a close examination of the deformities and motor activity of the child with polio should suggest the way to proceed. In all of these cases, the parent and/or patient needs to understand what can and cannot be done, as well as the ultimate expectations.

Management
Many African countries have few specialists capable of meeting the needs of the disabled children. If the specialists are available, they are almost never present in sufficient numbers. Poor families often lack sufficient funds to access the care, even if it is available. Many who do seek care come late—often too late.

The setting in which the patient presents, the level of expertise of the surgeon, the availability of materials, the investigative possibilities, the financial status of the patients, the ability to provide follow-up care, and various other factors often will dictate the potential management and outcome. The outcome in a limited-resource setting, although possibly far inferior to that anticipated in a sophisticated medical setting, might be considered quite acceptable to many in Africa. The expectations may be quite variable. Function, cosmesis, and/or practicality are all important; however, the expectations of the parents and/or the child should be ascertained prior to surgical care. A careful explanation of the procedure, the postoperative care, the need for appliances postoperatively, and the anticipated functional ability will assist in avoiding misunderstandings.

In the case of talipes, management should begin shortly after birth with manipulation and plaster. Early evaluation of the foot will allow the surgeon to explain the plan and the expectations to the parents. The Ponseti technique of serial casting and appropriate intervention will often avoid major surgical procedures. However, this technique demands that the parent bring the child early and cooperate in the care of the child. Such consistent care is often not possible for these children because the family does not understand the importance of the consistency of care, or they may live in a remote location without access to the health care workers needed to provide this care, or they cannot afford this level of care. Also, in reality, the regimen suggested by Ponseti is unknown to most of the health care workers of Africa, and, if known, cannot be provided due to a lack of training and/or supplies. In a a significant number of the children treated by this method major surgery will still be necessary.

Often in East Africa, children with club feet arrive for care when they are several years of age or even older; in most of these cases, there has been no previous orthopaedic care. First, the surgeon must decide

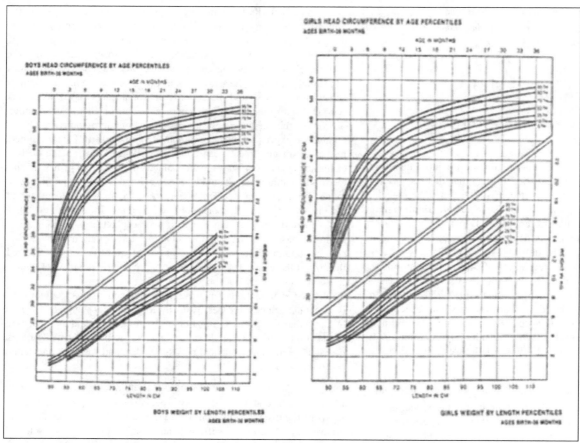

Figure 118.1: Growth charts for boys (left) and girls (right) from birth to 36 months: head circumference by age and weight by length.
Source: Modified from Hamill PV, et al. Physical growth: National Center for Health Statistics percentiles. Am J Clin Nutr 1979; 32(3):607–629.

whether any operation should be performed at that time, and, in the case of the immature foot, whether a soft tissue release should be done while delaying operations on the boney structures until the foot is more mature. One must seriously question whether the outcome will be a more functional foot, whether the child will wear a caliper (brace), and/ or whether the child will return for further care at an older age.

In cases of congenital pseudarthrosis of the tibia, once again, one must consider the setting. In the West, an amputation with prosthesis may be the preferred pathway; in an African setting, however, attempts at repairing the pseudarthrosis, even if it results in a short leg, may be preferred due to the lack of available prostheses, especially for a growing child, as well as the expense of providing these prostheses.

The late arrival for treatment of many children may dictate operative and nonoperative solutions that frequently are not described in most Western textbooks. Usually, Western medical texts assume that early care can be or has been provided. In the case of late presentation, the results of any attempt at treatment are often fraught with more complications and usually inferior to those to be expected if early care had been sought.

Some situations, possibly particularly in the case of polio deformities, may dictate consideration of remedial operations with, or without, bracing. Assuming inadequate follow-up and possibly poor compliance, a remedial operation may be the best option. A "perfect" operation without the use of a brace will often fail. Also, a growing child with a caliper will need to have the caliper replaced.

Obviously, the usual approaches and expectations must be modified when confronted by a 20-year-old with a cleft lip and palate, a 9-year-old with an untreated clubfoot, an 8-year-old with severe rickets, a 5-year-old with advanced hydrocephalus, or burn contractures untreated for decades. The contextualized treatment must consider not

only the surgical skills and treatment environment but also the abilities of the nonphysician staff to maximise the potential created by the surgical team. The ability to apply such modifications may allow the child to enjoy a much improved quality of life.

In some remote settings the health care workers (HCWs) may be the *last option* for many children. These HCWs often will be satisfied with less than "state-of-the-art" techniques, and many are just looking for a better "quality of life". Although such HCWs are not specialists, some who have some surgical experience may be put in a situations where the child has no other options. Many good books that are often considered remedial or out of date by the high-level specialist may offer good pictures and a description of the procedure that can be followed. These books (e.g., Lehman's *The Clubfoot*;[5] Goldstein's *Atlas of Orthopaedic Surgery*;[6] and Tachdjian's *Pediatric Orthopedics*[7]), often open and sitting by an operating table, lend support to the desperate surgeon. Many techniques of previous decades offer solutions that are quite satisfactory. Some books (e.g., Staheli's *Fundamentals of Pediatric Orthopedics*,[8] *Practice of Pediatric Orthopedics*,[9] and *Arthrogryposis: A Text Atlas*[10]) make difficult explanations simple enough for the generalist. Much of what is included in these books can also be obtained online.

Albright's *Operative Techniques in Pediatric Neurosurgery*[11] can be instructive for many surgeons. If one can shunt a child with hydrocephalus or close the back of a child with spina bifida, a large number of children can be assisted. Many varieties of ventriculoperitoneal shunt are available, with great variations in cost; Warf has found the Chhabra™ ventriculoperitoneal shunt to be equally successful to expensive Western shunts.[12] (In addition, the Chhabra shunt has been quite useful as an indwelling catheter in hypospadias repairs. It is soft silastic, inert, and of just the right size for the average older child.)

Postoperative Complications

When children with disabilities arrive late in the course of their disease, it is often more difficult to attain the desired endpoint. Too much done too quickly will often encourage complications. In the developing world, staged procedures may lead to fewer complications. The staged approach is often wisest with imperforate anus, hypospadias, neglected clubfeet, some polio deformities, osteogenesis imperfecta, spina bifida associated with hydrocephalus, and various other disabilities. For some disabilities, such as open spina bifida, infections will occur more commonly when the arrival of the child is delayed. In some cases, a further delay in surgical care to allow for improved preoperative preparation, intravenous antibiotics, and so forth may be best. Part of this preparation may include thorough cleansing of a dirty wound, the correction of anaemia, and malnutrition, and the preparation of the parent.

Also, having too few trained medical staff can lead to complications. When operative care includes plaster, the staff may either not be able to evaluate the extremities as often as desired, or not have adequate understanding of the importance of this task. Sometimes, it may be best to compromise by utilising a splint instead of a cylinder plaster.

Often, outcomes are compromised by a lack of specialised personnel. It is essential that an active therapy plan and program be in place following specialised operations on the hands of most burn victims. A planned, and sometimes painful, exercise program can make the difference between failure and success. Specialised personnel that are often helpful include orthopaedic technologists, speech therapists, occupational therapists, physiotherapists, and dentists.

Prognosis and Outcomes

Both prognosis and outcome are complicated by late presentation and preoperative conditions that contribute to poor outcomes. In addition to late presentation are the conditions dictated by the setting and expertise of those caring for the patients. Many of the factors expected in the West (e.g., surgical specialists and subspecialists in a wide variety of fields, greater expertise in nursing, good physiotherapy and occupational therapy, state-of-the-art orthotics and prostheses, sophisticated operative settings, and many other factors) are often not present in the developing world; perhaps contributing to less desirable outcomes. One might add that refugee status and a transient patient population also may contribute to poor outcomes. Often these patients do not understand the preoperative, operative and postoperative plans; some have no choice in their ability to regularly access appropriate medical care. The language barrier in many settings may promote unrealistic expectations on the part of the patient and parents and later disappointment.

In the midst of all of the difficulties, it is important for health care workers to become familiar with the pathways that may be acceptable to their patients and their families. A relatively crude therapy device that may be difficult to accept in the West is often quite acceptable in African settings. Werner's *Disabled Village Children*,[13] an important guide to the diagnosis and treatment pathways of various disabilities, also has designs for appliances that are quite effective.

In the case of cancer and the need for radiotherapy and/or chemotherapy, however, the cost is often prohibitive and specialised care is unavailable.

Prevention

Even though Western Hemisphere data suggests that polio has been eliminated there, this is not true in Africa. War, civil strife, and, in some cases, religious bias have led to fewer preventive measures in economies that may be oriented towards other goals. Within eastern and northeastern Africa, polio is more prevalent in Sudan, Ethiopia, and Somalia. Two decades ago, Uganda could have been included in this list due to its own civil strife. Immunisation, vitamin A, adequate teaching about various diseases, preconception folate, genetic counselling, antihelminthics, and appropriate iodine, as examples, would help in the prevention of various disabilities. One could easily add to this list clean, adequate water and soap as well as effective toilet facilities as contributing factors in a "preventive" program.

Ethical Issues

Children with disabilities often enter school later than other children. Unfortunately, many special schools are insufficiently staffed and are not equipped for the numbers and types of children coming for training. Most of these children need not only the normal education of children without disabilities, but also therapy and basic education in living skills. Few, if any, African countries have sufficient funding and expertise to provide such an educational experience for these children.

Some disabled children continue to be considered a "curse" on the African continent. They may be a shame to their family, their village, and/or their country. Consequently, many of these children are hidden from public view, sometimes for years. This attitude, a part of the cultures of many people, is more common in remote village settings where there is little education about medical issues and other problems. Such an attitude delays or prevents treatment. Often, when a choice—economic, cultural, or other—has to be made by the family, the child with a disability does not receive care. Frequently, this is due to economic issues within a poor family. Obviously, some disabilities are more overt and others are unseen. In general, the view that disabilities are a sign of a curse is still widespread in Africa.

In sub-Saharan Africa, where the economies of most countries are seriously compromised and there is an abundance of very poor people, the questions of what "should be done" often emerge. What are the circumstances that "allow" an investment in a child with hydrocephalus or spina bifida with all of the considerations that go along with their long-term care? What can the economy "afford" in its investment in disabled children in general? As physicians, what is our responsibility in pursuing the care of these children? These are issues for consideration; the answers likely will vary from country to country and from family to family.

Key Summary Points

1. Children with disabilities in Africa tend to arrive later in the course of their disease and will often need care and procedures not necessarily described in Western textbooks.

2. The parents of children should be carefully advised about the prognosis and expectations for their children.

3. When beginning work with children with hydrocephalus and spina bifida, the physician should select carefully the cases on which to operate. The physician should incorporate a team that includes an operating theatre technician, a physician with surgical skills, and a special nurse for pre- and postoperative care. A careful look at all of the ramifications of the care of these children is warranted.

4. Specialised surgeons are not available in most of Africa. Physicians must seek advice and do their best.

5. Regular follow-up is recommended for nearly all disabled children. Their needs will likely change as they get older.

6. The physician must recognise the setting and the audience and tailor the investigation and care to the patient's abilities. Although the hospital may not be "state-of-the-art", the patients also are likely to be poor.

7. Even older surgical textbooks are of value. They may include simpler operations that will help most of the children and have techniques that are much more inviting than those in sophisticated current textbooks.

8. The health care worker may be the only hope for many of the parents and their children.

9. Many specialists in the world might be willing to come to the local hospital and teach. Invite them.

References

1. Neufeldt V, Guralnik DB, eds. Webster's New World Dictionary of American English. Simon & Schuster, 1988, Pp 328, 390, 611.

2. World Bank WHO Statistics. Available at: http://web.worldbank.org/WBSITE/EXTERNAL/TOPICS/EXTSOCIALPROTECTION/EXTDISAB

3. Jones KL. Smith's Recognizable Patterns of Human Malformation. Saunders, 1997, P 722.

4. Berry RJ, Zhu L, Erickson JD, et al. Prevention of neural-tube defects with folic acid in China. NEJM 1999; 341(20):1485–1490.

5. Lehman WB, Torok G. The Clubfoot. JB Lippincott, 1980.

6. Goldstein LA, Dickerson RC. Atlas of Orthopedic Surgery. The CV Mosby, 1981.

7. Tachdjian MO. Pediatric Orthopedics, vol 2, 2nd ed. WB Saunders, 1990.

8. Staheli, LT. Fundamentals of Pediatric Orthopedics. Raven Press, 1992.

9. Staheli LT. Practice of Pediatric Orthopedics. Lippincott Williams & Wilkins, 2001.

10. Staheli LT, Hall JG, Jaffe KM, Paholke DO, eds. Arthrogryposis: a text atlas. Cambridge University Press, 1998.

11. Albright AL, Pollack IE, Adelson PD. Operative Techniques in Pediatric Neurosurgery. Thieme, 2001.

12. Warf BC. Comparison of one-year outcomes for the Chaabra™ and Codman Hakim Micro Precision™ shunt systems in Uganda: a prospective study in 195 children. J Neurosurgery (Pediatrics 4) 2005; 102:358–362.

13. Werner D. Disabled Village Children: A Guide for Community Health Workers, Rehabilitation Workers, and Families. The Hesperian Foundation, Berkeley, CA, 1987.

CHAPTER 119
NEURODISABILITY

Dan Poenaru
Nick Bauman

Introduction

Neurodisability is probably the most significant contributor to chronic surgical disability in African children. It involves primarily hydrocephalus (HC) and spina bifida (SB), which can occur in isolation or together. Other causes of neurodisability include encephaloceles, which are part of the spectrum of neural tube defects (NTDs). True cerebral palsy is primarily nonsurgical, and therefore not included in this chapter.

Hydrocephalus is the excessive accumulation of cerebrospinal fluid (CSF) within the cranial vault. Its management in developing nations is hindered by significant economic constraints and delays in treatment—most patients, in fact, do not present for several months after the onset of clinical symptoms. The management of hydrocephalus and the complications associated with its treatment require considerable surgical judgment and a lifelong approach to patient follow-up.

Spina bifida is the term used for a spectrum of congenital NTDs. Other terms used for these anomalies are spinal dysraphisms or myelodysplasias. NTDs are complex medical problems that challenge surgeons and paediatricians alike, both in their initial management and in their lifelong complications. Even though SB may become a vanishing disease in developed countries, it remains a very significant cause of morbidity and disability in the developing world.

Demographics

The prevalence and incidence of HC in developed nations is estimated at 0.9–1.2 per 1,000 and 0.2–0.6 per 1,000, respectively.[1] No reliable estimate is available in the African literature, but its incidence in Africa is likely higher due to untreated or poorly treated neonatal meningitis and nutritional deficiencies.

The key epidemiologic features of SB are wide regional and ethnic differences in prevalence, a worldwide decline in prevalence over the past three decades, and female preponderance.[2] The reasons behind the decline are unclear and most likely multifactorial, although folic acid supplementation and fortification and selective termination of pregnancies are probably key factors.[3] The range in prevalence in Western nations is roughly 0.1–1 per 1,000 live births; a few non-Western studies quote higher rates, widely spread.[4–6]

Aetiology/Pathophysiology

CSF is produced predominantly by the choroid plexus of the four cerebral ventricles, at a rate of 20 ml/hour. It flows via the foramina of Luschka and Magendie into the subarachnoid space, and it is absorbed by the arachnoid villi into the venous system via the superior saggital sinus.

HC has been categorised as communicating or noncommunicating. The former is due to the failure of CSF absorption by the arachnoid villi, whereas the latter involves obstruction of CSF flow into the subarachnoid space. A small minority of cases exhibit excessive production of CSF—most commonly secondary to a choroid plexus papilloma.

In developed nations, HC has historically been most commonly due to myelomeningocele, with the posthaemorrhagic hydrocephalus of prematurity becoming at least as common in recent years.[2] Some reports have suggested that the most common causes of hydrocephalus in central Africa are NTDs and congenital aqueductal stenosis. Similarly, in Zambia, the ratio of congenital to "postmeningitic" HC has been reported to be 2:1.[7] In contrast, well-documented prospective series in East Africa have shown the aetiology of HC to be 57% postinfectious, 29% non-postinfectious, and 13% myelomeningocele.[8] Thus, neonatal meningitis or ventriculitis is likely the most common cause of hydrocephalus in East Africa.[8]

SB may result either from failure of closure of the neural tube or from secondary reopening of a closed tube, although most of the evidence favours the former theory.[9] The aetiology of SB is multifactorial.[2] A genetic component is evidenced by the familial risk, which appears to be 20–50 per 1,000 if one child is affected, 100 per 1,000 if two children are affected, and 30 per 1,000 if the mother is older than 35 years of age.[3] Environmental factors include low socioeconomic factors, maternal hyperthermia, and medications–primarily carbamazepine, valproic acid, and folate. Mothers taking carbamazepine and valproic acid have a 1% risk of having infants with SB. Folic acid, conversely, has been conclusively shown to both prevent the first occurrence of SB defects in pregnant women and to cause a 70% reduction in recurrent SB in mothers who already had pregnancies with NTDs.[10]

Clinical Presentation

The clinical presentation of HC is characterised by signs and symptoms of increased intracranial pressure (ICP). Symptoms may include headache, vomiting, failing vision, drowsiness, fatigue, deteriorating mental function, and enlarged head circumference. Signs include wide tense fontanelle, papilloedema, reduced visual acuity, failure of upward gaze (the sunsetting sign), general clumsiness, dyspraxic gait, and increasing head circumference (Figure 119.1). Older children will not present with increased head circumference; they often complain of the classic triad: headache, vomiting, and lethargy.

The obvious (apparent) spinal defects include myelomeningoceles, meningoceles (together referred to as *spina bifida cystica*), and

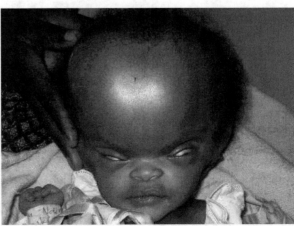

Figure 119.1: Severe congenital hydrocephalus with sunset eyes.

lipomeningoceles. Occult lesions include diastematomyelia (split cord), tight filum terminale, dorsal dermal sinus, and spinal lipoma. The term spina bifida occulta should be reserved for spinal bone fusion defects only.

The appearance of the spinal defect reveals its identity. Myelomeningoceles usually have a central "open" defect without normal skin, often with a visible placode (the open spinal cord). They may appear flat at birth, then often fill up with CSF. Older unoperated children will often have significant scarring, and the skin may indeed completely close the defect (Figure 119.2). Meningoceles and lipomeningoceles are fully skin-covered from birth, with the former typically cystic (Figures 119.3 and 119.4) and the latter fatty in consistency (Figures 119.5 and 119.6).

The distribution of the levels of SB depends on referral patterns and access to care, but usually about 40% are lumbosacral, 30% lumbar, and 30% thoracic or thoracolumbar.[11] The accurate assessment of the spinal cord function is critical. It must be kept in mind that the skin level of the defect may not accurately reflect the spinal level, that children may exhibit both upper and lower motor neuron lesions, and that the level may be asymmetrical. Areas of changed pigmentation, hairy patches, haemangiomas, lipomas, and deep skin pits in the thoracolumbar and sacral midline may belie an underlying NTD.

HC occurs in 80–90% of infants with spina bifida[1] (Figure 119.7), but may not be apparent until the spinal defect is closed. HC is less frequently seen in children with sacral defects. The authors' experience, as well as that reported elsewhere, points to a possible lower incidence of HC in developing countries.[11]

The associated Chiari II malformation may also cause specific hindbrain herniation symptoms in about 20% of children with SB. These symptoms include apnoea, a high-pitch cry, and swallowing difficulties.[3,9]

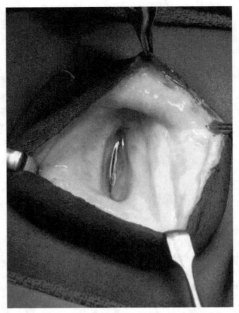

Figure 119.4: Intraoperative appearance of meningocele.

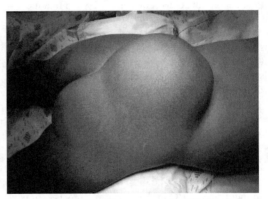

Figure 119.6: Intraoperative appearance of lipomeningocele, with adipose tissue invading dura and surrounding nerve fibres.

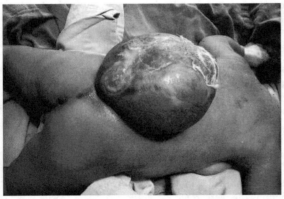

Figure 119.2: Late presentation of large myelomeningoceles with superinfection and partial scarring.

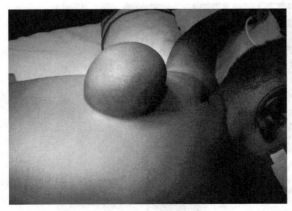

Figure 119.3: Thoracic meningocele with no neurological deficit.

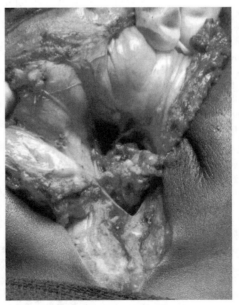

Figure 119.5: Large lipomeningocele.

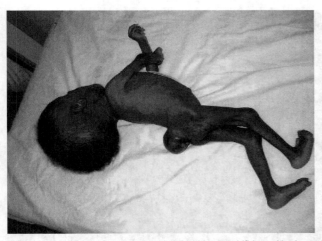

Figure 119.7: Severely malnourished child with spina bifida and hydrocephalus.

Investigations

The clinical exam is the most readily available investigation for the diagnosis of increased ICP. Cranial ultrasonography (US) is an essential diagnostic tool in developing countries; it can readily assess ventricular size with minimal training, and it is relatively inexpensive. Depending on operator skill, the size of the fourth ventricle can be assessed on US as a proxy indication of the patency of the aqueduct. This may be particularly relevant in stratifying patients for treatment with prosthetic shunts versus endoscopic third ventriculostomy (ETV).[8] Serial US imaging may be appropriate in patients with an equivocal presentation of ICP prior to subjecting them to shunt revision. All children with shunts should be followed up regularly, including a baseline US within 3 months of surgery. Although acute changes from baseline may help in the subsequent diagnosis of shunt failure, up to a third of patients will not exhibit any evidence of ventriculomegaly.[12]

Both computed tomography (CT) and magnetic resonance imaging (MRI) are excellent modalities, but their routine use is prohibitively costly in developing nations. Nevertheless, CT may be necessary in assessing the ventricular size in older children with closed fontanelles. Evidence of increased ICP in children with closed fontanelles can also be obtained through direct measurement of CSF pressure by lumbar puncture: the CSF column height is measured in a piece of IV tubing connected to the spinal needle via a three-way stopcock.

No immediate investigations are required in a regular case of SB. Spinal x-rays may reveal other occult dysraphisms in 10% of patients,[6] although this will likely not affect the management. High-resolution US of the spinal cord is as effective as MRI up to the age of 6 weeks, identifying diastematomyelia and tethered cord, and screening for dilatation of the urinary tract. MRI of the spine is frequently performed in developed nations, although rarely necessary routinely. US of the head for HC is useful, although the ventriculomegaly may not be evident until the CSF leak through the spinal defect is closed. Several investigations for the genitourinary system are discussed under the subheading "Urological Problems" later in this chapter.

Management

The definitive management of HC at present remains surgical. The diuretic acetazolamide has been shown to decrease CSF production in animal and human studies,[14] but it is of temporary benefit and should be used only in the palliative setting or in equivocal cases until a definitive diagnosis can be made. It has also been used in posthaemorrhagic HC of the newborn as a temporising measure to avoid shunting.[15]

The most common surgical intervention to treat HC is the insertion of a shunt through the skull and cortical mantle into the ventricle, with the distal catheter placed into a physiologic drainage basin, typically the peritoneal space (ventriculoperitoneal (VP) shunt). Other sites for CSF diversion include the right atrium and the pleural space. The advantage of a CSF shunt is that it is beneficial in nearly all types of HC, regardless of aetiology.

CSF Shunts

CSF shunts usually contain three parts: a ventricular catheter, a valve, and a distal catheter. Most valves are designed to allow for sampling via needle puncture. The so-called "differential pressure valves" use the gradient between the ventricle and the tip of the distal catheter to effect flow. Medium pressure valves are those that drain CSF if the pressure gradient is >10 mm Hg, and are used most commonly. Although many different valve designs exist, including siphon-limiting, flow-limiting, and programmable valves (whose settings can be changed by using an external magnet), there is limited evidence for their benefit. A large randomised trial has demonstrated no difference in time to first shunt failure with a standard differential pressure valve compared to two other higher-generation valves in the treatment of children with newly diagnosed HC.[15] Similarly, the use of an adjustable shunt was not shown to be of any benefit in terms of overall survival.[16] Finally, and of most relevance to the developing world, there is good evidence from a prospective randomised controlled trial demonstrating that the Chhabra® shunt (made by Surgiwear in India) is equivalent to its common Western counterpart in incidence of shunt complications, but sells for only about one-twentieth the cost.[17] The Chhabra shunts are available free to qualifying centres through the International Federation of Spina Bifida and Hydrocephalus (www.ifglobal.org) In extreme situations, a piece of IV tubing or a sterile Silastic® feeding catheter can be used as a VP shunt, but these nonvalved alternatives are associated with frequent complications and are not recommended.

Pleural Shunts

Pleural shunts are rarely required, but can be placed via the 4th to 6th intercostal space at the anterior axillary line into the pleural cavity, with care to avoid placement into lung parenchyma or the chest wall. The associated CSF effusion and iatrogenic pneumothorax resolve conservatively in most patients.

Ventriculoatrial Shunts

Ventriculoatrial shunts are rarely performed because of complications of cor pulmonale, shunt nephritis, and catheter embolisation. They require intraoperative US or fluoroscopy to document catheter placement into the atrium via the internal jugular vein. Their use is not recommended.

Endoscopic Third Ventriculostomy

The morbidity of the life-long shunt has created interest in the use of endoscopic third ventriculostomy (ETV), a procedure that can effectively treat HC without insertion of any foreign body. The principles of placement of an ETV include frontal access, ventricular cannulation, and insertion of a rigid or flexible neuroendoscope into the 3rd ventricle via the lateral ventricle and the foramen of Monroe. A fenestration is made in the base of the third ventricle between the infundibular recess and the mammillary bodies. This is commonly performed by using a combination of electrocautery and a balloon dilator, thus creating a cerebrospinal fluid fistula between the subarachnoid space and the 3rd ventricle.[18] More recently, the concurrent performance of cauterisation of the choroid plexus (CPC) has been added as a means of increasing shunt avoidance.

Classically, ETV was used for older children or adults with congenital aqueductal stenosis. Working in Uganda, Dr. Benjamin Warf has convincingly demonstrated, however, that ETV is a reasonable option for all children >1 year of age (irrespective of HC aetiology), with a shunt avoidance rate of 80%.[17] In addition, with the use of cranial US and direct endoscopic visualisation of the aqueduct, he stratified younger children based on aqueductal patency, and has demonstrated 70% success in those <1 year of age who have a post-infectious obstruction of the aqueduct. In addition, the use of ETV in combination with choroid plexus cauterisation has increased shunt avoidance from 35% to 76% in children with myelomeningocele, and from 20% to 71% in children <1 year of age with a non-postinfectious HC and an open aqueduct.

Performance of ETV is beyond the scope of this review, and requires adequate mentoring by an experienced surgical team and significant technical support for maintaining the endoscopic system. Although the avoidance of a shunt (and the accompanying morbidity and mortality of shunt failure) in the developing world is a reasonable goal, the additional safety of ETV has not yet been proven in the long term, and most authors counsel that the same life-long follow-up is required in either case.[1]

Spina Bifida Surgery

The management of a child with SB is lengthy and complex.[3,19] The closure of the spinal defect is the most obvious step, although it is by far not the most challenging one. In contrast, some older asymptomatic children presenting with relatively small defects that are fully skin-covered and mostly scarred may not need to have their defect "closed", especially as the surgery in those instances can be very difficult and dangerous. Such children will, however, need to be carefully followed up for the appearance of tethered cord symptoms and signs.

In the newborn with SB, the spinal defect should be closed ideally within the first 2 days, although delays within the first week of life while the child is on antibiotics do not seem to adversely affect the outcome.[2] In developing countries, children typically present after the first week of life,[11,20] and the defect is often grossly infected (see Figure 119.2). While preoperative intravenous antibiotics are the rule in all settings, there is little advantage to lengthy preoperative courses of antibiotics and dressings.

The standard repair of open SB includes the following steps:[3,9]

Step 1	The sac or the skin surrounding the placode is incised; the placode is isolated circumferentially with removal of all keratinized areas as well as the superficial granulation tissue.
Step 2	The placode is tubularised with a running monofilament fine suture to reduce the raw surface and re-create a tubular cord.
Step 3	All adhesions to the cord are lysed both proximally and distally.
Step 4	The dura is dissected circumferentially with overlying fatty tissue, down to the central region of the defect.
Step 5	A watertight dural closure is achieved with one layer of running fine monofilament suture.
Step 6	The skin and subcutaneous tissues is undermined widely laterally.
Step 7	The fascia is closed with interrupted absorbable sutures at the level of the original junction of the skin, dura, and defect covering. The skin is closed with no tension.

Variations to the above steps may include:

• no tubularization of the placode if it is technically difficult;

• division of a thickened filum terminale and correction of diastematomyelia, if found;

• resection of placode and transection of the cord in cases with full paraplegia, especially if infection is present and the cord is severely atrophic/dysplastic (Figure 119.8);

• irrigation and intrathecal injection of antibiotic (usually gentamycin); and

• transverse dural closure proximally only if the cord has been transected.

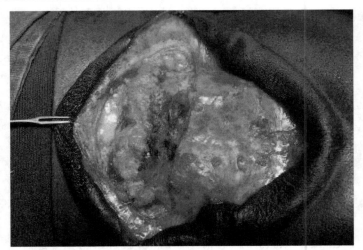

Figure 119.8: Proximal dural closure following cordotomy in thoracic-level myelomeningocele with paralytic lower extremities.

Postoperative Complications

Postoperative complications of shunt insertion can generally be classified as mechanical or infectious.

Mechanical Shunt Failure

Mechanical shunt failure can occur through proximal obstruction; distal obstruction; component separation, fracture, or migration; or excessive CSF drainage.

Proximal or distal obstruction generally presents with signs and symptoms of increased ICP, whereas infectious failure presents with fever, redness, or swelling at the surgical site, drainage of pus or CSF from the wound; nuchal rigidity; abdominal pain; or peritonitis. Shunt obstruction in older patients often presents with headache and is not associated with pain along the shunt tract. Although the signs and symptoms of shunt failure have been examined empirically, there is no ideal diagnostic test.

Revision of a noninfected but obstructed shunt should generally be approached from the cranial incision because obstruction is more common at the ventricular limb. Both ventricular and abdominal limbs can then be tested in sequence from this location after they have been disconnected from the valve. Nonfunctioning ventricular catheters that are adherent can be removed by gentle traction under most circumstances, but we do not advocate more aggressive measures; rather, a new shunt should be placed at an alternative site. Passage of a new peritoneal shunt down an established fibrous tract is occasionally possible as long as shunt infection has been ruled out preoperatively. Routine CSF culture in the absence of infectious signs or symptoms is not recommended because positive cultures in this setting are not predictive of subsequent infection.[21]

Shunt Infection

Shunt infection is widely believed to be caused by contamination at the time of surgery, with occasional infections caused by later wound breakdown either due to CSF fistulisation or skin breakdown over hardware (Figure 119.9). Most shunt infections usually present within 3 months of shunt insertion, and almost all within 6 months. The rate of shunt infection in North America is approximately 8–10%,[22] with some series reporting less than 1%,[23] but it is likely higher in Africa.[24] The most common organisms grown are consistently *Staphylococcus epidermidis* (~40%), followed by *S. aureus* (~20%).[25]

Risk factors for shunt infection include prematurity,[26,27] elaborate shunt configurations, multiple separate shunts, previous shunt infection, surgical inexperience, myelomeningocele, postoperative CSF leak, and longer duration of surgery.[28]

Common techniques to avoid shunt infection include the use of generous skin preparation, meticulous and consistent surgical technique, and preoperative prophylactic antibiotics.[29] Although there is significant worldwide heterogeneity with regard to choice of antibiotics,[30] we recommend ceftriaxone or cefazolin upon induction of anaesthesia. A Cochrane review in 2006 has supported the use of antibiotic prophylaxis in reducing shunt infection, with no evidence of benefit beyond 24 hours.[31]

As advocated by Faillace and colleagues, the avoidance of shunt-to-skin contact resulted in a three-fold decrease in shunt infection rates, from 9.1% to 2.9%.[32] As mentioned earlier, valve design does not appear to have any effect on shunt infection. The surgeon should develop a consistent routine by using the same equipment, and a meticulous approach; some authors have reported very low infection rates using similar techniques.[33] Finally, shunts should not be relegated to the most inexperienced member of the team. We agree with the author who suggested: "Although less glamorous than other neurosurgical cases, shunting procedures deserve no less attention to detail."[34]

Because conventional antimicrobial techniques are not effective in treating the bacterial biofilms that affect most neurosurgical-related device infections, all infected shunts should be removed.[35] This is to be combined with the insertion of an external ventricular drain with ongoing systemic and optional intrathecal antibiotics, with replacement of the shunt 10–14 days later with preoperative confirmation of a sterile CSF. Treatment with antibiotics alone has a high failure rate and probably is relevant only in the high-risk surgical patient. Vancomycin has poor CSF penetration by IV route, and thus preservative-free ventricular vancomycin has been commonly used to treat shunt infections, despite the incomplete understanding of its side effects and toxicity.[36]

Shuntalgia Syndrome

Shuntalgia syndrome is an unusual shunt complication that presents with focal discomfort around the shunt site *without* swelling, fluctuance or redness. There may be tenderness along the shunt itself, and there is usually a hard fibrotic sheath of scar tissue around the shunt. Shuntalgia syndrome is common in adolescents and should generally be treated with conservative measures, although narcotic analgesics have been required in some cases.

Shunt Separation, Fracture, or Migration

Shunts rarely may separate, fracture, and/or migrate within the first few months of surgery. Clinical examination and, if necessary, a shunt series of plain radiographs along the entire shunt tract are sufficient to confirm the diagnosis (Figure 119.10). The phenomenon of arrested HC (whereby a child develops true shunt independence) is infrequent: 80% of children who have stable ventricles despite a disconnected shunt have a raised ICP.[37] Therefore, most nonfunctioning shunts should be revised.

Hollow Viscus Perforation

Perforation of virtually every hollow viscus by the peritoneal catheter has been described, but is usually diagnosed by observation of the catheter protruding from the anus (Figure 119.11). The risk of hollow viscus perforation has been estimated at 1 per 1,000 shunt years.[38] Remarkably, peritonitis is *rarely* a presenting feature, likely due to the gradual erosion of the shunt through bowel. Treatment is similar to other cases of shunt infection and involves removal of the shunt in its entirety via a single valve-site incision in the cranium, external drainage for 10–14 days with intrathecal or intravenous (IV) antibiotics, followed by shunt replacement. Laparotomy is reserved for the rare case of peritonitis, but is not routinely required to remove the shunt.

Spina Bifida Problems

In spina bifida, wound problems are frequent, including infection, dehiscence, and necrosis.[11,39,40] They almost always can be managed conservatively with dressings, debridement, and sitz baths. CSF leaks may occur,[11] and although most will resolve with time and control of the CSF pressure (with shunting or acetazolamide), persistent leaks may require re-exploration.

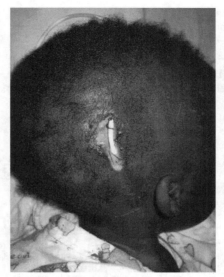

Figure 119.9: Ventriculoperitoneal shunt erosion.

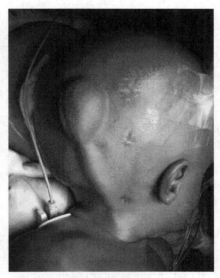

Figure 119.10: Perishunt CSF collection.

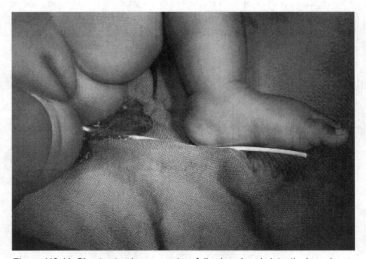

Figure 119.11: Shunt extrusion per rectum following chronic intestinal erosion.

Retethering of the cord at the repair site occurs in 15–20% of long-term cases[9] and requires prompt surgical untethering where there are progressive symptoms.

Chiari II Problems

Concomitant shunting for HC at the time of the neonatal spinal defect closure is standard in developed nations, but the approach must differ in the developing world. In the African experience, early shunting leads to frequent shunt infection and ventriculitis.[41] The authors' evidence-based practice is therefore to wait 5 days after the spinal closure for shunting, or longer if there is any evidence of wound infection. Mild, stable, HC with a cortical mantle of at least 3.5 cm can be observed safely for several months without deleterious effects.[3]

Other Chiari II symptoms and signs (e.g., apnoea, stridor, poor swallowing) are initially managed by decreasing the ICP through shunting.[9] Persistent symptoms may require a posterior fossa decompression,[3,9] although this procedure is challenging and should be referred to specialised centres.

Musculoskeletal Problems

Scoliosis and/or kyphosis are the most common orthopaedic associations of SB. They develop in up to 60% of children with SB,[11] especially in children with thoracic defects.[3] Seating appliances can help, but braces are of questionable value, and surgical management (spinal fusion) is very challenging.

Talipes equinovarus (TEV, or clubfoot) is the next most common orthopaedic problem.[11] Ideally, it is treated conservatively through casting in the neonatal period; later on, a posteromedial release may be required.[42] Other lower-extremity problems include high-arch foot deformity, leg-length discrepancy, flat foot, foot valgus, and congenital dislocation of the hip.[11]

Depending on the motor level, patients with SB may require a variety of orthotic devices to allow partial or full ambulation. These include above- and below-knee braces, crutches, walkers, and wheelchairs.[3] Traditional teaching states that independent ambulation is possible if the quadriceps are strong (L3–4), but long-term studies have shown that the mobility of children with SB decreases with age despite stable neurological status.[3,9]

Gastrointestinal Problems

Nutritional problems are frequent in the SB population. Whereas obesity from limited activity is common in developed nations, many children with SB in the developing world suffer from nutritional deficiencies.

Defecation problems are the main challenge in this population.[43,44] Constipation occurs predominantly in children with high lesions due to slow colonic transit, and in children with sacral lesions due to deficient rectal sensation.[45] Constipation may be managed through dietary manipulation combined with regular finger stimulation or manual evacuation.

Faecal incontinence is much more of a challenge, with at least half of children with SB being affected.[11,45] Children with lumbosacral lesions often have pellet-like stools from slow left colonic transit, evacuated without voluntary control despite fair sphincter function. They are best managed with intentional constipating foods and daily manual evacuation. School-age children who fail this regimen should first be tried on retrograde washouts every 1 to 3 days.[45,46] An enema device including a plastic "cone" used with an enema tube is an effective, easily produced, daily wash-out tool. The next step is the Malone antegrade continence enema (MACE) procedure.[46,47] In this procedure, the child's colon is cleaned daily with up to 500 ml water or saline administered through a cutaneous continent appendicostomy. In developed countries, this procedure has been modified to use a small cecostomy "button" device inserted under radiographic guidance.[48] The standard cutaneous appendicostomy, however, is quite effective and well-suited for the developing world.

Integumentary Problems

Decubitus ulcers occur frequently in patients with SB, especially those beyond the age of 5 years.[11] These ulcers represent therapeutic challenges. Similar to management of ulcers in other patients with neurological deficits, a conservative approach with saline dressings and avoidance of pressure areas is always warranted. Refractory ulcers can benefit from plastic surgical procedures, although recurrences are frequent.

Other ulcers in these patients are found in the perineal area and are caused by urinary and/or stool incontinence. These ulcers must be managed by attempting to address the underlying incontinence problems.

Latex Allergy

Latex allergy is an immunoglobulin E (IgE)-mediated problem leading to the spectrum of urticaria, bronchospasm, and anaphylaxis. Although latex allergy is a frequent (20-30%) complication in children with SB in developed countries,[49,50] it is rarely reported in the developing world. Some evidence from South Africa suggests a lower overall incidence compared to Western nations.[51]

Urological Problems

Spina bifida is the most common cause of neurogenic bladder dysfunction in Africa, although sacral agenesis, anorectal malformations, and sacrococcygeal teratoma also contribute. Neuropathic bladder leads to renal failure[52,53] in 50% of untreated patients by the age of 5 years, and this constitutes the main cause of mortality in this population.[54] Children with SB should be monitored from birth whenever possible—otherwise, late presentations may include palpable bladder, chronic renal failure, urinary tract infection (UTI), or urinary incontinence. Micturating cystourography (MCUG) and US may reveal a thick-walled bladder with hydronephrosis and vesicoureteric reflux (VUR).

The normal function of the bladder is to store urine at a safe pressure by coordinated relaxation of the detrusor muscle with tonic sphincter contraction, and to empty completely at low pressure on command by detrusor contraction with reflex sphincter relaxation. Failure of the sphincter tone leads to a low leak point pressure (LPP) and a wet child, but essentially a "safe" bladder. This may be assessed by examination of the anocutaneous reflex. If the anus is closed and contracts (winks) when the adjacent skin is scratched, this suggests an intact reflex arc and is usually matched by similar urinary sphincter competence. In contrast, the flaccid anus with no wink is usually associated with a low bladder outlet resistance.

An intact anocutaneous reflex, however, does not ensure coordinated detrusor sphincter activity, and lack of reflex sphincter relaxation during detrusor contraction (sphincter dyssynergia, or DSD) causes bladder outlet obstruction, often leading to detrusor hypertrophy and fibrosis. This, in turn, results in a poorly compliant bladder in which the pressure rises during filling until the leak pressure is overcome and the child is wet. If this pressure is high enough, reflux and renal damage ensue. Detrusor instability occurs as a result of primary nerve injury or secondary to bladder damage caused by the DSD. In some cases, however, the detrusor is of low tonicity, and the bladder will be large and low-pressure even with a low fixed-resistance sphincter. Whenever there is poor detrusor tone or DSD, voiding will not be complete and there will be a significant post-void residual (PVR); this reduces the functional capacity of the bladder and increases the infection risk.

In summary, there is an interplay between the bladder and sphincter muscles, which may be considered in three groups: synergic (both muscles acting in unison (19%); dyssynergic with or without detrusor hypertonicity (DSD) (45%), and denervated (36%). The basic urological work-up of patients with SB includes renal US with PVR measurement, serum creatinine, and volume urodynamics. This may be performed with disposable pressure sensors attached to a dedicated computer-based system, or, more appropriate to the African setting, using a simple burette and three-way stopcock apparatus.[55] Pressure measurement at 50% of estimated bladder capacity (8 ml/kg for infants or 30 ml/year of age), PVR and LPP are the most important guides. More sophisticated electromyography (EMG) urodynamics is rarely contributory to outcome or management.

The mainstay in the treatment of the neurogenic bladder of children with SB is clean intermittent catheterisation (CIC). This procedure is simple to perform and to teach in all patient groups; in addition, it is inexpensive, safe,[56] and very efficient. CIC has revolutionised urological care in SB and is well suited for resource-poor settings. It is most efficacious when started in infancy, although it can be started at any point in time. It is performed by the main caregiver of the child until the age of 6–7 years, after which self-catheterisation can be taught.[56]

Most European centres perform urodynamics early and at intervals of up to 5 yearly depending on individual assessment and management needs. Alternatively, a nonselective approach can be used, as performed at BethanyKids, volume urodynamics are performed 3 days after the closure of the spinal defect, and caregivers are then taught to perform CIC if the volumetric criteria are met (LPP ≥ 30 cm or a PVR ≥ 10 cc).[55] Other criteria used include laboratory evidence of renal dysfunction (abnormal renal US, creatinine, or urinalysis), recurrent UTIs, and the need to promote social continence in older children. A pressure rise of greater than 20 cm H_2O at 50% estimated bladder capacity has been associated with a poor renal outcome, and in developed countries is a relative indication for a bladder augmentation or diversion.

Antimuscarinics such as oxybutinin (administered either orally or intravesically) complement CIC by reducing detrusor overactivity; combined with CIC, these have been shown to significantly reduce the development of renal damage. CIC with or without medications will prevent renal deterioration in 90% of children with SB, and achieve social continence in about 85%.[3] Only a minority of patients should require urological procedures such as bladder augmentation, bladder neck reconstruction, or urinary diversion.[53,57,58] Augmentation cystoplasty and bladder neck repair have high revision and complication rates and should be performed only where ongoing surveillance and care can be guaranteed.

Long-term renal follow-up is essential in all SB patients, however. The authors advise twice yearly renal US initially, with void pattern and urodynamics at intervals depending on the assessment of risk and evidence of changing urological status. In developed countries, renal transplantation is ultimately the treatment of choice for renal failure,[54] but this is rarely an option in developing countries, underlining the importance of prevention of renal damage by good, early, assessment and management.

Prognosis and Outcomes

The mortality associated with shunt placement is about 0.1%, but shunt failure is more lethal—1–4%—especially in the African setting with its frequent difficult and delayed access to health care. The operative risk of ETV is still being defined, but perioperative mortality may approach 1%.[1] Shunts fail due to mechanical or infectious causes at a rate of 30–40% within the first year after placement,[22] 15% within the second year, and 1–7% per year thereafter. Shunt infection is associated with reduced intelligence quotient (IQ) and poor school performance, as well as a higher risk of future shunt infection.[59] Although the risk of ventriculitis is reduced after ETV, it is not zero.

The mortality in patients with SB appears to be 25–50% into adulthood,[3,50] and naturally higher in developing countries. Renal failure as well as sepsis and shunt complications are common causes of mortality.[60] According to a long-term Western study, more than 85% of SB patients have VP shunts, and most have undergone at least one revision.[50] A third of the patients have undergone a tethered cord release, and half have scoliosis. The same long-term Western study showed, however, that 85% of patients are attending or have graduated from high school and/or college, and more than 80% have social bladder continence.[50] A British study found a 50% mortality after 30 years; among the survivors, 70% had an IQ of 80 or more, 37% lived

independently in the community, 39% drove a car, 30% could walk more than 50 metres, and 26% were in formal employment.[61]

Results from developing countries are rather scanty. A Nigerian study found that 40% of children with myelomeningoceles were "functionally disabled" and could not be adequately rehabilitated because of limited resources.[39] The authors of that study therefore advocated selective management. A South African study revealed a 70% ambulation rate, 45% urinary continence, and a mean IQ of 80.[20] As expected, results were better in urban areas and in the higher socioeconomic groups. The authors' own experience in Kenya has shown that the quality of life of children with SB was quite acceptable, and was not related to the degree of the spinal defect.[62] Interestingly, quality of life in SB appears strongly influenced not only by neurological characteristics, but also by "soft" factors such as parental hope.[62]

Prevention

In East Africa, the single most common cause of hydrocephalus is infection of the CNS, usually via neonatal meningitis or ventriculitis. Neonatal sepsis is common and is exacerbated by the lack of skilled perinatal care for the majority of births in Africa.[8] Newborns presenting with febrile illness should ideally receive appropriate diagnostic tests and directed antibiotic therapy, and not just empiric therapy for presumed malaria. Efforts at improving perinatal care in developing countries will undoubtedly help to reduce the incidence of post-infectious HC.

Based on the overwhelming evidence for the importance of folic acid in preventing NTDs, folate supplementation of at least 400 μg daily has been uniformly recommended for all women of childbearing age. However, the difficulty in reaching this wide at-risk group makes food fortification, adopted in most developed countries, a much better method.[10] This policy, if implemented fully, is expected to result in a 50% reduction in NTDs. Unfortunately, only 10% of African countries have been able to implement this policy.[63]

Ethical Issues

There is a paucity of literature concerning the ethics of nontreatment of HC and the issues surrounding resource allocation in the treatment of this disease. Informed consent of the patient and family should address the need for lifelong ongoing surveillance of any child treated for HC, and the risks of shunt infection, shunt failure, and death. Families should be educated regarding signs of infection or shunt failure at the first admission.

Although we are not aware of any guidelines regarding assessment of medical futility in the setting of HC, we recommend extreme caution in shunting children with head circumferences >60 cm, or those who have nonhealing pressure sores on the skull. For many of these children, aggressive surgical intervention is futile, and family resources are challenged by lengthy or repeated admissions.

Similarly SB treatment is a long-term commitment, and the decision to operate must be carefully discussed with the family. Major associated congenital anomalies and prenatal large HC may lead to a palliative approach without surgery, but the level of the defect should not affect that decision. Although in the past some have advocated a selective approach to SB,[39,64] there is good evidence that a nonselective approach yields equally good results, while giving a chance for life to many more children.[3,62,65] In fact, the overall mortality and the IQs of the unselected groups compare favourably with those of the "best" infants from the selected group.[2] Looked at differently, 60% of the children from the selected group, who were allowed to die, would have been "competitive" if allowed to survive.[3]

Evidence-Based Research

Table 119.1 presents a prospective study of 195 Ugandan children that compares the Chhabra and Codman-Hakim Micro Precision shunt systems. Table 119.2 presents a trial study to evaluate the effect of folate supplementation periconceptionally in reducing foetal neural tube defects.

Table 119.1: Evidence-based research.

Title	Comparison of 1-year outcomes for the Chhabra and Codman-Hakim Micro Precision shunt systems in Uganda: a prospective study in 195 children
Authors	Warf BC
Institution	CURE Children's Hospital of Uganda, Mbale, Uganda
Reference	J Neurosurg (Pediatrics 4) 2005; 102:358–362
Problem	The high cost of commercial ventriculoperitoneal (VP) shunt systems is prohibitive in Africa.
Intervention	Insertion of VP shunts in hydrocephalic children.
Comparison/ control (quality of evidence)	Randomisation of 195 children between the Chhabra shunt system (cost: US$35) and Codman-Hakim Micro Precision Valve system (cost: US$650).
Outcome/ effect	No statistical difference was found in any shunt complication or overall outcome between the two shunt systems.
Historical significance/ comments	Classic, robust paper documenting the efficacy of appropriate simple technology for the African setting.

Table 119.2: Evidence-based research.

Title	Periconceptional supplementation with folate and/or multivitamins for preventing neural tube defects
Authors	Lumley J, Watson L, Watson M, Bower C
Institution	Cochrane Reviews
Reference	Cochrane Database Syst Rev 2001, Issue 3
Problem	The need to reduce the incidence of neural tube defects.
Intervention	Periconceptual folate supplementation.
Comparison/ control (quality of evidence)	Four trials including 6,425 women, all randomised between folate supplementation and control.
Outcome/ effect	Periconceptional folate supplementation reduced the incidence of neural tube defects (relative risk 0.28, 95% confidence interval 0.13–0.58). Folate supplementation did not significantly increase miscarriage, ectopic pregnancy, or stillbirth.
Historical significance/ comments	Critical Cochrane review documenting the clear positive effect of folate in reducing neural tube defects without any deleterious effects.

Key Summary Points

Hydrocephalus

1. Early treatment of HC with ventriculoperitoneal shunts remains the best method in Africa of preventing lifelong disability from increased intracranial pressure.

2. Clinical symptoms and signs and cranial ultrasound are sufficient for the diagnosis and management of children with HC.

3. Simple valved shunts, such as the Chhabra shunt, are as effective as more sophisticated devices and save significant resources.

4. Shunt placement must be a thoroughly sterile procedure performed by skilled, experienced surgeons.

5. Both mechanical and infectious shunt complications can be significantly reduced through meticulous technique and experience.

6. Children shunted for HC must be followed up for life and must have rapid access to health care facilities in case of complications.

7. Endoscopic third ventriculostomy shows significant promise for avoiding shunt morbidity in children with HC, but remains limited by technology and skill.

8. Besides early diagnosis, prevention of HC can be accomplished through efforts directed at the correct management of neonatal infections and folic acid supplementation for all women of child-bearing age.

Spina Bifida

1. Folic acid can prevent half of the cases of SB, and therefore efforts should be made to supplement folic acid in the diets of all women of child-bearing age. As this is very difficult in developing nations, policies for folic acid fortification of common foods should be actively pursued.

2. All children with SB should be thoroughly examined for associated conditions, including HC, musculoskeletal, genitourinary, gastrointestinal, and skin problems.

3. Initial investigations need include only head ultrasound and postoperative renal evaluation.

4. A nonselective approach to the treatment of SB leads to satisfactory results in developing nations and can be adopted if the resources are available.

5. Most SB defects in Africa present beyond 48 hours of life, and must therefore be considered infected.

6. Surgical repair may include transection of the cord, excision of the placode, and proximal dural closure in severe paraplegic cases.

7. Dural replacements and skin flaps must be avoided due to the risk of infection.

8. Shunting for HC, if needed, should be delayed by at least 5 days after the closure of the SB defect, due to the risk of infection.

9. The long-term management of children with SB is complex and requires multidisciplinary resources; therefore, these children should, as much as possible, be treated or referred to centres able to provide the necessary care.

10. The key impact on the long-term survival of children with SB is proper urological management, including urodynamic evaluation, clean intermittent catheterisation, and detrusor overactivity relaxants. Clean intermittent catheterisation is effective, inexpensive, and feasible in developing nations.

References

In addition to the following references, the reader is directed to the website for the International Federation for Spina Bifida and Hydrocephalus, www.ifglobal.org.

1. Garton H, Piatt J. Hydrocephalus. J Pediatr Clin NA 2004; 51:305–325.

2. Park TS. Myelomeningocele. In: Albright L, Pollack I, Adelson D, eds. Principles and Practice of Pediatric Neurosurgery. Thieme Medical Publishers, 1999, Pp 291–320.

3. Dias MS. Neurosurgical management of myelomeningocele (spina bifida). Pediatr Rev 2005; 26(2):50–60.

4. Airede KI. Neural tube defects in the middle belt of Nigeria. J Tropic Pediatr 1992; 38(1):27–30.

5. Kulkarni ML, Mathew MA, Reddy V. The range of neural tube defects in southern India. Arch Dis Child 1989; 64(2):201–204.

6. Msamati BC, Igbigbi PS, Chisi JE. The incidence of cleft lip, cleft palate, hydrocephalus and spina bifida at Queen Elizabeth Central Hospital, Blantyre, Malawi. Cent Afr J Med 2000; 46(11):292–296.

7. Adeloye A: Management of infantile hydrocephalus in Central Africa. Trop Doct 2001; 31:67–70.

8. Warf BC. Hydrocephalus in Uganda: the predominance of infectious origin and primary management with endoscopic third ventriculostomy. J Neurosurg (Pediatrics) 2005; 102:1–15.

9. Kaufman BA. Neural tube defects. Pediatr Clin N Amer 2004; 51(2):389–419.

10. Lumley J. Preconceptional supplementation with folate and/or multivitamins for preventing neural tube defects. Cochrane Database Syst Rev 2006;1.

11. Kumar R, Singh SN. Spinal dysraphism: trends in northern India. Pediatr Neurosurg 2003; 38(3):133–145.

12. Iantosca MR, Drake JM. Cerebrospinal fluid shunts. In: Albright AL, Pollack IF, Adelson PD, eds. Operative Techniques in Pediatric Neurosurgery. Thieme Medical Publishers, 2000, Pp 3–14.

13. Carrion E, Hertzog JH, Medlock MD, Hauser GJ, Dalton HJ. Use of acetazolamide to decrease cerebrospinal fluid production in chronically ventilated patients with ventriculopleural shunts. Arch Dis Child 2001; 84(1):68–71.

14. Libenson MH, Kaye EM, Rosman NP, Gilmore HE. Acetazolamide and furosemide for posthemorrhagic hydrocephalus of the newborn. Pediatr Neurol 1999; 20(3):185–191.

15. Kestle J, Drake J, Milner R, et al. Long-term follow-up data from the shunt design trial. Pediatr Neurosurg 2000; 33(5):230–236.

16. Pollack IF, Albright AL, Adelson PD. A randomized, controlled study of a programmable shunt valve versus a conventional valve for patients with hydrocephalus. Neurosurg 1999; 45:1399–1411.

17. Warf BC. Comparison of One-Year Outcomes for the Chhabra and Codman-Hakim Micro Precision shunt systems in Uganda: a prospective study in 195 children. J Neurosurg (Pediatrics 4) 2005; 102:358–362.

18. Pople, IK. Hydrocephalus. Surgery (Oxford) 2004: 22(3):60–63.

19. Dias L. Orthopaedic care in spina bifida: past, present, and future. Develop Med Child Neurol 2004; 46(9):579.

20. Buccimazza S, Molteno C, Dunne T. Pre-school follow-up of a cohort of children with myelomeningocele in Cape Town, South Africa. Ann Tropic Paediatr 1999; 19(3):245–252.

21. Steinbok P, Cochrane D, Kestle JR. The significance of bacteriologically positive ventriculoperitoneal shunt components in the absence of other signs of shunt infection. J Neurosurg 1996; 85(5):985–986.

22. Drake JM, Kestle JR, Milner R, et al. Randomized trial of cerebrospinal fluid shunt valve design in pediatric hydrocephalus. Neurosurg 1998; 43:294–305.

23. Choux M, et al. Shunt implantation: reducing the incidence of shunt infection. J Neurosurg 1992; 77:875–880.

24. Mwang'ombe NJ, Omulo T. Ventriculoperitoneal shunt surgery and shunt infections in children with non-tumour hydrocephalus at the Kenyatta National Hospital, Nairobi. East Afr Med J 2000; 77(7):386–390.

25. Turgut M, et al. Cerebrospinal fluid shunt infections in children. Pediatr Neurosurg 2005; 41:131–136.

26. Bruinsma N, et al. Subcutaneous ventricular catheter reservoir and ventriculoperitoneal drain-related infections in preterm infants and young children. Clin Microbiol Infect 2000; 6(4):202–206.

27. Kulkarni AV, et al. Cerebrospinal fluid shunt infection: a prospective study of risk factors. J Neurosurg 2001; 94:195–201.

28. Kontny U, Höfling B, Gutjahr P, et al. CSF shunt infections in children. Infection 1993; 21(2):89–92.

29. Haines SJ, Walters BC. Antibiotic prophylaxis for cerebrospinal fluid shunts: a metanalysis. Neurosurg 1994; 34(1):89–92.

30. Biyani N, Grisaru-Soen G, Steinbok P, et al. Prophylactic antibiotics in pediatric shunt surgery. Child Nerv Syst 2006; 22(11):1465–1471.

31. Ratilal B, Costa J, Sampaio C. Antibiotic prophylaxis for surgical introduction of intracranial ventricular shunts. Cochrane Database Syst Rev 2006; 3:CD005365.

32. Faillace WJ. A no-touch technique protocol to diminish cerebrospinal fluid shunt infection. Surg Neurol 1995; 43:344–350.

33. Choksey MS, Malik IA. Zero tolerance to shunt infections: can it be achieved? J Neurol Neurosurg Psychiatry 2004; 75(1):87–91.

34. Kanev PM, Sheehan JM. Reflections on shunt infection. Pediatr Neurosurg 2003; 39:285–290.

35. Braxton EE, et al. Role of biofilms in neurosurgal device-related infections. Neurosurg Rev 2005; 28(4):249–255.

36. Bafeltowska JJ et al. Therapeutic vancomycin monitoring in children with hydrocephalus during treatment of shunt infections. Surg Neurol 2004; 62(2):142–150.

37. Whittle IR, Johnston IH, Besser M. Intracranial pressure changes in arrested hydrocephalus. J Neurosurg 1985; 62:77–82.

38. Vinchon et al. Bowel perforation caused by peritoneal shunt catheters: diagnosis and treatment. Neurosurg 2006; 58(1 Suppl):ONS76-86.

39. Shehu BB, Ameh EA, Ismail NJ. Spina bifida cystica: selective management in Zaria, Nigeria. Ann Tropic Paediatr 2000; 20(3):239–242.

40. McLone DG, Dias MS. Complications of myelomeningocele closure. Pediatr Neurosurg 1991; 17(5):267–273.

41. Margaron F, Poenaru D, Bransford R, Albright L. Timing of ventriculoperitoneal shunt insertion following spina bifida closure in Kenya. Childs Nerv Sys (in print).

42. Flynn JM, Herrera-Soto JA, Ramirez NF, Fernandez-Feliberti R, Vilella F, Guzman J, et al. Clubfoot release in myelodysplasia. J Pediatr Orthopaed, Part B 2004; 13(4):259–262.

43. Doolin E. Bowel management for patients with myelodysplasia. Surg Clin N Am 2006; 86:505–514.

44. Lemelle JL. A multicentre study of the management of disorders of defecation in patients with spina bifida. Neurogastroenterol Motil 2006; 18:123–128.

45. Rintala RJ. Fecal incontinence in anorectal malformations, neuropathy, and miscellaneous conditions. Sem Pediatr Surg 2002; 11(2):75–82.

46. Christensen P, Kvitzau B, Krogh K, Buntzen S, Laurberg S, Christensen P, et al. Neurogenic colorectal dysfunction—use of new antegrade and retrograde colonic wash-out methods. Spinal Cord 2000; 38(4):255–261.

47. Ekmark E, Adams RC. The antegrade continence enema (ACE) surgical procedure: patient selection, outcomes, long-term patient management. Euro Jour Pediatr Surg 2000; 10(Suppl 1):49–51.

48. Chait PG, Shandling B, Richards HF. The cecostomy button. J Pediatr Surg 1997; 32(6):849–851.

49. Obojski A, Chodorski J, Barg W, Medrala W, Fal AM, Malolepszy J, et al. Latex allergy and sensitization in children with spina bifida. Pediatr Neurosurg 2002; 37(5):262–266.

50. Bowman RM, McLone DG, Grant JA, Tomita T, Ito JA. Spina bifida outcome: a 25-year prospective. Pediatr Neurosurg 2001; 34(3):114–120.

51. Johar A, Lim DL, Arif SA, Hawarden D, Toit GD, Weinberg EG, et al. Low prevalence of latex sensitivity in South African spina bifida children in Cape Town. Pediatr Allerg Immunol 2005; 16(2):165–170.

52. Carr MC. Bladder management for patients with myelodysplasia. Surg Clin N Am 2006; 86:515–523.

53. Lemelle JL, Guillemin F, Aubert D, Guys JM, Lottmann H, Lortat-Jacob S, et al. A multicenter evaluation of urinary incontinence management and outcome in spina bifida. J Urol 2006; 175(1):208–212.

54. Muller T, Arbeiter K, Aufricht C. Renal function in meningomyelocele: risk factors, chronic renal failure, renal replacement therapy and transplantation. Curr Opin Urol 2002; 12(6):479–484.

55. Jeruto A, Poenaru D, Bransford R. Clean intermittent catheterization: overview of results in 194 patients with spina bifida. Afr J Paed Surg 2004; 1(1):20–23.

56. Campbell JB, Moore KN, Voaklander DC, Mix LW. Complications associated with clean intermittent catheterization in children with spina bifida. J Urol 2004; 171(6, Pt 1):2420–2422.

57. Aslan AR, Kogan BA. Conservative management in neurogenic bladder dysfunction. Curr Opin Urol 2002; 12(6):473–477.

58. Gonzalez R, Schimke CM. Strategies in urological reconstruction in myelomeningocele. Curr Opin Urol 2002; 12(6):485–490.

59. Kanev PM, Park TS. The treatment of hydrocephalus. Neurosurg Clin N Am 1993; 4(4):611–619.

60. McDonnell GV, McCann JP. Why do adults with spina bifida and hydrocephalus die? A clinic-based study. Euro J Pediatr Surg 2000; 10(Suppl 1):31–32.

61. Oakeshott P, Hunt GM. Long-term outcome in open spina bifida. Brit J Gen Prac 2003; 53(493):632–636.

62. Cornege-Blokland E, Jansen HE, de Jong-de Vos van Steenwijk CCE, Poenaru D. Quality of life of children with spina bifida in Kenya is not related to the degree of the spinal defects. Tropical Med Int Health (in print). Trop Med Int Health 2011; 16 (1):30–36

63. UNICEF: The Micronutrient Initiative. Vitamin and mineral deficiency—a global damage assessment report. UNICEF, 2004.

64. Lorber J. Results of treatment of myelomeningocele. An analysis of 524 unselected cases, with special reference to possible selection for treatment. Develop Med Child Neurol 1971; 13(3):279–303.

65. Hunt GM. Open spina bifida: outcome for a complete cohort treated unselectively and followed into adulthood. Develop Med Child Neurol 1990; 32(2):108–118.

CHAPTER 120
COMMON PAEDIATRIC ORTHOPAEDIC DISEASES

Paul J. Moroz
Amaani K. Malima

Introduction

Globally, traumatic injuries are amongst the 10 leading causes of morbidity and mortality in children and adolescents, with most of the burden borne by low- and middle-income countries (LMICs), in particular in Africa, South-East Asia, and the Western Pacific Region.[1] Furthermore, for every injury-related death, an estimated four or five children with severe injury-related disabilities are a significant drain to their families and health systems troubled by already low resources.[2] Traumatic injury is estimated to get worse over time, in particular in the developing world, largely due to the increasing prevalence of road traffic injuries, especially in Africa.[3]

Most posttraumatic disabilities are due to injuries to the upper or lower extremities or to the spine.[4,5] For the sheer volume of musculoskeletal injuries seen everywhere in Africa, rural or urban, any hospital accepting all types of emergencies would require significant orthopaedic surgical services.[6] Furthermore, with more than 50% of the population under the age of 15 years in most developing countries, a specific familiarity with paediatric orthopaedic traumatic injuries would be required.

In most LMICs, very few orthopaedic surgeons are available to deal with these many surgical problems, and even fewer are formally trained *paediatric* orthopaedic surgeons. As such, most orthopaedic surgical services throughout Africa have been provided by general surgeons or orthopaedic clinical officers with some surgical training.[7] With the literature on the efficacy of African traditional bonesetters being limited, and in general negative,[8–10] it is likely that generalist surgeons and nonphysician clinical officers will continue to provide the vast majority of orthopaedic surgery in Africa for the foreseeable future.

Apart from the traumatic orthopaedic problems African children must endure are the additional surgical problems of congenital deformities, infections, and other conditions affecting the musculoskeletal system. Figure 120.1 presents data from Rwanda from what is probably the first national, population-based survey done in sub-Saharan Africa examining the extent of musculoskeletal impairment and treatment needs in children.[11] Beyond the sizeable burden of the acute traumatic issues already mentioned, data extrapolation from the results of this study estimates that 50,000 children in Rwanda are in need of orthopaedic surgery for *old* traumatic problems, neurological impairments, nontraumatic angular deformities (e.g., rickets), congenital anomalies (e.g., clubfoot), and bony infections.

The purpose of this chapter is to introduce newer, evidence-based approaches to some old and persistent orthopaedic surgical problems, not only in sub-Saharan Africa but also throughout the developing world. Bach[7] argues the traditional orthopaedic mantra of "Never close an open fracture nor open a closed one" in African centres, given improvements in sterilisation equipment, orthopaedic implants, availability of antibiotics, and so forth. Furthermore, failures of conservative orthopaedic care can result in significant disability. Utilisation of a public health, evidence-based approach to musculoskeletal surgical problems may reduce the sizeable morbidity of orthopaedic problems in African children. Specific problems discussed will include clubfoot, an approach to open fractures to reduce posttraumatic chronic osteomyelitis, and evidence to support an open surgical approach to supracondylar fractures of the paediatric elbow. Also addressed are angular deformities related to polio and nutritional rickets.

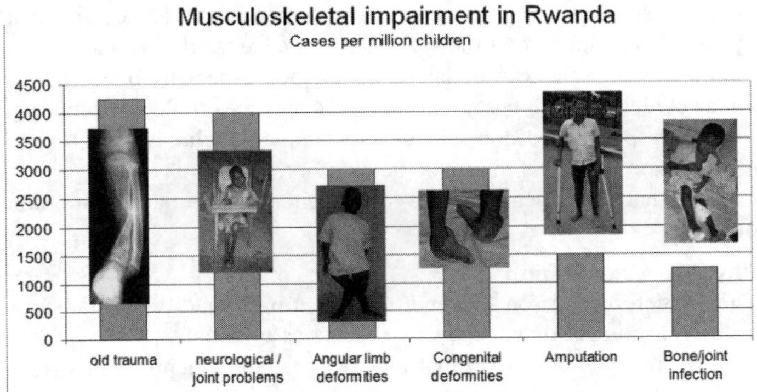

Musculoskeletal impairment in Rwanda
Cases per million children

Source: Atijosan O, Simms V, Kuper H, Rischewski D, Lavy C. The orthopedic needs of children in Rwanda: results from a national survey and orthopaedic service implications. J Pediatri Orthop 2009; 29:948–951.

Figure 120.1: The musculoskeletal problems that exist beyond the acute orthopaedic trauma needs for children in Rwanda. A major part of a public health–oriented, evidence-based approach to surgical problems is the need for accurate data to plan health services.

Congenital Idiopathic Clubfoot in Africa

Introduction

Clubfoot (CF) is perhaps the most prevalent, congenitally disabling musculoskeletal problem in the world today, leading to a lifetime of unnecessary morbidity if untreated. This condition always requires treatment, and in the past required a major surgical procedure from an experienced paediatric orthopaedic surgeon, with long-term follow-up. With few experienced surgeons and impoverished conditions, most CF in the developing world has been neglected, with resultant major disability. Over the last two decades, however, the developed world's evidence based movement in orthopaedic surgery has identified an essentially nonoperative clinical approach to CF called the Ponseti method.[12–14] An independent critical review of the available literature supports the Ponseti approach, and in Africa, Tindall and colleagues[15] have shown that even trained clinical officers (nondoctors, not just non-orthopaedists) can successfully manipulate idiopathic clubfeet using the Ponseti technique in Malawi. Similar findings elsewhere in Africa have demonstrated that a physiotherapist-delivered Ponseti programme can effectively manage CF in low-resource settings.[16]

Although not without some problems, the Ponseti method may significantly reduce the burden of this major orthopaedic disabler in many LMICs by reducing the need for major operative interventions.

Demographics

Clubfoot deformity is the most common congenital cause of ambulatory disability in the developing world, with a worldwide incidence of approximately 1 in 1,000 live births (1 in 500 in Malawi), the male-to-female ratio is 2:1, and it is bilateral in 50% of cases.[17] Omololu et al.[18] has shown, by a prospective study at the University of Ibadan, that the most common congenital orthopaedic malformations—more than 50% of all congenital musculoskeletal (MSK) malformations—were CF, with hip dysplasia accounting for only 2.2 % of all cases, for comparison.

Aetiology/Pathophysiology

Many theories exist regarding the aetiology of clubfoot, but none have been proven. These theories cite foetal development arrest, contracting fibrosis, and myogenic and neurogenic causes.

Clinical presentation

History

Clubfoot is not infrequently a component of an underlying syndrome, and therefore a complete history and physical are required. CF, for example, can be associated with hand anomalies, certain forms of dwarfism, arthrogryposis, myelomeningocele, and many other afflictions. Furthermore, the spine should be examined for evidence of spinal dysraphism at the base of the spine, such as a hairy tuft, haemangioma, lipoma, among others. A unilateral cavus foot, especially one that was not as evident at birth but has *developed* over time, could be secondary to an intraspinal condition such as a diastomatomyelia. A neurological examination is normal in idiopathic clubfoot.

Note that a significant genetic component exists for the transmission of CF.

Physical examination

The CF deformity is present and obvious at birth, and it is usually not a difficult clinical diagnosis. CF presents as a complex, three-dimensional congenital deformity that includes the components of hind-foot equinus, hind-foot varus, and mid-foot adductus and medial rotation (Figures 120.2 and 120.3). Another name for CF frequently seen in the literature is congenital talipes equinovarus (CTEV or TEV). It is the equinus component (the tight Achilles tendon) that differentiates it from severe metatarsus varus of the midfoot, another congenital foot anomaly evident at birth.

The CF deformity varies in severity, with classic or "idiopathic" clubfoot being most common. There is generalised hypoplasia of the entire leg on a limb affected with CF. The hind-foot, in particular the talus, is most dysplastic. The talar neck is shortened and angled medially and plantar-ward. The navicular articulates with the deformed medial head of the talus. All the hindfoot and midtarsal bones are hypoplastic, and the cartilage, ligaments, and muscles of the foot are hypoplastic and contracted.

The example of idiopathic clubfoot deformity in the newborn shown in Figure 120.2 is suitable for management with the Ponseti method. Treatment should begin immediately for best clinical outcomes. In contrast, neglected clubfoot is unsuitable for the Ponseti method of treatment and requires complex reconstructive surgery by an experienced surgeon. Functionality of the individual patient must be assessed carefully as it may be prudent to not submit the patient to difficult and somewhat risky surgical procedures. The child shown in Figure 120.3 would require several staged operations on each foot, and before this, he would likely need soft tissue releases for chronic knee contractures. This amount of surgery is beyond the capacity of most health systems in Africa. Clearly, treatment with the Ponseti method from birth would have prevented this chronic disability, and at a relatively low cost.

Currently, there is no widely used rating system for the severity of CF, but in general the more fixed a deformity, the greater the severity. The severity of clubfoot deformity is suggested by the extent of stiffness and size differentiation of the feet if unilateral.

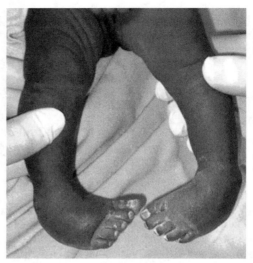

Source: Courtesy of Dr. Norgrove Penny, Senior Advisor for Physical Impairments, CBM International; Uganda Sustainable Clubfoot Care Project.

Figure 120.2: Bilateral clubfoot deformity in a newborn. Note the foot plantar flexion, hindfoot varus, and midfoot adductus.

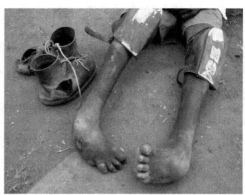

A

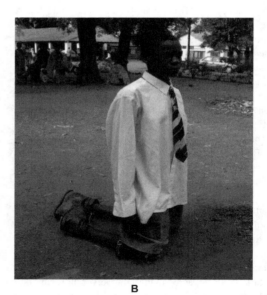

B

Source: Courtesy of Dr. Norgrove Penny, Senior Advisor for Physical Impairments, CBM International; Uganda Sustainable Clubfoot Care Project.

Figure 120.3: (A) An example of neglected clubfeet in an older child. (B) The foot deformity in this particular case is of such severity that sustained ambulation was too painful and it became easiest for the child to walk on his knees. Many children do ambulate upright on their deformed feet.

Investigations

Little consensus exists on the role of radiography in the diagnosis and management of idiopathic CF because the diagnosis in the newborn is readily made clinically. Ossification of the foot bones is slight even in healthy newborns, so the expenditure for radiographs would seem quite redundant. In neglected CF, radiographs may help the experienced surgeon to plan operative management; however, this is beyond the scope of this discussion.

Management

The general goal of management for CF of any kind and from any aetiology is to restore to the patient a pain-free, plantigrade foot. Here we discuss idiopathic CF diagnosed early, essentially after birth.

The Ponseti approach is a technique of serial manipulations and casting of the affected leg, beginning almost immediately after birth; most cases require a very minor surgical procedure—a percutaneous heel-cord tenotomy.[12] Ponseti demonstrated by using long-term studies spanning four decades, that his technique is so effective that the rate of primary operative treatment for clubfoot has decreased from more than 80% to less than 5% in many populations. Moreover, treatment results have been shown to be as effective as surgery in terms of overall function and reduction of risk of recurrence.

The clubfoot is manipulated through a series of sequential steps:

Step 1: The forefoot is supinated and the first metatarsal is dorsiflexed to correct the cavus deformity of the foot.

Step 2: While the forefoot remains in supination, the forefoot is abducted while counter pressure is applied to the head of the talus. This corrects the varus and medial deviation of the foot.

Step 3: Finally, dorsiflexion of the fully abducted foot corrects the equinus.

Step 4: The treatment consists of the application of serial casts to the manipulated foot, followed by orthotic management with a foot-ankle orthosis (FAO).

Treatment should begin immediately after birth, if possible. The clubfoot typically corrects after the application of four to five long-leg plaster casts that are applied to the manipulated foot with the knee at 90° (Figure 120.4). These casts are changed every 4 to 5 days. The final cast should be in a position of 70° of abduction and 20° of dorsiflexion. A percutaneous tenotomy of the Achilles tendon is necessary in 80% of the cases. If a tenotomy is performed, the last cast is worn for 3 weeks. After the removal of the final cast, an FAO is worn to prevent relapses. The FAO should be worn for 23 hours per day for the first 3 months and at naptime and nighttime only until 3–4 years of age. Relapses are correctable with the Ponseti method if caught early enough.[12,13]

The Ponseti treatment is *early* management of clubfoot and in general is not used in the clinical management of advanced neglected clubfoot. Neglected clubfoot treatment usually requires complex surgery, which cannot be taught to nonspecialists and should be referred to larger centres with experienced surgeons. However, some recent work in Brazil has shown some success in using low-cost Ponseti methods for treatment of neglected CF presenting after walking age, and more work may show less invasive techniques suitable for well-established cases of CF.[19]

Postoperative Complications

The stiffer the clubfoot, the less likely manipulation and casting by using the Ponseti technique will work. It is important to start treatment as soon as possible. If, after 3 months of Ponseti treatment, the foot is still not corrected, then a surgical procedure will likely be required at some point. Proper training on the Ponseti technique, with emphasis on the sequence of manipulation and casting being very

important, is required. Dr. Norgrove Penny, Senior Advisor for Physical Impairments, CBM International, Uganda Sustainable Clubfoot Care Project, has found that percutaneous tenotomy has a definite learning curve among trainees.

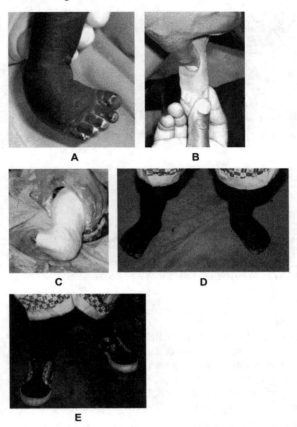

A   B

C   D

E

Source: Courtesy of Dr. Norgrove Penny, Senior Advisor for Physical Impairments, CBM International; Uganda Sustainable Clubfoot Care Project.

Figure 120.4 (A) A newborn idiopathic clubfoot deformity. (B) One step in the sequential Ponseti technique of serial manipulation of the clubfoot prior to (C) serial casting. All the sequences of the Ponseti method are not shown here. (D) A successful example of the general goal of all clubfoot care: a pain-free, plantigrade foot that can fit in normal shoes (E).

Prognosis and Outcomes

The Ponseti method achieved complete deformity correction in 95% of patients in a series by Morcuende et al.[20] Malawi has set up a Ponseti programme in 25 health districts and corrected 67% of cases to a functional plantigrade foot; however, difficulties with the supply of plaster and splints and patient compliance have affected the results, requiring more research.[17] Pirani et al.[21] have shown very impressive results in the management of idiopathic CF identified at birth. Their work in Uganda underscored the importance of ideal conditions. Due to the significant demand made on both the parents of affected children and the local health care systems, clinical success on a large scale may be more challenging than anticipated.

Prevention

In 2002, Uganda adopted a national strategy of clubfoot care as a public health prevention of disability programme. After six years, the Uganda Sustainable Clubfoot Care Project (USCCP) has collected data to suggest that the Ponseti clubfoot care approach is effective and sustainable.[21] Rural health care workers, including midwives and traditional birth attendants who come into regular contact with mothers and infants, were trained to diagnose CF and to refer infants with this deformity to local orthopaedic officers, who in turn were trained to treat these patients by the Ponseti method. A key to the programme was that orthopaedic officers and sensitized paramedical personnel were assigned to all district and regional hospitals. Early management is key to the success of the Ponseti method and part of the major challenge is community education to find the patients to start treatment (Figure 120.5).

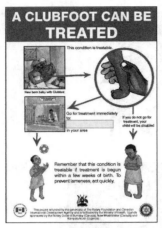

Figure 120.5. The Uganda Sustainable Clubfoot Care Project public education poster, which should be near every infirmary, birth site, hospital, and paediatric facility.

Ethical Issues

Every effort should be made to promote programmes such USCCP.[21] Surgeons, clinicians, and community leaders must advocate for the early diagnosis and referral to a centre providing Ponseti techniques and ongoing management (see Figure 120.5). It behooves surgeons and researchers to inform their respective health ministries and politicians of the success of programmes such as USCCP.

Secondary Prevention of Osteomyelitis Using Optimal Surgical Principles for Open Fractures

Introduction

Bickler et al.[22] showed that of all surgical conditions in the Gambia, osteomyelitis alone accounted for 15% of total hospital inpatient days, second only to burns. Although haematogenous osteomyelitis may be a more frequent cause of chronic bony infection in African children, posttraumatic osteomyelitis is also an important cause.[23] Indeed, from a surgeon's public-health-approach point of view, the open fracture is a more important cause because the surgeon can *secondarily* prevent posttraumatic osteomyelitis with an appropriate and timely surgical debridement. Haematogenous osteomyelitis can be prevented primarily through nonsurgical means, such as vaccination programmes,[24] improved nutrition, and poverty alleviation, which in general are not the purview of the African surgeon. From a cost-effectiveness point of view, the resources needed to treat an established posttraumatic osteomyelitis are likely much higher than those utilised to treat an acutely open fracture.[26]

It is the authors' contention that because open fractures are so common, many textbooks assume that their management is a readily available skill even in the primary health care worker's set of competencies. The sections on open fracture care in both King's *Primary Surgery*[26] or in the World Health Organization (WHO) *Surgical Care at the District Hospital*[27] each occupy less than half a page and suggest "careful wound toilet" without a detailed outline of the steps needed in appropriate debridement and irrigation and treatment of the open wound. It is the purpose of this section to give the salient details of open fracture management, in particular the precise factors important for optimum open fracture debridement.

Demographics

Ikem et al.[28] studied open fracture in Ile-Ife, Nigeria, and found the majority of open fractures were Gustilo type II or III open fractures (Table 120.1), indicating a higher risk of subsequent infection of lower-extremity fractures. Nearly half (45.8%) of these open fractures went on to fulminant infection, with delay in initial wound management being the major predisposing factor to subsequent infection.

Table 120.1: Gustilo classification of open fractures

Gustilo classification	Description
Type I	An open fracture with a wound <1 cm long and clean.
Type II	An open fracture with a laceration >1 cm long without extensive soft tissue damage, flaps, or avulsions.
Type III	Massive soft tissue damage, compromised vascularity, severe wound contamination, marked fracture instability.
Type IIIA	Adequate soft tissue coverage of fracture despite extensive soft tissue laceration or flaps, or high-energy trauma irrespective of the size of the wound.
Type IIIB	Extensive soft tissue injury loss with periosteal strippingand bone exposure; usually associated with massive contamination.
Type IIIC	Open fracture associated with arterial injury requiring repair.

Source: From Gustilo RB, Anderson JT. Prevention of infection in the treatment of 1,025 open fractures of long bones, retrospective and prospective analyses. J Bone Joint Surg 1976; 58-A:453–458.

Aetiology/Pathophysiology

Ikem and colleagues[28] found that in Nigeria *Staphylococcus aureus* and coagulase-negative staphylococci were the most common organisms associated with open fracture, and delay in initial wound management was a major predisposing factor to wound infection. Fortunately, these organisms are readily treated with antibiotics, but only if supplemented with surgical debridement.[25]

Clinical Presentation

History

The history of an injury resulting in an open fracture is important on a number of levels. The time from injury to treatment has been established as an important factor in the outcome of the injury. As important may be the mechanism of injury, with low-energy injuries (e.g., falls) usually resulting in a Gustilo type I or II fracture, and a high-energy trauma (e.g., motor vehicle crashes) resulting in a type III open fracture, with major tissue loss and possible vascular injury. One must always ask the extent of wound contamination at the injury site—for example, whether the contamination was from a farm, an environment notoriously bad for multiorganism and clostridium infections.

Comorbidities with the injury are also important in that a hypotensive patient cannot adequately perfuse injured tissue, making it more susceptible to inoculation by infecting organisms. Preinjury comorbidities, such as HIV, sickle cell anaemia, malaria, and malnutrition, can all affect susceptibility to infection in damaged tissue.[29]

The history should also include tetanus immunisation, as tetanus continues to be a problem in LMICs.[30] Allergy to antibiotics must also always be determined.

Physical examination

The accepted management of open fractures, where there is disruption of skin and soft tissue such that there is exposed bone to the environment, is surgical debridement and irrigation within 6 hours of the injury.[31]

In general, it is appropriate to consider type I and II fractures as low-energy wounds and type III fractures as high-energy wounds.[33]

Investigations

Plain radiographs can help the clinician decide the extent of debridement necessary and bony comminution (fragmentation of bone) within the fracture. Avascular pieces of bone will require removal from the wound during debridement because the avascularity of bone fragments will render them foci of infection in the wound if not removed.

Arguably, resources for taking and processing cultures of wounds in acute injuries should not be routinely utilized. Specimens for gram stain, culture, and sensitivity really play a role only in identifying organisms responsible for chronic infections in bone, such as established osteomyelitis.

Management

The goals of treatment for open fractures in children are to avoid infection, achieve soft tissue coverage and bony union and to restore function.

Presurgical management

Acute trauma resuscitation, tetanus prophylaxis, starting of antibiotics, removal of gross debris, sterile irrigation and sterile dressing, and immobilisation should be carried out initially. The theatre is prepared for surgery. Although general anaesthesia should be used ideally, in particular with type III fractures for more aggressive debridement, effective regional blocks of upper and lower extremities with local anaesthetic can be used for open fracture wound care. Lack of general anaesthetic capability should not be used as a reason not to wash out an open fracture. There is some evidence that early administration of antibiotics may protect against infection even if surgical debridement is delayed.[33]

Surgical management

Surgical management involves irrigation and debridement of open fractures. The necessary equipment includes a basic bone set (osteotome, curette, rongeur), 6–12 liters of normal saline, and wide-bore tubing for copious gravity irrigation as well as bulb and syringe for irrigation. The surgical procedure is as follows:

1. Open laceration is extended longitudinally to provide exposure.

2. Fracture ends are exposed.

3. Devitalised material is removed.

4. Bone ends are cleared of all debris, including haematoma (contaminated), with curette.

5. One litre of normal saline (or available solution) per centimeter of wound is used for irrigation.

6. Suture with 3-0 nylon.

7. Incisions are closed and the open wound is left open; if in doubt, the wound is left open but tendons, nerves, and vessels are covered.

A tourniquet can be applied for proximal vascular control, should it be required; however, the tourniquet should not be inflated in order to determine viability of tissue by bleeding. Any and all avascular tissue, including any bone fragments that no longer have soft tissue attachments (and hence blood supply) must be removed due to risks of becoming infectious foci.

Treatment of wounds by specific Gustilo type

For type I and II fractures, open wounds are opened further by longitudinal incisions proximal and distal to the open wound in order to expose the entire fracture site, (fragments and soft tissue) so that all areas can be inspected and debrided. A 1-cm wound, or even a puncture wound, more often than not hides a larger cavity below the surface. The sharp edge of the fractured bone usually has damaged muscle, leaving large cavities occupied by haematoma, which should be assumed contaminated until surgically debrided.

For type III fractures, principles similar to those for type I and II fractures apply. Sharp debridement is essential and does less damage than scraping healthy tissue with curettes. Wound debridement is done in a centripetal fashion,[34] and bony ends are delivered outside of the wound while the ends are meticulously cleaned of debris. The use of prophylactic fasciotomies should be considered. Repeat debridement is performed in 48–72 hours in order to excise devitalised tissue in type III fractures.

Types of solutions for irrigation

Normal saline is superior to other proposed irrigation agents because it is isotonic and does not disturb the body's natural healing processes.[32] The cost of sterile normal saline makes its availability a concern; a Cochrane Database Systematic Review[35] of tap water for cleansing has shown that in washing out open fractures, in the absence of potable water, boiled and cooled water or distilled water can be used as irrigation agents. Cyr and colleagues[36] studied the use of 5% sodium hypochlorite (Dakin's solution) in ground-derived field water, and showed that the treatment could virtually eliminate the bacterial burden and make the water useable.

Volume of solution for irrigation

Evidence for the optimum volume of solution to use in irrigation is minimal, but in general, the recommendation is 3 liters for a type I fracture, 6 liters for a type II fracture, and 9 liters for a type III fracture.[37] Another guideline is to use 3 liters of solution followed by 1 liter for each centimeter of open wound.

Solution delivery system for wound

High-pressure pulsatile lavage may injure already traumatised tissue and may drive bacteria deeper into the wound.[37] Low-pressure irrigation methods, such as continuous gravity irrigation or bulb syringe and suction irrigation, is efficacious in the removal of foreign material.[32]

Wound closure and fracture stabilisation

A soft tissue closure plan should be developed, but bone and wound coverage should not compromise excision of nonviable or contaminated tissue. A discussion on fracture stabilisation is beyond this review; however, protection of soft tissue should be the initial concern. Pain control is also important, and provisional stabilisation can always be revised. When in doubt, do not close the wound completely. In low-energy type I fractures that are treated less than 24 hours following the open injury, consideration can sometimes be made for primary closure. This is an approach used in the best of health care settings; it may not be realistic in the African setting. If in doubt, it is best to leave the wound open.

Antibiotics

The best "antibiotic" is an excellent wound debridement. In other words, no amount or duration of antibiotics can substitute for a timely and well-performed surgical debridement. Antibiotic prophylaxis for open fractures can depend on local factors and availabilities. In general, prophylaxis includes a first-generation cephalosporin, plus or minus an aminoglycoside, plus or minus penicillin, all depending on the type and extent of wound contamination.

Melvin et al.[32] have developed a detailed algorithm for management of open tibial fractures in the high-resource setting, but it still is useful to the low-income setting, in particular, in helping decision making for primary amputation following severe type III open fractures with neurovascular loss.

Postoperative Complications

The main adverse outcome of surgical debridement is ongoing infection and delayed union of the fracture. A low threshold for re-debridement of open wounds should be maintained at all times; for type III fractures, a routine re-debridement and irrigation at 48–72 hours after the first surgery should be considered almost routine.

Vascularity of tissue, including arterial supply and venous drainage, is the single most important determinant of complications following an open fracture.[34] Knowledge of watershed areas of blood supply to bone in the body is important, but is beyond the scope of this review.

Prognosis and Outcomes

Bach et al.[38] have shown in Malawi that modern management of open fractures in experienced hands can achieve clinical results similar to that seen in higher-income clinical settings. Chronic disability in their cohort of patients at a free-at source hospital was seen in only 12% of patients following open fractures. This work should stand as an indicator that much can be done in Africa to reduce the burden of posttraumatic osteomyelitis, as the prevalence of open fractures in children will likely increase with the increasing incidence of motor-vehicle crashes, in particular vehicles hitting children.[2]

Prevention

Prompt surgical intervention to remove the potential for infection in open fractures can be considered a form of *secondary* prevention. *Primary* prevention would be an intervention to avoid the traumatic event leading to the open fracture, such as streetlights at night so car-child impacts might be avoided. Secondary prevention by timely, aggressive, and extensive debridement and irrigation of an open fracture prevents the establishment of osteomyelitis.

Bach et al.[38] found that in Malawi only 72% of patients reached the hospital within 24 hours of their open fracture. Although the Gustilo and Anderson[31] recommendation of irrigation and debridement within 6 hours may be unrealistic at the present time for much of Africa, the most recent evidence from a North American setting suggests that chronic infection can be avoided following open fracture if the patient presents within a maximum of 24 hours.[39] However, an equally important factor is the quality of the debridement and irrigation.

Ethical Issues

The causes of delayed management of open fractures requires study, but little work has been done in this area in developing countries. Clearly, the effects of poverty, malnutrition, and clinical co-morbidities (e.g., human immunodeficiency virus (HIV), anaemia, sickle cell anaemia, malaria, tuberculosis (TB)) all will have profound effects on wound healing, bony union, and avoidance of infection.

Supracondylar Elbow Fracture in Children

Introduction

Supracondylar fractures (SCFs) in children are common injuries throughout the world and are also the most common injuries requiring surgical intervention. They also cause the most complications and poor outcomes if not adequately treated, in particular when suboptimally managed with poor local resources and expertise.[40] Every attempt should be made to manage these problematic fractures with closed reduction and percutaneous pinning, but there is an arguably growing consensus that the threshold for performing an open reduction should be lowered.[41] It is likely that a careful open reduction may be safer than multiple attempts at closed reduction and acceptance of a poorly reduced fracture. Furthermore, Howard[42] has described little difference in outcomes in closed versus open reductions, and the historical worries of excessive stiffness and heterotopic ossification following open reductions are likely unfounded.

In the developing world, other issues may favour open reduction, such as delayed presentation, where closed reductions of a type III displaced SCF after one week can be very difficult and perhaps even unsafe. Furthermore, it is the experience of one of the authors (PJM), working in Asia, that open reduction of SCF in the absence of x-ray assistance in the operating room (OR) can ensure anatomic reduction and accurate placement of percutaneous pins. Therefore, for practical reasons, open reduction of the paediatric supracondylar fracture in LMICs may be indicated, and it is the purpose of this section to briefly introduce the concept of open reduction via an anterior approach to the elbow for the typical extension-type supracondylar fracture.

It must be emphasized, however, that if an adequate closed reduction and percutaneous pinning can be achieved, it is the preferred management. However, in light of clear indications for open reduction and internal fixation (e.g., vascular or nerve deficit, irreducible fracture), an anterior approach as described herein aids in the vast majority of severe SCF of the paediatric elbow.

Demographics

Supracondylar fractures of the paediatric elbow are the most common operative fractures in children in both the developed[43] and developing[40] worlds. In the developing world, SCF often presents late and treatment is delayed, increasing the need for an open reduction.[44,45] Typically, more males have SCF, and the left elbow appears to be more at risk. The peak age of 5 to 8 years seems to correlate with the peak of hyperextensibility of the child's elbow.

Aetiology/Pathophysiology

Most SCFs displace in extension (95%), either posteromedially or posterolaterally, threatening important neurovascular structures as a result (Figures 120.6 and 120.7). Flexion injuries are far less common. The degree of fracture displacement likely indicates the risk to neurovascular structures.

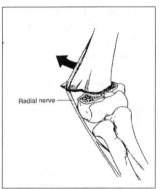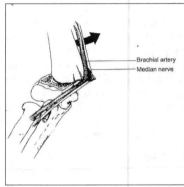

A	**B**

Source: Beaty JH, Kasser, JR, eds. Rockwood and Wilkins' Fractures in Children, 6th ed., Lippincott, Williams and Wilkins, 2006, with permission.

Figure 120.6: (A) In a posteromedial type III fracture, if the spike of bone from the leading edge of the proximal humeral fragment penetrates the brachialis muscle laterally, the radial nerve may be tethered. (B) In a posterolaterally displaced type III fracture, the spike can tether the median nerve and the brachial artery together.

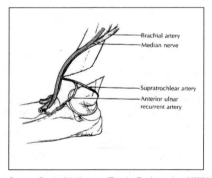

Source: Beaty JH, Kasser, JR, eds. Rockwood and Wilkins' Fractures in Children, 6th ed., Lippincott, Williams and Wilkins, 2006, with permission.

Figure 120.7: Mechanism of vascular injury to the brachial artery in typical extension-type supracondylar fracture of the elbow. Increasing displacement likely increases the extent of injury to the artery. Timely closed reduction, even in the emergency room, often will restore a feeble or absent radial pulse.

Clinical Presentation

History

Mechanism of injury details are important (e.g., how high was the fall? what was the position of the elbow during the fall?). Other injuries, especially ipsilateral shoulder/wrist/forearm injuries are important for management. The last meal, which hand is dominant, and previous injuries to the elbow may be important. Past immunisations and past general anaesthetic complications should be queried.

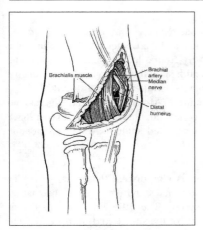

Source: Beaty JH, Kasser, JR, eds. Rockwood and Wilkins' Fractures in Children, 6th ed., Lippincott, Williams and Wilkins, 2006, with permission.

Figure 120.8: The anteromedial approach: A curvilinear anterior approach with the proximal arm of the incision being superomedial can address the neurovascular bundle (NVB) that is at risk in most type III SCFs. The proximal humeral fragment is often buttonholed through the brachialis muscle, and the NVB is tented over this. Because of the muscle damage anteriorly, the subcutaneous haematoma there can be used to guide the incision. Since most of the damage is done, direct visualisation allows for anatomic reduction and pinning of the fracture after the NVB is relieved or repaired.

Physical examination

The preoperative evaluation involves an obvious deformity with the elbow usually extended. Documentation of neurological status of the median, ulnar, and radial nerves as well as assessment of the pulse are important. A pulseless hand that is warm and with normal capillary filling can often be followed, but serial examination is important to ensure the hand remains viable despite an absent or weak pulse. Serial examination is important to watch for the evolution of a compartment syndrome. A cold, pulseless hand requires exploration of the brachial artery, as described in the Management section of this chapter. In 10–20% of cases there is a neurological deficit, the most common being the anterior interosseous nerve (AIN), which motors the deep flexor of the index finger and flexor polllicis longus.

A haematoma on the anterior elbow surface indicates muscle damage to the distal brachialis and biceps muscle and suggests the possibility of bone fragment invagination into muscle. An anterior haematoma on the skin is a good landmark to guide the anterior incision for an open approach to the fracture because following the skin incision, the deeper dissection is usually already done by the sharp fracture fragment, and just below the incision the fracture is often immediately accessible (Figure 120.8). Furthermore, the neurovascular structures (Figures 120.6–120.8) at risk for injury are easily found anteriorly.

Investigations

Plain anteroposterior (AP) and lateral radiographs suffice to show the type of fracture for classification purposes and for treatment. There are two types of fractures: the extension type (95%) and flexion type.

Gartland's classification for extension fractures recognizes that anterior cortex fails first with a resultant posterior displacement of the distal fragment:[46]

Management

Past concerns and reluctance to open the paediatric elbow due to concerns of stiffness are unfounded, and many authors have shown that open reduction is safe and effective.[47,48] Fleuri-Chateau et al.,[41] Gennari et al.,[49] and Beaty and Kasser[43] have demonstrated that open reduction of SCF is safe and effective and concluded that the threshold for open reduction should be lowered. It is the authors' contention that open reduction will likely be safer and more effective for severe, irreducible

fractures, in particular for the surgeon who deals relatively infrequently with these fractures. A brief review of the pertinent anatomy before surgery helps to appreciate the location of the neurovascular bundles demonstrated in Figures 120.6 and 120.7.

Open reduction improves the ability for satisfactory reduction in the absence of imaging intensification. With an anterior transverse incision, the fracture fragments can be pieced together and held with the fingers in position while K-wires are drilled retrograde from the distal into the proximal fragment. Without x-ray imaging, the position of the K-wires is appreciated because the surgeon can see where the K-wire is going into bone through the open wound.

Koudstaal et al.[50] demonstrated that the anterior approach to displaced extension type supracondylar fractures was preferable to other open techniques in terms of safety and simplicity. It is a compelling approach in that it exposes directly the threatened neurovascular bundle (see Figure 120.8) and the subcutaneous haematoma anterior to the elbow joint usually means the dissection deep to the skin incision down to bone has already been done by the proximal fracture sharp edge. Once skin is incised, exploration with the finger is often direct to bone.

Anterior approach to the paediatric elbow

Type I: nondisplaced fracture

Type II: displaced fracture with intact posterior cortex;

Type III: displaced fracture with no cortical contact (posteromedial > posterolateral)

1. A transverse incision is made just above the flexion crease of the elbow. Significant bruising often is seen where the incision is going. The incision can be extended distally on the ulnar aspect of the transverse incision and proximally on the radial side if needed (see Figure 120.8).

2. The NVB may be very superficial, and may disappear into the fracture site.

3. The brachial artery and median nerve are identified.

4. Dissection is proximal to distal.

5. Soft tissues (including periosteum) are removed from the anterior fracture site.

6. The fracture is reduced under direct vision.

7. The fracture is pinned in the usual fashion with 0.062 K-wires.

8. With a fracture, the reduced viability of the arm usually recovers whether or not the brachial artery is functioning. The collateral blood supply is usually adequate.

Following open reduction of the fracture the fracture can be easily reduced with no soft tissue interposition and can often be palpated to be anatomic. Thus, an image intensifier may not be required, although when present it should be used to assess the adequacy of reduction. Percutaneous pinning of the supracondylar fracture is then carried out, with two lateral pins usually; if still unstable, a supplementary medial pin is used.

Vascular injury

Note that the pulse often returns with a timely closed reduction, and this is the first approach to the displaced supracondylar fracture without a pulse.

Surgical exploration of an injured artery for the purposes of repair is a tertiary hospital activity by an experienced surgeon and is not practical in many African settings where supracondylar fractures occur. Fortunately, many pulseless hands with supracondylar fractures are warm and viable with very good capillary refill and do not require explorarion. Howard's review[42] of the best (level IV) evidence for this issue from the literature concludes that the pulseless, viable hand following supracondylar fracture should be treated by observation, with vascular interventions only when the pulseless hand appears cold and nonviable.

Postoperative Complications

Postoperative complications include the following:

- *Infection:* Pintract cellulitis, abscess, septic arthritis (especially if there are multiple lateral pins).

- *Nerve injury:* AIN injury is most common with a posterlateral type fracture; radial nerve injury is common with a posteromedial fracture displacement; and the ulnar nerve can be injured iatrogenically if a medial pin is used.

- *Compartment syndrome:* Watch for increased swelling, hard compartments, pain with passive flexion and extension of fingers, and often pain control. Close serial examination of the patient postoperatively is required, and a return to the theatre for compartmental fasciotomies must always be considered.

- *Growth disturbance:* This is rarely the cause of malalignment, which is usually due to malreduction.

- *Stiffness:* Patient may lose 10–20 degrees of terminal extension.

Prognosis and Outcomes

Farley et al.[51] have demonstrated that nonpaediatric orthopaedic physicians who treat SCF infrequently can manage these difficult fractures with outcomes and complication profiles similar to paediatric orthopaedists. Cubitus varus has an incidence of approximately 5% and is usually of cosmetic significance, usually with a good functional range of motion. The major poor outcome comes with compartment syndrome.

Prevention

Every district hospital and any moderately busy surgical centre in Africa—or anywhere in the world, for that matter—will see this common fracture, so local expertise should develop to deal with the most challenging aspects of these fractures. The anxiety with open SCF management should be reduced with the debunking of the concept that opening a paediatric elbow is somehow ill-advised or incompetent. Knowledge of the basic anatomical structures, as discussed in this section, makes this approach safe.

Ethical Issues

Two surgical Africa's exist: the bush hospital with no or minimal surgical resources and the slowly developing African district hospital surgical infrastructure, where an open approach to fractures is now safer, almost to the level of developed countries. In the former environment, open management is perhaps ill advised, whereas in the latter, basic surgical techniques should allow for safe and efficacious open reduction of SCF and the development of local expertise for management of this very common fracture, which is prone to a number of complications.

Poliomyelitis-Related Long Bone Angular Deformity

Despite decreasing rates of new cases of polio due to worldwide vaccination programmes, residual deformities secondary to polio continue to be common in Sub-Saharan Africa, India, and much of the developing world.[52] The literature on the orthopaedic management of polio is extensive and cannot be reviewed here other than to discuss some general principles. A detailed account of polio and the large number of procedures available to manage the musculoskeletal problems associated with this disease is available in the sizeable literature, in particular the classic surgical chapter by Tachdjian.[53] The emergence of "postpolio syndrome" (PPS), a condition that develops 20 to 30 years following the initial onset of polio, appears to be of increasing importance to clinicians and is reviewed briefly in this section. Although PPS has been recognized for more than 100 years, it appears important now because of the large epidemics of poliomyelitis that occurred in the 1940s and 1950s.

Demographics

WHO has indicated that polio has reemerged in a number of African countries, including Angola, Chad, and the Democratic Republic of the Congo, with increases due mostly from a lack of immunisations. The agency estimates that 75% of children on the African continent receive vaccines, and efforts are being taken to raise the number to 85%.[54]

As of 2010, in only four countries (Afghanistan, India, Nigeria, and Pakistan)[54] was polio endemic, compared with 125 countries in 1988.[55] It is important to note that unvaccinated adults traveling to endemic countries can contract polio.

Aetiology/Pathophysiology

Poliomyelitis is an acute infectious viral disease that initially invades the gastrointestinal and respiratory tracts and then spreads haematogenously to the central nervous system. The polio virus has a particular affinity for the anterior horn cells of the spinal cord, in particular the cervical and lumbar enlargements of the cord, and for specific motor nuclei of the brain stem.[53]

Clinical Presentation

History
The phases of polio

The course of polio is divided into acute, convalescent, and chronic phases, with the acute phase, lasting 5 to 10 days, being the period when paralysis may occur. The acute phase is considered terminated 48 hours following the return of normal temperature in the patient.

Following the acute phase of polio is the convalescent phase, or the recovery stage. Here, the acute symptoms and muscle tenderness disappear and the paralysed muscles start to recover. This stage can last for up to 2 years after the acute onset of polio. During this entire period, there is gradual recovery of the muscles, rapidly usually in the first 6 months, then more slowly. Motor power plateaus by 12 months in most patients.

The period after 18 to 24 months is called the residual-paralysis stage. No recovery of muscle power occurs in this stage, and deformities that occur are due to imbalance of muscle power and poor posture. There is also disuse atrophy of muscles and shortening of the leg due to interference with growth. In severely neglected cases, gross fixed deformities of the hip, knee, and foot occur with severe wasting of muscles (Figure 120.9).[56] Impoverished children with extensive paralysis and gross deformities literally have to crawl on all fours to move from place to place.

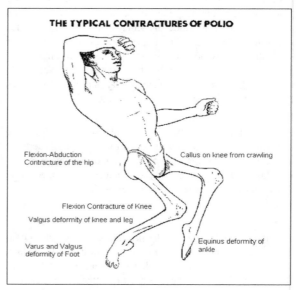

Source: Adapted from Vidyadhara S, Rao SK, Shetty MS, Gnanadoss JJ. Poliomyelitis. e-Medicine, updated 20 November 2008. Accessed 24 February 2010.

Figure 120.9: Contractures possible in polio after the chronic, residual phase with treatment addressing muscles and limbs generally neglected.

Postpolio Syndrome

Postpolio syndrome has received considerable attention recently with late manifestations of poliomyelitis developing in patients 20 to 30 years after the occurrence of the acute illness. An estimated 25–60% of the patients who had acute polio may experience these late effects of the disease.[56]

The specific cause or causes of PPS are unknown, with both pathophysiologic causes and functional causes. Pathophysiologic causes may include chronic poliovirus infection, death of the remaining motor neurons with aging, or damage to the remaining motor neurons caused by increased demands or secondary insults, and immune-mediated syndromes. Functional aetiologies for PPS include greater energy expenditure as a result of weight gain and muscle weakness caused by overuse or disuse.

Postpolio syndrome is characterised by neurologic, musculoskeletal, and general manifestations. Musculoskeletal manifestations include muscle pain, joint pain, spinal changes such as spondylosis and scoliosis, and secondary root and peripheral nerve compression. General manifestations include generalised fatigue and cold intolerance. The slowly progressive muscle weakness occurs in those muscle groups already involved, such as the quadriceps and calf muscles.

Physical examination

Physical examination of the limbs and joints is key in assessing the nature of extremity contractures, in particular the relationship of contractures to neighbouring joints and the spine. Experienced functional assessment skills by orthopaedic surgeons, orthopaedic clinical officers, physiotherapists, and occupational therapists are important to plan a comprehensive treatment plan for the polio patient.

Investigations

A history with a detailed orthopaedic and neurological clinical examination is essential to define the clinical problems to be addressed in the management of poliomyelitis. Depending on the stage of polio, serial examinations of the patient guide the therapeutic regimen. The rate and extent of muscle recovery is also appreciated only with serial examinations—monthly, if possible. When muscle power in a polio patient shows no improvement over a 3-month period, it is unlikely to recover any more functionally and serves as an important prognostic tool. At this point, appropriate orthotic treatment should be considered to improve function. If functional motor improvement is continuing, then orthotic/splint management may, in fact, thwart recovery.

Diagnostic criteria for postpolio syndrome include:

- A prior episode of paralytic poliomyelitis with residual motor neuron loss (which can be confirmed through a typical patient history, a neurologic examination, and, if needed, an electrodiagnostic examination, which in the African setting is unnecessary or unavailable.

- A period of neurologic recovery followed by an interval (usually 15 years or more) of neurologic and functional stability.

- A gradual or abrupt onset of new weakness or abnormal muscle fatigue (decreased endurance), muscle atrophy, or generalised fatigue.

- Exclusion of medical, orthopaedic, and neurologic conditions that may be causing the symptoms mentioned above.

Management

Treatment

Treatment in the acute stage is mainly medical, including general supportive treatment for fever and irritation, for the prevention of secondary respiratory infection, and for any respiratory paralysis. The paralyzed legs are supported by plaster splints or pillows and sandbags to keep the hip joints in slight flexion and in neutral rotation. The knee joint is held at 5° of flexion, and the foot is supported in a neutral, 90° position. Splinting relieves pain and spasm and prevents the development of deformities. Physiotherapy is needed to maintain range of motion and should be implemented from the very start of the acute phase of the disease. Prevention of joint contracture is much easier to treat, and less costly in dollars and manpower, than established joint contractures.

The general goals of management of poliomyelitis were established by the International Society of Prosthetics and Orthotics consensus conference on poliomyelitis at Hammamet, Tunisia, in 1997,[58] and include:

- overcoming the effects of paralysis;
- correcting deformities;
- restoring joint mobility;
- relieving pain; and
- restoring limb length discrepancy.

In low-resource settings, management is challenged by the need for a comprehensive treatment plan for each patient, with priorities focused on:

- addressing ambulation;
- prevention of deformity, especially during growth;
- decreasing the needs for bracing;
- addressing the upper extremity; and
- managing spinal deformity.

In the ideal setting, the orthopaedic physican/surgeon and the physiotherapist should be involved early with the polio patient in order to *prevent* many of the residual deformities that result from muscle imbalances, which result in the muscle and tendon contractures that impair function and produce joint contractures as well as the pain and disability associated with these.

Physiotherapy and rehabilitation

Physical therapy prevents or corrects deformity through passive stretching exercises and by increasing motor strength through active exercising of muscles that remain active following the chronic phase (after 18 months postexposure). Perhaps most important, physical therapy includes functional training, which enables the patient to learn methods to overcome the handicaps of physical disability from polio.

Orthotics and appliances

The primary objectives of orthotic management according to Tachdjian[53] include:

- supporting walking to increase functional activity;
- protecting a weak muscle from overstretching;
- augmenting weak muscles or substituting for absent muscles;
- preventing deformity and malposition; and
- correcting deformity by stretching contracted muscles.

In general, dynamic splinting is superior to static splinting; however, cost constraints preclude the manufacture of dynamic splints in many developing countries.

Surgery

Surgery is indicated when deformities interfere with the activities of daily living (ADLs), to stabilise joints that have become unstable due to chronic muscle imbalance, and to improve motor function via tendon transfer (Figure 120.10). A plethora of operative procedures, including fasciotomy, joint capsulotomy, tendon transfers, osteotomy, and bony arthrodesis, can be used to address the paralytic deformities of the upper or lower extremities seen in polio; however, a detailed account of these procedures is beyond the scope of this brief review. Leg length discrepancy is common in polio from shortening of the paralyzed leg, and many procedures are available to correct this. Patient selection is extremely important, requiring some surgical experience, and has been well described by Krul.[59]

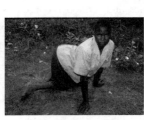
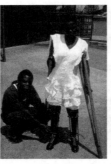

Figure 120.10: Large improvements in quality of life and productivity are seen following the management of postpolio paralysis. Resource-intensive care requires physiotherapy, appliances such as braces and walking aids, and also surgery; in this case, to relieve hip and knee contractures and lengthen tight heel-cords.

Postoperative Complications

The outstanding chapters in Tachdjian's *Pediatric Orthopedics*[53] describing surgery for all of the deformities related to polio and similar flaccid paralytic diseases include discussion of postoperative complications. Speigel[58] has also referenced many of the classic surgical articles for the management of polio.

Prognosis and Outcomes

Two primary factors are important when considering the prognosis of polio with ideal clinical management in place:

1. The severity of the initial paralysis: If total muscle paralysis persists beyond the second month, then severe motor cell destruction is likely; this is in contrast to partial paralysis, for which the prognosis is better.

2. The diffuseness of the regional distribution of paralysis: A weak muscle surrounded by paralyzed muscles is less likely to recover than if it were next to strong muscles.

Perhaps a larger factor in prognosis is scarcity of timely physical therapy resources to address contractures and provide range of motion for the patient. For this reason, Speigel[58] has stated that when resources are scarce, younger patients and those with lesser degrees of deformity should be prioritized.

Prevention

In recent years, some attention has focused on vaccine-associated paralytic poliomyelitis (VAPP), in which cases of poliomyelitis are caused by the oral vaccine. The risk of polio contraction from vaccine is extremely low, however, perhaps 1 case in 2.5 million doses, with those at risk including immunocompromised hosts and infants receiving their first dose. WHO has recommended that, to prevent this rare complication, children be inoculated first with inactivated vaccine, followed by oral attenuated vaccine.[60,61] The surgeon can act as community advocate in support of the widespread use of approved national vaccination programmes (Figure 120.11).

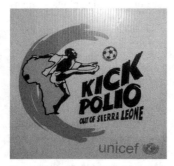

Source: Courtesy of UNICEF, with permission.
Figure 120.11: Poster promoting polio vaccine in Sierra Leone.

Ethical Issues

"Rehabilitation" surgery in the orthopaedic sense is meant to promote improvements in function.[20,58,59] Often, this surgery requires a very experienced surgeon; the clinical decision to operate is often a more difficult task than doing the actual operation itself. Furthermore, rehabilitation surgery should be performed only when there is patient access to physical therapy and orthotics. Resources are limited, thus limiting access to the benefits of this surgery to only a small number of Africans.

Nutritional Rickets and Angular Deformities in Orthopaedics

Introduction

Nutritional rickets (NR) constitutes a high burden of morbidity and mortality among children in Africa as the precursors of NR (i.e., poor socioeconomic status, low birth weight, protein-energy malnutrition, and common childhood infections) all continue to be common on the African subcontinent.[62] Surgeons and orthopaedic officers will likely not be providing the medical management of NR but will be referring children with significant angular deformities. This brief discussion of the orthopaedic management of NR will concentrate on the long bone angular deformities seen in the lower extremities.

Demographics

Nutritional rickets remains a public health problem in many countries, despite dramatic declines in the prevalence of the condition in many developed countries since the discoveries of vitamin D and the role of ultraviolet light in prevention. The disease continues to be problematic among infants in many communities, especially among infants who are exclusively breast-fed, infants and children of dark-skinned residents living in temperate climates, infants and their mothers in the Middle East, and infants and children in many developing countries in the tropics and subtropics, such as Nigeria, Ethiopia, Yemen, and Bangladesh.

Aetiology/Pathophysiology

Rickets has a long aetiological list; this discussion concentrates on NR, although the orthopaedic manifestations and surgical management may be similar for all aetiologies of ricketseal MSK disease. Rickets is caused by decreased levels of calcium or phosphate, leading to abnormal mineralisation of the skeleton. It occurs in growing children, and both the cartilage of the physes and the bones are involved.

Vitamin D deficiency is a major cause of rickets among young infants in many countries, because breast milk is low in vitamin D and its metabolites and social and religious customs and/or climatic conditions often prevent adequate ultraviolet light exposure. In sunny countries, such as Nigeria, South Africa, and Bangladesh, such factors may not apply.

Akpede et al.[63] showed that deficiency or reduced availability of dietary calcium may be of at least equal importance with vitamin D deficiency in the aetiology of NR in the Sahel savanna in Nigeria. In some parts of Africa, deficiency of calcium, phosphorus, or both in the diet may also lead to rickets, especially in societies where corn is predominant in the diet. Calcium and vitamin D intakes are also low in infants who are fed vegan diets, particularly lactovegans, and monitoring of their vitamin D status is essential. Dietary calcium deficiency and vitamin D deficiency represent two ends of the spectrum for the pathogenesis of nutritional rickets, with a combination of the two in the middle.

Clinical Presentation

History

By definition, rickets is observed only in growing children, although the effects may be observed later in life if untreated. No sexual predilection is noted. Agarwal et al.[64] showed that delayed walking in New Delhi children may be the initial manifestation of NR in children, and that the majority of ricketic nonwalkers will start to walk within 2 to 5 months of appropriate treatment.

Physical examination

Children affected with rickets present with short stature, often under the third percentile, as well as muscle weakness and frontal bossing of the skull with enlargement of suture lines. In more severe instances in children older than 2 years, vertebral softening can lead to kyphoscoliosis, the kyphotic segment known as the rachitic "catback" deformity. However, the physical ailment most disabling and that is most amenable to surgical intervention is the angular deformity of the lower extremity, either valgus or varus.

Weight bearing produces the angular deformities usually bowlegs (varus) and knock-knees (valgus). Oginni et al.[65] showed that children in Nigeria between the ages of 2 and 5 years with large angular deformities in their knees likely had rickets. They further showed that young children with NR generally had varus deformities at the knees. Children a bit older showed a more bimodal deformity presentation, either varus or valgus. Older children with NR were more likely to display valgus deformities (Figure 120.12).

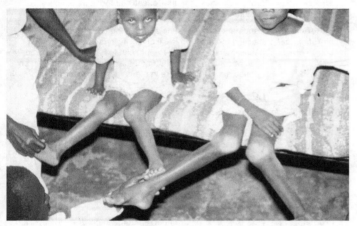

Source: Courtesy of Dr. Norgrove Penny, Senior Advisor for Physical Impairments, CBM International; Uganda Sustainable Clubfoot Care Project.

Figure 120.12: Two children with severe valgus (knock-kneed) deformities secondary to NR. Had they been younger walking children when their NR developed they would have more than likely had bowed, or varus, deformities. Correction of valgus deformities puts the peroneal nerves at risk and they must be mobilised surgically at the time of surgical correction to prevent postoperative drop-foot deformities.

In the chest, knobby deformities result in the rachitic rosary along the costochondral junctions. The weakened ribs pulled by muscles also produce flaring over the diaphragm, which is known as the Harrison groove. The sternum may be pulled into a pigeon-breast deformity.

Investigations

The biochemical diagnosis of NR is often the role of the paediatrician or medical consultant, and will not be discussed here. The treating surgeon will use x-rays largely to manage children with the MSK manifestations of NR. Radiographic findings of NR include widening of the metaphyses and the appearance of flaring or cupping at the physis (growth plate at the end of the long bone), in particular, those near the knee and the distal radius.

Management

Knowledge of the use of a variety of external fixation devices, from the circular frames developed by Ilizarov[66] in Russia to the uni- and multi-planar frames, is key for the surgeon managing the deformities of NR. Not all deformities require an external fixator, and the benefits of an acute correction via angular osteotomy include a one-time surgical procedure with the reduced risks of infection and other complications. Slow correction by external fixation, usually for more severe and complex deformities, requires considerable training and resources. A "one-time" osteotomy to correct a modest angular deformity may be

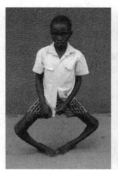
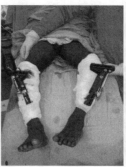
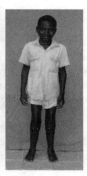

Source: Courtesy of Dr. Norgrove Penny, Senior Advisor for Physical Impairments, CBM International; Uganda Sustainable Clubfoot Care Project.

Figure 120.13:. A case of angular deformity from nutritional rickets in a young boy. A uniplanar external fixator, of a kind not readily available in Africa, was used to completely correct this child's gross angular deformity to a normal slight genu valgum.

appropriate in the district, "up-country" hospital, where ordinary orthopaedic hardware, such as plates or K-wires, can be used. However, the more severe and complex angular deformity, more suited for an external fixator, is more appropriate in the specialty hospital setting (Figure 120.13) due to the need for the complex frames.[20]

Considerable surgical experience is needed for the large, complex, sometimes three-dimensional (3D) deformities seen. Fortunately, most deformities from NR appear to be uniplanar, either valgus or varus, unlike the 3D deformities seen with posttraumatic malunions. Selection of internal versus external fixation is only one problem that must be solved in limb angular-deformity surgery. Another is the decision as to where exactly the "centre of rotational deformity" (CORA) lies in the long bone because this determines where the boney osteotomy will be performed.[67] Considerable preoperative planning is required here, and a detailed discussion of the appropriate use and intricacies of angular deformity surgery is beyond the scope of this chapter.

Postoperative Complications

The list of complications from surgery for angular deformity is lengthy and is beyond the scope of this chapter. With respect to complications affecting the efficacy of surgical management, the benefits of experience and preoperative planning cannot be underestimated.

Prognosis and Outcomes

There is a paucity of survey data on the types of paediatric orthopaedic conditions that require surgery and the factors influencing their outcome in most parts of sub-Saharan Africa. Akinyoola and colleagues[68] showed that the most common indications for surgery in Nigeria were angular knee deformities (from Blount's disease and rickets) and clubfoot. Wound infection was the most common postoperative complication (8.2%). The patient's age, length of preoperative hospital stay, length of operation, and intraoperative blood loss above 200 ml were statistically significant factors adversely affecting the surgical wound outcome. Most of these factors for poor outcome were patient- and environment-related and were considered preventable.

Prevention

The only systematic review of NR in Africa was carried out in Ethiopia in 2005,[62] and much work is needed to address nutritional, genetic, and clinical management issues with NR. Prevention of surgical issues of NR is best approached through primary care nutritional and poverty alleviation.

Thacher et al.[69] showed Nigerian children with rickets have a low intake of calcium and have a better response to treatment with calcium alone or in combination with vitamin D than to treatment with vitamin D alone. Since Nigerian children with rickets had low calcium intake, treatment should focus on dietary supplementation with calcium or a combination of calcium and vitamin D.

Ethical Issues

African mothers' awareness about rickets is still very low and is a major reason for late presentation or complete failure to seek treatment for rickettsial deformity. Lack of funds, poor compliance with treatment, prolonged treatment periods, and lack of information on where to seek treatment were among the important factors affecting completeness of treatment of knee deformity due to rickets in Nigeria.[70] Increased and sustained public health programmes are necessary for prevention, and it has been argued that health policy should incorporate free surgical fees for children with established rickettsial knee deformity to encourage community participation in the management of this preventable condition.

Evidence-Based Research

Table 120.2 presents results of a Rwandan national survey on the orthopaedic needs of children. Table 120.3 presents a USCCP training program for congenital clubfoot in Uganda. Table 120.4 presents a systematic review of treatment of open fractures of the tibia in children.

Table 120.2: Evidence-based research

Title	The orthopaedic needs of children in Rwanda: results from a national survey and orthopaedic service Implications
Authors	Atijosan O, Simms V, Kuper H, Rischewski D, Lavy C
Institution	Ministry of Health, Rwanda; Nuffield Orthopaedic Center, Oxford, UK; London School of Hygiene and Tropical Medicine, London, UK
Reference	J Pediatr Ortho 2009; 29:948–951
Problem	Lack of objective, population-based data on the magnitude of orthopaedic problems in Rwandan children and the types of services required, such as surgical services.
Intervention	A national survey of musculoskeletal impairment prevalence using cluster sampling techniques and an urban/rural demographic split matching national population distribution data.
Comparison/ control (quality of evidence)	The data are of high quality because this is a population-based survey. The weakness of the study is that some estimates are extrapolations. The survey also did not measure acute trauma, which any planning scheme would have to include.
Outcome/ effect	Establishment of benchmark data.
Historical significance/ comments	This study is possibly the first national-level, population-based study in sub-Saharan Africa to attempt to quantify the "global" burden of disease in children's orthopaedics for the purposes of treatment planning and provision. From a public health approach, disease surveillance is essential to determining burden levels for resource allocation planning. Very few benchmark studies exist for surgical problems in orthopaedics in developing countries.

Table 120.3: Evidence-based research

Title	Towards effective Ponseti clubfoot care: the Uganda Sustainable Clubfoot Care Project (USCCP)
Authors	Pirani S, Naddumba E, Mathias R, Konde-Lule J, Penny JN, Beyeza T, Mbonye B, Amone J, Franceschi F
Institution	Uganda Ministry of Health; University of British Columbia, Vancouver, Canada.
Reference	Clin Orthop Relat Res 2009; 467:1154–1163
Problem	Congenital clubfoot, one of the most common congenital musculoskeletal deformities worldwide.
Intervention	Ponseti technique of clubfoot care; not suitable for neglected cases of clubfoot.
Comparison/ control (quality of evidence)	Level IV, therapeutic study.
Outcome/ effect	USCCP has trained 798 healthcare professionals to treat foot deformities at birth. Ponseti clubfoot care is now available in 21 hospitals in Uganda.
Historical significance/ comments	Landmark programme to address the congenital deformity causing the most physical disability in the world. Ongoing assessment of USCCP-treated clubfoot cohort with a high level of evidence demonstrated that this programme can be applied almost anywhere in the developing world.

Table 120.4: Evidence-based research

Title	Open fractures of the tibia in the pediatric population: a systematic review
Authors	Baldwin KD, Babatunde OM, Huffman GR, Hosalkar HS
Institution	University of Pennsylvania, Children's Hospital of Philadelphia, Philadelphia, Pennsylvania, USA
Reference	J Child Orthop 2009; 3:199–208
Problem	How the treatment for open fractures in children has evolved over the past three decades, based on Gustilo type.
Intervention	Comparison of infection rates between different types of open fractures.
Comparison/ control (quality of evidence)	Systematic review of paediatric studies only with 14 studies with linear regression analysis insures level IV evidence.
Outcome/ effect	No significant difference in odds of infection between type I and type II fractures; type III fractures have 3.5-fold and 2.3-fold greater odds of infection than type I and type II fractures, respectively.
Historical significance/ comments	A strong relationship exists between Gustillo subtypes and odds of infection; union rates are delayed with increasing severity of injury.

Key Summary Points

Congenital Idiopathic Clubfoot

1. The Ponseti method of idiopathic clubfoot treatment can effectively treat clubfoot (CF) identified at birth with perhaps >90% effectiveness with only a small, percutaneous tenotomy required under local anaesthetic. This has changed the approach to CF worldwide and benefits low- and middle-income countries by relatively low-cost intervention.

2. African studies have shown that effective Ponseti treatment can be done with nonspecialist physicians and nonphysician health care workers.

3. Neglected clubfoot in older children will likely require surgery in experienced hands; however, some work suggests Posenti techniques may be used in neglected cases.

4. Percutaneous tenotomy is required in 80% of cases, and this outpatient procedure done under local anaesthetic can take some experience to master.

5. An important factor in effecting Ponseti treatment is bringing patients from rural settings to the district centres offering treatment. Community-based, public health approaches are needed.

Secondary Prevention of Osteomyelitis

1. Haematogenous osteomyelitis is probably the biggest cause of osteomyelitis in children in Africa; however, open fractures are another major cause, and open fractures are amenable to prevention by timely surgical techniques.

2. Surgeons can practise secondary prevention by immediate surgical debridement of open fractures.

3. Type I and II open fractures need urgent care and can be done with simple tools, such as local anaesthetic and simple, available, but copious solutions. Low-energy type I fractures can wait for surgery until the next morning, but should not be left until the following evening (i.e., should be treated within 24 hours).

4. Open fractures should not be treated without opening the wound. This is true even for what appears to be merely a puncture wound over the fracture site, since the cavity deep to the wound is often much larger than anticipated and can contain a haematoma that can become contaminated and the focus of a fulminant infection.

5. Type III open fractures require immediate surgical attention and antibiotics and, ideally, transfer to an experienced surgical facility where a secondary debridement should be planned almost routinely prior to or simultaneous to the definitive management of the fracture.

6. Work done in Africa shows that the disability from open fractures can be reduced almost to the level seen in developed countries when proper treatment is done.

Supracondylar Elbow Fracture

1. Open procedures on the paediatric elbow do not cause excessive stiffness or heterotopic ossification.

2. Open reduction of a paediatric supracondylar fracture (SCF) is safer than multiple attempts at reduction of a grossly displaced fracture and acceptance of a poor reduction.

3. An excellent approach to the typical type III extension SCF is a transverse anterior approach just above the flexor crease because once through the skin, much of the dissection has been done by the fracture and bone is easily seen, as are at-risk neurovascular structures.

4. Open reduction allows for anatomic reduction of fracture fragments by palpation, and appreciation of placement of K-wires, even without x-ray control or fluoroscopy.

5. A warm, pulseless, but viable hand associated with a type III SCF can be observed; a cold, pulseless hand needs immediate attempt at closed reduction to resume circulation and, if unsuccessful, then immediate open reduction.

Poliomyelitis-related Long Bone Angular Deformity

1. The emergence of postpolio syndrome, a condition that develops 20 to 30 years following the initial onset of polio, appears to be of increasing importance to orthopaedic surgeons.

2. Unvaccinated adults traveling to polio-endemic countries can contract polio.

3. Delay of referral of polio patients to the orthopaedic officer, physiotherapist, or surgeon is a major cause of severe joint contractures and the resulting severe functional impairment.

4. To be effective in polio patients, surgery requires dedicated pre- and postoperative physio- and occupational therapy.

5. Surgeons can also play important roles in their communities in advocating for preventative interventions, such as surveillance and immunisation programmes.

Nutritional Rickets and Angular Deformity

1. Nutritional rickets (NR) continues to be a significant problem in the developing world, although prevention interventions are effective.

2. Long bone angular deformity of the lower extremity is the primary problem dealt with by the orthopaedic officer or surgeon.

3. Surgeons and orthopaedic officers can play leading roles in their communities in advocating for prevention interventions for NR.

References

1. Hyder AA. World Health Report 2002: Reducing Risks, Promoting Healthy Life. World Health Organization, 2002.

2. Murray CL, Lopez AD. Global Patterns of Cause of Death and Burden of Disease in 1990, with projections to 2020. World Health Organization, 1996.

3. Peden M, Oyegbite K, Ozanne-Smith J, Hyder AA, Branche C, Rahman AKMF, et al, eds. World Report on Child Injury Prevention. World Health Organization, 2008.

4. Mock CN, Tiska M, Adu-Ampofo M, Boakye G. Improvements in pre-hospital trauma care in an African country with no formal emergency medical services. J Trauma 2002; 53:90–97.

5. Masiira-Mukasa N, Ombito BR. Surgical admissions to the Rift Valley Provincial General Hospital, Kenya. East Afr Med J 2002; 79:373–378.

6. Mock CN, Cherian MN. The global burden of musculoskeletal injuries. Clin Orthop Rel Res 2008; 466:2306–2316.

7. Bach O. Musculoskeletal trauma in an East African public hospital. Injury, Int J Care Injured 2004; 35:401–406.

8. Omololu AB, Ogunlade SO, Gopaldasani VK. The practice of traditional bonesetting: training algorithm. Clin Orthop Relat Res 2008; 466:2392–2398.

9. Omololu B, Ogunlade SO, Alonge TO. The complications seen from the treatment by traditional bonesetters. West Afr J Med 2002; 21:335–337.

10. Oyebola DD. Yoruba traditional bonesetters: the practice of orthopaedics in a primitive setting in Nigeria. J Trauma 1980; 20: 312–322.

11. Atijosan O, Simms V, Kuper H, Rischewski D, Lavy C. The orthopedic needs of children in Rwanda: results from a national survey and orthopaedic service implications. J Pediatri Orthop 2009; 29:948–951.

12. Ponseti IV. Congenital Clubfoot: Fundamentals of Treatment. New York: Oxford University Press, 1996.

13. Staheli L, ed. Ponseti Management of Clubfeet. Available at: Global-HELP.org.

14. Dietz FR. What is the best treatment for idiopathic clubfoot? In: Wright JG, ed. Evidence-Based Orthopaedics. The Best Answers to Clinical Questions. Saunders, Elsevier, 2009, P 265.

15. Tindall AJ, Steinlechner CW, Lavy CB, Mannion S, Mkandawire N. Results of manipulation of idiopathic clubfoot deformity in Malawi by orthopedic clinical officers using the Ponseti Method: a realistic alternative for the developing world? J Pediatr Orthop 2005; 25:627–629.

16. Shack N, Eastwood DM: Early results of physiotherapist-delivered Ponseti service for the management of idiopathic congential talipes equinovarus foot deformity. J Bone Joint Surg Br 2006; 88: 1085–1089.

17. Lavy CB, Mannion SJ, Mkandawire NC, Tindall A, Steinlechner C, Chimangeni S, Chipofya E. Club foot treatment in Malawi—a public health approach. Disabil Rehabil 2007; 29:857–862.

18. Omololu B, Ogunlade SO, Alonge TO. Pattern of congenital orthopaedic malformations in an African teaching hospital. West Afr J Med 2005; 24: 92–95.

19. Lourenco AF, Morcuendes correction of neglected idiopathic clubfoot by the Ponseti method. J Bone Joint Surg 2007; 89:378–381.

20. Morcuende JA, Dolan LA, Dietz FR, Ponseti IV. Radical reduction in the rate of extensive corrective surgery for clubfeet using the Ponseti method. Pediatr 2004; 113:376–380.

21. Pirani S, Naddumba E, Mathias R, Konde-Lule J, Penny JN, Beyeza T, Mbonye B, Amone J, Franceschi F. Towards effective Ponseti clubfoot care: the Uganda Sustainable Clubfoot Care Project. Clin Orthop Relat Res 2009; 467:1154–1163.

22. Bickler SW, Bickler, BS. Epidemiology of paediatric surgical admissions to a government referral hospital in the Gambia. Bulletin of the World Health Organization 2000; 78(11):1330–1336.

23. Onuba O. Coping with osteomyelitis. African Health 1992; 15:27–28.

24. Howard AW, Viskontas D, Sabbagh C. Reduction in osteomyelitis and septic arthritis related to Haemophilus influenzae type B vaccination. J Ped Orthop 1999; 19:705–709.

25. Museru LM, Mcharo CN. Chronic osteomyelitis: a continuing orthopaedic challenge in developing countries. Int. Orthop 2001; 25:127–131.

26. King M, ed. Primary Surgery, Vol. 2: Trauma. Oxford University Press, 1987.

27. Emmanuel JC. Surgical Care at the District Hospital. World Health Organization, 2004.

28. Ikem IC, Oginni LM, Bamgboye EA, Ako-Nai AK, Onipede AO. The bacteriology of open fractures in Ile-Ife, Nigeria. Niger J Med 2004; 13: 359–365.

29. Booker SR, Collins CM, Cover JA, Lavy CR, Brueton. Children's surgery cancelled due to malaria and anemia. Trop Doc 2007; 37:193.

30. Ajoye FO, Odusanya OO. Survival from adult tetanus in Lagos, Nigeria. Trop Doc 2009; 39:39–40.

31. Gustilo RB, Anderson JT. Prevention of infection in the treatment of 1025 open fractures of long bones, retrospective and prospective analyses. J Bone Joint Surg 1976; 58-A:453–458.

32. Melvin JS, Dombrowski DG, Torbert JT, Kovach JL, Esterhai JL, Mehta S. Open tibial shaft fractures: I. evaluation and initial wound management. J Amer Acad Orthop Surg 2010; 18:10–19.

33. Skaggs DL, Kautz SM, Kay RM, Tolo VT. Effect of delay of surgical treatment on rate of infection in open fractures in children. J Pediatr Orthop 2000; 20:183–188.

34. Zalavras CG, Marcus RE, Levin LS, Patzakis MJ. Management of open fractures and subsequent complications. J Bone Joint Surg Am 2007; 89:883–895.

35. Fernandez R, Griffiths R. Water for wound cleaning. Cochrane Database Syst Rev. 2008; 23(1):CDOO3861.

36. Cyr SJ, Hensley D, Benedetti GE. Treatment of field water with sodium hypochlorite for surgical irrigation. J Trauma 2004; 57:231–235.

37. Anglen JO. Wound irrigation in musculoskeletal injury. J Am Acad Orthop Surg 2001; 9:219–226.

38. Bach O, Hope MJ, Chaheka CV, Dzimbiri KM. Disability can be avoided after open fractures in Africa—results from Malawi. Injury 2004; 35:846–851.

39. Pollak AN, Jones AL, Castillo RC, Bosse MJ, MacKenzie EJ. The relationship between time to surgical debridement and incidence of infection after open high-energy lower extremity trauma. J Bone Joint Surg Am 2010; 92:7–15.

40. Gaudeuille A, Douzima PM, Makolati SB, Mandaba JL. Epidemiology of supracondylar fractures of the humerus in children in Bangui, Central African Republic. Med Trop (Mars) 1997; 57:68–70.

41. Fleuriau-Chateau P, McIntyre W, Letts M. An analysis of open reduction of irreducible supracondylar fractures of the humerus in children. Can J Surg 1998; 41:112–118.

42. Howard AW. How should we treat elbow fractures in children? In: Wright, JG, ed. Evidence based orthopedics: the best answers to clinical questions, 1st ed. Saunders, 2009, P 190.

43. Beaty JH, Kasser JR. Supracondylar fractures of the distal humerus. In: Beaty JH, Kasser JR, eds. Rockwood and Wilkins' Fractures in Children, 5th ed. Lippincott, Williams and Wilkins, 2001, Pp 577–615.

44. Reitman RD, Waters P, Millis M. Open reduction and internal fixation for supracondylar humerus fractures in children. J Pediatr Orthop 2001; 21:157–161.

45. Sibinski M, Sharma H, Bennet GC. Early versus delayed treatment of extension type-3 supracondylar fractures of the humerus in children. J Bone Joint Surg 2006; 88 Br;380–381.

46. Image available at: http://www.wheelessonline.com/image7/supr1.jpg.

47. Celiker O, Pestilci F, Tuzuner M. Supracondylar fractures of the humerus in children: analysis of the results in 142 patients. J Orthop Trauma 1990; 4:265–269.

48. Furrer M, Mark G, Ruedi T. Management of displaced supracondylar fractures of the humerus in children. Injury 1991; 22:259.

49. Gennari J, Merrot T, Piclet B, et al. Anterior approach versus posterior approach to surgical treatment of children's supracondylar fractures: comparative study of thirty cases in each series. J Pediatr Ortho 1998; 7:307–313.

50. Koudstaal MJ, De Ridder VA, De Lange S, Ulrich C. Pediatric supracondylar humerus fractures: the anterior approach. J Orthop Trauma 2002;16(6):409–412.

51. Farley FA, Patel P, Craig CL, Blakemore LC, Hensinger RN, Zhang L, Caird MS. Pediatric supracondylar humerus fractures: treatment by type of orthopedic surgeon. J Child Orthop 2008; 2:91–95.

52. Singh P, Das JK, Dutta PK. Eradicating polio: its feasibility in near future? J Commun Dis 2008; 40:225–232.

53. Tachdjian M. Poliomyelitis. In Herring JA, ed. Tachdjian's Pediatric Orthopedics, 3rd ed. WB Saunders, 2002, chap 26.

54. Data available at http://www.who.int/mediacentre/factsheets/fs114/en/index.html.

55. Dutta A. Epidemiology of poliomyelitis—options and update. Vaccine 2008; 26: 5767–5773.

56. Vidyadhara S, Rao SK, Shetty MS, Gnanadoss JJ. Poliomyelitis. e-Medicine Orthopedic Surgery; available at http://emedicine.medscape.com/article/1259213-overview (updated 29 September 2010; accessed 24 March 2011).

57. Perry J, Barnes G, Gronley JK. The postpolio syndrome. An overuse phenomenon. Clin Orthop Relat Res 1988; 233:145.

58. Spiegel DA. Bibliography of Orthopaedic Problems in Developing Countries. Global-HELP Publication, 2003, P 81.

59. Krul K, ed. Rehabilitation surgery for deformities due to poliomyelitis. Techniques for the district hospital. World Health Organization, 1993.

60. Minor P. Vaccine-derived poliovirus (VDPV): impact on poliomyelitis eradication. Vaccine 2009; 29:2649–2652.

61. World Health Organization. Polio reemerging in Africa. 15 December 2009. http://en.wikinews.org/wiki/WHO:_Polio_reemerging_in_Africa (accessed 24 February 2010).

62. Wondale Y, Shiferaw F, Lulseged S. A systematic review of nutritional rickets in Ethiopia: status and prospects. Ethiop Med J 2005; 43:203–210.

63. Akpede GO, Solomon EA, Jalo I, Addy EO, Banwo AI, Omotara BA. Nutritional rickets in young Nigerian children in the Sahel savanna. East Afr Med J 2001; 78:568–575.

64. Agarwal A, Gulati D, Rath S, Walia M. Rickets: a cause of delayed walking in toddlers. Indian J Pediatr 2009; 76:269–272.

65. Oginni LM, Badru OS, Sharp CA, Davie MW, Worsfold M. Knee angles and rickets in Nigerian children. J Ped Orthop 2004; 24:403–407.

66. Ilizarov GA. Transosseous osteosynthesis: theoretical and clinical aspects of the regeneration and growth of tissue. Springer-Verlag, 1998.

67. Paley D. Principles of Deformity Correction. Springer, 2002.

68. Akinyoola AL, Adegbehingbe OO, Ogundele OJ. Factors influencing the outcome of elective pediatric orthopedic operations in Ile-Ife, Nigeria. Tanzan J Health Res 2008; 10(2):68–72.

69. Thacher TD, Fischer PR, Pettifor JM, Lawson JO, Isichei CO, Reading JC, Chan GM. A comparison of calcium, vitamin D, or both for nutritional rickets in Nigerian children. N Engl J Med 1999; 341:602–604.

70. Adegbehingbe OO, Adegbenro CA, Awowole IO, Tomori PO, Oyelami OA. Perception and knowledge of mothers on causes and treatment of rickets associated knee deformity in Ile-Ife, Osun State, Nigeria. Tanzan J Health Res 2009; 11:40–45.

CHAPTER 121
PLASTIC AND RECONSTRUCTIVE SURGERY

Peter Nthumba

Introduction

In most parts of the African continent, plastic and reconstructive surgery remains among the least developed surgical specialties, with training opportunities available only abroad. As a result, this specialty still depends largely on the abilities of nongovernmental organisations (NGOs), philanthropic individuals, and organised surgical safaris/camps to meet the reconstructive needs of the majority of the populace. Because of the overwhelming needs for this service, general surgeons and the few paediatric surgeons provide this care. It is therefore essential that the surgeon managing paediatric reconstructive surgical problems be well informed on the spectrum of presenting pathologies, as well as the available options and resources for their treatment.

This chapter highlights the most common reconstructive topics peculiar to Africa. It is not intended to be a comprehensive text, and the reader is referred to appropriate texts, including those mentioned at the end of this chapter. Illiteracy, superstition, poverty, and armed conflicts continue to hamper the evolution of health care for all in Africa into the 21st century. In addition, children with disabilities or deformities are still hidden away from school and society. Most public transport, health, and education systems remain disability-unfriendly. Surgeons can become agents of change; by providing quality surgical care and educating the relatives and community, children with disabilities or deformities can become socially acceptable. Educational opportunities will give them the vehicles to self-actualisation.

A good understanding of embryology and anatomy are indispensable for the management of paediatric plastic and reconstructive surgical problems. Embryology is important because congenital aberrations and malformations form the majority of these problems; surgical restoration of form depends on a good knowledge of normal anatomy. As a caution to the surgeon, the patient and relatives of the patient, an appreciation of the limitations of current surgical techniques in achieving desired results is essential. Patients and their relatives must be involved in the decision-making process and informed on available options. Realistic goal-setting is a crucial part of reconstructive surgery. The physician must also gently inform the patient and relatives of the need for long-term follow-up and/or therapy. The surgeon seeks to restore form, function, and cosmesis, but this is not always possible, and part of the process of goal-setting must include agreeing on which of these aspects are the most feasible and most important to achieve. Staged procedures and their results should also be carefully relayed to the patients and relatives.

Whenever a congenital malformation is presented to the clinician, the history taken must include, amongst others:

- prenatal and postnatal history;
- maternal and paternal age;
- family medical history;
- consanguinity;
- previous maternal abortions; and
- teratogens.

A search must be made for other malformations in the child. Failure to diagnose a cardiac anomaly preoperatively may result in the death of a child from a non–life-saving procedure.

Skin Grafts

In many instances in surgical practice, relatively superficial or simple wounds cannot be closed primarily; skin grafts are a good choice for wound closure in such circumstances. Skin grafts may be split- or full-thickness (Table 121.1), depending on the amount of dermis included. Split-thickness grafts consist of the epidermis and varying amounts of dermis, whereas full-thickness grafts carry the entire dermis as well. Skin grafts carry with them adnexal structures.

Table 121.1: Features of split-thickness versus full-thickness grafts.

Parameters	Split-thickness graft	Full-thickness graft
Adnexal structures	Contains sweat glands, sebaceous glands	Contains sweat glands, sebaceous glands
Donor site	Donor sites heal primarily from skin adnexal structures	Requires closure or a split-thickness skin graft for closure
Available donor sites	Large amounts can be harvested	Limited donor sites. Size limited because of donor defect.
Graft "take"	Takes readily	Take is more precarious
Cosmesis of graft/color match	Poor	Fair to good
Primary contracture	Minimal	Significant
Secondary contracture	Significant (up to 40%)	Minimal

Primary contraction is the recoil of skin grafts immediately after harvest. It depends on the amount of elastin present in the dermis—the thicker the dermal layer, the greater the degree of contraction. This is not of clinical significance. Secondary contracture, in contrast, involves myofibroblastic activity. The thinner the graft, the greater the resulting secondary contracture.

The donor site must be well prepared to receive the skin graft for a successful "take". Skin grafts will not take on infected beds, exposed bone (without periosteum), cartilage (without perichondrium), or tendon (without paratenon). The only exception to this general rule is the facial skeleton. Skin grafts take well on temporal and orbital bones even without periosteum.

Meshing skin grafts increases the size of the available graft, but results in a poor cosmetic ("pebbled") appearance. The skin grafts must be well applied to the recipient bed. A moist environment enhances graft take, and thus wet bolster dressings should be applied to maintain close apposition, as well as to maintain a moist environment. Haematomas and seromas compromise skin grafts if not well immobilised.

If the recipient bed is bleeding excessively, the harvested skin may be stored in saline and applied the next day in the ward. This is an especially useful manoeuvre when operating time is limited. Skin stored in saline in a refrigerator is viable for up to one week.

Flaps

Unlike skin grafts, flaps have their own blood supply. For more complex, unstable, or deep wounds, skin grafts are inadequate. More tissue is required to fill these defects, and thus flaps are used. The flaps used may be pedicled or free, random or axial. Depending on the needs of the recipient, the defect, and available tissue, flaps may be cutaneous, myocutaneous, or even osteomyocutaneous.

Vacuum-Assisted Closure

Negative-pressure therapy, also called vacuum-assisted closure (VAC), was begun as a method of treatment of chronic wounds that were resistant to standard treatment modalities. Subsequent studies indicated that VAC therapy was a useful adjunct in the treatment of patients with lower-extremity injuries with exposed bone, tendon, and orthopaedic hardware. To date, negative-pressure therapy has been used for the management of all types of complex wounds and related conditions, including gastrointestinal fistulas, dehisced sternotomy, and abdominal wounds. Standard VAC therapy is expensive. VAC involves a piece of foam with an open-cell structure inserted into the wound, a drain placed on the foam, and the entire construct covered by a transparent adhesive plastic sheet secured to healthy wound margins. The drain is connected to a vacuum machine with a disposable reservoir.

The mechanism of action remains controversial, with many mechanisms proposed, including the acceleration of wound debridement, maintenance of a moist wound environment, and removal of oedema fluid. The VAC further improves wound perfusion, stimulates formation of healthy granulation tissue, and decreases bacterial colonisation.

The use of negative-pressure therapy significantly reduces the number of wound dressing changes as well as the associated pain.

Negative-pressure therapy is contraindicated in malignant wounds, grossly infected or necrotic wounds, and in wounds with inadequate haemostasis.

Because of the expense involved in procuring VAC kits, many hospitals in the developing world have developed novel negative-pressure therapy systems. Successful use of wall suction or suction machines (that must be turned on and off to simulate interrupted negative-pressure) therapy with gauzes packed into the wound and clean food-wrapping plastic available in the local supermarkets have been reported.

Tissue Expanders

Tissue expanders increase the surface area of local tissue, facilitating performance of reconstructive procedures and closure of defects that would otherwise require complicated procedures. Progressive inflation increases the overlying tissue and avoids the need for transfer of distant tissue, maximising aesthetic results.

Tissue expansion requires at least three stages: (1) the initial insertion; (2) an intermediate period of inflation to a predetermined size over a period of weeks; and (3) a final procedure, during which the prosthesis is removed, the flap is developed, and it is used to cover the defect. Leaving the injection port outside the skin avoids the pain of repeated injections through skin in subsequent visits. The amount instilled at each visit is determined by the amount that either blanches the skin or causes pain, whichever comes first.

Deformities resulting from burns, trauma, and irradiation, as well as congenital defects such as Poland's syndrome, are all amenable to coverage by use of tissue expansion. Myocutaneous flaps and full-thickness donor sites may all be pre-expanded to provide more tissue, both for the recipient site, as well as to facilitate primary donor closure, especially with free flaps. The resulting cosmesis is significantly enhanced. Unfortunately, tissue expanders are relatively expensive and have not yet found widespread use across Africa.

Several comments can be made regarding complications involved with tissue expansion.

- Infection may result, either from contamination of the prosthesis at the time of surgery, or later from exposure of the implant.

- Expander exposure is usually due to technical problems related to poor prosthesis placement or aggressive expansion. Remove the expander if exposure or infection occurs early in the course of expansion. If either occurs much later, the procedure is completed as planned.

- Discomfort and pain associated with expansion are usually transient and can be managed by using analgesics.

- The lower extremity, back, buttock, and neck are highly prone to complications.

- Skull deformation is temporary and resolves with time after the expander is removed.

- Implant deflation may occur if the prosthesis accidentally gets disconnected from the filling port.

- Seromas and haematomas are common, and are best prevented by the use of a closed/suction drain at the time of prosthesis insertion.

Vascular Lesions

Vascular lesions may be divided into haemangiomas and vascular malformations. Management of congenital vascular lesions remains a major challenge because their therapy carries a substantial risk of recurrence, morbidity, and—depending on location and size—even mortality. The wide spectrum of presentation extends from innocuous birthmarks to life-threatening conditions, such as the aggressive kaposiform haemangioendothelioma and tufted angioma (both associated with the Kasabach-Merritt phenomenon). Surgical extirpation is associated with significant bleeding, requiring massive transfusion. The lesions are therefore managed only in centres that are equipped to handle the expected difficulties and complications. Table 121.2 presents the most common sites and clinical evolution of vascular lesions.

Table 121.2: Vascular lesions.

Lesion	Most common sites	Clinical evolution
Haemangioma	Skin and viscera	Initial proliferation followed by involution. Size, location, and shunting are main concerns.
Kaposiform haemangioendothelioma	Skin and other tissues	Associated with Kasabach-Merritt phenomenon.
Tufted angioma	Skin	Slow growth. May present with tenderness or Kasabach-Merritt phenomenon.
Angiosarcoma	Skin and liver; pulmonary metastases possible	Degeneration of hepatic haemangioendothelioma or vascular malformation into angiosarcoma.
Congenital haemangioma	Skin	Spontaneous regression may occur; rarely, mild thrombocytopenia.
Eccrine angiomatous hamartoma	Skin (limbs)	Benign but painful.
Pyogenic granuloma	Oral, nasal cavities	Associated with trauma. Recurrence can occur in up to 15% upon excision.

Haemangiomas

Haemangiomas are the most common tumours of infancy and childhood, affecting approximately 12%, 1.4%, and 0.8% of Caucasian, African, and Asian infants, respectively, by the age of 1 year. The diagnosis is made from the patient's history and physical examination findings. There is a slight female predominance, and 60% of the lesions occur in the head and neck region.

Mulliken and Glowacki developed a biological classification of congenital vascular lesions based on the degree of cellular turnover, histology, clinical findings and natural history. They described two major groups: infantile haemangiomas and vascular malformations. The natural course of haemangiomas is defined by two distinct clinical stages: proliferation and involution. Except for the occasional precursor lesion, haemangiomas are not evident at birth. Proliferation occurs during the first 12 months of life, whereas involution begins at 1 year, peaks at 2 years, and gradually diminishes thereafter. Proliferation involves an increase in the size of the lesion. In contrast, involution occurs by cellular apoptosis, clinically characterised by a gradual decrease in size.

The behaviors of congenital haemangioma and noninvoluting haemangioma differ from that of classic haemangioma.

Significant complications may occur in up to 20% of patients with haemangiomas, including:

- ulceration (the most common complication);

- compression of vital structures, depending on location;

- high-output cardiac failure;

- bleeding; and

- Kasabach-Merritt syndrome.

Investigations

A full haemogram, chest radiograph with ultrasound (US) scan, computed tomography (CT) scan or magnetic resonance imaging (MRI) may be requested, as indicated and based on availability.

Management depends on the location of the lesion, its clinical effects, and the age of the child. Conservative management, consisting of observation, serial photographs, and regular review with reassurance, is the preferred mode of management.

Complicated haemangiomas may require any combination of the following:

- compression therapy;

- intralesional steroids (some response in 50–90% of cases);

- interferon α-2a;

- chemotherapy;

- intralesional sclerosing agents (hypertonic saline, glucose);

- cryotherapy;

- arterial embolisation;

- radiation therapy; and

- surgical intervention.

Surgical intervention is indicated in cases of rapid growth, ulceration, haemorrhage, or deterioration of haemodynamic status (as in high-output cardiac failure or in secondary ischaemic complications caused by high-flow arteriovenous shunting). The mass effect of a lesion due to its proximity to vital organs (e.g., orbit), or compression on the trachea or auditory canal are other indications for surgical intervention. A cosmetically severe deformity and intervention designed to improve quality of life (as in lesions located in eyelids, vermillion border, nasal tip (the so-called "Cyrano de Bergerac" deformity), and the eyebrow) would also be considered relative indications.

Resection is possible only in small lesions. Surgical debulking is all that can be performed in larger lesions. In much larger lesions, compartmentalisation is necessary. Multiple sutures are placed so as to create many segments, which are then subsequently injected with sclerosing agents, leading to a process of initial swelling, inflammation, and a gradual decrease in the size of the lesion.

Vascular Malformations

Vascular malformations are generally evident at birth and grow at a rate commensurate with the growth of the child. Vascular malformations include:

1. Capillary malformations, which remain present for life and have no tendency toward involution. Presentation depends on size and location.

2. Venous malformations, which are usually present at birth but may not be clinically apparent. They are bluish, soft, and easily compressible, presenting as diffuse and extensive or localised lesions. Small cutaneous lesions may be treated with intralesional injection with 1% sodium tetradecyl decanoate.

3. Intracranial arterial malformations, which are more common than extracranial lesions, and usually present in the head and neck region. They are usually present at birth, but may not be noticeable.

4. Lymphatic malformations, which are the most common congenital vascular aberrations. They may be the result of hypoplasia of lymphatic trunks and lymph nodes, presenting as lymphoedema, or may present as superficial or deep single or multiple cystic lymphatic malformations. The latter are divided into macrocystic (formerly cystic or cavernous hygromas) and microcystic (formerly lymphangioma or lymphangioma circumscriptum) lymphatic malformations. Cystic lymphatic malformations are always present at birth, but may not become apparent until later in life. Surgical excision is the mainstay of management.

5. Arteriovenous malformations, which are rare and clinically apparent at birth. They have a high propensity to bleeding and recurrence. Spontaneous rupture accompanied by life-threatening haemorrhage may also occur. Depending on size and location, embolisation followed by surgical excision is the best form of management.

6. Pyogenic granuloma (lobular capillary haemangioma), which is a benign lesion that occurs on skin and mucosal surfaces of the proximal aerodigestive tracts, but has also been reported to occur subcutaneously, intravenously, in the small bowel, colon, rectum, burn scar, and thigh. It may arise at any age, but is more common in childhood.

7. Nasopharyngeal angiofibroma, which is the most common benign tumour of the nasopharynx, and may present with recurrent epistaxis, nasal congestion, hearing loss, or even cranial nerve palsies, usually in prepubertal and adolescent males. A clinical exam with radiographic or CT/MRI scans will confirm the diagnosis. Embolisation followed by surgical excision is the standard mode of therapy, although radiotherapy and chemotherapy have also been used.

Other classifications divide vascular lesions into "low flow" (capillary, venous, and lymphatic) and "high flow" (arterial and arteriovenous) lesions.

Craniofacial Surgery

An appreciation of the dynamics of the growing skeleton is essential for the surgeon venturing into management of paediatric craniofacial pathology. A child is not a small adult; even though a child's anatomy may appear similar to that of an adult, the behavior and response of the growing skeleton to trauma, whether accidental or iatrogenic, is considerably different. Such trauma may thus result in poor craniofacial cosmesis, form, and function, including mastication and deglutition. An understanding of the importance of craniofacial anatomy and cosmesis, as well as the major role it plays in defining an individual's identity, is central to the success of craniofacial surgery. Where possible, a team approach in craniofacial surgery is recommended to obtain optimal results. This team may include the following specialists: a paediatrician, the surgeon, a neurosurgeon, a dentist, a speech therapist, and a nurse. Other specialists may be co-opted as needed. In practice, such a team is not feasible in most of Africa, and a more realistic approach would be to invest as many of the skills in the key members of the team—the surgeon and the nurse—as possible.

Most paediatric craniofacial problems are not merely surgical: they span the entire life of the individual, having their maximum impact in childhood and early adulthood. Appreciably, therefore, where possible, a team approach is required throughout life. Due counselling, with involvement of the patient and family in the decision-making process, is essential for the patient to gain self-esteem and fit into the various phases of life.

Definitions

Definitions of developmental aberrations will help in gaining a better understanding and appreciation of the need for a broad team approach in handling paediatric craniofacial problems.

- A *malformation* is a morphological defect of a part of the body consequent to an abnormal developmental process. Generally, malformations initiated late in foetal development are simple, whereas those initiated early (e.g., cleft lip, cleft palate, and microcephaly) are more complex and severe.

- *Deformation* is an abnormal form or position of a body part caused by nondisruptive mechanical forces. Deformations usually occur late in foetal development and may improve spontaneously once the deforming force is removed.

- *Disruption* is a defect of a part of the body resulting from mechanical interference with the normal developmental process (e.g., amniotic bands leading to amputations). The resulting defect depends on the timing of the mechanical insult. Disruptions are rare and occur sporadically.

- A *sequence* malformation is the result of multiple defects occurring consequent to a single presumed structural anomaly. An example is the Pierre Robin sequence, in which the primary event is thought to be a micrognathia resulting in a relative macroglossia, and consequently a failure of the palatal shelves to fuse.

- A *syndrome* encompasses groups of anomalies that contain multiple malformations and/or sequences, such as Treacher-Collins syndrome.

- An *association* is the nonrandom occurrence of a group of anomalies in multiple individuals. The constituent groups of anomalies must not be a sequence or syndrome. Examples are the CHARGE (Coloboma, Heart defect, Atresia choanae, Retarded growth, Genitourinary anomalies, Ear malformations) and VATER (Vertebral defects, imperforate Anus, Tracheo-Esophageal Fistula, and Renal) associations.

Airway Problems

Many congenital craniofacial anomalies have associated airway, hearing, and speech problems. Nasal obstruction is a major problem in infants younger than 3 months of age because at this stage in life they are obligate nose breathers. Affected infants have paradoxical cyanosis: cyanosis at rest with resolution upon crying. These babies need oral airways. Babies with micrognathia or maxillary hypoplasia should be nursed prone and with a nasopharyngeal airway. A tracheostomy may be performed as needed. Adenotonsillectomy may increase the size of the airway and improve ventilation.

Speech Problems

Speech disorders present mainly as hypernasality (as in velopharyngeal incompetence (VPI) and craniofacial anomalies associated with hearing loss); hyponasality (as in nasal obstruction); and hoarseness (as in VPI or after endotracheal intubation). These problems improve with speech therapy, or require surgery.

Common Presentations

Examples of common presentations include the following syndromes and sequences:

- The *Treacher-Collins syndrome* has an autosomal dominant inheri-

tance, with bilateral abnormalities of first and second branchial arches resulting in maxillary, mandibular, and zygomatic hyplasia. Affected children have downward-slanting eyes with colobomas of the lower eyelid and no eyelashes. Choanal atresia may be present, and airway control is therefore potentially difficult.

- The *Pierre Robin sequence* is a triad of micrognathia, glossoptosis, and cleft palate. Twenty percent of patients are syndromic and 80% are not. Airway management is a major concern, and failure of a nasopharyngeal airway may necessitate a tracheostomy.

- *Apert and Crouzon syndromes* are autosomal dominant and exhibit craniosynostosis, hypertelorism, exopthalmos, and maxillary hypoplasia. Whereas children with Crouzon syndrome have normal intellect and normal extremities, those with Apert syndrome have complex symmetrical syndactyly of the hands and feet as well as cervical vertebral anomalies, and they may be mentally retarded.

- The *Goldenhar syndrome* (the oculo-auriculo-vertebral complex) is defined by a unilateral craniofacial malformation involving the first and second branchial arches. Most cases occur sporadically. Clinically, these children have facial asymmetry, unilateral ear deformities, and vertebral malformations. They also have upper eyelid colobomas. Facial weakness occurs in 10–20%.

- The *Binder syndrome* (maxillofacial dysplasia) is characterised by a peculiar arrhinoid facies—affected children have no frontal sinus. They also have abnormal nasal bones with nasal mucosal atrophy, an absent anterior nasal spine, and maxillary hypoplasia with malocclusion.

- The *CHARGE association* involves four or more of the following presentations, from which it derives its name: coloboma, heart defect, choanal atresia, retarded growth, genitourinary anomalies, and ear malformations.

Cleft Lip and Palate

Cleft lip and palate have been described in more than 300 syndromes. Intrauterine diagnosis of cleft lips is possible from the second trimester of pregnancy. Cleft palates are more difficult to recognise with ultrasound. Postnatal diagnosis is clinical.

Other facial clefts have been described. The Tessier classification is the most commonly used system of classification. However, due to the rarity of these clefts, they will not be considered here.

Embryology

The primary palate is anterior to the incisive foramen and develops from mesodermal proliferation and fusion of the median nasal and maxillary processes during the 4th to 7th week of gestation. The secondary palate forms posterior to the incisive foramen in the 6th to 9th weeks of gestation. Palatal shelves change from a vertical to horizontal position and fuse in the midline. The tongue must first move antero-inferiorly to permit this fusion. Failure to move leads to palatal clefting, as in the Pierre-Robin sequence. A cleft lip may increase the likelihood of a cleft palate because the tongue may get trapped.

The secondary palate develops from the lateral maxillary processes that fuse in the midline. Thus, cleft lip and palate occur at 4–6 weeks of gestation, due to mesenchymal deficiency, whereas isolated cleft palate forms later, at 7–12 weeks, from partial or total failure of midline fusion.

Epidemiology

Most reports indicate that combined cleft lip and palate is the most common anomaly of this type (50%), followed by isolated cleft palates (30%), and isolated cleft lips (20%). Onyango and Noah reviewed 309 children managed in a single institution in Kenya and reported more isolated cleft lips than cleft palates. Accurate data for the African continent is lacking; however, estimates suggest there may be up to 400,000 children with clefts in Africa. Diabetic mothers and older paternity may be risk factors for the development of orofacial clefting.

Classification

Many different classifications are in use. The cleft lip may be unilateral or bilateral, complete or incomplete. Cleft lips occur as isolated anomalies or in combination with cleft palates. The cleft palate, likewise, may be uni- or bilateral, complete or incomplete. Submucous clefts and bifid uvulae are examples of incomplete palatal clefting.

Pathophysiology

The child with a cleft lip is unable to seal in air or fluid, when talking or eating. Malocclusion results from failure of lip seal, as well as due to intrinsic deformities of the alveolar process and teeth. In the child with a cleft palate, the nasal and oral cavities are in continuity, and air and fluid escape through the nose on attempted speech or drinking.

Associated problems

Children born with cleft lips and/or cleft palates are faced with the following potential problems: abnormal midface development, velopharyngeal incompetence, speech disorders, eustachian tube dysfunction with repeated middle ear infections, hearing and feeding difficulties, and malocclusion. Malocclusion occurs in almost all of these patients. Other significant dental anomalies include supernumerary teeth (20%), dystrophic teeth (30%), and missing teeth (50%). These problems contribute to poor cosmesis and may lead to a poor self image if not properly addressed, resulting in significant psychological difficulties.

Primary repair of cleft lip

Anatomically, there is lack of continuity of skin, muscle, and mucous membrane of the lip with associated nasal deformity. The skin, muscle, and mucous membrane should be repaired to restore lip continuity, symmetrical length, and function. Bilateral cleft lips are repaired simultaneously. In patients with cleft lip and palate, primary nose repair should include closure of the nasal floor. The use of presurgical orthodontics permits the palate to be moulded into anatomical position and may improve facial growth, leading to an easier and tensionless surgical repair.

Lip adhesion is a temporising measure that may improve breast-feeding as well as palatal anatomy; however, the definitive repair is more difficult because of scarring. This surgery is performed at about 2 weeks of age.

In primary cleft lip repair, the "rule of tens" is often used:

- 10 weeks of age;
- 10 pounds in weight, implying a healthy baby; and
- haemoglobin of 10 g/dl.

Early repair improves speech but may impair facial growth, leading to midfacial retrusion. Surgical repair alone, may improve VPI in up to 75% of patients. The rest require speech therapy, with surgical intervention being reserved for the few who fail to improve.

Although many procedures have been described, most surgeons use Millard's rotation-advancement flap technique. Common surgical complications include dehiscence, infection, and a prominent scar.

Primary repair of cleft palate

A palatal obturator may be used in high-risk cleft palate patients, in those who defer surgery, and in selected palatal fistulas that have repeated recurrences. The prosthesis is changed as the child grows.

Surgical repair is best performed around the age of 10 months, before development of intelligible speech. A number of techniques are currently in use, with the trend towards less scarring and less tension on the palate. Although push-back palatoplasty has been used widely, the Bardach or Veau-Wardill two-flap techniques are now popular. Scarring of the palate may cause impaired midfacial growth, leading to alveolar arch collapse, midface retrusion, and dental malocclusion. If surgery is delayed until the age of 18 months, facial growth may be less affected, but feeding, speech, and socialisation may suffer significantly.

Secondary procedures

Secondary procedures performed in cleft lip and palate patients, as indicated, include:

- *Pharyngoplasty* for velopharyngeal incompetence. The child may however develop stenotic side ports or continue to suffer from VPI. Of interest is the fact that some children with no VPI may develop incompetence after adenotonsillectomy.

- *Alveolar bone grafting* to close the palatal bony defect is delayed until the age of 6–12 years. The iliac crest is the most commonly used donor site. A palatal obturator may be used in patients with persistent fistulas.

- *Midfacial advancement* is achieved by using a *Le Forte osteotomy*. Potential complications include maxillary necrosis from vascular impairment, infection, and malocclusion.

- *Rhinoplasty* is used for the flattened nose and short columella, which frequently require secondary procedures.

Craniosynostosis

Craniosynostosis is the premature fusion of one or more cranial sutures, resulting in a partial or complete growth arrest of that suture, and leading to a skull deformity that is defined by the fused suture. Cranial growth is restricted perpendicular to the fused suture, leading to a corresponding compensatory growth parallel to this suture. The resultant cranial deformity causes a corresponding facial deformity. Some types of deformities are more common in certain populations than in others. In North Africans, for example, oxycephaly occurs with a high frequency.

Classification

Craniosynostosis syndromes (e.g., Crouzon, Apert, Pfeiffer, and Carpenter syndromes) are primarily due to genetic anomalies. Management of the child with syndromic craniosynostosis should include suspicion of hydrocephalus, increased intracranial pressure, mental retardation, and visual anomalies.

Table 121.3: Causes of secondary craniosynostosis disorders.

Disorder	Causes
Haematologic disorders	Sickle cell anaemia, thalassaemias
Metabolic disorders	Rickets, hyperthyroidism, mucopolysaccharidoses
Malformations	Microcephaly, shunted hydrocephalus, encephalocele
Teratogens	Valproic acid, diphenylhydantoin, etc.
Foetal head constraint	Uterine abnormalities, multiparous pregnancies

Table 121.4: Craniosynostoses classification.

Suture involved	Comments	Deformity
Metopic	Rare	Trigonocephaly and hypertelorism
Saggital	Most common form	Scaphocephaly
Coronal, unilateral		Frontal plagiocephaly
Coronal, bilateral		Brachycephaly/turricephaly
Lambdoid, unilateral or bilateral	Most posterior plagiocephaly due to deformational plagiocephaly	Posterior plagiocephaly
Multiple sutures	Rare	Cloverleaf deformity (Kleeblattschädel deformity)

Craniosynostosis can be primary or secondary. Primary craniosynostosis has no underlying identifiable abnormality, whereas secondary craniosynostosis occurs in association with other anomalies or identifiable causes (Table 121.3).

An anatomic classification of craniosynostosis by suture involved is shown in Table 121.4.

Management

The surgical procedure of choice for a specific type of craniosynostosis is age-dependent. The younger the patient, the less extensive or demanding the procedure. Strip craniectomies are generally performed in children younger than 6 months of age.

The differentiation between lambdoid craniosynostosis and deformational plagiocephaly is important, but may be a diagnostic difficulty. Deformational plagiocephaly, also called positional head deformity, is a benign cranial deformity resulting mainly from sleeping and nursing predominantly in one position (supine). There is no synostosis. There is a temporal association between increased deformational plagiocephaly and the "Back to Sleep" campaign in the West that was designed to combat sudden infant death syndrome (SIDS). Other causes include *in utero* compression and congenital torticollis. Most deformities are mild and resolve spontaneously, and the rest can be managed by the use of a moulding helmet.

Surgical intervention in craniosynostosis aims at correction of the craniofacial deformities and control of increased intracranial pressure, which is present in up to 30% of patients with two or more fused sutures.

Complications

Common complications of surgery for craniosynostosis include:

• *Haemorrhage:* Children do not tolerate blood loss well because of their small volumes, and loss must be replaced volume for volume.

• *Cerebrospinal fluid (CSF) leak:* Dural tears may occur. These should be sought for and repaired. If noted postoperatively, an initial conservative management may be attempted, but if this fails, definitive surgical repair must be performed.

• *Ocular complications:* Optic nerve injury or direct eye trauma is avoided by careful technique.

• *Infections:* These are rare, but potentially life-threatening should they occur.

• *Death:* Mortality should be rare.

Maxillofacial Trauma

In the management of paediatric maxillofacial trauma, tissue handling, both soft and especially bony, must be gentle, so as to ensure optimal restoration of mastication, deglutition, and cosmesis. The availability of resorbable plates and screws for use in craniofacial bone fixation has significantly reduced the morbidity associated with the need for hardware removal after fracture consolidation; however, the cost is prohibitive. Titanium plates and screws are the standard of care; however, wire fixation, although time consuming, is effective and affordable and does not require removal.

The craniofacial skeleton serves three main functions:

1. It offers structural support for muscles and other and soft tissues.

2. It protects important sensory organs.

3. Facial bones collapse from trauma and thus absorb most of the energy that would otherwise be transmitted to the brain.

In children younger than 5 years of age, the cranial skeleton is much larger than the facial skeleton; hence, there is a lower incidence of midfacial and mandibular fractures and a higher incidence of cranial injuries in this age group. With increasing age and facial growth, the midface and mandible become more prominent, with a concomitant increase in the incidence of facial fractures and a decrease in cranial injuries.

Incidence and aetiology

Social, cultural, and environmental factors vary from one country to another. These significantly influence the incidence and aetiology of craniofacial trauma. As examples, violence is the main cause of paediatric maxillofacial trauma in South Africa and Zimbabwe, and road traffic injuries account for 11% and 50% of paediatric craniofacial trauma in Zimbabwe and Libya, respectively.

Age-related activities in children also influence the incidence and aetiology of trauma. Younger (preschool) children usually sustain low-velocity trauma related to falls around the home, whereas school-age children are more likely to sustain high-velocity trauma, usually related to sports but also to road traffic injuries. Child abuse occurs in all cultures and across all paediatric ages.

Facial fractures in children occur less frequently than in adults. Facial fractures are frequently minimally displaced because of the thicker layer of adipose tissue, elastic bones, and flexible/deformable sutures. Lack of facial skeleton pneumatisation and the presence of tooth buds within the jaws are other contributing factors to a lower incidence of displaced fractures. However, as noted above, trauma to the growing skeleton may adversely affect long-term cosmesis. It is difficult to predict the long-term effects of any trauma because growth may serve to improve long-term results, as has been noted in occlusal realignment and compensatory condylar growth after condylar fractures.

Acute management

The initial presentation of a paediatric craniofacial injury may be so dramatic as to upset management priorities. The ABCs of trauma care must be recalled and used at all times; irrespective of the drama, these principles help save lives.

The ABCs of trauma care are:

A. Airway: Secure the airway and protect the cervical spine. This is especially important because craniofacial trauma may be associated with C-spine trauma (5–10%). Major facial trauma is also associated with the risk of upper airway obstruction. The obtunded patient will have no control of the tongue.

B. Breathing: Ensure adequate ventilation.

C. Circulation: Control bleeding. Life-threatening haemorrhage occurs in up to 5% of Le Fort fractures. Fracture reduction and direct pressure will generally control bleeding. Anterior and posterior nasal packing may be performed by using a urinary catheter passed through the nose into the nasopharynx, where it is inflated, then pulled back snugly.

D. Disability: Conduct a thorough neurological examination (e.g., Glasgow Coma Scale) to establish level of consciousness as well as any neurological deficits.

Administer tetanus toxoid to all trauma patients. Additionally, animal bite victims should be given the antirabies vaccine.

Cover avulsed tissues or organs (teeth, ears, nose, etc.) with saline-soaked gauze. Avulsed deciduous teeth may be discarded. Permanent teeth should be replaced and held in place for a little while. If a tooth has been out for more than 6 hours, it is unlikely to survive and may be discarded.

CT scans are the gold standard radiographic investigation in paediatric craniofacial trauma. Plain radiographs are not as helpful as they are in adults, particularly in the midface region, where poorly developed sinuses and tooth buds occupy space and obscure skeletal anatomic landmarks. The orthopantomogram (OPG) is a good tool in looking at mandibular fractures.

Because the plain radiograph may be the only tool available, paediatric radiograph atlases provide references for normal anatomy. Where radiographic examination is unavailable, clinical examination should reveal most of the injuries, with surgical exploration and repair as indicated. The index of suspicion is high, with clinical examination alone, however, and missed or untreated injuries are likely to result in significant morbidity, including poor facial cosmesis.

Nasal injuries

Nasal injuries may be associated with trauma to adjacent structures; thus, naso-ethmoid fractures may be missed if the apparent "simple" nasal injury is ignored. Also, septal perforation may complicate a missed septal haematoma that may also interfere with midfacial growth. Nasal fractures should be reduced and splinted at the earliest opportunity.

Mandibular trauma

Most mandibular fractures are simple, undisplaced or minimally displaced, and may be managed with maxilla-mandibular fixation. Minimal interference with the growing mandible and contained tooth buds will lead yield excellent results. The mandible is the final facial bone to complete growth, and injury to the condyle may result in facial asymmetry and malocclusion from arrested mandibular growth. Temporomandibular ankylosis and loss of mouth opening are further complications. If there are no other associated facial bone injuries, most condylar injuries are probably best managed conservatively, although this is controversial. There is currently no evidence that **open reduction, internal fixation** (ORIF) improves outcomes. Whatever the management, early institution of mouth-opening exercises are important to prevent temporomandibular joint (TMJ) fibrosis or ankylosis.

Maxillary trauma

Because sinuses develop between the ages of 6 and 12 years, the fracture patterns in children are different from those in adults. Thus, Le Fort fractures increase with increasing aeration of the maxillary and ethmoid sinuses. Displaced midfacial injuries, however, should be managed with open reduction and internal fixation, irrespective of age.

Orbital "blow out" fractures

Orbital "blow out" fractures are common in children. Failure to recognise and treat these injuries early will result in diplopia, enophthalmos, and extraocular muscle entrapment. These complications are difficult to treat. A high index of suspicion and early exploration and repair are mandatory due to the rapid rate of cicatrisation and consolidation seen in children.

Soft tissue trauma

As a general rule, soft tissue cuts and lacerations of the face and head (scalp) tend to bleed profusely. Because of good vascularity in this region, wounds heal well, and surgical wound infections are rare. Management consists of the following principles:

1. Wounds may be closed primarily safely, up to 24 hours after trauma.

2. Copious wound irrigation and minimal debridement are all that is required. Excessive debridement will lead to large defects that require skin grafts or other procedures, resulting in larger scars and inferior cosmetic results.

3. Degloved flaps that are still attached by a skin bridge should be preserved and replaced. Subsequent debridement will reveal how much of the flap is viable.

4. The suturing technique and material are equally important determinants of the scar. Intradermal sutures should be used to reduce tension on the skin sutures. Skin is closed by using a subcutaneous absorbable suture or with 5.0 monofilament, which must be removed on postoperative day 5 to avoid a "railroad" scar.

Animal bites are a common cause of facial trauma in children. The animal may bite off any of the parts of the face (ears, nose, or lips). At presentation, the piece of tissue may be missing or still attached. The same principles outlined above are used in managing animal bites, and if presentation is early, primary closure is attempted.

Complications

Problems commonly found in craniofacial trauma include:

• *CSF rhinorrhea,* which may be managed conservatively with head elevation at 30° to 45°.

• *Epistaxis,* for which, if anterior packing fails, additional posterior nasal packing should be done. Packing should not be left in for more than 48 hours because of a significant increase in infections. If packing needs to be left in for longer, then prophylactic antibiotics are used and the packing must be removed within 5 days.

• *Infraorbital nerve damage* may occur with Le Fort 3 fractures.

• *Facial nerve paralysis* may occur in petrous temporal bone fractures.

• *Subcutaneous emphysema* is evidence of fracture of one or more sinuses.

• *Anosmia* is the result of fracture of the cribriform plate.

• *Ocular and visual disturbances* occur from orbital fractures.

• *Epiphora* is evidence of damaged lacrimal ducts.

If surgical principles are followed, complications are very few because of the healing capacity of the craniofacial skeleton. Whereas nonunion is unlikely, malunion is the result of inadequate reduction. Most ocular trauma, brain injury, and death are causally related to the initial trauma.

In Africa, late presentation of patients is a particularly common occurrence. Reconstructive surgery must then be offered. This is frequently difficult and expensive, and it may require multiple stages. Referral to a competent centre may be preferable, as resources required at this stage may be unavailable locally.

Noma

Noma, variously known as gangrenous stomatitis or cancrum oris, primarily affects orofacial structures. There is a strong correlation between noma and poverty, malnutrition, poor oral hygiene, and infectious diseases (primarily malaria and measles). These conditions are widespread in sub-Saharan Africa, particularly within strife-ridden communities. It has thus been aptly called "the face of poverty", and afflicts mainly children in developing countries. The World Health Organization (WHO) estimates 140,000 new cases of noma each year, mostly from sub-Saharan Africa, with a mortality rate of up to 90%. The few reports from developed countries involve patients with debilitating diseases, including HIV, diabetes mellitus, and haematological disorders.

Aetiology

Although bacteriological studies are inconclusive on causative organisms, most experts agree that noma is the result of a mixed bacterial infection involving aerobic and anaerobic organisms. Fusiform bacilli such as *Fusiformis fusiformis* and *Borrelia vincenti* are frequent isolates. Other isolates include *Prevotella melaninogenica*, *Corynebacterium pyogenes*, *Fusobacterium nucleatum*, *Bacteroides fragilis*, *Bacillus cereus*, *Prevotella intermedia*, and *Fusobacterium necrophorum*.

To date, there is no effective mode of treatment, and thus prevention plus the treatment of noma sequelae remain the mainstay of care. Broader-spectrum antibiotics covering gingival flora, including aerobes and anaerobes, are now recommended, but the treatment has to be started as soon as possible.

Clinical evolution

Noma presents initially as a painful blister on the gingiva that becomes indurated, leading to massive oedema. Subsequent necrosis, ulceration, and slough separation leave underlying bone exposed. The slough is cone-shaped, with the base being in the oral cavity. This is an important consideration at the time of reconstruction because the size of the skin defect alone is misleading. The final result is an ugly midfacial defect that then scars and contracts with time if the patient does not succumb. Initial management in the acute stage consists of fluid resuscitation, nutritional rehabilitation, and administration of broad spectrum antibiotics. Any predisposing illnesses and/or infections are managed appropriately. Wound care consists of gentle debridement and dressing changes. Physiotherapy will help prevent trismus and the resulting TMJ ankylosis.

Survivors of the acute stage suffer severe destruction of the midface, including lips, cheeks, maxilla and mandible, nose, and occasionally the orbit. Progressive scarring, trismus, oral incontinence, and mandibulo-maxillary synostosis leave the patient malnourished, severely disfigured, and with speech difficulties. The psychosocial difficulties experienced by these children and their families should not be underestimated.

Surgical treatment

Reconstruction in noma surgery is a difficult undertaking; collaboration with a team versed with noma care is helpful. Modified Montandon's classification is a simple, comprehensive, and practical clinical classification. It is useful in formulating surgical intervention. The addition of a fifth grouping completes this classification:

1. Localised lip, commissure, or cheek defect
2. Upper lip and nose amputation
3. Lower lip and mandible amputation
4. Large defects (e.g., lips, cheek, palate, maxilla, orbital floor)
5. Bilateral defects (may be any combination of the above)

Free flaps offer the reconstructive surgeon considerable versatility. Single-stage reconstruction with appropriate tissue bulk and the avoidance of additional facial scars and incisions are important advantages. Free flaps, however, are labor- and technology-dependent, are expensive, and demand considerable technical skills. It is encouraging to note that microvascular reconstruction has been successfully performed in suboptimal environments, proving that these skills and technology can be modified to suit the operating theatre conditions found in most developing countries.

Loco-regional flaps provide excellent color match, minimise the number of surgical procedures, and are generally fail-safe, requiring simple postoperative care. Thus, although ideal, the use of free flaps for noma reconstruction is not essential, and loco-regional flaps can give very good results if well chosen.

It is important that the surgeon and patient realise that even though cosmesis may be improved significantly by surgery, functional outcomes may be poor at best.

Craniofacial Tumours of Bony Origin

Craniofacial tumours affecting children are too numerous to be discussed in this chapter, so only the most common bony lesions encountered in Africa are discussed here. The general subject of tumours is covered elsewhere in this book (Chapters 102–109).

Burkitt lymphoma

Burkitt lymphoma was initially described as "African jaw lymphoma". It affects children, shows rapid growth, and may involve the mandible or the maxilla. Burkitt is *not* a surgical disease—it is a purely medical disease, and is effectively treated using chemotherapeautic agents. It shows excellent response to prednisolone, with a rapid decrease in volume evident within 24 hours of administration. A fine needle aspirate for cytological analysis or a core biopsy is all that is required for diagnosis.

Dentigerous cyst

A dentigerous (follicular) cyst is the most common developmental cyst, comprising about 20% of all developmental cysts. On an OPG, it is a radioluscent lesion with well-defined, sclerotic margins encircling an unerupted tooth. Most of these cysts are asymptomatic, but when they are large, they may cause the displacement or resorption of adjacent teeth and cause pain. Drainage and marsupialisation or enucleation is done for large or symptomatic cysts.

Fibrous dysplasia

With fibrous dysplasia (FD), normal bone is replaced by fibrous connective tissue due to a defect in osteoblast differentiation and matura-

tion. This genetically based sporadic bone disease may affect single or multiple bones (monostotic or polyostotic, respectively). Twenty-five percent of monostotic FD occurs in the head and neck, and the maxilla is more often affected than the mandible. The polyostotic variant forms 15% of the total, and 50% of polyostotic lesions occur in the head and neck region. Cranial polyostotic FD may occur concurrent with café-au-lait spots and endocrinopathology (hyperthyroidism and precocious puberty in females), constituting McCune-Albright's syndrome.

FD clinically presents as a painless swelling with jaw asymmetry, usually in childhood or early adolescence, during the periods of greatest skeletal growth. Presentation depends on the specific site involved: hearing loss and facial palsy in temporal bone involvement; facial asymmetry and malocclusion with mandibular involvement; or pain, paraesthesia, and cranial nerve lesions with skull base involvement. Frontal bone involvement results in hypertelorism, with massive cranial bony involvement resulting in lionlike facies, known as "leontiasis ossea".

Cherubism, a variant of FD, is an autosomal-dominant disorder of variable penetrance. It is more severe in boys. The involvement of maxilla and mandible is symmetric. Some regression may occur after adolescence.

Radiologically, FD most commonly has a ground-glass pattern. FD lesions generally do not cross the midline and tend to be limited to one bone.

Management

Management of tumours of bony origin may consist of observation, conservative surgery involving shaping or contouring the dysplastic bone, or radical surgical excision and reconstruction. The choice depends on a combination of factors:

• age of the patient;

• growth rate of the lesion;

• extent and location;

• degree of cosmetic deformity; and

• level of functional impairment.

The aim of surgical treatment is to correct or prevent functional deficits and restore as near-normal facial cosmesis as possible. If possible, surgery should be deferred until skeletal maturity. Successful staged excision of extensive lesions, especially in the head and neck region, followed by multistaged reconstruction has been reported.

Accelerated growth or aggressive lesions require early surgical intervention with en bloc resection and bone graft reconstruction. The rate of transformation to malignancy is less than 1%, which has also been reported to occur after radiation therapy and is therefore contraindicated.

Chondrosarcomas and osteosarcomas are malignant lesions that occasionally affect the head and neck region. On the African continent, even in the best centres, these lesions generally have a poor prognosis.

Neurofibromatosis

Neurofibromatosis covers a number of distinct disorders that share many features but clearly differ from one another. These include neurofibromatosis type 1 (Nf1), neurofibromatosis type 2 (Nf2), and others, as recommended in 1987 by the National Institutes of Health (NIH) Consensus Conference on Neurofibromatosis.

Neurofibromas arise from nerve sheath cells and consist of a mixture of Schwann cells, fibroblasts, perineurial cells, and mast cells. Nf1, formerly known as von Recklinghausen disease, affects about 1 in 3,000 people. It has autosomal dominant inheritance with complete penetrance, variable expression, and a high rate of new mutation. The NIH Consensus Conference on Neurofibromatosis diagnostic criteria for Nf1 include neurofibromas, café-au-lait macules, skin-fold freckling, skeletal dysplasia, Lisch nodules, optic gliomas, and a first-degree relative with Nf1. A positive diagnosis is based on two or more of these signs.

Skeletal involvement in patients with Nf1 may include macrocephaly, dysplasia of the greater wing of the sphenoid, vertebral dysplasia, scoliosis, pseudoarthrosis, and a short stature, amongst others. About 50% of patients with Nf1 have learning disabilities as well as some behavioral problems. There is also a heightened risk of epilepsy and headaches. These patients have an increased risk for developing malignant tumours, such as malignant peripheral nerve sheath tumours, leukemia, and rhabdomyosarcoma.

Nf1 lesions that appear early in childhood can be disfiguring and cause psychological discomfort. Most are not resectable because of their diffuse nature. They are difficult to deal with even if only an agreeable cosmetic result is all that is desired. Conservative management is recommended unless a lesion presents with sudden enlargement, functional deficits, pain, or bleeding. In the craniofacial region, however, the smallest neurofibroma lesion produces a prominent abnormality, whereas the larger ones can result in hideous deformities in the child, leading to ostracisation from society. Surgical excision and reconstruction should be offered for lesions of the craniofacial region. Surgical debulking is associated with significant bleeding.

Lymphoedema

Lymphoedema is the accumulation of protein-rich interstitial fluid within the skin and subcutaneous tissues as a result of lymphatic dysfunction. The accumulated fluid provokes an intense fibrous reaction, further reducing lymphatic transport and leading to progressive swelling of the limb. Limb induration, fibrosis, and repeated attacks of cellulitis set up a vicious cycle that, untreated, leads to ulceration and chronic nonhealing wounds. Normal unidirectional lymph flow is due to a combination of factors: intrinsic lymphatic muscle contractions, muscle pump action, presence of valves, and negative intrathoracic pressure. The lymphatic system functions to clear proteins and lipids from the interstitial space into the vasculature by use of differential pressures. Lymph flows into the venous system at the neck. Lymphoedema results from a decrease in the number of functioning lymphatics below a critical level, or from an increased lymphatic load.

Lymphoedema is confined to the subcutaneous compartment; the deep muscle compartments remain uninvolved. The excess protein serves as a medium for bacterial multiplication, and the resultant infection adds to the lymphatic dysfunction. Recurrent soft tissue infection is one of the most troublesome aspects of chronic lymphoedema management.

Causes

Lymphoedema may be divided into primary or secondary, based on cause.

Primary lymphoedema is of unknown aetiology or congenital lymphatic dysfunction. Primary lymphatic obstruction may be caused by several anatomic abnormalities, including lymphatic hypoplasia and functional insufficiency or absence of lymphatic valves. It is further subclassified based on the age of onset or lymphangiographic findings (Table 121.5).

Table 121.5: Subclassification of primary lymphoedem

Age of onset	• Birth: lymphoedema congenita (e.g., Milroy's disease) • Adolescence: lymphoedema praecox • Adulthood: lymphoedema tarda
Lymphangiographic findings	• Lymphatic aplasia • Lymphatic hypoplasia • Varicosity of subcutaneous lymphatics

Secondary lymphoedema is more common and has a known precipitating cause. It may result from surgical, infectious, inflammatory, neoplastic, or traumatic causes. Filariasis is a common parasitic cause of lymphoedema in Africa, usually presenting in adulthood.

Clinical Presentation

The oedema generally begins distally and progresses proximally over months to years. Initially soft and pitting, it becomes nonpitting secondary to fibrosis. Peau d'orange changes in the skin (due to fibrosis), the Stemmer sign (inability to tent skin over the toes), and the blunted appearance of the digits of the involved extremity are the classic signs of lymphoedema.

Differential diagnoses include: chronic venous stasis, myxoedema, and lipoedema. These are distinguished on the basis of history and physical examination.

Management

It is important to discuss with the patient and guardians the fact that lymphoedema has no cure. Conservative management should be initiated immediately when the diagnosis is made. This should focus on the avoidance of infection and the application of compression to maintain or to reduce limb volume. Elastic compression garments, for example, have been shown to lead to a 30–40% reduction of oedema. Improved skin care avoids infection and prevents the development of associated skin changes.

Other nonsurgical therapies include treating infection with antibiotics and improving protein lymphatic transport by stimulating macrophage proteolysis (benzopyrones) and reducing oedema (diuretics), among other therapies. *Wuchereria bancrofti* and *Brugia malayi* infections should be eliminated with diethylcarbamazine, and antihistamine and/or anti-inflammatory agents may be used to control the allergic reactions to the dying parasite. Lymphangitis must be treated quickly when it occurs, and the patient may require lifelong antibiotic prophylaxis to prevent further episodes, which may occur in up to 25% of patients.

Surgical treatment options may be grouped together into:

• re-creation or imitation of lymphatic channels;

• bridging the lymphoedematous area to normal lymphatic areas; and

• resecting or debulking of lymphoedematous tissue.

The procedure may be physiologic, attempting to re-establish lymphatic drainage, or excisional—procedures that debulk the limb by removing excess skin and subcutaneous tissue. These procedures aim at improving the cosmetic appearance, preserving the function of a limb, and preventing infection episodes. Whereas the re-creation of lymphatics requires microsurgical capability, debulking is a much simpler surgical procedure.

The Homans' or modified Sistrunk procedure is easy to perform and results in up to a 50% reduction in limb volume. Excision of subcutaneous tissue is carried out in two stages over a 2- to 3-month period, excising half of the limb circumference at each stage. The skin and part of the subcutaneous tissue are preserved. The Charles procedure has no durable results and is mentioned here only for historical reasons.

Complications

Recurrent lymphangitis and cellulitis, progression of skin changes, oedema, fibrosis, and ulceration with chronic nonhealing wounds constitute the natural progression of untreated lymphoedema. The limb becomes heavy, may be painful, and in extreme cases, the patient may be unable to ambulate.

Genital lymphoedema is a significant problem in some patients. The management is similar to that of limb lymphoedema. Surgical excision is indicated only for cosmetic or functional reasons, such as where the lymphoedema interferes with micturition or causes significant discomfort with ambulation or dressing. Solitary lesions of any size may be excised.

Pressure Ulcers

Pressure ulcers involve tissue loss resulting from constant pressure. Decubitus ulcers occur in areas with underlying bony prominences—sacrum, trochanter, heel—when the subject is lying down. Three to 4.5% of all hospitalised patients will develop a pressure sore at some time during their hospitalisation. Geriatric nursing homes have the highest prevalence of pressure ulcers (35–64%). A number of theories have been proposed to explain pressure ulcer development. Currently, the accepted mechanism involves a direct effect by one or more extrinsic, or primary, factors (e.g., pressure, shear, friction), propitiated and modified by a number of intrinsic, or secondary, factors (e.g., infection, impaired mobility). Although bacteria do not cause pressure ulcers, they contribute to tissue breakdown and delayed healing. Keeping bacterial counts at less than 10^4 per gram of tissue allows for wound healing.

Aetiology

Patient immobility, resulting in prolonged contact with objects, may be due to long bone fractures, paralysis (congenital (e.g., spina bifida), trauma, neoplasm, infection, iatrogenic injury, or radiation), and loss of consciousness. Interestingly, cerebral palsy patients do not develop pressure sores, even when placed in wheelchairs for a long time.

Classification

Pressure ulcers are staged and graded depending on the depth of involved tissue (Tables 121.6 and 121.7). Whereas ulcer staging helps nursing planning to help reverse progression, ulcer grading aids in determining the type and volume of tissue required for the reconstruction.

Table 121.6: Pressure ulcer staging.

Stage	Lesion
I	Hyperaemia ≥ 1 hour after pressure relief
II	Blister or other break in the dermis with or without infection
III	Subcutaneous destruction into muscle with or without infection
IV	Involvement of bone or joint with or without infection

Table 121.7: Pressure ulcer grading.

Ulcer grade	Tissue involved
I	Limited to epidermis and superficial dermis
II	Adipose tissue
III	Muscle ± infection
IV	Bone and/or joint ± infection

Source: National Pressure Sore Advisory Panel Consensus Development Conference, 1989.

Management

Pressure ulcers add a significant burden in terms of cost of care and morbidity of the patient. Uncontrolled wound infection may lead to sepsis and death. Thus, prevention remains the most effective means of pressure ulcer management. Consequently, basic skin care and pressure dispersion by timely position changes must be taught to parents and guardians of those at risk. Also important is the use of topical antibiotics, such as silver sulfadiazine. Many paraplegic children remain ulcer-free until they start going to school. Thus, teachers and peers at school need to be taught about pressure ulcer prevention so that they can reinforce it at school.

Once an ulcer has developed, its management depends on several factors. As with all reconstructive surgical procedures, the setting of achievable goals, by both the patient/family and the surgeon, must form the first step in the process. For patients with potentially reversible underlying diseases in whom the goals are to restore normal function or prolong life, aggressive efforts at nutritional resuscitation, treatment of infection, physical therapy and surgical intervention are warranted. In contrast, for chronically or terminally ill patients with advanced or recurrent ulcers, the goal is to provide comfort only.

The severity of the ulcer is evidenced by its grade (see Table 121.7). Grade III and IV ulcers require flap coverage; skin grafts and primary closure will fail. Free flap coverage may be preferable, depending on skills and personnel.

Patient idiosyncrasies and family support in nursing care are important factors. The older child may develop depression because of low esteem, among other reasons. As a result, the child moves less, and thus develops a pressure ulcer. In contrast, the motivated and goal-oriented child is less likely to develop a pressure ulcer. Family interest and involvement form an important and integral part of patient care. Poor family support implies poor nursing care. Any surgery performed will therefore most certainly fail, and conservative management would be preferable.

The cost of managing a pressure ulcer is significant. To protect a flap after coverage, weight and pressure dispersion may require special equipment, including silicone pillows and wheelchairs. These issues must be discussed before initiating surgical treatment.

The goals of surgical intervention include the following:

- reduction of protein loss through the wound;
- prevention of progressive osteomyelitis and sepsis;
- avoidance of progression to secondary amyloidosis and renal failure;
- minimisation of rehabilitation costs;
- improved patient hygiene and appearance;
- simplification of nursing care, as well as improving patient capability for self-care in the future; and
- averting future development of Marjolin's ulcer.

Technique

The technique in treating pressure ulcers includes the following:

- excision of the ulcer, surrounding scar, underlying bursa, and soft tissue calcification, if any;
- radical removal of the underlying infected bone;
- padding of bone stumps and filling the dead space with fascia or muscle flaps;
- resurfacing with large regional pedicled flap or free flap as indicated;
- in flap design, never sacrificing muscles that are still innervated; and
- grafting the donor site of the flap with thick split skin, if needed.

In doing so, the following guidelines are important:

- Use the simplest, but appropriate method of closure.
- Design the flap as large as possible; place the suture line away from the area of direct pressure.
- Be sure the flap design does not violate adjacent flap territories.
- If sensate flap is available, use it.
- Always have a second, and third, coverage option, should the first fail.

Regional flap options are shown in Table 121.8.

Table 121.8: Regional flap options.

Ulcer regions	Flap options
Trochanteric ulcers	Tensor fascia lata (TFL), vastus lateralis, anterolateral thigh flap
Sacral ulcers	Gluteal flaps
Ischial ulcers	Gluteal flaps, V-Y hamstring flap, posterior thigh flap

Complications

Complications of surgical intervention for pressure ulcers include haematoma, infection, dehiscence, recurrence, and heterotopic ossification of muscle flaps.

Microsurgery in Africa

The African continent is replete with reconstructive surgical needs, but the manpower to meet this is either inadequate or totally lacking. The College of Surgeons of East, Central, and Southern Africa has made significant strides in helping to train surgeons in various specialties, including plastic and reconstructive surgery.

The operating microscope has revolutionalised reconstructive surgery and thus needs to be part of the skills that trainees develop. The immediate cost of the microscope is significant, but the benefits to the surgeon and patients are immense. Procedures that would normally require multiple stages are performed in a single stage, significantly saving the morbidity, cost, and time lost in otherwise multiple-staged procedures. Note that the skills and equipment are easily available on the Indian subcontinent, which has patients whose needs and financial capabilities are equivalent to those in Africa.

Key Summary Points

1. An understanding of embryology is critical to the management of paediatric congenital malformations.

2. Children are not "small adults"; their physiology and anatomy differ from that of adults in a number of significant ways.

3. In reconstructive surgical interventions, goal-setting with the patient and the patient's relatives and guardians is an essential part of the management.

4. Surgeons managing children with disabilities or congenital malformations should participate in and/or lead campaigns of community education and awareness to help these children become integrated into their individual communities.

5. The long-term cosmetic and functional results of neglected maxillofacial trauma in children can be devastating. An early referral or consultation is important. Mobile telephony and the Internet can be used well to this end.

Suggested Reading

Andreev A. The Bulgarian School for Diagnosis and Treatment of Vascular Malformations and the leading role of Stefan Belov. Int J Angiol 2002; 11:46–52.

Argenta LC, Morykwas MJ. Vacuum assisted closure: a new method for wound control and treatment: clinical experience. Ann Plast Surg 1997; 38: 563–577.

Banwell PE, Musgrave M. Topical negative pressure therapy: mechanisms and indications. Int Wound J 2004; 1:95–106.

Baratti-Mayer D, Pittet B, Montandon D, et al. Noma: an "infectious" disease of unknown aetiology. Lancet Infect Dis 2003; 3:419–431.

Bauer J, Phillips LG. MOC-PSSM CME article: pressure sores. Plast Reconstr Surg 2008; 121(1 Suppl):1–10.

Brown MD, Johnson TM. Complications of soft tissue expansion. J Dermatol Surg Oncol 1993; 19:1120–1122.

Chao JJ, Longaker MT, Zide BM. Expanding horizons in head and neck expansion. Oper Tech Plast Reconstr Surg 1998; 5:2–11.

Cheville AL, McGarvey CL, Petrek JA, Russo SA, Taylor ME, Thiadens SR. Lymphedema Management. Semin Radiat Oncol 2003; 13:290–301.

Chidzonga MM. HIV/AIDS orofacial lesions in 156 Zimbabwean patients at referral oral and maxillofacial surgical clinics. Oral Dis 2003; 9:317–322.

Crysdale WS, Gaffney RJ. Malformations and syndromes. In: Bluestone CD, Stool SE, Kenna MA, eds. Pediatric Otolaryngology, Vol I, 3rd ed. Saunders, 1995, Pp 51–70.

Damstra RJ, Mortimer PS. Diagnosis and therapy in children with lymphoedema. Phlebology 2008; 23:276–286.

Enweon WU. Epidemiological and biochemical studies of necrotizing ulcerative gingivitis and noma (cancrum oris) in Nigerian children. Arch Oral Biol 1972; 17:1357–1371.

Marchac D, Renier D. Craniosynostosis. World J Surg 1989; 13:358–365.

Millard DR. Cleft Craft, Vol 1. Little Brown, 1976, Pp 165–173.

Miraliakbari R, Mackay D. Skin grafts. Oper Tech Gen Surg 2006; 8:197–206.

Montandon D, Lehmann C, Chami N. The surgical treatment of noma. Plast Reconstr Surg 1991; 87:76–86.

Mooney MP, Siegel MI. Understanding craniofacial anomalies: etiopathogenesis of craniosynostoses and facial clefting. Wiley-Liss, 2002.

Msamati BC, Igbibi PS, Chisi JE. The incidence of cleft lip, cleft palate, hyrocephalus, and spina bifida at Queen Elizabeth Central Hospital, Blantyre, Malawi. Cent Afr J Med 2000; 46:292–296.

Mulliken JB, Glowacki J. Hemangiomas and vascular malformations in infants and children: a classification based on endothelial characteristics. Plast Reconstr Surg 1982; 69:412–420.

National Institutes of Health Consensus Development Conference Statement (1988), Neurofibromatosis. Arch Neurol 1988; 45:575–578.

Nicole M, Wymann E, Hölzle A, Zachariou Z, Iizuka T. Pediatric craniofacial trauma. J Oral Maxillofac Surg 2008; 66:58–64.

Nthumba PM. The donkey, the fox, the gun and a lip. Internet J Surg 2005; 6(2). Available at: http://www.ispub.com/ostia/index.php?xmlFilePath=journals/ijs/vol6n2/lip.xml.

Nthumba PM. Bilateral thigh flaps: a case report and review of literature. East & Cent Africa J Surg 2007; 12(2): 82-87.

Nthumba PM. Giant pyogenic granuloma of the thigh: a case report. J Med Case Reports 2008; March 31(2): 95.

Nthumba PM. "Blitz surgery": Redefining surgical needs, training and practice in Sub-Saharan Africa. World J Surg 2010; 34(3):433–437.

Nthumba PM, Bird G. Marjolin's ulcer in a spina bifida patient. A case report. East & Cent Afric J Surg 2010; 15(2):127-129.

Nthumba PM, Carter LL. Visor flap for total upper and lower lip reconstruction: a case report. J Med Case Reports 2009; June 9(3): 7312.

Odeku EL, Martinson FD, Akinosi JO. Craniofacial fibrous dysplasia in Nigerian Africans. Int Surg 1969; 51:170–182.

Onyango JF, Noah S. Pattern of clefts of the lip and palate managed over a three year period at a Nairobi hospital in Kenya. East Afr Med J 2005; 82:649–651.

Posnick JC, Costell BJ, Tiwana PS. Pediatric craniomaxillofacial fracture management. In: Miloro M, ed. Peterson's Principles of Oral and Maxillofacial Surgery. BC Decker, 2004, Chap 27, Pp 527–545.

Rockson SG. Lymphedema. Am J Med 2001; 110:288–295.

Ross JH, Kay R, Yetman RJ, Angermeier K. Primary lymphedema of the genitalia in children and adolescents. J Urol 1998; 160:1485–1489.

Ruggieri M. The different forms of neurofibromatosis. Childs Nerv Syst 1999; 15:295–308.

Sørensen JL, Jørgensen B, Gottrup F. Surgical treatment of pressure ulcers. Am J Surg 2004; 188:42S–51S.

Suleiman AM, Hamzah, ST, Abusalab, MA, Samaan, KT. Prevalence of cleft lip and palate in a hospital-based population in Sudan. Int J Paediatr Dent 2005; 15:185–189.

Tessier P. Anatomical classification of facial, cranio-facial and latero-facial clefts. J Maxillofac Surg 1976; 4:69–92.

Viljoen DL, Versfeld GA, Losken W, Beighton P, Optiz JM, Reynolds JF. Polyostotic fibrous dysplasia with cranial hyperostosis: new entity or most severe form of polyostotic fibrous dysplasia? Am J Med Genet 2005; 29:661–666.

SPECIAL TOPICS

CHAPTER 122
MINIMAL ACCESS SURGERY IN PAEDIATRIC PATIENTS

Nathan R. Zilbert
Daniel Sidler
Evan P. Nadler

Introduction

It is difficult to credit any one person for the development of minimal access surgery (MAS) (also referred to as minimally invansive surgery, or MIS, by some), but diagnostic laparoscopy has been used in various medical specialties since early in the 20th century. Laparoscopy was commonly used by gynecologists throughout the 1960s and 1970s. Semm performed the first laparoscopic appendectomy in 1980, and Mouret performed the first laparoscopic cholecystectomy in 1987, leading to the widespread application of this technology to general surgery.[1,2] In Africa, diagnostic laparoscopy is sometimes the only method to make or confirm a diagnosis because other, less invasive modalities, such as ultrasound (US), computed tomography (CT), and magnetic resonance imaging (MRI), often are not available. However, advanced laparoscopic techniques are being utilised only in select regions; other areas basically perform almost no minimal access surgery.

Minimal access operations have been developed for most adult general surgical procedures; however, technical limitations, such as the size of the scopes and instruments, have made the application to paediatric surgery more guarded. As smaller and more delicate instruments have been developed and minimal access techniques have become standard teaching in general surgical training programmes, there has been a greater number of children treated with laparoscopic or thoracoscopic operations.[3] This chapter briefly discusses the general concepts of laparoscopy and thoracoscopy and reviews the current applications of MAS in the paediatric population, with an emphasis on those basic procedures that may be the most relevant in Africa.

Demographics

It is difficult to determine the exact proportional use of laparoscopy in any one region; however, it is clear that at major academic centres around the world, the use of minimal access techniques is increasing. One centre in the Netherlands reported that, in 1998, 60% of all intraabdominal operations in infants and children were performed laparoscopically, and by 2005, this number had risen to 81%.[3,4] More generally, a 2004 survey of North American paediatric surgeons investigating the preferred technique for appendectomy showed that 11% of the 344 respondents use laparoscopy in every case, whereas 10.8% of respondents never use it.[5] In a similar survey of 94 paediatric surgeons regarding pyloromyotomy in the United Kingdom and Ireland in 2008, it was found that 15% use laparoscopy only, with an additional 5% using laparoscopy depending on the case.[6]

Rationale

The rationale for MAS has been defined largely in the adult general surgery population and covers a broad range of procedures.[7–10] In general, the advantages of MAS are (1) better focal visualisation for the surgeon and associated staff members, (2) shorter length of hospital stay, (3) reduced postoperative ileus, (4) decreased requirements for postoperative pain medication, (5) fewer wound complications, and (6) improved cosmetic results. Recently, children have been shown to

have the same benefits after laparoscopic surgery.[4,11] The advantages of the minimal access approach are outlined for specific procedures as they are mentioned throughout this chapter.

Physiological Changes

Laparoscopy

The physiological effects of carbon dioxide pneumoperitoneum can be divided into two categories: (1) gas-specific effects and (2) pressure-specific effects.[12] One of the most important gas-specific effects is due to carbon dioxide's rapid absorption across the peritoneal membrane into the circulation, potentially causing a respiratory acidosis by the generation of carbonic acid. The body's buffers absorb carbon dioxide to maintain a normal blood pH, minimising hypercarbia or respiratory acidosis during brief laparoscopic procedures. In fact, clinically significant acidosis is rare in procedures of less than 8 hours. Minimal access procedures of that duration are rare in children, with repair of large para-oesophageal hernias being a possible exception.[13]

In patients with normal respiratory function, the anaesthesiologist increases the ventilatory rate or vital capacity with the ventilator to compensate for any increase in end tidal carbon dioxide, although this is rarely needed in children.[14] In a situation where acidosis cannot be corrected by the anaesthesiologist, it is advisable to evacuate the pneumoperitoneum or reduce the intraabdominal pressure.[12] The preoperative assessment should include screening for cardiopulmonary dysfunction, which might increase the likelihood of developing a clinically significant acidosis; laparoscopy may be relatively contraindicated in patients with these conditions.[14] Mild respiratory acidosis probably is an insignificant problem, but more severe respiratory acidosis can lead to cardiac arrhythmias, which are rarely seen in children.[12]

Pressure-specific effects of pneumoperitoneum on cardiovascular physiology have also been documented.[12] In the hypovolaemic patient, excessive pneumoperitoneum may exert pressure on the inferior vena cava and cause decreased venous return and impaired cardiac output. Furthermore, increased pressure due to pneumoperitoneum is transmitted directly across the paralyzed diaphragm into the thoracic cavity, creating increased central venous pressure and increased filling pressures of the right and left sides of the heart. If the intraabdominal pressures are kept under 20 mm Hg, the cardiac output is usually well maintained; higher pressures, however, can impede venous return and decrease preload.[14] The direct effect of the pneumoperitoneum on increasing intrathoracic pressure is increased peak inspiratory pressure, pressure across the chest wall, and the potential for barotrauma.[12] Despite these concerns, disruption of blebs and consequent pneumothoraces are rare after uncomplicated laparoscopic surgery, and laparoscopic procedures in children usually do not result in significant hypotension or tachycardia.

Increased intraabdominal pressure may also decrease renal blood flow, glomerular filtration rate, and ultimately urine output.[12] These effects are likely mediated by direct pressure on the renal vein and kidney. Relative oliguria is common during laparoscopy, but the urine output is not a reflection of intravascular volume status. During an uncomplicated laparoscopic procedure, intravenous fluid administration should not be linked to urine output, and one must be judicious with the total volume of fluid given. The requisite for supplemental fluids is decreased, especially as fluid losses through the open abdomen are eliminated.

Thoracoscopy

The physiology of thoracoscopy is different from that of laparoscopy due to the rigid nature of the chest. The bony confines of the thorax render it unnecessary to use a significant amount of positive pressure when working in this body cavity. The disadvantages of positive pressure in the chest include decreased venous return, mediastinal shift, and the need to keep a firm seal at all trocar sites. However, visualisation of structures is greatly enhanced with a small degree of insufflation. In older children a double-lumen endotracheal tube may be placed so that the ipsilateral lung can be deflated to obtain a working space within the thorax. In smaller children (weighing less than 30–40 kg), double lumen tubes are unavailable, so the chest is usually insufflated in order to compress the ipsilateral lung.[14] Pressures of 4–6 mm Hg are sufficient to maintain visualisation of the operative field.

Equipment

A video system for MAS must have the following properties: illumination, resolution, and color. Without the first two attributes, video surgery is unsafe.[12] Currently, most imaging for laparoscopy, thoracoscopy, and subcutaneous surgery uses a rigid metal telescope containing a series of quartz optical rods with differing optical characteristics that provide a specific character to each telescope. The standard adult scopes are usually 30 cm in length, with smaller lengths used in paediatric surgery. These metal telescopes vary in diameter from 1 to 10 mm.[12,15,16] Rigid telescopes may provide a straight or oblique view, with the scope angle ranging from 0° to 70°.[12,15] Angled scopes allow greater ability to view the entire operative field.

Illumination is delivered to the laparoscope through a fibre-optic cable.[12] Due to the inefficiency of these light cables, an extremely bright light source (300 watts) is necessary to provide optimal visualisation for video endosurgery. The quality of the videoendoscopic image is only as good as the weakest component in the imaging chain. It is therefore important to use a video monitor that has a resolution equal to or greater than the camera being used. This is particularly important for the smaller telescopes used for laparoscopy on infants, for which a state-of-the-art video setup is required.[12,15]

Instruments for MAS usually are adaptations of conventional surgical instruments made longer, thinner, and smaller at the tip.[12] It is important to realise that laparoscopic grasping instruments apply a greater force over a smaller surface area, thereby increasing the risk for perforation or injury to an infant. Standard instruments are 5 mm in diameter and 30 cm in length, but smaller and shorter instruments are now available for neonatal and infant surgery, with a diameter as small as 2 mm and a length as short as 20 cm.[12,16] Some instruments, such as linear staplers and specimen retrieval bags, are not available in the 5-mm diameter size. A unique laparoscopic instrument is the monopolar electrical hook,[12] which may be configured with a suction and irrigation apparatus to eliminate smoke and blood from the operative field. The monopolar hook allows tenting of tissue over a bare metal wire with subsequent coagulation and division of the tissue.

Common Applications of MAS

One of the more common applications for MAS in both children and adults is appendectomy. The use of laparoscopy for the treatment of appendicitis was first described more than 20 years ago, but its use remains controversial.[17,18] As previously stated, a survey of North American paediatric surgeons showed that 11% of respondents use

laparoscopy for all appendectomies, and the same percentage of respondents never use it. In a large multicentre retrospective review from Europe, 1,506 laparoscopic appendectomies performed in children were compared to 826 open procedures.[19] Operative times and rates of complications were found to be similar, but the laparoscopic cohort had a shorter length of hospital stay for both acute and perforated appendicitis. In a review of 43 children with perforated appendicitis (Figure 122.1) who underwent laparoscopic appendectomy compared to 77 who underwent an open appendectomy, the infectious complication rate in the two groups was similar, but a lower overall complication rate was found in the laparoscopic group.[20] When interpreting these data, one must consider the learning curve required to master the laparoscopic approach. Statistically significant reductions in operative time, conversion rate, and presence of postoperative abscesses were observed when one group compared their experience between time periods before and after their learning curve.[21] The largest meta-analysis comparing laparoscopic (n=2789) versus open (n=3688) appendectomy in children revealed that there was a significantly decreased length of stay in the laparoscopic group, as well as lower rates of wound infection and postoperative ileus.[11] An advantage of a laparoscopic removal of a perforated appendicitis is also the ability to evacuate pus and fluid from the entire abdominal cavity (Figure 122.2). This might improve the outcome in African children who notoriously present late and with complicated appendicitis, although there are no hard data to support this contention.

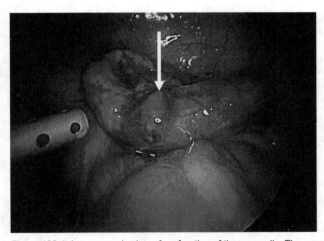

Figure 122.1: Laparoscopic view of perforation of the appendix. The arrow is pointing to pus extruding from the appendiceal lumen.

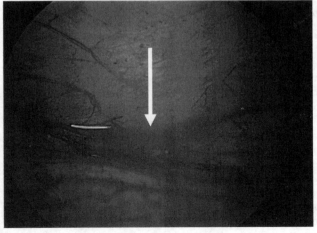

Figure 122.2: Laparoscopic view of pus (arrow) from a perforated appendix collecting in the left paracolic gutter.

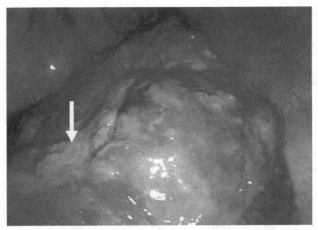

Figure 122.3: Thoracoscopic view of the left lung in an immunocompromised patient with fungal pneumonia. Fibrinous debris (arrow) was removed and lung biopsy was performed to confirm the diagnosis.

Table 122.1: Commonly performed paediatric MIS procedures.

Laparoscopic surgery	Thoracoscopic surgery
Oesophagomyotomy for achalasia	Lung biopsy
Fundoplication	Blebectomy
Gastrostomy	Lung resection
Pyloromyotomy	Debridement of empyema
Pyloroplasty	Lobectomy
Ladd's procedure	Tracheo-oesophageal fistula repair
Duodeno-duodenostomy	Aortopexy
Small bowel atresias	Mediastinal biopsy
Reduction of intussusception	Thymectomy
Appendectomy	Resection of mediastinal mass
Ileocolectomy	Diaphragmatic hernia repair or plication
Partial colectomy	Complex central venous access
Total abdominal colectomy	Patent ductus arteriosus (PDA) ligation
Pull-through for Hirschsprung's disease and anorectal malformations	Pectus excavatum
Cholecystectomy	
Kasai procedure	
Choledochojejunostomy	
Oncological procedures	
Splenectomy	
Nephrectomy	
Adrenalectomy	

The most common application of MAS in the thorax of paediatric patients is for debridement of empyemas (Figure 122.3). Pneumonia is one of the most common infections in the paediatric population, and parapneumonic effusions complicate 21–91% of cases.[22] When the pleural collections are simple (free flowing) the effusions often resolve with chest tube drainage and/or antibiotic therapy alone; however, a complicated effusion often requires pleural space drainage and sometimes decortication to facilitate recovery. Thoracoscopy has become the standard of care in North America for treating these conditions following the first report of its use in 1993.[23,24] Other options include thoracentesis, chest tube placement with instillation of fibrinolytics such as urokinase or tissue plasminogen activator, or antibiotics alone. Failure to treat these collections can lead to persistent pleural thickening and restrictive lung disease. This has led many to advocate for early surgery to treat complicated collections.[25–27] A number of small series have reported decreases in mean postoperative length when compared to thoracoscopy with the open technique.[2,28,29] A retrospective study comparing 54 children treated conservatively with 21 children treated with thoracoscopy found the mean length of stay was 15.4 days in the conservative group (chest tube and antibiotics alone) compared to 7.4 days in the thoracoscopy group, with no procedure-related complications in either case.[30] Clearly, these data show that using thoracoscopy can decrease hospital stay with significantly less morbidity. Although there is debate in the literature over the ideal timing of thoracoscopy and its efficacy compared to drainage with fibrinolysis, there is little doubt that thoracoscopy is the preferred surgical approach.[31–33]

Other Commonly Performed MAS Procedures

In addition to laparoscopic appendicitis and thoracoscopy, MAS has been applied to a large variety of procedures in both the abdomen and thorax (Table 122.1). As in the adult population, cholecystectomy is now routinely performed laparoscopically in children. In a retrospective review of 184 patients with a mean age of 14.1 years (range, 3–22 years) and a mean follow-up of 8.3 months, the only complications were one prolonged ileus and one wound infection.[34] Splenectomy is another operation performed frequently in children for a variety of haematological conditions, splenic cysts, complications of portal hypertension, and malignancies. For elective splenectomy, laparoscopy has become the standard, depending on the size of the spleen. In a retrospective study of 159 patients who underwent laparoscopic splenectomy at three centres,[35] eight cases were converted to open, one case required reoperation with laparoscopy for postoperative bleeding, and three generalised postoperative infections were noted.

Pyloric stenosis is now frequently treated laparoscopically in the United States and Europe, although its advantages are mainly cosmetic. A retrospective comparison of 52 open pyloromyotomies and 65 laparoscopic pyloromyotomies from a single institution found that operating time, incidence and time to postoperative emesis, time to full feedings, total costs, length of stay, and complication rates were not significantly different between the two groups.[36] A prospective randomised trial comparing the techniques revealed less postoperative pain and emesis with laparoscopy when compared to the open approach, with no difference in complication rate.[37] However, a French randomised trial failed to show any difference in postoperative emesis.[38] This French study compared the laparoscopic approach with an open umbilical approach, and found that laparoscopic pyloromyotomy does not decrease the incidence of postoperative vomiting, has a similar complication rate compared with the open umbilical approach, but may expose patients to a risk of inadequate pyloromyotomy.. The umbilical approach may provide improved cosmesis and could constitute an attractive approach in the African setting, although no data detail the cosmetic outcomes for any of the approaches to pyloromyotomy. Thus, the laparoscopic approach is far from universally accepted.[6]

Ladd's procedure for malrotation has also been performed laparoscopically.[39] In a series of 10 patients without midgut volvulus, ranging in age from 10 weeks to 25 years, operated on laparoscopically, the mean operative time was 111 minutes, mean length of stay was 3.6 days, and the only postoperative complication was an incisional hernia. One case was converted to open. This operation is also controversial because many believe that the laparoscopic approach will lead to fewer intraabdominal adhesions and perhaps a higher recurrence rate. However, no study directly comparing long-term outcomes for the laparoscopic and open Ladd's procedures has been published.

Laparoscopic Nissen fundoplication is routinely performed as an alternative to the open procedure in the United States. A retrospective study compared 150 open cases to 306 laparoscopic procedures.[40] Although reoperation was more common in the laparoscopic group (14% versus 8%), the laparoscopic group had significantly fewer complications, and mean length of stay was two days shorter. Another study comparing the hospital charges for 50 open fundoplications to 50 laparoscopic fundoplications found that the overall costs were similar between the two groups, with the shorter length of stay in the laparoscopic group offsetting higher costs in operating room time and equipment.[41] In fact, one study from South Africa has shown that select patients may be discharged on the day of surgery after laparoscopic Nissen fundoplication.[42] However, this practice has yet to be universally accepted.

A problem that is unique to developed nations but may be on the rise in other regions is morbid obesity. Laparoscopy is the preferred approach for bariatric procedures in adults; as adolescent obesity rates have risen in North America, similar procedures have been used in children.[43,44] These procedures should be reserved for only the most expert minimal access paediatric surgeons as part of a multidisciplinary weight-management team.

Minimal access techniques are now commonly used for colorectal surgery in the paediatric population. All three operations described for Hirschsprung's disease (Duhamel, Soave, and Swenson) have been successfully performed laparoscopically.[45] Laparoscopy allows for procurement of seromuscular biopsies to precisely identify the transition zone, and permits minimally invasive mobilisation of the colon, facilitating the pull-through procedures and ensuring a tension-free coloanal anastomosis. Similar techniques are used for colonic mobilisation when treating imperforate anus with mainly high rectourethral fistulas where a laparotomy might be needed in conjunction with the Pena posterior sagittal ano-rectoplasty.[46] A recent article compares laparoscopic-assisted and posterior sagittal anorectoplasty.[47] Laparoscopic-assisted proctocolectomy with J-pouch reconstruction has also been successfully performed in children with ulcerative colitis or familial adenopolyposis.[48]

Advanced thoracoscopic procedures are also being safely performed. In a review from six institutions of 104 patients with oesophageal atresia or tracheo-oesophageal fistula repaired thoracoscopically, the mean age at the time of surgery was 1.2 days and the mean operative time was 129.9 minutes.[49] Early leak or stricture developed in 11.5% of patients, at least one oesophageal dilatation was required in 31.7%, and 4.8% of the procedures were converted to thoracotomy. Three patients died, one related to oesophageal atresia/tracheo-oesophageal fistula (OA/TEF) on the 20th postoperative day. These complications were similar to the authors' experience with open repairs.

Thoracoscopy may also be used to treat pulmonary malignancies in children.[50] In a retrospective review of 55 thoracoscopy cases (31 pulmonary resections, 19 biopsies, 5 resections of mediastinal tumours), there were two cases of trocar site infections and no other complications. Congenital pulmonary malformations are also amenable to the thoracoscopic approach. A retrospective comparison of 12 patients with congenital cystic adenomatous malformations (CCAM) treated with thoracoscopy with 24 open resections found that the thoracoscopy group had a significantly shorter length of stay and that hospital costs were similar overall.[51]

Investigations and Management

Minimal access procedures rarely require a preoperative evaluation different than open procedures for the same conditions. Similarly, management is based on the disease being treated and can be derived from experience with the open approach. However, with MAS, the return of bowel function may be expedited and the duration and need for pain medication may be reduced.

Complications

Many of the known complications that may occur with open surgery also are common when using laparoscopic or thoracoscopic techniques. Some complications, however, such as trocar and Veress needle injuries, are unique to MAS, but these are rare in the hands of an experienced surgeon.[52] The most common injuries after placing trocars in the abdomen are injuries to the small bowel, colon, liver, and vascular structures. With the closed technique, a Veress needle is inserted into the abdomen blindly to deliver carbon dioxide, and subsequently, the umbilical trocar is placed. The placement of a needle blindly into the abdomen may result in injury to the intraabdominal viscera. It is due to this risk that many advocate an open technique. In the open, or Hasson, technique, an umbilical incision is made and the fascia is identified and incised. A blunt trocar is then placed through this incision, and the abdomen is insufflated. Although this approach may be safer, bowel and vascular injury may still occur.[53] In a large retrospective review comparing more than 400,000 closed laparoscopies and 12,000 open procedures, a statistically significantly higher rate of visceral and vascular injuries were found in the closed group. Hernias can develop at trocar sites. It is important that all subsequent trocar insertions and removals be watched under direct vision, to prevent iatrogenic injuries.[54]

Laparoscopy also increases the risk of electrothermal injuries. Monopolar, biploar, and ultrasonic instruments are all used routinely in MAS.[55–57] Overall, the incidence of electrothermal injuries is about 2–5 per 1,000 cases, with inadvertent perforation of the bowel occurring in 0.6–3 per 1,000 cases.[54,55] These numbers may be underreported, however. In addition to bowel perforation, electrosurgical injuries may lead to biliary, uretheral, and anal strictures; hydroureter; or fistula formation in the genitourinary tract.[56] Electrothermal injury can come from inadvertent direct application of the probe to tissue, a defect in the insulation of an instrument, direct coupling (unintended contact between the probe and a noninsulated instrument such as the scope or a grasper), or capacitive coupling (current passing from the probe through intact insulation to the tissue, which occurs when an active probe is in a trocar).[55,56] It is important to note that 75% of all electrothermal burns to the bowel go unrecognised at the time of initial surgery.[57] Thus, a high index of suspicion is paramount. In general, missed injuries present with signs and symptoms of peritonitis 4–10 days after the initial surgery and require emergent reoperation. Minimising electrothermal injuries is achieved via regular training of surgical staff and routine thorough equipment maintenance. The surgeon must ensure that the electrosurgical unit is activated only when the entire conducting component of the instrument is in view. Short bursts of the electrosurgical unit allow tissue to cool and may reduce the incidence and severity of electrothermal injuries as well. Thus, most units are designed to deliver short bursts of energy regardless of the intentions of the user.[55] In general, bipolar electrosurgical systems have a more limited area of thermal spread than monopolar systems, as well as a decreased risk of capacitive coupling.[55,56]

The ultrasonic coagulating shears (harmonic scalpel) work by converting electrical energy into mechanical vibrations (ultrasonic energy).[55] A lower temperature is reached in the jaws of this instrument than in traditional electrosurgical probes, resulting in less lateral tissue injury.[55,57] This device can safely seal vessels up to 3 mm in diameter, but comes in only 5- or 10-mm versions, and thus often is not used for MAS in infants. The electrothermal bipolar vessel sealer (LigaSure™)

can seal vessels up to 7 mm in size and also has a reduced thermal spread compared to traditional electrosurgical units.

Port-site metastases are another complication unique to laparoscopic or thoracoscopic techniques, but these are rare and occur when malignant cells implant on port sites during minimally invasive oncologic resections. This complication has been reported in children, but is not usually of major concern.[58] A survey of the Japanese Society of Paediatric Endosurgeons, designed specifically to identify the incidence of port-site metastasis, found no cases following 129 laparoscopic or thoracoscopic cancer operations.[59] Obviously, this relatively small sample size was unable to capture the true incidence of port-site recurrences, but suggests that port-site metastasis is not a common event. In general, the use of plastic bags for the removal of surgical specimens to decrease the contact between malignant cells and the port site and thus decrease the incidence of port-site metastasis is recommended.

Ethical Considerations

It is clear that minimal access techniques are becoming increasingly used for a variety of surgical diseases in children, but it is unclear which indications best warrant such technology in societies with limited resources. When basic health care needs cannot be met, it is difficult to justify the capital costs associated with purchasing the equipment necessary for MAS and training the surgical and ancillary staff to use it. However, there is no doubt that there are advantages to laparoscopic surgery with its smaller incisions, decreased pain, shorter hospital stay, and reduced complication rates. African children should have the same rights to these benefits as children from developed countries. Thus the chappenge is presented of finding new ways of collaboration where the strengths of both worlds could be integrated to help improve the service to all children.

This type of surgery has minimum basic requirements that should not be taken for granted within developing regions. An alternative approach should always be available in case of sudden loss of electricity. Furthermore, laparoscopic or thoracoscopic surgery should not be undertaken unless the surgeon is trained in the techniques and has ample experience with the open approach. We recommend that critical and honest data acquisition be a part of any program where MAS is to be used. Due to the lack of research infrastructure throughout many parts of Africa, however, this may be more difficult than it appears.

Quality control is not the sole responsibility of the operative surgeon—the hospital must also participate in this overall goal. It is of great importance that there be clearly designated responsibility for maintenance of the equipment, its safe storage, its postoperative cleaning, and its replacement and repair if broken. The surgical and nursing staff should attend ongoing training on handling the very sensitive equipment. We advise a clear and strict policy outlining the reuse of disposable equipment, taking note of all potential complications associated with such reuse. This policy is particularly important, considering the African context and the high prevalence of human immunodeficiency virus (HIV).

It may be that "minimally invasive" surgery as defined by laparoscopy and thoracoscopy may not be ideal in regions where resources are limited. Alternatives exist that apply the concept of MAS without utilising the highly sophisticated and expensive technology of videoscopic surgery. Suitable options for children in Africa include the transanal approach for Hirschsprung's disease, the Tan-Bianchi periumbilical incision and its variations[60] for hypertrophic pyloric stenosis, extended to other intraabdominal procedures such as for intestinal atresia repairs.[61] Surgery within the African context may be viewed as a challenge conducive for innovation and development.

Evidence-Based Research

No prospective randomised controlled trials compare open appendectomy to laparoscopic appendectomy or thoracoscopic debridement to thoracotomy for parapneumonic effusions in the paediatric population. Decisions therefore must be made by using retrospective studies as well as expert opinion and professional society guidelines. A retrospective study for laparoscopic appendectomy is presented in Table 122.2.

Several papers demonstrate the benefits of using thoracoscopy early in a child's course with complicated pneumonia. Table 122.3 presents a retrospective study for parapenumonic effusions or empyemas.

Table 122.2: Evidence-based research.

Title	Laparoscopic versus open appendectomy in children: a meta-analysis
Authors	Aziz O, Athanasiou T, Tekkis PP, et al.
Institution	Imperial College of Science, Technology and Medicine, Department of Surgical Oncology and Technology, St. Mary's Hospital, London, UK
Reference	Ann Surg 2006; 243(1):17-27
Problem	Surgical approach in treating appendicitis in children: laparoscopic versus open appendectomy.
Intervention	Laparoscopic versus open appendectomy.
Comparison/ control (quality of evidence)	Meta-analysis of 23 studies comparing a total of 2,789 laparoscopic appendectomies to 3,688 open appendectomies.
Outcome/ effect	The outcomes analysed were postoperative fever, ileus, wound infection, intraabdominal abscess formation, operative time, and postoperative hospital stay. Wound infection was significantly reduced with laparoscopic versus open appendectomy (1.5% versus 5%; OR = 0.45, 95% CI = 0.27–0.75), as was ileus (1.3% versus 2.8%; OR = 0.5, 95% CI = 0.29–0.86). Postoperative stay was significantly shorter in the laparoscopic group (weighted mean difference, 0.48; 95% CI = 0.65–0.31). Intraabdominal abscess formation was more common following laparoscopic surgery, although this was not statistically significant. There was no statistically significant difference in operative time or postoperative fever.
Historical significance/ comments	This large meta-analysis of 23 studies and almost 6,500 children represents the largest data set comparing laparoscopic and open appendectomy in the paediatric population. The results of this study demonstrate a lower incidence of wound infection and postoperative ileus and a shorter length of stay in the laparoscopic group. The finding of a decreased number of wound infections is seen in almost every procedure that is done laparoscopically when compared to its open counterpart. Regarding postoperative ileus, it is suggested that this may be reduced in laparoscopic surgery due to decreased handling of the bowel, reduced opiate requirements, and earlier mobilisation. Clearly, these same factors would affect postoperative length of stay. Additional benefits of laparoscopy are the ability to examine the entire abdomen prior to performing appendectomy, which is particularly useful when the diagnosis of appendicitis is in question. This study is a meta-analysis, which makes it imperfect in many ways. First, different studies may have had slightly different defining criteria for the outcome measures of interest, and this was not always clearly identified, according to the authors. The authors also point out the importance of nonpublication bias, as meta-analytic research is based only on published studies. Generally, meta-analyses are only as good as the studies included in the analysis. Thus, if the original studies are flawed, so is the meta-analysis. Despite these concerns, the conclusions drawn from this manuscript suggest a decreased length of stay, fewer wound infections, and a reduction in postoperative ileus in the laparoscopic group.

Table 122.3: Evidence-based research.

Title	Comparative analysis of chest tube thoracostomy and video-assisted thoracoscopic surgery in empyema and parapneumonic effusion associated with pneumonia in children
Authors	Aziz A, Healy JM, Qureshi F, Kane TD, Kurland G, Green M, Hackam DJ
Institution	Divisions of Pediatric Surgery, Pediatric Pulmonology, and Pediatric Infectious Disease, Children's Hospital of Pittsburgh and the University of Pittsburgh School of Medicine, Pittsburgh, Pennsylvania, USA.
Reference	Surg Infect 2008; 9(3):317–323
Problem	Conservative versus operative management of parapneumonic effusions and empyemas.
Intervention	Chest tube drainage versus thoracoscopic debridement.
Comparison/ control (quality of evidence)	Forty-nine paediatric patients with pneumonia complicated by parapneumonic effusion or empyema treated between 1997 and 2003 were divided into three groups: primary chest tube (n=21), chest tube followed by thoracoscopy (n=15), or primary thoracoscopy (n=13).
Outcome/ effect	The following data were obtained: Sex, age, presenting symptoms, duration of symptoms, comorbidities and history of empyema, vital signs on presentation, chest radiographic findings, antibiotic treatment, surgical procedure, pleural fluid content, intensive care unit stay, total days in hospital, and total hospital charges. All groups were similar with respect to demographics and initial antibiotic usage. Patients undergoing primary thoracoscopy had a higher initial temperature, whereas radiographic findings of mediastinal shift and air bronchograms were more likely to be found in patients who underwent primary chest tube placement. Patients undergoing primary thoracoscopy demonstrated a significantly shorter total hospital stay and lower hospital charges than the other groups. Forty percent of children started on chest tube therapy required subsequent thoracoscopy, necessitating a significantly longer hospital course (18±3 versus 11±0.8 days; p<0.05) and higher hospital charges ($50,000±$7,000 versus $29,000±$1,000) than those having primary thoracoscopy.
Historical significance/ comments	This study is certainly limited due to the fact that it is retrospective and has a relatively small sample size. However, the analysis performed was extensive and the results are striking for a significantly reduced length of stay and total hospital charges when primary thoracoscopy is the approach used. The fact that there were no significant differences across groups in regard to demographics, initial vital signs, or initial antibiotic course strengthens these results. The authors' conclusions advocate for this approach for all children presenting with parapneumonic effusions or empyemas. The authors suggest that one of the factors predisposing to failure of chest tube drainage is that the tubes placed by interventional radiology are smaller and may be more prone to obstruction compared to the larger caliber tubes placed in the operating room. Another factor that may increase the benefit of thoracoscopy is the improved visualisation, allowing for complete evacuation of debris and earlier expansion of the lung. Clearly, a prospective trial would be helpful in determining which patients are best treated surgically and which could be successfully managed with chest tube drainage alone.

Key Summary Points

1. Minimal access surgery for adults has been widely practiced by general surgeons for two decades; more recent technical advances have led to this technology being applied to the care of infants and children.

2. A large number of reports exist in the literature on minimal access techniques being successfully and safely applied to the care of infants and children for surgical disease in the abdomen and chest.

3. Laparoscopic appendectomy results in decreased incidence of wound infections and postoperative ileus as well as shorter length of hospital stay when compared to the open procedure.

4. Laparoscopic appendectomy can be performed safely for both acute and perforated appendicitis.

5. Thoracoscopic debridement of empyemas following complicated pneumonia has become standard in many centres. Early intervention has been shown to decrease hospital stay and total costs.

6. Thoracoscopic debridement for complicated pneumonia may be the most appropriate application of minimal access surgery to resource-limited African communities.

7. Complications unique to minimal access surgery include Veress needle and trocar injuries as well as electrothermal injuries. Early recognition and immediate treatment of vascular or visceral injuries improves outcome.

8. Controversy remains over the most appropriate applications of minimally invasive techniques in the paediatric population; these may differ, depending on the geographic location in question.

9. In resource-limited communities of Africa that are considering establishing a minimal access surgery program, attention must be paid not only to operative technique but also to equipment maintenance and storage, training of ancillary staff in equipment use, and critical acquisition of outcomes.

References

1. Litynski GS. Kurt Semm and the fight against skepticism: endoscopic hemostasis, laparoscopic appendectomy, and Semm's impact on the "laparoscopic revolution". JSLS 1998; 2(3):309–313.

2. Polychronidis A, Laftsidis P, Bounovas A, Simopoulos C. Twenty years of laparoscopic cholecystectomy: Philippe Mouret—March 17, 1987. JSLS 2008; 12(1):109–111.

3. Ure BM, Bax NM, van der Zee DC. Laparoscopy in infants and children: a prospective study on feasibility and the impact on routine surgery. J Pediatr Surg 2000; 35(8):1170–1173.

4. te Velde EA, Bax NM, Tytgat SH, de Jong JR, Travassos DV, Kramer WL, van der Zee DC. Minimally invasive pediatric surgery: increasing implementation in daily practice and resident's training. Surg Endosc 2008; 22(1):163–166.

5. Muehlstedt SG, Pham TQ, Schmeling DJ. The management of pediatric appendicitis: a survey of North American Pediatric Surgeons. J Pediatr Surg 2004; 39(6):875–879.

6. Mullassery D, Perry D, Goyal A, Jesudason EC, Losty PD. Surgical practice for infantile hypertrophic pyloric stenosis in the United Kingdom and Ireland—a survey of members of the British Association of Paediatric Surgeons. J Pediatr Surg 2008; 43(6):1227–1229.

7. Garbutt JM, Soper NJ, Shannon WD, Botero A, Littenberg B. Meta-analysis of randomized controlled trials comparing laparoscopic and open appendectomy. Surg Laparosc Endosc 1999; 9(1):17–26.

8. Winslow ER, Brunt LM. Perioperative outcomes of laparoscopic versus open splenectomy: a meta-analysis with an emphasis on complications. Surgery 2003; 134(4):647–653; discussion 654–655.

9. Keus F, de Jong JA, Gooszen HG, van Laarhoven CJ. Laparoscopic versus open cholecystectomy for patients with symptomatic cholecystolithiasis. Cochrane Database Syst Rev 2006; (4):CD006231.

10. Tjandra JJ, Chan MK. Systematic review on the short-term outcome of laparoscopic resection for colon and rectosigmoid cancer. Colorectal Dis 2006; 8(5):375–388.

11. Aziz O, Athanasiou T, Tekkis PP, Purkayastha S, Haddow J, Malinovski V, Paraskeva P, Darzi A. Laparoscopic versus open appendectomy in children: a meta-analysis. Ann Surg 2006; 243(1):17–27.

12. Jobe BA, Hunter GG. Minimally invasive surgery. In: Brunicardi FC, Andersen DK, Billiar TR, Dunn DL, Hunter JG, Mathews JB, Pollock RE, Schwartz SI, eds. Schwartz's Principles of Surgery, 8th ed. McGraw-Hill Scientific, Technical & Medical, 2004.

13. Bettolli M, Rubin SZ, Gutauskas A. Large paraesophageal hernias in children. Early experience with laparoscopic repair. Eur J Pediatr Surg 2008; 18(2):72–74.

14. Siedman L. Anesthesia for pediatric minimally invasive surgery. Lobe TE, ed. Pediatric Laparoscopy. Landes Bioscience, 2003.

15. Lobe TE. Mini-laparoscopy in infants and children. In: Lobe TE, ed. Pediatric Laparoscopy. Landes Bioscience, 2003.

16. Bax KNMA. Instrumentation in pediatric endoscopic surgery. In: Lobe TE, ed. Pediatric Laparoscopy. Landes Bioscience, 2003.

17. Agresta F, De Simone P, Michelet I, Bedin N. Laparoscopic appendectomy: why it should be done. JSLS 2003; 7(4):347–352.

18. Little DC, Custer MD, May BH, Blalock SE, Cooney DR. Laparoscopic appendectomy: an unnecessary and expensive procedure in children? J Pediatr Surg 2002; 37(3):310–317.

19. Esposito C, Borzi P, Valla JS, Mekki M, Nouri A, Becmeur F, Allal H, Settimi A, Shier F, Sabin MG, Mastroianni L. Laparoscopic versus open appendectomy in children: a retrospective comparative study of 2,332 cases. World J Surg 2007; 31(4):750–755.

20. Nadler EP, Reblock KK, Qureshi FG, Hackam DJ, Gaines BA, Kane TD. Laparoscopic appendectomy in children with perforated appendicitis. J Laparoendosc Adv Surg Tech A 2006; 16(2):159–163.

21. Phillips S, Walton JM, Chin I, Farrokhyar F, Fitzgerald P, Cameron B. Ten-year experience with pediatric laparoscopic appendectomy—are we getting better? J Pediatr Surg 2005; 40(5):842–845.

22. Padman R, King KA, Iqbal S, Wolfson PJ. Parapneumonic effusion and empyema in children: retrospective review of the duPont experience. Clin Pediatr (Phila) 2007; 46(6):518–522.

23. Cohen E, Weinstein M, Fisman DN. Cost-effectiveness of competing strategies for the treatment of pediatric empyema. Pediatrics 2008; 121(5):e1250–e1257.

24. Kern JA, Rodgers BM. Thoracoscopy in the management of empyema in children. J Pediatr Surg 1993; 28(9):1128–1132.

25. Kohn GL, Walston C, Feldstein J, Warner BW, Succop P, Hardie WD. Persistent abnormal lung function after childhood empyema. Am J Respir Med 2002; 1(6):441–445.

26. Merry CM, Bufo AJ, Shah RS, Schropp KP, Lobe TE. Early definitive intervention by thoracoscopy in pediatric empyema. J Pediatr Surg 1999; 34(1):178–180; discussion 180–181.

27. Chan W, Keyser-Gauvin E, Davis GM, Nguyen LT, Laberge JM. Empyema thoracis in children: a 26-year review of the Montreal Children's Hospital experience. J Pediatr Surg 1997; 32(6):870–872.

28. Stovroff M, Teague G, Heiss KF, Parker P, Ricketts RR. Thoracoscopy in the management of pediatric empyema. J Pediatr Surg 1995; 30(8):1211–1215.

29. Silen ML, Weber TR. Thoracoscopic debridement of loculated empyema thoracis in children. Ann Thorac Surg 1995; 59(5):1166–1168.

30. Cohen G, Hjortdal V, Ricci M, Jaffe A, Wallis C, Dinwiddie R, Elliott MJ, de Leval MR. Primary thoracoscopic treatment of empyema in children. J Thorac Cardiovasc Surg 2003; 125(1):79–83.

31. Kalfa N, Allal H, Montes-Tapia F, Lopez M, Forgues D, Guibal MP, Counil F, Galifer RB. Ideal timing of thoracoscopic decortication and drainage for empyema in children. Surg Endosc 2004; 18(3):472–477.

32. Cremonesini D, Thomson AH. How should we manage empyema: antibiotics alone, fibrinolytics, or primary video-assisted thoracoscopic surgery (VATS)? Semin Respir Crit Care Med 2007; 28(3):322–332.

33. Aziz A, Healey JM, Qureshi F, Kane TD, Kurland G, Green M, Hackam DJ. Comparative analysis of chest tube thoracostomy and video-assisted thoracoscopic surgery in empyema and parapneumonic effusion associated with pneumonia in children. Surg Infect (Larchmt) 2008; 9(3):317–323.

34. Siddiqui S, Newbrough S, Alterman D, Anderson A, Kennedy A Jr. Efficacy of laparoscopic cholecystectomy in the pediatric population. J Pediatr Surg 2008; 43(1):109–113.

35. Murawski M, Patkowski D, Korlacki W, Czauderna P, Sroka M, Makarewicz W, Czernik J, Dzielicki J. Laparoscopic splenectomy in children—a multicenter experience. J Pediatr Surg 2008; 43(5):951–954.

36. Campbell BT, McLean K, Barnhart DC, Drongowski RA, Hirschl RB. A comparison of laparoscopic and open pyloromyotomy at a teaching hospital. J Pediatr Surg 2002; 37(7):1068–1071.

37. St Peter SD, Holcomb GW 3rd, Calkins CM, Murphy JP, Andrews WS, Sharp RJ, Snyder CL, Ostlie DJ. Open versus laparoscopic pyloromyotomy for pyloric stenosis: a prospective, randomized trial. Ann Surg 2006; 244(3):363–370.

38. Leclair MD, Plattner V, Mirallie E, Lejus C, Nguyen JM, Podevin G, Heloury Y. Laparoscopic pyloromyotomy for hypertrophic pyloric stenosis: a prospective, randomized controlled trial. J Pediatr Surg 2007; 42(4):692–698.

39. Draus JM Jr, Foley DS, Bond SJ. Laparoscopic Ladd procedure: a minimally invasive approach to malrotation without midgut volvulus. Am Surg 2007; 73(7):693–696.

40. Diaz DM, Gibbons TE, Heiss K, Wulkan ML, Ricketts RR, Gold BD. Antireflux surgery outcomes in pediatric gastroesophageal reflux disease. Am J Gastroenterol 2005; 100(8):1844–1852.

41. Ostlie DJ, St Peter SD, Snyder CL, Sharp RJ, Andrews WS, Holcomb GW 3rd. A financial analysis of pediatric laparoscopic versus open fundoplication. J Laparoendosc Adv Surg Tech A 2007; 17(4):493–496.

42. Banieghbal B, Beale P. Day-case laparoscopic Nissen fundoplication in children. J Laparoendosc Adv Surg Tech A 2007; 17(3):350–352.

43. Nadler EP, Youn HA, Ren CJ, Fielding GA. An update on 73 US obese pediatric patients treated with laparoscopic adjustable gastric banding: comorbidity resolution and compliance data. J Pediatr Surg 2008; 43(1):141–146.

44. Lawson ML, Kirk S, Mitchell T, Chen MK, Loux TJ, Daniels SR, Harmon CM, Clements RH, Garcia VF, Inge TH. Pediatric Bariatric Study Group. One-year outcomes of Roux-en-Y gastric bypass for morbidly obese adolescents: a multicenter study from the Pediatric Bariatric Study Group. J Pediatr Surg 2006; 41(1):137–143; discussion 137–143.

45. Zilbert N, Nadler EP. Laparoscopic-assisted procedures for the treatment of Hirschprung's disease: review of the literature and technical report. Chin J Minim Invasive Surg 2008; 8(3):225–229.

46. Georgeson KE, Inge TH, Albanese CT. Laparoscopically assisted anorectal pull-through for high imperforate anus—a new technique. J Pediatr Surg 2000; 35(6):927–930.

47. deVos C, Arnold M, Moore SW. A comparision of the laparoscopic assisted (LAARP) and posterior saggital (PSARP) ano-rectoplasty in the outcome of intermediate and high anorectal malformations. SAJS (in press).

48. Meier AH, Roth L, Cilley RE, Dillon PW. Completely minimally invasive approach to restorative total proctocolectomy with J-pouch construction in children. Surg Laparosc Endosc Percutan Tech 2007; 17(5):418–421.

49. Holcomb GW 3rd, Rothenberg SS, Bax KM, Martinez-Ferro M, Albanese CT, Ostlie DJ, van Der Zee DC, Yeung CK. Thoracoscopic repair of esophageal atresia and tracheoesophageal fistula: a multi-institutional analysis. Ann Surg 2005; 242(3):422–428; discussion 428–430.

50. Esposito C, Lima M, Mattioli G, Mastroianni L, Riccipetitoni G, Monguzzi G, Zanon G, Cecchetto G, Settimi A, Jasonni V. Thoracoscopic surgery in the management of pediatric malignancies: a multicentric survey of the Italian Society of Videosurgery in Infancy. Surg Endosc 2007; 21(10):1772–1775.

51. Vu LT, Farmer DL, Nobuhara KK, Miniati D, Lee H. Thoracoscopic versus open resection for congenital cystic adenomatoid malformations of the lung. J Pediatr Surg 2008; 43(1):35–39.

52. Schäfer M, Lauper M, Krähenbühl L. Trocar and Veress needle injuries during laparoscopy. Surg Endosc 2001; 15(3):275–280.

53. Bonjer HJ, Hazebroek EJ, Kazemier G, Giuffrida MC, Meijer WS, Lange JF. Open versus closed establishment of pneumoperitoneum in laparoscopic surgery. Br J Surg 1997; 84(5):599–602.

54. Chen MK, Schropp KP, Lobe TE. Complications of minimal-access surgery in children. J Pediatr Surg 1996; 31(8):1161–1165.

55. Harrell AG, Kercher KW, Heniford BT. Energy sources in laparoscopy. Semin Laparosc Surg 2004; 11(3):201–209.

56. Wu MP, Ou CS, Chen SL, Yen EY, Rowbotham R. Complications and recommended practices for electrosurgery in laparoscopy. Am J Surg 2000; 179(1):67–73.

57. Birch DW, Park A, Shuhaibar H. Acute thermal injury to the canine jejunal free flap: electrocautery versus ultrasonic dissection. Am Surg 1999; 65(4):334–337.

58. Sartorelli KH, Partrick D, Meagher DP Jr. Port-site recurrence after thoracoscopic resection of pulmonary metastasis owing to osteogenic sarcoma. J Pediatr Surg 1996; 31(10):1443–1444.

59. Iwanaka T, Arai M, Yamamoto H, Fukuzawa M, Kubota A, Kouchi K, Nio M, Satomi A, Sasaki F, Yoneda A, Ohhama Y, Takehara H, Morikawa Y, Miyano T. No incidence of port-site recurrence after endosurgical procedure for pediatric malignancies. Pediatr Surg Int 2003; 19(3):200–203.

60. Tan KC, Bianchi A. Circumumbilical incision for pyloromyotomy. Br J Surg 1986; 73:399.

61. Banieghbal B, Beale PG. Minimal access approach to jejunal atresia. J Pediatr Surg 2007; 42(8):1362–1364.

CHAPTER 123
PRENATAL DIAGNOSIS AND FOETAL THERAPY

Kokila Lakhoo

Introduction

Prenatal diagnosis and foetal therapy are rare in Africa except for the presentation of polyhydraminios in foetal bowel obstruction. This chapter therefore covers prenatal diagnosis and therapy as practised in resourced countries.

Expertise in surgical correction of congenital malformations may favourably influence the perinatal management of prenatally diagnosed anomalies, by changing the site of delivery for immediate postnatal treatment; altering the mode of delivery to prevent obstructed labour or haemorrhage; early delivery to prevent ongoing foetal organ damage; or treatment in utero to prevent, minimise or reverse foetal organ injury as a result of a structural defect. The referral base for a paediatric surgeon now includes the perinatal period.

The diagnosis and management of complex foetal anomalies require a team effort by obstetricians, neonatologists, genetecists, paediatricians, and paediatric surgeons to deal with all the maternal and foetal complexities involved in diagnosis of a structural defect. This team should be able to provide information to prospective parents on foetal outcomes; possible interventions; appropriate setting, time, and route of delivery; and expected postnatal outcomes. The role of the surgical consultant in this team is to present information regarding the prenatal and postnatal natural history of an anomaly, its surgical management, and the expected long-term outcome.

Congenital Malformations

Congenital malformations account for one of the major causes of perinatal mortality and morbidity. Single major birth defects affect 3% of newborns, and 0.7% of babies have multiple defects. The prenatal hidden mortality is higher because the majority abort spontaneously. Despite improvements in perinatal care, serious birth defects still account for 20% of all deaths in the newborn period and an even greater percentage of serious morbidity later in infancy and childhood. The major causes of congenital malformation are chromosomal abnormalities, mutant genes, multifactorial disorders, and teratogenic agents.

Prenatal Diagnosis

Prenatal diagnosis has remarkably improved our understanding of surgically correctable congenital malformations. It has allowed us to influence the delivery of the baby, offer prenatal surgical management, and discuss the options of termination of pregnancy for seriously handicapping or lethal conditions. Screening for Down syndrome may now be offered in the first trimester (e.g., nuchal scan combined test) (Figure 123.1) or second trimester (e.g., triple blood test). Better resolution and increased experience with ultrasound (US) scans have led to the recognition of US soft markers, which have increased the detection rate of foetal anomalies albeit at the expense of higher false positive rates.

Routine US screening identifies anomalies and places these pregnancies in the high-risk categories with maternal diabetes, hypertension, genetic disorders, and raised alpha foetoprotein, among others. Parents with high-risk pregnancies may be offered further invasive diagnostic investigations, such as amniocentesis or chorionic villous sampling. Structural abnormalities that are difficult

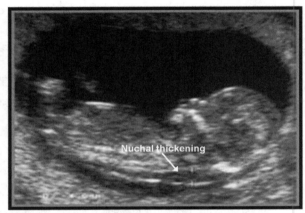

Figure 123.1: Nuchal thickening on scan.

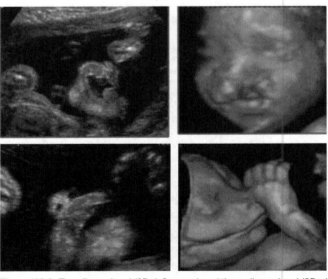

Figure 123.2: Two-dimensional (2D; left panes) and three-dimensional (3D; right panes) scan of facial banding.

to define on US, such as hindbrain lesions or those in the presence of oligohydramnios, are better imaged on ultrafast magnetic resonance imaging (MRI). With the increasing range of options and sophistication of diagnostic methods (Figure 123.2), parents today are faced with more information, choices, and decisions than ever before, which can create as well as help to solve dilemmas.

Specific Surgical Conditions

Congenital Diaphragmatic Hernia

Congenital diaphragmatic hernia (CDH; Figure 123.3) accounts for 1 in 3,000 live births worldwide and challenges the neonatologist and paediatric surgeon in the management of this high-risk condition. Mortality remains high (>60%) when the "hidden" mortality of in utero death and termination of pregnancy are taken into account. Lung hypoplasia and pulmonary hypertension account for most deaths in isolated CDH newborns. Associated anomalies (30–40%) signify a grave prognosis with a survival rate of less than 10%.

In the United Kingdom, most cases of CDH are diagnosed at the 20-week anomaly scan, with a detection rate approaching 60%. MRI has a useful role in accurately differentiating CDH from cystic lung lesions and may be useful in measuring foetal lung volumes as a predictor of outcome. Cardiac anomalies (20%); chromosomal anomalies of trisomy 13 and 18 (20%); and urinary, gastrointestinal, and neurological anomalies (33%) can coexist with CDH. These associated anomalies and, in isolated lesions, early detection, liver in the chest, polyhydramnios, and foetal lung-head ratio (LHR) of less than 1 are implicated as poor predictors of outcome. In these patients with poor prognostic signs, foetal surgery for CDH over the last two decades has been disappointing; however, benefit from foetal endoscopic with tracheal occlusion (FETO) awaits randomised studies. Favourable outcomes in CDH with the use of antenatal steroids has not been resolved in clinical settings. Elective delivery at a specialised centre is recommended with no benefit from caesarean section.

Cystic Lung Lesions

Congenital cystic adenomatous malformations (CCAMs), bronchopulmonary sequestrations (BPSs), or "hybrid" lesions containing features of both are common cystic lung lesions noted on prenatal scans. Less common lung anomalies include bronchogenic cysts, congenital lobar emphysema, and bronchial atresia. Congenital cystic lung lesions (Figure 123.4) are rare anomalies, with an incidence of 1 in 10,000 to 1 in 35,000.

The prenatal detection rate of lung cysts at the routine 18- 20-week scan is almost 100%; this scan may be the most common mode of actual presentation. Most of these lesions are easily distinguished from CDH; however, sonographic features of CCAM or BPS are not sufficiently accurate and correlate poorly with histology. MRI, although not routinely used, may provide better definition for this condition; however, inaccuracies have been reported in 11% of cases.

Bilateral disease and hydrops foetalis are indicators of poor outcome, whereas mediastinal shift, polyhydramnios, and early detection are not poor prognostic signs. In the absence of termination, the natural foetal demise of antenatally diagnosed cystic lung disease is 28%. It is well documented that spontaneous involution of cystic lung lesions can occur, but complete postnatal resolution is rare, and apparent spontaneous "disappearance" of antenatally diagnosed lesions should be interpreted with care because nearly half of these cases subsequently require surgery.

In only 10% of cases does the need for foetal intervention arise. The spectrum of intervention includes simple centesis of amniotic fluid, thoracoamniotic shunt placement, percutaneous laser ablation, and open foetal surgical resection. Maternal steroid administration has also been reported to have a beneficial effect on some CCAMs, although the mechanism is unclear. A large cystic mass and hydrops in isolated cystic lung lesions are the only real indications for foetal intervention.

Normal vaginal delivery is recommended unless the maternal condition indicates otherwise. Large lesions are predicted to become symptomatic shortly after birth; thus, delivery at a specialised centre would be appropriate. Smaller lesions are less likely to be symptomatic at birth, however, and could be delivered at the referring institution with follow-up in a paediatric surgery clinic.

Abdominal Wall Defects

Exomphalos and gastroschisis are both common but distinct abdominal wall defects with an unclear aetiology and a controversial prognosis. Attention may be drawn to their presence during the second trimester because of raised maternal serum alpha foetoprotein level, or abnormal US scan.

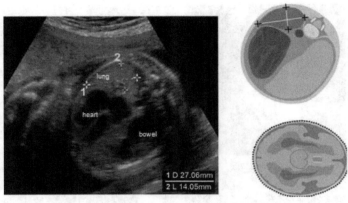

Figure 123.3: Diaphragmatic hernia.

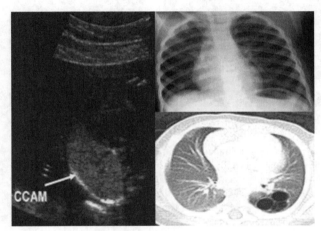

Figure 123.4: Congenital lung cyst.

Exomphalos

Exomphalos (Figure 123.5) is characteristically a midline defect, usually near the insertion point of the umbilical cord, with a viable sac composed of amnion and peritoneum containing herniated abdominal contents. Incidence is known to be 1 in 4,000 live births worldwide. Associated major abnormalities, which include trisomy 13, 18, and 21; Beckwith-Wiedemann syndrome (macroglossia, gigantism, exomphalos); pentalogy of Cantrell (sternal, pericardial, cardiac, abdominal wall, and diaphragmatic defects); and cardiac, gastrointestinal, and renal abnormalities are noted in 60–70% of cases. Thus, karyotyping, in addition to detailed sonographic review and foetal echocardiogram, is essential for complete prenatal screening. Foetal intervention is unlikely in this condition. If termination is not considered, normal vaginal delivery at a centre with neonatal surgical expertise is recommended, and delivery by caesarean section is reserved only for large exomphalos with exteriorised liver, to prevent damage.

Gastroschisis

Gastroschisis (Figure 123.6) is an isolated lesion that usually occurs on the right side of the umbilical defect with evisceration of the abdominal contents directly into the amniotic cavity. The incidence has increased from 1.66 per 10,000 births to 4.6 per 10,000 births worldwide and in the last 10-15 years, affecting mainly mothers younger than 20 years of age. Associated anomalies are noted in only 5–24% of cases, with bowel atresia the most common coexisting abnormality. On prenatal scan, with a detection rate of 100%, the bowel appears to be free floating, and the loops may appear to be thickened due to damage by amniotic fluid exposure, causing a "peel" formation. Dilated loops of bowel (see Figure 123.3) may be seen from obstruction, secondary to protrusion from a defect or atresia due to intestinal ischaemia.

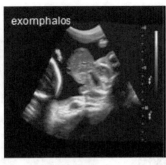
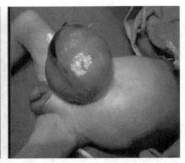

Figure 123.5: Exomphalos.

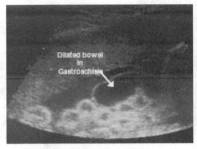
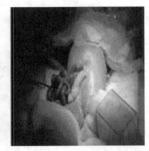

Figure 123.6: Gastroschisis.

Predicting outcomes in foetuses with gastroschisis based on prenatal US findings remains a challenge. There is some evidence that maximum small bowel diameter may be predictive; however, thickened matted bowel and Doppler measurements of the superior mesenteric artery are not accurate predictors of outcome. To reduce the rate of third-trimester foetal loss, serial US scans are performed to monitor the development of bowel obstruction, and delivery at around 37 weeks is recommended, preferably at a centre with neonatal surgical expertise.

Tracheo-Oesophageal Fistula and Oesophageal Atresia
Repair of tracheo-oesophageal fistula and oesophageal atresia (TOF/OA) measures the skill of paediatric surgeons from trainee to independent surgeon. The incidence of TOF/OA is estimated at 1 in 3,000 births worldwide. Prenatally, the condition may be suspected from maternal polyhydramnios and absence of a foetal stomach bubble at the 20-week anomaly scan. Prenatal scan diagnosis of TOF/OA is estimated to be less than 42% sensitive with a positive predicted value of 56%. Additional diagnostic clues are provided by associated anomalies such as trisomy (13, 18, 21), the VACTERAL (vertebral, anorectal, cardiac, tracheo-oesophageal, renal, limbs) sequence, and CHARGE (coloboma, heart defects, atresia choanae, retarded development, genital hypoplasia, ear abnormality) association. These associated anomalies are present in more than 50% of TOF/OA cases and worsen the prognosis; thus, prenatal karyotyping is essential. Duodenal atresia may coexist with TOF/OA. The risk of recurrence in subsequent pregnancies for isolated TOF/OA is less than 1%. Delivery is advised to be at a specialised centre with neonatal surgical input.

Gastrointestinal Lesions
The presence of dilated loops of bowel (>15 mm in length and 7 mm in diameter) on prenatal US scan is indicative of bowel obstruction.

Duodenal atresia has a characteristic "double-bubble" appearance on prenatal scan, resulting from the simultaneous dilatation of the stomach and proximal duodenum. The detection rate on a second-trimester anomaly scan is almost 100% in the presence of polyhydramnios and the double-bubble sign. Associated anomalies are present in approximately 50% of cases, with trisomy 21 most notably in 30% of cases, cardiac anomalies in 20%, and the presence of the VACTERL association.

The incidence of duodenal atresia is 1 in 5,000 live births worldwide. The postnatal survival rate is >95% with associated anomalies, low birth weight, and prematurity contributing to the <5% mortality. Temporary delay in enteral feeding occurs due to dysmotility in the dilated stomach and duodenum.

There are many bowel abnormalities that may be noted on prenatal scanning (dilated bowel, ascites, cystic masses, hyperparistalsis, poyhydramnios, and echogenic bowel); however, none is absolutely predictive of postnatal outcome. Patients with obstruction frequently have findings (especially in the third trimester) of bowel dilatation, polyhydramnios, and hyperparistalsis, but US is much less sensitive in diagnosing large bowel anomalies than those in the small bowel. The large bowel is mostly a reservoir with no physiologic function in utero, so defects in this region, such as anorectal malformations or Hirshsprung's disease, are very difficult to detect. Bowel dilatation and echogenic bowel may be associated with cystic fibrosis; therefore, all such foetuses should undergo postnatal evaluation for this disease. Prenatally diagnosed small bowel atresia does not select for a group with a worse prognosis, and survival rates are 95–100%.

Sacrococcygeal Teratoma
Sacrococcygeal teratoma (SCT; Figure 123.7) is the most common neonatal tumour, affecting 1 in 35,000 to 40,000 births worldwide. Four types of SCT have been defined:

Type 1:   External tumour with a small presacral component.

Type 2:   External tumour with a large presacral component.

Type 3:   Predominantly presacral with a small external component.

Type 4:   Entirely presacral.

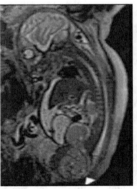
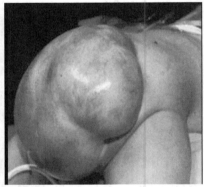

Figure 123.7: Sacrococcygeal teratoma (left: MRI).

Types 3 and 4 carry the worst prognosis due to delay in diagnosis and malignant presentation. Doppler US is the diagnostic tool; however, foetal MRI provides a better definition of the intrapelvic component. SCT is a highly vascular tumour, and the foetus may develop high cardiac output failure, anaemia, and ultimately hydrops, with a mortality of almost 100%. Foetal treatment of tumour resection or ablation of the feeding vessel has been attempted in hydropic patients. Caesarean section may be offered to patients with large tumours to avoid the risk of bleeding during delivery. Postnatal outcomes following surgery in type 1 and 2 lesions are favourable; however, type 3 and 4 tumours may present with urological problems and less favourable outcomes. Long-term follow-up with alpha foetoprotein and serial pelvic US scans are mandatory to exclude recurrence of the disease.

Renal Anomalies
Urogenital abnormalities are among the most common disorders seen in the perinatal period, accounting for almost 20% of all prenatally diagnosed anomalies. The routine use of antenatal US scans has resulted in the early detection of these conditions, and in selected cases this has

led to the development of management strategies including foetal intervention aimed at preservation of renal function. Two major issues are the indications for intervention in bladder outlet obstruction and early pyeloplasty in infancy in cases with hydronephrosis.

Prenatal evaluation of a dilated urinary tract is based on serial US scans as well as measurement of urinary electrolytes. US provides measurements of the renal pelvis, assessment of the renal parenchyma, and the detection of cysts in the cortex. In severe disease, lack of amniotic fluid may make US assessment of the renal tract difficult, and MRI may be helpful. Oligohydramnios is indicative of poor renal function and poor prognosis due to the associated pulmonary hypoplasia. Urogenital anomalies coexist with many other congenital abnormalities, and amniocentesis should be offered in appropriate cases. It is estimated that 3% of infants will have an abnormality of the urogenital system and half of these will require some form of surgical intervention.

Upper Urinary Tract Obstruction

Antenatal hydronephrosis is present in 0.6–0.65% of pregnancies. The most common cause of prenatal hydronephrosis is pelviureteric junction (PUJ) obstruction; others include transient hydronephrosis, physiological hydronephrosis, multicystic kidney, posterior urethral valves, ureterocoele, and ectopic ureter. The prognosis of antenatally diagnosed hydronephrosis in unilateral disease and with renal pelvic diameter of <10 mm is excellent. Spontaneous resolution is noted in 20% of patients at birth and 80% at 3 years of age. Only 17% of prenatally diagnosed hydronephrosis cases need surgical intervention.

Lower Urinary Tract Obstruction

Posterior urethral valves (PUVs; Figure 123.8) are the most common causes for lower urinary tract obstruction in boys, with an incidence

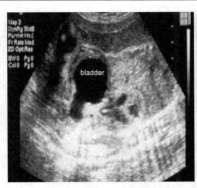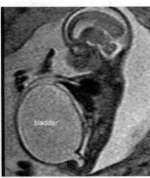

Figure 123.8: US scan (left) and MRI (right) of posterior urethral valves.

of 1 in 2,000 to 4,000 live male births worldwide. The diagnosis of PUV is suspected on a prenatal US finding of bilateral hydronephrosis associated with a thickened bladder and decreased amniotic fluid volume. Serial foetal urine analysis may provide prognostic information on renal function. Prenatal diagnosis for patients with PUV is a poor prognostic sign, with 64% incidence of renal failure and transient pulmonary failure, compared to 33% in postnatally diagnosed patients. Pulmonary hypoplasia secondary to oligohydramnios largely contributes to the morbidity and mortality from foetal urethral obstruction. Outcomes of foetal intervention with vescicoamniotic shunting or foetal cystoscopic ablation of the urethal valve are still under review and await a multicentre trial.

Key Summary Points

1. The boundaries of paediatric surgical practice have been extended by prenatal diagnosis.

2. The care of patients with surgically correctable defects can now be planned prenatally with the collaborative effort of obstetricians, geneticists, neonatologists, and paediatric surgeons.

3. Understanding the specific surgical condition's prenatal natural history is essential.

4. Prenatal diagnosis has its limitations.

5. Associated anomalies need to be detected.

6. Understanding the risks and indications of foetal intervention programmes and postnatal outcomes is essential.

7. Prenatal counselling is an essential component of paediatric surgical practice and should be ensured in the training programme for future paediatric surgeons.

Suggested Reading

Black R, Boyd P. What's new in prenatal diagnosis? Trends in Urology. Gynaecol Sexual Health 2004; 9:9–11.

Boyd PA, Keeling JW. Congenital abnormalities, prenatal diagnosis and screening. In: Keeling JW, ed. Fetal and Neonatal Pathology. Springer-Verlag, 2007.

Lakhoo K. Fetal counselling for congenital malformations. Pediatr Surg Int 2007; 23:509–519.

Lakhoo K, et al. Best clinical practice: surgical conditions of the fetus and newborn. Early Human Dev 2006; 82:281–324.

CHAPTER 124
CONJOINED AND PARASITIC TWINS

Alastair J.W. Millar

Introduction

The birth of conjoined twins has always fascinated mankind, with the public's view of malformed children greatly influenced by the prevailing culture and religious beliefs. In prehistoric times, conjoined twins were depicted in cave drawings, on pottery, or as figurines. In folklore, they were often regarded as an omen of impending disaster, eliciting strong emotions ranging from wonder and admiration to rejection and hostility. Although malformed children were treated compassionately at times, historical records show that infanticide was frequently practiced and the mother was often held responsible for causing the malformation.

Demographics

Although the worldwide incidence of monozygotic twinning is the same in all ethnic groups, the incidence of conjoined twins appears to be higher in sub-Saharan Africa, ranging from 1 in 50,000 to 1 in 100,000 live births, or 1 in 400 monozygotic twin births. The natural history that follows a prenatal diagnosis of conjoined twins confirms that a large number of infants die either in utero (28%) or immediately after birth (54%); in fact, only around 20% survive.

Aetiology and Pathophysiology

Conjoined twins are monozygotic, monoamniotic, and monochorionic. They are always of the same gender, with a 3:1 female preponderance. Their formation results either from failure of separation of the embryonic plate between 15 and 17 days gestation, or from secondary union of two separate embryonic discs at the dorsal neural tube or ventral yolk sac areas at 3 to 4 weeks gestation.

Spencer's extensive embryological studies appear to favour the latter theory, but this remains controversial. Although genetically identical, one of the conjoined twins is almost always weaker or smaller than the other and may have additional congenital defects. These twins also develop dissimilar personalities from an early age. Conjoined twins are individual and deformed but symmetrical and proportional.

Classification

Conjoined twins are always joined at homologous sites, and the clinical classification is based on the most prominent site of union, combined with the suffix "pagus" meaning "that which is fixed". There are eight recognized configurations, as shown in Figure 124.1: thoracopagus (chest), omphalopagus (umbilicus), pygopagus (rump), ischiopagus (hip), craniopagus (cranium), parapagus (side), cephalopagus (head), and rachipagus (spine).

Conjoined twins can be further described as symmetrical or asymmetrical. Asymmetrical, or incomplete, conjoined twins result from the demise of one twin with remnant structures attached to the complete twin, with the junction remaining at or near one of the common sites of union (Figure 124.2). Fetus-in-feto refers to asymmetrical monozygotic diamniotic intraparasitic twins. Conjoined triplets are exceptionally rare, and their pathogenesis remains even more obscure.

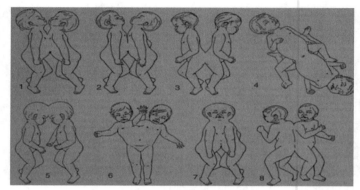

Figure 124.1: Different types of conjoined twins described according to their site of conjunction: (1) thoracopagus, (2) omphalopagus, (3) pygopagus, (4) ischiopagus tetrapus (four legs), (5) craniopagus, (6) paragagus dipus (two legs), (7) cephalopagus, (8) rachipagus.

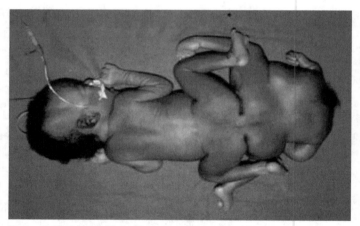

Figure 124.2: Asymmetric ischiopagus tetrapus twins with an anencephalic parasite but extensive perineal conjunction.

Management

This section includes descriptions of the lessons learned at one hospital over a period of 42 years, supplemented by a literature review. These descriptions encompass prenatal diagnosis, obstetric intervention, special investigations, postnatal management, anaesthetic considerations, and surgical strategies, with the major focus on thoracopagus conjunction.

Prenatal Diagnosis

In developed countries, antenatal diagnosis is usually made by ultrasound (US) scan. Once the diagnosis is suspected, echocardiography and ultrafast foetal magnetic resonance imaging (MRI) may be used to confirm the diagnosis. The mother is referred for advice either to plan the mode of delivery because of obstetric implications or for consideration of termination of the pregnancy with the attendant ethical and moral considerations.

Diagnosis has been made as early as the 9th week of gestation. Diagnostic US criteria for conjoined twins include the relative fixed position of the two foetuses. These may be facing each other, as in thoracopagus, with hyperextension of the cervical spine. Continuity of the skin and mirror-image body parts with limbs close together may be noted. The presence of a single heart and fused liver, fused spine, or even absence of a limb in tripus cases would confirm the diagnosis.

Obstetric Intervention

The birth of conjoined twins is often unexpected, resulting in obstructive labour with difficult transvaginal delivery or emergency caesarean section (CS). These complications can be avoided by planned CS at 36 to 38 weeks gestation, once the foetal lungs have reached maturity. The high rate of stillbirths and dystocia support planned CS. Children weighing less than 3 kg, including thoracopagus and ischiopagus conjunction, have been born vaginally. Most children born normally do not sustain any damage to the connecting sites (bridges), except where there is an omphalocoele associated with thoraco-omphalopagus conjunction. Rupture of the exomphalos and evisceration of liver and bowel may occur. Maternal mortality during labour has also been reported.

Ideally, the immediate perinatal management of the babies is also planned, and in one case in which a twin with a normal heart perfused the co-twin with a rudimentary heart, the ex utero intrapartum treatment (EXIT) procedure was utilised due to concern that the normal twin would suffer immediate cardiac decompensation at birth. This EXIT to separation strategy allowed prompt control of the airway and circulation before clamping the umbilical cord and optimised management of a potentially lethal situation with survival of the normal twin.

Once born, the twins should be referred for appropriate investigation and surgical management. The therapeutic options to be considered range from conservative, nonsurgical management to emergency or planned surgery (see next subsection).

Special Investigations

Investigations should be directed towards identifying the anatomy of conjunction and consequently the viability of separation. The areas of fusion largely determine the imaging modalities chosen. Skeletal surveys, echocardiography, US, computed tomography (CT), MRI, and angiography provide excellent anatomical detail, demonstrating organ position, shared viscera, and vascular anatomy. Contrast imaging evaluates the gastrointestinal and urinary systems, and endoscopy is of further help in the urogenital assessment. Radioisotope scanning can assess regional perfusion fields.

Twins with no reasonable chance of survival, largely due to cardiac anomalies incompatible with life, and those with irreversible postnatal diseases such as necrotising enterocolitis totalis, should receive only palliative treatment and are not considered for separation. Where separation is clearly not possible without the inevitable death or unacceptable mutilation of both twins, it is perfectly reasonable to accept this situation and to provide counselling and all possible support for their future growth and development.

Emergency surgery is indicated when there is damage to the connecting bridge or when correctable anomalies threaten the survival of one or both twins and there is the possibility of saving at least one of the twins. Elective surgery is best scheduled for when the infants are thriving and all investigations have been completed, providing a comprehensive and functional description of normal and fused anatomy. Improved survival rates for conjoined twins are due to advances in perinatal and postnatal diagnostic techniques, meticulous interpretation of the special investigations, and correct anaesthetic and surgical management carried out by an experienced multidisciplinary team. The anatomical configurations encountered are often complex, with unexpected anatomic variations frequently identified during surgery despite all the extensive preoperative investigatons (Figure 124.3).

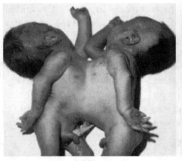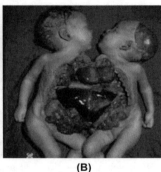

(A)   (B)

Figure 124.3 (A) A set of thoraco-omphalopagus twins with typical cervical extension position. (B) Another set of conjoined twins with similar conjunction, at postmortem. Note the single conjoined heart (cause of death) and extensive hepatic fusion with separate gastrointestinal tracts (GITs).

Table 124.1: Evaluation of conjoined twins.

System	Evaluation
Cardiorespiratory	Electrocardiogram (ECG)
	Echocardiography/Doppler ultrasound
	MRI/CT with contrast
	Angiogram
Alimentary tract	Contrast meal and enema
	Ultrasound
	Radioisotope scans (liver); technetium Tc99m-(Sn) colloid and excretion Tc99m mebrofenin
	Radioisotope scintigraphy
Genitourinary	Ultrasound
	Isotope renography
	Micturating cystourethrography
	Genitogram
Skeletal system	Radiography
	MRI (spinal cord)
	Ultrasound
Vascular	Doppler ultrasound
	Angiography
Cross-circulation	Radioisotope scan Tc99m-DMSA

Many examples exist of conjoined twins living full and productive lives without separation. The case for this acceptance is most eloquently made in the book *One of Us* by Alice Dreger.

The investigations used to fully evaluate conjoined twins are listed in Table 124.1. Prior meticulous clinical examination is conducted with necessary examination under anaesthetic and placement of catheters for later contrast radiological studies.

Postnatal Management

Immediate postnatal management consists of resuscitation and stabilisation of the twins. This is followed by a thorough physical examination with special investigations to define the relevant anatomy. If emergency surgery is anticipated, all twins should undergo echocardiography and plain roentgenography, which provide limited but essential information. The site of conjunction will determine the type and order of special investigations. The information obtained will determine the surgical approach, the timing of separation, the allocation of organs and structures, and the eventual prognosis regarding survival and functional outcome. Important structures to evaluate are the cardiac, hepatobiliary, intestinal, urogenital, and spinal systems. The use of diagrams, three-dimensional (3D) organ models, and surgical rehearsal of the procedure will ensure the best possible outcome. Despite all these investigations and careful analysis of findings, however, preoperative interpretation may still be difficult, with incorrect conclusions drawn.

Emergency separation has resulted in up to a 70% mortality rate compared to 20% for elective procedures, emphasizing the need to stabilise the infants initially and to postpone surgery until the basic investigations have been completed. In the author's experience, emergency surgery was necessary to alleviate intestinal obstruction, to treat necrotising enterocolitis, to manage a ruptured exomphalos, and for deteriorating cardiac-respiratory status threatening survival of one or both twins. Delaying separation into early childhood may result in increased postnatal deformities and psychological problems. If separation is possible and desirable, surgery should be performed within the first 6 to 9 months, before the twins develop an awareness of their condition. Motor skills, sensory integration, and personality need to develop in separated twins.

Anaesthetic Considerations

Anaesthesia for separation of conjoined twins is a complex, demanding procedure that is facilitated by having two colour-coded anaesthetic teams representing each child. The author's experience has highlighted the following anaesthetic considerations. The infants are often premature with pre-existing cardiac and pulmonary dysfunction, and the induction of anaesthesia is often compromised by the abnormal positions and proximity of the twins. During surgery, difficulties with vascular access, haemodynamic stability, and temperature control can be considerable.

To maintain haemodynamic stability, blood volumes transfused may range from 10% to 450% of the estimated blood volume. Blood loss can be especially extensive in thoracopagus and ischiopagus separations, and relative changes in position of the two infants during surgery lead to significant shifts in blood volumes. Due to cross-circulation, pharmacokinetics and pharmacodynamics are inconsistent, especially in thoracopagus twins, and altered drug responses must be expected. Anticipated postseparation problems include respiratory insufficiency, haemodynamic instability, fluid balance, temperature control, sepsis, wound closure difficulties with staged closure if necessary, and residual organ dysfunction.

Surgical Strategies

The first successful surgical separation took place in 1689 and more than 1,200 cases had been reported in the literature by 2000. The surgical separation of conjoined twins presents a great challenge and undoubtedly requires a multidisciplinary team. An unequal external union, variations in internal anatomy, and discordant anomalies mandate thorough elucidation of the anatomy of conjunction before planning the surgical procedure required to separate and individualise the twins.

Many descriptions of surgical procedures to separate the various types of conjoined twins have been published. Technical details are determined by the anatomy of conjunction, the allocation of sharing of organs and structures, and the planned reconstruction. Standard approaches are normally utilized, but variations may demand a novel surgical approach or alternative techniques.

Major factors that will govern successful separation include the order of separation, the distribution of organs between the twins, meticulous aseptic surgical techniques, the reconstruction of divided organs and structures, and wound closure. It is also necessary to distinguish between structures that are shared by both twins and those belonging only to one individual. Allocation of shared organs usually involves the anus, rectum, genitourinary tract, lower spine, and spinal cord. Unexpected anatomical variations are often encountered, including previously unrecognised cardiac, gastrointestinal, hepatobiliary, spinal, and genitourinary anomalies. Operation time is prolonged with the separation of the more complex thoracopagus and ischiopagus twins, and is in the order of 7–13 hours and 13–19 hours, respectively.

Skin closure

Whenever there is extensive sharing of body surface areas (e.g., thoracopagus and ischiopagus), closure of the disconnected surfaces may pose major problems, especially when separation is undertaken as an emergency. Subcutaneous tissue expansion is used to provide tissue for reconstruction or closure where insufficient natural tissue exists (Figure 124.4). This allows for primary tension-free closure, thereby minimising respiratory and wound complications. Closure under tension is poorly tolerated, and it is preferred that the body cavities (both chest and abdomen, if necessary) are left open for later staged closure with plastic reconstruction using skin and muscle flaps or split skin grafting onto granulation tissue. Vacuum dressings may assist a more rapid healing, earlier grafting, and wound closure. Unfortunately, tissue expansion is not always possible and has a nearly 60% incidence of complications due to factors such as placement over bony areas with little subcutaneous tissue, wound sepsis, and skin necrosis. Skin expanders must be correctly sited; placements are best tolerated in older infants. It takes 6 to 8 weeks to gain maximum advantage.

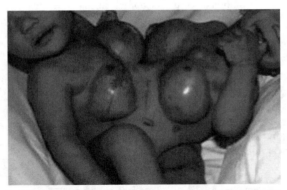

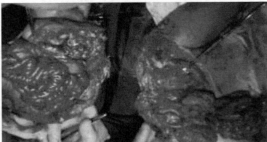

Figure 124.4: Tissue expanders inserted in omphalo-ischiopagus twins prior to separation (top) and the extensive open wound at separation (bottom). Wound closure is facilitated by use of the skin and tissue gained from the expanders and by posterior iliac osteotomies with medial rotation of the acetabular component and figure-of-eight suture of the symphysis pubis of each.

Cardiovascular system

Experience with 22 thoracopagus sets of twins has shown that evaluation requires the use of every tool available—from clinical evaluation to angiography. The ECG is generally unreliable because two separate ECGs do not rule out significant sharing of cardiac structures. The mainstay of the evaluation is echocardiography, generally best accomplished by a pair of investigators who meticulously double-check each other's findings. The investigators may be left with apical and suprasternal views only. Tracheo-oesophageal echo is frequently not possible, given the size of the infants. The newer multislice CT scanning and modern MRI machines will clearly have roles to play in future evaluations, despite the radiation exposure and the need for a general anaesthetic.

In the author's experience, an MRI investigation resulted in "overcalling" ventricular sharing. Angiography under general anaesthetic may still be needed, but it remains a high-risk procedure with an unpredictable response to anaesthesia. In a set of twins with venous-pole sharing, induction of anaesthesia resulted in asystole in the twin with a myopathic ventricle, resulting in brain death and an emergency separation. Prior to separation, the surgeon may still not know the exact nature of venous connections, coronary arterial anatomy, the branching anatomy of the head and neck vessels, and the true size of the right ventricle.

No twins with ventricular conjunction have ever been successfully separated with both twins surviving; however, there is a report of successful separation of thoracopagus twins with two normal hearts joined by a myocardial bridge. In a situation where one twin is acardiac or where the twins share ventricles, successful separation is impossible without sacrificing one infant. The chest wall and skin of the sacrificed twin are used to obtain skin cover and to create a firm structure to protect the protuberant fused single heart, as any dislocation of the heart from its natural position is likely to cause disturbance of function. All the main inflow and outflow vessels from the sacrificed twin have to be disconnected from the heart, and the whole cardiac complex is then assigned to the infant selected to survive. In two cases of infants surviving a sacrifice procedure, one survived 30 days and died from aspiration and the other is a long-term survivor of nearly 15 years. Subsequent reconstruction of the deformed chest is possible at a later stage. Thoracopagus conjoined twins may be classified according to the degree of cardiac conjunction.

Hepatobiliary system
The liver is shared in almost all ventral forms of conjoined twins. Ultrasound, CT scanning, and radio nucleotide scanning provide the best overall picture of hepatic conjunction, the biliary drainage system including the gallbladder, and configuration of the pancreas. For successful hepatic division, each liver has to have an inferior vena cava to its own heart. Hepatic conjunction is along an oblique plane, and venous connections may consist of a labyrinth of small venous channels that may bleed excessively during surgery. In the author's experience, hepatic division has always been possible. Cardiac disconnection must be accomplished before hepatic division because a large volume of blood can circulate through the liver, creating a false impression that both hearts are able to sustain independent life. The anatomy of the extra hepatic biliary system (EHBS) needs to be confirmed, which may require intraoperative cholangiography. Two gallbladders do not always equate with two EHBSs, especially if there is fusion of the proximal duodenum, which may be demonstrated by upper contrast radiography. However, two gallbladders and two duodenums usually indicate two separate extrahepatic bile ducts. Bile drainage is imperative, and in the presence of a single EHBS, one twin should be allocated the EHBS, while every attempt should be made to establish bile drainage through a Roux-en-Y hepaticojejunostomy in the other twin. Anatomically, the pancreas belongs to the duodenum, and is best left with the EHBS.

Gastrointestinal system
The intraabdominal gastrointestinal tract is frequently shared in ventral and caudal types of junction and usually follows one of two patterns. In the first, duodenal junction is often encountered in thoracopagus twins. The junction can extend distal to the duodenum and involve the upper small bowel up to the level of Meckel's point, where it divides again into two separate distal ilea. The second type of GIT sharing (ileocolic or, rarely, only colonic) is commonly encountered in ischiopagus twins. The single ileocolon, resembling a conjoined organ, opens into a single anus. A double blood supply may facilitate longitudinal division of the colon, thus preserving an anatomically normal or foreshortened colon for each child. Alternatively, one child can be allocated the ileocecal valve and the other the anus, with both sharing the divided colon. Pygopagus twins always have a common anal canal. It is the author's practice to reconstruct the anorectal region at the time of primary division. A previously placed colostomy, however, demands a different type of allocation and reconstruction.

Urogenital tract
Complex and variable urogenital abnormalities accompany pelvic fusion and are restricted to symmetrical and asymmetrical ischiopagus and pygopagus twins. These are less commonly seen in thoracopagus conjunction. The incidence of shared pelvic organs is on the order of 15% for pygopagus to 50% or more for ischiopagus twins. An unobstructed continent urinary system with a physically acceptable and functional genital system is the primary goal. Essential in the workup of urogenital abnormalities are genitourinary US, isotope renography, micturating cystourethrography, and endoscopy.

The kidneys may vary in number, size, ectopia, degree of fusion, and the course of the ureters. Most ischiopagus twins have four kidneys and two bladders, with one ureter crossing to the ipsilateral and one to the contralateral bladder. One or two bladders may be present, lying side by side or fused in the midline with one draining into the other. In most cases, despite these variations, a functional bladder can be reconstructed. The presence of spinal fusion in its various forms complicates the situation by introducing a neuropathic element into the behaviour of the bladder, which has a significant influence on future management. Crucial decisions regarding assignment are therefore required when shared organs that cannot be divided are present.

The genital pattern varies widely, and every effort should be made to achieve functional reconstruction, which may require an individual approach. In females, urogenital sinuses or even cloacal abnormalities are often present, requiring careful consideration during division, allocation of organs, and reconstruction. In males, the status of the external genitalia, urethra, and testes are important. Twins with two sets of external genitalia can undergo successful separation; secondary reconstructive genitoplasty may be required if only one set of external genitalia is present. Staged procedures may be required to achieve optimum outcome.

Central nervous system
Neurosurgical interest in conjoined twins has tended to focus on craniopagus twins, who comprise only 2–6 % of all conjoined twins but present some of the greatest challenges in separation. A recent review proposes a practical four-category classification based on the angle of union (vertical or angular) and the degree to which the dural venous sinuses are shared. Conjoined cerebral tissue may present an important technical challenge, but preservation of the venous drainage of the brain has emerged as one of the most critical determinants of outcome following separation. Various surgical approaches have been reported.

Bony abnormalities of the spine, such as haemivertebrae remote from the area of conjunction, put twins at risk for progressive spinal deformity and scoliosis after separation.

Musculoskeletal system
The orthopaedic surgeon is predominantly involved early in the separation of ischiopagus twins. Three-dimensional reconstruction CT of the pelvis is most helpful in ascertaining the anatomical configuration of the pelvic ring and the possible junction of the vertebral columns. In ischiopagus twins, the conjunction is at the pelvis with the twins lying on their backs. The legs of each of the twins are widely separate with the hips at right angles to the median plane. Diastasis of the pelvis is due to external rotation of the posterior segment. Posterior osteotomies of the iliac bones allow for medial rotation of the acetabula and symphysis pubes, which restores the whole pelvic ring into normal alignment

and facilitates anterior abdominal wall closure and urogenital closure, rendering stability to the perineum. Although osteotomy rarely prevents rediastasis of the symphysis pubis, it helps early reconstruction of the pelvic anatomy and corrects acetabular retroversion to anteversion. The commonly encountered postoperative flexion deformities of the hips of 30°–50° usually resolve within 6 months. Associated with ischiopagus twins are spinal and cord abnormalities and lower limb abnormalities in nearly two-thirds of cases. Correction of the pelvic abnormalities ensured that all six ischiopagus children operated on at the author's institution became community walkers.

Separation of asymmetric heteropagus twins requires the same detailed investigative approach and may also be a considerable surgical endeavour, but only one patient is at risk and thus skin cover can be supplied from the parasite and any organ conjunction is divided in favour of the autosite.

As mentioned previously, children with hemivertebrae, asymmetrical or diminutive chest cavities, and even those with caudal junction are prone to develop scoliosis. Progressive scoliosis in nonparalytic patients will not affect the hips—it is more a cosmetic deformity or affects respiratory capacity. Long-term follow-up is mandatory because rotational abnormalities, contractures, and dislocation of the hips, together with progressive scoliosis, can occur.

Postoperative Management

Cardiovascular and respiratory failures remain the most frequent causes of death in the immediate postoperative period. Further operations may be required for secondary wound closure or dehiscences and skin grafting. There is also hidden long-term morbidity and mortality. A number of infants have died later from factors such as unresolved aspiration from gastro-oesophageal reflux, bronchopneumonia aggravated by poor diaphragmatic function (particularly with thoracopagus), cerebral anoxia, gastroenteritis, urinary tract infections, biliary sepsis, and even malaria.

Prognosis and Outcomes

Inevitably, the ultimate prognosis will depend on the state of the conjoined organs and the potential for successful separation. Tragically in some, separation will not be possible. Detailed preoperative assessment is essential to determine the best surgical approach, reconstruction methods, and ultimate outcome. Despite successful separation, some children are left crippled and disabled, requiring lifelong follow-up and care. The overall survival for symmetrical twins is 33.3%, but it is 64.7% for those who underwent surgery. Emergency surgery had a dismal outcome with only around 33% surviving. Asymmetrical separation had a 92% survival rate.

Prevention

Better preconceptual maternal nutrition with folic acid supplementation is likely to reduce the incidence as it has the incidence of twinning abnormalities and spina bifida. If the diagnosis is made antenatally, then the decision to terminate the pregnancy may be taken after detailed evaluation and counselling.

Ethical Issues

Ethical considerations, which need to reconcile the best options for the twins and their parents, are playing an increasing role in present-day decision making. The sacrifice of one twin due to the inability to sustain life alone is the controversy that evokes the most anguish. The decision on whether to operate is rendered more complex by those surviving conjoined twins who consciously elect not to be separated and report that they have lived socially acceptable lives. Equal controversy surrounds those few conjoined twins who have survived to adulthood and then decide that separation should be attempted despite the operative risks and the potential for significant long-term morbidity as separate individuals.

Being conjoined does not necessarily negate individual development. Religious views may support only minimal surgical interference, especially when one twin has a high risk of dying at surgery. "We cannot accept one baby must die so that the other one may live. It is not God's will", which differs from the legal opinion "Why I must order twin baby to die"—both quotations were recorded in the press in a case in the United Kingdom when parents did not give consent to separation but doctors asked for legal support for separation. In the words of Eliza Chulkhurst, one of the most famous conjoined twins of the premedical era, "As we came together, we will also go together".

From a practical point of view, the Great Ormond Street Ethical Guidelines for Conjoined Twin Separation have been widely accepted:

- Where separation is feasible with a reasonable chance of success, it should be carried out.

- When surgery is not possible, custodial care should be offered and nature allowed to take its course.

- Where one twin is dead or has a lethal abnormality and cannot survive independently from its normal twin and if unoperated both twins could die, separation to save the healthy twin should be attempted.

I acknowledge huge contributions of the teams of surgeons, anaesthetists, intensivists, nurses, social workers, physiotherapists and occupational therapists who, over the last 50 years, have so successfully managed our series of patients at the Red Cross War Memorial Children's Hospital in Cape Town. Separation surgery was pioneered at this hospital by Sidney Cywes and Jannie Louw and continued by my colleague Heinz Rode.

Key Summary Points

1. Conjoined twins are usually symmetrical, of the same gender, and, in addition to the areas of conjunction, have an increased incidence of other congenital malformations.

2. Separation should be delayed for several months after birth, if possible.

3. Separation is not always possible nor indeed mandatory.

4. Success is achieved with meticulous attention to detail with a multidisciplinary team approach.

5. Long-term follow-up is always required to manage, in particular, musculoskeletal deformity and urogenital anomalies.

6. Expertise around the world can and should be shared.

Suggested Reading

Bratton MQ, Chetwynd SB. Clinical ethics: one into two will not go: conceptualising conjoined twins. J Med Ethics 2004; 30:270–285.

Cywes S, Davies MRQ, Rode H. Conjoined twins—the Red Cross War Memorial Children's Hospital experience. SAJ Surg 1982; 20(2):105–118.

Cywes S, Millar AJW, Rode H, Brown RA. Conjoined twins—the Cape Town experience. Pediatr Surg Int 1997; 12:234–248.

Dreger AD. One of us. Conjoined twins and the future of normal. Harvard University Press, 2004.

Kaufman MH. The embryology of conjoined twins. Childs Nerv Syst 2004; 20:508–525.

MacKenzie TC, Crombleholme TM, Johnson MP, Schnaufer L, Flake AW, Hedrick HL, Howell LJ, Adzick NS. The natural history of prenatally diagnosed conjoined twins. J Pediatr Surg 2002; 37:303–309.

O'Neill JA. Conjoined twins. In: O'Neill JA, Rowe M, Grosfeld JL, Fonkalsrud EW, Coran AG, eds. Pediatric Surgery, 5th ed. Mosby St. Louis, 1998, Chap 127, Pp 1925-1938.

Spencer R. Theoretical and analytical embryology of conjoined twins, part 1: embryogenesis. Clin Anat 2000; 13:36–53.

Spencer R. Theoretical and analytical embryology of conjoined twins, part 2: adjustments to union. Clin Anat 2000; 13:97–120.

Spitz L. Surgery for conjoined twins. Hunterian Lecture. Ann R Coll Surg Engl 2003; 85:230–235.

CHAPTER 125
OTORHINOLARYNGOLOGY

Frank Agada
Manali Amin
Andrew Coatesworth

Introduction

This chapter covers the common diseases of the ear, nose, and throat (ENT). The aim is to present a brief but practical insight into the common childhood otorhinolaryngology (ORL) diseases in Africa. ORL diseases are among the least understood in Africa because ORL does not feature prominently in the syllabus of many medical schools, and many countries have only a handful of practicing ORL specialists.[1–3] It is therefore important to highlight common problems that can be treated by the paediatric surgeon in the absence of an ENT specialist.

EAR

Hearing Assessment

Assessment of hearing in a young child can be challenging. Otoacoustic emissions (OAEs) and auditory brainstem response (ABR) are objective tests, which require little to no interaction from a child. OAE is used routinely in newborn screening in most developed countries, but for most African countries, the challenge is obtaining resources and funding for such programs. In the absence of such universal screening programs, practicing clinicians in Africa depend on behavioural hearing tests, which are subjective and generally not possible prior to the age of 6–7 months. Behavioural hearing tests include:

- *Distraction testing:* A frequency-specific sound is presented to the child. The child is observed for head turning. This test is inexpensive and quick, when compared to visual reinforcement audiometry, which is also a variant of the distraction test.

- *Visual reinforcement audiometry (VRA):* A sound is presented in the environment or through earphones or headphones. The child is observed for a response and is rewarded with a lighted toy when he or she responds.

- *Conditioned play audiometry (CPA):* A child is nonverbally instructed to wait, listen, and respond with a repetitive task when he or she hears a sound. The response is a play task, such as placing blocks in a box.

- *Conventional audiogram:* An auditory stimulus is presented through headphones, and the child is asked to raise the hand on the side of the sound presentation.

Conductive Hearing Loss

Once a conductive hearing loss (CHL) has been identified, its aetiology may be determined. In cases of cerumen impaction and foreign bodies, removal of the offending object will resolve the problem.

Otitis media

Otitis media (OM) is the leading cause of hearing loss in African children.[4–5] OM presents with pain, fever, chills, perforation of the tympanic membrane, and drainage. A higher prevalence is seen in males and in young children (birth to 5 years of age).[6]

The organisms responsible for OM vary, depending on the region and the human immunodeficiency virus (HIV) status of the child:

- Nigeria, HIV-negative children: *Streptococcus*, *Klebsiella*, and *Pseudomonas*

- Nigeria, HIV-positive children: *Klebsiella*, *Proteus*, *Staphylococcus*, and *Pseudomonas*

- Sudan: *Proteus*, *Klebsiella*, *Staphylococcus aureus*, *Pseudomonas*, and *Escherichia coli*

In developed countries, day care attendance, exposures to second-hand smoke, and adenoid hypertrophy are often correlated with high rates of OM. In West African countries, low social status and malnutrition are more highly correlated with developing chronic OM.[7] Without treatment, OM may result in significant morbidity and even mortality.

Treatment of OM consists of (1) removing otorrhea with suctioning, wicking, or irrigations, and (2) topical antimicrobials and antiseptics if there is fluid/inflammatory changes in the ear canal; (3) systemic antibiotics. Surgical treatment, such as a tympanomastoidectomy, may be required with acute infections that have resulted in mastoiditis and in chronic infections that do not respond to antibiotic therapy. "Ear camps" have been established in Namibia and other countries to help with treatment.

Prevention of OM infections may be accomplished through widespread use of vaccinations, improving nutrition, and increasing education and health care access.

Otitis externa

Otitis externa (OE) is inflammation of the external auditory canal. It presents with otalgia, otorrhea, itching, and CHL. In addition to the bacterial aetiologies mentioned above, OE may also be caused by fungal infections. Malnourished children and males are at higher risk of developing otomycosis.[8] In Nigeria, the most commonly isolated fungi are *Aspergillus* species, *Candida*, and *Mucor*.

Treatment consists of debridement and application of 1% clotrimazole cream.[9] Bacterial OE is generally treated with suctioning of the ear canal as well as topical and occasionally systemic antibmicrobials. Malignant OE, a condition typically seen in diabetic patients, is sometimes seen in malnourished, nondiabetic children younger than 2 years of age.[10] Malignant OE is considered a medical emergency and should be treated aggressively with debridement and intravenous (IV) antibiotic therapy. Left untreated, it may result in death.

OE may be prevented in some instances by keeping fingers and objects out of the ear canal, as local trauma may introduce bacteria into the skin.

Congenital anomalies

Less common reasons for a CHL include congenital anomalies. Congenital malformations of the ear can include one or multiple parts of the ear and are dependent upon the timing of the insult, which results in arrested development during embryogenesis.

Microtia

Microtia is evident upon examination at birth and is variable in presentation. In its mildest form, a fully developed ear is present, but it is noted to be smaller in size than the opposite, normal ear. In its extreme forms, only a small rudimentary skin tag or no ear (anotia) is present. Microtia and anotia are often associated with auditory canal atresia or stenosis, varying degrees of ossicular malformation, and CHL. In utero exposures to thalidomide, retinoid, and mycophenolate mofetil, among other agents, have been implicated.[11–12] Microtia is more commonly seen in males and more often affects the right ear in unilateral cases. It results in a CHL, which can significantly impact a child's ability to develop socially and academically. Nonsurgical options include sign language and/or bone conduction hearing aids. Surgical options are a bone-anchored hearing aid (BAHA) or atresia repair with ossicular reconstruction. Prior to consideration of aural atresia repair, a computed tomography (CT) scan to evaluate the anatomy and an audiogram to confirm the existence of cochlear function are recommended.

Ossicular malformations

While microtia, anotia, and canal atresia are evident on physical examination, ossicular abnormalities cannot be identified without high-resolution CT scan imaging. Isolated ossicular abnormalities must be considered in an individual with CHL and no evidence of middle ear dysfunction. The ossicles begin to develop at around 5 weeks gestational age and are usually completed by 24 weeks. Of the three ossicles, the stapes is most likely to be affected because its development occurs over a longer time period than the malleus and incus. Nonsurgical treatment involves hearing aids. If the canal is patent, a conventional hearing aid may be used. Surgically, the ossicular chain may be reconstructed.

Sensorineural hearing loss

Sensorineural hearing loss (SNHL) continues to remain a challenging problem for most developing countries. It may be congenital or acquired, hereditary or nonhereditary, and syndromic or nonsyndromic.

Genetic mutations, intrauterine exposure to viruses, intrauterine exposure to toxoplasma gondii, and perinatal anoxia are a few of the identifiable aetiologic agents for congenital hearing loss. Acquired losses are often the result of bacterial meningitis and cochlear ossification. Meningococcal meningitis epidemics have been reported in parts of Africa with subsequent SNHL noted in 25% of the cases.[13]

Children with a hearing loss may appear socially disinterested and lag behind their peers in the development of speech and language skills. The prevalence of childhood SNHL has been reported to be as high as 14%;[14] however, the prevalence is likely to be much higher. Given the limited health care resources in Africa, diagnosis is often delayed and sometimes not made at all.

Treatment depends upon the severity of the hearing loss. With a mild, unilateral hearing loss, no treatment may be needed. Amplification with conventional hearing aids is helpful for many losses. In the case of bilateral profound hearing loss, a child should be taught sign language. Cochlear implantation is an alternative, but not one that is readily accessible for most African children.

In the developing world, emphasis must be placed on early diagnosis of hearing loss and prevention. Some countries are advocating universal hearing screening of newborns.[14] More important, prevention of acquired causes of hearing loss may be implemented in the short term. Widespread immunisation against viruses such as measles, mumps, and rubella would help to curb some of the viral causes of SNHL. Similarly, education regarding hygiene and proper handling and cooking of meats may help decrease the incidence of congenital toxoplasmosis, one of the causes of SNHL.

Nose

Nasal Airway Obstruction in the Infant

Presentation

Infants are obligate nasal breathers up to approximately 6 months of age; therefore, nasal obstruction can be life threatening. Infants may present with difficulty feeding, stertor, cyanosis, and apnoea. If purulent secretions are also present, an infectious aetiology may be suspected.

Diagnosis

Examination may be completed by placing an otoscope in the nostrils. A quick examination of airflow may be accomplished by placing a small mirror beneath each nostril. In addition, a suction catheter may be placed through each nostril to confirm patency of the choanae. A flexible nasopharyngoscope, if available, can be used for a more comprehensive examination.

Differential diagnosis and treatment

A diagnosis of *rhinitis of infancy and gastroespophageal reflux disease* (GERD) may be considered in the absence of anatomic abnormalities, purulent discharge, or cough. Treatment is with a short course of topical decongestants or topical steroids. Improvement in symptoms with H_2-blocker or proton pump inhibitor therapy supports the diagnosis of GERD.

Infections are characterised by rhinorrhea, fevers, and cough. Clear secretions suggest viral infection. Purulent secretions are often bacterial. Chlamydia in the newborn period presents with congestion, purulent nasal discharge, and cough in the absence of a fever. If chlamydial infection is suspected, the child should be treated empirically with a macrolide antibiotic. In contrast, congenital syphilis presents with clear, watery rhinorrhea and may be diagnosed with serologic testing. If diagnosed, the child should be treated with penicillin.

Choanal atresia (CA) has been reported to have an incidence of 1 in 3,100 in certain parts of Northern Africa.[15] An atresia may be bony, membranous, or a combination of both. Unilateral atresia is more common than bilateral (Figure 125.1). CA may be suspected in a child in whom no airflow is noted on a mirror placed under the nostril and in whom a catheter does not pass through the nostril. Definitive diagnosis is made with flexible endoscopy and CT scanning. Temporising measures include placement of an oral airway or intubation. In the long run, surgical correction is recommended. CA may be corrected through an endoscopic approach or a transpalatal approach. Intranasal stents are placed postoperatively to prevent stenosis. Stents must be cleaned meticulously to keep them open during the healing period. This involves use of nasal saline and suctioning. Revision procedures are sometimes needed to keep the choanae patent.

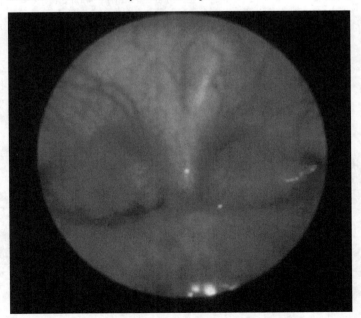

Source: With kind permission of Dr. Bruce Benjamin, University of Sydney, Australia.
Figure 125.1. Bilateral choanal atresia.

Pyriform aperture stenosis (PAS) is less common than CA. It is a narrowing of the nostril anteriorly at the pyriform aperture. It may be seen with other anomalies, notably holoprosencephaly and megaincisors. The stenotic region may be visible with an otoscope or flexible endoscope. If a catheter can be passed through the stenotic segment, it will pass into the nasopharynx. Definitive diagnosis is on CT scanning. A temporising measure is placement of a nasal airway. In some cases, a child with this anomaly may be observed expectantly—the child can be observed indefinitely and with growth will have a large enough nasal airway to not require surgical intervention. Conservative management includes the use of nasal saline and topical decongestants and steroids as needed. Surgical correction is reserved for those children in whom breathing difficulties lead to slow growth or cyanotic episodes. A stent is placed postoperatively for approximately 1 week.

A small pit or hair extending from the nasal dorsum should lead one to suspect an *intranasal dermoid*. If a dermoid is suspected, a CT scan or magnetic resonance imaging (MRI) would be recommended to delineate the extent of the cyst and assess for an intracranial component. If the lesion is small, excision can be undertaken by making an elliptical incision around the pit or hair and dissecting around the cyst.

Intranasal encephaloceles are a herniation of brain tissue through the foramen caecum. If the neural tissue is not in continuity with the brain, it is considered a *glioma*. In addition to an intranasal mass, one might see widening of the nasal dorsum and lateral displacement of the medial canthi. In Dakar, fronto-ethmoidal encephaloceles account for approximately 10% of all encephaloceles.[16] Surgical removal may be approached endoscopically in cases of smaller gliomas. A combined neurosurgical approach is necessary for larger fronto-ethmoidal encephaloceles.

Nasal Airway Obstruction in the Child

Presentation of nasal airway obstruction may be unilateral or bilateral; differential diagnosis and treatment for specific presentations follows.

Unilateral obstruction

A child with unilateral congestion should be suspected of having a foreign body or unilateral CA. Diagnosis is made by examination. If a unilateral CA is suspected, work-up and treatment should proceed as discussed earlier in this chapter for infants. If a foreign body is noted, removal may be accomplished with the use of small tools such as a suction or ear curette. In rare instances, an object is too large to remove through the nostril, and a lateral rhinotomy may be required. Note that alkaline batteries must be removed as quickly as possible because they can result in significant intranasal necrosis, scarring, and subsequent stenosis. Necrotic tissue may need to be debrided with multiple surgical procedures.

Allergic rhinitis

Congestion associated with clear rhinorrhea, sneezing, and cough are most consistent with a viral upper respiratory tract infection or allergic rhinitis (AR). If symptoms are short lived and resolve spontaneously, the likely aetiology is viral. If symptoms are chronic and associated with itchy, watery eyes, however, the diagnosis may be allergic rhinitis. Individuals with AR may also have a personal or family history of eczema or asthma. Dust mites and cockroaches are the most common allergens in the Ivory Coast.[17] In Egypt, 40% of school children have AR. It is more common in children attending state-run schools, in boys, and in children exposed to cigarette smoke.[18] Definitive diagnosis is made with allergy testing. Alternatively, successful treatment of suspected AR with antihistamines and nasal steroids may help to establish the diagnosis.

Bacterial rhinosinusitis

Nasal congestion associated with mucopurulent rhinitis and a cough, especially a nocturnal cough, suggests bacterial rhinosinusitis. Chronic mucopurulent rhinitis may be seen with HIV infections.[19] Bacterial rhinosinusitis is treated with antibiotics. Commonly identified bacteria by geographic location are:

- Ethiopia: *Streptococcus pneumonia* and *Hemophilus influenza*[20]
- Sudan: *Staphylococci, Streptococci*, and *Escherichia coli*[21]
- South Africa: *Streptococcus milleri* and *Hemophilus influenza*[22]

The choice of antibiotics is based upon the most common pathogens and resistance patterns in an area.[23] When antibiotics do not resolve the infection or if a complication of acute bacterial sinusitis occurs, surgical intervention is warranted. Prior to surgical intervention, ideally a CT scan should be obtained (Figure 125.2).

In the case of a complication such as a subperiosteal periorbital abscess or orbital abscess (Figure 125.3), an ethmoidectomy and drainage of abscess would be advocated. To determine the proper timing and selection of patients requiring ethmoidectomy, South African otolaryngologists studied patients with orbital complications. Those patients with only cellulitis were successfully treated with intravenous antibiotics alone. Those with cellulitis and proptosis with or without eye movement limitation fared better with surgical intervention.[24] Endoscopic sinus surgery has largely replaced open surgical procedures. Either would be appropriate, however, depending upon the extent of disease and the skills of the surgeon. Complications of surgery include injury to the eyes or brain with possible double vision, loss of vision, CSF rhinorrhea, loss of sense of smell, and intraorbital haematoma.

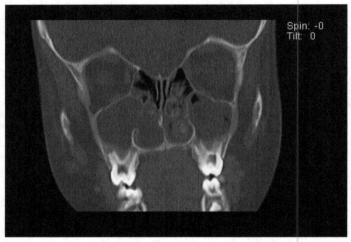

Figure 125.2: Choronal CT scan showing diseases in the maxillary and anterior ethmoidal sinus (chronic sinusitis).

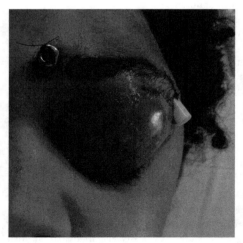

Figure 125.3: Orbital abscess.

Fungal rhinosinusitis

Fungal infections are commonly seen in parts of Africa. The most common presenting symptom of nasosinus aspergillosis is congestion secondary to nasal polyposis. Infection with *Aspergillus flavus* is a common form of sinusitis in Sudan.[25] Unlike bacterial infections, fungal infections must be treated with surgical debridement followed by antimicrobial treatment such as itraconazole. Recurrence is seen in approximately 10% of patients and is generally the result of incomplete antifungal treatment following surgery.

Cystic fibrosis

In addition to a work-up for fungal infections, nasal polyposis in any child should prompt a work-up for cystic fibrosis (CF). The prevalence of CF in African populations remains largely unknown. Mutations of the cystic fibrosis transmembrane regulator (CFTR) gene have been identified in Egyptian, Algerian, Tunisian, and other Northern African populations.[26–28] Presentation is quite variable and can include recurrent respiratory problems, recurrent sinusitis, failure to thrive, steatorrhea, diarrhoea, and jaundice. Sweat chloride testing and genetic testing for CFTR mutations are two ways of diagnosing the disease. Sinusitis in patients with CF is treated with a combination of medical therapy and surgical intervention. Patients may be treated with steroids to reduce inflammation, antibiotic irrigations, and surgery.

Burkitt lymphoma

Burkitt lymphoma (BL) is endemic in certain parts of Africa. In Nigeria, it accounts for nearly 40% of all childhood malignancies.[29] It is a B-cell, non-Hodgkin's lymphoma seen primarily in children. Infection with Epstein-Barr virus (EBV) and plasmodium falciparum malaria have been implicated in the pathogenesis of this disease.[30–32] Children with HIV infections are also at higher risk of developing BL.[30–31] Nearly three-quarters of all cases present in the head and neck region. The male-to-female distribution is 3:1, and peak presentation is often in the first decade of life. The paranasal sinuses are the second most common site of presentation after the jaw. When presenting in the paranasal sinuses, BL may present as nasal congestion, epistaxis, loose teeth, trismus, proptosis, and a mass in the maxilla. Diagnosis is made with a biopsy. Treatment generally consists of a combination of chemotherapeutic drugs. The protocol in Nigeria includes cyclophosphamide, oncovin, methotrexate, and prednisolone. In Kenya and Uganda, cyclophosphamide, doxyrubicin, vincristine, methotrexate, and prednisolone are in use.[33] The treatment protocols are very expensive and, in many cases, too toxic for malnourished children. As a result, physicians in Cameroon and Malawi have advocated using a regimen of cyclophosphamide and intrathecal methotrexate with comparable results, reserving vincristine for those who relapse.[33] Drug resistance is seen in 2% of patients in certain parts of Africa.[29] Despite treatment, mortality remains high. Three-year survival is only 61%.[34] There is evidence to suggest that malaria prevention with the use of mosquito nets may help to reduce the risk of developing BL.[30,31]

Nasopharyngeal carcinoma

Nasopharyngeal carcinoma (NPC) has a high prevalence in Northern Africa, especially in Tunisia, Algeria, and Morocco. In Uganda, the disease is more prevalent in the Nilotic and Para-Nilotic tribes of the north compared to the Sudanic and Bantu tribes of the south.[35] In Northern Africa, NPC has a bimodal age distribution, including one peak between the ages of 10 and 20 years.[36] In addition to a genetic predisposition, exposure to EBV and other environmental factors, such as consumption of rancid butter, rancid sheep fat, and cured meats, may increase the likelihood of developing NPC.[37] In Kenya, exposure to carcinogenic hydrocarbons generated from burning of wood in wattle and mud huts has been associated with a higher incidence of NPC.[35] Avoidance of these environmental factors may help to reduce the incidence of the disease.

NPC may present with nasal congestion, epistaxis, otitis media, otalgia, cranial nerve palsies, headache, and a neck mass from metastasis. Examination of the nasopharynx by using either a flexible fibre-optic endoscope or a nasopharyngeal mirror will reveal a mass in the nasopharynx. Imaging studies such as an MRI or CT scan help to determine the extent of disease and may assist in differentiating it from a juvenile nasopharyngeal angiofibroma (JNA). NPC, similar to BL, is diagnosed by a biopsy. There are three distinct forms, as described by the World Health Organization (WHO): type I is the keratinising form, type II is nonkeratinising, and type III is undifferentiated. In addition, serologic testing for antibodies to EBV may assist in making the diagnosis.[35] Treatment consists of concurrent radiation therapy and chemotherapy with cisplatin.[38] In the past, it was felt that the location of the tumour prevented surgical intervention. In certain situations, however, an NPC may be surgically removed. Overall disease-free survival at 5 years is reported at just under 70%.[39]

Juvenile nasopharyngeal angiofibroma

Seen only in prepubertal and adolescent males, JNA presents with nasal congestion and epistaxis. It is an idiopathic, benign tumour that originates near the sphenopalatine foramen. It is highly vascular and can be locally aggressive and extend intracranially (Figure 125.4). Without treatment, JNA can result in significant morbidity from bleeding. The primary treatment is preoperative embolisation of feeding vessels followed by surgical excision. The approach to excision varies based upon the size and extent of the tumour. This includes an endoscopic approach, a transpalatal approach, a midface degloving, or lateral rhinotomy. Tumours that extend intracranially may require a combined neurosurgical approach. Radiation therapy has been used in selective "inoperable" cases in the past. In general, if this benign tumour can be removed, radiation should be avoided due to concerns of future malignancy.[40]

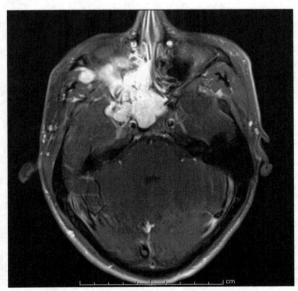

Figure 125.4: Axial view of CT showing an extensive JNA.

Epistaxis

Epistaxis (nose bleed) is a common occurrence in children of all ages. The aetiology varies from minor trauma to large skull-base tumours.

Demographics

Epistaxis patterns in Africa are as follows

• Zaire: up to 50% of children younger than 13 years of age with sickle cell anaemia[41]

• Ethiopia: 20% of children infected with louse-born relapsing fever[42]

- Zimbabwe: common presentation of autoimmune thrombocytopenic purpura[43]

- Other regions: seen with immune thrombocytopenic purpura and onyalai[44-45]

Investigations

Laboratory examinations may be useful in the diagnosis of some of the infectious and haematologic disorders listed.

Treatment

Conservative treatment for epistaxis includes topical pressure and vasoconstrictive medications such as topical phenylephrine or topical oxymetazoline. Common procedures involve nasal packing and cauterisation using silver nitrate or electrocautery. In refractory cases, the treatment is embolisation or arterial ligation. Arterial ligation of the sphenopalatine artery in children may be performed endoscopically. Transantral ligation of the internal maxillary artery may be difficult due to the lack of midface development and poor maxillary pneumatisation at younger ages.

The Pharynx: Tonsillitis

In children, the common diseases of the pharynx are due to infection. Infection of the tonsils accounts for most pharyngeal infections. In Africa, due to the common complaint of sore throat and presence of other significant infectious diseases, adequate recognition and treatment of tonsillitis is not often achieved. The other diseases include the common cold, infectious mononucleosis, candidiasis, HIV, diphtheria, Vincent's angina, and acute leukaemia.

A study from a tertiary centre in Benin, Nigeria, has shown that tonsillitis accounts for 10.5% of children with acute admission for febrile illness.[47] It is therefore a significant workload for paediatricians. The widespread practice of uvulectomy by traditionalists for "sore throat", with its fatal outcome in some children,[48,49] exemplifies the challenges for paediatricians and surgeons in Africa with regard to management of pharyngeal infections.

Aetiology

The palatine tonsils are part of Waldeyer's ring of lymphoid tissue surrounding the oropharynx and nasopharynx. The palatine tonsils are covered by stratified squamous epithelium, which extends deep into the tonsillar tissue, resulting in crypts. Desquamated epithelium can get stuck in the pits; this has been implicated in the aetiology of infection of the tonsils.

Group A beta haemolytic streptococcus accounts for the majority of tonsillitis. In Africa, it appears that this strain type has a predilection to the heart and kidneys, as there is a high rate of rheumatic heart disease from tonsillitis and pharyngitis.[50-52]

Clinical Presentation

Tonsillitis presents as an acute episode that is characterised by sore throat associated with odynophagia, and sometimes secondary otalgia and a febrile illness. In the acute phase, the tonsils are enlarged and red, with associated erythema of the tonsillar pillars. There may be pus within the tonsil crypts. The jugulodiagastric nodes are often enlarged and tender.

Children often present with recurrent episodes of tonsillitis. This can have significant implications in children with sickle cell anaemia or those who are at a risk of developing rheumatic heart disease.

Investigation

Diagnosis is based on clinical evaluation. Microbiology of throat swabs is generally not helpful.

Management

Management is supportive, with antibiotics. Children who are not pyrexic and complain only of sore throat should be given analgesia and adequate hydration, whereas those with fever and failure to eat should also be treated with antibiotics. Penicillin remains the first choice of antibiotics to be used.[53] The use of antibiotics for all should be discouraged, however, because sore throat is a common complaint from nonbacterial infection. Amoxicillin is contraindicated in patients with mononucleosis.

When to Offer Tonsillectomy

In the United Kingdom, children who have five episodes or more of tonsillitis per year are offered tonsillectomy. In Africa, however, a lower threshold of three or more in a year with a significant history of febrile illness should be considered for tonsillectomy[54] due to the higher risk of developing rheumatic heart disease from beta haemolytic streptococcus infection, and issues of access to a specialist.

Affected children should be screened for sickle cell anaemia, and adequate preparation must be made before tonsillectomy of children with sickle cell disease. These children presenting for elective tonsillectomy should be transfused to reduce the haemoglobin S ratio to less than 40% in an attempt to reduce postoperative complications.[55-58] In addition, aggressive hydration is important in these children. If possible, such children should be managed in centres that have a good paediatric anaesthetist who is familiar with sickle cell disease. Otherwise, a team approach among surgeons, anaesthetist, and paediatricians should be developed.

Complications

Nonsuppurative complications of tonsillitis include scarlet fever, rheumatic fever, and glomerulonephritis. Suppurative complications include peritonsillar, parapharyngeal, and retropharanyngeal abscesses.

Peritonsillar abscess

Peritonsillar abscess is common in the adolescent age group but rarely occurs in younger children. Patients present with poor intake or inability to eat. Drooling of saliva and trismus associated with high fever are some of the clinical features. The uvula may be deviated to the opposite side. Younger children and adolescents who cannot tolerate aspiration or incision and drainage under local anaesthesia should be offered tonsillectomy.

Parapharyngeal abscess

Parapharyngeal abscess is characterised by a toxic-appearing child, trismus, dysphasia, and increasing airway difficulties. Urgent US or CT scans should be followed by either an internal or external drainage of the abscess. Intravenous antibiotics are also administered.

Retropharyngeal abscess

Retropharyngeal abscess is rare and seen mainly in children younger than 5 years of age.

The Larynx

A multidisciplinary approach in the management of children with airway disease offers the best outcome; therefore, each local hospital should strive to form a team among paediatric nurses, anaesthetist, paediatricians, and paediatric surgeons.

Congenital Laryngeal Lesions

The incidence of congenital laryngeal lesions in Africa is not known. Worldwide, it is thought to be in the region of 1 in 10,000 to 1 in 50,000 live births.[59,60] It is important to recognise laryngeal abnormalities early.

Laryngomalacia

The most common (60%) of all laryngeal abnormalities is laryngomlacia, with a male-to-female ratio of 2:1. The aetiology involves redundant posterior arytenoids tissue, laryngopharyngeal reflux disease,[61] or poor development of the cartilage.[62]

Patients present within 1 to 2 weeks after birth with a history of noisy breathing. Symptoms include inspiratory stridor, retractions, cyanotic episodes, growth disturbance, or any combination of these. Symptoms are worse in a supine position, during feeding, and when the

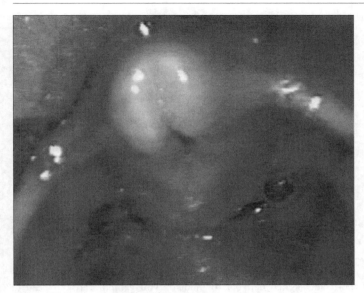

Figure 125.5: Laryngomalacia with the classic "omega-shaped" epiglottis and short aryepiglottic folds.

child is agitated. Prone and lateral decubitus positioning relieves the symptoms. The cry is normal.

Examination by a flexible laryngoscopy, transnasal or oral, in clinic is often satisfactory.[63] Children with severe stridor should have a microlaryngoscopy and bronchoscopy. A bronchoscopy should also be considered in a child whose symptoms are out of proportion to the degree of laryngomalacia or whose symptoms are atypical (e.g., biphasic stridor) because a small but substantial number of patients (18%) will have a second airway lesion.[64]

Examination reveals an omega-shaped epiglottis and short aryepiglottic folds (Figure 125.5). Redundant posterior arytenoid tissue, which on inspiration is prolapsed anteromedially, is also present.

Most laryngomalacias are self-limiting and require only assurance to the parents. A few require an aryepiglottoplasty,[65] which is generally reserved for those children with cyanosis or growth delays secondary to excessive calories used for the increased work of breathing.

Complications from laryngomalacia are rare and are generally the result of untreated severe laryngomalacia (e.g., recurrent cyanotic attacks, obstructive apnoea, pulmonary hypertension, right heart failure, and failure to thrive).

Vocal cord paralysis

Vocal cord paralysis is the second most common congenital anomaly of the larynx. It accounts for 15–20% of all cases.[66] It has a male-to-female ratio of 1:1. The aetiology is multifactorial, including Idiopathic causes; central neuromuscular immaturity; lesions in the central nervous system (including Arnold-Chiari malformation[67,68]; cerebral palsy; hydrocephalus; myelomeningocele; spina bifida; hypoxia;[67,69] lesions in the mediastinum (e.g., tumours or vascular malformations); and birth trauma. Even though birth trauma is an acquired cause, it is included because it is a major problem in Africa, which has a high number of forceps deliveries and poor maternal services. Iatrogenic vocal cord paralysis from cardiac surgery, such as patent ductus arteriosus (PDA) ligation, is rare in Africa.

Congenital vocal cord palsy is often a bilateral palsy characterised by inspiratory stridor that is present at rest but made worse by agitation and can quickly lead to airway obstruction. This can rapidly progress to an emergency requiring airway intervention. Aspiration may present with recurrent chest infection. This is common with bilateral vocal fold paralysis. Unilateral vocal fold paralysis may manifest during the first few weeks of life, or it may go unnoticed. Symptoms are a hoarse, breathy cry that is aggravated by agitation. Feeding difficulties and aspiration may also occur.

On examination, the stable child has minimal symptoms and does not appear to be in significant respiratory distress. The unstable child, in contrast, presents in respiratory distress (nasal flaring, supraclavicular or intercostal recession, cyanosis).

Flexible endoscopy usually elucidates the diagnosis. Direct laryngoscopy and rigid bronchoscopy are often necessary to confirm the diagnosis and to evaluate the airway for other anomalies.[70]

Other investigations include a CT scan of the neck and chest. Where available, laryngeal electromyography has been used for both evaluation and management.

Reassurance is all that is required in a child who has a stable airway and no aspiration. This is more common in those with unilateral vocal cord palsy.

A child with an unstable airway requires urgent endotracheal intubation followed by tracheostomy.

The suitability of a child for decannulation is undertaken by laryngoscopy and bronchoscopy, processes that also help to remove granulation above the tracheostomy. The child may be decannulated if there is sufficient airway size or when there is recovery of the palsy. This is commonly after the ago of 2 years.[71]

Children who fail to recover would require vocal cord lateralisation procedures, which can be either arytenoidectomy or endoscopic laser cordotomy.

Congenital subglottic stenosis

Congenital subglottic stenosis is the third most common congenital anomaly of the larynx, with a male-to-female ratio of 2:1. It is the most common indication for tracheostomy in infants. Two types of congenital subglottic stenosis are recognised: membranous (the most common) and cartilaginous.

The aetiology of this anomaly is incomplete recanalisation of the laryngotracheal tube.

An inflammatory process tends to initiate symptoms. Biphasic stridor with or without symptoms of respiratory distress is the most common presenting symptom. The presentation of congenital subglottic stenosis is similar to croup, but the cry is normal. Recurrent croup-like symptoms commonly are seen in children with subglottic stenosis.

Flexible endoscopy under local anaesthesia is inadequate to make a diagnosis; therefore, a rigid bronchoscopy under general anaesthesia is required.

Spontaneous resolution occurs in most cases as the child grows. If there is significant airway obstruction, however, management is by endotracheal intubation followed by tracheostomy.[72] Decannulation can be performed when the subglottic space widens, by about age 3–4 years.[73] Laryngotracheoplasty is reserved for severe cases of subglottic stenosis.

Laryngeal Infection

Laryngeal infection in children is a life-threatening disease. This is because a child's laryngeal diameter is very small, and any degree of oedema would narrow the laryngeal diameter significantly. For example, the neonate subglottic cross-sectional area is about 4 mm, compared to that of an adult, which may be 14 mm. Therefore, 1 mm of subglottic oedema at that level would result in approximately 65% reduction of the airway area in a neonate, compared to approximately 25% reduction in adults.

It is important to recognise early signs of laryngeal inflammation and aggressively treat children. The two common but dangerous infections of the larynx in children are acute epiglottitis and laryngotracheobronchitis (LTB, or croup). Other important differential diagnoses that are common in Africa include laryngeal candidiasis and tuberculosis. These infections have been attributed to the high prevalence of HIV infection in children in Africa,[74] and they should be considered if a child presents with unusual symptoms.

Table 125.1: Key features of acute epiglottitis and laryngotracheobronchitis.

Key Features	Acute Epiglottitis	Laryngotracheobronchitis
Age	3 years and older	3 months to 3 years
Onset	Abrupt	Gradual
Progression	Rapid	Gradual
Cough	None	Barking
Hoarseness	Yes	More from barking cough
Stridor	Inspiratory	Inspiratory or biphasic
Posture	Sitting and leaning forward	Supine
Drooling	Yes, with odynophagia	No
Soft tissue neck x-ray	Thumb sign (enlarged epiglottis), on lateral view (X-ray not recommended)	Steeple sign (narrowed subglottis), on AP view
Aetiology	*Haemophilus influenza* type B	Viral (parainfluenza virus in two-thirds of cases)
Findings	Red swollen epiglottis (cherry red)	
Treatment	• Examine in the operating theatre and secure airway by endotracheal intubation. Convert to nasotracheal intubation, if possible. • Under no circumstances should a child with a suspected diagnosis of epiglottitis be disturbed until the team is ready to evaluate the child in the theatre. • Cephalosporins/ chloramphenicol. • Steroids.	• Supportive (oxygen/steroids/ antibiotics/). • Steroids: dexamethasone (0.6 mg/kg) or nebulised budesonide. • Antibiotics are indicated if associated bronchial pneumonia or pyerixia or aetiology is thought to be bacterial LTB. • Note that in Africa prognosis is poor when infection follows measles; early airway support should be considered. • The Westley croup score system can be used to determine the severity and need for airway support.

Diphtheria of the larynx is another infection that remains a concern. Immunisation remains the key to its eradication. Sadly, this is still a public health problem in a number of African countries. It is important to note that laryngeal diphtheria tends to occur after a pharyngeal infection.

Other differential diagnoses for laryngeal infection are foreign body aspiration, acute laryngeal trauma, angioneurotic oedema, and retropharyngeal abscess. A good history often leads to the diagnosis of any of these differentials.

In Africa, acute epiglottitis and LTB remain challenges as a result of poor immunisation and a significantly poor socioeconomic living standard for children. Table 125.1 summarises the key features of acute epiglottitis and LTB and their management.

Hoarseness

Hoarseness is underestimated in children, and in Africa it does not receive adequate attention. This situation has been attributed to several factors, such as the changing pitch in normally growing children and a poor understanding of children's voice dynamics, among others.

Reports from many centres in Africa, for example, show a high rate of emergency tracheostomy for laryngeal papillomatosis in children due to late presentation. The need to increase awareness is challenging but necessary. A coordinated approach to dealing with children with hoarseness is key.

The causes of voice changes (dysphonia) in children are commonly due to vocal nodules and functional voice disorders, laryngeal papillamatosis, intubation injuries, or vocal cord paralysis.

Vocal nodules and functional voice disorders

The most common cause of dysphonia in children is vocal nodules and functional voice disorders. Diagnosis is usually by flexible laryngoscopy; however, rigid laryngoscopy under anaesthesia may be required if a child is unable or unwilling to cooperate. Voice therapy is the main treatment. Surgery for nodules is not recommended in children, but it can be considered after failed response to adequate voice therapy and after puberty. Antireflux medications are also recommended.

Laryngeal papillamatosis

Laryngeal papillamatosis is also referred to as juvenile onset recurrent respiratory papillamatosis (RRP). It is due to the human papilloma virus, mainly types 6, 11, and rarely 16. Types 6 and 11 are associated with genital warts.

The peak age of presentation is 3 to 4 years. Firstborn children are more likely to be affected by laryngeal papillamatosis, and children born via vaginal delivery to mothers with genital warts are said to have a relative risk of developing the disease. No current evidence, however, supports caesarian section delivery as a means of prevention of laryngeal papillamatosis.

Commonly, RRP patients present with a history of hoarseness, chronic cough, and a gradual but progressive history of stridor. In Africa, a large number of children are diagnosed only when they present with stridor because RRP is often misdiagnosed as croup. Studies from Nigeria show that RRP is the most common cause of airway obstruction in children.[75] Late presentation accounts for the high incidence of emergency trachestomies in this population.

Any child with hoarseness that has not resolved within three weeks should have a laryngeal examination. Transnasal flexible laryngoscopy is recommended in children who can cooperate. If this is not possible, direct laryngoscopy under anaesthesia should be carried out.

The use of a powered microdebrider is a recent advancement in RRP treatment and is replacing laser ablation (CO₂, KTP, ND:YAG), the current gold standard. The use of a powered microdebrider might be a more affordable tool than laser for many centres in Africa. Other treatments include photodynamic therapy and adjuvant use of interferon, cidofouvir, acyclovir, indole-3-carbinol, and cimetidine.

Tracheostomy is indicated only for a child with severe diseases, where it is a life-saving procedure. This should be used as a last resort, however, especially in Africa, where management of trachestomy in children is very challenging. Furthermore, a tracheostomy in these children may result in seeding of the trachea.

Intubation injuries

Intubation injuries often present as vocal cord granulation of the posterior larynx. In neonates, it can present as an acquired subglottic cyst or subglottic stenosis.

Vocal cord paralysis

Unilateral vocal cord palsy presents with hoarseness and aspiration. Bilateral vocal cord paralysis has been described in this chapter in the subsection "Congenital Laryngeal Lesions".

Key Summary Points

Ears

1. Children with a hearing loss may appear socially disinterested and lag behind their peers in the development of speech and language skills.

2. In the absence of universal screening programs, practicing clinicians in Africa should do a behavioural hearing test for any child with a hearing impairment

3. Otitis media (OM) is the leading cause of hearing loss in African children.

4. Low social status and malnutrition correlates with developing chronic OM.

Nose

5. Epistaxis (nose bleed) is a common occurrence in children of all ages.

6. Conservative treatment for epistaxis includes topical pressure and vasoconstrictive medications such as topical phenylephrine or topical oxymetazoline, Common procedures involve nasal packing and cauterisation using silver nitrate or electrocautery.

Larynx

7. Laryngeal abnormalities should be recognised early.

8. Noisy breathing or stridor in a child should be taken seriously; if in doubt, referral to an appropriate centre is urgently recommended.

9. Flexible laryngoscopy (transnasal or oral), microlaryngoscopy, or bronchoscopy, when appropriate, often confirms the diagnosis of congenital subglottic stenosis.

Oropharynx

10. Other congenital anomalies of the larynx that are rare include congenital subglottic cyst, laryngeal webs, and subglottic haemangioma, among others.

11. Sore throat is a common complaint, not always due to tonsillitis.

12. A majority of sore throats can be treated with supportive measures.

13. Penicillin remains the drug of choice for tonsillitis.

14. There is a low threshold for tonsillectomy for children in Africa due to the high prevalence of rheumatic heart disease and nephritic disease from beta haemolytic streptococcus infection.

15. Children should be screened for sickle cell anaemia before surgery for tonsillitis, and adequate pre- and postoperative management should be planned for children with sickle cell disease.

References

1. Alberti PW. Pediatric ear, nose and throat services' demands and resources: a global perspective. Int J Pediatr Otorhinolaryngol 1999; 49(Suppl 1):S1–S9.

2. Oburra HO. Ear, nose and throat/head and neck medical services in developing countries: challenges and future perspectives. East Afr Med J 1998; 75(6):317–318.

3. Amadasun JEO Editorial: our aim and objectives in the way ahead. West African Newsletter of Oto-Rhino-Laryngology, Head and Neck Surgery 1997; 1(1):1–2.

4. Smith A, Hatcher J. Preventing deafness in Africa's children. Afr Health 1992; 15(1):33–35.

5. Smith A, Hatcher J, MacKenzie I, et al. Randomised controlled trial of treatment of chronic suppurative otitis media in Kenyan schoolchildren. Lancet 1996; 348:1128–1133.

6. Obi CL, Enweani IB, Giwa JO. Bacterial agents causing chronic suppurative otitis media. East Afr Med 1995; 72(6):370–372.

7. Lasisi AO, Olaniyan FA, Muibi SA, et al. Clinical and demographic risk factors associated with chronic suppurative otitis media. Int J Ped Otorhinolaryngol 2007; 71: 1549–1554.

8. Enweani IB, Igumbor H. Prevalence of otomycosis in malnourished children in Edo State, Nigeria. Mycopathologia 1998; 140:85–87.

9. Ologe FE, Nwabuisi C. Treatment outcome of otomycosis in Ilorin. West Afr J Med 2002; 21(1):34–36.

10. Akre EE, Akre A, Tanon MJ. Necrotizing external otitis in children in Abidjan (Ivory Coast). Rev Laryngol Otol Rhinol (Bord) 2002; 123(4):225–230.

11. Eavey RD. Microtia and significant auricular malformation. Arch Otolaryngol Head Neck Surg 1995; 121:57–62.

12. Tekin M, Oztürkmen A, Fitoz S, et al. Homozygous FGF3 mutations result in congenital deafness with inner ear agenesis, microtia, and microdontia. Clin Genet 2008; 73(6):554–565.

13. Melaku A. Sensorineural hearing loss in children with epidemic meningococcal meningitis at Tikur Anbessa Hospital. Ethiop Med J 2003; 41(2):113–121.

14. Lasisi OA, Ayodele JK, Ijaduola GTA. Challenges in management of childhood sensorineural hearing loss in sub-Saharan Africa, Nigeria. Int J Ped Otorhinolaryngol 2006; 70:625–629.

15. Mir NA, Grewal BS, Kishan J, et al. Congenital choanal atresia in North African infants. Ann Trop Paediatr 1986; 6(2):141–144.

16. Ba MC, Kabre A, Badiane SB, et al. Fronto-ethmoidal encephaloceles in Dakar. Report of 9 cases. Dakar Med 2003; 48(2):131–133.

17. Ngom AS, Koffi N, Blessey M, Aka-Danguy E. Prevalence of allergy to cockroaches in African intertropical zone. Review of the literature. Allerg Immunol (Paris) 1999; 31(10):351–356.

18. Georgy V, Fahim HI, Gaafary EI, Walters S. Prevalence and socioeconomic associations of asthma and allergic rhinitis in northern Africa. Eur Respir J 2006; 28:756–762.

19. Nkrumah FK, Choto RG, Emmanuel J, Kumar R. Clinical presentation of symptomatic human immuno-deficiency virus in children. Cent Afr J Med 1990; 36(5):116–120.

20. Mohammed E, Muhe L, Geyid A, et al. Prevalence of bacterial pathogens in children with acute respiratory infection in Addis Ababa. Ethiop Med J 2000; 38(3):165–174.

21. Yagi H. Sinusitis in Sudanese patients: a clinical review. East Afr Med J 1991; 68(12):944–947.

22. Mortimore S, Wormald PJ, Oliver S. Antibiotic choice in acute and complicated sinusitis. J Laryngol Otol 1998; 112(3):264–268.

23. Brink AJ, Cotton MF, Feldman C, et al. Guideline for the management of upper respiratory tract infections. S Afr Med J 2004; 94(6, Pt 2):475–483.

24. Singh B. The management of sinogenic orbital complications. J Laryngol Otol 1995; 109(4):300–303.

25. Yagi HI, Gumaa SA, Shumo AI, et al. Nasosinus aspergillosis in Sudanese patients: clinical features, pathology, diagnosis and treatment. J Otolaryngol 1999; 28(2):90–94.

26. Lakeman P, Gille J, Dankert-Roelse J, et al. CFTR mutations in Turkish and North African cystic fibrosis patients in Europe: implications for screening. Genet Test 2008; 12(1):25–35.

27. Loumi O, Ferec C, Mercier B. CFTR mutations in the Algerian population. J Cyst Fibros 2008; 7(1):54–59.

28. Naguib ML, Schrijver I, Gardner P, et al. Cystic fibrosis detection in high-risk Egyptian children and CFTR mutation analysis. J Cyst Fibros 2007; 6(2):111–116.

29. Amusa YB, Adediran IA, Akinpelu VO, et al. Burkitt's lymphoma of the head and neck region in a Nigerian tertiary hospital. West Afr J Med 2005; 24(2):139–142.

30. Mutalima N, Molyneux E, Jaffe H, et al. Associations between Burkitt lymphoma among children in Malawi and infection with HIV, EBV and malaria: results from a case-control study. PLoS ONE 2008; 3(6):e2505.

31. Orem J, Mbidde EK, Weiderpass E. Current investigations and treatment of Burkitt's lymphoma in Africa. Trop Doct 2008; 38(1):7–11.

32. Rainey JJ, Rochford R, Sumba PO, et al. Family environment is associated with endemic Burkitt lymphoma: a population-based case-control study. Am J Trop Med Hyg 2008; 78(2):338–343.

33. Hesseling PB, Molyneux E, Tchintseme F, et al. Treating Burkitt's lymphoma in Malawi, Cameroon and Ghana. Lancet Oncol 2008; 9(6):512–513.

34. Ribiero RC, Sandlund JT. Burkitt lymphoma in African children: a priority for the global health agenda? Pediatr Blood Cancer 2008; 50:1125–1126.

35. McDermott AL, Dutt SN, Watkinson JC. The aetiology of nasopharyngeal carcinoma. Clin Otolaryngol 2001; 26:82–92.

36. Khabir A, Sellami A, Sakka M, et al. Contrasted frequencies of p53 accumulation in the two age groups of North African nasopharyngeal carcinomas. Clin Cancer Res 2001; 7(1):220.

37. Feng BJ, Jalbout M, Ayoub WB, et al. Dietary risk factors for nasopharyngeal carcinoma in Maghrebian countries. Int J Cancer 2007; 121:1550–1555.

38. M'Rabati H, Sbiti Y, Afquir S, et al. Chemotherapy in nasopharyngeal carcinoma. Ann Otolaryngol Chir Cervicofac 2006; 123(2):59–64.

39. Jmal A, Bouseen H, Ghanem A, et al. Nasopharyngeal carcinoma in Tunisian children: retrospective epidemiological, clinical and biological study about 48 cases. Bull Cancer 2005; 92(11):977–981.

40. Maharaj D, Fernandes CM. Surgical experience with juvenile nasopharyngeal angiofibroma. Ann Otol Rhinol Laryngol 1989; 98(4, Pt 1):269–272.

41. Tshilolo L, Mukendi R, Girot R. Sickle cell anemia in the south of Zaire. Study of two series of 251 and 340 patients followed-up 1988–1992. Arch Pediatr 1996; 3(2):104–111.

42. Borgnolo G, Denku B, Chiabrera F, Hailu B. Louse-born relapsing fever in Ethiopian children: a clinical study. Ann Trop Pediatr 1993; 13(2):165–171.

43. Mukiibi JM. Autoimmune thrombocytopenic purpura (AITP) in Zimbabwe. Trop Georg Med 1989; 41(4):326–330.

44. Bedri A, Abebe E. Idiopathic thrombocytopenic purpura (ITP) in Ethiopian children: clinical findings and response to therapy. Ethiop Med J 1995; 33(2):75–81.

45. Hesseling PB. Onyalai in Namibia. Clinical manifestations, haematological findings, course and management of 103 patients in the Kavango territory. Trans R Soc Trop Med Hyg 1987; 81(2):193–196.

46. Isaacson G, Monge JM. Arterial ligation for pediatric epistaxis: developmental anatomy. Am J Rhinol 2003; 17(2):75–81.

47. Obi JO, Ejeheri NA, Alakija W. Childhood febrile seizures (Benin City experience). Ann Trop Paediatr 1994; 14(3):211–214.

48. Einterz EM, Einterz RM, Bates ME. Traditional uvulectomy in northern Cameroon. Lancet 1994; 343(8913):1644.

49. Hartley BE, Rowe-Jones J. Uvulectomy to prevent throat infections. J Laryngol Otol 1994; 108(1):65–66.

50. Zentralbl Bakteriol Mikrobiol. The concurrent associations of group A streptococcal serotypes in children with acute rheumatic fever or pharyngitis-associated glomerulonephritis and their families in Kuwait. Hyg 1986; 262(3):346–356.

51. Majeed HA, Khuffash FA, Yousof AM, Farwana SS, Chugh TD, Moussa MA, Rotta J, Havlickova H. The concurrent associations of group A streptococcal serotypes in children with acute rheumatic fever or pharyngitis-associated glomerulonephritis and their families in Kuwait. Zentralbl Bakteriol Mikrobiol Hyg [A] 1986; 262(3):346–356.

52. Tewodros W, Kronvall G. M protein gene (emm type) analysis of group A beta-hemolytic streptococci from Ethiopia reveals unique patterns. J Clin Microbiol 2005; 43(9):4369–4376.

53. Brink AJ, Cotton MF, Feldman C, Geffen L, Hendson W, Hockman MH, Maartens G, Madhi SA, Mutua-Mpungu M, Swingler GH. Working Group of the Infectious Diseases Society of South Africa guideline for the management of upper respiratory tract infections. S Afr Med J 2004; 94(6, Pt 2):475–483.

54. Okafor BC. Tonsillectomy: an appraisal of indications in developing countries. Acta Otolaryngol 1983; 96(5–6):517–522.

55. Akinyanju O, Johnson AO. Acute illness in Nigerian children with sickle cell anaemia. Ann Trop Paediatr 1987; 7(3):181–186.

56. Halvorson DJ, McKie V, McKie K, Ashmore PE, Porubsky ES. Sickle cell disease and tonsillectomy. Preoperative management and postoperative complications. Arch Otolaryngol Head Neck Surg 1997; 123(7):689–692.

57. Duke RL, Scott JP, Panepinto JA, Flanary VA. Perioperative management of sickle cell disease children undergoing adenotonsillectomy. Otolaryngol Head Neck Surg 2006; 134(3):370–373.

58. Derkay CS, Bray G, Milmoe GJ, Grundfast KM. Adenotonsillectomy in children with sickle cell disease. South Med J 1991; 84(2):205–208.

59. Van den Broek P, Brinkman WF. Congenital laryngeal defects. Int J Pediatr Otorhinolaryngol 1979; 1(1):71–78.

60. Ahmad SM, Soliman AM. Congenital anomalies of the larynx. Otolaryngol Clin N Amer 2007; 40(1):177–191.

61. Daniel SJ. The upper airway: congenital malformations. Paediatr Respir Rev 2006; 7(Suppl 1):S260–S263. Epub 6 June 2006. Review.

62. Iyer VK, Pearman K, Raafat F. Laryngeal mucosal histology in laryngomalacia: the evidence for gastro-oesophageal reflux laryngitis. Int J Pediatr Otorhinolaryngol 1999; 49(3):225–230.

63. Lima TM, Gonçalves DU, Gonçalves LV, Reis PA, Lana AB, Guimarães FF. Flexible nasolaryngoscopy accuracy in laryngomalacia diagnosis. Rev Bras Otorrinolaringol (Engl Ed) 2008; 74(1):29–32.

64. Mancuso RF, Choi SS, Zalzal GH, Grundfast KM. Laryngomalacia. The search for the second lesion. Arch Otolaryngol Head Neck Surg 1996; 122(3):302–306.

65. Olney DR, Greinwald JH Jr, Smith RJ, Bauman NM. Laryngomalacia and its treatment. Laryngoscope 1999; 109(11):1770–1775.

66. Hasniah AL, Asiah K, Mariana D, Anida AR, Norzila MZ, Sahrir S. Congenital bilateral vocal cord paralysis. Med J Malaysia 2006; 61(5):626–629.

67. Omland T, Brøndbo K. Paradoxical vocal cord movement in newborn and congenital idiopathic vocal cord paralysis: two of a kind? Eur Arch Otorhinolaryngol 2008; 265(7):803–807. Epub 18 April 2008.

68. Miyamoto RC, Parikh SR, Gellad W, Licameli GR. Bilateral congenital vocal cord paralysis: a 16-year institutional review. Otolaryngol Head Neck Surg 2005; 133(2):241–245.

69. Holinger LD, Holinger PC, Holinger PH. Etiology of bilateral abductor vocal cord paralysis: a review of 389 cases. Ann Otol Rhinol Laryngol 1976; 85(4, Pt 1):428–436.

70. Kaushal M, Upadhyay A, Aggarwal R, Deorari AK. Congenital stridor due to bilateral vocal cord palsy. Indian J Pediatr 2005; 72(5):443–444.

71. Berkowitz RG. Natural history of tracheostomy-dependent idiopathic congenital bilateral vocal fold paralysis. Otolaryngol Head Neck Surg 2007; 136(4):649–652.

72. Healy GB. Subglottic stenosis. Otol Clin North Am 1989; 22:599.

73. Cotton RT. Pediatric laryngotracheal stenosis. J Pediatr Surg 1984; 19(6):699–704.

74. Jeena PM, Bobat R, Kindra G, Pillay P, Ramji S, Coovadia HM. The impact of human immunodeficency virus 1 on laryngeal airway obstruction in children. Arch Dis Child 2002; 87(3):212–214.

75. Nwaorgu OG, Bakari AA, Onakoya PA, Ayodele KJ. Recurrent respiratory papillomatosis in Ibadan, Nigeria. Niger J Med 2004; 13(3):235–238. Erratum in: Niger J Med 2005; 14(4):459.

CHAPTER 126
PAEDIATRIC TRANSPLANTATION

Hesham M. Abdelkader
Khaled M. El-Asmar
Alaa F.Hamza

Introduction

Paediatric transplantation is still considered a difficult task in the African continent. Lack of resources, cadaveric programs, and technical facilities, as well as delayed referral of cases are among the important obstacles that need to be overcome in order to start transplantation programs. South Africa has a well-established cadaveric program for kidneys and liver, and success related to both is found in Egypt and some North African countries. The progress of immune suppression, intensive care, and nutritional support will lead to improvement in more African countries in the near future.

Liver Transplantation

Liver transplantation is now the standard treatment for end-stage liver disease (ESLD) in children. Children had paved the way for transplantation since the beginning of the procedure; the initial cases were performed by Thomas E. Starzl on two children in 1963 and 1968. Now, more than 500 paediatric patients recieve transplants every year; this number of transplant procedures has been relatively stable since the mid-1990s, but there has been a shift to utilisation of an increasing number of "partial" liver grafts from cadaveric and living donors. Due to organ scarcity and size problems, paediatric liver transplantation is considered a challenge. Donors younger than the age of 5 years comprise only 26% of the paediatric cadaveric donors. As a consequence, split-liver, living-related, and—much less now—reduced liver techniques are important in paediatric transplantation. Survival has been significantly improved and now approaches 90% at 1 year and 80% at 5 years. Many children survive into adolescence and adulthood with good quality of life (QOL) as a consequence of technical improvements, intensive care unit (ICU) advances, early transplantation, and the huge changes in immune suppression.

Indications

The most common indications of childhood transplantation are currently classified into groups:

- ESLD due to cholestatic and noncholestatic causes of cirrhosis;

- acute hepatic failure;

- stable liver disease with remarkable morbidity and/or a known mortality;

- some metabolic liver diseases;

- select tumours; and

- a variety of miscellaneous indications.

One of the major indications in children is liver disease that limits long-term survival or quality of life or markedly impairs normal growth and development. Cirrhosis alone is not an indication for transplantation because many of these patients can be medically managed for a prolonged period before decompensation. In acute liver failure, the development of clear symptoms such as refractory coagulopathy, acidosis, and cerebral oedema that correlate with a poor prognosis for spontaneous recovery of liver function is an indication for transplantation. Otherwise, medical support in those patients with a better prognosis is provided until liver function returns to normal.

Children usually present with decompensation of hepatocellular function or portal hypertension, including progressive jaundice, coagulopathy, protein-calorie malnutrition and growth retardation, impaired cognitive development, encephalopathy, hypersplenism, variceal haemorrhage, and advanced or refractory ascites. The majority of patients undergoing transplantation in this population are deeply jaundiced due to secondary or primary biliary cirrhosis from long-standing intrahepatic and/or extrahepatic biliary obstruction. On physical examination, these patients often have muscle wasting; an enlarged spleen; a hard, palpable liver; abdominal distention from ascites; and peripheral oedema. With decompensation, long-term survival without liver transplantation is limited; referral for transplantation must be made before decompensation.

Neonatal Cholestatic Liver Diseases

Cholestatic liver disorders—the most common being biliary atresia—are the most common indications for transplantation in children. Biliary atresia accounts for 70% of this cholestatic group, which itself represents 60% of all transplanted children per year. The management of biliary atresia rests on early diagnosis and portoenterostomy if diagnosis precedes the development of cirrhosis, usually before 3 months of age. Although long-term results from portoenterostorny are optimal if it is peformed before 8 weeks of age, only 20–25% of all atresia patients will not need transplantation. In many cases, however, portoenterostomy allows reasonable growth and development so that transplantation is forestalled until the child is older and larger. Liver transplantation is indicated when the diagnosis is made in infants older than 3 months of age, when ESLD is clearly present at any age, or after a portoenterostomy failure. Jaundice and malnutrition are the problems with most of these children, who present in very bad condition (especially in the African continent). Preparation for transplantation is therefore extremely difficult and many children could die while awaiting the procedure.

Other uncommon causes of cholestatic liver injury and cirrhosis include familial paucity of intrahepatic bile ducts, which exists in syndromic (e.g., Alagille syndrome) and nonsyndromic forms; familial cholestatic syndromes (progressive familial intrahepatic cholestasis); primary or secondary sclerosing cholangitis; and uncorrectable choledochal cyst disease, including Caroli's disease. All of these conditions proceed to jaundice, cirrhosis, and portal hypertension.

Noncholestatic cirrhosis

Causes of cirrhosis and ESLD include autoimmune hepatitis, neonatal hepatitis, chronic viral (B or C) hepatitis, and cryptogenic cirrhosis.

Fulminant hepatic failure

Fulminant hepatic failure is encephalopathy within 28 days after the onset of jaundice in a patient with acute liver failure without evidence of chronic liver disease. Acute liver failure of an undefined type makes up the largest group within fulminant hepatic failure, followed by drug toxicity, toxin exposure, and previously unrecognised metabolic disease. Acute liver failure includes profound coagulopathy, acidosis, hypoglycaemia, and progressive hyperbilirubinaemia. These patients can develop acute renal failure, multiorgan failure syndrome, or cerebral oedema progressing to herniation. Deterioration in coagulation is one of the major parameters to indicate transplantation in these conditions. Transplantation should be done before the patient develops coma stage IV, when the prognosis is extremely dire.

Metabolic liver disease
Metabolic liver disease disorders have in common an enzyme deficiency or some other defect in hepatocellular function. This impairment can result in progressive fibrosis or cirrhosis (e.g., cystic fibrosis, chronic Wilson's disease, and neonatal iron storage disease) with a typical presentation of ESLD. In other cases, the liver is structurally normal but harmful by-products of metabolism accumulate to cause neurologic injury (e.g., Crigler-Najjar syndrome, ornithine transcarbamylase deficiency, and Wilson's` disease); cardiovascular disease (e.g., familial hypercholesterolaemia); or renal injury (familial hyperoxaluriain, in which case both kidney and liver should both be transplanted). Some disorders are associated with the development of malignancies, such as tyrosinaemia, and transplantation should be considered preemptively.

Tumours
Hepatoblastoma is now considered a good indication for transplantation in cases of an unresectable tumour with no extrahepatic spread and initial good response to chemotherapy. Living-related transplantation with removal of the vena cava has been reported with good results in few sporadic cases. Hepatocellular carcinoma is primarily seen in older children with viral hepatitis or in association with cirrhosis from other causes. Nonmetastatic malignancies in paediatric patients are managed by surgical resection unless tumour size and/or location preclude resection. The long-term survival after liver transplantation for hepatoblastoma is approximately 60%, whereas outcomes from hepatocellular carcinoma are not nearly as good. The major issue that remains to be resolved is whether transplantation should be attempted for large hepatoblastomas primarily or as salvage after recurrence postresection. Data from Europe suggest a worse outcome when liver transplantation is performed as a salvage procedure. The most common benign tumour of the liver is haemangioendothelioma; and although the vast majority regresses with growth and medical therapy, occasionally heart failure or mass effect warrants transplantation.

Miscellaneous
Other conditions that may indicate transplantation include diagnoses such as Budd-Chiari syndrome, trauma, and biliary cirrhosis secondary to intestinal failure and long-term use of total parenteral nutrition.

Contraindications to Transplantation
Contraindications to transplantation include HIV-positive serology patients, extrahepatic malignancy, metastatic liver malignancy, terminal nonhepatic pathology, uncontrolled systemic sepsis, and irreversible neurological damage.

Pretransplant Care
Many problems present in cases with evidence of ESLD who are candidates for liver transplantation. Most cases are below the fifth percentile with regard to weight and height, and those with ascites, malnutrition, bad coagulation profile, and haematemesis are very difficult to handle. Vaccination is another issue that should be dealt with before transplantation because living attenuated vaccine cannot be used posttransplantation due to immune suppression. Therefore, most presenting children receive nutritional support, oral decontamination, and a full battery of investigations. Radiology is used to assess the patency of vessels (the portal vein in cases of biliary atresia), the presence of port-caval shunts, and the vascular anatomy of the recipient. Another problem is timing—at the time a paediatric donor is available, a size-matched paediatric recipient may not be available. This, of course, is not the case in living-related liver transplantation (LRLT), when scheduled transplantation is the case and the problem of being put on a waiting list is removed.

In 2002, the Pediatric End-stage Liver Disease (PELD) score was implemented to allocate organs based on the "sickest first" paradigm. The PELD score consists of five variables:

1. International Normalised Ratio;

2. total serum bilirubin concentration;

3. serum albumin level;

4. growth retardation (= 2 standard deviations below the median height or weight for age); and

5. young age (much less than 1 year, or 1 to 2 years of age).

Status I is used to designate patients with fulminant hepatic failure, primary graft nonfunction after transplantation, early hepatic artery thrombosis, and miscellaneous acute conditions. Unlike the case for adults, paediatric ESLD patients requiring care in an ICU for any reason are listed as status I because their mortality is high despite a minimal change in PELD score. In an effort to ameliorate the shortage of potential organs, the livers of all donors 18 years of age and younger are preferentially allocated to paediatric recipients. This protocol, combined with the widespread use of split-liver transplantation, has markedly reduced waiting times and positively impacted waiting list mortality.

The Surgical Procedure

The donor hepatectomy
The use of organs from cadaveric donors in paediatric liver transplantation involves selecting an appropriate quality- and size-matched donor, organising an experienced transplant harvest team, and performing a precise technical operation that recognises arterial anatomic variants and allows for multiorgan procurement. The advent of segmental liver transplantation has expanded the acceptable donor age to approximately 40 years. Preharvest donor management should focus on maintenance of haemodynamic stability with adequate but not excessive volume loading, minimising the use of vasopressors, optimising oxygenation without excessive use of positive end expiratory pressure (PEEP), and correcting hypernatraemia that results from diabetes insipidus. In the stable donor, once these goals are achieved, the procurement operation can be performed. In the properly selected unstable donor, unnecessary delays are to be avoided because expedient hypothermic perfusion and cold storage only help to minimise the ongoing organ ischaemia.

1. The donor operation begins with midline laparotomy and median sternotomy for wide exposure.

2. The abdominal great vessels are exposed by a medial visceral rotation of the right colon and small intestine, and the aorta and inferior mesenteric vein are cannulated.

3. The liver quality is assessed, and the biliary tree is flushed via the gallbladder.

4. After full systemic heparinisation, the supraceliac aorta is cross-clamped and the intrapericardial inferior vena cava is incised to exsanguinate the donor.

5. Cold-organ perfusion is then initiated through the previously placed cannulas, and the abdominal cavity is immersed in ice in an attempt to achieve a liver core temperature of 4°C.

The University of Wisconsin (UW) solution has been used as the standard preservation solution in the United States since 1987, when it was developed by Belzer and Southhard. This solution extends the limit of preservation to as long as 12–18 hours, after which the incidence of primary graft failure increases substantially. However, the acceptable preservation time depends on numerous donor and recipient variables and should still be minimised when possible. This is especially important in instances of reduced size or split-liver transplantation. The UW solution is a hyperkalemic, hyperosmolar solution that prevents cellular swelling, maintains stable transmembrane electrical gradients upon reperfusion by preventing efflux of intracellular potassium during storage, and contains a variety of oxygen-free radical scavengers. Recently, some centres have employed a histidine-tryptophan-ketoglutarate solution because of its low potassium content and viscosity. Once the donor organ is procured, the harvest team typically transports the liver graft to the transplant centre and prepares it for engraftment by a separate recipient team.

Segmental liver transplantation

Segmental liver transplantation can be of three kinds: living-donor, reduced-size, and split-liver.

Living-related transplantation

In living-related transplantation, the donor is investigated preoperatively with extensive radiologic evaluation regarding vascular anatomy as well as biliary and volumetry of the liver lobes. The choice of the graft depends on the expected volume in relation to recipient weight. Segments 2 and 3 (left lateral segment, or LLS) are usually suitable for children who weigh less than 25 kg. Older children can have segments 2, 3, and 4, or even the right lobe in adolescents. The ratio between liver weight and recipient weight should be above 1% to avoid a small-for-size graft. Grafts of more than 5% of body weight, however, have a bad prognosis due to the large size of the graft in relation to the child's abdomen and the compartmental syndrome that might occur.

Reduced-size transplantation

Due to the small but real risk of safety in a healthy donor, reduced-size transplantation was simultaneously developed as an alternative method. It involves resecting the LLS graft before or after cold-organ perfusion and discarding the remaining liver. Obviously, this benefits the paediatric recipient but wastes an organ that could be used by an adult recipient.

Split-liver transplantation

Splitting the whole organ into a right trisegrnent and an LLS graft to utilise in an adult and paediatric recipient, respectively, was first described by Pichlmayr in Hanover, Germany, in 1988. This can be done either before cold-organ perfusion (in situ technique) or after cold-organ perfusion and removal of the liver from the donor (ex vivo technique). This technique provides a suitable graft for the paediatric population without worsening the already severe organ shortage in the adult population.

The recipient operation

The procedure for total hepatectomy is the same for living-related and cadaveric transplantation, except for vena cava removal, which is not done in living-related or split-liver procedures.

This procedure for total hepatectomy has changed little over the past two decades. Whereas there are tremendous individual and institutional differences in the subtleties of using certain techniques, the basic steps in the procedure remain the same. The procedure can roughly be divided into four major phases, each with its own anatomic and physiologic challenges: hepatectomy phase, anhepatic phase with engraftment, reperfusion with arterialisation, and biliary reconstruction.

Perhaps the most challenging step during liver transplantation is the hepatectomy. Coagulopathy, portal hypertension, and poor liver and renal function create a surgical environment in which continuous bleeding is possible. During this phase, the anaesthesiologist plays a key role in maintaining volume and rapid transfusion, correcting coagulopathy and fibrinolysis, and maintaining body temperature. The goal of this phase is to devascularise the liver by ligating and dividing the hepatic artery and portal vein as well as mobilising the suprahepatic and infrahepatic vena cava to enable removal. At the authors' institution, the strategy is to leave at least one hepatic artery perfusing the liver until the graft is ready, and to ligate it just before removing the liver. This procedure has been found to reduce the lactacidosis during the anhepatic phase. These goals are achieved while leaving in the recipient adequate lengths of each vessel for later implantation of the donor graft. In the majority of paediatric liver transplant operations,

the rettohepatic vena cava is retained as the liver is dissected off the vena cava by dividing the tributaries from the right and caudate lobes; often, only partial occlusion of the vena cava is necessary. Meticulous but expedient surgical technique is essential during the hepatectomy in ensuring optimal patient outcome. During the anhepatic phase, the anaesthesiologist must support certain aspects of hepatic function to prevent or treat acidaemia, hypothermia, coagulopathy, and occasionally fibrinolysis. In addition, the anaesthesiologist must ensure adequate circulating volume and maintain haemodynamic stability. Veno-venous bypass is rarely used in children.

1. While the patient is anhepatic, the liver graft is removed from hypothermic storage and engrafted. The insertion of the graft begins with the suprahepatic vena caval followed by the infrahepatic vena caval in cases of cadaveric full liver.

2. If the retrohepatic cava was retained, the "piggyback" technique is used, in which the hepatic vein of the graft is sewn to the cloacae created from the confluence of the recipient hepatic veins.

3. Next is portal vein anastomosis with careful suturing to avoid twisting, adding a growth factor to the sutures to avoid stenosis.

4. Before reperfusion the liver is flushed with a cold colloid or albumin solution via the donor portal vein to reduce the risk of potential reperfusion-associated complications.

5. Reperfusion is undertaken in a controlled manner by first removing the suprahepatic vena cava clamp, then the infrahepatic vena cava clamp, and lastly the portal venous clamp; or, in case of LRLT, the hepatic venous then portal anastomoses, respectively.

Communication between the surgical and anaesthesia teams at the time of reperfusion is essential to allow the anaesthesiologist time to institute preparative and preventive measures.

As blood is reintroduced into the liver allograft and allowed to drain into the right atria, many serious and potentially life-threatening complications can develop. The major challenges encountered by the anaesthesiologist at this point are life-threatening hyperkalaemia, acidosis, arrhythmias, and haemodynamic instability with or without surgical or coagulopathic bleeding. A contributing factor is the return of cold, acidotic, and hyperkalemic blood directly into the right atrium. It is at this point that maintenance of physiologic stability by the surgeon and anaesthesiologist in the preceding phases, the preoperative state of the recipient, and the intrinsic quality of the graft converge to determine early graft function as well as the course of the remainder of the operation. Without a doubt, this is one of the most hazardous portions of the liver transplant procedure.

1. The hepatic arterial anastomosis is then performed. In some cases, when the arteries are small calibre (<3 mm), the arterial anastomosis is performed before reperfusion. In general, though, arterial inflow is obtained from one of the branches of the celiac trunk. In some instances, however, inflow from these vessels is not adequate, necessitating the use of aortic conduits. A conduit can be placed either on the supraceliac or infrarenal aorta.

2. The biliary tree is then reconstructed by choledochocholedochostomy or by Roux-en-Y choledochojejunostomy, the latter being more common in biliary atresia cases, in small children, and used exclusively in partial liver grafts because of the size of the donor duct.

3. After ensuring sufficient haemostasis, drains are placed, and the abdominal cavity is closed. In cases of large-for-size grafts, those with a graft weight-to-recipient's body weight ratio (GRWR) >4–5, the abdomen is closed over a synthetic prosthesis only so as not to kink the vessels and compromise the graft; this prosthesis can be removed a few days later.

4. The patient is then transferred directly to the ICU.

Postoperative Care

Very close follow up is the mainstay of posttransplant care in children. Most of the patients will have a very short period of ventilation unless there is pulmonary hypertension, and some of the patients are extubated in the theatre. Regular laboratory investigations to detect early manifestations of sepsis, rejection, or vascular insult are mandatory, even in asymptomatic patients. Duplex study is done daily in the first 2 weeks to detect vascular flow, changes in wave patterns, areas of congestion, and biliary radicles.

Graft function can be assessed in many ways. Physiologic and clinical assessment can be done almost immediately. A warm, arousable, and haemodynamically stable patient with a graft producing "golden-brown" bile is the hallmark of a functional graft. Failure of a graft without vascular compromise (primary nonfunction) requires retransplantation in almost all cases, with the outcome directly related to the time to retransplantation. The incidence of primary nonfunction in paediatric patients is 5–10%. Renal functions should be assessed accurately, and the possibility of systemic hypertension and diabetes due to immune suppression is assessed.

Technical Complications

Technical complications can be divided into vascular, biliary, and general surgical complications. In the early postoperative period, infectious and general surgical complications of liver transplantation today are similar to those that occur after any major abdominal operation. However, the incidence of fungal infection is higher and the incidence of bowel perforation in paediatric recipients is as high as 19% in some series.

Vascular complications

Major vascular complications include hepatic artery thrombosis, portal vein thrombosis, and vena caval thrombosis or stenosis. Intravenous low-dose unfractionated heparin is used for prophylaxis to prevent vascular thromboses in some centres. In the authors' unit, aspirin is the only drug used for its antiplatelet effect. Early detection is essential. For rapid management, duplex ultrasonography (US) is usually the first line for diagnosis because it is done routinely. Computed tomography (CT) or conventional angiography are accepted means of diagnosis.

Hepatic artery thrombosis (HAT) is the most common vascular complication, with an incidence that varies from 5% to 18%, depending on patient age and type of graft. Early vascular complications are usually technical in nature, whereas immunologic and infectious (e.g., cytomegalovirus, or CMV) causes have been ascribed to those occurring months after transplantation. HAT occurring in the first week after liver transplantation is commonly associated with graft nonfunction and biliary necrosis or leak. Those instances occurring later do not necessarily affect graft function immediately but can produce biliary complications, including intrahepatic biliary abscesses, biliary anastomotic stricture, and sclerosing cholangitis with sepsis, all of which lead to significant morbidity.

If diagnosed early, some patients can be managed by thrombectomy and surgical revision. However, most patients with early HAT require urgent retransplantation. Late HAT with preserved graft function can be managed by radiologic interventional techniques, and the patient can undergo retransplantation remote from the time of the initial transplant procedure. Thrombosis of the portal vein occurs in 2–4% of paediatric liver transplant procedures and is usually associated with loss of the graft. Prompt retransplantation is required for patient salvage. Late portal vein thrombosis usually presents as recurrent variceal bleeding or ascites and can be managed medically, endoscopically, or surgically with either shunting or retransplantation. Vena caval or hepatic vein thrombosis or stenosis occurs in 3–6% of paediatric liver transplant patients and is manifested with ascites or pleural effusion; it is usually best managed with balloon dilatation in an interventional radiology unit.

Biliary complications

Biliary complications that are not associated with HAT occur in 3–20% of patients, depending on the type of graft and whether a choledochojejunostomy was employed. These complications usually result from technical errors, but occasionally warm ischaemia or immunologic and infectious factors can be implicated (e.g., CMV). Diagnosis is achieved by cholangiography, and treatment can be by endoscopic or radiologic intervention or by surgical revision.

Immunosuppressive therapy and rejection

Immunosuppression for liver transplantation in the modern era rests on a class of drugs known as calcineurin inhibitors (CNI), the prototype of which is cyclosporine. Cyclosporine—especially its microemulsion formulation, which allows better bioavailability and more consistent therapeutic levels—revolutionised organ transplantation by reducing the incidence of rejection in all solid organs. The second-generation CNI tacrolimus was first used clinically in 1990. The greater potency of tacrolimus allowed for a further reduction in the early incidence of rejection after liver transplantation while also allowing earlier weaning of corticosteroid therapy. Initial reports of a higher incidence of opportunistic infections and posttransplant lymphoproliferative disorders have been refuted by modem data. Currently, most liver transplantation centres utilise a tacrolimus-based regimen combined with corticosteroid therapy with or without adjunctive agents such as mycophenolate mofetil (MMF).

Cyclosporine and tacrolimus share certain acute and long-term side effects while having some that are unique to each agent. The most important of these is nephrotoxicity, which occurs in an acute variety from vasoconstriction of the afferent renal arterioles and is reversible, as well as a more chronic variety marked by tubular atrophy, interstitial fibrosis, and glomerulosclerosis. The chronic variety is variably reversible, depending on the degree of disease. To minimise acute toxicity and to allow lower early CNI levels, especially with pretransplant renal insufficiency, a purine antimetabolite mycophenolate mofetil is sometimes used as an adjunctive agent.

The newest class of immunosuppressive agents are the inhibitors of the mammalian target of rapamycin, the prototype of which is sirolimus. This agent has been used sparingly in paediatric liver transplantation, and only preliminary data regarding its efficacy are available. Although this drug has no nephrotoxicity, it is associated with other long-term sequelae, such as hypercholesterolaemia. At present, there are no perfect immunosuppressive agents available.

Acute rejection is common in paediatric liver transplantation, with the peak incidence occurring within the first 6 months; 30–50% of patients experience at least one episode. Acute rejection is less common after the first posttransplantation year, occurring in less than 10% of cases. Diagnosis of acute rejection is suspected when elevated aspartate or alanine transaminase levels or elevated alkaline phosphatase levels and gamma-glutamyl transferase levels are observed. Acute rejection is an alloantigen specific, T-cell-mediated inflammatory process that targets vascular endothelium and biliary epithelium but not hepatocytes. This is related to the greater expression of donor human leukocyte antigens on the former cell types. The histologic hallmark of acute rejection is a mixed inflammatory cell infiltrate (polymorphonuclear cells, lymphocytes, and eosinophils) in the portal triad with evidence of endothelitis and/or biliary epithelial injury. Rejection is graded as mild, moderate, or severe, depending on the proportion of involved portal triads, the degree of infiltrate and injury, and the presence of central vein endothelitis, which is a sign of severe acute rejection.

Treatment of acute rejection is centred on a high-dose methylprednisolone bolus, but unresponsive cases may require use of antibody therapy (OKT-3, ATG). Acute rejection does not influence long-term graft survival in adults or children unless it occurs in multiple or corticosteroid refractory episodes. Acute rejection accounts for less than 3% of overall patient and graft loss. However, treatment of acute rejection is an important risk factor for the development of cytomegalovirus (CMV) and Epstein-Barr virus (EBV) infections in children. The latter is then a risk factor for the development of posttransplant lymphoproliferative disorder. Therefore, a balance between adequate immunosuppression to prevent acute rejection and over-immunosuppression to avoid toxicity is necessary. Currently, long-term morbidity from immunosuppressive drug therapy is the major challenge facing long-term survival and QOL in the paediatric solid organ transplantation population.

Chronic rejection is a common cause of late graft loss in children; disease recurrence is uncommon. Chronic rejection is not entirely alloantigen driven and may be due to a number of factors that share a final common pathway of graft injury. The hallmark of chronic rejection is the intrahepatic loss of bile ducts, which has been termed "vanishing bile duct syndrome" owing to this histological finding noted on biopsy. Rejection is suspected by the presence of progressive jaundice and a rising serum alkaline phosphatase level. Currently, there is no prophylactic or therapeutic agent available to treat chronic rejection, although progression of graft fibrosis may be forestalled by sirolimus, based on animal data. The only accepted treatment when decompensated graft failure occurs is retransplantation.

Infectious complications

Posttransplant infections are the most common cause of morbidity and mortality after liver transplantation. The highest incidence of bacterial and fungal infections occurs in the first month after transplantation.

Table 126.1: Agents responsible for infectious morbidity, their presentation, diagnosis, and treatment.

Organism	Presentation	Methods of diagnosis	Antimicrobials
Cytomegalovirus (CMV)	Infection results from: reactivation of virus; blood transfusion; infected transplanted organ. Mild viral, "flu-like" syndrome. Invasive tissue infection (retinitis, pneumonitis, myocarditis, enterocolitis, hepatitis, central nervous system)	Quantitative CMV-DNA PCR. PP-65 antigen. Tissue cultures. Blood or fluid cultures. Biopsy with immunostains	Prophylaxis: intravenous ganciclovir, oral valganciclovir. Therapy: intravenous ganciclovir with or without CMV immunoglobulin
Epstein-Barr virus (EBV)	Spectrum: infectious mononucleosis to lymphoproliferative disease to lymphoma to EBV-associated soft tissue tumours. Occurs with EBV and immunosuppression, 10% to 15% infant liver transplantation. Gastrointestinal tract, neck, thorax, central nervous system	Quantitative EBV-DNA PCR. Blood smear. Biopsy with immunostains. CT scans of suspected sites	Prophylaxis: intravenous ganciclovir, oral valganciclovir. Therapy: acyclovir, reduction or withdrawal of immunosuppression. Possible use of systemic chemotherapy for lymphoproliferative disorders or lymphoma
Herpes simplex virus (HSV)	Skin lesions, gastrointestinal tract disseminated herpes: fever, fatigue, abnormal liver functions, hepatitis, pneumonia	HSV-1 and HSV-2 antibodies. Biopsy with viral cultures	Acyclovir
Pneumocystis	Atypical pneumonia, can progress to life-threatening pneumonitis	Bronchoalveolar lavage, lung biopsy	Prophylaxis: Low-dose oral trimethoprim/ sulfamethoxazole, dapsone, or pentamidine. Therapy: High-dose intravenous trimethoprim/ sulfamethoxazole
Candida	Local mucous membrane, invasive tissue infection, fungemia	Blood, fluid, and tissue cultures, fundoscopic examination	Prophylaxis: Fluconazole, in very-high-risk patients possibly lipid formulation of amphotericin B. Therapy: Fluconazole (for sensitive candidal species) or lipid formulation of amphotericin B, caspofungin, or voriconazole (insensitive Candida or Aspergillus)
Aspergillus	Entry via upper or lower respiratory tract with metastatic spread (central nervous system, intraabdominal, solid organ)	Blood, fluid, and tissue cultures, Bronchoalveolar lavage, CT scans	
Bacteria	Gram-negative: Enterobacteriaceae, Escherichia coli, Pseudomonas. Gram-positive: Enterococcus, Staphylococcus	Blood, fluid, and tissue cultures. Bronchoalveolar lavage, CT scans, surgical exploration	Varies

Fungal infections occurring months to years after transplantation are unusual and are more commonly the atypical or endemic organisms, such as *Cryptococcus, Mucor, Blastomyces,* or *Coccidioides* species. Viral infections are the most common infections after the early posttransplant period. CMV and EBV infections account for the vast majority of opportunistic viral infections. Overall reduction and more selective immunosuppression and prophylaxis with ganciclovir have reduced the incidence and morbidity of these infections. The other agents responsible for infectious morbidity, their presentation, diagnosis, and treatment are included in Table 126.1.

Of particular importance in children is the prophylaxis and effective treatment of EBV. This is associated with the development of numerous malignant consequences, the most common of which is a diffuse proliferation of lymphoid tissue known as posttransplant lymphoproliferative disorder. This disorder can present as a mononucleosis-like syndrome with diffuse lymphadenopathy or as lymphoma involving any organ. A variety of other tumours are also associated with EBV infections. The general therapy for posttransplant lymphoproliferative disorder is reduction or elimination of immunosuppression and, occasionally, surgical intervention and/or chemotherapy. The complete discussion of these disorders is beyond the scope of this chapter.

Outcome

Numerous factors are known to impact patient and graft survival in children after liver transplantation. Overall, survival has improved, with 1-year and 5-year patient survival approaching 90% and 80%, respectively, in patients younger than 18 years of age. Age, nutritional status, urgency of transplantation, the indication for transplantation, and presence of renal dysfunction are all major factors that determine outcome. Whereas early data have suggested that patients with biliary atresia have worse outcomes due to their often malnourished state, young age, and previous surgical intervention, more recent data suggest that this difference is not significant. Patients with metabolic disease do exceedingly well because they often are older, do not have liver failure and its sequelae, and have not previously undergone an abdominal operation. Finally, transplantation for malignancy in children is associated with survival that is substantially below average but much better than the natural history of the disease. Numerous large series exist in the literature detailing the improvement in outcome with experience.

Although outcomes have improved, many issues remain to be resolved. The first and foremost is organ shortage. The number of listed patients awaiting liver transplantation is increasing steadily, whereas the number of suitable donors, even with segmental liver transplantation, has plateaued. Strategies aimed at expanding the donor pool and allocating organs to those patients who have not only the greatest survival benefit compared with pretransplant survival but also the greatest chance of optimal posttransplant outcome are essential. National policies aimed at effectively identifying donors amenable for organ splitting and development of local, regional, and national sharing of split grafts still await refinement.

Finally, the development of gene therapy or optimisation of hepatocyte transplantation as alternatives to whole organ transplantation for metabolic diseases may alleviate some of the current organ shortage.

Another important challenge for the liver transplantation community is the perfection of immunosuppression. Currently, all immunosuppressive agents have long-term side effects that result in impaired growth and development, infectious morbidity, malignancies, and numerous medical complications, including renal failure. The development of drug therapy that minimises or eliminates these complications is essential. Furthermore, a better understanding of the immunology of peripheral T-cell tolerance and chronic rejection is important. Although the past decade has witnessed improvements in many technical and immunosuppressive aspects of liver transplantation, improvements

in survival and QOL in the next decade will rest firmly on a better understanding of the human immune system on cellular and molecular levels. The quest to achieve immunotolerance has been elusive.

Intestinal Transplantation

Patients with intestinal failure (IF) will not be able to maintain a normal state of nutrition, fluid and electrolyte balance, nor normal growth and development. Because total parenteral nutrition (TPN) is only a supportive modality that does not restore normal intestinal function, it is not a cure for IF. Besides, TPN is an expensive modality and has many serious long-term complications.

The prognosis for patients who develop severe complications from parenteral nutrition is poor. In this category of patients, it should be stressed that intestinal transplantation (ITx) is the only life-saving treatment with an unequivocal and well-proven survival advantage. The problem, however, is that all too often, transplant surgeons are confronted with patients being referred to ITx too late and in extremely bad general condition.

Historical Aspect

The experimental era of ITx was initiated by Lellehei and associates in 1959, and the transplantation of a multivisceral composite graft was performed by Thomas E. Starzl in 1960. The 1960s and 1970s saw nine published attempts of human ITx under the standard immunosuppression of that era (steroids, azathioprine, antilymphocyte globulin), but with disheartening outcomes.

Under the era of cyclosporine, the first successful human multivisceral transplantation by Starzl and associates was performed in 1987. Then, in 1988, the transplantation of the first isolated intestinal allograft from a live donor was performed, followed by the first combined liver-intestinal transplantation by Grant and colleagues.

In 1989, with the use of tacrolimus, reports of series of patients undergoing successful ITx were first published. Today, tacrolimus is considered the mainstay of most immunotherapeutic regimens for recipients of ITx.

Indications for Small Bowel Transplantation

Intestinal failure can have life-threatening complications, have high morbidity and poor QOL, or result in early death despite optimal parenteral nutrition (PN). Indications for transplantation due to these consequences are the following:

- Intestinal failure with life-threatening complications:
  - TPN-induced liver disease;
  - recurring catheter related sepsis;
  - impending loss of central venous access; or
  - frequent episodes of severe dehydration despite intravenous fluid in addition to home parenteral nutrition (HPN).
- Intestinal failure with high morbidity and poor QOL:
  - frequent/chronic hospitalisations;
  - narcotic dependency;
  - inability to function (i.e., pseudo-obstruction, high output stoma); or
  - patient's unwillingness to accept long-term HPN.
- Intestinal failure virtually resulting in early death despite optimal PN:
  - extremely short bowel syndrome;
  - congenital intractable mucosal disorder; or
  - desmoid tumours associated with familial adenomatous polyposis.

Contraindications for Small Bowel Transplantation

Contraindications for small bowel transplantation can be absolute or relative. Absolute contraindications include:

- nonresectable malignancy (local or metastatic);

- severe congenital or acquired immunological deficiencies;

- advanced cardiopulmonary disease;

- advanced neurological dysfunction;

- major psychiatric illness;

- sepsis with multisystem organ failure;

- multisystem autoimmune diseases;

- life-threatening and other noncorrectable illnesses not related to the digestive system;

- demonstrated patient noncompliance with medical recommendations; and

- insufficient vascular patency for central venous access for up to 6 months following ITx.

Relative contraindications include:

- history of cancer in the past 5 years;

- physical debilitation;

- lack of family support;

- infants weighing less than 5 kg; and

- multiple previous abdominal surgical procedures.

Donor Selection and Preparation

The selection of a donor for ITx is based on ABO blood type, organ size compatibility, and virus serological results. Human leukocyte antigen (HLA) typing and cytotoxic crossmatch have not been universally adopted to the selection criteria. Preparation of the graft is done by administration of gut decontaminant solution (amphotericin B, polymixin B, gentamycin) through a nasogastric tube and intravenous antibiotics; this should be done as soon as possible.

Candidate Evaluation

A thorough and comprehensive multidisciplinary evaluation of patients with intestinal failure is essential to assess appropriate candidacy for transplantation and provide the best possible outcome for these complex patients. Candidates must be assessed from surgical, medical, and psychosocial perspectives by the transplant team and various consultants.

Living-Donor Intestinal Transplantation

The role of living-donor intestinal transplantation (LDITx) is not as well defined, mostly due to limited experience with the procedure.

The potential advantages of LDITx include the elimination of waiting time; minimisation of cold ischaemia time; better preservation of mucosal integrity; reduction of the risk of systemic sepsis from bacterial translocation; better HLA matching, reducing the risk of acute rejection; an elective surgery setting with shorter hospitalisation stays; and fewer hospital readmissions than reported following cadaveric ITx. The main disadvantage is the operative risk for the donor and the potential problems associated with the use of a shorter graft.

The donor's safety is the most important consideration in LDITx. The operative risk of a healthy adult undergoing elective segmental bowel resection is quite low—surely comparable to the risks taken by a living kidney donor for elective nephrectomy, and inferior to the risk of right hepatectomy for adult-to-adult living-donor liver transplant.

Operative Procedures

The fundamental strategy of multivisceral organ retrieval focuses on isolating the organs that will be procured for each individual recipient, and core cooling them with an infusion of a preservation solution (the University of Wisconsin solution). Multivisceral on-block retrieval, which includes the stomach, duodenum, pancreas, liver, and small intestine, is the parent operation, which bases its blood supply on the celiac and superior mesenteric arteries.

Five general graft options are available for ITx candidates, depending on the integrity of the remnant gastrointestinal tract and the status of the other visceral organs:

- isolated bowel consisting of all or part of the jejunoileum;

- combined liver and intestinal graft;

- multivisceral graft consisting of the liver, stomach, pancreas, duodenum, and jejunoileum;

- modified multivisceral graft to include the previous option without the liver; or

- isolated liver graft.

Isolated intestinal transplant

The basic steps for an isolated intestinal transplant procedure are as follows:

Step 1: Donor operation (organ procurement, cadaveric):

- The aorta and inferior vena cava (IVC) and mesentery root are exposed retroperitoneal.

- The infrarenal aorta is cannulated and systemic heparinisation is carried out.

- The IVC above the diaphragm is sectioned and the thoracic aorta is cross-clamped.

- The visceral organs are perfused with cold preservation solution.

- The entire intestine is mobilised and the duodenum and distal ileum are stapled.

- The superior mesenteric artery (SMA) and superior mesenteric vein (SMV) are dissected and divided.

- The liver, small bowel (SB), pancreas, and spleen are removed en bloc.

Step 2: Back-table preparation and core cooling with an infusion of the preservation solution:

- The liver is separated.

- The SMA is dissected until the first jejunal branch.

- The celiac trunk is dissected and the splenic artery is divided.

- The bile duct is divided at the superior aspect of the head of the pancreas.

- The SMV and portal vein are dissected.

- The neck of the pancreas is divided.

- The splenic vein is ligated and divided.

- The anterior surface of the portal vein and distal end of the bowel are marked.

Step 3: Recipient operation (implantation of the graft with establishment of vascular anastomosis and gastrointestinal tract (GIT) reconstruction) involves the following:

- arterial inflow: SMA versus infrarenal aorta;

- venous outflow: portal (SMV or portal vein) versus systemic (IVC or left renal vein);

- GIT reconstruction: proximal and distal anastomosis with creation of a proximal stoma;

- biliary reconstruction; and

- a double lumen gastrojejunostomy tube.

Combined liver and intestinal transplant

The basic steps for a combined liver and intestinal transplant procedure are as follows:

Step 1: Donor operation (organ procurement):

- The organs are procured en bloc with preservation of the celiac artery and SMA with a Carrel patch of the aorta.

- IVC is divided just above the diaphragm suprahepatic and just above the renal veins infrahepatic.

Step 2: Back-table operation and core cooling with an infusion of the preservation solution:

- The Carrel patch is anastomosed to a conduit of the donor thoracic aorta.

Step 3: Recipient operation (implantation of the graft with establishment of vascular anastomosis and GIT reconstruction) involves the following:

- removing the diseased organs;
- donor aortic conduit anastomosed end-to-side with recipient aorta;
- donor suprahepatic IVC anastomosed to recipient hepatic veins;
- portal vein anastomosis;
- reperfusion; and
- GIT and biliary reconstruction.

Multivisceral transplantation

Multivisceral transplantation has the following features:

- The abdominal exenteration results in a larger cavity for the new graft.
- There are fewer vascular and enteric anastomoses.
- The vascular inflow to the multivisceral graft can be obtained either from the infra- or suprarenal aorta.
- The outflow of the graft is via the suprahepatic vena cava of the donor.

For a living-related donor for intestinal transplantation, the procedure includes:

- A 150–180-cm graft of small bowel is measured, starting 20 cm from the ileocaecal valve (ICV), making sure to leave at least 60% of the small bowel for the donor.
- Arterial inflow is through the terminal branch of the SMA just distal to the take-off of the ileocaecal branch, with its vein next to it.

Postoperative Management

Medical

Immediately postoperative, the patient is transferred to the paediatric intensive care unit (PICU) where meticulous assessment should include respiratory status, oxygenation and ventilation, fluid status, cardiovascular status, renal function, neurological status, electrolyte balance, surgical dressings and drains, any bleeding, pain management, and medication administration. Frequent monitoring of vital signs and obtaining blood for laboratory tests is also done. Doppler US is routinely performed on postoperative day 1 to assess vessel patency or as clinically indicated.

The intermediate phase of care begins approximately 7 or 8 days after transplantation. By this time, most patients have been extubated, have had most monitoring lines removed, and have been stabilised enough to transfer to the paediatric step-down unit. The assessment continues to cover the major organ systems.

Immunosuppression

Over the past decade, new potent immunosuppressives have become available. The introduction of tacrolimus has improved patient and graft survival rates and continues to be the cornerstone of most immunosuppressive regimens after ITx.

Most successful immunosuppressive regimens currently are based on tacrolimus and steroid therapy. Several centres are adding third agents to this cocktail to improve success. Still, rejection, infection, and immunosuppressive-related side effects are common. These issues have driven efforts towards the development of newer, novel immunotherapeutic protocols. The most promising current protocols involve the addition of the interleukin-2 receptor antagonist, sirolimus, rabbit antithymocyte globulin, and alemtuzumab.

Monitoring of the graft function

Monitoring of the graft function is clinically in the first line. Symptoms of graft dysfunction are ballooned abdomen, abdominal pain, liquid diarrhoea, vomiting or ileus, and dark purple color of graft mucosa. Further diagnostic examination contains an endoscopic inspection of the graft with serial biopsies. Endoscopic access is via the grafts ileostomy. During the early postoperative phase, graft endoscopies are performed twice weekly.

A helpful development was the introduction of zoom endoscopy, which allows better macroscopic inspection of the villus. An intestinal contrast media passage is performed at postoperative day 4 or 5 to verify patency of the gastrointestinal anastomoses. At present, specific parameters for monitoring of intestinal graft function are currently not available. Thus, laboratory chemistry is restricted to routine parameters.

Postoperative Complications

Rejection

After sepsis, rejection is the second most common cause of death in small bowel transplant recipients, but it is the primary reason for graft loss. In practice, rejection and infection often occur simultaneously, and it may be difficult to determine which one is the dominant pathologic process.

Higher immunosuppressive maintenance therapy in the intestinal transplanted patient increases the risk of infection, tacrolimus-induced nephrotoxicity, and posttransplant lymphoproliferative disorder (PTLD).

The clinical presentations of acute rejection include fever, diarrhoea, malabsorption, bloody ostomy drainage, paralytic ileus, or an increase in liver function tests. Fever is the most common presentation. Diarrhoea is also a common manifestation of acute rejection. The amount of ostomy output should be monitored closely. A significant decrease in ostomy output, however, can also reflect rejection because bowel motility can be suppressed by rejection, similar to paralytic ileus.

Acute episodes of rejection occur early posttransplant, mostly within the first 6 months, and then decline rapidly with very few episodes observed past 2 years after transplant.

An assessment of acute rejection in ITx is based primarily on pathological findings found on multiple biopsies taken during endoscopic survey. Endoscopy and biopsies should be performed twice weekly during the patient's initial 2-3 weeks posttransplant hospitalisation, then weekly over the next 3 months, and then monthly until stoma closure. During the course of any rejection, biopsies should be performed at least twice a week.

Prevention and treatment of rejection are the most difficult and most important dilemmas in clinical intestinal transplantation. Early detection of rejection and timely initiation of treatment are critically important for intestinal transplant recipients. The recent introduction of daclizumab as a third agent to be administered with corticosteroids and tacrolimus for induction therapy has improved early postoperative outcomes.

Treatments for acute rejection include augmentation with steroids, upward adjustment of the tacrolimus level, or the use of antilymphocyte antibody immunosuppression, such as OKT-3.

Infections

Infection is a significant postoperative complication with any solid organ transplant patient due to the use of immunosuppressive medication to control rejection. As noted earlier, immunosuppression is kept at higher levels within these intestinal transplanted patients to decrease episodes and severity of rejection. This increases the risk of infection. The literature reports that 91% of transplant recipients developed infectious complications within the first year of transplantation.

Posttransplant lymphoproliferative disease

PTLD is the most common cause of late graft loss in ITx. This high incidence of PTLD in ITx recipients is likely related to the high level of immunosuppression in these patients and possibly from the high lymphoid cell content in the intestinal allograft.

The term "EBV-associated PTLD" is used to include all clinical syndromes associated with EBV-driven lymphoproliferation, ranging from a benign self-limited form of polyclonal proliferation to true malignancies containing clonal chromosomal abnormalities. Pathology remains the gold standard for PTLD diagnosis.

In the absence of reliably effective therapy for all stages of PTLD, the optimal strategy for management is currently focused on prevention. Recommended strategies for prevention are identification of the patient at high risk for PTLD development prior to transplant to be adequately monitored. Aggressive immunosuppression should be employed only in the presence of biopsy-proven acute rejectiManagement includes reducing immunosuppression, surgical resection, local irradiation, antiviral agents (acyclovir, ganciclovir), and passive antibody (intravenous immunoglobulin, or IVIG). When reduction in immunosuppression fails, anti-CD20 antibody (e.g., rituximab) represents an attractive second-line therapeutic option because of its low toxicity.

Graft versus host disease

Graft versus host disease (GVHD) occurs when immunocompetent donor lymphoid cells damage recipient tissues after allogeneic transplantation. The major targets are epithelial cells of the skin, intestine, and liver. This complication had been anticipated after clinical intestinal transplantation because the large inoculum of lymphoid cells in a small bowel graft was predicted to increase the likelihood of this disease. The diagnosis of GVHD is based on clinical presentation and includes a skin biopsy for histopathological confirmation.

The development of GVHD is almost always associated with a low level of immunosuppressive agents, and patients usually respond well to the augmented immunosuppression.

Other postoperative complications

Other postoperative complications include recurrence of the original disease and preservation and reperfusion injury.

Surgical Complications

Surgical complications that need emergency operations are graft duodenal stump leaks, spontaneous small bowel perforations, abdominal compartment syndrome, acute bowel obstruction, wound dehiscence, biliary stricture, reflux at esophagogastrostomy, pancreatitis, intraabdominal haemorrhage, intraabdominal abscess, and anastomotic leaks occurring at the coloanal and esophageal anastomosis leading to peritonitis. Graft-associated vascular complications include hepatic artery thrombosis, disruption of the aortic anastomosis, portal vein stenosis, and chylous ascites.

Outcome and Quality of Life

The University of Pittsburgh Medical Center has the largest single experience in transplantation worldwide; the present transplant rate exceeds 60 cases per year. Their latest reported figures showed a 1-year patient survival of 92% in 89 patients transplanted between 2001 and 2003. The numbers of successful intestinal transplants that are now more than 10 years posttransplant are accumulating, with the longest survivor now approaching 15 years posttransplant.

Following transplantation, overall QOL improved significantly; there was an average improvement in all the parameters in patients following transplantation; and significant improvements were seen in psychological, physical, and social aspects.

Survival of intestinal transplant recipients can be expected to improve further with earlier referral, as the procedure is more successful when patients are transplanted from home. Successful outcome should not be judged on survival alone, however. It is reasonable to know whether the quality of the extended life is good, thus justifying the stress of further surgery and hospitalisation.

Evidence-Based Research

Table 126.2 presents a study on health-related quality of life (HRQOL) for liver transplantation children younger than 5 years of age, comparing those with living-related and cadaveric donor liver transplantation (CDLT).

Table 126.2: Evidence-based research.

Title	Impact of liver transplantation on HRQOL in children less than 5 years old
Authors	Cole CR, Bucuvalas JC, Hornung RW, Ryckman FC, et al.
Reference	Pediatric Transplantation 2004; 8:222–227
Problem	Assess health-related quality of life (HRQOL) score in comparison to type of liver transplantation whether cadaveric or living-related.
Intervention	adaveric donor liver transplantation (CDLT), living-related liver transplantation (LRLT)
Comparison/ control (quality of evidence)	HRQOL scores were determined before and one year after transplantation. In addition, demographic and clinical factors associated with QOL were assessed during the period of the study, which was between October 1997 and January 2002.
Outcome/ effect	The baseline infant-toddler health status questionnaire (ITHQ) subscale score was greatest for global mental health (GlobalMH); the score improved significantly during the first 6 months after transplantation, and the score steadily improved over the rest of the first year. The ITHQ subscale score at baseline was similar for children receiving CDLT and those receiving LRLT. Children with biliary atresia had lower baseline scores than those with other diagnoses. Multivariant analysis conducted to identify independent predictors of the ITHQ subscale score revealed that donor type had no effect on QOL parameters.
Historical significance/ comments	This report on assessment of HRQOL in children younger than 5 years of age receiving liver transplantation emphasized that the functional health of children who received LDLT was similar to that of children who received CDLT.

Further analysis showed that functional health improves with time elapsed since transplantation in both groups. These results are similar to those obtained in older children (>5 years of age) who underwent liver transplantation. In this study, age at transplant had a negative effect on the impact of the illness on the patient. Age at transplantation did not affect any of the other scales of ITHQ. GlobalMH improved with an increase in the number of inpatient hospital days.

The study had several limitations: (1) basing the study on the experience of a single paediatric liver transplant program limited its sample size and statistical power; (2) all demographic characteristics of families are representative of the population referred to that institution for transplantation but may not reflect those at other centres; and (3) the bias of the parents in completing the questionnaire.

The authors concluded that HRQOL improves after transplantation in all of their patients irrespective of the donor type. As the number of paediatric patients who receive liver transplantation increases, it is important for health care providers and families to be aware of HRQOL improvements. Functional health, clinical outcome and cost must be part of the discussion between caregivers, health professionals, policy makers, and third-party payers.

Assessment of HRQOL should be an integral part of the care of liver transplant patients and their caregivers. |

Key Summary Points

1. Paediatric transplantation is considered one of the difficult tasks to be achieved in the African continent due to lack of resources, cadaveric programs, and technical facilities, as well as delayed referral of cases.

2. Liver transplantation is now the standard treatment for end-stage liver disease in children.

3. Extrahepatic biliary atresia is the main indication for paediatric liver transplantation, constituting 60–70% of the indications.

4. Malnutrition, vaccination problems, and long waiting lists are major pretransplant issues still to be addressed.

5. Small-sized vessels, donor-recipient size mismatch, and previous surgeries are all technical difficulties unique to paediatric liver transplantation.

6. Vascular complications, especially hepatic artery thrombosis, are not still considered a major problem.

7. Although biliary complications are frequent in paediatric living-related transplantation, they are not associated with decreased patient survival.

8. In children, morbidity and mortality rates from infections exceed those from rejection after transplant, and immunosuppression can hinder growth, renal function, and graft tolerance.

9. Intestinal transplantation is a more advanced procedure, with mainly cadaveric donors.

10. Liver and intestine or en bloc transplantation has better results than intestinal alone.

11. Both infection and rejection contribute to the lower success rate of combined liver and intestine or en bloc transplantation compared to liver transplantation.

Suggested Reading

Abu-Elmagd K, Bond G, Mazariegos G, et al. A new tolergenic immunosuppressive strategy for human intestinal transplantation. Transplantation 2004; 78:58.

Andersen D, DeVoll-Zabrocki A, Brown C, et al. Intestinal Transplantation in pediatric patients: a nursing challenge, part two: intestinal transplantation and the immediate postoperative period. Society of Gastroenterology Nurses & Associates, 2000; 23(5):201–209.

Barshes NR, Lee TC, Udell IW, O'Mahoney CA, Karpen SJ, Carter BA, et al. The pediatric end-stage liver disease (PELD) model as a predictor of survival benefit and posttransplant survival in pediatric liver transplant recipients. Liver Transplantation 2006; 12:475–480.

Beath SV, Goyet JV, Kelly DA, et al. Current opinion in organ risk factors for death and graft loss after small bowel transplantation. Transplant 2003; 8:195–201.

Benedetti E, Testa G. Living donor intestinal transplantation in pediatric recipients. Curr Opin Organ Transplant 2006; 11:543–545.

Braun F, Broering D, Faendrich F. Small intestine transplantation today. Arch Surg 2007; 392:227–238.

Braun F, Platz K, Faendrich F, et al. Dünndarmtransplantation. In: Siewert JR, Rothmund M, Schumpelick V, eds. Praxis der Viszeralchirurgie. Springer, 2006; Pp 415–429.

Bueno J, Abu-Elmagd K, Mazariegos G, et al. Composite liver-small bowel allografts with preservation of donor duodenum and hepatic biliary system in children. J Pediatr Surg 2000; 35:291–296.

Busuttil RW, Farmer DG, Yersiz H, Hiatt JR, McDiarmid SV, Goldstein LI, et al. Analysis of long-term outcomes of 3200 liver transplantations over two decades: a single-center experience. Ann Surg 2005; 241:905–916.

Carmody IC, Farmer DG. Indications for small bowel transplantation in the new millennium. Curr Opin Organ Transplant 2003; 8:190–194.

Cockfield SM. Identifying the patient at risk for post-transplant lymphoproliferative disorder. Transpl Infect Dis 2001; 3:70–78.

Colombani PM, Dunn SP, Harmon WB, et al. Pediatric transplantation. Am Transplant 2003; 3(Suppl 4):53–63.

Deltz E, Schroeder P, Gebhard H, et al. Successful clinical small bowel transplantation: report of a case. Clin Transplant 1989; 21: 89–91.

Farmer DG. Clinical immunosuppression for intestinal transplantation. Curr Opin Organ Transplant 2004; 9:214–219.

Farmer DG, Gordon SA. Intestinal transplantation. In: O'Neill JA, Coran AG, Fonkalsrud E, Grosfeld JL, eds. Pediatric Surgery. Elsevier, 2006; Pp 742–753.

Farmer DG, Venick RS, McDiarmid SV, Ghobrial RM, Gordon SA, Yersiz H, et al. Predictors of outcomes after pediatric liver transplantation: an analysis of more than 800 cases performed at a single institution. J Am Coll Surg 2007; 204:904–914.

Fishbein TM, Matsumoto CS. Regimens for intestinal transplant immunosuppression. Curr Opin Organ Transplant 2005; 10:120–123.

Fishbein TM, Gondolesi GE, Kaufman SS. Intestinal transplantation for gut failure. Gastroenterol 2003; 124:1615–1628.

Fryer JP. Intestinal transplantation: an update. Curr Opin Gastroenterol 2005; 21:162–168.

Ganschow R, Nolkemper D, Helmke K, Harps E, Commentz JC, Broering DC, et al. Intensive care management after pediatric liver transplant: a single-center experience. Pediatr Transplant 2000; 4:273–279.

Goss JA, Shackleton CR, McDiarmid SV, et al. Long-term results of pediatric liver transplantation: an analysis of 569 transplants. Ann Surg 1998; 228:411–420.

Grant D, Wall W, Mineualt R, et al. Successful small bowel/liver transplantation. Lancet 1990; 335:181–184.

Green M. Management of Epstein-Barr virus–induced post-transplant lymphoproliferative disease in recipients of solid organ transplantation. Am J Transplant 2001; 1:103–108.

Karakayali H, Boyvat F, Sevmiş S, Dalgiç A, Moray G, Emiroğlu R, et al. Biliary complications and their management in pediatric liver transplantations: one center's experience. Transplant Proc 2005; 37: 3174–3176.

Kato T. New techniques for prevention and treatment of rejection in intestinal transplantation. Curr Opin Organ Transplant 2000; 5:284–289.

Kato T, Ruiz P, Thompson JF, et al. Intestinal and multivisceral transplantation. World J Surg 2002; 26:226–237.

Kato T, Tzakis A, Selvaggi G, et al. Surgical techniques used in intestinal transplantation. Curr Opinion Organ Transplant 2004; 9:207–213.

Lee RG, Nakamura K, Tsamandas AC, et al. Pathology of human intestinal transplantation. Gastroenterol 1996; 110:1820–1834.

Mazariegos GV, Abu-Elmagd K, Jaffe R, et al. Graft versus host disease in intestinal transplantation. Am J Transpl 2004; 4:1459–1465.

McAllister VC; Grant DR. Clinical small bowel transplantation. In: Grant DR, Woods RFM, eds. Small Bowel Transplantation. Edward Arnold, 1994, Pp 121–132.

Nalesnik MA. The diverse pathology of post-transplant lymphoproliferative disorders: the importance of a standardized approach. Transpl Infect Dis 2001; 3:88–96.

O'Keefe S, Emerling M, Koritsky D, et al. Nutrition and quality of life following small intestinal transplantation. Am J Gastroenterol 2007; 102:1093–1100.

Oertel SHK, Verschuuren E, Reinke P, et al. Effect of anti-CD 20 antibody rituximab in patients with post-transplant lymphoproliferative disorder (PTLD). Am J Transpl 2005; 5:2901–2906.

Paya CV, Fung JJ, Nalesnik MA, et al. Epstein-Barr virus–induced posttransplant lymphoproliferative disorders. ASTS/ASTP EBV-PTLD Task Force and The Mayo Clinic Organized International Consensus Development Meeting. Transplantation 1999; 68:1517–1525.

Pirenne J, Hoffman I, Miserez M, et al. Selection criteria and outcome of patients referred to intestinal transplantation: an European center experience. Transplant Proc 2006; 38:1671–1672.

Pirenne J, Koshiba T, Coosemans W, et al. Recent advances and future prospects in intestinal and multi-visceral transplantation. Pediatr Transplant 2001; 5:452–456.

Pironi L, Hébuterne X, Gossum AV, et al.; Candidates for intestinal transplantation: a multicenter survey in Europe. Am J Gastroenterol 2006; 101:1633–1643.

Preiksaitis JK, Keay S. Diagnosis and management of posttransplant lymphoproliferative disorder in solid-organ transplant recipients. Clin Infect Dis 2001; 33:38–46.

Reyes J, Bueno J, Kocoshis S, et al. Current status of intestinal transplantation in children. J Pediatr Surg 1998; 33:243–254.

Reyes J, Green M, Bueno J, et al. Epstein-Barr virus associated posttransplant lymphoproliferative disease after intestinal transplantation. Transplant Proc 1996; 28: 2768–2769.

Reyes J, Mazariegos GV, Bond GMD, et al. Pediatric intestinal transplantation: Historical notes, principles and controversies. Pediatr Transplant 2002; 6:193–207.

Schafer DF. Liver transplantation. Looking back, looking forward. In: Maddrey WC, Schiff ER, Sorrell MF, eds. Transplantation of the Liver. Lippincott, Williams, & Wilkins, 2001, Pp 1244–1360.

Selvaggi G, Kato T, Gaynor JJ, et al. Analysis of rejection episodes in over 100 pediatric intestinal transplant recipients. Transplant Proc 2006; 38:1711–1712.

Starzl TE, Rowe MI, Todo S, et al. Transplantation of multiple abdominal viscera. JAMA 1989; 261:1449–1458.

Testa G, Panaro F, Schena S, et al. Living related small bowel transplantation donor surgical technique. Ann Surg 2004; 240:779–784.

Tzakis AG, Kato T, Levi DM, et al. 100 multivisceral transplants at a single center. Ann Surg 2005; 242:480–493.

CHAPTER 127
TELEMEDICINE AND E-HEALTH

Franklin C. Margaron
David A. Lanning
Dan Poenaru
Maurice Mars
Ronald Merrell

Introduction

The challenges facing Africa in delivering high-quality paediatric surgical care during the next century are great. Overcoming poverty, difficult access to medical care, governmental instability, lack of trained physicians, and a large burden of existing and emerging diseases all appear at times insurmountable. In September 2000, the largest gathering of heads of state ever held, including leaders from 189 countries, adopted the Millennium Declaration with eight Millennium Development Goals (MDGs) as a blueprint to accomplish by the year 2015.[1] These include progress in ending poverty and hunger; addressing universal education, gender equality, child health, and maternal health; combatting HIV/AIDS; and working toward environmental sustainability and global partnership. The MDG update report for 2008 shows that Africa continues to have the largest need of any continent in the world, and is making only minimal progress in meeting its goals.[2]

Medical diagnostics and therapeutics are becoming more advanced daily, creating a larger gap between services possible in the industrialised world and those available to most Africans. The physician in Africa is forced to work between two worlds: one of technologic advancement and voluminous medical information and one of limited resources and profound medical need. How can the modern African surgeon bridge this gap? Appropriately applied technology can provide part of the solution. Information and communication technologies continue to undergo a revolution, making instant access to remote locations easier and less expensive. Telemedicine utilises these technologies to bring medical information and services to geographically or physically isolated people who would not otherwise be able to reach a physician. Perhaps the greatest utility of these technologies is in the developing world, where the disparity between access and need is the largest. The World Health Organization (WHO) has recognised the capacity of telemedicine to increase health care information and delivery. WHO recommends that all their member states should:

> integrate the appropriate use of health telematics in the overall policy and strategy for the attainment of health for all in the 21st century, thus fulfilling the vision of a world in which the benefits of science, technology and public health development are made equitably available to all people everywhere.[3]

The Africa Health Infoway is the current initiative of WHO to provide a technology platform that supports the collection of subnational health data and statistics for analysis, dissemination, and use to facilitate decision making in health and to strengthen the capacity of African countries to use information in decision making.[4] WHO is working in collaboration with the International Telecommunication Union (ITU), Digital Solidarity Fund, Telemedicine Task Force, and others to establish telemedicine infrastructure, district health information systems, and e-health applications to improve health care delivery in Africa. Specific emphasis is being directed to remote areas. Having an understanding of the terminology, functioning, and applications of telemedicine is of great importance for the African surgeon. This chapter is written as an introduction to that knowledge.

Definition of Telemedicine

Telemedicine is the delivery of health care and the exchange of health care information across distances.[5] Information, rather than the individuals, is moved from one place to another. Analog voice and video are fading from use, although we may continue to rely upon handwritten messages—the modern information mode is digital. The capture and exchange of digital information is enabled by the targeted use of medical recording devices and communication technologies. Telemedicine is not a new form of medicine or a separate specialty; rather, it is technology applied to the entire scope of current medical activities to link one location to another. Telemedicine finds application in clinical evaluation of patients, physician consultation, continuing education for health care providers and the public, administrative tasks, and research. The term "telecare" refers to telemedical applications to deliver services to chronic or debilitated patients at home or in specialised care centres. An argument has been made for utilisation of the term "telehealth" to include public health ventures and other health professionals such as community health workers and psychologists.[6,7] The term "e-health" has also gained some favor to include medical applications utilising the Internet.[8]

History

Over the years, telemedicine has mirrored the development of communications technology. In the mid-19th century, the telegraph was utilised to convey casualty information and order medical supplies during the American Civil War.[5] The telephone was introduced in the late 19th century, and it immediately found widespread telemedical application. Radio medical consultation occurred as early as 1920 through the Seaman's Church Institute of New York to provide medical advice to seafarers. The International Radio Medical Centre (CIRM), which was set up in 1935, became the largest organisation to provide maritime radio telemedicine. In its first 60 years, CIRM gave medical assistance to more than 42,000 patients at sea.[9]

The introduction of the television became a new source of inspiration for distance medicine. In the United States in 1964, the Nebraska Psychiatric Institute in Omaha set up a two-way closed-circuit television link to Norfolk State Hospital, 180 km away.[10] This was utilised for education and consultations between specialists and general practitioners. Another example was the Massachusetts General Hospital/Logan International Airport Medical Station established in 1967, which accomplished a two-way microwave link for medical care of passengers and airport employees 24 hours a day.[11] Satellite communications were first utilised in 1971 by the Alaska ATS-6 Biomedical Demonstration, which worked to improve village health in Alaska by using satellite-mediated video consultation.[12]

Initially, telemedical applications were expensive and required the funding of large high-tech ventures such as the space explorations of the National Aeronautics and Space Administration (NASA) in the United States. These applications were targeted for the monitoring and care of their own astronauts, but were also expanded very early to meet the medical needs of rural populations, such as the Papago Indian Reservation in Arizona in 1972.[13] NASA was also involved in the first international telemedicine programme in 1989 through the Space Bridge to Armenia and Ufa.[7] This project was initiated following a massive earthquake that hit the Soviet Republic of Armenia. It demonstrated the utility of telemedicine to cross geographic, cultural, political, and economic distances. Four medical centres in the United States utilised video, voice, and facsimile to deliver telemedicine consultations over a satellite network.

The contributions of many other individuals and organisations, combined with the rapid development of communications technologies, have led to the international explosion of interest and experience with telemedicine over the past 30 years. African telemedicine has seen several successful initiatives, but is still in its infancy. Perhaps the most established telemedicine system in Africa is the Réseau en Afrique Francophone pour la Télémédecine (RAFT).[14] Formed in 2000, RAFT now broadcasts weekly continuing educational sessions, coordinates videoconferences, and facilitates teleconsultations to 10 French-speaking African countries. The future of telemedicine and e-health in Africa is full of promise.

Classification

Telemedicine can be classified by the people involved in the connection, the types of interactions, and the information conveyed. Typical forms of people interactions include clinical evaluation between doctor and patient, clinical consultation between physician and expert, and education between professor and student. Many other forms of communication are possible, such as conferencing for strategic planning or administrative tasks.

Interactions can be either asynchronous (also called store-and-forward) or synchronous (real-time). These forms have their respective benefits and drawbacks.

Asynchronous Telemedicine

Asynchronous applications rely on storing prerecorded digital data, which can be accessed at any time by the recipient. One example is email, which is sent to and stored at a regional network server. Asynchronous telemedicine can be very convenient for both parties because it eliminates the need to coordinate complex schedules, sometimes across time zones, for a live consultation. The systems infrastructure to support it is relatively simple, generally requiring less bandwidth and fewer technical components than synchronous telemedicine. Asynchronous telemedicine also has much lower costs associated with its utility compared to live interactions. Teleradiology, teledermatology, and telepathology are fields of medicine that lend themselves well to this form, as they rely mainly on static images, which can be easily digitised and transferred. Electronic medical records (EMRs) and data reports are also conveyed well asynchronously. Asynchronous technologies have been shown to be feasible, clinically useful, sustainable, and scalable for the developing world.[15,16] Disadvantages of asynchronous telemedicine include delay in response to the question, the impersonal nature of the communication, and the inability for the consultant to affect or manipulate how the data are acquired. Asynchronous technology cannot be the primary modality for emergent situations.

Synchronous Telemedicine

Synchronous telemedicine involves a real-time connection with continuous streaming of data. One simple example of real-time audio telemedicine is through the use of the telephone. This has been widely used for patient evaluation, follow-up, and education. The current advances in mobile phone technologies are exciting, with many potential applications to telemedicine. Mobile phones have already been utilised effectively to convey digital images and electrocardiograms (ECGs). Another example, which many associate most readily with telemedicine, is videoconferencing. This form of telemedicine is effective in

terms of patient consultation and has good patient satisfaction.[17,18] It allows immediate results, and consultants can request missing data with instant response. Real-time consultation also enables greater education to be conveyed from the expert to the recipient. Bergmo has estimated that a general practitioner in rural Norway was able to reduce his referral rate to an ear, nose, and throat (ENT) specialist by 50% in one year based on the improved knowledge acquired through weekly interactions.[19] Drawbacks to videoconferencing technologies include scheduling difficulties, high costs for system acquisition and upkeep, and the larger bandwidth required to support the application.

Types of Telemedicine Data

Data conveyed through telemedicine can be classified into text documents, audio, still images, and video images. All of these forms can be utilised by synchronous or asynchronous technologies. Text documents can be recorded in digital form on an EMR or digitised from paper forms with a document scanner. Audio applications include voice recording through radio, telephone, or video as well as digitised stethoscopes, which can be effective in evaluating heart tones. Still images can include radiographs, ECG tracings, digital photos, pathology slides, and other medical reports. Low-cost digital cameras can be invaluable in data recording. Diagnostic agreement between teledermatology consultations using digital still images and face-to-face consultations have been found to be between 51% and 95%, which is similar to levels of agreement between dermatologists in separate face-to-face examinations.[20] Prerecorded telepathology images have been shown to have a high degree of agreement (97%) versus examination at the microscope.[21] Radiology already has wide applications in telemedicine, and well-established DITEC standards of image quality.[22] Videos are useful for patient exam, and for medical study data such as ultrasound, teaching, and operative recording.

Distance Information Transfer

Transfer of digital data requires a recording device at one end that can encode the information for transfer, a transfer path or "backbone", and a receiving device that can decode the information and display it. Many different technologies have been developed and continue to emerge to facilitate these three phases of distance information transfer.

Data Technology

Digital data are transferred in quantities called bytes (B) and bits (b). A byte of information corresponds roughly to a single character of alphabetical text. Each byte is represented in the computer by 8 binary digits (either 0 or 1) called bits. Thus 5,000 bytes (5 kB) is equivalent to 40,000 bits (40 kb). Telecommunication networks are evaluated by how much data-carrying capacity they have, or their bandwidth, which is measured in bits per second (bps). Bandwidth can range from 1,200 bps for certain mobile phones to more than 1,000 Mbps (1,000 million bps) for fibre-optic cables.[5] The speed of data transmission is based on how much bandwidth is available. As more connections are made through the same server simultaneously, the amount of bandwidth available to any single user decreases. To speed data transfer or accommodate bandwidth, digital data can be compressed to smaller amounts by using algorithms such as those employed by commercial videoconferencing units. This, however, may lower the quality of the video image in order for it to be transmitted in real time. If higher quality is required, either more bandwidth is required for real-time functions or data can be sent asynchronously over a longer time. For many telemedical applications, however, data of adequate quality can be conveyed at very low bandwidth.[23] Compression devices must be compatible on both ends of the link. International standards have been adopted through the ITU to ensure that videoconferencing units from different manufacturers can operate with one another. The common intermediate format (CIF) provides compatibility between the National Television Standards Committee (NTSC) broadcast TV video standards utilised in Japan and

North America and the phase-alternating line (PAL) used in Europe, despite the different display characteristics in these systems.

For a telemedicine connection to be functional, it needs to have adequate bandwidth and be sufficiently reliable. Many possible solutions to the means of data transfer have been developed. The following discussion of the subtypes of data transfer is intended to show that a technical solution to the information problem can exist anywhere in the world. Some technologies lend themselves more strongly to the solution in certain areas.

Standard telephone

Standard older telephone lines operate on an analogue-based public-switched telephone network (PSTN). This technology sets up a one-to-one connection between the ends of the link but has low bandwidth (56 kbps) and is not reliable due to complex mechanisms required for electromechanical switching. In addition, analogue data are lost based on the distance the information has to travel.

Digital data transfer

The advance to digital data transfer used in Integrated Services Digital Networks (ISDN) in many areas of the industrialised world preserved the one-to-one connection of PSTN lines while solving some of its problems. Digital data are not lost or corrupted across distance, do not require electromechanical switching, and offer higher bandwidth. Basic-rate ISDN lines offer a bandwidth of 128 kbps in two separate 64 kbps channels, which are capable of operating basic commercial video-conferencing systems. Three ISDN lines can be aggregated together in a cable to provide bandwidth of 384 kbps, and primary-rate ISDN lines offer a bandwidth of 2 Mbps. ISDN lines are very useful for telemedicine because they are reliable, secure, and have sufficient bandwidth. However, they are not available in most areas of Africa, require significant cables to be run over large distances, and are expensive to operate. Telemedicine can employ such technology only when demand has been created by a wide range of commercial users. Due to these limitations, this is likely not the best solution for development of telemedicine infrastructure for Africa.

Satellite

Satellite connection offers bandwidth similar to that of ISDN and has global coverage with good utility in remote locations. Satellite has traditionally been very expensive to establish and operate, but as technology improves, costs decrease. The Telemedicine Task Force, composed of various African organisations, WHO, the European Commission (EC), and the European Space Agency (ESA) completed an evaluation in sub-Saharan Africa in 2007, finding it the most disenfranchised region in the world with regard to Internet access.[24] The Task Force concluded that complete telemedical coverage of the region could be accomplished by complementing the existing terrestrial infrastructure with satellite communications.

Broadband

With reference to standard telephony, the digital subscriber line (DSL) is often referred to as broadband and provides the user with an Internet protocol (IP) address. It utilises the same copper wires as a telephone to establish a higher bandwidth connection. One limitation is that the connection must be within 5 km of the telephone company switch, as speed drops off with distance. Also, the bandwidth to receive data is much higher than what is available to send data, so it has limited application for videoconferencing.

Wireless

Wireless technology is already finding widespread application in Africa through mobile phones. Currently, digital data transfer on this technology is limited by low bandwidth, similar to the situation with PSTN. Even at this bandwidth, some telemedicine applications are possible. Mobile phone technology has already been used to effectively transmit computed tomography (CT) scans[25] and ECGs,[26,27] evaluate

soft tissue injury,[28] and monitor glucose levels and insulin therapy in diabetics.[29] As mobile third-generation (3G) networks that offer higher bandwidth become established, more applications will be forthcoming. The development of fourth-generation (4G) networks carry bandwidth potential of 100 Mbps or perhaps a Gbps (1,000 Mbps). This can provide comprehensive Internet, voice, text, and video transmission wirelessly, where available. One special aspect of wireless is that it relies on line-of-sight transmission, so there must be a regular tower to pass on the signals. Wireless cannot go through walls unless the transmission energy is appropriately strong. Wireless can bridge back to a satellite transponder or to a suitable fibre-optic cable in larger cities. In terms of cost and utility for rapid telemedicine systems development, wireless technology will likely be the most appropriate solution in developing nations, rather than expanding traditional terrestrial forms such as ISDN. In currently available WiMAX (worldwide interoperability for microwave access) configurations, transmission rates for wireless easily reach a megabit per second (a million bps). WiMAX technology, a telecommunications protocol that provides fixed and fully mobile Internet access, is already available in many parts of Africa, with deep penetration in South Africa and Uganda. We can anticipate significant gains toward at least WiMax, and eventually 4G, for coverage of the continent with dependable and affordable telecommunications.

Asynchronous Transfer Mode takes advantage of fibre-optic cables for very high bandwidth transmission (gigabits per second). Usually this is used for the backbone for major telecommunications carriers for data transfer over large distances. It is not available for user application.

Internet

The Internet is a collection of interconnected worldwide web (WWW) servers that store data for subsequent distribution to users. It is accessed via a modem at the bandwidth of the lines through which it operates. The Internet has limitless application for telemedicine. One of the difficulties with the Internet is limiting access to secured information. Virtual private networks (VPN) or private secure connections between two sites can be established. The limitation is the bandwidth available locally through the Internet service provider (ISP). In 2008, most of the world switched to the next protocol iteration standard, called IPv6. In this Internet agreement, delay at routers is much reduced, and privacy is greatly enhanced by encryption technology inherent to the format. The Internet can easily be made broadband by additional fibre links and can be accessed by satellite.

Voice-over-IP technology is the intersection of Internet and telephony and can convey voice and imaging with great fidelity. Simple Internet access can assure participation in the global knowledge pool of medicine, which doubles every several years. Internet means that medical innovation need not remain out of reach until someone actually travels to the site of the innovation and participates in expensive courses.

Internet email means that the community of medicine can be truly collegial. It allows physicians to contact peers in the region to accumulate information on disease burden or epidemics. Certainly, local experience is pertinent and may be paramount in seeking solutions for one patient or a population. Digitising data allows smaller areas to pool data into larger databases, which may have a higher impact on understanding regional disease patterns. Sometimes it is much more reasonable to contact the surgeon in the next district who shares the same issues and challenges rather than to look for advice from Europe or the United States. However, paediatric surgery is a specialty with certain diseases and congenital malformations that present infrequently. Many of these rarities can be easily treated with the right guidance. Internet email allows a doctor anywhere to contact the best medical centres with the most advanced technology to seek advice on difficult cases.

Implementing a Successful Telemedicine System

Many barriers and problems can exist when implementing a telemedicine system. Programmes have been started with excitement only to see expensive equipment sit idle. Careful planning, clearly defined objectives, and perseverance are necessary for success.[30] A list of helpful guidelines for anyone considering telemedicine applications follows:

1. Be sure technology supports a defined medical need. Purchasing expensive videoconferencing technology is wasteful if the objectives can be met through a simpler technology. American surgical teams visiting Africa have shown low-bandwidth store-and-forward patient descriptions and digital photos have high accuracy and utility for adult and paediatric surgical prescreening.[31] These simple and inexpensive technologies should be the starting point for teleconsultation and network building in the developing world.

2. Become familiar with technology and terminology and facile with such computer applications as Microsoft® Word, Excel, and PowerPoint. Be able to speak authoritatively with decision makers about plans and purchases. Telemedicine input is just as important as advice on the purchase of a new medical device or stocking a new drug. Be the champion and not the victim.

3. Utilise electronic means to record and track your own practice. Electronic charts and digital photos provide a great data resource for patient follow-up, can easily be transferred to email communication for consultation, and can be incorporated into data bases, papers, and presentations.

4. Identify committed individuals at both locations in the consultation link who will champion the effort. If the desire and work is unidirectional, unanswered communication can cause frustration and system failure.

5. Make technology infrastructure simple to use and reliable. All individuals directly involved need to have adequate training on the operating systems. Technical support should also be available. Apprehension about unknown and confusing technology can be a large barrier to some medical professionals becoming involved in telemedicine.

6. Develop good relationships with local government, surrounding hospitals, and remote sites. This is essential. The telecommunications backbone often requires upkeep and upgrading at the governmental level. Be open and honest about intentions and needs.

7. Involve an expert when planning a budget for the project. Expenses for equipment acquisition and setup, communications charges, education, personnel, and data-recording devices need to be included. Reimbursement for services should be established with the consultant. Make clear which expenses are the responsibility of the remote site. Many private and public grants and initiatives for telemedicine are currently targeting sub-Saharan Africa. With clearly defined goals and needs assessments, money can be available to initiate these programmes. This is especially helpful in the initial start-up phase, when the majority of the financial burden exists for equipment acquisition and setup.

8. Look for international efforts that seem to be helpful. If short-term volunteer groups are coming to the area, make the best use of their time by store-and-forward consultation ahead of time to set up an operative plan and list of equipment needs. These groups are an excellent resource for future collaboration and consultation on difficult cases. Make sure that you build relationships through progress reports and follow-up on patients these teams cared for.

9. Take advantage of the many opportunities for virtual networking. Get email addresses of colleagues in the region and communicate frequently, anecdotally and even quantitatively, as you share your experiences, problems, and joy of practice in a virtual community. Contact a professional society with a question. Try the Swinfen Trust for consultation. Send an email to the corresponding author on a paper. Join a telemedicine society.

Tele-education

The Internet provides a platform of instant access to up-to-date medical information, continuing education, video instruction, medical societies, and research. Online publishing is unregulated, so care must be taken to gather information from reputable, peer-reviewed sources of information. Online access to medical societies, full medical texts, and journal articles has in the past been limited in Africa due to the cost of subscriptions.

Health InterNetwork Access to Research Initiative

The Health InterNetwork Access to Research Initiative (HINARI) gives the developing world free or very low-cost online access to peer-reviewed journals in biomedical and related social sciences. HINARI was launched in 2002 by WHO in collaboration with major publishers as well as public and private partners to strengthen public health services by providing access to high-quality, relevant, and timely health information via the Internet to public health workers, researchers, and policy makers.[32] Local, not-for-profit institutions can register for access to journals through HINARI with cost based on the country's annual gross national income (GNI, World Bank figures). Those countries with GNI per capita below US$1,250, which includes many African nations, are eligible for free access. Those institutions in countries with a GNI of US$1,250–3,500 pay a fee of $1,000 per year per institution. The programme has more than 2,500 participating members in 113 countries. More than 100 publishers now give access to more than 5,500 full-text journal titles. The Internet also offers webinars and other websites for information. Because Internet data are not officially regulated, however, not all information is reliable. Professional societies are usually reliable and provide links on their websites to other good resources.

Instructional and continuing education sessions can be established through a real-time video or audio link. This access can provide expertise that would otherwise rarely be available in remote settings.

Information and Communication Technologies

Although widespread adoption of the use of information and communication technologies (ICT) has not occurred in sub-Saharan Africa, isolated examples of sustained use of ICT in health education do exist, which serve as models of what is achievable. The Internet, WWW, and videoconferencing offer seemingly simple solutions to the provision of, and access to, information and teaching for countries with a shortage of doctors. They also offer the potential of telemedicine and learning through case discussion.

Several reasons exist for the lack of technology on the African continent, including restrictive telecommunications' legislation, lack of basic infrastructure, and high telecommunication costs. Although every sub-Saharan African country has Internet access, this is presently mainly in the urban areas. Rural areas, where it is estimated that approximately two-thirds of sub-Saharan Africa's population lives,[33] have only limited access. Internet penetration for the continent is 11%, and for sub-Saharan Africa, it is 7%.[34] Broadband penetration is about 1%, with fixed line broadband access less than 0.1%.[35] Internet access costs are high. The ITU has developed an ICT Price Basket and ranks 161 countries on the basis of a set of standardized fixed phone line telephony, mobile cellular, and broadband services, and describes these in terms of relative cost expressed as a percentage of the average monthly GNI per capita. Nineteen of the 20 most expensive services are in sub-Saharan African countries.

Broadband costs vary greatly. In the Central African Republic, Ethiopia, and Malawi, the monthly cost of the ITU bundle for fixed broadband services is 39, 21, and 20 times the average per capita GNI per month, respectively. Broadband access exceeds the monthly GNI in 19 African countries.[36] Satellite connectivity costs in Africa also are higher than in the developed world. The average annual satellite Internet licence fee for African universities in 40 countries was US$13,553, compared to US$426 for European Union universities.[37] Even though prices have come down, they remain higher than terrestrial links.[38]

Significantly more bandwidth has become available to Africa with the completion of the TEAMS, Seacom, and EASSY undersea cables that have been laid around the East coast of Africa, with landfall sites in South Africa, Mozambique, Tanzania, Kenya, Somalia, Djibouti, Eritrea, Sudan, and Madagascar. West Africa, which has long been dependent on the SAT3 cable for terrestrial bandwidth, will have another four undersea cables operational in 2011. Several countries have commenced laying a fibre-optic backbone between cities and into larger towns. Expectations are that bandwidth costs may fall by as much as 90%, but this has yet to realised.[39] O3b, which stands for the "other three billion people" who do not have Internet access, is a company that announced an ambitious plan to position 16 satellites over the developing world to offer low-cost, high-speed access to the Internet. More cost-effective Internet-based communication may soon become a reality in Africa.

The Future

The anticipated gradual deregulation of the telecommunication industries in Africa, reduction in bandwidth cost, and an associated increase in bandwidth provision will allow expansion of existing projects and the implementation of new projects. Internet penetration will, however, probably still remain low due to hardware setup costs. Internet access using mobile phones may increase penetration, but this is presently an expensive option. Videoconferencing hardware will remain expensive, but the alternative of desktop videoconferencing offers great promise for the African setting, especially if it is accomplished by using free and open source software.

Africa has a rapidly developing cellular telephone industry, with cellular telephone penetration in the region of 37%, as opposed to 7% for Internet penetration. Cellular telephony is set to grow in Africa. In 2007, the GSM Users Association pledged US$50 billion to the development of cell phone infrastructure in Africa over the next four years, to which the World Bank added US$5 billion. Cell phone coverage will far exceed Internet coverage in rural areas. Rapid advances are being made in migrating e-Learning to m-Learning (mobile learning) on smart phones and personal digital assistants (PDAs). Surgeons have been leaders in the use of technology in medicine, and it is probable that Africa will leapfrog what the developed world has taken for granted in terms of PC-based access to the Internet and the WWW and join in the cellular phone environment.

Conclusion

The medical needs of Africa are great, and many entities are committed to its improvement. Telemedicine can be utilised to bring high-quality information and medical care to locations previously limited by lack of finance, inadequate training, and geographic distance. Adherence to the principles described in this chapter can aid the development of successful telemedicine programmes throughout the African continent. WHO and many developed countries aim to aid Africa in its efforts to develop a functional telemedicine infrastructure that will ultimately have a major impact on the health of its children.

Helpful Resources

- PubMed: The National Library of Medicine's MEDLINE access (http://www.ncbi.nlm.nih.gov/PubMed) is a search engine offering free access to abstracts and many full-text articles for all medical literature indexed by the National Library of Medicine since 1966.

- Telemedicine Information Exchange (TIE; http://tie.telemed.org) is the largest and most comprehensive online source of information on telemedicine. It offers a bibliographic database to more than 15,000 telemedicine publications, information on more than 150 major international telemedicine programmes, lists of telemedicine meetings and conferences internationally, information on vendors of telemedicine equipment, and an extensive list of links to other telemedicine resources.

- Google.com is one of the largest and best search engines on the Internet.

- The International Society for Telemedicine and ehealth (ISfTeH; http://isft.net) is an NGO in official relation with WHO that exists as an international umbrella for national telemedicine groups and functions to disseminate knowledge and experience in telemedicine and e-health worldwide.

- The American Telemedicine Association (ATA; http://www.americantelemed.org) sponsors an international special interest group.

- The Swinfen Charitable Trust (http://www.swinfencharitabletrust.org runs a system that can be used in Africa for simple e-mail consultation.

References

1. Information available at: www.un.org/millenniumgoals/.

2. United Nations. The Millennium Development Goals Report 2008.

3. World Health Organization. A Health Telematics Policy (document DGO/98.1). WHO, 1998.

4. World Health Organization. The Africa Health Infoway: A District-based Public Health Information Network for African Health. Available at: www.who.int/kms/initiatives/ahi/en/.

5. Wootton R, Craig J, Patterson V. Introduction to Telemedicine, 2nd ed. Royal Society of Medicine Press, 2006.

6. Mitchell J. Fragmentation to Integration: National Scoping Study for the Telemedicine Industry in Australia. Department of Industry, Science and Tourism, Canberra, ACT, 1998.

7. Norris AC. Essentials of Telemedicine and Telecare. John Wiley & Sons, 2002.

8. Goldstein DE. E-Healthcare: Harnessing the Power of Internet, E-Commerce and E-Care. Aspen, 2000.

9. Amenta F, Rizzo N. Maritime radiomedical services. In: Wootton R, ed. European Telemedicine 1998/99. Kensington Publications, 1999, Pp 125–126.

10. Benschoter RA, Wittson CL, Ingham CG. Teaching and consultation by television: I. Closed-circuit collaboration. J Hosp Commun Psychiat 1965; 16: 99–100.

11. Murphy RLH, Bird KT. Telediagnosis: a new community health resource. Observations on the feasibility of telediagnosis based on 1000 patient transactions. Am J Public Health 1974; 64:113–119.

12. Foote D, Hudson H, Parker EB. Telemedicine in Alaska: The ATS-6 Satellite Biomedical Demonstration. National Technical Information Service (NTIS). US Department of Commerce, 1976.

13. Bashshur R. Technology Serves the People: The Story of a Cooperative Telemedicine Project by NASA, the Indian Health Service and the Papago People. US Government Printing Office, 1980.

14. Geissbuhler A, Bagayoko CO, Ly O. The RAFT network: 5 years of distance continuing medical education and tele-consultations over the Internet in French-speaking Africa. Int J of Med Informatics 2007; 76:351–356.

15. Wootton R. Telemedicine support for the developing world. J Telemd Telecare 2008; 14:109–114.

16. Wootton R, Prospective case review of a global e-health system for doctors in developing countries. J Telemed Telecare 2004; 10(S1):94–96.

17. Hailey D, Ohinmaa A, Roine R. Study quality and evidence of benefit in recent assessments of telemedicine. J Telemed Telecare 2004; 10:318–324.

18. Mair F, Whitten P. Systematic review of studies of patient satisfaction with telemedicine. BMJ 2000; 320:1517–1520.

19. Bergmo TS. An economic analysis of teleconsultation in otorhinolaryngology. J Telemed Telecare 1997; 3:194–198.

20. Whited JD. Teledermatology. Current status and future directions. Am J Clin Dermatol 2001; 2:59–64.

21. Williams BH, Mullick FG, Butler DR, Herring RF, O'Leary TH. Clinical evaluation of an international static image-based telepathology service. Hum Pathol 2001; 32:1309–1317.

22. Ruggiero C. Teleradiology: a review. J Telemed Telecare 1998; 4:25–35.

23. Rosser Jr JC, Bell RL, Harnett B, Rodas E, Murayama M, Merrell R. Use of mobile low-bandwidth telemedical techniques for extreme telemedicine applications. J Am Coll Surg 1999; 189;397–404.

24. Telemedicine Initiative for Sub-Saharan Africa: Pilot Projects Proposal. European Space Agency, 20 March 2007. Available at: www.telecom.esa.int.

25. Reponen J, Ilkko E, Jyrkinen L, et al. Initial experience with a wireless personal digital assistant as a teleradiology terminal for reporting emergency computerized tomography scans. J Telemed Telecare 2000; 6:45–49.

26. Freedman SB. Direct transmission of electrocardiograms to a mobile phone for management of a patient with acute myocardial infarction. J Telemed Telecare 1999; 5:67–69.

27. Adams GL, Campbell PT, Adams JM, Strauss DG, Wall K, Patterson J, Shuping KB, Maynard C, Young D, Corey C, Thompson A, Lee BA, Wagner GS. Effectiveness of prehospital wireless transmission of electrocardiograms to a cardiologist via hand-held device for patients with acute myocardial infarction (from the Timely Intervention in Myocardial Emergency, NorthEast Experience [TIME-NE]). Am J Cardiol 2006; 98(9):1160–1164.

28. Hsieh CH, Tsai HH, Yin JW, Chen CY, Yang JC, Jeng SF. Teleconsultation with the mobile camera-phone in digital soft-tissue injury: a feasibility study. Plast Reconstr Surg 2004; 114(7):1776–1782.

29. Kollmann A, Riedl M, Kastner P, Schreier G, Ludvik B. Feasibility of a mobile phone-based service for functional insulin treatment of type 1 diabetes mellitus patients. J Med Internet Res 2007; 9(5):36.

30. Latifi, Rifat. Current Principles and Practices of Telemedicine and e-Health. IOS Press, 2008.

31. Lee S, Broderick TJ, Haynes J, Bagwell C, Doarn CR, Merrell RC. The role of low-bandwidth telemedicine in surgical prescreening. J Pediatr Surg 2003; 38(9):1281–1283. Information available at: www.who.int/hinari.

32. World Health Organization. World Health Statistics 2010. WHO Press, 2010.

33. Internet usage statistics for Africa. Internet World Stats. Available at: http://www.internetworldstats.com/stats1.htm (accessed 23 November 2010).

34. Information society statistical profiles 2009 (Africa). International Telecommunication Union, 2009, 1-66. Available at: http://www.itu.int/dms_pub/itu-d/opb/ind/D-IND-RPM.AF-2009-PDF-E.pdf (accessed 23 November 2010)

35. Measuring the information society 2010. International Telecommunication Union, 2009, 1-108. Available at: http://www.itu.int/ITU-D/ict/publications/idi/2010/index.html (accessed 23 November 2010)

36. Hawkins R. Enhancing research and education connectivity for Africa—the findings of the African Tertiary Institution Connectivity Study (ATICS) and Lessons for the Future of Campus Networks. World Bank. Available at: http://www.oecd.org/dataoecd/49/48/35765204.pdf (accessed 23 November 2010).

37. Pehrson B, Comstedt A. Connecting West and Central Africa to the global research and education infrastructure. Available at: http://www.feast-project.org/documents/aauf-fibre-final-report-2009-08-07.pdf (accessed 23 November 2010)

38. ICTWorks. Why Internet bandwidth prices are still high. Available at: http://www.ictworks.org/news/2010/05/05/why-african-internet-bandwidth-prices-are-still-high (accessed 23 November 2010).

CHAPTER 128
PAEDIATRIC SURGERY EDUCATION IN SUB-SAHARAN AFRICA

Maurice Mars

A major problem with paediatric surgery care in developing countries is that there is a general lack of knowledge regarding the care of children with surgical disease.[1]

Paediatric surgery is part of the far greater problems facing health care and delivery in sub-Saharan Africa. The World Health Organizaton (WHO) World Health Report of 2006 summarises these:

The WHO Region of the Americas with 10% of the global burden of disease, has 37% of the world's health workers spending more than 50% of the world's health financing, whereas the African Region has 24% of the burden but only 3% of health workers commanding less than 1% of world health expenditure. The exodus of skilled professionals in the midst of so much unmet health need places Africa at the epicentre of the global health workforce crisis.[2]

Despite the ravages of tuberculosis (TB), malaria, and human immunodeficiency virus (HIV), the population of Africa is forecast to increase from 967 million people in 2008 to 1,998 billion people in 2050.[3] That means more than 1 billion children will be born in Africa over the next 42 years. This will place an additional strain on the continent's already overburdened and underresourced health services. With an estimated cumulative risk of 85% for all surgical conditions by age 15 years, the demand for surgical care of children will continue to increase.[4]

Who will provide this care? Currently, 44% (426 million people) of sub-Saharan Africa's population are 14 years of age or younger.[3] In 2002, only 39 paediatric surgeons were reported to be in sub-Saharan Africa. That number is probably now nearer 100, with the majority in Nigeria and South Africa. This gives a rough ratio of about 1 paediatric surgeon to 5 million children. Few African children will directly benefit from the services of a paediatric surgeon unless a large number of paediatric surgeons are trained. There is the unfortunate paradox: the developed world, with an aging population and falling birthrate, having a relative oversupply and overproduction of paediatric surgeons, and sub-Saharan Africa, with its fast-growing young population, not being able to service its paediatric surgical needs.[5]

The need for subspecialty training in paediatric surgery in Africa has been questioned. There is a strong argument for the general surgeon to return to being a true "general" surgeon with additional training in paediatric surgery. In the overall context of Africa, this additional training should also include neuro-, plastic, and obstetric surgery. This approach makes the assumption that there are or will be enough general surgeons, but there are not (Table 128.1).

Most sub-Saharan African countries have less than one surgeon per 100,000 people; in contrast, the United States has 5.7 general surgeons per 100,000 people.[6] It is estimated that the availability of surgical services in sub-Saharan Africa is "at least ten times below the minimal needs".[7] Just as for paediatric surgeons, production of general surgeons in sub-Saharan Africa is not keeping pace with demand and migration, nor is the production of doctors.[8,9]

The shortage of doctors in sub-Saharan Africa is acute. WHO suggests that at least 20 doctors per 100,000 people are required to provide minimum basic health services.[2] Thirty-five sub-Saharan African countries fail to meet this criterion, and 28 countries have 10 or fewer doctors per 100,000 people.[10] For comparison, the number of doctors per 100,000 people in other countries is: Germany, 350; USA, 270; England, 210; Brazil, 170; and Australia, 100. The African shortage is largely due to undersupply and migration to the developed world.[2]

One solution is to produce more doctors. It is often forgotten that when there is a shortage of doctors, there is also a shortage of doctors to train doctors. Africa has 121 medical schools, a ratio of 1 per 7.6 million people, compared to the developed world norm of 1 per 2 million people. Of the 121 African medical schools, 87 are in sub-Saharan Africa, and four countries do not have a medical school.[11] Although there is a trend for medical schools to increase their output, they are not meeting needs. Producing more doctors, however, is not always a solution; Kenya has trained more doctors than it can afford to hire in the public sector.[7] The need to return to practical surgical training at African medical schools has been suggested, with students being expected to "have performed numbers of simple, frequently required operations".[12]

Even were the human resource deficiencies to be corrected, the problem of under-resourced facilities remains. Fifty-three percent of people in sub-Saharan African countries live on less than US$1 per day.[10] Poverty is extreme. The gross national income of these countries is low, and governments budget a smaller percentage of an already

Table 128.1: Total number of general surgeons, number of general surgeons and doctors per 100,000 population, and the percentage of doctors who are surgeons, for some sub-Saharan African countries.

Country	Number of surgeons	Number of surgeons per 100,000 population	Number of doctors per 100,000 population	Percentage of doctors who are surgeons
Kenya	230	0.7	13.2	5.3
Malawi	9	0.1	1.1	9.1
Mozambique	35	0.2	2.4	8.3
South Africa	954	2.1	69.2	3.0
Tanzania	105	0.3	2.2	13.6
Uganda	63	0.4	4.7	8.5
Zambia	50	0.5	6.9	7.2

small national budget on health, compared to developing countries. The cost of providing minimum health care in Africa is estimated at about US$34 per capita per annum. Nevertheless, 29 countries spend less than US$20 per capita per annum, with an average expenditure for all of Africa of US$34 and a median of US$14.[10] As a result, district hospitals and rural clinics are poorly equipped, and staff are poorly remunerated. To add to the problem, power supply in many countries, and more particularly in the rural areas, is sporadic.

Despite all these obstacles, surgery continues in the rural and district hospitals in the absence of surgeons and paediatric surgeons. Although not specific to paediatric surgery, a recent study from Uganda reported 1,505 general surgical operations were performed in a year in four public general or district hospitals at which there were no general surgeons or anaesthetists.[9] A similar report from a rural hospital in Nigeria indicates that 95% of the surgical procedures were considered simple enough to be performed by general practitioners with general surgery experience. There are no data on the percentage of these patients who were children.[12] Loefler, citing personal experience, noted that about half of the patients he had operated on in peripheral hospitals around Africa were children.[12] Even with surgery being performed by medical officers and general practitioners, the demand for surgery is not being met. In rural areas of developing countries, only an estimated one-third of injured patients are seen at a health facility.[7]

The problem of the shortage of human resources is not new, and the comments of Wasunna, made in 1987, are still relevant:

> There is a shortage of surgical manpower all over Africa. … Current training and recruitment programmes are inadequate in correcting existing manpower deficiencies. The situation is further aggravated by a gross maldistribution of available manpower in favour of large urban centres. In many parts of rural Africa, minor surgical procedures are carried out by suitably trained, non-physician health workers, but facilities and resources for surgery outside urban centres are generally inadequate.[13]

Some countries—notably, Mozambique, Tanzania, and Malawi—have successfully trained nonphysicians in surgery, and these individuals perform up to 90% of the surgery undertaken outside the major cities. The standard and duration of training differs among countries. In Mozambique, the nonphysician surgeons (*tecnicos de chirurgia*) undergo a three-year training programme leading to a bachelor's degree, followed by two years of supervised work in a major teaching institution.

Other countries reject this approach. Although Kenya does not train nonphysician surgeons, it relies heavily on nurse anaesthetists and registered clinical officer anaesthetists.

Issues Facing Paediatric Surgery Education and Training

• What is the role of the paediatric surgeon in sub-Saharan Africa?

• Which health care workers should be trained of those who make up the surgical team: surgeons, anaesthetists, nurses, laboratory technicians, and radiographers, among others?

• What should be the scope of their training in and practice of paediatric surgery?

• Where should they be trained, and by whom?

The Role of the Paediatric Surgeon
A paediatric surgeon has been defined as a surgeon "whose practice is largely or wholly concerned with the diagnosis and management of the diseases and disorders of childhood and who has received special training in the management of these diseases and disorders".[5] The role of the paediatric surgeon in Africa is to set the standards for the surgical

care of children, to teach, and to undertake research. Teaching should include training general surgeons and other health care workers in aspects of paediatric surgery and perioperative care.[5] Setting standards of care should also include (1) developing protocols for the management of uncomplicated cases; (2) setting criteria for referral; and (3) determining which procedures are appropriate at different levels of health care and which should be performed by the different cadres of practitioner.

Who Should Be Trained
For the foreseeable future in sub-Saharan Africa, there will be a need to train different levels of doctors and health care workers. Despite the misgivings of some that subspecialisation has been detrimental to surgery in Africa,[14] there is a need to train paediatric surgeons. Without them, who will train the general surgeons, manage those conditions that would not normally be handled by a general surgeon, and maintain and improve the standards of surgical care of children? General practitioners and medical officers wishing to perform routine low-risk surgery should also be required to undergo further training and initial practice under supervision.

The nonphysician surgeon is anathema to many medical practitioners and especially to surgeons. In well-regulated and controlled environments, nonphysician surgeons appear to play important roles in the provision of surgical services, which should include basic procedures on children. Less contentious is the training of nurse or clinical assistant anaesthetists.

The surgical management of a child depends on a large team, all of whom require training. These include the midwife or birth attendant; the clinic- and district-level primary care team of doctors and nurses who diagnose, treat, or refer paediatric surgical conditions; those responsible for neonatal and infant transportation; and those responsible for anaesthetic and perioperative care.

A major role player who is often ignored is the traditional healer. There is a need to engage with, and raise awareness of, traditional healers with regard to paediatric surgical conditions. They are the primary practitioners of many patients. Some medical schools are beginning to acknowledge the role of these health providers, which is heartening.[5]

Training in paediatric surgery should not occur in isolation. Training to ensure adequate provision of ancillary services, such as radiography and basic laboratory services, needs to be addressed, if necessary.

Scope of Training and Practice
Ideally, training in any developing country should be relevant to the disease patterns specific to the region and should take into account late presentation, advanced pathology, available services, infrastructure, and resources such as the availability of medicines, while keeping abreast of the management of conditions not commonly seen. It is not generally useful to send trainees from Africa to the developed world for surgical training because they will meet a different patient and disease profile, different resource base, and different organisational structure. Furthermore, attempts to duplicate services provided in the developed world have led to the impression that the surgical care of children is too expensive to be supported.[1]

Few data are available about the burden of disease attributable to the surgical conditions seen in sub-Saharan Africa and the spectrum of paediatric surgical pathology seen in different regions. Reports of surgery on children in the rural setting include activities that might not necessarily be performed by a paediatric surgeon in the developed world, such as minor wound toilet and suture, incision and drainage of minor soft tissue infections, treatment of osteomyelitis, and sequestrectomy.

Bickler et al. identified the need to define an "essential package of paediatric surgical services for developing countries".[1] From available data, this would include management of trauma, surgical infections, congenital abnormalities, malignancy, circumcision, and inguinal hernias. Training should be relevant to the level of the trainee and the environment in which the trainee will practice.

Where and by Whom Surgeons Should Be Trained

This topic may seem to be irrelevant to those in the developed world. As has been stated, there is not only a shortage of doctors in Africa, there is a shortage of doctors to train doctors. In an address to the Association of Surgeons of East Africa in 1999, Loefler noted that the most successful surgeons are in major cities and that not enough use has been made of their skills in surgical training. He contended that the best hospitals, including mission hospitals, are not used for training; he said, "environments of the teaching hospitals are not conducive to learning of high standards", and called for the reintroduction of practical surgery in the undergraduate medical curriculum.[12]

The growing requirement of medical schools in sub-Saharan Africa that clinical faculty must have a PhD or equivalent degree is a barrier to the appointment of skilled surgeons who do not have a research background; this restrictive requirement should be reconsidered. Another obstacle at some teaching hospitals is lack of equipment. Training should take place at a site where there is adequate supervision and the spectrum of clinical practice is appropriate. Training at medical schools may be supplemented with training by surgeons in private practice and take place in private or nongovernmental hospitals, where facilities and equipment often are better, and completed with training in district and regional hospitals with experienced staff.

In some countries, training and examination for accreditation of surgeons and paediatric surgeons has been controlled by medical schools through master of medicine in surgery programmes; in others, it has been controlled by colleges. The West African College of Surgeons serves five Anglophone countries in West Africa and offers a fellowship in general surgery. The College of Surgeons of East, Central and Southern Africa (COSECSA) offers fellowships in general surgery and orthopaedics for 10 member countries. The Colleges of Medicine of South Africa, through its various colleges, offer fellowships in general, paediatric, cardiothoracic, neuro-, orthopaedic, and plastic surgery as well as in ophthalmology and urology. All colleges identify suitable training institutes, determine curricula, and examine candidates for registration as specialist surgeons.

Educational Initiatives in Sub-Saharan Africa Based on Information and Communication Technologies

Surgery in Africa is an initiative of the Office of International Surgery at the University of Toronto and COSECSA. Surgery in Africa offers an online, journal-based course for candidates preparing for the fellowship examination, with monthly review articles relevant to the African setting, and Fellow of the College of Surgeons (FCS) degree syllabus and full text, book, and journal references.[15] The Ptolemy Project, a partnership of the University of Toronto, the Association of Surgeons of East Africa, COSECSA, and the Canadian Institutes of Health Research, aims to foster both research and research capacity development in East and Central Africa through access to and dissemination of information over the Internet.[16]

Since 2000, the RAFT (Resau en Afrique Francophone pour la Telemedicine) Project, based at the Hopitaux Universitaires de Geneva, has been offering two-hour-long weekly education programme using V-Sat satellite technology. The project involves interactive webcasting at low bandwidth to 18 sites in Francophone West Africa.[17] In Kenya, the African Medical and Research Foundation (AMREF) has commenced a large project to improve the skills of up to 22,000 nurses, some of whom are receiving their education as e-learning from compact disc (CD)-based material.[18] The National School of Public Health in Rwanda offers modules in an asynchronous format using Adobe® Presenter.

The University of KwaZulu-Natal in South Africa has been providing videoconferenced seminars in a range of specialties since 2001. In paediatric surgery, the weekly seminar, which is part of the academic training programme at the University of KwaZulu-Natal, started in the second semester of 2005 and has been shared with up to three other sites by interactive videoconference by using Integrated Services Digital Networks (ISDN) links. Only three paediatric surgeons and on average 10 trainees and medical students are present in the teaching hospital at each teaching session. Videoconferencing extends the sessions to three other sites: a satellite teaching hospital, a medical school in another province, and a regional hospital in another province.[19] Over the first four and a half years of the programme, 217 sessions have been held, with an average of 76 people participating in each session, 63 of whom are at distant sites. Surgeons from several other African countries have requested to be included in the videoconference programme. In the absence of videoconferencing infrastructure at other medical schools in Africa, the videoconferenced seminars in Durban have been recorded to digital video disc (DVD) and mailed to four medical schools in Central and East Africa. They have been incorporated into the postgraduate training programmes of surgeons and paediatric surgeons and also used in undergraduate medical training. An additional 140 people have acces to the seminars through this programme.

Key Summary Points

1. Africa's population will increase by more than 1 billion by 2050.

2. The existing shortage of health care professionals in Africa will not be redressed in the near future.

3. A need exists to develop an essential package of paediatric surgical service for developing countries.

4. The role of paediatric surgeons in sub-Saharan Africa needs to be defined.

5. The majority of surgical procedures on children in sub-Saharan Africa are performed by general surgeons and medical officers. These providers require further training by paediatric surgeons in paediatric surgery and the perioperative needs of children.

6. Paediatric surgery cannot take place without anaesthetic and other basic laboratory services, and the training needs of these ancillary services must be considered concurrently with training in paediatric surgery.

7. The place of the "nonphysician surgeon" needs to be considered.

8. Information and communication technologies offer promise for decentralized and shared education programmes in the future.

References

1. Bickler SW, Kyambi J, Rode H. Pediatric surgery in sub-Saharan Africa. Pediatr Surg Int 2001; 17(5-6):442–447.

2. World Health Report 2006. Available at: http://www.who.int/whr/2006/en/ (accessed 23 November 2010).

3. 2008 Africa population data sheet. Population Reference Bureau and African Population & Health Research Center. Available at: http://www.prb.org/pdf08/africadatasheet2008.pdf (accessed 23 November 2010).

4. Bickler SW, Rode H. Surgical services in developing countries. Bull World Health Organ 2002; 80(10):829-835.

5. Hadley GP. The paediatric surgeon in Africa: luxury or necessity? East Cent Afric J Surg 2004; 9(2):103–109.

6. Lynge DC, Larson EH, Thompson MJ, Rosenblatt RA, Hart LG. A longitudinal analysis of the general surgery workforce in the United States, 1981–2005. Arch Surg 2008; 143(4):345–350.

7. Bellagio Essential Surgery Group. Increasing access to surgical services in resource-constrained settings in sub-Saharan Africa. 2007; 1-13. Available at: http://www.google.co.za/#hl=en&source=hp&biw=926&bih=831&q=Increasuing+Access+to+surigical+services+in+resource&btnG=Google+Search&aq=f&aqi=&aql=&oq=Increasuing+Access+to+surigical+services+in+resource&gs_rfai=&fp=dbc0fb07035912d4 (accessed 23 November 2010).

8. Mahande M, Tharaney M, Kirumbi E, Ngirawamungu E, Geneau R, Tapert L, Courtright P. Uptake of trichiasis surgical services in Tanzania through two village-based approaches. Br J Ophthalmol 2007; 91(2):139–142.

9. Ozgediz D, Galukande M, Mabweijano J, Kijjambu S, Mijumbi C, Dubowitz G, Kaggwa S, Luboga S. The neglect of the global surgical workforce: experience and evidence from Uganda. World J Surg 2008; 32(6):1208–1215.

10. World Health Organization. World Health Statistics 2010. WHO Press, 2010.

11. Institute for International Medical Education,_Database of Medical Schools. Available at: http://www.iime.org/database/africa/index.htm (accessed 23 November 2010).

12. Loefler I. The future of surgery in East Africa. Association of Surgeons of East Africa. Available at: http://www.asea.org.mz/Future_Surgery_East_Africa.htm (accessed 8 November 2008).

13. Wasunna AE. Surgical manpower in Africa. Bull Am Coll Surg 1987; 72(6):18–19.

14. Loefler IJ. The drawbacks of overspecialisation. J R Coll Surg Edinb 1999; 44(1):11–12.

15. Office of International Surgery, University of Toronto. Surgery in Africa. Available at: http://www.utoronto.ca/ois/SIA.htm (accessed 23 November 2010).

16. Office of International Surgery, University of Toronto. The Ptolemy Project. Available at: http://www.ptolemy.ca/ (accessed 23 November 2010).

17. Geissbuhler A, Bagayoko C, Ly O. The RAFT network: 5 years of distance continuing medical education and tele-consultations over the Internet in French-speaking Africa. Intl J Med Informatics 2007; 76(5–6):351–356.

18. Train health workers. African Medical Research Foundation. Available at: http://www.amref.org/what-we-do/train-health-workers/ (accessed 23 November 2010).

19. Hadley GP, Mars M. Postgraduate medical education in paediatric surgery: videoconferencing—a possible solution for Africa? Pediatr Surg Int 2008; 24(2):223–226.

ACRONYMS

3D	three-dimensional		BOO	bladder outlet obstruction
A&E	accident and emergency (department)		BP	blood pressure
AAS	Association for Academic Surgery		BPS	bronchopulmonary sequestration
ABL	allowable blood loss		BPSU	British Paediatric Surveillance Unit
ABR	auditory brainstem response		BRRI	Building and Roads Research Institute (Ghana)
ACE	antegrade continent enema			
ACS	American College of Surgeons		BSA	body surface area
ACTH	adrenocorticotropic hormone		BSO	bilateral salpingo-oophorectomy
ADA	adenosine deaminase		BWS	Beckwith-Weidemann syndrome
ADH	antidiuretic hormone		BXO	balanitis xerotica obliterans
ADL	African degenerative leiomyopathy		CA	condylomata acuminatum; choanal atresia
ADPKD	autosomal dominant polycystic kidney disease			
			CAEBV	chronic active Epstein-Barr virus
AER	air enema reduction		CAH	congenital adrenal hyperplasia
AF	anal fissure (fissure-in-ano)		CAIS	complete androgen insensitivity syndrome
AFB	acid-fast bacilli			
AFP	alpha-foetoprotein		CBF	cerebral blood flow
AFS	American Fertility Society		CCAM	congenital cystic adenomatous malformation (lung)
AGA	average for gestational age			
AIDS	acquired immune deficiency syndrome		CD	cluster of differentiation; Crohn's disease; compact disc
AIN	anterior interosseous nerve			
AIS	Abbreviated Injury Scale		CDH	congenital diaphragmatic hernia
AJOL	African Journals Online		CDLT	cadaveric donor liver transplantation
ALL	acute lymphocytic leukaemia		CECT	contrast-enhanced computed tomography
ALT	aspartate transaminase; akternative lengthening of telomeres			
			CESP	Confederation of European Specialists in Paediatrics
ALTE	acute life-threatening events			
AML	acute myelogenous leukaemia		CF	cystic fibrosis
AMREF	African Medical and Research Foundation		CFP 10	culture filtrate protein 10
AP	anteroposterior; Anatomical Profile		CFS	congenital fibrosarcoma
APC	adenomatous polyposis coli (gene)		CFTR	cystic fibrosis transmembrane (conductance) regulator
APSA	American Paediatric Surgical Association			
AR	androgen receptor; allergic rhinitis		CHARGE	Coloboma, Heart defect, Atresia choanae, Retarded growth and development, Genital hypoplasia, Ear anomalies/deafness (syndrome)
ARM	anorectal malformation			
ARPKD	autosomal recessive polycystic kidney disease			
			CHD	congenital heart disease
ART	antiretroviral treatment		CHEOPS	Children's Hospital of Eastern Ontario Pain Scale
ASA	American Society of Anesthesiologists			
ASCOT	A Severity Characterization Of Trauma		CHL	conductive hearing loss
ASSC	acute splenic sequestration crisis		CIC	clean intermittent catheterisation
AST	alanine transaminase		CIE	counterimmunoelectrophoresis
ATLS	Advanced Trauma Life Support		CIF	common intermediate format
ATRD	African Trauma Registry Database		CIIP	chronic idiopathic intestinal pseudo-obstruction
ATT	antitubercular treatment			
AVM	arteriovenous malformation		CIRM	International Radio Medical Centre
AVPU	alert, verbal, painful, unresponsive (method to assess level of consciousness)		CLD	chronic liver disease
			CLE	congenital lobar emphysema
AXR	abdominal x-ray; abdominal radiograph		CLO	congenital lobar overinflation
BA	biliary atresia		CMT	congenital muscular torticollis
BAC	bronchioloalveolar carcinoma		CMV	conventional mechanical ventilation; cytomegalovirus
BAHA	bone-anchored hearing aid			
BAPS	British Association of Paediatric Surgeons		CNI	calcineurin inhibitors
BCG	bacille Calmette-Guérin		CNS	central nervous system
b.d.	twice daily		CO	cardiac output
β-hCG	β-human chorionic gonadotropin		COPUM	congenital obstructive posterior urethral membrane
BMI	body mass index			

CORA	centre of rotational deformity	EIA	enzyme-linked immunosorbent assay
COSECSA	College of Surgeons of East, Central and Southern Africa	EIS	endoscopic injection sclerotherapy
		ELISA	enzyme-linked immunosorbent assay
CPA	conditioned play audiometry	EMG	electromyography
CPAM	cystic pulmonary adenomatous malformation (lung)	EMLA	eutectic mixture of local anaesthetics
		EMR	electronic medical record
CPAP	continuous positive airway pressure	ENT	ear, nose, and throat
CPC	cauterisation of the choroid plexus	ERCP	endoscopic retrograde cholangiopancreatography
CPP	cerebral perfusion pressure		
CPR	cardiopulmonary resuscitation	ERP	endorectal pull-through
CR	capillary refill	ESAT6	early secretory antigenic target-6
CRP	C-reactive protein	ESFT	Ewing's sarcoma family of tumours
CSF	cerebrospinal fluid	ESLD	end-stage liver disease
CT	computed tomography (scan)	ESPE	European Society for Paediatric Endocrinology
CTEV	congenital talipes equinovarus (CTEV)		
CVA	central venous access	ESR	erythrocyte sedimentation rate
CVP	central venous pressure	ESRD	end-stage renal disease
CXR	chest x-ray	ESRF	end-stage renal failure
DA	duodenal atresia	ESWL	extracorporeal shock-wave lithotripsy
DALYs	disability-adjusted life years	ET	empyema thoracis
DCS	dynamic compression system	ETF	enteral tube feeding
DDH	developmental dysplasia of the hip	ETRS	embryonic testicular regression syndrome
DEC	diethylcarbamazine	ETV	endoscopic third ventriculostomy
DES	diethylstilbesterol	EUS	endoscopic ultrasonography
DIC	disseminated intravascular coagulation	EUSOL	Edinburgh University solution of lime
DGE	delayed gastric emptying	EVD	external ventricular drainage
DHT	dihydrotestosterone	EWS/ETS	Ewing sarcoma breakpoint region/ erythroblastosis virus E26 oncogene transcription factor fusion gene
DJ	duodenojejunal		
DMSA	dimercaptosuccinic acid		
DNA	deoxyribonucleic acid	EXIT	ex-utero intrapartum treatment
DOA	dead on arrival	FAC	familial adenomatosis coli
DOT	directly observed therapy	FAO	foot-ankle orthosis
DPG	diphosphsglycerate	FAP	familial adenomatosis polyposis
DPL	diagnostic peritoneal lavage	FAST	focused abdominal sonography for trauma
DPPC	dipalmitoylphosphatidyl choline	FBC	full blood count
DRE	digital rectal examination	FDA	Food and Drug Administration (US)
DSA	digital substraction angiography	FEF	forced expiratory flow
DSD	disorders of sex differentiation; detrusor sphincter dyssynergia	FETO	fetal endoscopic tracheal occlusion
		FEV	forced expiratory volume
DSL	digital subscriber line	FFP	fresh frozen plasma
DTPA	diethylenetriamine penta-acetic acid	FGC	female genital cutting
DVD	digital video disc	FIA	fistula-in-ano
DYG	double-Y glanuloplasty	FLACS	Faces, Legs, Activity and Consolability Scale
EBV	Epstein-Barr virus		
ECG	electrocardiogram	fMRI	functional Magnetic Resonance Imaging
ECM	extracellular matrix	FNA	fine needle aspiration
ECMO	extracorporeal membrane oxygenation	FNAB	fine-needle aspiration biopsy
ECW	extracellular water	FNH	focal nodular hyperplasia
ED	Emergency Department (of a hospital)	FRC	functional residual capacity
EDNRB	endothelin B receptor gene	FSH	follicle-stimulating hormone
EF	examining finger	FVC	forced vital capacity
EFD	estimated (preoperative) fluid deficit	GA	general anaesthesia
EFR	estimated fluid requirement (maintenance fluids)	GABHS	group A beta-hemolytic streptococcal
		GCRG	giant cell reparative granuloma
EGD	oesophagogastroduodenoscopy	GCS	Glasgow Coma Scale
EGF	epidermal growth factor	GDNF	glial (cell line) derived neurotrophic factor
eGFR	estimated glomerular filtration rate	GDP	gross domestic product
EHBS	extra hepatic biliary system	GF	growth factor

GFR	glomerular filtration rate		ID	immunodiffusion
GGT	gamma-glutaml transpeptidase		IDA	iminodiacetic acid
GI	gastrointestinal		IF	intestinal failure
GID	gastrointestinal duplication		IFN-g	interferon gamma release protein
GIEESC	Global Initiative for Emergency and Essential Surgical Care		IgA, IgE, IgG, IgM	immunoglobulin A, E, G, M
GIT	gastrointestinal tract		IGF	insulin growth factor
GOR	gastro-oesophageal reflux		IH	inguinal hernia
GORD	gastro-oesophageal reflux disease		IHA	indirect haemogglutination antibody
GOS	Glasgow Outcome Scale		IHPS	infantile hypertrophic pyloric stenosis
GRWR	graft weight-to-recipient's body weight ratio (transplantation)		IJV	internal jugular vein
			IL	insensible losses (fluids)
GVHD	graft versus host disease		IM	intramuscular
GWD	guinea worm disease		INR	international normalization ratio
Gy	gray (radiation dose)		INSS	International Neuroblastoma Staging System
H&E	haematoxylin and eosin (staining)		IO	intraosseous
HAART	highly active antiretroviral therapy		IOM	Institute of Medicine
HAEC	Hirschsprung's-associated enterocolitis		IP	Internet protocol
HB	hepatoblastoma		IPAA	ileal-pouch anal anastomosis
HbAS	sickle cell trait		IQR	interquartile range
HbS/β thal	sickle cell thalassemia disease		IRA	ileorectal anastomosis
HbSC	sickle cell haemoglobin C disease		IRIS	immune reconstitution inflammatory syndrome
HbSS	homozygous sickle cell anaemia		IRS	Intergroup Rhabdomyosarcoma Study Group
HC	hydrocephalus			
HCC	hepatocellular carcinoma		INH	isoniazid
hCG	human chorionic gonadotropin		ISDN	Integrated Services Digital Networks
HCMV	human cytomegalovirus		ISfTeH	International Society for Telemedicine and ehealth
HCW	health care worker			
HD	Hirschsprung's disease		ISP	Internet service provider
HHML	hemihyperplasia-multiple lipomatosis syndrome		ISS	Injury Severity Score
			ITP	idiopathic thrombocytopaenic purpura
HIDA	hepato-iminodiacetic acid		ITU	International Telecommunication Union
HINARI	Health InterNetwork Access to Research Initiative		ITx	intestinal transplantation
			IV	intravenous
HIT	hydrodistention-implantation technique		IVA	ifosfamide, vincristine, and actinomycin D
HIV	human immunodeficiency virus			
HLA	human leukocyte antigen		IVC	inferior vena cavography; inferior vena cava
HMS	hyperactive malarial splenomegaly			
HO	hematogenous osteomyelitis		IVF	in vitro fertilisation
HPF	high-power fields		IVIG	intravenous immunoglobulin
HPN	home parenteral nutrition		IVU	intravenous urography
HPZ	high pressure zone		JCV	John Cunningham virus (but just say JC virus)
HR	heart rate			
HSCR	Hirschsprung's disease		JNA	juvenile nasopharyngeal angiofibroma
HSP	Henoch-Schönlein purpura		KS	Kaposi sarcoma
H-TOF	H-type tracheo-oesophageal fistula		KSHV	Kaposi sarcoma-associated herpes virus
HVA	homovallinic acid			
IBCA	isobutyl cyanoacrylate		KTS	Kampala Trauma Score
IBD	inflammatory bowel disease		LAD	leukocyte adhesion deficiency
IBI	intralesional bleomycin injection		LATS	long-acting thyroid stimulating (hormones)
ICCS	International Children's Continence Society			
			LB flap	lateral-based flap
ICP	intracranial pressure		LDH	lactate dehydrogenase
ICT	information and communication technologies		LDITx	living-donor intestinal transplantation
			LF	lymphatic filariasis
ICU	intensive care unit		LFT	liver function test
ICV	ileocaecal valve		LGA	large for gestational age
ICW	intracellular water			

LHR	lung-head ratio (foetal)
LLS	left lateral segment (liver)
LMA	laryngeal mask airway
LMIC	low- and middle-income country
LOH	loss of heterozygosity
LOS	length of (hospital) stay; lower oesophageal sphincter
LPD	lymphoproliferative disorder
LPP	leak point pressure
LPU	lower pole ureter
LRLT	living-related liver transplantation
L/S	lecithin/spingomyelin (ratio)
LTB	laryngotracheobronchitis
LWAT	location without advanced technology
LWPES	Lawson Wilkins Pediatric Endocrine Society
MACE	Malone antegrade continence enema
MAG3	mercaptoacetyltriglycine
MAGPI	meatal advancement and glanuloplasty incorporated
MAP	mean airway pressure; mean arterial pressure; mutYH-associated-polyposis (gene)
MC&S	microscopy, culture, and sensitivities
MCDK	multicystic dysplastic kidney; multicystic diseased kidney
MCUG	micturating cystourethrogram; micturating cystourethrography
MD	Meckel's diverticulum
MDGs	Millennium Development Goals
MDR	multidrug-resistant
MEN2	multiple endocrine neoplasia type 2
MFH	malignant fibrous histiocytoma
MIBG	metiodobenzylgaunidine (scan)
MIP	mega-meatus intact prepuce
MIR	minimally invasive repair
MIS	Müllerian-inhibiting substance; minimally invasive surgery
MMF	mycophenolate mofetil
MMP	matrix metalloproteinases
MMR	measles-mumps-rubella (vaccine)
MSP	manual separation with prophylaxis
MRA	magnetic resonance angiography
MRCP	magnetic resonance cholangiopancreatography
MRI	magnetic resonance imaging
MRKH	Mayer-Rokitansky-Kuster-Hauser (syndrome)
MSK	musculoskeletal
MSP	manual separation with prophylaxis
MTC	medullary thyroid carcinoma
mTOR	mammalian target of rapamycin
MTOS	Major Trauma Outcome Study
NASA	National Aeronautics and Space Administration (USA)
NBCA	n-butyl cyanoacrylate
Nd:YAG	neodymium:yttrium aluminium garnet (laser)

NEC	necrotizing enterocolitis
NF	necrotising fasciitis
NGO	nongovernmental organisation
NGT	nasogastric tube
NHL	non-Hodgkin's lymphoma
NICU	neonatal intensive care unit
NIO	neonatal intestinal obstruction
NJT	nasojejunal tube
NK	natural killer (cell)
NMDA	N-methyl-d-aspartate
NNBSD	nonneurogenic bladder sphincter dysfunction
NNIS	National Nosocomial Infection Surveillance (index)
NOR	nonoperative reduction
NPC	nasopharyngeal carcinoma
NPO	nothing by mouth, literally nil per os
NPWT	negative pressure wound therapy
NR	nephrogenic rests; nutritional rickets
NRC	National Research Council (US)
NRSTS	nonrhabdomyosarcoma soft tissue sarcoma
NS	normal saline
NSAIDS	nonsteroidal anti-inflammatory drugs
NSS	normal saline solution
NTD	neural tube defect
NTSC	National Television Standards Committee
NVB	neurovascular bundle
NWTSG	National Wilms' Tumour Study Group
OA	oesophageal atresia
OAE	otoacoustic emission
OGD	oesophago-gastric-duodenoscopy
ONS	oral nutritional supplements
OPG	orthopantomogram
OPSI	overwhelming postsplenectomy infection
OR	operating room
ORIF	open reduction, internal fixation
ORL	otorhinolaryngology
ORS	ovarian remnant syndrome
PA	pulmonary artery
PAA	perianal abscess
PACU	postanaesthetic care unit
PADUA	progressive augmentation by dilating the urethra anterior
PAIR	percutaneous aspiration, instillation, and reaspiration
PAIS	partial androgen insensitivity syndrome
PAL	phase alternating line
PAPSA	Pan African Paediatric Surgical Association
PAS	para-aminosalicylic acid; pyriform aperture stenosis
PAX/FKHR	Paxillin [Drosophila melanogaster])/ (forkhead box O1 [Homo sapiens]) fusion gene
PBM	pancreaticobiliary malunion
PC	phosphatidyl choline (lecithin)
PCA	patient-controlled analgesia

PCEA	patient-controlled epidural analgesia	RBC	red blood cells; red blood count
PCR	polymerase chain reaction	RBF	renal blood flow
PDS	polydioxanone	RCT	randomised controlled trial
PE	pleural effusion; pectus excavatum	rDNA	ribosomal DNA
PEB	cisplatin, etoposide, and bleomycin	RDS	respiratory distress syndrome
PEEP	positive end expiratory pressure	REAL	Revised Euro-American Lymphoma
PEG	percutaneous endoscopic gastrostomy	RET	REarranged during Transfection (gene)
PELD	Pediatric End-stage Liver Disease	RL	Ringer's lactate
PEP	post exposure prophylaxis	RMS	rhabdomyosarcoma
PEPFAR	President's Emergency Plan for AIDS Relief	RPC	recurrent parotitis in children
		RPL	recurrent pregnancy loss
PET	positron emission tomography (scan)	RR	respiratory rate
PFC	persistent foetal circulation	RRP	recurrent respiratory papillamatosis
PFIC	progressive familial intrahepatic cholestasis	RSV	respiratory syncytial virus
		RTS	Revised Trauma Score
PHT	portal hypertension	RUT	rapid urease test
PIC	percutaneously(or peripherally) inserted central (venous)	RVF	rectovaginal fistulae
		SARS	sacral anterior root stimulation
PICU	paediatric intensive care unit	SB	spina bifida; small bowel
PLP	pathological lead point	SBO	small bowel obstruction
PN	parenteral nutrition	SBP	systolic blood pressure
PNET	primitive neuroectodermal tumour	SC	sickle cell hemoglobin in sickle cell disease
PO	per os (by mouth, orally)		
PPD	purified protein derivative	SCD	sickle cell disease
PPF	periportal fibrosis	SCF	supracondylar fracture
PPHN	persistent pulmonary hypertension of the newborn	SCIWORA	spinal cord injury without radiographic abnormality
		SCT	sacrococcygeal teratoma
PPI	proton pump nhibitor	SCV	subclavian vein
PPS	post-polio syndrome	SEER	Surveillance, Epidemiology and End Results (U.S. program)
PPV	patent processus vaginalis		
P(s)	probability of survival	SENIC	Study on the Efficacy of Nosocomial Infection Control (CDC)
PSARP	posterior sagittal anorectoplasty		
PSE	passive stretching exercise	SGA	small for gestational age
PSI	pleural space infection	SHML	sinus histiocytosis with massive lymphadenopathy
PSS	postsplenectomy sepsis		
PSTN	public switched telephone network	SIDS	sudden infant death syndrome
PSVT	Paroxysmal supraventricular tachycardia	SIOP	Société Internationale d'Oncologie Pédiatrique (International Society of Pediatric Oncology)
PT	prothrombin time		
PTEN	phosphatase/tensin		
PTFE	polytetrafluoroethylene		
PTH	parathormone	SIRS	systemic inflammatory response syndrome
PTLD	posttransplant lymphoproliferative disorder	SIS	small intestinal submucosa
PTS	Paediatric Trauma Score	SLE	systemic lupus erythematosus
PTSD	posttraumatic stress disorder	SM	streptomycin
PTT	partial thromboplastin time	SMA	superior mesenteric artery
PUD	peptic ulcer disease	SMT	sternomastoid tumour
PUJ	pelviuretic junction. (see also UPJ)	SMV	superior mesenteric vein
PUV	posterior urethral valve	SNHL	sensorineural hearing loss
PV	processus vaginalis	SNS	sympathetic nervous system
PVO	portal vein occlusion	SOMI	sterno-occipito-mandibular immobilization
PVR	post-void residual	SPE	streptococcal pyrogenic exotoxins
PVT	portal vein thrombosis	SS	sickle cell hemoglobin in sickle cell disease
PZA	pyrazinamide		
QOL	quality of life	SSI	surgical site infection
RA	regional anaesthesia	STD	sexually transmitted disease
RAFT	Réseau en Afrique Francophone pour la Télémédecine	StAR	steroidogenic acute regulatory (protein function)
Rb	retinoblastoma (gene)	STEP	serial transverse enteroplasty procedure

STING	subureteric Teflon injection
StrepTSS	streptococcal NF associated with toxic shock syndrome
STS	soft tissue sarcoma
SVT	supraventricular tachycardia
TAP	tunica albuginea plication
TB	tuberculosis
TBA	traditional birth attendants
TCA	total colonic aganglionosis
TEV	talipes equinovarus
TFL	tensor fascia lata
TGD	total gastric dissociation
TGF	transforming growth factor
TIP	typhoid intestinal perforation; tubularised incised plate
TIPSS	transjugular intrahepatic portosystemic stent shunt
TLOSR	transient lower oesophageal sphincter relaxation
TMJ	temporomandibular joint
TNF	tumour necrosis factor
TNM	tumour, nodes, metastases (staging system)
TOF	tracheo-oesophageal fistula; tetralogy of Fallot
TORCH	Toxoplasmosis, Rubella, Cytomegalovirus, Herpes
TPA	tissue plasminogen activator
TPPPS	Toddler-Preschooler Postoperative Pain Scale
TPN	total parenteral nutrition
TR	trauma registry
TRH	thyrotropin-releasing hormone
TRISS	Trauma and Injury Severity Score
T-RTS	Triage RTS
TS	Trauma Score
TSH	thyroid-stimulating hormone
TSPY	testis-specific protein Y-encoded
TSS	toxic shock syndrome
TST	tuberculin skin test
TV	tunica vaginalis

UC	ulcerative colitis
UDT	undescended testis
UGI	upper gastrointestinal
ULE	unilateral limb enlargement
UNFPA	United Nations Population Fund
UNICEF	United Nations Children's Fund
UPJ	ureteropelvic junction (see also PUJ)
UPU	upper pole ureter
URTI	upper respiratory tract infection
US	United States; ultrasound, ultrasonography
UVJ	ureterovesical junction; see also VUJ
UTI	urinary tract infection
VAC	vacuum-assisted closure; vincristin, actinomycin D, and cyclophosphamide
VACTERL	Vertebral and spinal cord, Anorectal, Cardiac, TracheoEsophageal, Renal and other urinary tract, Limb
VAPP	vaccine-associated paralytic poliomyelitis
VATER	Vertebrae, Anus, Trachea, Esophagus, and Renal (association)
VATS	video-assisted thoracic surgery
VCUG	voiding cystourethrogram
VDRL	Venereal Disease Research Laboratory
VEPTR	vertical expandable prosthetic titanium rib
VCUG	voiding cystourethogram
VLBW	very low birth weight
VMA	vanillylmandelic acid
VP	ventriculoperitoneal (shunt)
VPI	velopharyngeal incompetence
VSD	ventricular septal defect
VUJ	vesicoureteric junction; see also UVJ
VUR	vesicoureteric reflux; vesicouretal reflux
WAGR	an acronym for WT, Aniridia, Genito-urinary malformations, mental Retardation
WBC	white blood cells
WHO	World Health Organisation
WT	Wilms' tumour
WWW	worldwide web
XRT	x-ray therapy
YTP	inverted-Y tubularised plate

INDEX

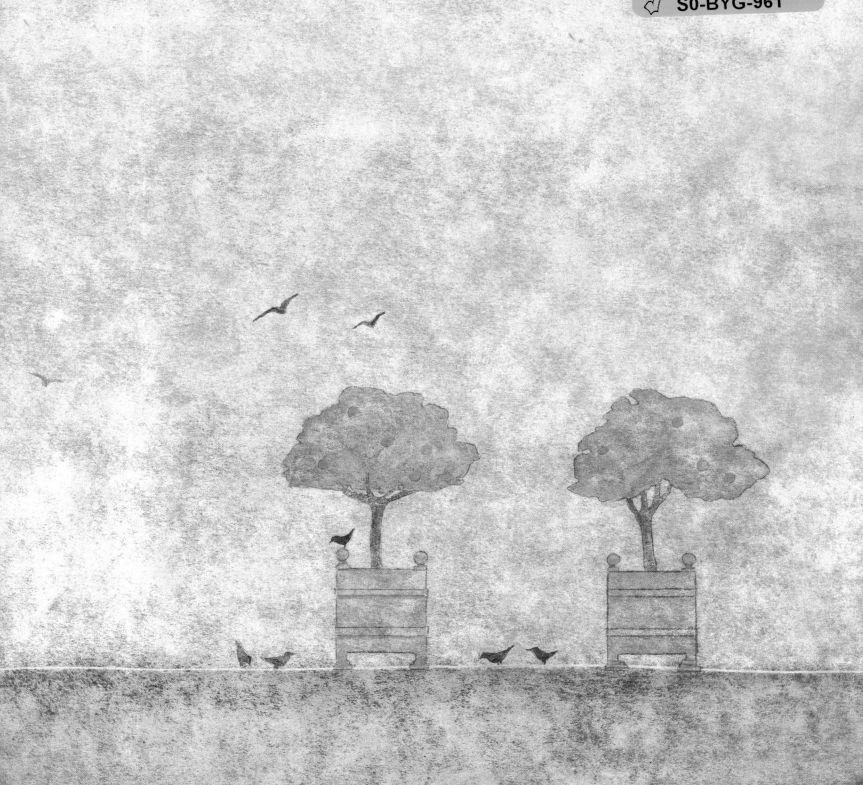

Brave Babette & Sly Tom

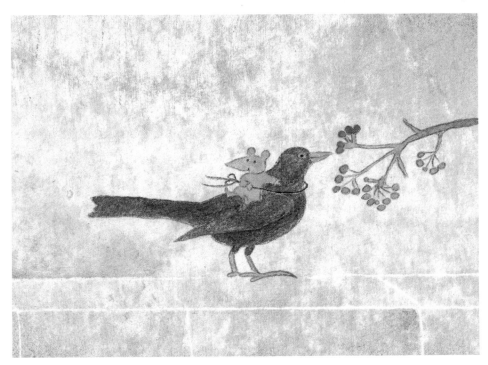

written and illustrated by Elzbieta

Dial Books for Young Readers
NEW YORK

In the middle of Paris
there is a beautiful park called the Luxembourg Gardens.
Since the park was first made,
it has been the site of many wonderful stories:
royal stories, extraordinary stories,
and stories that few people know.
I'm going to tell you the story
of how a blackbird found a mouse in his nest.

It happened like this:

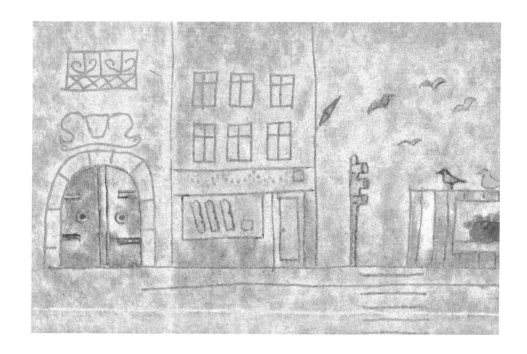

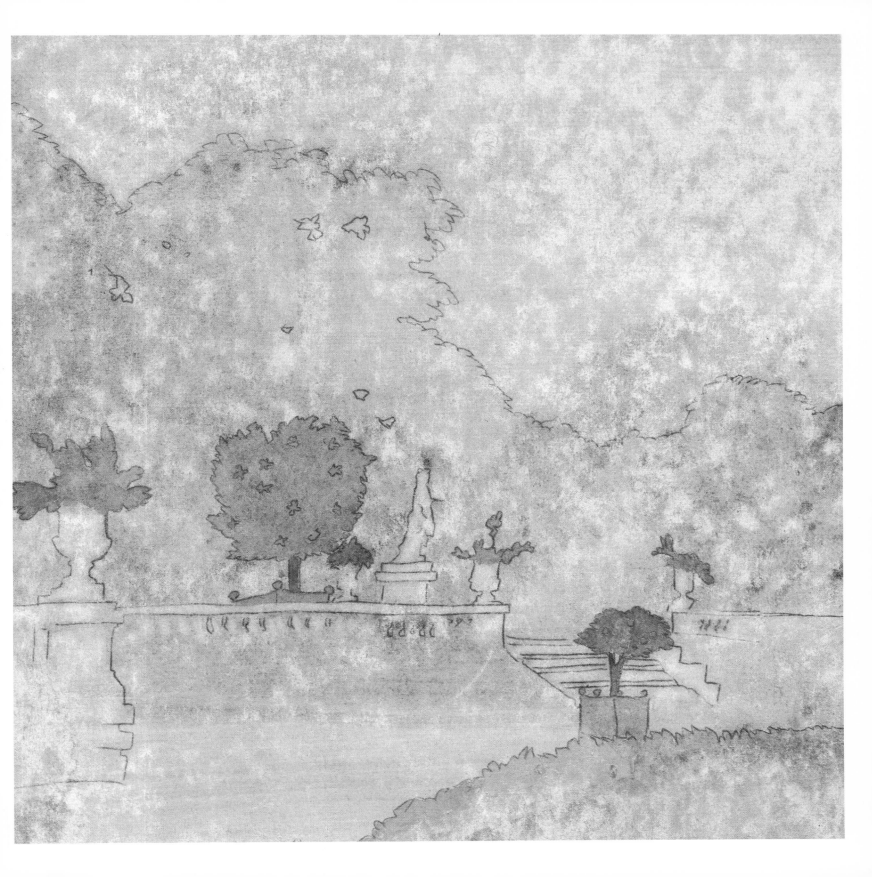

One winter's day
a mouse came scurrying across Paris.
She was pregnant right up to her whiskers.
As night fell, she reached the park.
The huge gates with golden spikes had just swung shut.
The ponies, who had spent the day taking children
for rides under the chestnut trees, had all gone.
The keys had been turned in the locks
and the goldfish slept at the bottom of the pool.
Everything was quiet.

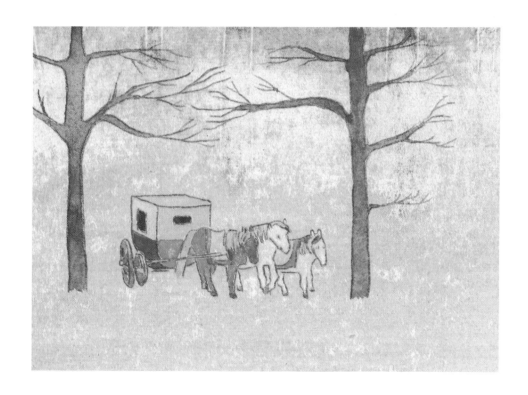

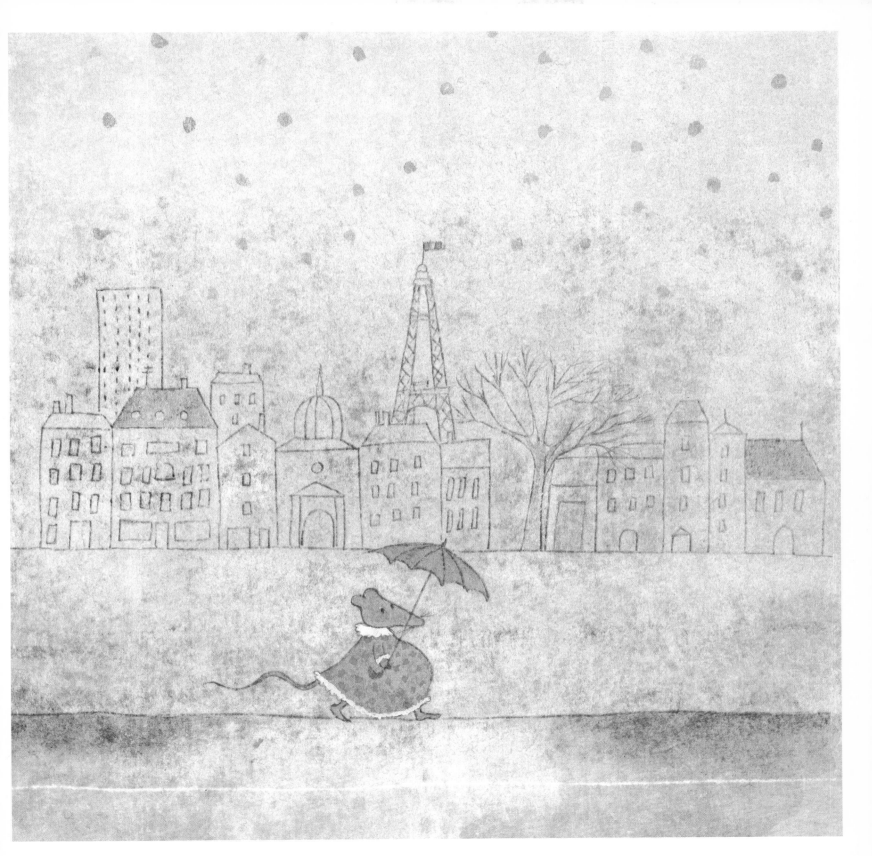

The park was so lovely, so big, and so peaceful
that the mouse said to herself,
"I will give birth to my child here.
She will grow up in this park and be happy."
No sooner had she said this
than the mouse climbed up a tree
till she reached a blackbird's nest and there
she gave birth to the loveliest of baby mice.
"I shall call you Babette," she said.

The little mouse had only just been born
when snow began to fall on the park and into the nest.
The mouse kissed her baby and said to her,
"Don't be frightened, Babette, I'm just going to fetch
my umbrella from the foot of the tree.
I'll be back very soon. Be good."

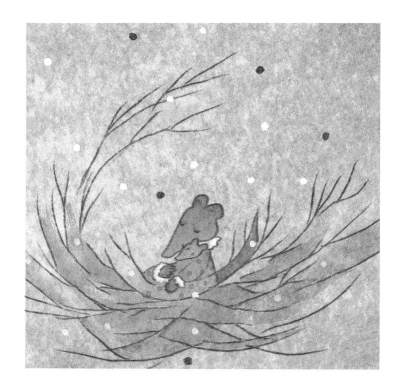

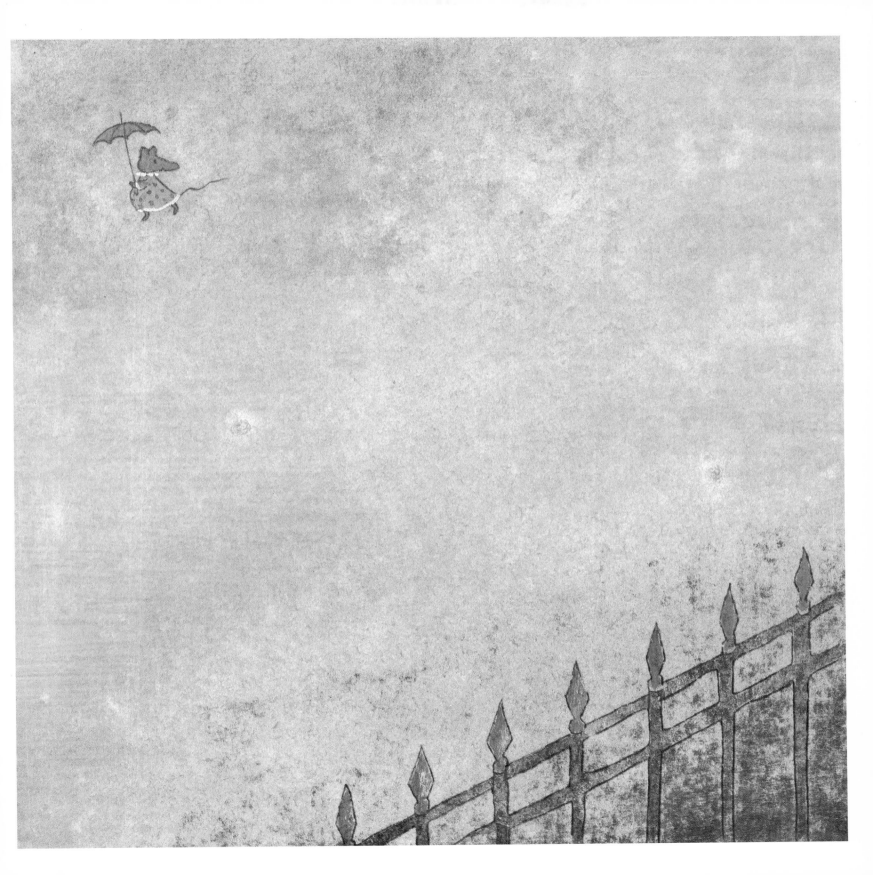

Now, at that time
a dreadful monster was terrorizing
the park and the streets around it.
He was an enormous cat who was named Sly Tom
because he moved without a sound.

Sly Tom stole chops from the butcher.
He scratched babies who tried to stroke his back.
And in the park the animals grew silent
with fear at the very mention of his name.

Just that day over by the merry-go-round
he had swallowed a sparrow.
Then he had gone to the fountain
and gulped down a goldfish.
Then he went to the lawn where he pounced on a pigeon,
leaving nothing but a few feathers on the green grass.

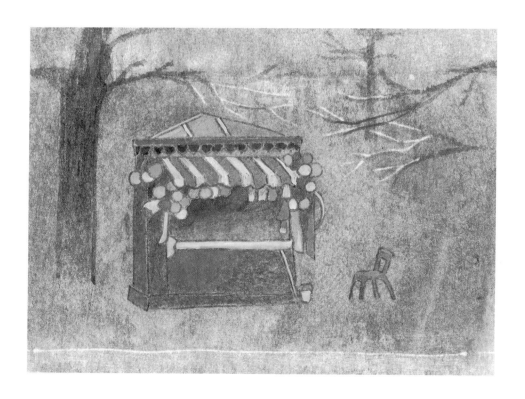

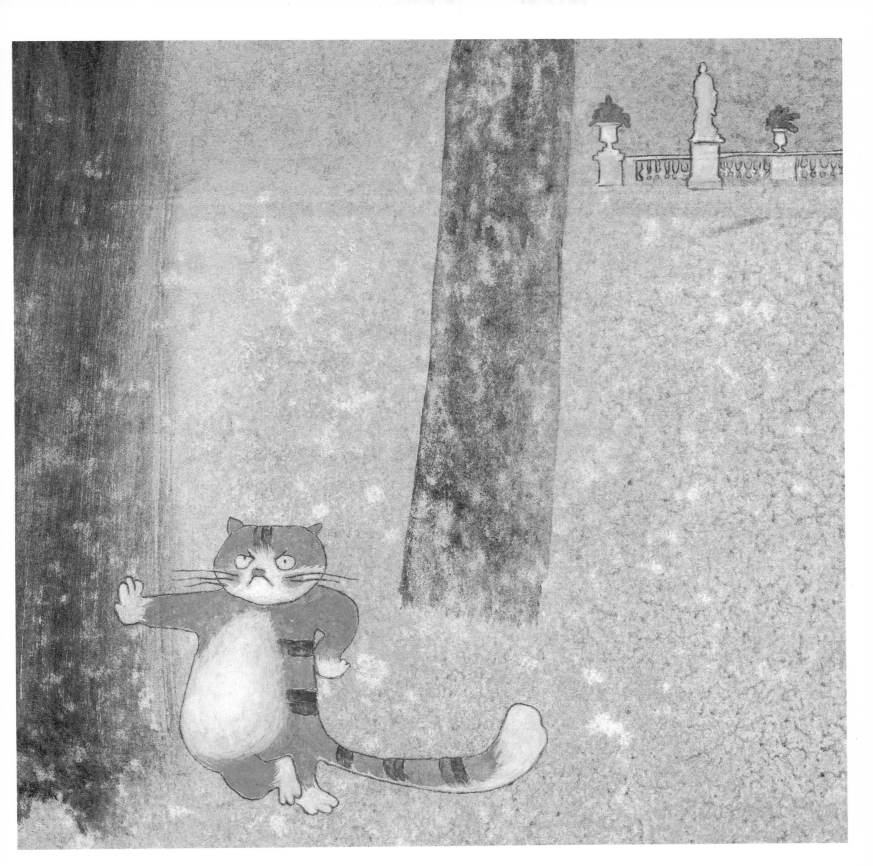

At dusk Sly Tom was still roaming about
looking for dessert.
When he spied the mouse,
he jumped at her like lightning.
The little mouse dropped her umbrella
and ran away as fast as her legs would carry her.
She even managed to climb a tree.
But Sly Tom was not far behind,
and when she got to the top, she thought all was lost.
"Babette, my little Babette, just born and already an orphan,"
she cried in despair.
"Good-bye, good-bye, the cat is going to eat me."

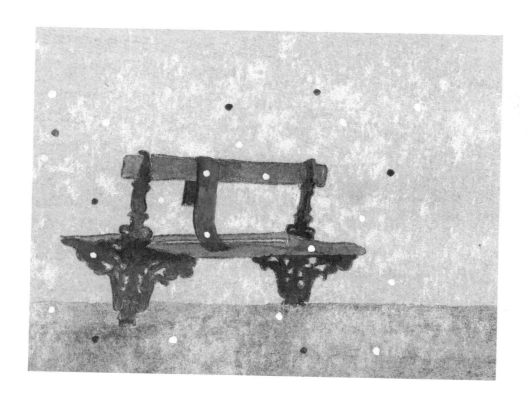

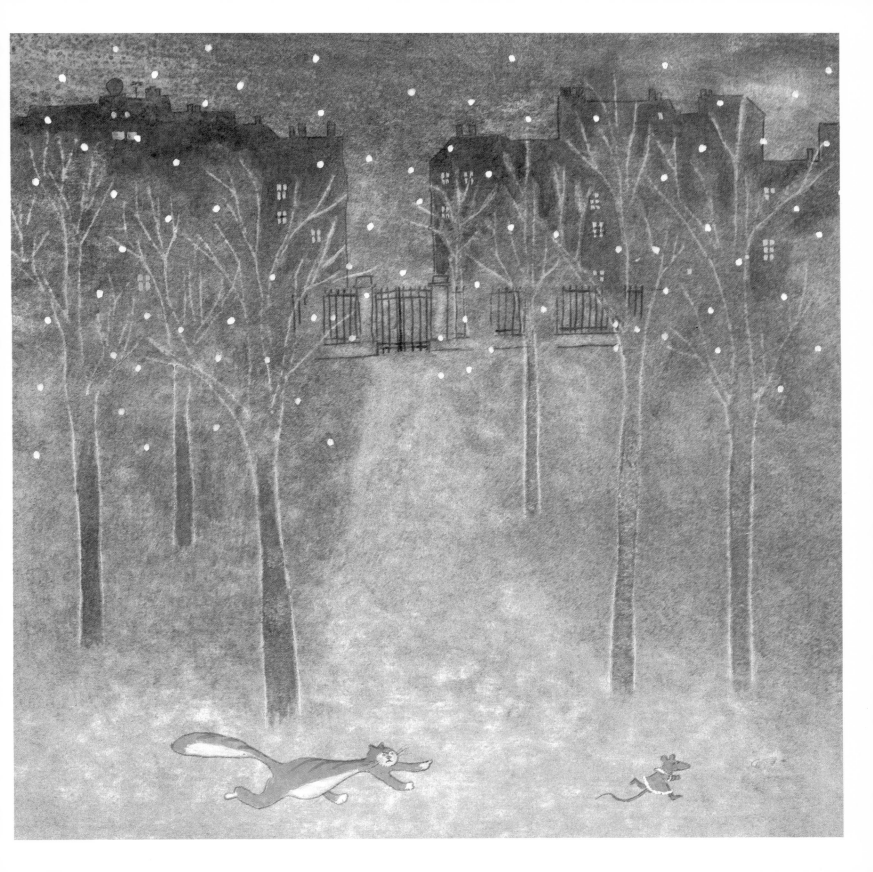

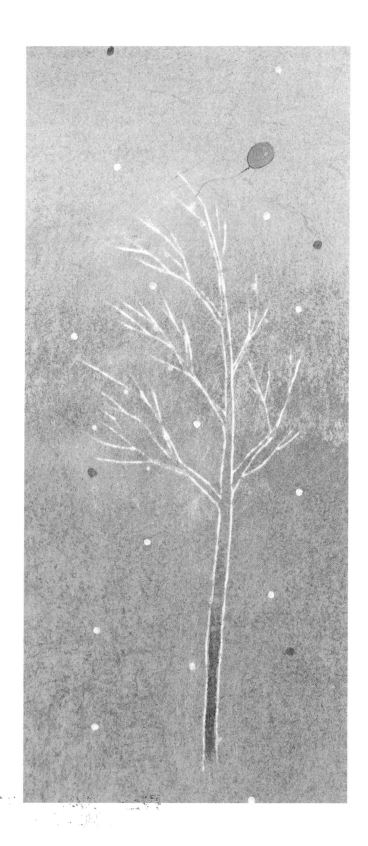

But she was in luck.
There,
tangled up in the highest branches,
was a red balloon that had escaped
from the fingers of a little boy
that morning.
Sly Tom opened his mouth
to gobble up the mouse
when just in time,
she managed to free the string
and float away
toward the snow clouds.
"Birds, bees, and goldfish
of the Luxembourg Gardens,
look after my child.
Babette, Babette,
I shall be back soon."

But the wind was strong.
It blew the mouse's words far away.
No one heard her
and no one saw her disappear
over the rooftops.

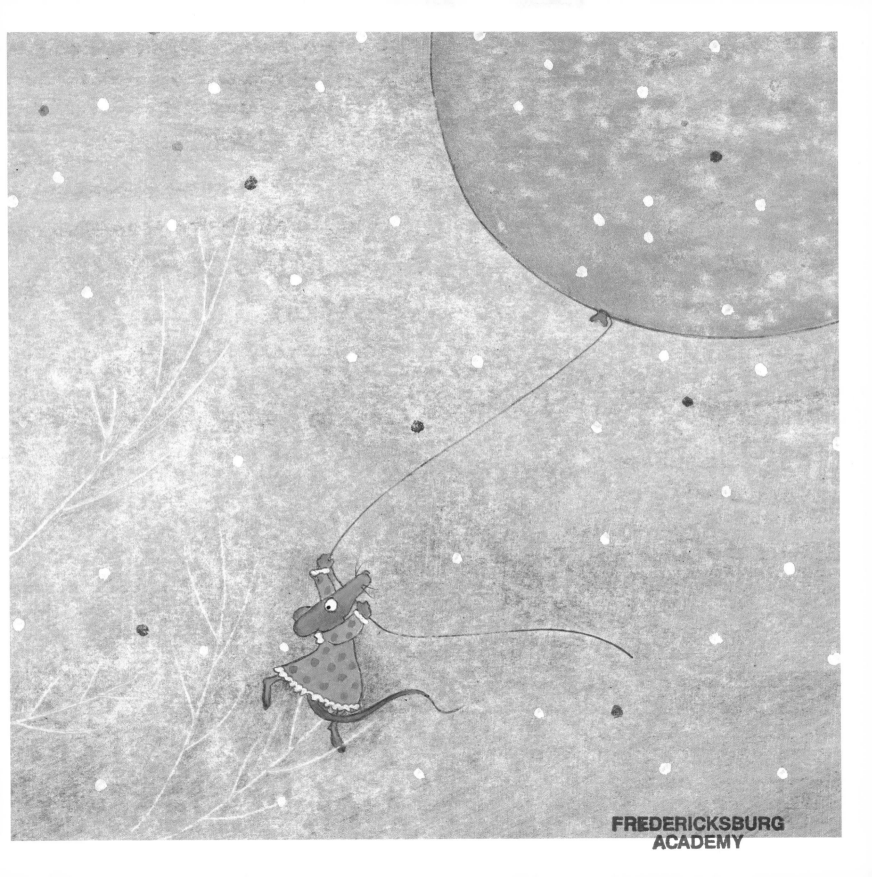

FREDERICKSBURG
ACADEMY

A little later a blackbird swooped down over the trees
and settled on the edge of his nest.
"There's something in my nest!" he exclaimed.
"In fact there's someONE in my nest!"

The blackbird looked about.
Under the tree he found the mouse's umbrella
and her footsteps in the snow.
Then he saw Sly Tom's claw marks
and he knew that Babette was alone in the world.

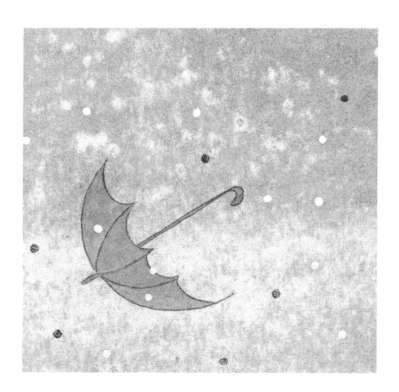

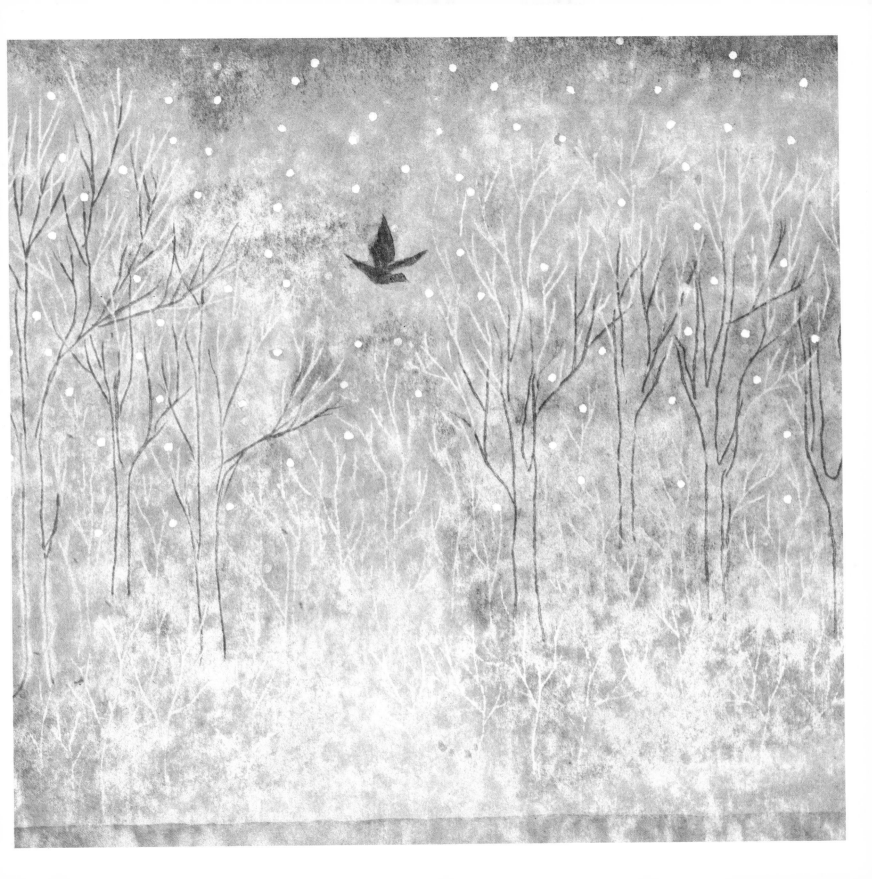

So he leaned over the abandoned mouse
and sheltered her with his wing.
"I never thought I'd have a child," he murmured softly,
"and now I've found a tiny mouse in my nest—cute as a cuckoo."

From that moment the blackbird
looked after her like a father.
He took care of her so well in his feather-lined nest
that the little mouse really thought she was a bird.
She had no fear of the tree's high branches and would
talk back to any bird that said she didn't belong.

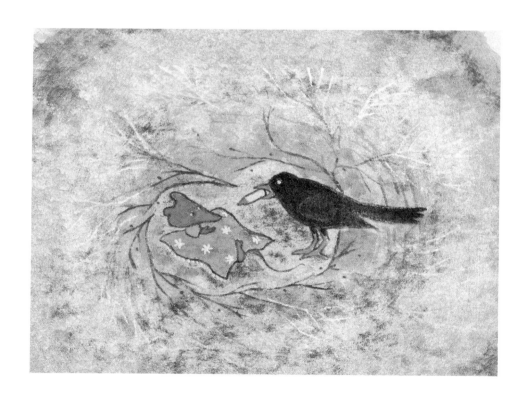

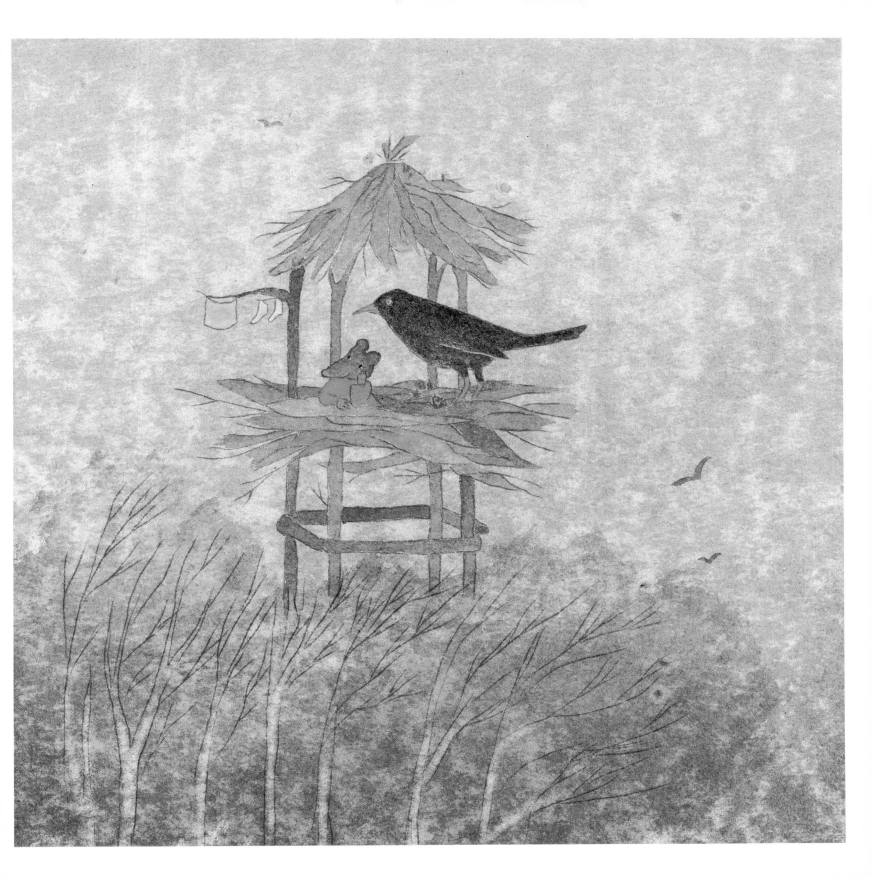

But one day she asked,
"Papa Blackbird, when will I have a beak
and feathers and wings and everything?
And when will I be able to fly?"

Then the blackbird told her everything he knew about her.

When she found out that she wasn't a little bird,
Babette was furious and hurt.
The blackbird told her that she had
beautiful whiskers, lovely soft fur, and pretty little ears,
but she stamped her feet and shouted,
"It's not true! I don't want them!
I want feathers! I want wings!"

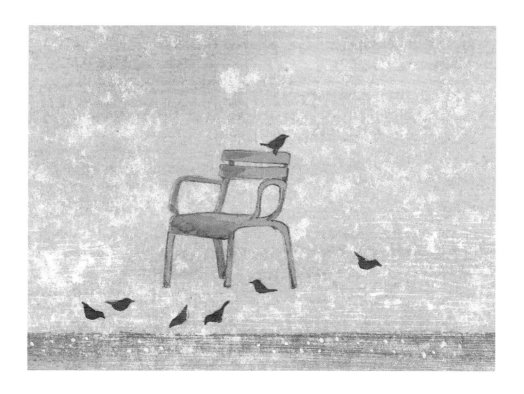

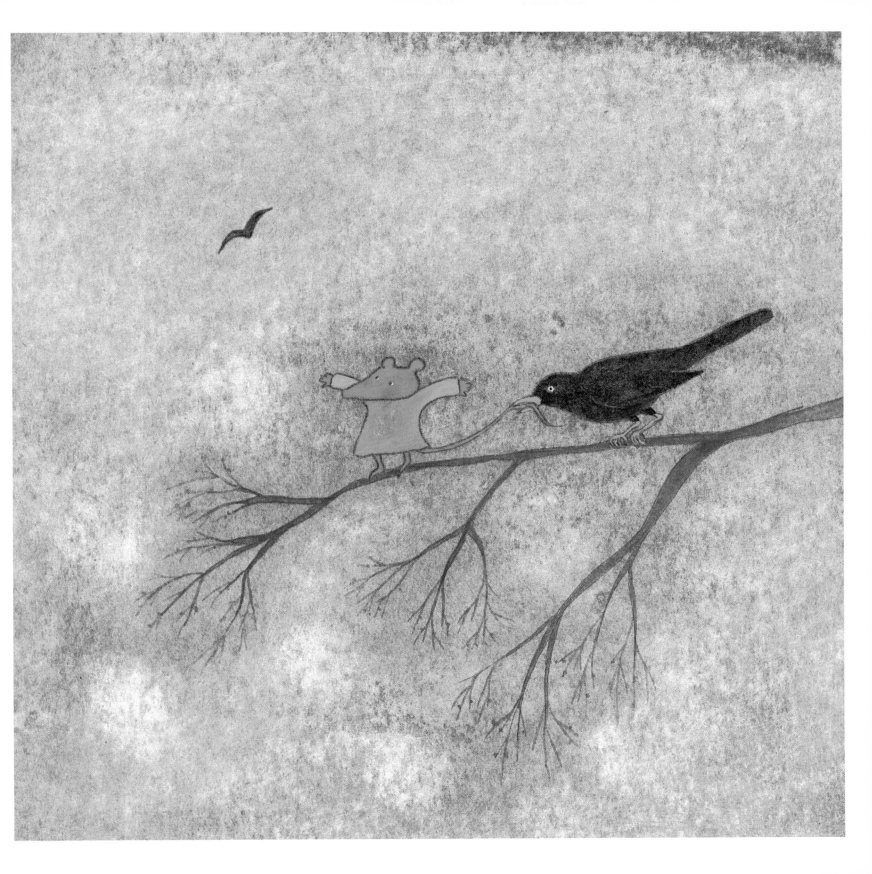

When night came, still in a painful rage,
Babette did something absolutely forbidden—
she went off to walk alone by the light of the moon.
Sly Tom saw her instantly.
"I'm going to eat you up," he said to her.
"That would surprise me," answered Babette,
her eyes glittering with anger.
"Oh, really?" said Sly Tom, "and why is that?"
"Because of my magic powers. I shall change you
into a Thingamagig," she said, looking very fierce.
Sly Tom went pale. No one had ever threatened *him* before.
"Don't do that," he said, his voice trembling.
"Yes!" said Babette, "I'm going to."
Sly Tom threw himself at her feet.
"I have another idea. Listen to me," he begged.
"You could *tame* me."

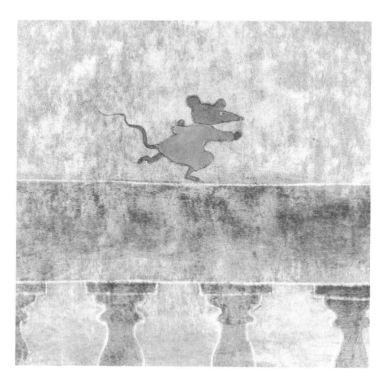

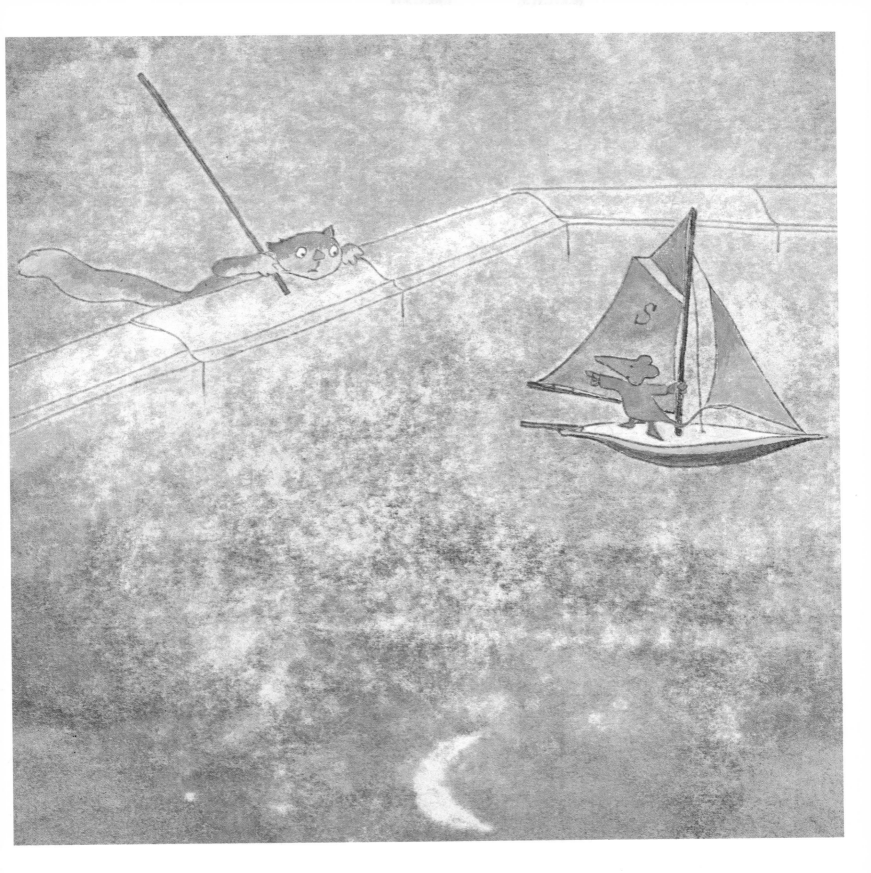

"Tame you?" said Babette.
"Yes. You could have a little whip and a cape.
I'd stand on a platform and look really fierce
and I'd do everything you said.
The crowds would clap and you'd be rich."
"And you wouldn't say anything if I cracked the whip?"
"No, I promise."
"And you wouldn't bite me if I put my head between your jaws?"
"No, no, NO!" promised Sly Tom.
"Well in that case," said Babette severely,
"I will give you one last chance. Tomorrow I shall tame you."

The next day the first of Babette's shows took place:
BABETTE THE BRAVE,
THE TOMCAT TAMER

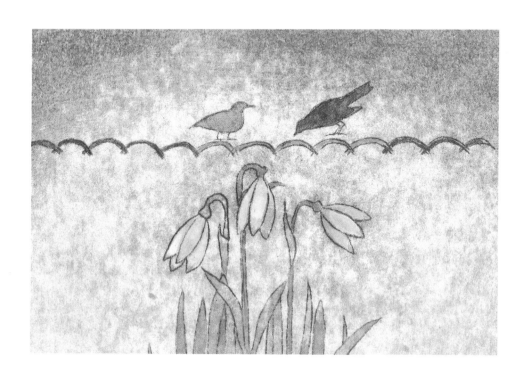

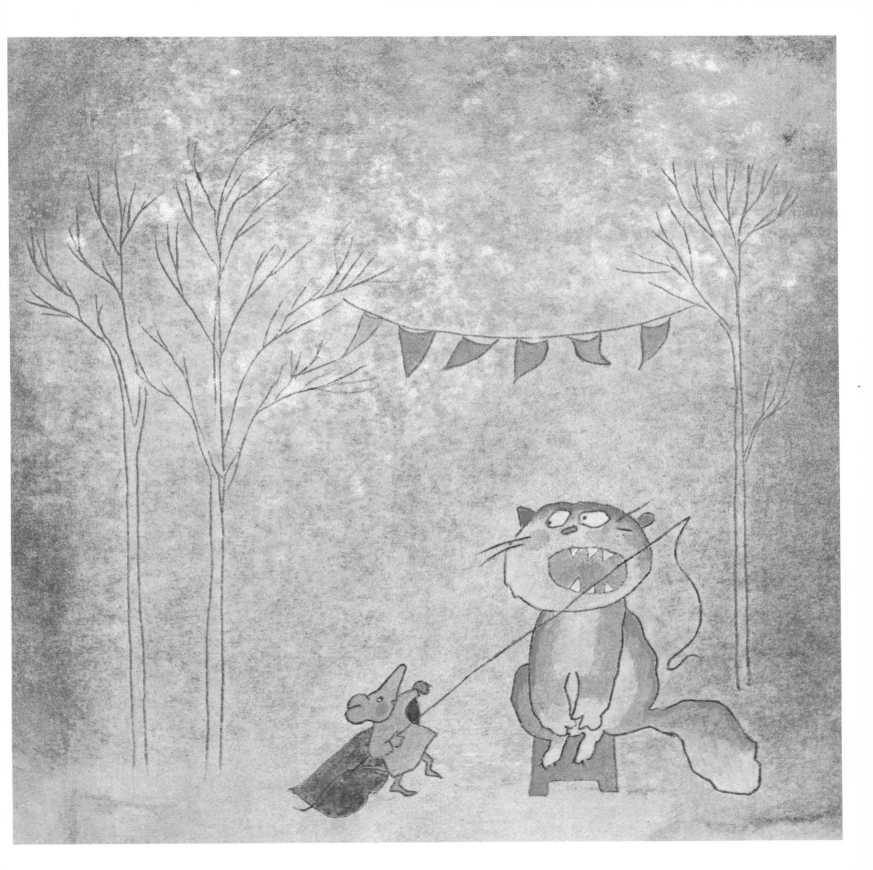

She was a huge success.
From then on people came running from all over Paris
to see the show.

One Sunday afternoon
while a huge crowd gathered for the show,
a red balloon floated down into the park.

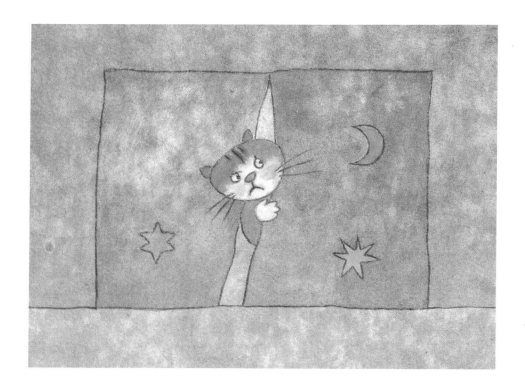

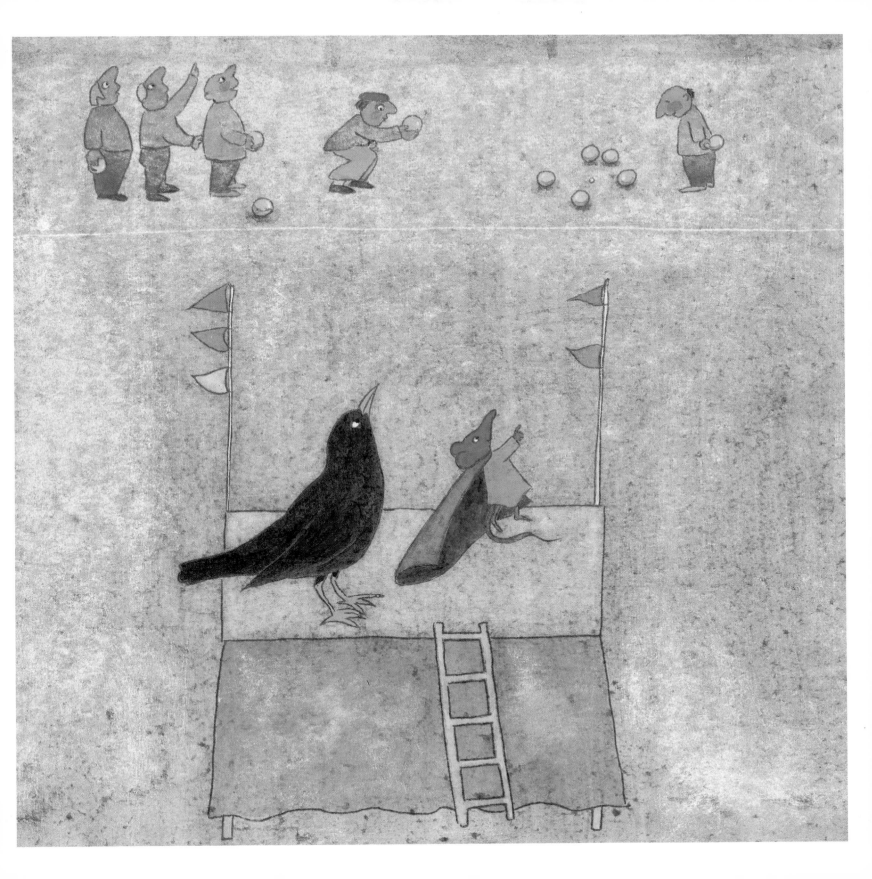

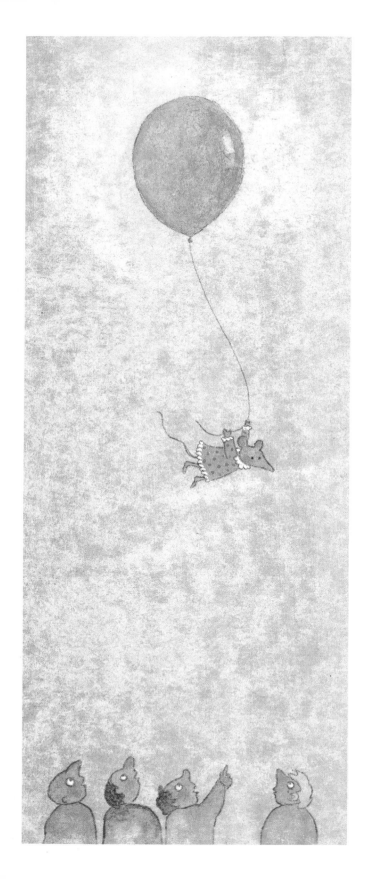

Clinging to the end of the string
was Babette's mother!
The wind had blown her this way and that,
all the way around the world,
before bringing her back to her child.

Babette's mother married the blackbird
and together they all built a huge nest
in one of the trees by the fountain.
And if you ever visit the Luxembourg Gardens,
perhaps you'll see them,
because they are still living there,
comfortable and happy.

Sly Tom was a terrible
Cowardly cat—
Brave Babette tamed him
And that was that.

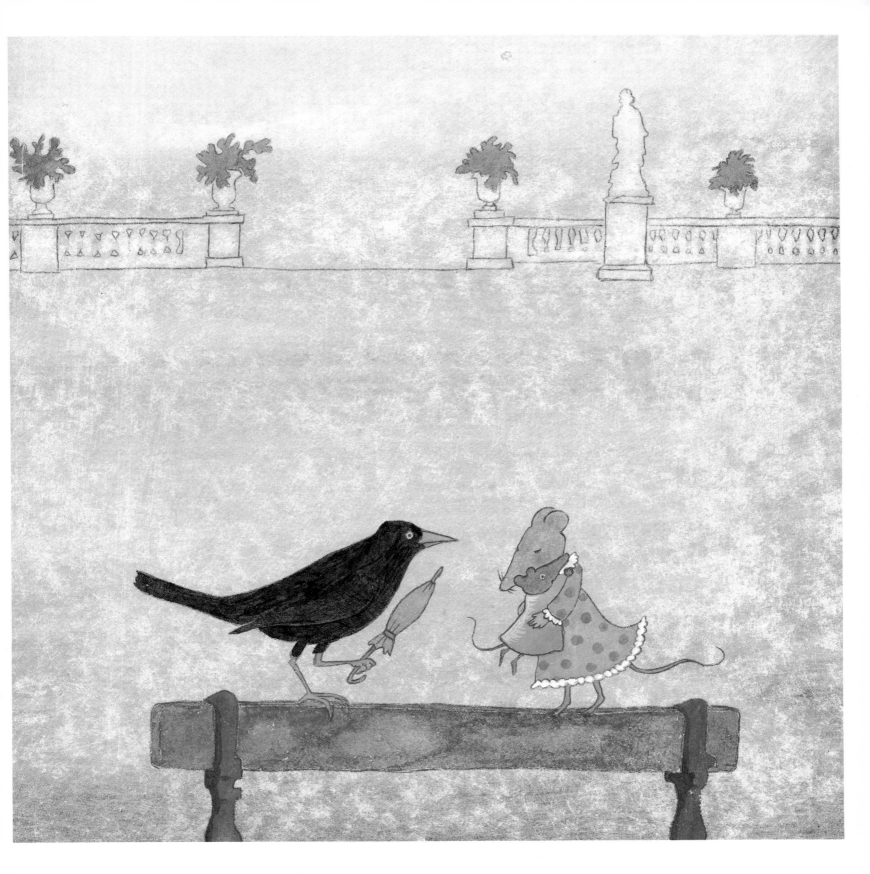

For Hassan Jouad

First published in the United States 1989
by Dial Books for Young Readers
A Division of NAL Penguin Inc.
2 Park Avenue
New York, New York 10016

Published in Belgium 1988 by Pastel,
an imprint of l'école des loisirs,
as *Larirette & Catimini*
Copyright © 1988 by l'école des loisirs, Paris
American text copyright © 1989
by Dial Books for Young Readers
All rights reserved / Typography by Amelia Lau Carling
Printed in Belgium
First Edition
(c)
1 3 5 7 9 10 8 6 4 2

Library of Congress Cataloging in Publication Data
Elzbieta. Brave Babette and Sly Tom.
Translation of: Larirette & Catimini.
Summary: Adopted by a kindly blackbird after her
mother is chased away by a nasty tomcat,
Babette the mouse eventually manages to turn
the tables on the cat in an unusual manner.
[1. Mice—Fiction. 2. Cats—Fiction.
3. Birds—Fiction.] I. Title.
PZ7.E563Br 1989 [E] 88-20392
ISBN 0-8037-0633-2